Infectious Diseases
In Women

Infectious Diseases in Women

Sebastian Faro, M.D., Ph.D.
The Woman's Hospital of Texas
Houston, Texas
Visiting Professor
Rush Medical College and Rush-Presbyterian-
   St. Luke's Medical Center
Chicago, Illinois

David E. Soper, M.D.
Professor
Department of Obstetrics and Gynecology and
   Medicine, Division of Infectious Diseases
Medical University of South Carolina
Charleston, South Carolina

In consultation with Mark G. Martens, M.D.

W.B. SAUNDERS COMPANY
A Harcourt Health Sciences Company
Philadelphia   London   New York   St. Louis   Sydney   Toronto

W.B. SAUNDERS COMPANY
A Harcourt Health Sciences Company

The Curtis Center
Independence Square West
Philadelphia, Pennsylvania 19106

Library of Congress Cataloging-in-Publication Data

Infectious diseases in women / [edited by] Sebastian Faro, David Soper.—1st ed.

p.   cm.

ISBN 0–7216–7379–1

1. Communicable diseases.   2. Women—Diseases.   3. Women—Health and
  hygiene.   4. Generative organs, Female—Infections. I. Faro, Sebastian.
  II. Soper, David.
[DNLM: 1. Genital Diseases, Female.   2. Infection.   3. Pregnancy
Complications, Infectious.   4. Women's Health.   WP 145 I43 2001]

RC112.I4625 2001   616.9′082—dc21   00–030110

Acquisitions Editor: Judith Fletcher
Project Manager: Gina Scala
Production Manager: Norman Stellander
Illustration Specialist: Robert Quinn
Book Designer: Jonel Sofian

INFECTIOUS DISEASES IN WOMEN   ISBN 0–7216–7379–1

Printed in the United States of America.

Last digit is the print number: 9   8   7   6   5   4   3   2   1

To all the women who granted us the privilege
of delivering care during their illness
and allowing us to develop an understanding
of infectious diseases affecting women.

Sebastian Faro
David E. Soper

Contributors ■ ▼ ◗

Javier A. Adachi, M.D.
Center for Infectious Diseases, University of Texas–Houston Medical School and School of Public Health, Houston, Texas
INFECTIOUS DIARRHEA

Stuart P. Adler, M.D.
Professor, Department of Pediatrics, Division of Infectious Diseases, Medical College of Virginia of Virginia Commonwealth University; Attending Physician, Department of Pediatrics, Medical College of Virginia Hospitals, Richmond, Virginia
PARVOVIRUS

Marvin S. Amstey, M.D.
Professor of Obstetrics and Gynecology, University of Rochester School of Medicine and Dentistry; Senior Attending, The Genesee Hospital, Rochester, New York
VARICELLA-ZOSTER

Vincent T. Andriole, M.D.
Professor of Medicine, Yale University School of Medicine, New Haven, Connecticut
URINARY TRACT INFECTIONS

Joseph Apuzzio, M.D.
Professor, Obstetrics, Gynecology and Women's Health; Director, Maternal-Fetal Medicine, New Jersey Medical School, Newark, New Jersey
PYELONEPHRITIS; AMINOGLYCOSIDES

Kevin A. Ault, M.D.
Assistant Professor, Department of Obstetrics and Gynecology, University of Iowa, Iowa City, Iowa
INFECTION AND INFERTILITY

David A. Baker, M.D.
Professor, Obstetrics, Gynecology and Reproductive Medicine, Health Sciences Center, State University of New York at Stony Brook, Stony Brook, New York
GENERAL MICROBIOLOGY: VIROLOGY; HERPES; ANTIVIRALS

Susanne L. Bathgate, M.D.
Assistant Professor, Department of Obstetrics and Gynecology, The George Washington University; Attending Physician, The George Washington University Hospital, Washington, D.C.
GROUP B STREPTOCOCCAL INFECTIONS IN PREGNANCY

Roger E. Bawdon, M.S., Ph.D.
Clinical Professor, University of Texas Southwestern Medical Center, Department of Obstetrics and Gynecology, Dallas, Texas
PLACENTAL PHARMACOKINETICS AND ANTI-HIV COMPOUNDS

Jorge D. Blanco, M.D.
Department of Obstetrics and Gynecology, University of Florida—Pensacola Division; Medical Director, Sacred Heart Women's Hospital, Pensacola, Florida
SEPTIC PELVIC THROMBOPHLEBITIS

Karen J. Brasel, M.D., M.P.H.
Assistant Professor, Medical College of Wisconsin, Milwaukee, Wisconsin
INTRA-ABDOMINAL INFECTIONS

Brian M. Casey, M.D.
Assistant Professor, University of Texas Southwestern Medical Center, Dallas, Texas
PLACENTAL PHARMACOKINETICS AND ANTI-HIV COMPOUNDS.

Susan M. Cox, M.D.
Assistant Dean for Professional Education, Associate Professor, Obstetrics and Gynecology, Director, Maternal-Fetal Medicine Fellowship, University of Texas Southwestern Medical Center, Dallas, Texas
INTRA-AMNIOTIC INFECTION

William R. Crombleholme, M.D.
Professor and Vice-Chair, Department of Obstetrics and Gynecology and Reproductive Sciences, University of Pittsburgh School of Medicine; Director, OB-GYN Residency Program, Magee-Women's Hospital, Pittsburgh, Pennsylvania
HUMAN IMMUNODEFICIENCY VIRUS IN PREGNANCY

Louise-Marie Dembry, M.D.
Associate Professor of Medicine and Epidemiology, Yale University School of Medicine, New Haven, Connecticut
URINARY TRACT INFECTIONS

Geraldo Duarte, M.D., Ph.D.
Associate Professor, Department of Obstetrics and Gynecology, and Director, Perinatology, University of Sao Paulo School of Medicine at Ribeirao Preto, Brazil
HUMAN IMMUNODEFICIENCY VIRUS IN PREGNANCY

Herbert L. DuPont, M.D.
Clinical Professor of Medicine, University of
  Texas–Houston Medical School and Baylor College
  of Medicine; Chief, Internal Medicine, St. Luke's
  Episcopal Hospital, Houston, Texas
INFECTIOUS DIARRHEA

J. M. Ernest, M.D.
Associate Professor, Department of Obstetrics and
  Gynecology, Wake Forest University School of
  Medicine, Winston-Salem, North Carolina
RUBELLA

Sebastian Faro, M.D., Ph.D.
The Woman's Hospital of Texas, Houston, Texas;
  Visiting Professor, Rush Medical College and Rush-
  Presbyterian-St. Luke's Medical Center, Chicago,
  Illinois
GENERAL MICROBIOLOGY: BACTERIOLOGY; MYCOLOGY: GENERAL
MYCOLOGY AND FUNGAL DISEASE; LYME DISEASE; PREMATURE
LABOR AND INFECTION; CHORIOAMNIONITIS; POSTPARTUM
ENDOMETRITIS; TRICHOMONAS VAGINALIS; HIDRADENITIS SUPPURATIVA;
RESPIRATORY INFECTIONS; DERMATOLOGIC CONDITIONS;
CHLAMYDIA TRACHOMATIS; PENICILLINS; CEPHALOSPORINS;
CARBAPENEMS; MACROLIDES; ANTIFUNGAL AGENTS; ANTIVIRALS

Janice I. French, CNR, MS
Research Associate, Denver Health, Denver, Colorado
BACTERIAL VAGINOSIS

Stanley A. Gall, M.D.
Professor of Obstetrics and Gynecology and Director,
  OB-GYN Residency Program, University of
  Louisville School of Medicine; Chief, Department
  of Obstetrics and Gynecology, University of
  Louisville Hospital, Louisville, Kentucky
HUMAN PAPILLOMAVIRUS

Pamela Gilmore, M.D.
Past Chief Resident, University of Rochester School of
  Medicine and Dentistry, Rochester, New York
VARICELLA-ZOSTER

Larry C. Gilstrap III, M.D.
Emma Sue Hightower Professor in Obstetrics and
  Gynecology, and Chair, Department of Obstetrics,
  Gynecology and Reproductive Sciences, The
  University of Texas-Houston Medical School,
  Houston, Texas
EPISIOTOMY INFECTIONS

Bernard Gonik, M.D.
Professor and Associate Chairman, Department of
  Obstetrics and Gynecology, Wayne State University
  School of Medicine; Chief, Department of
  Obstetrics and Gynecology, Sinai-Grace Hospital,
  Detroit, Michigan
SEPTIC SHOCK

David Gonzalez, M.D.
Instructor, Obstetrics, Gynecology and Women's
  Health, New Jersey Medical School, Newark;
  Monmouth Medical Centers, Long Branch, New
  Jersey
PYELONEPHRITIS; AMINOGLYCOSIDES

Jennifer Gunter, M.D.
Assistant Professor, Department of Obstetrics and
  Gynecology, The University of Kansas Medical
  Center, Kansas City, Kansas
METRONIDAZOLE; QUINOLONES

W. David Hager, M.D., F.A.C.O.G.
Professor, Department of Obstetrics and Gynecology,
  University of Kentucky College of Medicine;
  Director, U.K.-Affiliated Residency Training
  Program, Central Baptist Hospital, Lexington,
  Kentucky
MASTITIS

Gerri S. Hall, Ph.D.
Sandy, Utah
SPECIMEN COLLECTION AND DIAGNOSTIC PROCEDURES FOR THE
LABORATORY DIAGNOSIS OF INFECTIONS IN FEMALES

James H. Harger, M.D.
Professor of Obstetrics and Gynecology, University of
  Pittsburgh, School of Medicine, Magee-Women's
  Hospital, Pittsburgh, Pennsylvania
PARVOVIRUS

Cathleen M. Harris, M.D.
Assistant Professor, University of Chicago; Associate
  Medical Director, Phoenix Perinatal Associates,
  Phoenix, Arizona
WOUND INFECTION

David L. Hemsell, M.D.
Professor, and Director, Division of Gynecology,
  Department of Obstetrics and Gynecology,
  University of Texas Southwestern Medical School:
  Attending Physician, Parkland Health and Hospital
  Systems, Dallas, Texas
POSTHYSTERECTOMY INFECTIONS

Lisa M. Hollier, M.D., M.P.H.
Assistant Professor, Obstetrics and Gynecology, The University of Texas–Houston Medical School, Houston, Texas
INTRA-AMNIOTIC INFECTION

Melisa M. Holmes, M.D.
Associate Professor, Departments of Obstetrics and Gynecology and Pediatrics, Medical University of South Carolina, Charleston, South Carolina
PEDIATRIC VULVOVAGINITIS

Michael J. Hussey, M.D.
Assistant Professor, Rush Medical College, Chicago, Illinois
DERMATOLOGIC CONDITIONS

Mahmoud A. Ismail, M.D.
Professor of Obstetrics and Gynecology, Section of Maternal Fetal Medicine, University of Chicago, Chicago, Illinois
WOUND INFECTION

Tammie T. Ismail, B.A.
Pending MA in Social Science, University of Chicago, Chicago, Illinois
WOUND INFECTION

William C. Koch, M.D.
Associate Professor, Department of Pediatrics, Division of Infectious Diseases, Medical College of Virginia of Virginia Commonwealth University; Attending Physician, Department of Pediatrics, Medical College of Virginia Hospitals, Richmond, Virginia
PARVOVIRUS

Daniel V. Landers, M.D.
Professor and Director, Division of Reproductive Infectious Diseases and Immunology, Department of Obstetrics and Gynecology, University of Pittsburgh, Chief, Infectious Diseases, Magee-Women's Hospital, Pittsburgh, Pennsylvania
HUMAN IMMUNODEFICIENCY VIRUS IN PREGNANCY

John W. Larsen, M.D.
Oscar I. and Mildred S. Dodek, Professor and Interim Chairman, Department of Obstetrics and Gynecology, The George Washington University; Attending Physician, The George Washington University Hospital, Washington, D.C.
GROUP B STREPTOCOCCAL INFECTIONS IN PREGNANCY

Michael R. Leonardi, M.D.
Clinical Assistant Professor of Obstetrics and Gynecology, and Residency Director, University of Illinois at Chicago College of Medicine at Peoria; Perinatologist, OSF/St. Francis Medical Center, Peoria, Illinois
SEPTIC SHOCK

Oliver Liesenfeld, M.D.
Senior Research Fellow, Department of Medical Microbiology and Immunology of Infection, Free University of Berlin, Berlin, Germany
TOXOPLASMOSIS

Charles H. Livengood, III, M.D.
Associate Professor (tenured), Department of Obstetrics and Gynecology, Duke University Medical Center; Director, Chlamydia Laboratory, Duke Hospital, Durham, North Carolina
SYPHILIS

Maurizio L. Maccato, M.D.
Assistant Professor, Baylor College of Medicine, Houston, Texas
RESPIRATORY INFECTIONS

James A. McGregor, M.D.C.M.
Professor of Obstetrics and Gynecology, University of Colorado School of Medicine; Senior Physician, Denver Health, Denver, Colorado
BACTERIAL VAGINOSIS

Susan M. Mou, M.D.
Highland Hospital, Rochester, New York
TRICHOMONAS VAGINALIS

Jorma Paavonen, M.D., Ph.D.
Professor, Department of Obstetrics and Gynecology, University of Helsinki, Helsinki, Finland
CERVICITIS

Joseph G. Pastorek, II, M.D.
The Woman's Consultant, Metairie, Louisiana
GENERAL MICROBIOLOGY: PARASITOLOGY; HEPATITIS A TO E; ECTOPARASITES

Mark D. Pearlman, M.D.
Vice Chair and Associate Professor, Department of Obstetrics and Gynecology, Associate Professor, Department of Surgery, Assistant Chief of Staff, University of Michigan Health Systems, Ann Arbor, Michigan
SEPTIC ABORTION

Lou Ellen Phillips-Smith, Ph.D., F.A.A.M.

Project Manager, Concepts in Pharmaceutical
    Research, Inc., Vero Beach, Florida

SPECIMEN COLLECTION AND DIAGNOSTIC PROCEDURES FOR THE
LABORATORY DIAGNOSIS OF INFECTIONS IN FEMALES

Kate Pierce, R.N., B.S.N., I.B.C.L.C.

President and CEO, Lactation Station, Inc.
    International Board Certified Lactation Consultant
    Previously, Director of Lactation Services at Central
    Baptist Hospital, Lexington, Kentucky

MASTITIS

Phillip Pinell, M.D.

Department of Obstetrics and Gynecology, Houston
    Perinatal Associates, Houston, Texas

SULFONAMIDES; VANCOMYCIN

Sanjay Ram, M.D.

Department of Infectious Diseases, Boston Medical
    Center, Boston, Massachusetts

GONOCOCCAL INFECTIONS

Jack S. Remington, M.D.

Professor, Department of Medicine, Division of
    Infectious Diseases and Geographic Medicine,
    Stanford University Medical Center, Stanford;
    Chairman, Department of Immunology and
    Infectious Diseases, Research Institute, Palo Alto
    Medical Foundation, Palo Alto, California

TOXOPLASMOSIS

Peter A. Rice, M.D.

Department of Infectious Diseases, Boston Medical
    Center, Boston, Massachusetts

GONOCOCCAL INFECTIONS

John W. Riggs, M.D.

Associate Professor, Department of Obstetrics and
    Gynecology, University of Texas–Houston Medical
    School, Lyndon B. Johnson General Hospital,
    Houston, Texas

SEPTIC PELVIC THROMBOPHLEBITIS

Scott W. Roberts, M.D.

Assistant Professor, Department of Obstetrics and
    Gynecology, and Director of Maternal-Fetal
    Medicine, University of Kansas School of Medicine,
    Wichita, Kansas

CEPHALOSPORINS

George P. Schmid, M.D.

Medical Epidemiologist, Division of STD Prevention,
    Centers for Disease Control and Prevention,
    Atlanta, Georgia

EPIDEMIOLOGY OF SEXUALLY TRANSMITTED INFECTIONS; GENITAL
ULCER DISEASE

John L. Sever, M.D., Ph.D.

Professor of Pediatrics, Obstetrics and Gynecology,
    Microbiology, and Immunology, George Washington
    University School of Medicine and Health Sciences;
    Professor of Pediatrics, Obstetrics and Gynecology,
    Microbiology, and Immunology, Children's National
    Medical Center, Washington, DC

CYTOMEGALOVIRUS INFECTIONS IN WOMEN, PREGNANCY, AND THE
NEONATE

Antonio V. Sison, M.D.

Director, OB/GYN Residency Program and Medical
    Education, Department of Obstetrics and
    Gynecology, Albert Einstein Medical Center,
    Philadelphia, Pennsylvania

CYTOMEGALOVIRUS INFECTIONS IN WOMEN, PREGNANCY, AND THE
NEONATE

Jack D. Sobel, M.D.

Professor of Internal Medicine, of Microbiology and
    Immunology, and of Obstetrics and Gynecology,
    Wayne State University School of Medicine; Chief,
    Division of Infectious Diseases, Detroit Medical
    Center, Detroit, Michigan

MYCOLOGY: CANDIDA VAGINITIS

David E. Soper, M.D.

Professor, Department of Obstetrics and Gynecology
    and Medicine, Division of Infectious Diseases,
    Medical University of South Carolina, Charleston,
    South Carolina

PELVIC INFLAMMATORY DISEASE; NECROTIZING FASCIITIS;
CLINDAMYCIN

John A. Weigelt, M.D., D.V.M.

Professor of Surgery, and Vice Chair, Medical College
    of Wisconsin, Milwaukee, Wisconsin

INTRA-ABDOMINAL INFECTIONS

Raul Yordan-Jovet, M.D.

Assistant Professor of Obstetrics and Gynecology,
    Uniformed Services University of the Health
    Sciences, F. Edward Hebert School of Medicine,
    Bethesda, Maryland. Chief, Urogynecology and
    Reconstructive Pelvic Surgery, Wilford Hall USAF
    Medical Center, Brook Army Medical Center, San
    Antonio Uniformed Services Health Education
    Consortium, San Antonio, Texas

HEPATITIS A TO E

Preface ■ ▼ ◗

Infectious diseases continue to be a major cause of morbidity and mortality, and there are no boundaries with regard to when and where infection will strike. This book was conceived as a single resource for busy physicians who treat women. Hopefully, obstetrician/gynecologists, surgeons, internists, family physicians, pediatricians treating adolescent girls, residents, nurse practitioners, and midwives will find this book to be a useful resource.

Infectious Diseases in Women is a major contribution to the infectious disease literature. The list of contributors is extensive. Each contributing author focused on a specific area with an emphasis on women. The approach to infectious disease in women may—on the surface—be no different from the approach to infectious disease in men; however, there are unique circumstances regarding infections in women. Where disease similarities exist between men and women, these similarities will be readily apparent. When there are situations and conditions unique to diagnosis, treatment, and management in women, these situations and conditions will also become readily apparent.

Our goal is to incorporate basic microbiology into the content of the medical information. This blending should enable the reader to understand how the basic principles facilitate the understanding of the micropathophysiology, and lead the physician to establish a correct diagnosis by employing techniques and diagnostic aides. The end result should be the proper choice of antibiotic therapy and, hopefully, a decrease

in the misuse of antibiotic therapy. Not only should physicians be concerned with treating the patient and achieving a cure, but also we should not contribute to the development of resistant microorganisms. Such resistance would lead to a decrease in successful therapy and an increase in morbidity and mortality.

Again, the ultimate goal of this book is to provide a single resource for the practicing physician caring for women with infection. This book provides an appreciation and foundation for a specific area of women's health—infectious diseases. The book was conceived by obstetrician/gynecologists who have devoted their careers to the area of infectious disease specifically involving women.

We are especially indebted to Mrs. Donna Roth, who has devoted innumerable hours and has also made a true commitment to facilitating completion of this book. This project has consumed a great deal of her time and energy. Mrs. Roth has ensured not only that this project would reach a successful conclusion, but that it is of the highest quality. We would also like to thank Dr. Mark Martens for his contribution. Finally, we would like to thank Cathy Carroll, our Developmental Editor at Saunders, for her patience, understanding, and guidance.

SEBASTIAN FARO, M.D., Ph.D.
DAVID E. SOPER, M.D.
EDITORS

Contents ■ ▼ ▶

Introduction

1

General Microbiology
Bacteriology

SEBASTIAN FARO

Bacteria of importance to women constitute a large number of organisms. Some exist in a commensal relation with the individual, some function synergistically, and some have the potential to cause infection. Bacteria are unique life forms in that they are, for the most part, unicellular; however, they are not eukaryotic cells, but prokaryotes. Bacteria do not have a nucleus that is confined by a nuclear membrane. Thus, bacteria belong to the kingdom Procaryotae.

Bacteria reproduce by binary fission. Most bacteria are capable of performing all tasks necessary for the maintenance of life. Members of the families Chlamydiae and Rickettsiae are true obligate parasites. Bacteria do not contain 80S ribosomes but do contain 70S ribosomes or intracellular organelles; for example, nucleus, mitochondria, lysosomes, endoplasmic reticulum, Golgi bodies, or typical cilia or flagella made up of 9 + 2 fibrils found in eukaryotic cells. Bacteria contain a single circular chromosome that is not encased in a membrane and does not replicate by mitosis. The bacterial cell is surrounded by a cytoplasmic membrane that consists of ester-linked lipids. The cell membrane of bacteria is a structure that not only contains the intracellular cytoplasms, ribosomes, and chromosomes but also carries out transport and biosynthetic functions. Most bacteria, except for *Mycoplasma* and *Ureaplasma*, have a cell wall. The cell walls of all bacteria are not the same. This difference enables some bacteria to retain Gram's reagent, thus staining blue and being classified as gram-positive bacteria, whereas others are not able to retain Gram's reagents and stain red, gram-negative. Some bacteria produce appendages that project from the cell surface, referred to as pili or fimbriae. These appendages serve as adhesive structures that enable the bacterium to adhere to epithelial cells or other bacteria.

Bacterial species are defined by their phenotypic and biochemical characteristics. A bacterial strain is derived from a single colony that has been established in a pure culture. Species are defined by (1) shape, size, specific type of movement, resting stage, Gram stain reaction, and macroscopic growth characteristics, (2) biochemical and nutritional characteristics, (3) physiologic traits relative to oxygen, temperature, pH, and response to antibacterial agents, (4) ecologic characteristics, and (5) DNA base composition, homology, and genetic traits.[1]

All bacteria are placed in the kingdom Procaryotae, and the system of bacterial classification is based on *Bergey's Manual of Systematic Bacteriology.* The kingdom Procaryotae contains four divisions: I, Gracilicutes, the gram-negative bacteria; II, Firmicutes, the gram-positive bacteria; III, Tenericutes, the cell wall–less bacteria; IV, Mendosicutes (Archaeobacteria), bacteria that are predominantly terrestrial and aquatic, found in anaerobic, hypersaline, and hydrothermally or geothermally heated environments.[1] The organization of bacterial classification utilized in *Bergey's Manual* is divided into sections or groups (Table 1–1).[2]

There is an extremely large number of bacteria, but

TABLE 1–1 ▸ GROUPS OF MAJOR BACTERIA

Group 1. Spirochetes
Group 2. Aerobic/microaerophilic, motile, helical/vibrioid gram-negative
Group 3. Nonmotile, gram-negative bacteria
Group 4. Gram-negative aerobic/microaerophilic rods and cocci
Group 5. Facultatively anaerobic gram-negative rods
Group 6. Gram-negative, anaerobic, straight, curved, and helical rods
Group 7. Dissimilatory sulfate- or sulfur-reducing bacteria
Group 8. Anaerobic gram-negative cocci
Group 9. *Rickettsia* and *Chlamydia*
Group 10. Anoxygenic phototropic bacteria
Group 11. Oxygenic phototrophic bacteria
Group 12. Aerobic chemolithotrophic bacteria and associated organisms
Group 13. Budding and/or appendaged bacteria
Group 14. Sheathed bacteria
Group 15. Nonphotosynthetic, nonfruiting gliding bacteria
Group 16. Fruiting gliding bacteria: the *Myxobacterium*
Group 17. Gram-positive cocci
Group 18. Endospore-forming gram-positive rods and cocci
Group 19. Regular, nonsporing gram-positive rods
Group 20. Irregular, nonsporing gram-positive rods
Group 21. *Mycobacterium*
Groups 22–29. *Actinomyces*
Group 30. *Mycoplasma*
Group 31. Methanogens
Group 32. Archeal sulfate reducers
Group 33. *Halobacterium*
Group 34. Cell wall–less Archaeobacteria
Group 35. Extremely thermophilic and hyperthermophilic sulfur-metabolizers

only those that can cause infection in women will be listed. There has been a change in the categories, facultative anaerobic gram-negative bacilli is currently aerobic gram-negative bacilli, the Enterobacteriaceae (fermenters of sugars) and the Nonenterobacteriaceae (nonfermenters). Facultative anaerobic bacteria grow well in an environment that contains oxygen as well as an environment that lacks it. The current recommended classification is divided into nine groups (Table 1–2).[3, 4]

BACTERIAL STRUCTURE

Bacteria range in size from 0.4 μm (*Rickettsia* and *Mycoplasma*) to 0.5 to 10 μm (*Escherichia coli* and *Bacillus anthracis*). Most bacteria are encapsulated by an outer cell wall (except *Mycoplasma*). The chemical structure of the bacterial cell envelope has characteristics that enable it to react specifically with Gram's reagents and acid-fast stain. The bacteria can be divided into gram-positive and gram-negative acid-fast organisms. These organisms differ in the content of lipids, polysaccharides, proteins, and ultrastructure (Table 1–3).

The cell wall of eubacteria consists of cross-linked peptidoglycan. The glycan component consists of alternating beta-1-4- linked *N*-acetyl-D-glucosamine and *N*-acetyl-D-muramic acid. The glycan polymers consist of less than 10 to more than 170 disaccharide repeating

---

TABLE 1–2 ▶ BACTERIAL CLASSIFICATION*

Aerobic Gram-Positive Cocci
  Catalase-Positive
    Staphylococcus aureus
    S. epidermidis
    S. saccharolyticus (*Peptococcus saccharolyticus*)
  Catalase-Negative
    Enterococcus faecalis
    Enterococcus faecium
    Streptococcus agalactiae
    Streptococcus pyogenes
    Viridans streptococci
Aerobic Gram-Negative Cocci
    Moraxella catarrhalis
    Neisseria gonorrhoeae
    N. meningitidis
Aerobic Gram-Positive Bacilli
    Actinomyces israelii
    Corynebacterium diphtheriae
    Lactobacillus acidophilus
    Lactobacillus casei
    Lactobacillus gasseri
    Listeria monocytogenes
    Mycobacterium tuberculosis
    Nocardia asteroides
Aerobic Gram-Negative Bacilli: Enterobacteriaceae
    Citrobacter freundii
    Enterobacter aerogenes
    Enterobacter cloacae
    Escherichia coli
    Klebsiella pneumoniae
    Proteus mirabilis
    Proteus vulgaris
    Providencia rettgeri
    Providencia stuartii
    Salmonella sp.
    Serratia sp.
    Shigella sp.
    Yersinia sp.
Aerobic Gram-Negative Bacilli: Nonenterobacteriaceae (Fermenters)
    Aeromonas sp.
    Pasteurella sp.
    Vibrio sp.
Aerobic Gram-Negative Bacilli: Nonenterobacteriaceae (Nonfermenters)
    Acinetobacter sp.
    Alcaligenes sp.
    Moraxella sp.
    Pseudomonas aeruginosa
    Pseudomonas sp.

Aerobic Gram-Negative Coccobacilli
    Bordetella pertussis
    Brucella abortus
    Calymmatobacterium granulomatis
    Campylobacter sp.
    Chlamydia pneumoniae
    Chlamydia psittaci
    Chlamydia trachomatis
    Haemophilus ducreyi
    Haemophilus influenzae
    Haemophilus parainfluenzae
    Helicobacter pylori
    Legionella sp.
    Rickettsia sp.
Mycoplasma
    Mycoplasma genitalium
    M. hominis
    M. pneumoniae
    Ureaplasma urealyticum
Treponemataceae
    Borrelia burgdorferi
    Borrelia crocidurae
    Borrelia graingeri
    Leptospira sp.
    Treponema pallidum
Anaerobic Gram-Negative Bacilli
    Bacteroides distasonis
    Bacteroides fragilis
    Bacteroides ovatus
    Bacteroides thetaiotaomicron
    Bacteroides vulgatus
    Bacteroides capillosus
    Bacteroides ureolyticus
    Fusobacterium necrophorum
    Fusobacterium nucleatum
    Prevotella bivia
    Prevotella disiens
    Prevotella intermedia
    Prevotella melaninogenica
Non-Spore Forming Gram-Positive Bacilli
    Actinomyces sp.
    Mobiluncus curtisii
    M. mulieris
    Propionibacterium acnes
Endospore-Forming Gram-Positive Bacilli
    Clostridium sp.
Gram-Positive Cocci
    Peptostreptococcus anaerobius

*The above list does not include all bacteria that can cause infection, but represents only those that are more commonly associated with infections in women.

TABLE 1-3 ▶ CHEMICAL CONSTITUENTS OF THE THREE TYPES OF BACTERIAL CELL ENVELOPES		
Gram-Positive	**Gram-Negative**	**Acid-Fast Bacteria**
Peptidoglycan (multilayered)	Peptidoglycan (bilayered)	Peptidoglycan (trilayered)
Proteins	Lipoproteins	Polypeptides
Lipoteichoic acids	Outer membrane	Mycolic acid–glycolipids
Teichoic acids	Lipopolysaccharides	Arabinogalactans Arabinomannans
Teichuronic acid	Proteins	Cord factor
Polysaccharides	Polysaccharides	Sulfolipids Mycocides Lipooligosaccharides

Adapted from Wheat RW: Composition, structure, and biosynthesis of bacterial cell envelope and energy storage polymers. In: Joklik WK, Willet HP, Amos DB, Wilfert CM (eds): Zinsser Microbiology. East Norwalk, CT, Appleton & Lange, 1992, pp 76–93.

units. The glycan chains that are layered in parallel rows are cross-linked through peptide units via lactic acid carboxyl groups of the muramic acid to the amino acid and of a tetrapeptide (L-alanine-D-glutamic acid-D, L-diaminopimelic acid-D-alanine). A continuous framework of glycotetrapeptides is formed via cross-linkage of tetrapeptide units.[5]

The cell wall contains three major groups of lytic enzymes: (1) endo-beta-1,4-N-acetylhexosamidases, (2) endopeptidases, and (3) amidases. The endo-beta-1,4-N-acetylhexosamidases cleave the glycan polymers between N-acetylmuramic acid and N-acetylglucosamine or acetylglucosamine–muramic acid glucosidic linkages. Endopeptidases hydrolyze the interpeptide linkages. The amidases hydrolyze the glycan-peptide bond between N-acetylmuramic acid and L-alanine.[6]

Several components of the bacterial cell wall have the capability to stimulate the immune response. N-Acetylmuramyl-L-alanyl-D-isoglutamine, referred to as muramyldipeptide (MDP), is pyrogenic.[7] Group A polysaccharide found in Streptococcus pyogenes has been shown to induce endogenous pyrogens, such as interleukin-1 (IL-1), inflammatory arthritic joint disease, granulomatous liver disease, and inflammatory bowel disease,

The outer membrane (OM) is found only in gram-negative bacteria and contains phospholipids, lipopolysaccharides (LPS), and a variety of proteins (pore proteins or porins and lipoproteins). The outer membrane is bilayered; the LPS is found in the outer layer, and the phospholipid resides in the inner layer. The outer membrane serves multiple functions (Table 1–4).[8]

Porins (pore proteins) are proteins that form stable openings, or pores, in the outer membrane that permit the diffusion of small molecules across the OM into the cell.[9, 10] Among Procaryotae, porins are found only in gram-negative bacteria and may demonstrate either specific or nonspecific activity with regard to the pas-

TABLE 1-4 ▶ FUNCTIONS OF THE OUTER MEMBRANE
A barrier to hydrophobic barrier
A molecular differentiating barrier to water-soluble molecules
Has receptors for attachment of bacteriophage and bacterial conjugation
Contains a variety of compounds (enzymes, aggressins, evasins, and toxins) to enhance pathogenesis
Protects the bacterial cell from environmental poisons
Encloses the cellular contents
Releases LPS and proteins

sage of molecules. Some porins function mainly as receptors; for example, the OM protein A (OmpA) functions as the F-pilus receptor in conjunction with porins and has low activity with regard to regulating the passage of molecules into the cell.

The OM also functions as a barrier, especially in bacteria that exist in environments that are hyperosmotic, for example, bile salts, chemical, and digestive enzymes. The OM also blocks the entrance of various compounds (e.g., antimicrobial agents, macromolecules). The barrier function is most evident among the enteric bacteria.

Lipopolysaccharide lipid contains lipid A (endotoxin), which is found in gram-negative bacteria. Lipopolysaccharide is amphiphilic; that is, one end is hydrophilic and the other end is hydrophobic. Basically, LPS consists, in most instances, of three regions: (1) O-specific polysaccharide, referred to as region I; (2) core polysaccharide, region II; and (3) lipid A, region III. All gram-negative bacteria produce identical lipid A components of LPS. Not all gram-negative bacteria (e.g., Neisseria and Haemophilus species), produce region I polysaccharides. These bacteria produce a shorter region II polysaccharide called lipolyoligosaccharides (LOS).

Lipopolysaccharide lipid A, or endotoxin, is a powerful compound that has a variety of pathophysiologic effects associated with gram-negative infection (Table 1–5). Endotoxin causes release of cytokines (e.g., IL-1, tumor necrosis factor [TNF], IL-6), leukocytosis, a rise in plasma cortisol, hypoferremia, hypozinemia, hypertriglyceridemia, hypoglycemia, production of colony-stimulating growth factor, alterations in liver enzymes, presence of fibrin polymers, and synthesis of serum amyloid.[11] Endotoxin stimulates macrophages to produce endogenous pyrogens. IL-1, IL-6, and TNF-α in-

TABLE 1-5 ▶ PATHOPHYSIOLOGIC EFFECTS OF ENDOTOXIN	
Fever	Hypotension
Hematologic changes	Disseminated intravascular
Changes in the immune response	coagulation (DIC)
Endocrinologic alterations	Shock
Metabolic changes	Death

duce the production of prostaglandins (e.g., PGE$_2$), which act on the hypothalamus. Other pyrogenic compounds produced are macrophage inflammation factor-1-alpha (MIF-1-alpha) and MIF-1-beta.

The cell walls of the gram-positive bacteria are much thicker than those of the gram-negative bacteria. The M protein, the virulence factor of group A *Streptococcus*, forms a diffuse, thick layer external to the cell wall. The cell walls of gram-positive bacteria do not contain LPS or endotoxin, as do those of the gram-negative bacteria. The difference in thickness separates the gram-positive bacteria from the gram-negative bacteria with regard to their reaction to Gram's reagents.

The Bayer junctions, or adhesions sites, seen in gram-negative cells are found internally. External adhesion sites function as points of attachment for bacteriophage and complement-mediated lysis. The internal Bayer junctions are considered to be growth sites, translocation of secretory protein, OM proteins, LPS, capsular polysaccharides, and emergence sites for sex pili and flagella.[12]

The periplasm lies in the space between the inner membrane and the outer membrane. The periplasm is usually present and can be detected in gram-negative bacteria but may not be readily detected in gram-positive bacteria.[13] The periplasm contains membrane-derived oligosaccharides, and hydrolytic enzymes (proteases, nucleases, beta-lactamases, protein-binding sugars, amino acids, and ions).

The bacterial cell membrane contains most of the cell protein and up to 40% of the cell lipid. The major lipids are phosphatidylethanolamine, phosphatidylglycerol, and glycolipids. The bacterial cell membranes also house energy-producing cytochrome and oxidative phosphorylating enzymes. The bacterial cell membrane also plays a role in regulating the passage of material into and out of the cell. In addition, polymer-synthesizing enzymes are also found on the cell membrane.

Mesosomes are membrane cytoplasmic sacs found in gram-positive bacteria. The mesosome contains lamellar, tubular, or vesicular structures. The mesosomes are involved with the development of division septa. The mesosome appears to be attached to the DNA chromatin and cell membrane.

The bacterial DNA does not exist as a discrete nucleus, as is found in eukaryotic cells, but as a fibril that lies parallel to the axis of the cell. During bacterial multiplication, the DNA does form a structure resembling a chromosome but remains as a diffuse bacterial cell containing a chromatin fibrillar network.

The bacterial cell contains a 70S ribosome that can be dissociated into 30S and 50S subunits. The ribosomes form aggregates or chains of 70S ribosomes attached to messenger RNA. Rapid, actively growing bacteria contain a larger number of ribosomes than slowly growing bacterial cells. Only the fimbriated strains of *Neisseria gonorrhoeae* are infectious. The M protein of group A *Streptococcus* is an adhesin that enables the organism to colonize host epithelium.[14] The M protein also functions as an evasin, preventing phagocytosis, and is leukocytal, thus functioning as an aggressin or toxin.[12]

Specific microfibrils are present on gram-negative bacteria, known as common pili or sex pili. These pili may also be present with other pili and are usually not present in abundant numbers. For example, there may be up to 200 fimbriae per cell, whereas there are usually 1 to 4 sex pili present on the same bacterial cell.[15, 16] The pili attach to a receptor on the receiving cell, and genetic material is transferred to the cell.

The bacterial cell typically reproduces by cellular division. The growth time is dependent on the particular species; for example, *Escherichia coli* reproduces every 60 minutes. Cell division and DNA replication are closely timed to ensure that each cell receives an identical amount of genetic material. In *E. coli*, replication of DNA takes approximately 40 minutes and cell division takes about 20 minutes. Cell division occurs following replication of DNA.[17, 18]

There are three stages in the replication of bacterial DNA. The initial stage, referred to as "initiation," begins at a specific site on the genome, known as oriC. Activation of oriC requires a specific protein that is synthesized by a *dnaA* gene. Activation occurs when the activator protein binds to oriC, which, in turn, facilitates the binding of a second protein (helicase) synthesized by a *dnaB* gene. The enzyme helicase is responsible for unwinding the DNA near the origin, which allows DNA polymerase to initiate replication.[19, 20]

The second stage is elongation. Following initiation, the DNA unwinds and replication of both single strands begins in opposite directions, resulting in duplication of the bacterial genome. DNA polymerase is the enzyme responsible for adding nucleoside residues in the 5'3' direction for chain growth. *Escherichia coli* possesses three DNA polymerases: DNA polymerase I is responsible for repairing gaps; DNA polymerase II is responsible for DNA repair; and DNA polymerase III is responsible for DNA synthesis.[19, 21]

DNA repair occurs only in the 5'3' direction; this is referred to as the leading strand, and because the two parental strands are in an antiparallel position, the opposite strand (lagging strand) is replicated in a manner different from that of the 5'3' strand. Replication of the lagging strand occurs in segments, or discontinuous retrograde patches, referred to as Okazaki fragments. Once a fragment is completed, it is united to an adjacent fragment by DNA ligase.

The third stage in DNA replication is termination. There are four identical DNA sequences that function to block replication. The terminus region is located at approximately the middle portion of the DNA chromosome.

REFERENCES

1. Wheat RW: The classification and identification of bacteria. In: Joklik WK, Willet HP, Amos DB, Wilfert CM (eds): Zinsser Microbiology. East Norwalk, CT, Appleton & Lange, 1992, pp 8–17.
2. Holt JG, Kreig NR, Sneath PHA, et al: Bergey's Manual of Determinative Bacteriology. Baltimore, Williams & Wilkins, 1994, pp 17–21.
3. Bruckner DA, Colonna P: Nomenclature for aerobic and facultative bacteria. Clin Infect Dis 1997; 25:1.
4. Jousimies-Somer H, Summanen P: Microbiology terminology update: Clinically significant anaerobic gram-positive and gram-negative bacteria (excluding spirochetes). Clin Infect Dis 1997; 25:11.
5. Wheat RW: Composition, structure, and biosynthesis of bacterial cell envelope and energy storage polymers. In: Joklik WK, Willet HP, Amos DB, Wilfert CM (eds): Zinsser Microbiology. East Norwalk, CT, Appleton & Lange, 1992, pp 76–93.
6. Ghuysen JM: Use of bacteriolytic enzymes in determination of wall structure and their role in cell metabolism. Bacteriol Rev 1968; 32:425.
7. Chetty C, Klapper DG, Schwab JH: Soluble peptidoglycan-polysaccharide fragments of the bacterial cell wall induce acute inflammation. Infect Immun 1982; 38:1010.
8. Inouye M (ed): Bacterial Outer Membranes: Biogenesis and Functions. New York, Wiley, 1979.
9. Nikaido H: Outer membrane barrier as a mechanism of antimicrobial resistance. Antimicrob Agents Chemother 1989; 33:1831.
10. Nikaido H, Vaara M: Molecular basis of bacterial outer membrane permeability. Microbiol Rev 1985; 49:1.
11. Vogel SN, Hogan MM: Role of cytokines in endotoxin-mediated host responses. In: Oppenheim JJ, Shevach E (eds): Immunophysiology: Role of Cells and Cytokines in Immunity and Inflammation. New York, University of Oxford Press, 1990, p 238.
12. Wheat RW: Bacterial morphology and ultrastructure. In: Joklik WK, Willett HP, Amos DB, Wilfert CM (eds): Zinsser Microbiology. East Norwalk, CT, Appleton & Lange, 1992, pp 18–30.
13. Cook WR, McAlister TJ, Rothfield LI: Compartmentalization of the periplasmic space at division sites in gram-negative bacteria. J Bacteriol 1986; 168:1430.
14. Beachey EH: Bacterial adherence: Adhesin-receptor interactions mediating the attachment of bacteria to mucosal surfaces. J Infect Dis 1981; 143:325.
15. Clegg S, Gerlach GF: Enterobacterial fimbriae. J Bacteriol 1987; 169:934.
16. Gaastra W, de Graaf FK: Host-specific fimbrial adhesins of noninvasive enterotoxigenic Escherichia coli strains. Microbiol Rev 1982; 46:129.
17. Cooper S, Helmstetter CE: Chromosome replication and the division cycle of Escherichia coli. Br J Mol Biol 1968; 31:519.
18. Clark DJ: Regulation of deoxyribonucleic acid replication and cell division in E. coli. Br J Bacteriol 1968; 96:1214.
19. Jacob F, Brenner S, Cuzin F: On regulation of DNA replication in bacteria. Cold Springs Habor Symp Quant Biol 1963; 28:329.
20. Meselen M, Stahl FW: The replication of DNA in Escherichia coli. Proc Natl Acad Sci 1958; 44:671.
21. Jacob F, Brenner S, Cuzin F: On regulation of DNA replication in bacteria. Cold Springs Harbor Symp Quant Biol 1963; 28:329.
22. Meselson M, Stahl FW: The replication of DNA in Escherichia coli. Proc Natl Acad Sci USA 1958; 44:671.

Virology

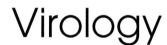

DAVID A. BAKER

Of major impact to women is infection and the disease caused by viruses. Over the last three decades,[1] the incidence of sexually transmitted bacterial infections has decreased in the United States. However, there has been a marked, prolonged, and major increase in viral sexually transmitted diseases that affect women.

The classification and structure of viral infections into individual viral families relies on whether the virus is composed of either RNA or DNA, the protein coat of the virus called the capsid and whether the capsid is surrounded by a lipid envelope.[2] The classification of viruses currently has approximately 19 distinct families and has become complex and has expanded with the discovery of new viruses that infect humans.[3]

Infection of the cell by a virus requires many events and can lead to cell death or can produce latent or dormant viral infections. There must be initial viral attachment to the cell surface in order for the virus to infect the cell and produce disease.[4] Much work and research has elaborated the viral cell attachment proc-

ess. It appears that many viruses may attach by specific proteins or specific receptors either produced by the virus or found on the cell surface. Viruses that possess a lipid envelope may require this structure for viral attachment. Research into antiviral compounds that prevent or inhibit viral cell attachment holds great promise.

Once attachment is completed, the infecting virus must penetrate the cellular member.[5] The entry into the cell again is complex, and there may be varied mechanisms by which different viruses penetrate the cell membrane. Once the virus has penetrated into the cell, it exhibits elaborate mechanisms and the ability to use cellular structures and function to replicate its RNA or DNA as well as its required proteins.[6] In many cases, the virus produces specific viral coated proteins or enzymes that are required for viral multiplication and for the virus to successfully complete its life cycle. This basic research into the mechanisms by which viruses replicate intracellularly has led to the production of potent antiviral agents.[7] All that remains for the virus is assembly and exit from the cell. Many viruses produce a lytic cycle in which there is cell destruction and release of many viral particles, whereas others allow the cell to remain relatively intact, with production of continuous viral particles at low levels. This leads to the concepts of acute and chronic viral infections: in the former, the virus causes the host's death; in the latter, the virus is latent or dormant for periods, with infection causing sporadic disease.

The pathogenesis of viral infections is the process by which a virus produces disease in the host. Different viruses have different degrees of virulence, which implies the ability of the virus to produce significant illness or death. There are numerous and varied ways by which viruses are transmitted to humans. Certainly the most common are as follows: the virus enters the respiratory tract, the virus directly enters into the gastrointestinal tract, and vertical transmission from mother to fetus or newborn. One of the most common modes of viral infection in women is through sexual contact. It is clear from numerous studies that the female is at significantly greater risk for viral infection than is the male during sexual intercourse: the female has greater surface area that can be exposed to viral infections, with a greater potential for a large inoculum of virus to contact a mucosal surface.

After infection of the specific target site, the virus disseminates via the lymphatic system, blood stream, or nervous system. Of the specific pathogens that pose significant problems for women, herpes simplex virus is considered neurotrophic, and spread of this virus can occur via the nervous system. Hematogenous dissemination is a major factor in the spread of specific viral infections. There may be direct entry into the patient's blood stream via transfusion of blood or blood products, or by invasion of tissue after replication at a primary site. Most primary viral infections produce viremia, which results in systemic manifestations of the infection that could include fatigue, myalgia, lethargy, and fever. Of major concern is when the female host is pregnant: the viremia could produce infection of the fetus. It is clear that transmission or transport of virus in the blood stream may involve either the cell-free plasma or specific cells of the blood stream infected with the particular organism.[8] An example of this mechanism by which virus survives and is transported within the host by macrophages is seen with human immunodeficiency virus (HIV). In the majority of viral infections, there is a short period of time during which virus appears in the blood stream. In the significantly immunocompromised patient, there may be a marked increase in the duration as well as in the quantity of virus found within the blood stream. Numerous viral infections incorporate many routes for facilitating the spread of the virus. A prime

example of this is varicella-zoster virus. With this pathogen, there is initial infection and spread within the lung, and then subsequent viremia and transmission to the host's skin. From the skin, infection proceeds to sensory neurons, resulting in a latent virus infection located in the dorsal root ganglia.[9] Many other factors influence pathogenesis and virulence, including tissue trophism in which only specific viral types infect specific tissues. A principal example of this is human papillomavirus: only specific types of this virus infect the male and female genital tracts. Continued research is directed specifically at how viral proteins interact with the host cell genome. In addition, the basic genetic make-up of the host may play a significant part in determining the ability of the virus to infect the specific host and produce disease.

Health care providers must appreciate the specific prevalence of infection and risk that sexually active patients face with regard to acquiring these viral infections. Therefore, clinicians must be alert to the incidence of specific viral infections in their patients' communities and offer appropriate counseling, education, and therapeutic and preventive interventions for their patients. A complete and frank history elicited from the patient is a necessity in providing the best patient care. The history includes a comprehensive and detailed sexual history, with the realization that oral-genital contact can transmit these organisms into the oral or genital mucosa.[10, 11] The clinician needs to inquire about anal intercourse and other sexual practices in addition to any history of symptomatic disease in the patient's sexual partner. Knowing the incubation period of the specific infection is important. The mean incubation period for primary genital herpes is short—approximately 6 days.[12] For genital warts, the incubation is significantly greater, approximately 1 to 3 months; for molluscum contagiosum, it is 2 to 26 weeks.[13] Additional history is important in determining the specific risks of sexually transmitted diseases (STDs), including specific viral STDs. This additional information includes residence and travel outside of the United States.

The specific clinical presentation of the disease may be varied and atypical, especially in patients with an underlying immunodeficiency. Recurrent severe genital herpes is one of the initial presentations of HIV infection.[14] Although many of these viral STDs are acquired without clinical symptoms and may be present and transmitted subclinically, many patients present with specific complaints. Certainly, investigation for viral STDs may be appropriate in patients presenting with vaginal discharge, pain, and pruritus and with the presentation of typical or atypical lesions. Therefore, a careful clinical inspection of the external and internal genital tract should be performed, with an emphasis on proper lighting and magnification to determine whether there are any vesicular, ulcerative, papular, or verrucous lesions. In addition, careful inspection of the perianal region should be performed on all patients. Only with a heightened sense of awareness and careful attention to history, examination, and ordering appropriate laboratory testing can this epidemic of viral STDs be managed.

This book deals specifically with the most common viral STDs, including HIV, human papillomavirus, and herpes simplex virus infections. There is emphasis on these specific infections because of their high incidence in and easy transmission to susceptible women.

REFERENCES

1. Centers for Disease Control: Sexually Transmitted Disease Surveillance 1997. 1998, 5:64.
2. Harrison S: Principles of virus structure. In: Fields BN (ed): Virology. New York, Raven Press, 1990.
3. Tyler KL, Fields BN: Introduction to viruses and viral disease. In: Mandell GL, Bennett JE, Dolin R (eds): Principles and Practice of Infectious Diseases. New York, Churchill Livingstone, 1995.
4. Lonberg-Holm K: Attachment of animal viruses to cells: An introduction. In: Lonberg-Holm K, Philipson L (eds): Virus Receptors, Part 2. London, Chapman & Hall, 1981, pp 3–20.
5. Simons K, Garoff H, Helenius A: How an animal virus gets into and out of its host cell. Sci Am 1982; 246:58.
6. Fields BN, Knipe DM (eds): Fields Virology, 2nd ed. New York, Raven Press, 1990.
7. Galasso GJ, Merigan TC, Buchanan RA (eds): Antiviral Agents and Viral Disease of Man, 3rd ed. New York, Raven Press, 1990.
8. Tyler KL, Fields BN: Pathogenesis of viral infections. In: Fields BN, Knipe DM (eds): Fields Virology. New York, Raven Press, 1990, pp 191–240.
9. Gelb LDB: Varicella-zoster virus. In: Fields BN (ed): Virology. New York, Raven Press, 1990, pp 2011–2054.
10. Choukass NC, Toto PD: Condyloma accuminatum of the oral cavity. Oral Surg 1982; 54:480.
11. Mertz GJ: Genital herpes simplex virus infections. Med Clin North Am 1990; 74:1433.
12. Corey L, Adams HG, Brown ZA, et al: Genital herpes simplex infection: Clinical manifestations, course, and complications. Ann Intern Med 1983; 98:958.
13. Margolis S: Genital warts and molluscum contagiosum. Urol Clin North Am 1984; 11:163.
14. Siegal FP, Lopez C, Hammer GS, et al: Severe acquired immunodeficiency in male homosexuals manifested by chronic perianal herpes simplex lesions. N Engl J Med 1981; 305:1439.

Parasitology

JOSEPH G. PASTOREK, II

The physician practicing in a "developed" country, working within a modern urban environment, driving to the hospital or clinic in an air-conditioned automobile, scrubbing for surgery with clean running water, rarely thinks of the diseases caused by the various protozoan parasites. Unless he is traveling out of the country and is warned to take medications for malaria prophylaxis, for example, the gynecologist in the civilized world simply addresses the ever-present *Trichomonas* infection (addressed in Chapter 20 in this text), or counsels a patient here or there on the risk of contracting toxoplasmosis (covered in Chapter 3 as well) during pregnancy, and relegates the bulk of his tropical medicine and parasitology training to some seldom-used corridor of his brain. Why should someone in New York City, so far from the jungles of equatorial Africa, worry about malaria, after all? Why would someone in the Wisconsin suburbs, with modern water treatment plants and running water, worry about a water supply contaminated with protozoa? Indeed!

Well, dear reader, the era of "emerging disease" is upon us. Illnesses, especially infectious diseases, which had been driven almost to extinction in our parts of the world are making a comeback. Because of world travel, because of a large reservoir of immunocompromised individuals, because of massive political migrations, and, yes, because of war, microorganisms are hitch-hiking on humans and animals to return to areas from which they had been exterminated.

Take malaria in the United States, for example. As of the 1950s, malaria had been considered to be eradicated from this country, save for an occasional imported case. That is, someone infected elsewhere (e.g., Africa) happens to get off an airplane in the U.S. before his disease is recognized and treated. However, in the past decade, there have been several episodes of locally acquired malaria in areas of the U.S. with dense populations and appropriate mosquito infestations, including New York City, Houston, and suburban New Jersey.[1] Similarly, in 1993, a "modern" water supply, namely a Milwaukee water works plant, was responsible for 400,000 cases of intestinal *Cryptosporidium* infection, which resulted in some deaths despite the fact that the water was properly treated and filtered following accepted protocols.[2]

Thus, the modern physician, even in the most advanced of countries, cannot turn a deaf ear to discussions of protozoan disease. His patients, and even he and his family, may be the next "victims" of his ignorance.

AMEBIASIS

Epidemiology

The causative agent of human intestinal and extraintestinal amebiasis is the protozoan organism *Entamoeba histolytica.* Other species of amebae may inhabit the human intestinal tract, such as *E. coli, E. gingivalis, E. polecki, Endolimax nana, Dientamoeba fragilis* (possibly a pathogen), and *Iodamoeba bütschlii.*[3] Further, *E. histolytica* is thought to have pathogenic and nonpathogenic strains, those nonpathogens separated into a distinct *Entamoeba dispar.*[4] Therefore, estimates of the true prevalence of *E. histolytica* infection are less than accurate, since older reports did not necessarily distinguish between the nonpathogenic amebae and the *E. histolytica.*[5] It is estimated, however, that intestinal carriage of *Entamoeba* affects roughly 10% of the world's population (approximately 500 to 600 million persons), but in only 10% of these cases is the organism pathogenic, i.e., *E. histolytica.* Further, the prevalence of amebic liver disease is much lower. Even so, the combination of either colitis or hepatic abscesses is estimated to occur in only 7% to 8% of cases of amebiasis.[6] It has been calculated that complicated amebiasis, as opposed to simple intestinal carriage, is responsible for more than 40,000 deaths annually.[7]

The invasive form of *E. histolytica* is the trophozoite, which may invade the colonic mucosa and from there occasionally travel elsewhere in the host (e.g., the liver). However, trophozoites quickly die outside of the body. Therefore, it is the cyst form of the organism, produced in the colon and excreted in the feces, which may remain viable in a suitable moist environment for months. Fecal contamination is thus almost a prerequisite for amebiasis, and for this reason amebiasis is primarily a disease of the poor, the overcrowded, and the institutionalized. Close communal living, in the setting of inadequate plumbing, facilitates the spread of the protozoan. In addition, male homosexual behavior presumably spreads the organism by anal contact. The illness itself, once the organism has been acquired, is more severe in neonates and children, pregnant and postpartum women, patients with malignancies, patients treated with corticosteroids and other immunosuppressive medications, and the malnourished.[8]

Clinical Manifestations

The majority of persons infected with *E. histolytica* at any given time are asymptomatic. If invasion of the colonic mucosa occurs, it may be of varying degrees, with various clinical signs and symptoms present. It is helpful to conceptualize amebic infections as existing along a spectrum: the clinician will place the individual patient into one category or another according to her presentation and the results of ancillary tests.

Entamoeba histolytica *Infection*

INTESTINAL AMEBIASIS

- ▶ Asymptomatic infection
- ▶ Symptomatic infection, noninvasive
- ▶ Amebic dysentery (usually colon or rectum)
- ▶ Fulminant colitis with perforation
- ▶ Toxic megacolon
- ▶ Chronic colitis
- ▶ Ameboma
- ▶ Perianal ulceration

EXTRAINTESTINAL AMEBIASIS

- ▶ Lung abscess
- ▶ Liver abscess (with or without peritonitis, empyema, pericarditis)
- ▶ Brain abscess
- ▶ Genitourinary amebiasis (e.g., rectovaginal fistula)

Quite obviously, the patient with amebiasis may present with anything from nonspecific colic to fulminant, catastrophic illness. What is incumbent on the physician is to be aware of the possibility of amebiasis in any patient with the appropriate constellation of symptoms and possibility of infection, and to perform the appropriate testing (see later) so that the diagnosis may be made without any untoward delay.

The pregnant woman with amebiasis may be at risk for more invasive infection, owing to increased cortisol and increased circulating levels of cholesterol (utilized for parasite growth), and also because of relatively depressed T-cell immunity.[8, 9] However, amebic liver abscess appears less common during pregnancy, perhaps because of the protective effect of estrogen. Also, transplacental infection with amebae has not been reported.

Pathophysiology

The *E. histolytica* trophozoite may live in the crypts of the colonic mucosa without causing disease. However, when invasion occurs, it is an apparent lytic effect (hence, the name) on the colonic epithelium that allows the organism to produce the characteristic ulcerations and invade further. In animal models, it has been determined that the mucus layer insulates the colonic epithelium from invasion by the ameba.[10] Thus, one can speculate as to the nature of the circumstances that would interrupt the colonic mucus in a previously asymptomatic carrier and lead to invasive disease; for example, malnutrition, other causes of dysentery, and trauma (anal intercourse).

Invasive disease thus occurs in the setting of (1) adherence of the protozoan to the colonic cell wall; (2) cytolytic and/or proteolytic effects on the host cell; and (3) resistance by the organism to the host's defense mechanisms.[11] The host immune mechanisms operative in amebic infection are still incompletely understood, and obviously there are some mechanical factors in play (e.g., mucus layer). However, repeat infection is rare, and human antibody is cidal to normal trophozoites (as distinguished from trophozoites in patients with amebic liver abscess). Therefore, it is apparent that at least some humoral protection is operative after an immune response against the organism has been mounted. Such is the basis for hopes of a vaccine against *E. histolytica*.[8]

Diagnosis

Serologic studies or stool studies of populations may give an overall numerical figure of amebic colonization, but this does not accurately identify the individual who is acutely or chronically suffering from clinical amebiasis, since the majority of patients with intestinal amebiasis are asymptomatic. Therefore, it is problematic to match a patient with some complaint or other with a positive fecal smear or biopsy, and declare it a case of amebiasis. The Centers for Disease Control and Prevention have therefore published a case definition for use in determining whether a given patient indeed constitutes a case of clinical amebiasis:

Clinical Description:
Infection of the large intestine by *E. histolytica* may result in an illness of variable severity ranging from mild, chronic diarrhea to fulminant dysentery. Infection also may be asymptomatic. Extraintestinal infection also can occur (e.g., hepatic abscess).

Intestinal Amebiasis:
▶ Demonstration of cysts or trophozoites of *E. histolytica* in stool or
▶ Demonstration of trophozoites in tissue biopsy or ulcer scrapings by culture or histopathology (Fig. 1–1)

Case Classification:
▶ Confirmed, intestinal amebiasis: a clinically compatible illness that is laboratory confirmed
▶ Confirmed, extraintestinal amebiasis: a parasitologically confirmed infection of extraintestinal tissue, or among symptomatic persons (with clinical or radiographic findings consistent with extraintestinal infection), demonstration of specific antibody against *E. histolytica* as measured by indirect hemagglutination or other reliable immunodiagnostic test (e.g., enzyme-linked immunosorbent assay).[12]

Treatment and Prevention

Eradication of fecal contamination of water sources and foodstuffs is of paramount importance in the prevention of amebiasis. Most commonly, vegetables that are exposed to feces above ground (e.g., lettuce) and water sources that allow sewage contamination are the culprits in such infection. On the other hand, purposeful fecal contact (i.e., anal intercourse) may also be a source of contamination. Thus, avoidance of these is mandatory. Boiling of water and washing of vegetables with strong detergent (and of course the abandonment of use of human feces for fertilization) are recommended.

Treatment of amebiasis depends on where in the spectrum of disease the patient's condition lies. One set of recommendations is presented in Table 1–6.[8] Of note for use in pregnancy: Metronidazole is extensively used (after the first trimester of pregnancy) and has been shown not to be teratogenic[13]; paromomycin is an aminoglycoside that, though toxic when given parenterally, is not absorbed when given orally[14]; chlo-

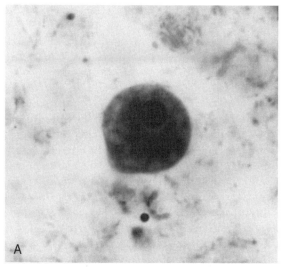
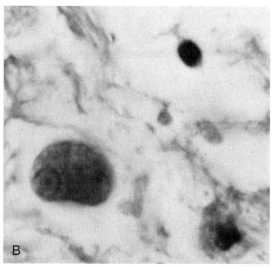

FIGURE 1–1 ▶ Histologic section of *Entamoeba histolytica* trophozoites invading tissue.

TABLE 1-6 ▶ RECOMMENDED TREATMENT SCHEDULES FOR VARIOUS STAGES OF AMEBIASIS

Stage	Drug	Dosage	Duration	Efficacy (%)
Intraluminal	Diloxanide	500 mg tid	10 days	87–96
	Paromomycin	30 mg/kg/day	5–10 days	85–90
	Tetracycline	250 mg qid	10 days	95
	followed by			
	Diiodohydroxyquin	650 mg tid	20 days	
	Metronidazole	750 mg tid	10 days	90
Invasive colitis	Metronidazole	750 mg tid	5–10 days	>90
		or		
		2.4 g qd	2–3 days	>90
		or		
		50 mg/kg	One dose	86
		plus		
	Diloxanide or paromomycin (for intraluminal eradication)			
	Tetracycline	250 mg qid	15 days	94
	plus			
	Chloroquine base	600 mg once, 300 mg once then, 150 mg tid for 14 days	14 days	
	Dehydroemetine	1–1.5 mg/kg/day IM	5 days	90
		plus		
	Diloxanide or paromomycin (for intraluminal eradication)			
Liver abscess	Metronidazole	750 mg tid	5–10 days	95
		or		
		2.4 g qd	1–2 days	
		plus		
	Diloxanide or paromomycin (for intraluminal eradication)			
	Dehydroemetine	1–1.5 mg/kg/day IM	5 days	90
		plus		
	Diloxanide or paromomycin (for intraluminal eradication)			
	Chloroquine base	600 mg once, 300 mg once then, 150 mg tid for 14 days	14 days	60
	(can be added to other drugs, rather than used alone)			

Adapted from Ravdin JI, Petri WA: *Entamoeba histolytica* (amebiasis). In: Mandell GL, Bennett JE, Dolin R (eds): Principles and Practice of Infectious Diseases, 4th ed. New York, Churchill Livingstone, 1995.

roquine has been extensively used for malaria during pregnancy and is considered safe.

BABESIOSIS

Epidemiology

The various species of the intraerythrocytic parasitic protozoan *Babesia* are found extensively in animals, particularly in tropical and subtropical areas. Some species cause significant economic losses in farm animals. In fact, the plague that decimated the cattle of the Pharaoh Rameses the Second in the Bible's book of Genesis was possibly babesiosis,[15] and "Texas cattle fever," caused by a species of *Babesia*, was the first disease demonstrated to be arthropod-borne, in 1893. However, babesiosis in humans has been formally recognized only since 1957, when a human case was reported from Yugoslavia.[16]

In the United States, human babesiosis is caused primarily by *Babesia microti*, but also occasionally *B. bigemina*; in Europe, *B. divergens* and *B. bovis* (which may be the same species) are seen. What these infections have in common is the proximity of humans to an animal reservoir (especially the white-footed deer mouse in North America, and cattle in Europe), and the presence of a suitable arthropod vector, namely, ticks of the genus *Ixodes* (*I. dammini*, also called *I. scapularis*, in the U.S., and *I. ricinus* in Europe) (Fig. 1–2). Thus, in the U.S., the documented human cases of babesiosis have occurred in the context of campers, hunters, and other vacationers encountering ticks in areas endemic to the rodent vectors, such as the New England states and states farther south on the U.S. Atlantic coast, as well as Wisconsin, Minnesota, Washington state, and Mexico. In Europe, exposure to cattle (and their ticks) was implicated in Yugoslavia, Russia, France, and the British Isles. Further, *B. divergens/bovis* infections in Europe are encountered almost entirely in splenectomized individuals.[17]

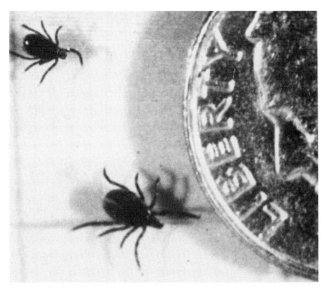

FIGURE 1-2 ▶ Male deer tick, *Ixodes dammini* (*I. scapularis*).

Clinical Manifestations

The clinical presentation of human babesiosis depends in large part on the clinical situation; that is, the particular species of *Babesia* and whether the human victim has an intact spleen and competent immune system. Infection with *B. microti*, in the United States, generally manifests as a mild, self-limiting illness with onset 1 to 3 weeks after the bite of the infected tick nymph. In the elderly, or in immunocompromised individuals (including those without spleens), however, the infection may be severe, leading to massive hemolysis, shock, renal shut-down, and adult respiratory distress syndrome (ARDS), all of which is similar to the usual presentation of *B. divergens* infection in Europe, where infection almost always occurs in splenectomized individuals.

Fortunately, the majority of cases of babesiosis in the U.S. represent a nonspecific syndrome complex of malaise, fatigue, fever, headache, myalgia, arthralgia, nausea, vomiting, and other constitutional symptoms. Rash has been noted, but there is a high probability that patients infected with *Babesia* have also been infected with the agent of Lyme disease, so that the rash may be secondary to borreliosis, rather than babesiosis. The illness has been thought to be self-limited, although a recent report indicates that chronic parasitemia may occur in a significant proportion of cases, especially if untreated or improperly treated.[18]

Babesiosis has been described in pregnancy, although not with great enough frequency to determine the course of the disease (i.e., is it different from infection in the nonpregnant individual?), whether the organism crosses the human placenta, or whether the fetus suffers any direct ill effects.[19] Extrapolating from infection in animals, it is expected that occasional fetal infection will cause hydropic hemolytic disease not unlike that seen, for example, with human parvovirus B19.[20]

Pathophysiology

The sporozoite of the *Babesia* protozoan resides in the salivary glands of the tick. At a prolonged blood meal, the sporozoites are ultimately injected into the mammalian host's blood steam, where they penetrate the erythrocyte, transforming into trophozoites. Trophozoites reproduce by asexual budding, dividing into two or four daughter merozoites (Fig. 1-3). The division (schizogony) is asynchronous, and *Babesia* organisms exit their erythrocyte hosts in more of a steady stream, unlike that of malarial organisms. Therefore there are no periodic bouts of fever or massive hemolysis due to large, discrete waves of merozoites being released. As the merozoites exit the erythrocyte, the plasma membrane is damaged, perforated, and otherwise deformed, ultimately leading to cell disruption (hemolysis).

Deformed, infected erythrocytes are sequestered in the spleen, where macrophages can ingest the infected cells and control the infection. Otherwise, the parasitized erythrocytes simply circulate through the body, shedding merozoites to perpetuate and amplify the infection. This is presumably the reason splenectomized patients fare much worse during a bout of babesiosis.[17]

Diagnosis

Any patient with a febrile or constitutional illness who may have been exposed to ticks should be evaluated for babesiosis. Thick or thin blood smears processed with Giemsa stain is the diagnostic method of choice (see Fig. 1-3). One drawback is the possibility that an erythrocyte parasitized with *Babesia* could be mistaken for one parasitized by *Plasmodium* (malaria). Beyond

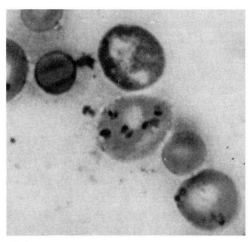

FIGURE 1-3 ▶ Intraerythrocytic parasites of *Babesia* infection.

that, inoculation in laboratory animals (rodents such as hamsters or gerbils, who demonstrate infection several weeks after inoculation) and serology (via indirect immunofluorescence testing available from the Centers for Disease Control and Prevention in Atlanta, GA) may aid in the diagnostic process if organisms are not seen on blood smear. Antibody titers of 1:256 or higher are diagnostic of *B. microti* infection.[21] As with many infections, newer polymerase chain reaction techniques are being developed for use in situations of low parasite load (amniotic fluid eventually?).[22]

Treatment and Prevention

Babesiosis in immunocompetent, younger patients appears to be a mild, self-limited illness, even though the fatigue may last for a couple of months. Previously, expectant management was often recommended (assuming that the diagnosis was even made to begin with, in the minimally symptomatic patient). This philosophy may need to be rethought, when one considers the possibility of chronic parasitemia, which has apparently become more recognized.[18] A number of antimicrobials are effective against *Babesia* species. First and foremost, however, is prevention of babesiosis by the avoidance of ticks and their bites in the first place.

Severe infection should be treated with the combination of clindamycin, 300 to 600 mg every 6 hours parenterally, and oral quinine, 650 mg every 6 to 8 hours. This regimen should be continued for 7 to 10 days.[23] This regimen is not foolproof, however. Pentamidine and trimethoprim-sulfa has been used to treat a case of *B. divergens* infection in a splenectomized patient in Europe,[24] and in severe cases exchange transfusion has been used to reduce the parasite load and remove other toxic hematologic and immunologic factors.[25]

CRYPTOSPORIDIOSIS

Epidemiology

Since 1907, the various species of *Cryptosporidium* have been known to infect animals.[26] However, only in 1976 was human infection recognized. Thereafter, from the early 1980s on, the explosion of patients with HIV infection caused *Cryptosporidium* to become a well-publicized opportunistic infection that figured in the clinical definition of acquired immunodeficiency syndrome (AIDS). The usual cause of cryptosporidiosis in humans is *C. parvum*, which is found in humans and other mammals. *Cryptosporidium muris* also occasionally causes human disease. *Cryptosporidium* is found in mammals and other animals throughout the world; so, cryptosporidiosis is a common zoonosis among those who deal closely with livestock. Cryptosporidiosis has also been identified as a causative

factor in outbreaks of childhood diarrhea in day care center situations, owing to the fecal-oral nature of spread.[27] Also, as mentioned previously, contaminated water supplies have been responsible for large outbreaks of intestinal illness due to the organism, since contaminated water is an important avenue of infection and chlorination and filtration do not kill or remove the tiny spores (Fig. 1–4).[2]

Clinical Manifestations

Because *Cryptosporidium* damages the brush border of intestinal epithelial cells, the primary clinical syndrome caused by the organism is a profuse, watery diarrhea, due to malabsorption and aberrant osmotic fluid flux.[28] Occasionally, there is cramping, nausea, and vomiting, and low-grade fever (Table 1–7). However, in immunocompetent individuals, the illness lasts for several weeks, but is self-limited. In immunocompromised patients, such as AIDS patients, the diarrhea may be severe and dehydration may be troublesome. Also, in these patients, the illness becomes chronic and persistent, at least until such time as the immunocompromised condition is corrected or resolves, depending on its etiology. Beyond the intestine itself, cryptosporidiosis may cause cholecystitis, hepatitis, pancreatitis, reactive arthritis, and respiratory disease.

More severe disease is seen in HIV-infected individuals, the very young, the very old, and patients receiving immunosuppressive drugs, such as steroids. Although poorly understood, both B- and T-lymphocyte processes are important in the defense against this organism. Thus, both patients with T-cell disease (e.g., AIDS) and those with B-cell disease (e.g., agammaglobulinemia) are more susceptible to cryptosporidiosis.[27]

Pathophysiology

The life cycle of *Cryptosporidium*, unlike that of some other human pathogenic protozoa, is completed

TABLE 1–7 ▶ SYMPTOMS OF 205 PATIENTS WITH CONFIRMED CRYPTOSPORIDIOSIS DURING THE MILWAUKEE OUTBREAK

Symptom	Prevalence (%)
Watery diarrhea	93
mean = 12/d; med = 9/d (1–55 d)	
mean = 19/d; med = 12/d (1–90 d)	
39% recurred after 2 d free	
Abdominal cramps	84
Weight loss	75
med = 10 lb (1–40 lb)	
Fever	57
med = 38.3°C (37.2°–40.5°C)	
Vomiting	48

From Guerrant RL: Cryptosporidiosis: An emerging, highly infectious threat. Emerg Infect Dis 3(1):51–57, 1997.

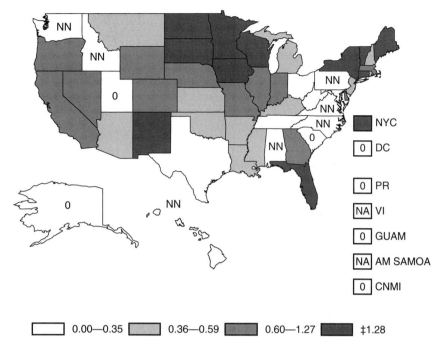

	NYC
0	DC
0	PR
NA	VI
0	GUAM
NA	AM SAMOA
0	CNMI

| 0.00—0.35 | 0.36—0.59 | 0.60—1.27 | ‡1.28 |

FIGURE 1-4 ▶ Cryptosporidiosis—reported cases per 100,000 population, United States and territories, 1997. (From Guerrant RL: Cryptosporidiosis: An emerging, highly infectious threat. Emerg Infect Dis 1997; 3[1]:51–57.)

within a single host. Oocysts are ingested and release sporozoites, which adhere to the cell wall of an epithelial cell, presumably within the bowel. The organism then resides in an extracytoplasmic, but intracellular, vacuole, made up of two membranes derived from the host cell and two derived from the parasite.[29] The sporozoites develop asexually into meronts, which release merozoites into the bowel lumen. Merozoites may immediately reinfect the same host, or may develop through sexual maturation into zygotes or oocytes, which then may excyst to autoinfect the same host, or may be excreted into the environment, where they may remain infectious for many months.[28] The double cycle of autoinfection is one reason that very few organisms are needed to initiate a severe infection, and also the reason that persistent disease may develop in the setting of immunoincompetence.

Diagnosis

Classically, small bowel biopsy specimens were necessary for diagnosing cryptosporidiosis. This procedure was, of course, relatively invasive, and not very sensitive. Cryptosporidiosis may now be diagnosed with the use of acid-fast or immunofluorescence staining on unconcentrated fecal smears. Detection can be enhanced by concentration methods when small numbers of oocysts are present; however, some methods (e.g., formalin–ethyl acetate concentration) may cause the loss of significant percentages of oocysts, thus ob-

scuring the diagnosis.[30, 31] Currently, a number of enzyme-linked immunosorbent assay (ELISA) methods are available for the detection of fecal cryptosporidial antigen with sensitivities in the 83% to 95% range in diarrheal specimens. These methods are less sensitive in formed specimens and time-consuming. Microscopy that uses immunofluorescence antibody is slightly more sensitive and may be faster,[32, 33] and polymerase chain reaction techniques are being developed, primarily for research purposes.[34]

Treatment and Prevention

There has been very little headway made in finding antimicrobial agents efficacious against *Cryptosporidium*. Most medications active against other protozoans are not active against this one. Although paromomycin does not eradicate the parasite from the gut, it has been shown to improve symptoms significantly in AIDS patients with cryptosporidiosis.[35] Treatment with zidovudine, perhaps because of relative restoration of the immune system, has also been shown to have a beneficial effect in the setting of cryptosporidiosis in AIDS patients.[35]

The major difficulty in avoiding cryptosporidiosis remains the hardiness and the elusiveness of the *Cryptosporidium* oocyte against chlorination and filtration methods. Therefore, enteric precautions and avoidance of infected animals are recommended. In fact, patients with AIDS or other significant immunosuppression should drink only pure bottled water, since the municipal purifications regimens are so ineffective generally at sterilizing water contaminated with *Cryptosporidium*.

LEISHMANIASIS

Epidemiology

Leishmaniasis, infection with the various species of the protozoan *Leishmania*, can be separated into three major clinical syndromes, depending on the invasiveness of the infection: cutaneous leishmaniasis (including the variant of leishmaniasis recidivans), mucocutaneous leishmaniasis, and visceral leishmaniasis. Humans usually contract the infection by the bite of a sandfly that has previously fed on an infected carrier animal. In 1994, the worldwide annual incidence of visceral leishmaniasis was estimated to be 500,000 cases, and that of cutaneous leishmaniasis thought to be between 1 and 1.5 million, making leishmaniasis a significant global health problem caused by flies.[36]

Cutaneous leishmaniasis is classically divided into New and Old World forms, the former endemic in South and Central America and usually caused by members of the *L. mexicana* complex (*L. mexicana, L. amazonensis,* and *L. venezuelensis*) and the *L. brasiliensis* complex (*L. brasiliensis, L. panamensis,* and *L. guyanensis*).[37, 38] In the United States, a few cases of New World disease have also been reported in Texas.[38] In general, the reservoir of New World cutaneous leishmaniasis consists of small sylvatic rodents. Local synonyms for the disease include uta, pian bois (bush yaws), and chiclero ulcer.[3] Outbreaks have occurred when large areas of forest have been cleared, thereby flushing rodents into contact with humans, and when the military or travelers enter an endemic area.[39]

Old World cutaneous leishmaniasis, most frequently caused by *L. major, L. tropica,* or *L. aethiopica,* occurs throughout the tropical and subtropical regions of Asia Minor, the Mediterranean basin, Eastern Asia, and Africa. Occasionally, reservoirs of *L. major* are desert rodents; *L. tropica* is found in dogs and humans, and *L. aethiopica* resides primarily in species of hyrax. Old World cutaneous leishmaniasis is usually a sporadic disease, but it may occur in an epidemic pattern when large numbers of susceptible persons suddenly gather in an endemic area (e.g., travelers, military personnel, or refugees).[39]

The visceral form of leishmaniasis in India and Africa is usually caused by *L. donovani,* while *L. infantum* causes the illness in the Mediterranean region; *L. chagasi* is etiologic in Latin America. Occasionally, species more commonly associated with cutaneous disease (e.g., *L. mexicana* and *L. major*) present as classic visceral disease. Rodents and the small mammals that eat them are the usual reservoirs for *L. donovani,* while *L. infantum* and *L. chagasi* are carried by dogs, foxes, and humans.[40]

Clinical Manifestations

In New World leishmaniasis, the spectrum of disease ranges from a single, localized cutaneous ulcer (in cutaneous leishmaniasis) to disseminated nodules (in diffuse cutaneous leishmaniasis) to mucocutaneous involvement (in mucocutaneous leishmaniasis) to visceral involvement (visceral leishmaniasis). In the case of localized cutaneous disease, the initial lesion usually appears 2 to 8 weeks after the bite of a sandfly. Initially, an erythematous papule develops at the site where promastigotes were inoculated. The lesion then progresses to a leishmaniotic ulcer, which may persist for months to years. The ulcer is characteristically round with an indurated border.[39]

Leishmania brasiliensis infection may manifest as regional lymphadenopathy for a week to several months before skin lesions appear. As the ulcer enlarges, the lymphadenopathy resolves. Fever, malaise, anorexia, and weight loss occur in a variable percentage of patients.[39]

Diffuse cutaneous leishmaniasis, which has been associated with *L. amazonensis, L. aethiopica,* and *L. mexicana* infection, is the manifestation of cutaneous leishmaniasis in the anergic host.[40, 41] In diffuse cutaneous leishmaniasis, large numbers of parasites are present in the skin owing to an ineffective cell-mediated immune response, similar conceptually to lepromatous leprosy.

A small percentage of persons infected with *L. brasiliensis,* and rarely with others of the genus, develop mucocutaneous leishmaniasis (locally called "espundia"). While mucocutaneous leishmaniasis is rarely fatal, there is significant morbidity attached to the infection.[40] The illness is characterized by disfiguring mucosal lesions of the nose, mouth, pharynx, or larynx months to years after the skin lesion heals. This can present as nasal obstruction, congestion, discharge, or nosebleeds resulting from soft tissue, cartilage, and bone destruction. Half the time, mucocutaneous leishmaniasis occurs within 2 years of development of cutaneous disease, but the interval may be as short as 1 month or as long as 24 years. Some patients with mucocutaneous leishmaniasis have coexisting skin lesions (12% to 28%) or no evidence of previous cutaneous disease at all (8% to 16%).[41]

The clinical presentation of localized Old World cutaneous leishmaniasis depends on the *Leishmania* species involved and the host's immune response. The incubation period ranges from 2 weeks to several months. Similar to that with New World cutaneous leishmaniasis, the initial lesion is a papule that ultimately enlarges and ulcerates, and occasionally is accompanied by regional lymphadenopathy. After several months to a year, the ulcer heals, leaving a flat, atrophic scar. This classic single, chronic ulcerative lesion is known by other names in various areas of the Old World, such as bouton d'orient, bouton de Crete, bouton d'Alep, bouton de Biskra, Aleppo evil, oriental sore, Baghdad boil, and Delhi boil. Previous immunologic experience with the organism is associated with a high level of resistance to reinfection by the homologous species.[39]

Like its New World counterpart, Old World cutaneous leishmaniasis can present as diffuse cutaneous disease, in which a nonulcerating papule progresses to disseminated nodules on the face, arms, and legs. Another form is leishmaniasis recidivans, the variant of cutaneous leishmaniasis in a hyperergic patient (also termed *chronic relapsing cutaneous leishmaniasis*). Parasites are present in low numbers, and lesions appear as isolated or grouped tubercles over or around scars of healed cutaneous lesions. Both syndromes are chronic, often persisting for 20 years or more. In Old World leishmaniasis, diffuse cutaneous disease is associated with *L. aethiopica,* while leishmaniasis recidivans is associated with *L. tropica.*[41]

The local names for visceral leishmaniasis include kala-azar, Assam fever, Dumdum fever, or infantile splenomegaly. The incubation period is usually 3 to 8 months, but it can be as short as 10 days or as long as 34 months.[40] The onset of signs and symptoms of visceral leishmaniasis may be gradual or sudden, and the clinical features represent a spectrum of disease. The wide range of disease presentations and prognoses of symptomatic visceral leishmaniasis appears to depend on the host's immune response as well as the virulence of the infecting *Leishmania* species.

Classic visceral leishmaniasis presents as fever, malaise, weight loss, hepatosplenomegaly, lymphadenopathy, pancytopenia, and hypergammaglobulinemia. The clinical picture is often complicated, as patients from endemic areas often have multiple other coexistent illnesses, including various infections and infestations. Symptomatic visceral leishmaniasis is often fatal if untreated, although many individuals with asymptomatic or relatively mild infections recover without treatment, a condition sometimes referred to as viscerotropic leishmaniasis. For example, small numbers of American soldiers who served in Operation Desert Storm developed malaise, fatigue, chronic low-grade fever, and, in some instances, diarrhea. Each individual was infected with *L. tropica,* previously associated with cutaneous disease. Similar presentations have been described in Brazilian children: Among those with positive antibody titers, 44% did not develop classic visceral disease but had a chronic illness characterized by intermittent cough, diarrhea, and low-grade fever with spontaneous recovery in 2 to 4 years.[42]

The AIDS epidemic has underscored the phenomenon that immunosuppression can result in development of symptomatic visceral leishmaniasis. Symptoms appear almost exclusively in HIV-infected patients with CD4+ counts less than $200/mm^3$. Patients with visceral disease and concurrent HIV may present with classic findings, but atypical presentations are not uncommon. The opportunistic behavior of the *Leishmania* is similar to that of *Mycobacterium tuberculosis* when coexisting with HIV. Like tuberculosis, leishmaniasis may occur as a primary infection as well as reactivation of a latent infection. Exclusive cutaneous involvement is uncommon in *Leishmania*–HIV coinfection.[38, 43]

Pathophysiology

Leishmania species have a dimorphic life cycle, living as intracellular amastigotes in the phagocytes of mammalian hosts. Sandflies of the genera *Lutzomyia* in the New World and *Phlebotomus* in the Old World feed on an infected animal or human, allowing the amastigotes access to the sandfly's gut, where conversion to the promastigote form occurs, followed by replication and migration to the fly's proboscis. In cutaneous leishmaniasis, the amastigote multiplies in macrophages within the skin, causing lysis of the mammalian cell and local spread. Visceral leishmaniasis occurs when amastigotes spread via the reticuloendothelial system throughout the body.[42]

At the bite of the appropriate vector, promastigotes are phagocytosed by macrophages and cause a lymphocytic and plasma cell response. Epithelioid cells and giant cells may appear, indicating delayed hypersensitivity. The host may then eradicate the amastigotes from the skin, resulting in complete immunity to that strain of *Leishmania.* On the other hand, variations in the immune response dictate whether infection is self-limited, or whether some variety of progressive or invasive infection follows.[44]

Diagnosis

Leishmaniasis should always be considered in the differential diagnosis of persons who have traveled to or live in endemic areas and present with appropriate symptomatology. The diagnosis is often delayed in the U.S., owing to lack of familiarity with the disease, and may be missed in immigrants or returning travelers. Moreover, the diagnosis may be confusing in the absence of classic signs and symptoms (e.g., HIV patients).

The gold standard of the diagnosis of leishmaniasis is the visualization of amastigotes in tissue or the growing of promastigotes in culture. The growth of the organism is beneficial in that it permits species identification, although tissue staining with monoclonal antibody allows identification of species if appropriate antibodies are available (usually only in research facilities).

In both cutaneous and mucocutaneous disease, smears are taken from the base of the ulcer, from punch biopsies or small incisions, or from aspirates of the border of the ulcer. Species such as *L. donovani* and *L. mexicana* may be cultured. In chronic cutaneous lesions due to *L. aethiopica*, organisms may be scarce and hard to detect by any method. Instead, aspiration of enlarged lymph nodes, if present, may be undertaken.[45] With visceral disease, bone marrow aspiration is diagnostic in 54% to 86% of cases.[46]

Recent interest in serologic testing, skin testing, and the polymerase chain reaction technique has attempted to eliminate the need for tissue samples. Serologic tests are not particularly sensitive in cutaneous disease, owing to the low level of circulating antibodies—sensitivities (67% to 76%) and specificities are low. Antibodies to *Leishmania* may not be detectable in HIV patients. On the other hand, immunodiagnosis is promising in diagnosing visceral and mucocutaneous disease when there is a large parasite load. Visceral disease presents a problem, however, as some leishmanial antigens cross-react with antigens of *Trypanosoma, Mycobacterium, Plasmodium,* and *Schistosoma*. Intradermal skin testing permits the evaluation of the delayed-type hypersensitivity response to leishmanial antigens, although the reagents are not licensed for use in the U.S. In addition, as in many areas of infectious disease, and medicine in general, the polymerase chain reaction technique has generated some interest in the diagnosis of leishmaniasis. If this method proves successful for routine use with blood products (as opposed to other methods that use tissue) for the diagnosis of the species responsible for visceral leishmaniasis, it may replace direct parasite identification and culture. For the diagnosis of cutaneous disease, further studies will be needed to demonstrate its practicality over classic techniques.[42]

Treatment and Prevention

Pentavalent antimony (Sb) compounds were first used for the treatment of leishmaniasis in the early 1900s and are the drugs of choice for cutaneous and visceral leishmaniasis. The mechanism of action of these drugs is unknown, but it is thought to be related to the inhibition of the organism's energy metabolism.[47] The agents used today are stibogluconate sodium and meglumine antimoniate. Only stibogluconate sodium is available in the U.S., from the Centers for Disease Control and Prevention (Table 1–8).

Cutaneous leishmaniasis does not necessarily require treatment, depending on factors such as disfigurement or functional impairment and whether the causative agent is suspected to be the more dangerous *L. brasiliensis*. Thus, patients with New World cutaneous disease should be informed about the possibility of developing mucocutaneous leishmaniasis, even after therapy, and all cases of mucocutaneous leishmaniasis should be treated, although the response of mucocuta-

TABLE 1–8 ▶ TREATMENT REGIMENS FOR LEISHMANIASIS	
Leishmania **Species**	**Antimicrobial Regimen**
Visceral Leishmaniasis	
India, Africa *L. donovani*	Antimony, 20 mg/kg/day for 28 days
Mediterranean basin *L. infantum*	Amphotericin B, 0.5 mg/kg qod for 14 injections, or 1 mg/kg/day for 20 injections
	Secondary regimens:
Latin America *L. chagasi*	Pentamidine, 4 mg/kg tid for 15–25 injections
L. amazonensis *L. tropica*	Paromomycin, 15 mg/kg/day for 20 days
	Interferon, 100 µg/m² qod *plus* antimony 20 mg/kg/day for 20–28 days
Cutaneous Leishmaniasis	
Old World: *L. major, L. tropica*	Antimony, 20 mg/kg/day for 20 days
L. donovani, L. infantum *L. aethiopica*	Pentamidine, 2 mg/kg qod for 7 injections
	or
	3 mg/kg qod for 4 injections
New World: *L. brasiliensis, L. mexicana* *L. amazonensis, L. panamensis*	
L. peruviana, L. guyanensis *L. garnhami, L. venezuelensis* *L. chagasi, L. pifanoi*	*Topical:* Paromomycin/methylbenzethonium chloride bid for 10 days
	Intralesional antimony weekly for 5 injections
Mucocutaneous Leishmaniasis	
Central, South America *L. brasiliensis*	Antimony, 20 mg/kg/day for 28 days
	Amphotericin B, 1 mg/kg qod for 20–30 injections

Data modified from Lee MB, Gilbert HM: Current approaches to leishmaniasis. Infect Med 1999; 16:34–45.

neous disease to antimonial agents is often poor.[48] Failures also frequently occur in cases of diffuse disease and leishmaniasis recidivans.

The response to antimony is generally not dramatic in visceral disease: lack of response to the initial treatment is 10% in most areas, a rate that seems to be increasing. Failures are especially common in persons with HIV coinfection, and the prognosis is poor. Antimony remains effective in Africa and probably Brazil, but in India there is likely to be resistance to antimonial therapy; therefore, the treatment of choice is amphotericin B.[37]

Toxicity from pentavalent antimonial agents is significant, but most patients tolerate this treatment fairly well. However, amphotericin B has been found to be a much more potent drug in vitro. Amphotericin B formulations are currently more widely used in the treatment of visceral disease than they were previously, owing to an increase in visceral leishmaniasis–causing organisms that are resistant to antimony and pentamidine. Further, there is now greater availability of less-toxic lipid-associated amphotericin B preparations.[42]

Pentamidine isethionate has been extensively studied in India for the treatment of visceral leishmaniasis. Although the cure rate seems to reflect the duration of treatment (77% after 5 weeks of therapy, rising to 94% after 9 weeks), this rate has declined over the recent decade, indicating increasing clinical resistance of the organism. Pentamidine is therefore considered a second-line agent for the treatment of visceral leishmaniasis. Adverse effects are greater when higher doses and longer courses of therapy are employed. Therefore, pentamidine should be used only when it is likely to be more effective than antimony.[42]

Given the uncertain results of antimicrobial therapy in some cases, the best treatment for leishmaniasis is its prevention. Mild visceral infections found in the veterans of Operation Desert Storm indicate that travelers to endemic areas are at risk for leishmaniasis, and there is no commercially available prophylaxis. A 1993 report of the epidemiologic features of 59 U.S. travelers who developed cutaneous disease showed that ignorance of risk, lack of use of personal protective measures, delay in diagnosis, and inappropriate clinical management were major problems.[49] Thus, it is important to educate travelers about minimizing sandfly bites by covering exposed skin, using permethrin-impregnated clothing, using permethrin-impregnated fine-mesh bed nets, and applying effective repellents on the skin. Cheaper repellents (e.g., lemon essential oils and 2% neem oil) are also effective.[38]

GIARDIASIS

Epidemiology

The flagellated protozoan *Giardia lamblia* (also known variously as *G. intestinalis*, *G. duodenalis*, and *Lamblia intestinalis*) is perhaps the most common intestinal protozoan parasite in humans. *Giardia* enjoys worldwide distribution, and it is perhaps the first enteric pathogen to infect infants during childhood, especially in developing countries. The reservoir of *Giardia* in the wild is not clearly known, although some mammals (e.g., beavers) have been shown to carry the organism. It is clear, however, that human sewage contaminating food or water supplies is a major source of outbreaks.[50]

Giardiasis is frequently implicated in diarrheal disease in travelers, since the organism can be found in water that has not been properly processed, and it survives well in cold well water. In the 20 years from 1965 to 1984, giardiasis was the leading waterborne disease in the United States, infecting more than 23,000 individuals in 90 separate outbreaks.[51] But besides improperly treated and unfiltered water, *Giardia* is transmitted through fecal-oral contact, commonly between children in day care centers, institutionalized persons, male homosexuals, and members of overcrowded, poor populations. However, more and more reports of giardiasis transmission in restaurants, office party settings, and other small gatherings indicate an increasing importance of "regular" food and hand-to-hand spread.[50]

Clinical Manifestations

Infection with *G. lamblia* causes a spectrum of illness ranging from asymptomatic carriage in 5% to 15% of infected persons, to acute diarrheal illness in 25% to 50%, to a chronic syndrome of diarrhea and weight loss from malabsorption in as many as 35% to 70% of victims (Table 1–9). The diarrheal syndrome may last up to several weeks, but may clear spontaneously even without antibiotic therapy. The chronic form of the disease may wax and wane until spontaneous or antibiotic-associated resolution. However, even chronic asymptomatic carriage has been documented to last more than 6 months in children.[52]

Pathophysiology

Giardiasis occurs after ingestion of *Giardia* cysts, which then pass into the upper small bowel and release trophozoites, which adhere to the enteric brush border cells and cause their effects. Although the pathogenesis is not completely clear, the organism may cause disease manifestations by disruption of the brush border, by invasion of the mucosal cells, by production of an enterotoxin, or by inciting an inflammatory reaction.[53]

Both humoral and cellular immune responses are apparently important in the host interaction with *G. lamblia*, and a systemic antibody response ensues when a human is infected. In fact, chronic disease may, in some cases, be caused by a failure of the host to mount a local gut IgA response to specific *Giardia* antigens.[54]

TABLE 1–9 ▶ RELATIVE SYMPTOMS OF ACUTE GIARDIASIS

Symptom	Average Incidence (%)	Range (%)
Diarrhea	89	64–100
Malaise	84	72–97
Flatulence	74	35–97
Foul-smelling, greasy stools	72	57–79
Abdominal cramping	70	44–85
Abdominal bloating	69	42–97
Nausea	68	59–79
Anorexia	64	41–82
Weight loss	64	56–73
Vomiting	27	17–36
Fever	13	0–21
Urticaria	9	4–14
Constipation	9	0–17

Data adapted from Hill DR: Giardia lamblia. In: Mandell GL, Bennett JE, Dolin R (eds): Principles and Practice of Infectious Diseases, 4th ed. New York, Churchill Livingstone, 1995.

Further evidence that gut immunity is protective comes from the observation that breast milk with antigiardial antibody protects against neonatal infection.[55]

Diagnosis

Giardiasis should be in the differential diagnosis of all patients with prolonged diarrhea, especially if it is foul-smelling and associated with weight loss and malabsorption. Travel to endemic areas or exposure through institutions (e.g., child care centers) makes the diagnosis more likely. Traditionally, the search for cysts or trophozoites in the stool has been the primary mode of diagnosis (Fig. 1–5). Currently, antigen techniques may be used on stool specimens as well. Both immunofluorescence and ELISA are available for detecting *Giardia* antigen in clinical specimens. Antigen assays are not much more expensive than the usual stool examination and have a sensitivity of approximately 85% to 98% and a specificity of 90% to 100%.[56]

For research purposes, polymerase chain reaction techniques and gene probes are available for research purposes. Serologic testing for giardiasis is useful in epidemiologic studies, but not particularly useful clinically, save for anti-*Giardia* IgM, which may distinguish acute from past disease, if that is clinically important.[57]

Treatment and Prevention

Avoidance of fecal-oral contamination and proper chlorination and filtration of public water supplies are important measures in controlling outbreaks of giardiasis. During foreign travel, all water should be suspect (including ice) and should be either boiled or treated with some commercially available halogen preparation (e.g., chlorine, iodine).[58]

Quinacrine has long been the drug of choice for the treatment of giardiasis, at least in adults (it is poorly tolerated in children) (Table 1–10). It is, however, not readily obtainable nowadays because of discontinued production. Currently, metronidazole is the most common drug used for this purpose in the U.S. As mentioned earlier in this chapter, metronidazole

TABLE 1–10 ▶ TREATMENT REGIMENS FOR *GIARDIA LAMBLIA* INFECTION	
Medication	**Dosage Regimen**
Quinacrine	100 mg tid for 5–7 days
Metronidazole	250 mg tid for 5–7 days
Furazolidone	100 mg qid for 7–10 days
Paromomycin	25–30 mg/kg/day in 3 doses for 7–10 days
Tinidazole, ornidazole, nitromidazine	None available in U.S.

has never been shown to cause problems in pregnancy[13]; thus, it is probably the best drug for use during pregnancy. Alternatively, the luminal aminoglycoside paromomycin may be used, as it is not systemically absorbed. However, paromomycin is not extremely effective at eliminating *Giardia* from the stool, even though it causes improvement in clinical symptoms. Furazolidone, a nitrofuran drug, is often used in pediatric patients because it is available as a liquid.[50]

MALARIA

Epidemiology

Malaria, infection with members of the genus *Plasmodium*, has been clinically recognized since the dawn of recorded history. Chinese writers from 1700 BC, Egyptian papyri from 1570 BC, the writings of Homer, and so on, all have variously described the fever and splenomegaly and their relationship to the bad air, *malaria*, of the marshlands, whence came the mosquito vectors about which we know so much today.[59]

The mosquito is the usual vector and definitive host of *Plasmodium*; humans are merely an intermediate host and reservoir. Female mosquitoes become infected only if they take a blood meal from a person whose blood contains mature male and female gametocytes. Thereafter, a complex cycle begins with union of the male and female gametocytes in the stomach of the mosquito, ending with sporozoites in the vector's salivary glands (Fig. 1–6). This is where the human becomes infected, when the mosquito bites. The sporogonic cycle, or the time required for maturation of the parasite in the mosquito, is variable, depending on the species of *Plasmodium* and on the ambient temperature. Only anophelines who live longer after an appropriate blood meal than the sporogonic cycle can transmit malaria, since sporozoites must be produced for the mosquito to become infective. Thus, environmental factors that help determine the lifespan of the female anopheline (e.g., temperature, humidity, and rainfall) in large part determine whether infection can be successfully transmitted in a particular geographic locale.

Anophelines feed at night; thus, transmission generally occurs between sunset and dawn. When an in-

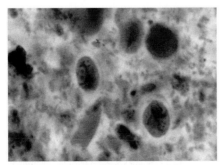

FIGURE 1–5 ▶ *Giardia lamblia* cyst in stool specimen (trichrome stain).

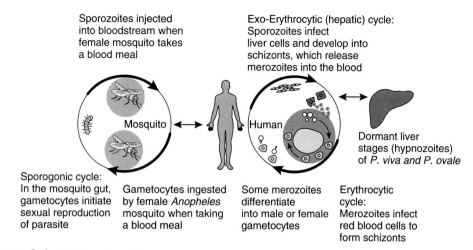

Sporozoites injected into bloodstream when female mosquito takes a blood meal

Exo-Erythrocytic (hepatic) cycle: Sporozoites infect liver cells and develop into schizonts, which release merozoites into the blood

Mosquito

Human

Dormant liver stages (hypnozoites) of *P. viva and P. ovale*

Sporogonic cycle: In the mosquito gut, gametocytes initiate sexual reproduction of parasite

Gametocytes ingested by female *Anopheles* mosquito when taking a blood meal

Some merozoites differentiate into male or female gametocytes

Erythrocytic cycle: Merozoites infect red blood cells to form schizonts

FIGURE 1-6 ▶ Life cycle of *Plasmodium* species through human transmission. (From Zucker JR: Changing patterns of autochthonous malaria transmission in the United States: A review of recent outbreak. Emerg Infect Dis 2[1]:37–43, 1996.)

fected mosquito feeds, sporozoites are injected from its salivary glands into the victim's blood stream, thereafter infecting hepatocytes and beginning a process of development and multiplication. The life cycle is completed when another mosquito ingests a blood meal from this newly infected intermediate host and ingests male and female gametocytes, allowing for sexual reproduction and a repeat of the entire process.[1]

Historically, malaria has been a scourge of Western man, through his exploration of the world from the fifteenth and sixteenth centuries. Wherever travelers encountered climate and geography that supported the *Anopheles* mosquito, the protozoan *Plasmodium* could be passed between infected host and new victim. Tropical and subtropical, moist climates were particularly favorable to the development of malaria, as well as other mosquito-borne diseases (e.g., yellow fever). However, in recent years, malaria has been considered a disease primarily of tropical and subtropical *developing countries*, as the U.S. (and other industrialized nations) had effectively eliminated the disease by the 1950s through mosquito control.[1] In fact, it might be noted that the Centers for Disease Control and Prevention was originally the Office of Malaria Control, so prevalent had been the disease in the U.S. (and Canada) since the U.S. Revolutionary War.[60]

However, because of world travel, and particularly because of war in Southeast Asia and the resultant flux of soldiers and refugees to and from that endemic area, increases in the numbers of cases of malaria were seen in the U.S. in the late 1960s on through to the 1980s[61] (Fig. 1–7). This is not the alarming problem,

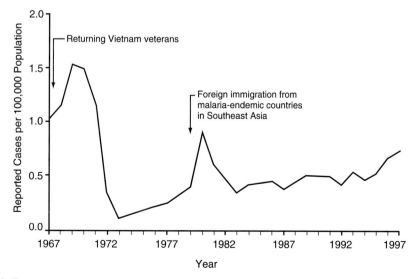

FIGURE 1-7 ▶ Malaria—by year, United States, 1967–1997. (From the Centers for Disease Control and Prevention: Summary of notifiable diseases, United States, 1997. MMWR 46[54]:43, 1997.)

however. In the past 10 years or so, it has become apparent that the anopheline mosquitoes indigenous to the United States, *Anopheles quadrimaculatus, An. freeborni,* and *An. hermsi,* are present in sufficient density, and still have significant available infected targets: Locally acquired, autochthonous (mosquito-borne) malaria in this country has been on the rise. Just in the past decade, three significant local outbreaks have occurred in the U.S., as mentioned previously.[1] In fact, malaria has been reported across the country, from New York to California (Fig. 1–8).

Therefore, as we approach the millennium (whether one wishes to accept the year 2000 or the year 2001 as the actual start of the twenty-first century), physicians in the U.S., Canada, and other developed countries must once again give proper attention to this age-old disease, malaria, which is making a comeback.

Clinical Manifestations

The classic presentation of malaria is cyclical high fever, chills, and rigors. The syndrome is associated with the release of merozoites from schizont rupture and lysis of erythrocytes. This characteristic presentation may be divided into three stages: (1) the "cold" stage, in which the patient is cold and suffers shaking chills, lasting from a quarter of an hour to several hours; (2) the "hot" stage, in which the patient's temperature may rise to as high as 40°C (>140°F), with tachycardia, hypotension, backache, headache, cough, abdominal pain, nausea, vomiting, and altered sensorium, and with the possibility of hyperthermic convulsions and ultimate brain damage, and (3) the "sweat-

ing" stage, with diaphoresis, defervescence, and exhaustion. The cause of the fever is still unknown, although it may be secondary to the elaboration of TNF-alpha from macrophages.[62]

The cyclical fever characteristic of malaria is dependent on the cycling release of parasite. The several *Plasmodium* species have slightly different life cycles; thus there are different intervals between their fever spikes. *Plasmodium vivax* and *P. ovale* cause fevers that occur every 48 hours (so-called tertian malaria), and *P. malariae* causes fever spikes every 72 hours (so-called quartan malaria). *Plamodium falciparum* has a parasite cycle of 48 hours but, practically speaking, has more of an irregular cycle, with irregularly intermittent fever spikes.[60]

If there is massive hemolysis during a paroxysmal malaria crisis, there may be significant anemia and hemoglobinuria (so-called black water fever) and compromised tissue oxygenation. With *falciparum* malaria especially, microvascular compromise occurs when parasitized red blood cells adhere en masse to small blood vessels throughout the body, causing sludging and further tissue hypoxemia. Other complications of malarial paroxysms are seizures and coma from cerebral malaria (especially with *P. falciparum*), acute renal impairment, pulmonary edema, splenomegaly (even with late splenic rupture, with *P. vivax*), and immune complex glomerulonephritis (with *P. malariae*). In general, *P. falciparum* incites a symptom complex that is more severe than those of the other three species. However, in persons partially immune to *P. falciparum*, symptoms of parasitemia may be few, while an immunologically naive individual may actually sicken and die with the

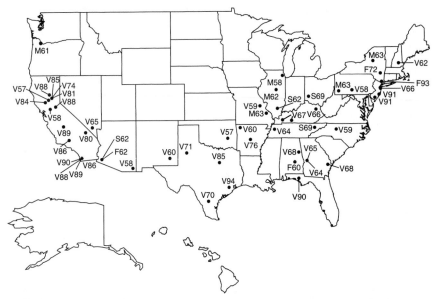

FIGURE 1–8 ▶ Location of presumed mosquito-borne malaria cases reported in the United States from 1957 to 1994. Each point denotes the location of the case; the species identified (V = *Plasmodium vivax*; F = *P. falciparum*; M = *P. malariae*; and S = *P.* sp.); and year of occurrence is given. (From Zucker JR: Changing patterns of autochthonous malaria transmission in the United States: A review of recent outbreak. Emerg Infect Dis 2[1]:37–43, 1996.)

same parasite load of *P. falciparum.* The immunology behind this difference has not yet been completely elucidated.

Pregnant women may be more susceptible to malaria because of the decrease in immunity that accompanies pregnancy. During a malarial attack, anemia may become particularly severe in the gravida.[63] Further, the fetus may suffer growth restriction or even death owing to the effects of the parasite on the placenta.[64] Also, adequate maternal therapy may not always protect the fetus from infection, as the placenta appears to be a favorite spot for parasite sequestration and avoidance of chemotherapeutic agents.[65]

Pathophysiology

As noted previously, a mosquito suitably primed by having sporozoites in the salivary glands takes a blood meal from a victim, thereby injecting sporozoites within the body of the new host. These sporozoites travel through the vasculature to the liver, where they mature into hepatic (tissue) schizonts, which may rupture, releasing merozoites that shower the blood stream, infecting erythrocytes. Alternatively, some hepatic schizonts remain dormant within the liver as hypnozoites (with *P. vivax* and *P. ovale* only), emerging as tissue schizonts 6 to 11 months later, heralding a relapse.

Within the erythrocytes, the merozoites mature into the ring, trophozoite, and schizont stages, all asexual parasites. These schizonts then rupture, releasing merozoites, to start this process again. However, some intraerythrocytic parasites develop into male and female gametocytes, which lay in wait for another mosquito vector to return and phlebotomize the host, allowing for sexual reproduction within the gut of the mosquito, completing the reproductive cycle.

All stages of this life cycle appear to be, in most part, benign to the human host except for the lysis of red cells and the release of merozoites, which causes the clinical disease previously catalogued. Immunologic and/or parasitic byproducts, and infected and adherent erythrocytes, incite the fever and other manifestations of the illness. And in the case of *P. vivax* and *P. ovale,* the dormant liver stage sets the patient up for a recurrent bout of disease even after appropriate chemotherapy.

Diagnosis

The clinical presentation of an acute malarial paroxysm, especially if it is not the first one, is so characteristic that in endemic areas no further diagnostic testing is necessary for the diagnosis to be made with some confidence. However, other sources of high fever and hemolysis must be considered, especially if the history is not absolutely clear or the geographic or demographic picture is not typical. The hallmark of the diagnosis of malaria is the demonstration of the parasite on thin or thick blood films. The four different species are so morphologically distinct in the erythrocyte host that they may be differentiated microscopically by any competent pathologist or other trained individual. It may be necessary, however, to obtain repeated smears over a day's time to ensure that some organisms are eventually seen. Ancillary laboratory testing will simply verify the manifestations of the illness (e.g., anemia, hemoglobinuria, and microvascular disease of the liver). Serologic testing is not helpful acutely.[66]

Treatment and Prevention

The best preventive measure for malaria is avoidance of areas where mosquitoes are likely to be infective. However, as noted at the outset, this is becoming more and more difficult, even in the United States. For those traveling into endemic areas or who otherwise feel at risk, antimalarial prophylaxis is in order. Prophylaxis should begin 1 week before travel and continue for 4 weeks after leaving the endemic area. If chloroquine-resistant *P. falciparum* is *not* a problem in the target area, chloroquine is the drug of choice, even for pregnant women. Otherwise, mefloquine is preferred over pyrimethamine-sulfadiazine, doxycycline, and chloroquine plus proguanil, which are more likely to produce side effects or are less efficacious[60, 66] (see Table 1–11).

Therapy for established malaria also depends on the species of *Plasmodium* involved, and whether chloroquine-resistance is known or suspected. It should also be noted that the hypnozoite forms of *P. ovale* and *P. vivax* are not affected by antimalarial agents, thus opening the door for spontaneous recurrent disease months later despite proper initial therapy. During pregnancy, chloroquine is safe, mefloquine is possibly safe[67] (although clinical experience is limited), and quinine, though abortifacent at higher dosages, had demonstrated clinical benefit when used in pregnant women[68]—this being stated with the understanding that malaria during pregnancy may be severe and the fetus may be adversely affected (see Table 1–12).

TABLE 1–11 ▶	PROPHYLACTIC REGIMENS FOR MALARIA PREVENTION	
Medication	**Dosage**
Chloroquine phosphate*	300 mg (base) PO weekly
Mefloquine†	250 mg PO once/wk
Doxycycline	100 mg PO daily
Proguanil (given with weekly chloroquine)	200 mg PO daily

*Safe in pregnancy.
†Apparently safe in pregnancy (limited experience).

TABLE 1-12 ▶ TREATMENT REGIMENS FOR MALARIA

Indication	Medication	Dosage Regimen
General use	Chloroquine*	600 mg PO initially, 300 mg PO 6 h later 300 mg PO on days 2 and 3
Chloroquine-resistant *P. falciparum*	Quinine‡	650 mg PO q8h for 3–7 days *plus*
	Pyrimethamine-sulfadiazine	3 tabs PO on the last day of quinine administration
	or Quinine‡ followed by Tetracycline	250 mg PO qid for 7 days
	or Quinine‡ followed by Clindamycin*	900 mg PO tid for 3 days
	Mefloquine†	1,250 mg PO single dose
	Halofantrine	500 mg PO q6h for 3 doses, repeat 1 wk later
Prevention of relapse from *P. ovale* or *vivax*	Primaquine	15 mg PO daily for 14 days
Parenteral drug therapy	Quinidine	10 mg loading dose IV (saline) over 1–2 h, then 0.02 mg/kg/min until able to take PO meds
	Quinidine	20 mg salt/kg IV (5% dextrose) over 4 h, then 10 mg/kg q8h until able to take PO meds

*Safe for use in pregnancy.
†Apparently safe for use in pregnancy (limited experience).
‡Possibly beneficial in pregnancy at antimalarial dosages.

REFERENCES

1. Zucker JR: Changing patterns of autochthonous malaria transmission in the United States: A review of recent outbreak. Emerg Infect Dis 1996; 2:37.
2. Guerrant RL: Cryptosporidiosis: An emerging, highly infectious threat. Emerg Infect Dis 1997; 3:51.
3. Botero D: Nonpathogenic amebae. In: Goldsmith R, Heyneman D (eds): Tropical Medicine and Parasitology. East Norwalk, CT, Appleton & Lange, 1989.
4. Diamond LS, Clark CG: A redescription of *Entamoeba histolytica* Schaudinn. 1903 (Emended Walker, 1911), separating it from *Entamoeba dispar* Brumpt. 1925. J Eukaryotic Microbiol 1993; 40:340.
5. Ravdin JI: Amebiasis. Clin Infect Dis 1995; 20:1453.
6. Botero D: Intestinal protozoan disease. In: Goldsmith R, Heyneman D (eds): Tropical Medicine and Parasitology. East Norwalk, CT, Appleton & Lange, 1989.
7. Walsh JA: Problems in recognition and diagnosis of amebiasis: Estimation of the global magnitude of morbidity and mortality. Rev Infect Dis 1986; 8:228.
8. Ravdin JI, Petri WA: *Entamoeba histolytica* (amebiasis). In: Mandell GL, Bennett JE, Dolin R (eds): Principles and Practice of Infectious Diseases, 4th ed. New York, Churchill Livingstone, 1995.
9. Armon PJ: Amoebiasis in pregnancy and the puerperium. Br J Obstet Gynaecol 1978; 85:264.
10. Leitch GJ, Dickey AD, Udenzulu IA, et al: *Entamoeba histolytica* trophozoites in the lumen and mucus blanket of rat colons studied in vivo. Infect Immun 1985; 47:68.
11. Ravdin JI: *Entamoeba histolytica*: Pathogenic mechanisms, human immune response, and vaccine development. Clin Res 1990; 38:215.
12. Centers for Disease Control and Prevention: Case definitions for infectious conditions under public health surveillance. MMWR 1997; 46(No.RR-10):43.
13. Burtin P, Taddio A, Ariburnu O, et al: Safety of metronidazole in pregnancy: A meta-analysis. Obstet Gynecol 1995; 172:525.
14. Nicolau DP, Quintiliani R: Aminoglycosides. In: Yu VL, Merigan TC, Barriere SL (eds): Antimicrobial Therapy and Vaccines. Baltimore, Williams & Wilkins, 1999.
15. Dammin GJ: Babesiosis. In: Seminars in Infectious Disease. Weinstein L, Fields B (eds): New York, Stratton, 1978, pp 169–199.
16. Smith T, Kilbourne FL: Investigation into the nature, causation and prevention of Texas or south cattle fever. USDA Bureau Animal Ind Bull 1893; 1:1.
17. Gelfand JA: Babesia. In: Mandell GL, Bennett JE, Dolin R (eds): Principles and Practice of Infectious Diseases, 4th ed. New York, Churchill Livingstone, 1995.
18. Krause PJ, Spielman A, Telford SR, et al: Persistent parasitemia after acute babesiosis. N Engl J Med 1998; 339:160.
19. Raucher HS, Jaffin H, Glass JL: Babesiosis in pregnancy. Obstet Gynecol 1984; 63:7S.
20. Erbsloh JK: Babesiosis in the newborn foal. J Reprod Fertil 1975; 23:725.
21. Krause PJ, Telford SR, Ryan R, et al: Geographical and temporal distribution of babesial infection in Connecticut. J Clin Microbiol 1991; 29:1.
22. Persing HD, Mathiesen D, Marshall WF, et al: Detection of *Babesia microti* by polymerase chain reaction. J Clin Microbiol 1992; 30:2097.
23. Wittner M, Rowin KS, Tanowitz HB, et al: Successful chemotherapy of transfusion babesiosis. Ann Intern Med 1982; 96:601.
24. Raoult D, Soulayrol L, Toga B, et al: Babesiosis, pentamidine, and cotrimoxazole. Ann Intern Med 1987; 107:944.
25. Jacoby GA, Hunt JV, Kosinoski KS, et al: Treatment of transfusion-transmitted babesiosis by exchange transfusion. N Engl J Med 1980; 303:1098.
26. Tyzzer EE: A sporozoan found in the peptic glands of the common mouse. Proc Soc Exp Biol Med 1907; 5:12.
27. Craft JC: Nonamebic protozoal enteritides. In: Hoeprich PD, Jordan MC, Ronald AR (eds): Infectious Diseases: A Treatise of Infectious Processes, 5th ed. Philadelphia, JB Lippincott, 1994.
28. Current WL, Garcia LS: Cryptosporidiosis. Clin Microbiol Rev 1991; 4:325.
29. Marcial MA, Madara JL: *Cryptosporidium*: Cellular localization, structural analysis of absorptive cell-parasite membrane-membrane interactions in guinea pigs, and suggestion of protozoan transport by M cells. Gastroenterology 1986; 90:583.
30. Wuhib T, Silva TM, Newman RD, et al: Cryptosporidial and

microsporidial infections in human immunodeficiency virus–infected patients in northeastern Brazil. J Infect Dis 1994; 170:494.

31. Weber R, Bryan RT, Bishop HS, et al: Threshold of detection of *Cryptosporidium* oocysts in human stool specimens: Evidence for low sensitivity of current diagnostic methods. J Clin Microbiol 1991; 29:1323.

32. Newman RD, Jaeger KL, Wuhib T, et al: Evaluation of an antigen capture enzyme-linked immunosorbent assay for detection of *Cryptosporidium* oocysts. J Clin Microbiol 1993; 31:2080.

33. Kehl KS, Cicirello H, Havens PL: Comparison of four different methods for detection of *Cryptosporidium* species. J Clin Microbiol 1995; 33:416.

34. Laxer MA, Timblin BK, Patel RJ: DNA sequences for the specific detection of *Cryptosporidium parvum* by the polymerase chain reaction. Am J Trop Med Hyg 1991; 45:688.

35. Petersen C: Cryptosporidiosis in patients infected with the human immunodeficiency virus. Clin Infect Dis 1992; 15:903.

36. Division of Communicable Disease Prevention and Control, Communicable Disease Program, HPC/HCT, PAHO: Leishmaniasis in the Americas. Epidemiol Bull 1994; 15:8.

37. Berman JD: Human leishmaniasis: Clinical, diagnostic, and chemotherapeutic developments in the last 10 years. Clin Infect Dis 1997; 24:648.

38. Magill AJ: Epidemiology of the leishmaniasis. Dermatol Clin 1995; 13:505.

39. Pearson RD, de Queiroz Sousa A: *Leishmania* species: Visceral (kala-azar), cutaneous, and mucosal leishmaniasis. In: Mandell GL, Bennett JE, Dolin R (eds): Principles and Practice of Infectious Diseases, 4th ed. New York, Churchill Livingstone, 1995.

40. Pearson RD, de Queiroz Sousa A: Clinical spectrum of leishmaniasis. Clin Infect Dis 1996; 22:1.

41. Melby PC, Kreutzer RD, McMahon-Pratt D, et al: Cutaneous leishmaniasis: Review of 59 cases seen at the National Institutes of Health. Clin Infect Dis 1992; 15:924.

42. Lee MB, Gilbert HM: Current approaches to leishmaniasis. Infect Med 1999; 16:34.

43. Alvar J, Canavate C, Gutierrez-Solar B, et al: Leishmania and human immunodeficiency virus coinfection: The first 10 years. Clin Microbiol Rev 1997; 10:298.

44. Manson-Bahr PEC: Leishmaniasis. In: Hoeprich PD, Jordan MC, Ronald AR (eds): Infectious Diseases: A Treatise on Infectious Processes, 5th ed. Philadelphia, JB Lippincott, 1994.

45. Barral A, Guerreiro J, Bomfim G, et al: Lymphadenopathy as the first sign of human cutaneous infection by *Leishmania braziliensis*. Am J Trop Med Hyg 1995; 53:256.

46. Report of the informal meeting on the chemotherapy of visceral leishmaniasis. UNDP/World Bank/WHO Special Programme for Research and Training in Tropical Diseases. Nairobi, Kenya, June 1982.

47. Herwaldt BL, Berman JD: Recommendations for treating leishmaniasis with sodium stibogluconate (Pentostam) and review of pertinent clinical studies. Am J Trop Med Hyg 1992; 46:296.

48. Berman JD: Chemotherapy for leishmaniasis: Biochemical mechanisms, clinical efficacy, and future strategies. Rev Infect Dis 1988; 10:560.

49. Herwaldt B: American cutaneous leishmaniasis in US travelers. Ann Intern Med 1993; 118:779.

50. Hill DR: Giardia lamblia. In: Mandell GL, Bennett JE, Dolin R (eds): Principles and Practice of Infectious Diseases, 4th ed. New York, Churchill Livingstone, 1995.

51. Craun GF: Waterborne giardiasis in the United States 1965–1984. Lancet 1986; 2:523.

52. Pickering LK, Woodward WE, DuPont HL, Sullivan P: Occurrence of *Giardia lamblia* in children in day care centers. J Pediatr 1984; 104:522.

53. Farthing MJ: Diarrhoeal disease: Current concepts and future challenges. Pathogenesis of giardiasis. Trans R Soc Trop Med Hyg 1993; 87(suppl 3):17.

54. Char S, Cervallos AM, Yamson P, et al: Impaired IgA response to *Giardia* heat shock antigen in children with persistent diarrhoea and giardiasis. Gut 1993; 34:38.

55. Walterspier JN, Morrow AL, Guerrero MI, et al: Secretory *anti–Giardia lamblia* antibodies in human milk: Protective effect against diarrhea. Pediatrics 1994; 93:28.

56. Wolfe MS: Giardiasis. Clin Microbiol Rev 1992; 5:93.

57. Sullivan PB, Neale G, Cevallos AM, et al: Evaluation of specific serum anti-*Giardia* IgM antibody response in diagnosis in children. Trans R Soc Trop Med Hyg 1991; 85:748.

58. Ongerth JE, Johnson RL, MacDonald SC, et al: Backcountry water treatment to prevent giardiasis. Am J Public Health 1989; 79:1633.

59. Bruce-Chwatt LJ: History of malaria from prehistory to eradication. In: Wernsdorfer WH, MacGregor IA (eds): Malaria: Principles and Practice of Malariology. London, Churchill Livingstone, 1988, pp 1–59.

60. Krogstad DJ: *Plasmodium* species (malaria). In: Mandell GL, Bennett JE, Dolin R (eds): Principles and Practice of Infectious Diseases, 4th ed. New York, Churchill Livingstone, 1995.

61. Centers for Disease Control and Prevention: Summary of notifiable diseases, United States, 1997. MMWR 1997; 46:43.

62. Kwiatkowski D, Cannon JG, Manogue KR, et al: Tumor necrosis factor production in falciparum malaria and its association with schizont rupture. Clin Exp Immunol 1989; 77:361.

63. Gilles HM, Lawson JB, Sibelas M, et al: Malaria, anemia, and pregnancy. Ann Trop Med Parsitol 1969; 63:245.

64. Watkinson M, Rushton DI: Plasmodial pigmentation of placenta and outcome of pregnancy in West African mothers. Br Med J 1983; 287:251.

65. Bray RS, Sinder RE: The sequestration of *Plasmodium falciparum* infected erythrocytes in the placenta. Trans R Soc Trop Med Hyg 1979; 73:716.

66. Redd SC, Campbell CC: Malaria. In: Hoeprich PD, Jordan MC, Ronald AR (eds): Infectious Diseases: A Treatise on Infectious Processes, 5th ed. Philadelphia, JB Lippincott, 1994.

67. Steketee RW, Wirima JJ, Slutsker L, et al: Malaria prevention in pregnancy: The effects of treatment and chemoprophylaxis on placental malaria infection, low birth weight and fetal, infant and child survival. CDC-ARTS Publication 099-4048. Washington, DC: U.S. Department of Health and Human Services; 1994.

68. Looareesuwan S, Phillips RE, White NJ, et al: Quinine in severe falciparum malaria in late pregnancy. Lancet 1985; 2:4.

2

Mycology
General Mycology and Fungal Disease

SEBASTIAN FARO

INTRODUCTION

The fungi consist of approximately 50,000 species, with fewer than 300 causing disease in humans. In order for fungi, which are primarily saprophytic organisms, to become pathogenic, major adaptations in metabolism had to occur. Although approximately 300 species have been implicated in human disease, 90% of all fungal infections can be attributed to 20 that cause systemic infection, 20 that are responsible for cutaneous disease, and 12 that cause severe, localized, subcutaneous infection.

CHARACTERISTICS

Fungi are true eukaryotic organisms: each cell contains at least one nucleus, a nuclear membrane, an endoplasmic reticulum, and mitochondria. The fungal cell is surrounded by a rigid cell wall made up of polymers of glucose or N-acetylglucosamine, or mannan (Table 2–1).

Fungi typically inhabit water, soil, or decaying organic matter and are either obligate or facultative aerobes. Therefore, in order to assume the role of a pathogen, the fungi had to adapt to the human host by evolving alternative mechanisms of metabolism. Fungi initiate growth by secreting enzymes into their environment, thereby degrading organic material into soluble nutrients that are absorbed by the fungal cell.

Fungi grow as either yeast or filamentous forms. The fungal filamentous colony is made up of hyphae that grow at its tip. Typically, a hypha branches at regular intervals. There are two basic hyphal forms. The substrate hyphae form the flat, matted colony and sink strands, or individual hypha, into the substrate. The aerial hyphae support the asexual reproductive structures, spores or conidia. These spores are usually contained within a membranous-like structure, which forms a sporangium. When conditions are appropriate, the sporangium breaks, liberating asexual spores that travel on air currents or the appendages of insects or animals. When these spores are provided the appropriate nutrients, they germinate and begin the asexual

life cycle of the organism. In fungi that possess a sexual cycle, opposite mating types must come into contact to initiate the sexual part of the life cycle.

The asexual life cycle of filamentous fungi is observed daily when one notes the growth of green or black mold on cheese or bread. Typically, this is *Penicillium*, *Rhizopus*, or *Aspergillus*. These fungi grow as filamentous colonies, and the surface hyphae tend to be white, giving the colony a cotton-like character. The colored part of the colony is caused by the high concentration of pigmented spores housed on the aerial hyphae that form the sporangium or conidiophore.

Yeast are unicellular and either spherical or elliptical, and vary in size from 3 to 15 μm.[1] Reproduction of yeast occurs through budding, although a few reproduce by binary fission. Budding occurs via lysis of a localized area of the cell wall. The dissolution of a point in the cell wall results in the cytoplasmic membrane of the mother cell distending outwardly and

TABLE 2–1 ▶ CARBOHYDRATE CONSTITUENTS OF FUNGAL CELL WALLS

Polymer	Monomer	Organism
Cellulose	D-Glucose, via beta-1–4 linkages	Aquatic fungi
Chitin	N-Acetylglucosamine, beta-1–4 linkages	Zygomycetes
Beta-glucans	D-Glucose, beta-1–4 linkages	Ascomycetous yeast
Mannans	D-Mannose, alpha-1–6 linkages with alpha-1–2 and alpha-1–3 linked branches	
Chitin Basidiomycetous Mannans		Yeast
Chitin	N-Acetylglucosamine, beta-1–4 linkages	Fungi with septate hyphae
Beta-glucans	D-Glucose, beta-1–3 linked backbone with beta-1–6 linkages at branch points	

From Mitchell TG: General characteristics of fungi. In: Joklik WK, Willet HP, Amos DB, Wilfert CM (eds): Zinsser Microbiology. East Norwalk, CT, Appleton & Lange, 1992, pp 1073.

26

increasing in size, forming a daughter cell. The nucleus divides via mitosis, with one nucleus migrating into the daughter cell. The progeny cell continues to grow in size, with the production of a new cell wall to heal the defect created in the process of reproduction. Eventually, the progeny breaks off and can repeat the process. A scar remains at the site where the new cell developed. Some yeast form multiple cells before separating from the parent cell, thus producing a hyphal-like structure, referred to as a pseudohypha.

Some fungi have the capacity to grow as either the yeast or the filamentous form; this ability is referred to as dimorphism. These fungi are able to alter their growth pattern in response to pH, carbon dioxide concentration, temperature, or glucose concentration.[2, 3] This ability to alter their growth pattern and metabolism has enabled some fungi to become pathogenic.

PATHOGENICITY

The ability of fungi to cause infection requires that the organism penetrate the host and gain entrance to deeper tissues. The fungal cell wall possesses sites that enable the organism to attach to host cells, epithelial cells, and endothelial cells.[4, 5] Fungal cell wall surface ligands and receptors enable the fungal cell to avoid the host defenses, thus allowing the organism to invade, colonize, and subsequently establish an infection. Evasion of host cell defense can occur because the fungal cell (e.g., *Candida albicans*), possesses a cell wall protein that resembles the mammalian CR3 receptor for iC3b. In addition, other lectin proteins recognize sugars, such as fucose and glucosamine, on epithelial cell membranes, while fungal cell wall mannans can facilitate adherence to fibrinogen, fibronectin, and laminin.[1]

Humans are constantly exposed to fungal elements, but infection of the healthy, immunocompetent individual is infrequent. The most common fungal infections, in nonendemic areas, occurring in immunocompetent individuals are typically those of the skin and genital area. Fungal infections can be classified as (1) allergic responses, caused by inhalation of fungal spores; (2) mycotoxicoses, resulting from ingestion of toxic substances; and (3) mycoses, that is, invasion of the host and growth of the fungus.

Humans are constantly exposed to aerosolized spores or conidia, which generally does not pose a problem until the spore count exceeds $10^9/m^3$. Concentrations above $10^9/m^3$ can sensitize the individual, who subsequently becomes allergic to the particular fungus or group of fungi that share similar antigens. Allergic individuals present with symptoms such as rhinitis and bronchial asthma. Individuals who are immunocompromised may develop more serious disease (Table 2–2).

TABLE 2–2 ▶ RESPIRATORY DISEASE CAUSED BY FUNGAL INFECTION		
Allergy	**Source**	**Etiology**
Cheese washer's lung	Cheese	*Penicillium casei*
Malt-worker's lung	Barley malt	*Aspergillus clavatus*
Maple-bark stripper's lung	Maple tree bark	*Cryptostroma corticale*
Sequoiosis	Redwood sawdust	*Aureobasidium pullulans, Graphium*
Suberosis	Cork	*Penicillium frequentans*
Wood-pulp worker's disease	Wood pulp	*Alternaria*
Farmer's lung	Stored hay	*Faenia rectivirgula,* Thermoactinomyces vulgaris
Bagassosis	Sugar cane	Thermoactinomyces sacchari
Humidifier lung	Humidifiers, air conditioners	Thermoactinomyces vulgaris Thermoactinomyces candidus

Adapted from Mitchell TG: Principles of fungus diseases. In: Joklik WK, Willet HP, Amos DB, Wilfert CM (eds): Zinsser Microbiology. East Norwalk, CT, 1992, pp 1081–1090.

Fungi produce substances that are very toxic to humans and animals. Mushrooms primarily produce these substances. Unfortunately, many individuals ingest poisonous mushrooms that not only can make them severely ill but also can be lethal. *Amanita* produces several toxins: phalloidin, phallin, and alpha-, beta-, and gamma-amanitin, which affect the liver and interfere with protein synthesis as well as destroy the endoplasmic reticulum.[6] However, mycotoxins are not solely produced by mushrooms: filamentous fungi can also produce toxins, which are referred to as aflatoxins. The most potent aflatoxins, B_1 and G_1, are produced by *Aspergillus flavus*.

The mycoses, the most common form of fungal diseases, present as either topical infections (e.g., dermophytoses or candidiasis) or systemic infections. The infection may have manifestations of both dermal and systemic components. The most common mycoses are aspergillosis, mucormycosis, blastomycosis, candidiasis, coccidioidomycoses, cryptococcoses, and histoplasmoses.

Coccidioidomycosis, blastomycosis, paracoccidioidomycosis, and histoplasmosis are caused by organisms that can grow dimorphically in response to temperature. Coccidioidomycosis and histoplasmosis are found in dry soil mixed with guano in the southwestern and midwestern-northeastern United States, respectively.[7-13] Coccidioidomycosis is caused by *Coccidioides immitis*, a dimorphic fungus. Four distinct morphologic structures are produced during the life cycle, depending on environmental conditions. *Coccidioides immitis* typically grows as a filamentous organism when observed in nature or in the laboratory. The hyphae are septated and branched, and when the culture ages arthroconidia are produced, which can be separated from the hypha and characteristically are unicellular and barrel shaped. Arthroconidia are resistant to desiccation and elevated temperatures and can survive periods of starvation.

Arthroconidia can be inhaled and, when in the host, assume a spherical shape, referred to as spherules. These are thick-walled structures containing numerous endospores. On rupture of the spherule wall, the endospores are released into adjacent tissue or into the blood stream. The endocondia then form sporules to repeat the cycle. The arthroconidium is the main infectious agent of *Coccidioides immitis*. The cell wall of the arthroconidium is composed of three layers that contain potent antigens. These antigens are released when the arthroconidium is converted into a spherule. Once in the host, the arthroconidium is stimulated by the temperature (37°C) and the carbon dioxide concentration to develop into a spherule. The presence of arthroconidia or endospores in lung tissue stimulates the migration of macrophages and phagocytosis. However, the fusion of a lysosome with a phagosome containing the fungus is inhibited. Activation of macrophages with immune T cells or lymphokines results in phagosome-lysosome fusion and, subsequently, killing of *Coccidioides immitis*.[14, 15]

The incubation period of primary respiratory *Coccidioides immitis*, 10 to 16 days, is usually asymptomatic, but the patient may exhibit chest pain, fever, cough, or weight loss.[16] The clinical spectrum of disease caused by *Coccidioides immitis* can be divided into the following categories[17]:

I. Primary Coccidioidomycosis
  A. Pulmonary Disease
    1. Asymptomatic: Diagnosis is made by skin test. Individuals suspected of having contracted the disease are subjected to an intradermal injection of coccidioidin.
    2. Symptomatic: Affected individuals develop flu-like symptoms or can develop severe pulmonary disease. Incubation is usually 10 to 16 days; some individuals may experience an incubation period of 7 to 28 days.
      a. Fever: No specific pattern of temperature elevations. The fever course is diurnal. The fever can persist for several months and may be associated with night sweats. Individuals may develop spontaneous resolution and experience a recrudescence in temperature elevation that indicates that the disease has become disseminated. However, dissemination of the infection can occur in the absence of a temperature elevation.
      b. Pain: Chest pain is a frequent complaint and is the initial symptom in approximately 90% of infected individuals who develop symptomatic disease. The pain is usually mild but may resemble the pain associated with myocardial infarction, or acute cholecystitis. Auscultation of the chest may reveal the presence of a friction rub. The patient's breathing is shallow because the pain is increased with deep respiration or coughing. If the individual develops a spontaneous pneumothorax, respiratory distress occurs. Some patients develop a dry, nonproductive cough. Individuals who develop a productive cough often have purulent sputum that can be blood tinged. The sputum should be mixed with potassium hydroxide, which destroys all material in the sputum except the fungus because the chitin in the cell wall is resistant to strong alkaline solutions.
      c. Anorexia: Infected individuals may lose 20 to 30 pounds within a 3-week period. Patients with disseminated disease may become cachectic.
  B. Cutaneous Infection: This is a rare manifestation of coccidioidomycosis. Cutaneous infection occurs following injury to the skin, allowing conidia or spherules to enter the dermis.[18–20] The lesion begins as an indurated nodule, which develops central necrosis, resembling a chancre. The lesion is painless.
II. Secondary Coccidioidomycosis
  A. Pulmonary Complications
    1. Benign Chronic Disease
      a. Nodular Disease: A common occurrence following coccidioidal pneumonia. Nodules are spherical and dense and reside in the middle lung fields, usually within 5 cm of the hila. The fungus is found within these nodules and remains viable.[21]
      b. Cavitary Disease: This occurs in association with primary infection and typically is not associated with chronic disease. Cavitation may occur within the first 10 days of the disease, and it typically develops as a thin-walled vesicle containing fluid. The most common associated finding is hemoptysis. Spontaneous rupture of the cavity can result in dissemination of the infection, pleural effusion, empyema, pneumothorax, or bronchopulmonary fistula. In approximately 50% of cases, cavitary lesions do not spontaneously resolve after successful an-

tifungal therapy and must be surgically removed. Cavitary lesions that persist place the patient at risk for secondary infections with other fungi or bacteria.

2. Progressive Disease: Typically, residual pulmonary disease can be chronic and stable, but it may become progressive and disseminated. Progressive, disseminated, or systemic disease occurs primarily in immunocompromised patients and is associated with a 50% mortality rate.[22]

B. Extrapulmonary Involvement
1. Meningitis: This is the most serious complication of disseminated disease. If meningitis goes untreated, death occurs within 2 years.[23] Cultures of cerebrospinal fluid tend to be negative, and the diagnosis is dependent on the presence of complement fixation antibodies.
2. Chronic Cutaneous Disease: The skin is the most common extrapulmonary site of involvement. Lesions range from papules to verrucae to subcutaneous abscessed nodules, and draining sinuses originate from abscesses in deep tissue.
3. Systemic Disease: Genitourinary tract infection is not an uncommon form of disseminated disease. Renal involvement was found in 50% of 95 patients at the time of autopsy.[24] In addition, infection has been documented in the prostate gland, epididymis, fallopian tubes, ovaries, and endometrium.[25–28]

Disseminated coccidioidomycosis is a common complication associated with acquired immunodeficiency syndrome (AIDS), particularly in patients living in endemic areas.[29] Approximately 70% of the patients have chest radiographs demonstrating diffuse reticulonodular infiltrates and hilar adenopathy as well as pleural effusions.[30, 31] The fungus can be isolated from lymph nodes, blood, urine, and cutaneous lesions from patients with disseminated disease. Dissemination is more common in men than in women, except if the infection occurs during the third trimester of pregnancy.[32]

DIAGNOSIS: SKIN TEST

Skin testing is conducted with a crude extract of the culture filtrate. A positive test result occurs when an area of induration larger than 5 mm is raised on the skin at the site of injection of coccidioidin. This hypersensitivity reaction occurs 2 weeks after the onset of symptoms and prior to the development of precipitins and complement-fixing antibodies.[16] Interpretation of the test relies on knowing the patient's history. A positive test result is meaningful only if the patient

was known to be previously negative, unless the diagnosis can be supported by additional clinical data. A negative test result in an immunocompetent patient rules out coccidioidomycosis. However, if the patient is anergic, a negative test result is associated with significant mortality.

The diagnosis is established when spherules of *C. immitis* are found in sputum or other specimens. The spherules can be demonstrated by subjecting the specimen to 20% potassium hydroxide (KOH) or staining tissue with hematoxylin and eosin. The specimen should be plated out on Sabouraud's agar medium containing cycloheximide, chloramphenicol, and gentamicin to inhibit the growth of bacteria as well as saprophytic fungi. The diagnosis can also be made by the detection of specific antibodies to *C. immitis*. Within 2 weeks of the onset of infection, IgM antibodies (precipitins) can be detected in 90% of patients. The IgM antibodies will disappear 4 months after the appearance of symptoms and signs of infection. Precipitins are heat stable in temperatures up to 60°C.

IgG antibodies to *C. immitis* can be detected by the complement fixation test. These antibodies to coccidioidin persist for much longer than the precipitins (IgM) and reflect either active infection or recovery.[33–35] It is beneficial to obtain multiple serum samples, at least 1 to 2 weeks apart, to determine the acuity of the disease. A rising IgM (precipitin) and a low IgG indicate a recent infection. Serial specimens will reflect a decreasing level of IgM and an increasing level of IgG over time. Low IgG titers (≤ 1:16) suggest a nondisseminated infection, whereas titers above 1:32 indicate the presence of disseminated disease. A low titer rules out the presence of coccidioidomycosis meningitis. If disseminated disease is suspected, assessment of the spinal fluid should be performed. Patients with coccidioidomycosis meningitis will usually have a positive complement fixation test or IgG present in the spinal fluid.[36]

TREATMENT

The treatment of coccidioidomycosis rests basically with the use of ketoconazole, Diflucan (fluconazole), and amphotericin B. Patients with asymptomatic pulmonary disease or acute pulmonary disease that is not severe can be treated with oral agents (e.g., miconazole, ketoconazole, or fluconazole). If the patient has severe primary pulmonary disease or complications of pulmonary disease, intravenous amphotericin B should be administered. Patients with documented meningitis should receive intrathecal amphotericin B.[37]

Patients with meningitis have been treated with ketoconazole, and improvement was reported in a few individuals.[38, 39] The relatively poor outcome is related to the inadequate penetration of ketoconazole into the cerebrospinal fluid. In order to achieve therapeutic levels of ketoconazole in the cerebrospinal fluid, a dose of 1,200 to 2,000 mg/day must be administered.

HISTOPLASMOSIS

Histoplasmosis is the most prevalent fungal infection of the respiratory tract in humans. It is caused by *Histoplasma capsulatum*, a dimorphic fungus. On culture media, the organism grows as a white-to-brownish cotton-like (mycelial) colony, whereas in the lung it grows as a yeast. The fungus is acquired by inhalation of conidia. Approximately 95% of the infections are asymptomatic, or subclinical, and diagnosed by chest radiograph. The telltale sign on x-ray film is the presence of pulmonary calcifications. The diagnosis is confirmed by a positive histoplasmin skin test. The organism is disseminated in the guano of birds, such as starlings, chickens, and pigeons, and of bats.[41–45] The most cases reported in the United States are from the Ohio-Mississippi River Valley, with Missouri, Kentucky, Tennessee, southern Illinois, Indiana, and Ohio being the most endemic areas.

Infection by *Histoplasma capsulatum* takes on one of two forms, benign or opportunistic. Individuals who inhale a low inoculum usually develop subclinical infection, and infection is detected by the presence of pulmonary calcifications on chest radiograph (Fig. 2–1*A* and *B*) and a positive skin test result. These patients may develop flu-like symptoms, which have been termed *fungus flu*. This is a moderately severe form of the disease and is characterized by the presence of fever, night sweats, and weight loss. The patient may also develop hemoptysis, and the organism can frequently be cultured from this fluid.

Another benign form of this disease is cutaneous infection, which is rare. The patient may have been inadvertently injected with contaminated material or, conceivably, may have become inoculated if there was a break in the skin and this area came into contact with soil containing a significant number of conidia. The lesion begins as an indolent chancriform ulcer, with inflammation of the regional lymph nodes. In the nonimmunosuppressed patient, the lesion usually heals spontaneously within 2 to 3 months. However, in the immunosuppressed patient, the disease tends to become progressive.[46, 47]

Histoplasmosis is also seen in an epidemic form, which occurs in the person exposed to a large inocula of conidia. If the individual has not had previous exposure to the fungus, an incubation period of 10 to 18 days ensues. The patient then manifests a flu-like syndrome: fever, malaise, myalgias, and chills. Individuals who have been previously exposed to the fungus can develop infection, referred to as reinfection histoplasmosis. Patients who develop primary and reinfection histoplasmosis can develop disseminated disease.

However, all lesions tend to heal, as do lesions in the lungs, leaving behind calcifications. The individuals at risk for disseminated disease are the immunosuppressed.

Histoplasmosis is diagnosed by the detection of yeast cells on clinical specimens, with subsequent culturing of the organism. Individuals who have been exposed to the fungus convert to a positive skin test within 2 weeks of the initial exposure. The antigen, histoplasmin, is injected intradermally, and a negative test result in an immunocompetent individual can rule out infection. Testing in anergic patients yields a false-negative result. A positive test result, in the absence of a previously negative test result, is of no benefit in making the diagnosis. Thus, a conversion from negative to positive is of help in arriving at the diagnosis. The complement fixation test is reliable in detecting the presence of antibodies to *Histoplasma capsulatum*, especially in individuals who have active disease. A titer of 1:8 or more indicates the presence of disease. If the titer is 1:32 and persists or rises, the patient should be considered to have active disease.[48] However, cross-reactivity to cryptococcosis, blastomycosis, and, in rare instances, coccidioidomycosis has been demonstrated.[49–51]

Individuals who have a positive complement-fixation test to more than one fungus should be tested with the immunodiffusion method. This procedure is performed in Ouchterlony plates that contain wells surrounded by agar. The antigen and patients sera are placed in separate wells and allowed to diffuse toward each other (Fig. 2–2).[53, 54] A positive test result is established by the formation of a line when antibody and antigen come into contact. An individual who has had the disease will test positive but, over time, will revert to negative. A line usually develops closer to the patient's serum, which has been termed the *m line*. Individuals with acute infection usually develop a line closer to the well containing the antigen: this line has been termed the *h line*. The immunodiffusion test is the most reliable method for establishing a diagnosis of histoplasmosis.

Treatment

Histoplasmosis typically is asymptomatic and resolves spontaneously, leaving behind the calcifications seen on radiograph as the telltale sign that the individual has had the disease. However, individuals who develop progressive, symptomatic disease require treatment. The treatment of choice is amphotericin B. Initially, 1 to 5 mg/day is administered intravenously; the dosage is increased 0.3 to 0.6 mg/kg of body weight per day in 5% glucose with mannitol. The total dose administered should not exceed 3 g. The patient's blood urea nitrogen (BUN) and creatinine should be monitored closely. Toxic side effects include renal failure, throm-

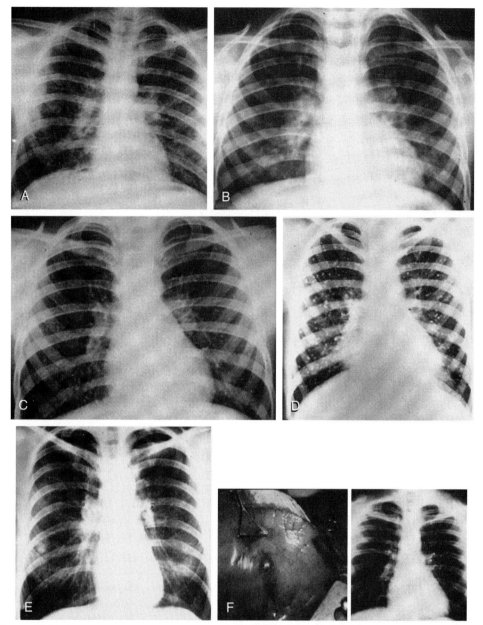

Figure 2-1 ▶ Radiologic aspects of histoplasmosis. *A*, Diffuse interstitial and nodular infiltrates are seen in both lungs and are associated with hilar and mediastinal involvement. This is symptomatic primary histoplasmosis, or "fungus flu." *B*, Multiple miliary nodules in both lungs of a child associated with hilar and mediastinal adenopathy, summer sickness of children. *C*, Two years later, there are multiple calcified densities through both lung fields. *D*, Epidemic primary disease. Numerous small, calcified areas in lung parenchyma. Bilateral involvement. (Courtesy of J. Fennessy.) *E*, A well-circumscribed peripheral nodule in the right middle lobe associated with enlarged hilar nodes; a residual coin lesion. *F*, Well-circumscribed peripheral nodule in right lower lobe and appearance of the lesion at surgery. (Courtesy of F. Kittle.) (From Rippon JW: Medical Mycology: The Pathogenic Fungi and the Pathogenic Actinomycetes, 2nd ed. Philadelphia, WB Saunders, 1982, pp 154–248.)

bophlebitis, hypokalemia, anemia, chills, fever, headache, and anorexia.

BLASTOMYCOSIS

Blastomycosis is a chronic infection acquired via inhalation of conidia of *Blastomyces dermatitidis*. This dimorphic fungus grows in a mycelial form, producing septate hyphae and conidia. The reservoir for this organism has not been established. It has been isolated from soil and fresh water and is associated with contact with chickens and other animals. The organism causes systemic infection, which involves the skin, and pulmonary infection, which involves other organ systems.

Blastomycosis has a reported incidence of up to 4 cases per 100,000 population per year, with most cases occurring in states surrounding the Mississippi and Ohio Rivers. The largest concentration of cases has

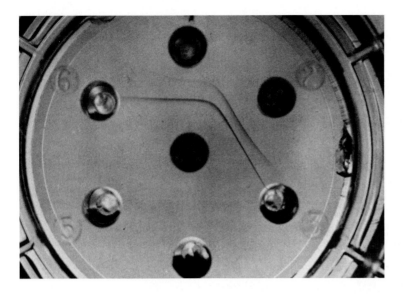

Figure 2–2 ▶ Histoplasmosis. Immunodiffusion plate with a known positive serum in one outer well and an unknown one in an adjacent well. The antigen is in the center well. Note the lines of identity in the two tests. The h line is the finer line near the serum-containing well. The m line is near the antigen-containing well. (From Rippon JW: Medical Mycology: The Pathogenic Fungi and the Pathogenic Actinomycetes, 3rd ed. Philadelphia, WB Saunders, 1988, p 409.)

been reported from Kentucky, Mississippi, Arkansas, North Carolina, Tennessee, Louisiana, Illinois, and Wisconsin.[54] Originally, the organism *Blastomyces dermatitidis* was believed to be endemic only to North America, being termed *North American blastomycosis*, and to be separate and distinct from South American blastomycosis. However, this view is no longer held to be valid because cases of blastomycosis have been reported with increasing frequency from other continents.[55, 56] South American blastomycosis is actually caused by another organism, *Paracoccidioides brasiliensis*. There have been nine epidemics reported in the United States. These have occurred in North Carolina, Illinois, Minnesota, Wisconsin, and Virginia.[57–65] Although all these cases have been associated with outdoor activities and the organism has been found in soil and water, the isolation of *Blastomyces dermatitidis* has been difficult. The problem with determining the true niche of this fungus is that not only is it difficult to isolate it with some degree of regularity, but also it has been isolated from animals, birds, and their droppings.

Infection originates via the inhalation of spores. The organism, once in the lung, undergoes a metamorphosis into the yeast phase and is disseminated by lymphohematogenous spread. The initial reaction to infection is a migration of numerous polymorphonuclear leukocytes. The area then becomes infiltrated with lymphocytes and monocyte-derived macrophages, ultimately producing a granuloma.[66]

The major host defense is cellular immunity, not humoral immunity. Evidence for this lies in the demonstration that individuals with hypogammaglobulinemia are quite capable of handling fungal infections.[67] The important role of cellular immunity in fighting fungal infections has also been demonstrated in infections caused by *Histoplasma capsulatum*, *Paracoccidioides brasiliensis*, and *Coccidioides immitis*.[68–70]

Clinical Characteristics

Males are more commonly infected than females, 4:1 to 15:1. The symptoms of infection are weight loss, fever, fatigue, and malaise. The patient initially presents with a clinical picture of a flu-like illness.[71, 72] The lung is the most common site of infection, with pulmonary infiltrates being the initial finding. The infiltrate appears as an alveolar or mass-like infiltrate.[66] The patient with pulmonary blastomycosis can present with acute pneumonia or chronic pneumonia, or may be totally asymptomatic.

The patient with acute pneumonia typically presents with manifestations like those of any other patient with pneumonia, exhibiting fever, chills, and productive cough with purulent sputum. These signs and symptoms may be mistaken for bacterial pneumonia, and administration of antibiotics will be unsuccessful. Spontaneous resolution of the pneumonia has been

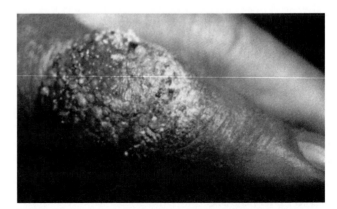

Figure 2–3 ▶ Verrucous form of skin involvement with blastomycosis. The peripherally spreading, crusting, nodular appearance with a sharp border at the margin of the lesion is typical of the lesions seen in blastomycosis. (From Bradsher RW: Systemic fungal infections: Diagnosis and treatment. I. Blastomycosis. Infect Dis Clin North Am 2[4]:887, 1988.)

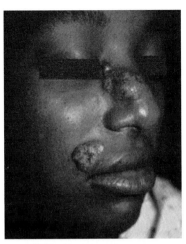

Figure 2–4 ▶ Two facial lesions due to blastomycosis. The fungating appearance with an irregular elevation is typical of the verrucous form of this infection. The exudate seen on the surface of the lower lesion is evidence of the underlying disease. (From Bradsher RW: Systemic fungal infections: Diagnosis and Treatment. I. Blastomycosis. Infect Dis Clin North Am 2[4]:887, 1988.)

reported.[73–75] Chronic pneumonia lasts up to 6 months and is accompanied by weight loss, night sweats, fever, cough, purulent sputum, and chest pain.[66] It is not uncommon for these patients to be treated as if they had tuberculosis. Patients found to have asymptomatic pneumonia frequently have pulmonary infiltrates, which are seen on x-ray film obtained for other purposes, for example, chest radiograph during routine physical examination.

Blastomycosis may present as a skin lesion, verrucoid or ulcerative. The verrucous lesion usually presents as a crusted, raised lesion over a subcutaneous abscess (Figs. 2–3 and 2–4). The border of the lesion is sharp, with central papillomatosis.[76] An ulcerative lesion may be a coincident finding, indicating that the disease involves other areas as well. Faro and colleagues[77] reported a case of blastomycosis that presented in a

woman with an ulcerative lesion (Fig. 2–5) on the thigh and irregular uterine bleeding. The patient was seen in the emergency room for heavy irregular uterine bleeding. A specimen was obtained from the ulcer, an endometrial biopsy was performed, and a culture for fungi was taken. Both specimens grew *Blastomyces dermatitidis* (Fig. 2–6). The genitourinary tract is a relatively common site of involvement, resulting in prostatitis and epididymo-orchitis.[78–81] Transmission of the fungus can occur during sexual intercourse, resulting in endometrial infection, tubo-ovarian abscess, and uterine infection.[82] Although blastomycosis is most frequently found to cause pulmonary infection, any organ system can be infected. The skin is the next most common site of infection, followed by bone, the genitourinary tract, and the nervous system.

Diagnosis

The diagnosis is established by identifying the organism in tissue or exudate and subsequently isolating the fungus in culture. The identification of the fungus is concrete evidence of blastomycotic infection. This fungus does not appear as a contaminant, as is the case with other fungi (e.g., *Candida* and *Aspergillus*). Diagnostic tests are available (e.g., complement fixation antibodies [CF], enzyme-linked immunoassay [EIA] antibodies, immunodiffusion precipitin bands, and delayed-hypersensitivity skin testing with blastomycin), but these tests are not as reliable as identification of the fungus in tissue or sputum specimens and culture.[63, 83–85] There is also cross-reactivity to other antigens (e.g., between *B. dermatitidis* and *H. capsulatum*).[86, 87]

Treatment

Pulmonary infection tends to resolve spontaneously, and patients found to have pneumonia secondary to

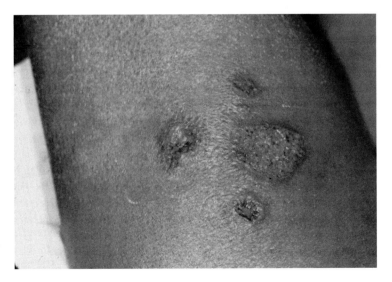

Figure 2–5 ▶ Cutaneous lesions of the thigh caused by *Blastomyces dermatitidis*. Note the erythematous, clean base and the raised margin.

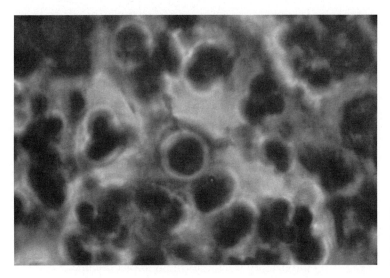

Figure 2-6 ▶ *Blastomyces dermatitidis.* Note the yeast cell on a hematoxylin and eosin stain of tissue specimen obtained from endometrial biopsy. The yeast is in the center of the illustration. A clear zone appears between the cell well and the shrunken cytoplasm.

blastomycosis can be observed for 1 to 2 weeks.[63, 75, 83, 88] Another approach in the patient with a solitary pulmonary infection is to surgically resect the involved lung tissue, if no other disease is present. With any other forms of the disease, or with progressive pulmonary disease, the patient should be treated with antifungal therapy.

Amphotericin B continues to be an excellent antifungal agent for the treatment of blastomycosis. The drug is administered intravenously in increasing dosage until 1 to 3 g has been administered. Amphotericin B is administered in a dose of 0.3 to 0.6 mg/kg per day in 5% glucose with mannitol until a total dose of up to 3 g is reached. The patient's BUN and creatinine level must be monitored. The adverse effects of amphotericin are renal toxicity, thrombophlebitis, hypokalemia, anemia, chills, fever, headache, nausea, and anorexia.

The development of other antifungal agents, such as miconazole, ketoconazole, fluconazole, and itraconazole, all of which are less toxic than amphotericin B, affords the clinician with the opportunity to treat pulmonary blastomycosis.[71, 89–90] Patients treated with any of these agents should be monitored for signs of relapse. Patients with systemic disease who are very ill should be treated with amphotericin B. Once they have improved, a change can be made to complete the treatment course with ketoconazole, 400 mg/day for 6 months.[89, 91]

Another systemic fungal infection is paracoccidioidomycosis (South American blastomycosis), in which the etiologic agent is *Paracoccidioides brasiliensis.*

The following are considered opportunistic infections, but they can cause systemic disease:

Candidiasis
Cryptococcosis
Aspergillosis
Mucormycosis
Trichosporosis
Geotrichosis

Subcutaneous fungal infections include the following:

Sporotrichosis
Chromomycosis
Phaeohyphomycosis
Mycetoma
Rhinosporidiosis
Lobomycosis
Rhinoentomophthoromycosis
Phycomycosis

Fungi that cause skin infections (dermatophytes) are as follows:

Epidermophyton floccosum
Microsporum canis var. *canis, M. canis* var. *distortum, M. cookei, M. ferrugineum, M. gallinae, M. gypseum, M. nanum, M. vanbreuseghemii*
Trichophyton ajelloi, T. equinum, T. megninii, T. mentagrophytes, T. rubrum, T. schoenleinii, T. tonsurans, T. verrucosum, and *T. violaceum*

SPOROTRICHOSIS

Sporotrichosis is caused by *Sporothrix schenckii*, a dimorphic fungus that gains entrance through a break in the skin. *Sporothrix schenckii* is found in soil and on plants. Common mechanisms for acquiring the fungus are a thorn prick (e.g., rose thorn) and being pricked by a splinter. A nodule develops at the site of entrance or trauma, and the organism advances via the lymphatics draining the site of injury. Although it rarely happens, the fungus can gain entrance to other organs causing systemic disease.

Sporothrix schenckii can cause upper respiratory tract disease via inhalation. Infection of the vocal cords and larynx has been reported in women working in a sphagnum moss packing plant.[92] Sinus infection has also been reported secondary to *S. schenckii*, with the subsequent development of endophthalmitis.[93] Pulmonary sporotrichosis has been reported and can arise either via inhalation of the fungal spores or secondary to dissemination from cutaneous infection. Individuals who develop pulmonary disease usually have underlying disease (e.g., chronic obstructive pulmonary disease), are long-time smokers, or have a history of alcohol abuse.[94] Patients who develop pulmonary disease, although it is usually limited, have evidence of being immunocompromised; for example, pulmonary tuberculosis, sarcoidosis, chronic obstructive lung disease, or chronic steroid use.[94–96] Patients typically present with pneumonitis and may demonstrate hilar or paratracheal lymphadenopathy.[97, 98]

Sporotrichosis has been reported to cause arthritis, which is thought to arise from hematogenous dissemination. The disease is indolent and progresses very slowly, affecting weight-bearing joints, especially the knee.[99, 100] Patients at high risk are those in occupations in which the organism is endemic (e.g., gardening, forestry, wood product development) and those who have underlying disease. The disease tends to be monoarticular, but multiple joints can be involved.[101]

Genitourinary tract disease is rare. Infections of kidneys, epididymis, and testes have been reported.[102, 103] Infection of the female reproductive tract has not been reported. Disseminated disease, including involvement of the central nervous system, is extremely rare. One case has been reported of disseminated cutaneous and subcutaneous sporotrichosis in a woman who was not immunocompromised.[104]

The diagnosis of sporotrichosis is initially dependent on strong clinical suspicion. The typical cutaneous lesions are granulomas. Histologically, the granulomas contain histiocytes and polymorphonuclear leukocytes.[105] The presence of an asteroid body is pathognomonic of sporotrichosis; the body is usually found in the center of a granuloma and is surrounded by eosin-stained material.[106] The organism is difficult to identify in tissue, but use of a modified periodic acid–Schiff (PAS) stain can enhance identification of the fungus in tissue specimens.[107, 108] Specimens should be obtained for culture, isolation, and identification of the fungus. Serologic tests can be used to assist in establishing a diagnosis.

Skin testing is available but is not very helpful in establishing a diagnosis. Skin testing is more applicable to epidemiologic studies. The latex agglutination–slide test is a suitable test that does not cross-react with other fungal antigens.[109] The absolute level of antibodies does not correlate with the duration of infection; a titer of more than 80 is indicative of infection.[106] Other tests that correlate well with the agglutination test are the slide–latex agglutination test and the enzyme-linked immunosorbent assay (ELISA). The latter test is particularly useful in the testing of serum and cerebrospinal fluid.[110]

A variety of approaches have been used to treat sporotrichosis. Since the organism is temperature sensitive, local applications of heat have been used to treat pregnant patients.[111, 112] This approach appears to be satisfactory when the disease is limited.

Patients with pulmonary disease may require surgical resection of the involved tissue.[113] Individuals with joint and bone involvement may require surgical intervention, excision of involved tissue, and/or drainage.

Medical management includes the administration of potassium iodide (up to 1.8 g/day) for treatment of cutaneous and lymphangitic cutaneous disease.[106] The patient receiving potassium iodide must be monitored for gastrointestinal and thyroid toxicity. Alternatives are administration of amphotericin B and/or 5-fluorocytosine.[94, 103, 114, 115] Miconazole was effective in treating one individual with pulmonary sporotrichosis.[116] Itraconazole appears to be effective in the treatment of cutaneous and lymphangitic sporotrichosis.[117]

DERMATOPHYTOSIS

The dermatophytes cause infection of the skin, hair, and nails. These fungi secrete keratinases that allow the fungus to invade the nonliving keratinized tissue. This group of fungi—approximately 50 have been identified—are the most prevalent in the world. The typical infection is commonly referred to as ringworm. The three genera that cause this infection are *Trichophyton*, *Microsporum*, and *Epidermophyton*:

Tinea capitis (scalp infection)—*Trichophyton tonsurans, T. violaceum, T. verrucosum, Microsporum audouinii, M. ferrugineum, M. canis, M. gypseum*

Tinea favosa (scalp and torso infection)—*T. schoenleinii, T. violaceum*

Tinea barbae (facial hair infection)—*T. rubrum, T. verrucosum*

Tinea corpori (extremities, torso infection)—*T. rubrum, T. mentagrophytes, M. canis*

Tinea cruris (genitocrural folds)—*T. rubrum, T. mentagrophytes, Epidermophyton floccosum*

Tinea pedis and manus (hands and feet infection)—*T. rubrum, T. mentagrophytes*

Tinea unguium (infection of the nails)—*T. rubrum, T. mentagrophytes, E. floccosum*

Tinea imbricata (infection of the torso)—*T. concentricum*

The dermatophytes are extremely common, and very likely dermatophytoses are the most common infections in the world. Dermatophytic infections are commonly found among individuals living in crowded conditions. Most dermatophytic infections are acquired from the external environment, and dermatophytes live as saprophytes. The dermatophytic fungi appear to evolve to a state where they develop a benign relationship with the host. The host has become the natural reservoir for most dermatophytes. Probably the most common dermatophytic infections of women are tinea corporis (ringworm of the body), tinea cruris (ringworm of the groin), and tinea unguium (ringworm of the nail). *Trichophyton rubrum*, *T. mentagrophytes*, *T. tonsurans*, *Microsporum canis*, and *M. audouinii* cause tinea corporis, or ringworm of the body.

Trichophyton rubrum, *T. mentagrophytes*, *Epidermophyton floccosum*, and *T. verrucosum* cause tinea corporis in adults. The infection can result in two types of lesions: *T. rubrum* and *E. floccosum* produce a dry, scaly annular lesion, and *T. mentagrophytes* and *T. verrucosum* produce vesicles. Typically, *T. rubrum* produces a lesion con-

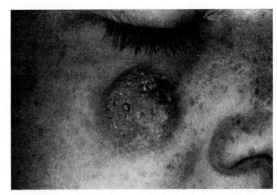

Figure 2–8 ▶ Tinea corporis (tinea faciei). Vesicular-type lesion. Vesicles and crusts are seen over the entire area (T. verrucosum). The infection was acquired from a cow. (From Rippon JW: Medical Mycology: The Pathogenic Fungi and the Pathogenic Actinomycetes, 3rd ed. Philadelphia, WB Saunders, 1988, p 201.)

sisting of concentric rings. The edge appears erythematous, and the central area is covered with scales. *Epidermophyton floccosum* appears as a maculopapular rash with a serpiginous border and a hyperemic central area[118] (Fig. 2–7). The lesion produced by *T. mentagrophytes* and *T. verrucosum* has an elevated, advancing border. Vesicles are found throughout the lesion (Fig. 2–8).

Clinically, the dermatophytoses were termed ringworm because they formed raised, circular lesions; however, these lesions are not caused by worms. The host contracts the fungus when the skin is traumatized and comes into contact with dermatophytes in soil (geophilic species) or on animals (zoophilic species). The fungus can also be contracted when the host comes into contact with dermatophytes found on fomites or another infected human (anthropophilic species). A variety of conditions have been associated with an increased risk of contracting a cutaneous fungal infection (Table 2–3).

Dermatophytes infecting the skin can be diagnosed with the assistance of a Wood's light (ultraviolet light). The patient is placed in a darkened room and a Wood's light is placed over the suspected area. If *Trichophyton* or *Microsporum* is present, it will emit a greenish fluorescence. Scrapings of the suspected area can be obtained and placed in 10% to 20% KOH and examined microscopically for fungal elements. Patients who have a negative microscopic analysis and culture can be diagnosed by determining their immunologic status to the dermatophytes. This is accomplished by

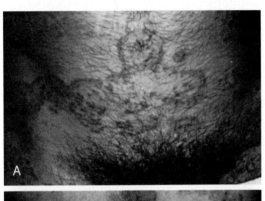
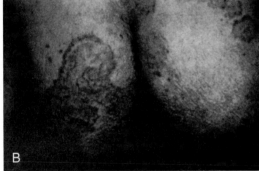
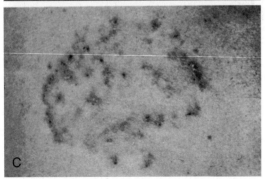

Figure 2–7 ▶ Tinea corporis. Annular appearance of lesions on trunk *(A)* and on gluteal area *(B)*. (Courtesy of S. Lamberg.) *C,* Annular lesion on the thigh. Such concentric rings are the most commonly encountered acute form of tinea corporis caused by *T. rubrum*. (From Rippon JW: Medical Mycology: The Pathogenic Fungi and the Pathogenic Actinomycetes, 3rd ed. Philadelphia, WB Saunders, 1988, p 200.)

TABLE 2–3 ▶	CHARACTERISTICS ASSOCIATED WITH INCREASED RISK OF INFECTION
Moisture	Large inoculum
Increased temperature	Crowded living conditions
Sebum	Immunodeficiency
Perspiration	Familial endocrinopathies

intradermally inoculating trichophytins, a mixture of fungal proteins, glycoproteins, and carbohydrates. Typically, the patient has an immediate skin reaction and an elevated IgE titer. Sera obtained from patients with chronic infection inhibit cell-mediated immunity. Patients with acute infection have a normal immune response. Patients with chronic and acute infection develop normal titers of IgG antibody to the fungal antigens.

Treatment of the dermatophytoses consists mainly of topical application of antifungal agents. The agent is applied three or four times a day for several weeks. Oral treatment can be accomplished with the administration of griseofulvin, 500 mg daily. Skin infections require up to 6 weeks of treatment, whereas nail infections require up to 12 months of treatment. Oral ketoconazole and fluconazole may be effective in the treatment of dermatophytoses.

Another infection of the skin, referred to as tinea versicolor or pityriasis versicolor, is caused by *Malassezia furfur*. The infection is characterized by discrete, serpentine, hyperpigmented and, in some cases, hypo- to depigmented maculae occurring on the thorax, abdomen, or arms. Hairs can also become infected, resulting in folliculitis.

The infection is prominent in areas where the temperature is warm and the humidity remains high. Patients who are immunosuppressed are more likely to develop severe infection, inflammatory folliculitis. Individuals receiving total peripheral nutrition or other forms of parenteral nutrition with lipid emulsions are at risk for developing systemic infection. Treatment is removal of the catheter, since the infection is usually acquired via a contaminated catheter and/or administration of amphotericin B. The lipid emulsion should also be examined and cultured for the fungus.

Skin infections can be diagnosed with the aid of a Wood's light, with the clinician looking for a golden-yellow fluorescence. The lesion is scraped, and the specimen is mixed with 10% KOH and then examined microscopically for the presence of fungal elements. Culturing the organism may not be significant, since the fungus can be isolated from the skin of uninfected individuals. The treatment is the application of 2.5% selenium sulfide for 10 minutes daily for 7 days. Alternative treatment is the application of topical antifungal agents, such as miconazole or ketoconazole, or oral ketoconazole and itraconazole.

REFERENCES

1. Mitchell TG: General characteristics of fungi. In: Joklik WK, Willet HP, Amos DB, Wilfert CM (eds): Zinsser Microbiology. East Norwalk, CT, Appleton & Lange, 1992, pp 1071–1080.
2. Cabib E, Farkas V: The control of morphogenesis: An enzymatic mechanism for the initiation of septum formation in yeast. Proc Natl Acad Sci USA 1971; 68:2052.
3. Ruiz-Herrera J, Lopez-Romero E, Bartnicki-Garcia S: Properties of chitin synthetase in isolated chitosomes from yeast cells of *Mucor rouxii*. J Biol Chem 1977; 252:3338.
4. Calderone RA, Braun PC: Adherence and receptor relationships of *Candida albicans*. Microbiol Rev 1991; 55:1.
5. Domer JE: *Candida* cell wall mannan: A polysaccharide with diverse immunologic properties. Crit Rev Microbiol 1989; 17:33.
6. Mitchell TG: Principles of fungus diseases. In: Joklik WK, Willet HP, Amos DB, Wilfert CM (eds): Zinsser Microbiology. East Norwalk, CT, Appleton & Lange, 1992, pp 1081–1090.
7. Drutz DJ, Cantanzaro A: Coccidioidomycosis. Part I. Am Rev Respir Dis 1978; 117:559.
8. Drutz DJ, Cantanzaro A: Coccidioidomycosis. Part II. Am Rev Respir Dis 1978; 117:727.
9. Edwards LB, Palmer C: Prevalence of sensitivity to coccidiodin, with special reference to specific and nonspecific reactions to coccidiodin and histoplasmin. Dis Chest 1957; 31:35.
10. Symmers WS: An Australian case of coccidioidomycosis. Pathology 1971; 3:1.
11. Gaur PK, Lickwardt RW: Preliminary visual screening of soil samples for the presumptive presence of *Histoplasma capsulatum*. Mycologia 1980; 72:259.
12. Wilcox KR: The Walworth, Wisconsin, epidemic of histoplasmosis. Ann Intern Med 1958; 49:388.
13. Zeidberg LD, Ajello L, Dillon A, Runyon LC: Isolation of *Histoplasma capsulatum* from soil. Am J Public Health 1952; 42:930.
14. Ampl NM, Wieden MA, Galvani JN: Coccidioidomycosis: Clinical update. Rev Infect Dis 1989; 11:897.
15. Berman L, Benjamin E, Pappagianis D: Activation of macrophages by lymphokines: Enhancement of phagosome-lysosome fusion and killing of *Coccidioides immitis*. Infect Immun 1983; 39:1201.
16. Mitchell TG: Systemic mycosis. In: Joklik WK, Willett HP, Amos DB, Wilfert CM (eds): Zinsser Microbiology. East Norwalk, CT, Appleton & Lange, 1992, pp 1091–1112.
17. Rippon JW: Medical Mycology: The Pathogenic Fungi and the Pathogenic Actinomycetes. Philadelphia, WB Saunders, 1982, pp 396–397.
18. Guy WH, Jacob FM: Granuloma coccidioides. Arch Dermatol 1927; 16:308.
19. Trimble JR, Doucette J: Primary cutaneous coccidioidomycosis: Report of a case of laboratory infection. Arch Dermatol 1956; 74:405.
20. Wilson JW, Smith CE, Plunkett OA: Primary cutaneous coccidioidomycosis: The criteria for diagnosis. Calif Med 1953; 79:233.
21. Cox AJ, Smith CE: Arrested pulmonary coccidioidal granuloma. Arch Pathol 1939; 27:717.
22. Salkin D: Clinical examples of reinfection in coccidioidomycosis. Am Rev Respir Dis 1967; 95:603.
23. Winn WA: The treatment of coccidioidal meningitis. Calif Med 1964; 101:78.
24. Forbus WD, Berstebreurtje AM: Coccidioidomycosis: A study of 95 cases of the disseminated type with special reference to the pathogenesis of disease. Milit Surg 1946; 99:653.
25. Bylund DJ, Nanfro JJ, Marsh WL Jr: Coccidioidomycosis of the female genital tract. Arch Pathol Lab Med 1986; 110:232.
26. Chen KT: Coccidioidomycosis of the epididymis. J Urol 1983; 130:978.
27. Conner WT, Drach GW, Bucher WC: Genitourinary aspects of disseminated coccidioidomycosis. J Urol 1975; 113:82.
28. Sung JP, Sun SS, Crutchlow PF: Coccidioidomycosis of the prostate gland and its therapy. J Urol 1979; 121:127.
29. Sobonya RE, Barbee RA, Wiens J, Trego D: Detection of fungi and other pathogens in immunocompromised patients by bronchoalveolar lavage in an area endemic for coccidioidomycosis. Chest 1990; 97:1349.
30. Fish DG, Ampel NM, Calgiani JN, et al: Coccidioidomycosis during HIV infection: A review of 77 patients. Medicine 1990; 69:384.
31. Murray JF, Mills J: Pulmonary infectious complications of HIV infection (part II). Am Rev Respir Dis 1990; 141:1582.
32. Pappagianis D: Epidemiology of coccidioidomycosis. In: Stevens DA (ed): Coccidioidomycosis: A Text. New York, Plenum Publishing, 1980, p 80.
33. Huppert M, Krasnow I, Vukovich KR, et al: Comparison of

coccidioidin and spherulin in complement fixation test for coccidioidomycosis. J Clin Microbiol 1977; 6:33.

34. Huppert M: Serology of coccidioidomycosis. Mycopathol Mycol Applicata 1970; 41:107.

35. Pappagianis D, Zimmer BL: Serology of coccidioidomycosis. Clin Microbiol Rev 1990; 3:247.

36. Bouza E, Dreyer JS, Hewitt WL, Meyer RD: Coccidioidal meningitis: An analysis of thirty-one cases and review of the literature. Medicine 1981; 60:139.

37. Labadie EL, Hamilton RG: Survival improvement in coccidioidal meningitis by high-dose intrathecal amphotericin B. Arch Intern Med 1986; 146:2013.

38. Craven PC, Graybill JR, Jorgensen JH, et al: High-dose ketoconazole for the treatment of fungal infections of the central nervous system. Ann Intern Med 1983; 98:160.

39. Goodpasture HC, Hershberger RE, Barnett AM, Peterie JD: Treatment of central nervous system fungal infection with ketoconazole. Arch Intern Med 1985; 145:879.

40. Graybill JR, Stevens DA, Galgiani JN, et al: Ketoconazole treatment of coccidioidal meningitis. Ann NY Acad Sci 1988; 544:488.

41. Ajello L, Manson-Bahr PEC, Moore JC: Amboni caves, Tanganyika: A new endemic area for *Histoplasma capsulatum.* Am J Trop Med Hyg 1960; 9:633.

42. DiSalvo AF, Johnson WM: Histoplasmosis in South Carolina: Support for the microfocus concept. Am J Epidemiol 1979; 109:480.

43. DiSalvo AF, Ajello L, Palmer JW Jr, et al: Isolation of *Histoplasma capsulatum* from Arizona bats. Am J Epidemiol 1969; 89:606.

44. Gaur PK, Lichtwardt RW: Preliminary visual screening of soil samples for the presumptive presence of *Histoplasma capsulatum.* Mycologia 1980; 72:259.

45. Zeidberg LD, Ajello L, Dillon A, Runyon LC, et al: Isolation of *Histoplasma capsulatum* from soil. Am J Public Health 1952; 42:930.

46. Cott GR, Smith TW, Hinthron DR, Liu C: Primary cutaneous histoplasmosis in immunosuppressed patients. JAMA 1979; 242:456.

47. Giessel M, Rau JM: Primary cutaneous histoplasmosis: A new presentation. Cutis 1980; 25:152.

48. Wheat J, French ML, Kohler RB, et al: The diagnostic laboratory tests for histoplasmosis: Analysis of experience in a large urban outbreak. Ann Intern Med 1982; 97:680.

49. Campbell CC: Serology in the respiratory mycosis. Sabouraudia 1967; 5:240.

50. Campbell CC: History of the development of serologic test for histoplasmosis. In: Ajello L, Chick EW, et al (eds): Histoplasmosis. Proceedings of the Second National Conference. Springfield IL, Charles C Thomas, 1971 (Chapter 42).

51. Campbell CC, Hill GB, Falgout BT: *Histoplasma capsulatum* isolated from a feather pillow associated with histoplasmosis in an infant. Science 1962; 136:1050.

52. Kaufman L, Blumer S: Occurrence of serotypes among *Histoplasma capsulatum* strains. J Bacteriol 1966; 91:1434.

53. Larsh HW, Bartels PA: Serology of histoplasmosis. Mycopathol Mycol Applicata 1970; 41:115.

54. Furcolow ML, Chick EW, Busey JF, Menges RW: Prevalence and incidence studies of human and canine blastomycosis. 1. Cases in the United States, 1885–1968. Am Rev Respir Dis 1970; 102:60.

55. Berkowitz I, Diamond TH: Disseminated *Blastomyces dermatitidis* infection in a non-endemic area: A case report. S Afr Med J 1987; 71:717.

56. Fragoyannis S, van Wyk G, de Beer M: North American blastomycosis in South Africa: A case report. S Afr Med J 1977; 51:169.

57. Centers for Disease Control: Blastomycosis—North Carolina. MMWR 1976; 25:205.

58. Smith JR Jr, Harris JS, Conant NF, et al: An epidemic of North American blastomycosis. JAMA 1951; 158:641.

59. Tosh FE, Hammerman KJ, Weeks RJ, Sarosi GA: A common source epidemic of North American blastomycosis. Am Rev Respir Dis 1974; 109:525.

60. Sarosi GA, King RA: Apparent diminution of the blastomycin skin test: Follow-up of an epidemic of blastomycosis. Am Rev Respir Dis 1977; 116:785.

61. Kitchen MS, Reiber CD, Eastin GB: An urban epidemic of North American blastomycosis. Am Rev Respir Dis 1977; 115:1063.

62. Klein BS, Vergeront JM, DiSalvo AF, et al: Two outbreaks of blastomycosis along rivers in Wisconsin: Isolation of *Blastomyces dermatitidis* from riverbank soil and evidence of its transmission along waterways. Am Rev Respir Dis 1987; 136:1333.

63. Klein BS, Vergeront JM, Weeks RJ, et al: Isolation of *Blastomyces dermatitidis* in soil associated with a large outbreak of blastomycosis in Wisconsin. N Engl J Med 1986; 314:529.

64. Armstrong CW, Jenkins SR, Kaufman L, et al: Common source of outbreak of blastomycosis in hunters and their dogs. J Infect Dis 1987; 155:568.

65. Cockerill FR III, Roberts GD, Rosenblatt JE, et al: Epidemic of pulmonary blastomycosis (Namekagon fever) in Wisconsin canoeists. Chest 1984; 86:688.

66. Bradsher RW: Systemic fungal infections: Diagnosis and treatment. I. Blastomycosis. Infect Dis Clin North Am 1988; 2:877.

67. Biggar WD, Meuwissen HJ, Good RA: Successful defense against *Histoplasma capsulatum* in hypogammaglobulinemia. Arch Intern Med 1971; 128:585.

68. Alford RH, Goodwin RA: Variation in lymphocyte reactivity to histoplasmin during the course of chronic histoplasmosis. Am Rev Respir Dis 1973; 108:85.

69. Cox RA, Vivas JR, Gross A, et al: In vivo and in vitro cell-mediated responses in coccidioidomycosis. I. Immunologic responses of persons with primary, asymptomatic infections. Am Rev Respir Dis 1976; 114:937.

70. Musatti CC, Rezkallah MT, Mendes E, Mendes NF: In vivo and in vitro evaluation of cell-mediated immunity in patients with paracoccidioidomycosis. Cell Immunol 1976; 24:365.

71. Parker JD, Doto IL, Tosh FE: A decade of experience with blastomycosis and its treatment with amphotericin B. Am Rev Respir Dis 1969; 99:895.

72. Sarosi GA, Davies SF, Klein BS, et al: Recent developments in blastomycosis. Am Rev Respir Dis 1986; 134:817.

73. Bradsher RW, Balk RA, Jacobs RF: Growth inhibition of *Blastomyces dermatitidis* in alveolar and peripheral macrophages from patients with blastomycosis. Am Rev Respir Dis 1987; 135:412.

74. Bradsher RW: Development of specific immunity in patients with pulmonary or extrapulmonary blastomycosis. Am Rev Respir Dis 1984; 129:430.

75. Recht LD, Philips JR, Eckman MR, Sarosi GA: Self-limited blastomycosis: A report of 13 cases. Am Rev Respir Dis 1979; 120:1109.

76. Barr CC, Gamel JW: Blastomycosis of the eyelid. Arch Ophthalmol 1986; 104:96.

77. Faro S, Pastorek JG III, Collins J, et al: Severe uterine hemorrhage from blastomycosis of the endometrium: A case report. J Reprod Med 1987; 32:247.

78. Farber ER, Leahy MS, Meadows TR: Endometrial blastomycosis acquired by sexual contact. Obstet Gynecol 1968; 32:195.

79. Watts EA, Gard PD Jr, Tuthill SW: First reported case of intrauterine transmission of blastomycosis. Pediatr Infect Dis 1983; 2:308.

80. Inoshita T, Youngberg GA, Boelen LJ, Langston J: Blastomycosis presenting with prostatic involvement: Report of 2 cases and review of the literature. J Urol 1983; 130:160.

81. Short KL, Harty JI, Amin M, Short LF: The use of ketoconazole to treat systemic blastomycosis presenting as acute epididymitis. J Urol 1983; 129:382.

82. Murray JJ, Clark CA, Lands RH, et al: Reactivation blastomycosis presenting as a tubo-ovarian abscess. Obstet Gynecol 1984; 64:828.

83. Furcolow ML, Busey JF, Menges RW, et al: Prevalence and incidence studies of human and canine *Blastomyces*. II. Yearly incidence studies in three states, 1960–1967. Am J Epidemiol 1970; 92:121.

84. Furcolow ML, Chick EW, Busey JF, Menges RW: Prevalence and incidence studies of human and canine blastomycosis. I.

Cases in the United States, 1885–1968. Am Rev Respir Dis 1970; 102:60.

85. Klein BS, Vergeront JM, Weeks RJ, et al: Isolation of *Blastomyces dermatitidis* in soil associated with a large outbreak of blastomycosis in Wisconsin. N Engl J Med 1986; 314:529.

86. Davies SF, Sarosi GA: Serodiagnosis of histoplasmosis and blastomycosis. Am Rev Respir Dis 1987; 136:254.

87. Sarosi GA, Davies SF: Blastomycosis. Am Rev Respir Dis 1979; 120:911.

88. Edson RS, Keys TF: Treatment of primary pulmonary blastomycosis. Mayo Clin Proc 1981; 56:683.

89. Anonymous: Treatment of blastomycosis and histoplasmosis with ketoconazole: Results of a prospective, randomized clinical trial. Ann Intern Med 1985; 103(6 pt 1):861.

90. McManus EJ, Jones JM: The use of ketoconazole in the treatment of blastomycosis. Am Rev Respir Dis 1986; 133:141.

91. Bradsher RW, Rice DC, Abernathy RS: Ketoconazole therapy of endemic blastomycosis. Ann Intern Med 1985; 103(6 pt 1):872.

92. Agger WA, Seager GM: Granulomas of the vocal cords caused by *Sporothrix schenckii*. Laryngoscope 1985; 95:595.

93. Agger WA, Caplan RH, Maki DG: Ocular sporotrichosis mimicking mucormycosis in a diabetic. Ann Ophthalmol 1978; 10:767.

94. Pluss JL, Opal SM: Pulmonary sporotrichosis: Review and treatment and outcome. Medicine 1986; 65:143.

95. England DM, Hochholzer L: Primary pulmonary sporotrichosis: Report of eight cases with clinicopathologic review. Am J Surg Pathol 1985; 9:193.

96. Jay SJ, Platt MR, Reynolds RC: Primary pulmonary sporotrichosis. Am Rev Respir Dis 1977; 115:1051.

97. Michelson E: Primary pulmonary sporotrichosis. Ann Thorac Surg 1977; 24:83.

98. Ridgeway NA, Whitcomb FC, Erickson EE, et al: Primary pulmonary sporotrichosis. Am J Med 1962; 32:153.

99. Chang AC, Destouet JM, Murphy WA: Musculoskeletal sporotrichosis. Skeletal Radiol 1984; 12:23.

100. Weitzner R, Mak E, Lertratanakul Y: Articular sporotrichosis. Ann Intern Med 1977; 87:382.

101. Molstad B, Strom R: Multiarticular sporotrichosis. JAMA 1978; 240:556.

102. Selman SH, Hampel N: Systemic sporotrichosis: Diagnosis through biopsy of epididymal mass. Urology 1982; 20:620.

103. Wilson DE, Mann JJ, Benett JE, Utz JP: Clinical features of extracutaneous sporotrichosis. Medicine 1967; 46:265.

104. Kluge RM, Hornick RB: Sporotrichosis: An unusual disseminated cutaneous case and fatal pulmonary case. South Med J 1976; 69:855.

105. Lurie HI: Histopathology of sporotrichosis. Arch Pathol 1963; 75:421.

106. Winn RE: Systemic fungal infections: Diagnosis and treatment. I. Sporotrichosis. Infect Dis Clin North Am 1988; 2:899.

107. Fetter BF, Tindall JP: Cutaneous sporotrichosis. Arch Pathol 1964; 78:613.

108. Smith LM: Sporotrichosis: Report of four clinically atypical cases. South Med J 1945; 38:504.

109. Welsh RD, Dolan CT: *Sporothrix* whole yeast agglutination test: Low-titer reactions of sera of subjects not known to have sporotrichosis. Am J Clin Pathol 1973; 59:82.

110. Aram H: Sporotrichosis: A historical approach. Int J Dermatol 1986; 25:203.

111. Romig DA, Voth DW, Liu C: Facial sporotrichosis during pregnancy: A therapeutic dilemma. Arch Intern Med 1972; 130:910.

112. Vanderveen EE, Messenger AL, Voorhees JJ: Sporotrichosis in pregnancy. Cutis 1982; 30:761.

113. Jung JY, Almond CH, Campbell DC, et al: Role of surgery in the management of pulmonary sporotrichosis. J Thorac Cardiovasc Surg 1979; 77:234.

114. Beardmore GL: Recalcitrant sporotrichosis: A report of a patient treated with various therapies including oral miconazole and 5-fluorocytosine. Aust J Dermatol 1979; 20:10.

115. Shelley WB, Sica PA Jr: Disseminate sporotrichosis of skin and bone cured with 5-fluorocytosine: Photosensitivity as a complication. J Am Acad Dermatol 1983; 8:229.

116. Rohwedder JJ, Archer G: Pulmonary sporotrichosis: Treatment with miconazole. Annu Rev Respir Dis 1976; 114:403.

117. Restrepo A, Robledo J, Gomez I, et al: Itraconazole therapy in lymphangitic and cutaneous sporotrichosis. Arch Dermatol 1986; 122:413.

118. Rippon JW: Medical Mycology: The Pathogenic Fungi and the Pathogenic Actinomycetes, 2nd ed. Philadelphia, WB Saunders, 1982, pp 154–248.

Candida Vaginitis

JACK D. SOBEL

EPIDEMIOLOGY

The incidence of *Candida* vaginitis (CV) is poorly documented, particularly since CV is not a reportable entity. Furthermore, collecting data on CV is hampered by inaccuracies of diagnosis of the condition. Regrettably, CV is routinely diagnosed without benefit of microscopy or culture, and as many as half the women so diagnosed may be normal or have other conditions.[1] Data on incidence, where diagnostic data are based on definite clinical and mycologic findings, are exceptional. Moreover, most studies have been carried out in sexually transmitted disease (STD) clinics and family

planning or student health clinics, largely ignoring the private sector and older women. The availability of over-the-counter (OTC) antifungal medications and the potential for widespread abuse of these agents in the community may seriously impair future epidemiologic studies. Most studies suggest a CV prevalence of 5% to 15%, depending on the population studied.[2]

CV affects most females at least once during their lives, at an estimated rate of 70% to 75%, of whom 40% to 50% will experience a recurrence.[3–5] A small subpopulation of probably fewer than 5% of all adult women have recurrent, often intractable episodes of CV.[6] Diagnosis and treatment of CV, together with lost productivity, result in an estimated cost of 1 billion dollars annually in the United States.[7] Statistical data in the United Kingdom derived from patients whose conditions were diagnosed at genitourinary medicine centers show a sharp increase in the annual incidence of CV, from 118 per 100,000 women to 200 per 100,000 women during the last decade.[8] In the United States, CV is currently the second most common cause of vaginal infections, with bacterial vaginosis (BV) the most common diagnostic entity.[9, 10] Based on the number of prescriptions written for treating yeast infections between 1980 and 1990, the incidence of CV almost doubled; these numbered approximately 13 million in 1990.

Point-prevalence studies indicate that *Candida* spp. may be isolated from the lower genital tract of approximately 20% (occasional studies set upper limit at 55%) of asymptomatic healthy women without abnormal vaginal discharge.[11–13] Among women with symptoms of vulvovaginitis, 29.8% had yeast isolated, confirming the diagnosis of CV.[14] Most studies indicate that CV is a frequent diagnosis among young women, affecting as many as 15% to 30% of symptomatic women visiting a clinician. By age 25 years, half of all college women will have experienced at least one physician-diagnosed episode of CV.[3]

MICROBIOLOGY

Between 85% and 90% of yeast strains isolated from the vagina belong to the species of *Candida albicans*. The remainder are non-*albicans* species, the commonest of which is (*Torulopsis*) *Candida glabrata*. Non-*albicans* species can also induce vaginitis, which is clinically indistinguishable from that caused by *C. albicans*; moreover, they are often more resistant to therapy.[2, 4, 13, 15, 16]

It has been claimed, but not proved, that the percentage of vaginal *Candida* infections caused by non-*albicans* strains is dramatically rising.[17–20] Single-dose, oral and topical regimens, together with the popularity of low-dosage azole maintenance regimens and the availability of OTC antimycotics, have been blamed for the appearance of non-*albicans* species, given their lesser susceptibility to azole agents. Nevertheless, recent multicenter studies failed to demonstrate any increase in the prevalence of CV caused by non-*albicans* species.[21] It is of interest that anecdotal reports occasionally describe a natural high-frequency of non-*albicans* CV, often exceeding 50%.[22] After *C. albicans*, *C. glabrata* is by far the next most frequent cause of acute and chronic vulvovaginitis. Other infrequent causes of fungal vaginitis include *C. parapsilosis* and *C. tropicalis*, although virtually every species of *Candida* has been associated with vaginitis.

In earlier epidemiologic studies directed at identifying strains with specific tropism for the vagina, no such tropism was identified.[23] Similarly, no evidence emerged of vaginopathic strains of *C. albicans* demonstrating greater or lesser virulence, which might explain why some women remain heavily colonized with *Candida* spp. despite being entirely asymptomatic, whereas other women develop severe symptomatic vaginitis. DNA typing has provided a more reliable and reproducible method of answering these questions. Using computer-assisted DNA-probe typing and also Southern blots, Soll and co-workers[24] have presented data to support the concept of "vaginal tropism," in which selected organisms demonstrate adaptation to unique anatomic niches that facilitates persistence and survival at certain anatomic sites, including the vagina.

Candida organisms are dimorphic, in that they may be found in humans in different phenotypic phases. In general, blastospores (blastoconidia) represent the phenotype responsible for transmission or spread, and are associated with asymptomatic colonization of the vagina. In contrast, germinated yeast with the production of mycelia most commonly (but not exclusively) constitute a tissue-invasive form, usually identified in the presence of symptomatic disease together with larger numbers of blastospores.

CANDIDA VIRULENCE FACTORS

In order for species of *Candida* to colonize the vagina, they must first adhere to vaginal epithelial cells. *Candida albicans* adheres to such cells in numbers significantly higher than those of *C. tropicalis*, *C. krusei*, and *C. kefyr*.[25] This may explain the relative infrequency of the latter species causing vaginitis. All *C. albicans* strains appear to adhere equally well to both exfoliated vaginal and buccal epithelial cells. In contrast, there is considerable person-to-person variation in vaginal epithelial cell receptivity to *Candida* organisms in adherence assays.[26]

Germination of *Candida* cells enhances colonization[27] and facilitates tissue invasion. Using a mutant strain of *C. albicans* that failed to germinate at 37°C, Sobel and co-workers[27] demonstrated in vivo that nongerminating mutants were incapable of inducing experimental vulvovaginal candidiasis. The implications of this observation are that factors that enhance or facilitate germination might tend to promote symptomatic vaginitis, whereas measures that inhibit germination may prevent vaginitis in women who are asymptomatic carriers of yeast.[28]

Little is known regarding the role of candidal proteolytic enzymes, toxins, and phospholipase in determining the virulence of the organisms. A secreted aspartyl proteinase elaborated by pathogenic *Candida* spp. has been identified in vaginal secretions and is detected in women with symptomatic vaginitis, but not in those with asymptomatic colonization.[29] These proteolytic enzymes with broad substrate specificity destroy free and cell-bound proteins that impair fungal colonization and invasion. Levels of proteinase secreted by vaginal *C. albicans* isolates were greater in isolates obtained from symptomatic women than in those from asymptomatic carriers.[29] Several genes governing proteinase production have been cloned, and a strong correlation exists both in vitro and in experimental vaginitis between gene expression, aspartyl proteinase secretion, and the ability to cause disease.[30] Mycotoxin (e.g., gliotoxin) may act to inhibit chemotaxis or phagocytic activity or may suppress the local immune system. Gliotoxin has been found in vaginal secretions.[31]

High-frequency, heritable switching occurs in the colony morphology of most *Candida* spp. grown on amino acid–rich agar in vitro at 24°C.[32] The variant phenotypes contain a variable capacity to form mycelia spontaneously and to express other virulence factors, such as drug resistance, adherence, and capacity to invade and survive in diverse body sites as well as to cause disease. Although currently there is incomplete evidence that phenotypic switching occurs in vivo at 37°C, this is an attractive hypothesis for explaining spontaneous in vivo transformation from asymptomatic colonization to symptomatic vaginitis. Fresh clinical vaginal isolates obtained from women with acute vaginitis have been found to be in a high-frequency mode of switching. These multiple phenotypes at a given site represent the same or related genetic strains.[33–35] Phenotypic transition occurs spontaneously but is facilitated by exogenous factors, such as temperature and as yet unknown factors.

Overall adaptability of *C. albicans* to different microenvironments itself represents a factor of virulence. Using a DNA probe with sensitive discriminatory ability, investigators have shown that even though the same strain may persist for a long period in the vagina, nevertheless a certain degree of yeast genetic instability exists, especially in the setting of repeated courses of antifungal therapy.[36]

Iron binding by *Candida* organisms has been shown to facilitate their virulence.[37] The ready availability of erythrocytes and hemoglobin in the vagina creates an ideal niche for yeast possessing erythrocyte-binding surface receptors.

PATHOGENESIS

Candida organisms gain access to the vaginal lumen and secretions predominantly from the adjacent perianal area.[38] Vulvovaginal candidiasis is seen predominantly in women of childbearing age, and in the majority of cases a precipitating factor is not identified for explaining the transformation from asymptomatic carriage to symptomatic vaginitis.

Hurley and associates[4, 6] have fostered the view that *C. albicans* is never a commensal in the vagina, in that

clinicians could almost always detect vaginal pathology even in asymptomatic patients from whom such strains have been isolated. Subsequent investigators, however, have not corroborated this view, and have demonstrated that many women carry *C. albicans* in the vagina without symptoms or signs of vaginitis, usually with low concentrations of yeast organism.[11] These observations are compatible with the view that *C. albicans* may be a commensal or a pathogen in the vagina, and that changes in the host vaginal environment are usually necessary before the organism induces pathologic effects. This concept has been challenged as simplistic and excludes a primary role of the commensal organism in inducing symptomatic infection due to spontaneous phenotype switching.[34]

Two fundamental questions are critical in understanding the pathogenesis of vulvovaginal candidiasis. The first relates to the mechanism by which asymptomatic colonization of the vagina changes to symptomatic vulvovaginal candidiasis. The second concerns the mechanism by which some women suffer from repeated and chronic vulvovaginal candidiasis.

PREDISPOSING FACTORS (Fig. 2–9)

Age appears to be an important factor in the overall incidence of vulvovaginal candidiasis. While the condi-

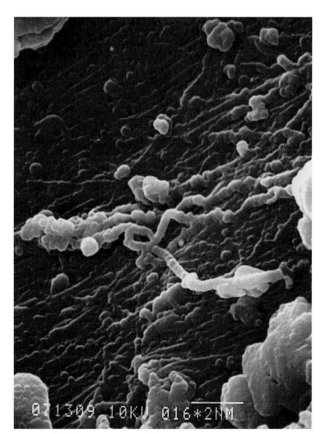

Figure 2–9 ▶ Scanning electron micrograph of *Candida albicans* hyphae invading the vaginal epithelial surface.

tion is extremely rare prior to menarche, the annual incidence increases dramatically toward the end of the second decade of life and peaks over the next two decades. The occurrence of CV may vary by racial group and behavioral factors. Among college women, CV is more common among black than among white women[5] and is associated with initiation of sexual activity.[3] The increased use of estrogen hormone replacement therapy (HRT) in postmenopausal women has recently been suggested as a contributory factor in late-onset CV; however, supportive data are not available.

Pregnancy

During pregnancy, the vagina shows an increased susceptibility to infection by *Candida*, resulting in both a higher prevalence of vaginal colonization and a higher rate of symptomatic vaginitis.[39] The rate of symptomatic vaginitis is maximally increased in the third trimester, and symptomatic recurrences are also more common during pregnancy.[16, 39] High levels of reproductive hormones provide an excellent carbon source for *Candida* organisms by providing a higher glycogen content in the vaginal tissue.[40] A more complex mechanism is likely, in that estrogen enhances adherence of yeast cells to the vaginal mucosa. A cytosol receptor or binding system for female reproductive hormones has been documented in *Candida albicans*.[41] Several investigators demonstrated in vitro binding of female sex hormones to *Candida* organisms as well as the capacity of certain hormones to enhance yeast mycelial formation and hence virulence.[42] Not surprisingly, therefore, rates of cure of CV are significantly lower during pregnancy.[39] Despite the prevailing views on the epidemiology and nature of CV in pregnancy, it should be noted that no recent studies have been performed and the original studies[39] suffered a variety of methodologic flaws.

Contraceptives

Many small, poorly controlled studies have contributed to conflicting conclusions regarding the risk associated with the use of oral contraceptives. Some have shown increased vaginal colonization with species of *Candida* and symptomatic episodes following the use of high-estrogen oral contraceptives.[2, 5, 43] Almost certainly, the same mechanism operative in pregnancy applies to these subjects. Other studies in women utilizing low-estrogen oral contraceptives have not found an increase in CV.[44–47] Nevertheless, many investigators continue to identify oral contraceptives as predisposing to recurrent vulvovaginal candidiasis. Rahman and co-workers[48] reported that users of any contraceptive method were more likely to harbor *Candida* organisms than are nonusers. Several studies found increased carriage of such yeasts in those who use intrauterine

devices (IUDs).[47, 49, 50] Peddie and co-workers[51] found increased *Candida* carriage in diaphragm and condom users with or without use of spermicide. On the other hand, Barbone and colleagues[47] as well as Hooton and co-workers[52] reported an increased colonization associated with use of nonoxinol 9. In the Hooton study, sexual intercourse with the use of a diaphragm and spermicide in the preceding 3 days was found to be associated with a marked increase in the rate of candidal colonization.[55] An association between spermicide use and frank CV has not been confirmed.[51] Other risk factors may include the contraceptive sponge, whereas in an extensive study of risk factors in college students, Foxman[46] identified no difference in risk between users of no birth control method versus users of oral contraceptives, diaphragms, condoms, and spermicides.[46]

Diabetes Mellitus

Vaginal colonization with *Candida* organisms is more frequent in diabetic women. Although uncontrolled diabetes predisposes to symptomatic vaginitis, most diabetics are not afflicted by such repeated infections.[1] It has become traditional to perform glucose tolerance tests in all women with recurrent CV. The yield of these expensive studies is extremely low; therefore, testing is not justified in premenopausal women. Occasionally, women prone to CV describe an association between "candy binges" and exacerbation of symptomatic vaginitis. However, for the most part, dietary restrictions have no place in the routine management of yeast vaginitis.

Antibiotics

The onset of symptomatic CV is frequently observed during courses of systemic and topical antibiotics. Broad-spectrum antibiotics, such as tetracycline and beta-lactams, are mainly responsible for exacerbation of symptoms.[53] Vaginal colonization rates increase from approximately 10% to 30%.[54] Antibiotics are thought to facilitate CV by eliminating the protective vaginal bacterial flora. Thus, the natural flora is thought to provide a colonization resistance as well as preventing germination and hence superficial mucosal invasion.[55] In particular, aerobic and anaerobic resident lactobacilli have been singled out as providing such a protective function. Auger and Joly[56] found low numbers of lactobacilli in vaginal cultures obtained from women with symptomatic CV. Current concepts of a lactobacilli–yeast cell interaction include competition for nutrients, as well as stearic interference by lactobacilli of receptor sites on vaginal epithelial cells for *Candida* organisms.[26] Other mechanisms include the elaboration of bacteriocins by lactobacilli that inhibit yeast proliferation and germination, as well as a direct antibiotic-induced stimulatory effect on the growth of *Candida* spp. Nevertheless, a clear association between lack or loss of vaginal lactobacilli, hydrogen peroxide production, and susceptibility to CV has not been established in women who develop infections while taking antibiotics.[57] It should be emphasized that most women who receive antibiotics do not develop symptomatic vaginitis. Moreover, the overwhelming majority of women with acute CV have not been the recent recipient of antibiotics. It would appear that a subpopulation of women only, already colonized by potentially virulent species of *Candida*, are at risk for developing vaginitis following antimicrobial therapy and do so on a fairly predictable basis.[57]

Behavioral Factors

The incidence of CV increases dramatically in the second decade, corresponding to the onset of sexual activity, and peaks in the third and fourth decades, declining in females older than 40 years, until the hypothesized permissive effect of HRT becomes apparent. Sexual transmission of *Candida* organisms occurs during vaginal intercourse, although the relative role of sexual and nonsexual practices in introducing *Candida* organisms into the lower genital region has not been appraised.[23, 59, 60] Other studies have provided conflicting evidence as to the role, if any, of sexual behavior in causing symptomatic CV.[37, 46–49] The likelihood that sexual behavior may play a role in CV is logical, but epidemiologic evidence is limited.[61] Some authors suggest that recent sexual intercourse frequency correlates with acute vaginitis[48]; however, individual episodes of CV do not appear to be related to lifetime numbers of sexual partners or frequency of intercourse.[5, 61, 62] Engaging in and the frequency of receptive orogenital contact does appear to increase risk.[5, 62, 63] Despite anecdotal evidence, Foxman[46] also found no epidemiologic evidence incriminating female hygiene habits as risk factors for CV.

Miscellaneous

Among the putative factors that have contributed to the increased incidence of CV in Western societies has been the use of tight, restricting, poorly ventilated clothing and nylon underclothing, with increased local, perineal moisture and temperature.[2, 64] The use of well-ventilated clothing and cotton underwear may be of value in preventing infection.[65] On the other hand, Foxman[46] found no increased risk of CV among wearers of tight clothing or noncotton underwear. There is no evidence confirming that iron deficiency predisposes to infection.[65] Anecdotal evidence suggests that the use of commercial douches, perfumed toilet paper, chlorinated swimming pools, and feminine hygiene sprays contributes to symptomatic vaginitis. Chemical contact and local allergy or hypersensitivity reactions may alter the vaginal milieu and permit the transformation from asymptomatic colonization to symptomatic vaginitis.

SOURCES OF INFECTION

Intestinal Reservoir

Although the gastrointestinal tract may well be the initial source of colonization of the vagina by *Candida* organisms,[66] there is considerable controversy regarding the role of the intestinal tract as a source of reinfection in women with recurrent CV.[15]

Species of *Candida* were recovered on rectal culture from 100% of women with recurrent CV.[67] This observation has been the basis of the concept of a persistent intestinal reservoir. Reinoculation of the vagina occurs from the persistent rectal focus following apparent eradication of vaginal yeast by topical therapy. This hypothesis has been criticized, as several authors have found much lower concordances between rectal and vaginal cultures in patients with recurrent CV.[23] The high rate of positive anorectal cultures in some studies probably reflects perineal and perianal contamination from the vaginal discharge. In women, CV recurred frequently in the absence of simultaneously positive rectal cultures. Two controlled studies using oral nystatin treatment, which reduces intestinal yeast carriage, failed to prevent symptomatic recurrence of CV.[68, 69] Furthermore, some women had persistent intestinal yeast carriage and failed to develop vaginal colonization. Nevertheless, despite mounting skepticism, the possibility that persistent gastrointestinal tract carriage is a source of vaginal reinfection cannot be entirely dismissed, especially since the majority of *Candida* strains isolated from the rectum and the vagina are identical.[15, 70] Women prone to recurrent CV are not known to suffer from perianal or rectal candidiasis.

Sexual Transmission (see behavioral factors)

Penile colonization with *Candida* organisms is present in approximately 20% of male partners of women with recurrent CV.[59, 60] *Candida* organisms are most commonly found in uncircumcised, usually asymptomatic males in the vicinity of the coronal sulcus. Asymptomatic male genital colonization with species of *Candida* is four times more common in male sexual partners of infected women.[59] Infected partners usually carry identical strains.[23] Despite the aforementioned evidence indicating that sexual transmission does occur, the contribution of sexual transmission to the pathogenesis of infection remains unknown. Based on the prevalence of positive penile and urethral cultures, the role of sexual spread appears limited.

Vaginal Relapse

After conventional antifungal therapy for CV, resultant negative vaginal *Candida* cultures once more turn positive within 30 days in 20% to 25% of women, strongly supporting the hypothesis that yeast persistence and vaginal relapse is responsible for recurrent CV.[2] Strains isolated before and after therapy are of identical type in more than two thirds of recurrences.[23] Symptomatic relief after clinically successful topical therapy for symptomatic vaginitis is accompanied by a drastic reduction in the number of viable yeast cells in the vagina. Small numbers of the microorganisms persist, however, within the vaginal lumen, generally in numbers too small to be detected by conventional vaginal cultures.[71] It is also conceivable that small numbers of *Candida* organisms might sojourn temporarily within superficial cervical or vaginal epithelial cells, only to reemerge some weeks or months later.[72]

VAGINAL DEFENSE MECHANISMS

Humoral System

Patients with profound immunoglobulin deficiencies show no increase in susceptibility to vaginal yeast infections. Following acute CV, systemic (IgM and IgG) and local (S-IgA) responses are elicited.[73, 74] A protective role for vaginal anti-*Candida* antibodies has been suggested.[75] Patients with recurrent infection, however, do not lack antibody.[76] Lower antibodies titers have been described during active vaginal infections, which may reflect an adsorption effect. Using an experimental animal model of vaginitis, Polonelli and co-workers[77] provided supportive evidence for a protective role of specific antibodies induced by immunization. Elevated serum and vaginal IgE antibodies to *Candida* organisms were detected in some women with recurrent vulvovaginal candidiasis,[78, 79] even though the total IgE levels were normal.[79]

Phagocytic System

Although both polymorphonuclear leukocytes and monocytes play an important role in limiting systemic candidal infection and deep-tissue invasion, these phagocytic cells are characteristically absent from vaginal fluid during CV. Accordingly, these phagocytic cells are not thought to play a role in influencing mucosal colonization or even preventing superficial invasion of the vaginal epithelium by *Candida* organisms. In the rat model of experimental CV, as in humans, the histology of the vagina fails to demonstrate leukocytes in the vaginal fluid or stratified squamous epithelium. Polymorphonuclear cells can be seen concentrating within the underlying lamina propria, but it appears that they are not presented with a chemotactic signal to induce migration into more superficial layers or vaginal fluid.

Cell-Mediated Immunity

Oral thrush, which correlates well with depressed cell-mediated immunity, is frequently seen in debilitated or immunosuppressed patients. This is particularly evident in patients with chronic mucocutaneous candidiasis or with AIDS. In this context, *Candida* organisms are typically opportunistic pathogens. Accordingly, one might anticipate that lymphocytes similarly contribute to normal vaginal defense mechanisms, preventing mucosal invasion by such organisms, possibly by the elaboration of cytokines such as interferon-gamma, which inhibits germ tube formation.[80]

The role of cell-mediated immunity is further emphasized by studies that investigated the role of impaired cell-mediated immunity in predisposing women to idiopathic recurrent CV. Virtually all adult women have positive cutaneous delayed-hypersensitivity reactions as well as in vitro lymphoblast proliferation response to *Candida* antigens. Earlier studies reported cutaneous anergy and depressed lymphoblastic response to *Candida* antigens in women with recurrent CV.[81, 82, 84] The possibility of a subpopulation of suppressor lymphocytes[83] or cytokine switch-inducing suppression of local vaginal cell-mediated immunity has been postulated.[84] Recent studies[84] using a variety of *Candida* antigens and measurement of cytokine elaboration demonstrated a normal systemic cell-mediated immune response in this population, and the previously reported cutaneous anergy was shown to be only transient and the consequence—not the cause—of recurrent vulvovaginal candidiasis, hence, impaired systemic cell-mediated immunity was not involved in the pathogenesis of recurrent vulvovaginal candidiasis. Several additional studies by Fidel and colleagues,[85–88] using the mouse vaginitis model, determined that systemic cell-mediated immunity has only a minor role in providing a normal defense function at the level of the vaginal mucosa. These studies also demonstrated that local and systemic immunity to infection by *Candida* organisms could be induced by vaginal sensitization with *Candida* antigens and that the local vaginal cell-mediated immunity is partially protective. Compartmentalization of the cell-mediated immune response was apparent.[86, 87]

The studies by Fidel[84–88] did not exclude the possibility of an acquired defect in local vaginal cell-mediated immunity predisposing to recurrent CV. In this regard, Witkin and co-workers[89, 90] reported in vitro studies supporting impaired cell-mediated immunity in women with recurrent CV. They postulated that local elaboration of prostaglandin E_2 by a patient's macrophages blocked local protective lymphocyte function, possibly by inhibiting interleukin-2 production.[91] According to this hypothesis, abnormal macrophage function could be either the result of local IgE antibodies to *C. albicans* in the vagina of women with recurrent CV or the result of inhibitory serum factors.[92] The exact protective mechanism of vaginal T lymphocytes has yet to be explained but appears to conform to a Th-1 profile.[86] Recent studies indicate unique subpopulations of vagina-specific lymphocytes.[88]

Vaginal Flora

Probably the most important defense against both candidal colonization and symptomatic inflammation is the normal natural bacterial flora. Any newly arrived *Candida* organism, in order to survive and persist, must initially adhere to epithelial cells and then grow, proliferate, and germinate to successfully colonize the vaginal mucosa. Although microbial competition for nutrients has long been considered the most important source of competition, animal studies suggest that lactobacilli and *Candida* organisms frequently survive side by side.[93] The role of bacteriocins in inhibiting yeast growth and germination requires additional investigation (see the section on antibiotics).

Miscellaneous Defense Mechanisms

Although not studied in the vagina, various natural secretions have been shown to possess considerable antifungal activity. Pollack and co-workers[94] reported fungistatic and fungicidal activity against *C. albicans* of human parotid salivary histidine-rich polypeptides.

MECHANISMS INVOLVED IN INVASION AND INFLAMMATORY RESPONSE

The mechanism by which *Candida* induces inflammation has not yet been established. Yeast cells are capable of producing several extracellular proteases as well as phospholipase. The paucity of phagocytic cells in the inflammatory exudate possibly reflects the lack of or inhibition of chemotactic substances elaborated. Both blastoconidia and pseudohyphae are capable of destroying superficial cells by direct invasion.

During the symptomatic episode, there is the conspicuous appearance of the germinated or filamentous forms of *Candida* cells. Germinated organisms not only enhance colonization but also represent the dominant invasive phase capable of penetrating intact epithelial cells (Fig. 2–10) and invading the vaginal epithelium, although only the very superficial layers are involved[95] (see Fig. 2–10). Symptoms are not strictly related to the yeast load; nevertheless, CV does tend to be associated with greater numbers of *Candida* organisms and with the germinated yeast phase.[95] Approximately 10^3 to 10^4 *Candida* cells per milliliter of vaginal fluid may be recovered in both the symptomatic and the asymptomatic states.[2]

The clinical spectrum varies from an acute florid exudative form, with thick, white vaginal discharge and large numbers of germinated yeast cells, to the other extreme of absent or minimal discharge, fewer organisms, and yet severe pruritus. Based on this, it is suggested that more than one pathogenic mechanism may exist. In the presence of pruritus alone, hypersensitivity or immune mechanisms are likely to be involved.[96–98]

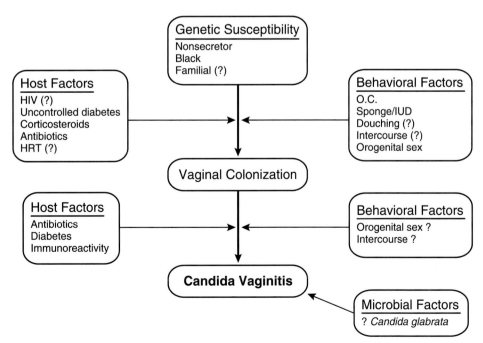

Figure 2–10 ▶ Factors predisposing to vaginal colonization with *Candida* species and responsible for transformation to symptomatic *Candida* vaginitis.

Hence, uncertainty exists regarding the relative contribution of the microorganisms with their capacity to induce inflammation versus the host immune response in the causation of the clinical syndrome. Not infrequently, male partners of asymptomatic female carriers of *Candida* develop postcoital penile erythema and pruritus, which usually last only several hours.

CLINICAL MANIFESTATIONS

Acute pruritus and vaginal discharge are the usual presenting complaints, but neither symptom is specific to CV and neither is invariably associated with disease. The most frequent symptom is that of vulvar pruritus. Vaginal discharge is not invariably present and is frequently minimal. Although described as typically cottage cheese–like in character, the discharge may vary from watery to homogeneously thick. Vaginal soreness, irritation, vulvar burning, dyspareunia, and external dysuria are commonly present. Odor, if present, is minimal and nonoffensive. Examination frequently reveals erythema and swelling of the labia and vulva, often with discrete pustulopapular peripheral lesions and fissure formation (Fig. 2–11). The cervix is normal, and vaginal erythema is present, together with

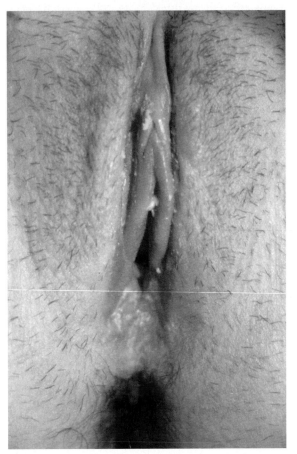

Figure 2-11 ▶ Acute *Candida* vaginitis. Note the presence of edema and erythema of the labia minora. No external discharge is apparent.

adherent whitish discharge. Characteristically, symptoms are exacerbated in the week preceding the onset of menstrual flow.

It is apparent that a clinical spectrum of CV exists. In some patients, a more exudative picture is apparent, with copious discharge and white plaques satisfying the traditional description of vaginal thrush. At the other end of the spectrum are patients with minimal discharge and severe erythema, particularly with extensive vulvar involvement often extending into the inguinal and perianal regions. In general, a quantitative relationship exists between the signs and the symptoms of CV and the numbers of organisms found on culture.

Although *Candida* species occasionally cause extensive balanoposthitis in male partners of women with vaginal candidiasis, a more frequent event is a transient rash, erythema, and pruritus or a burning sensation of the penis that develops minutes or hours after unprotected intercourse. The symptoms are self-limited and frequently disappear after showering. A history of postcoital penile rash is reported in approximately 20% of the partners of women with recurrent CV.

DIAGNOSIS

The lack of specificity of symptoms and signs of CV precludes a diagnosis that is based on history and physical examination only. Clinical signs and symptoms alone should not be regarded as a satisfactory basis for diagnosis.[99] Regrettably, both approaches are common in practice, as myriad infections and noninfections may cause patients to present with identical signs and symptoms; hence, the need for laboratory confirmation. Bergman and colleagues[100] emphasized that a patient's symptoms are of little practical value in predicting CV. The most specific symptom in genital *Candida* infection is pruritus without discharge, and even this criterion correctly predicted CV in only 38% of patients.[100] This situation has been made worse by the growing role of self-diagnosis as a basis for purchasing OTC antimycotics. Although few data are available regarding the reliability of self-diagnosis, most women have been poorly educated in the limitations of self-diagnosis. In a study of self-diagnosed CV, Ferris and co-workers[101] found that more than half of the patients did not have *Candida* confirmed as the etiology.

Most patients with symptomatic vaginitis may be readily diagnosed on the basis of microscopic examination of vaginal secretions (Fig. 2–12*A* and *B*). Accordingly, a wet mount or saline preparation should routinely be done, not only to identify the presence of yeast cells and mycelia but also to exclude the presence of "clue cells" and motile trichomonads. Large numbers of white cells are also invariably absent and, when present, should suggest a mixed infection. The 10% KOH preparation is extremely valuable and even more sensitive in identifying germinated yeast (65% to 85%).

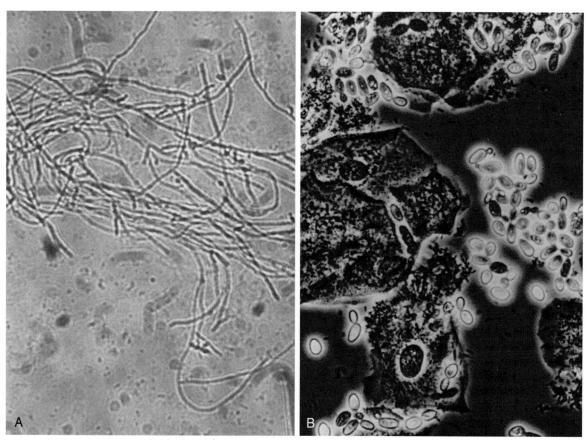

Figure 2-12 ▶ *A*, Photomicrograph of large numbers of *Candida albicans* hyphal elements seen on saline wet preparation *(low power)*. *B*, *Candida glabrata* infection coexists with bacterial vaginosis, and large numbers of yeast singlets and budding yeast are present.

Similarly, vaginal pH estimations reveal a normal pH (4.0 to 4.5) in CV, and the finding of a vaginal pH in excess of 5.0 usually indicates bacterial vaginosis, trichomoniasis, or a mixed infection.

Despite the value of direct microscopy, several studies have consistently revealed that as many as 50% of patients with culture-positive symptomatic CV (responding to antimycotic therapy) will have negative microscopy.[38] Thus, although routine cultures are unnecessary if the wet-mount of KOH preparations shows yeast and mycelia, vaginal culture should be performed in the presence of negative microscopy if CV is suspected on the basis of symptoms or signs (Fig. 2–13). Reliable clinical cultures can also be obtained with Nickerson's medium or semiquantitative "slide-stix" cultures. The Papanicolaou (Pap) smear is unreliable as a diagnostic modality, being positive in only about 25% of cases.[102] Although vaginal culture is the most sensitive method currently available for detecting *Candida* cells, a positive culture does not necessarily indicate that the yeast is responsible for the vaginal symptoms. Merson-Davies and colleagues[103] have shown that a positive microscopic examination usually correlates with relatively high yeast concentrations in vaginal secretions, as confirmed by quantitative vaginal cultures. Their studies also suggested that in most women the

yeast cell numbers correlate with severity of clinical signs and symptoms, and finally that commensal yeast vaginal carriage tends to be associated with lower numbers of vaginal yeast. Diagnosis of CV requires a correlation of clinical findings, microscopic examination, and vaginal culture. Although some prefer to use a selective medium, there is no advantage in using anything but Sabouraud's agar. Vaginal culture for yeast is an underutilized diagnostic test for patients with negative microscopy and normal pH estimation. There is no reliable serologic technique for the diagnosis of CV.

Success has been reported in achieving rapid and reliable diagnosis of CV, utilizing a latex agglutination–slide technique employing polyclonal antibodies reactive with multiple species of *Candida* and directed against yeast mannan.[104] One reported study revealed a sensitivity of 81% with a specificity of 98.5%.[104] Additional testing under clinical conditions confirmed reasonable sensitivity of this test but nevertheless found that it had no advantage over standard microscopy.[105]

Most clinicians consider only trichomoniasis and bacterial vaginosis in the differential diagnosis of CV. Given the profound differences in pH, polymorphonuclear count, and Gram stain appearance, these three common clinical infectious entities are easy to differentiate. More consideration is needed in the symptomatic

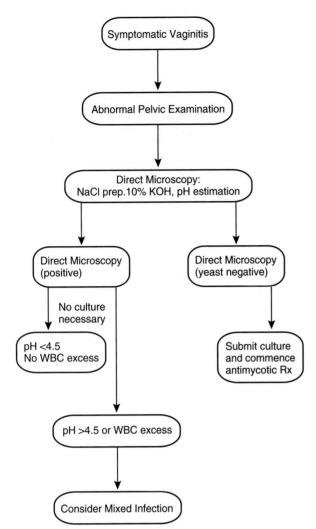

Figure 2-13 ▶ Diagnostic algorithm for symptomatic women with suspected *Candida* vaginitis.

patient in whom these three conditions have been excluded. Among the possibilities in the differential diagnosis of vulvovaginitis in the presence of normal PH and polymorphonuclear leukocyte count and negative yeast cultures are numerous noninfectious causes, including hypersensitivity, irritant and allergic vulvovaginitis, idiopathic focal vulvovestibulitis, cytolytic vaginosis, and physiologic leukorrhea.

TREATMENT

Acute Vaginitis

Highly effective topical azole agents are now available in a variety of formulations[106, 107] (Table 2–4). No strong evidence exists that any one formulation results in superior cure rates; neither is there convincing evidence of the superiority of any specific azole over another azole in the treatment of CV.[107] Overall cure rates for topical azole agents, defined as eradication of symptoms and negative mycologic cultures, are of the

order of 80% to 90%. Oral systemic azole agents achieve comparable or marginally higher therapeutic cure rates, and patients enjoy the convenience of oral administration, which eliminates local side effects and messiness. On the other hand, oral azoles suffer the drawback of potential systemic toxicity, which has limited the use of ketoconazole, although toxicity is a lesser consideration in prescribing intraconazole and fluconazole. Despite the wide therapeutic armamentarium available to practitioners, numerous management issues, some highly controversial, continue to permeate the clinical arena. None of the available agents or regimens fits all the desired properties of the ideal vaginal antifungal agents. None of the agents are fungicidal (achieving a greater than 99.9% killing of all *Candida* organisms isolates within 24 hours). Although capable of killing organisms, azoles are by strict definition fungistatic agents. This point may be irrelevant when one deals with *C. albicans* strains, but in the presence of non-*albicans* species, including *C. tropicalis*, *C. parapsilosis*, and particularly *C. glabrata*, organisms inherently less susceptible[108] to all azoles, clinical failure is by no means infrequent.[19]

Several surveys have consistently shown that most women prefer the convenience of oral therapy.[109] Of the three oral azoles, ketoconazole, although the first effective systemic imidazole, is unlikely to gain widespread usage in CV because of rare but serious hepatotoxicity.[110] Both itraconazole, 200 mg twice a day (for a single day), and fluconazole, 150 mg (single dose), are highly effective triazoles, although neither achieves substantially higher cure rates than those of topical

TABLE 2-4 ▶	THERAPY FOR VAGINAL CANDIDIASIS	
Drug	**Formulation**	**Dosage**
Topical Agents		
Butoconazole	2% cream	5 g × 3 days
*Clotrimazole	1% cream	5 g × 7–14 days
	100-mg vag tab	1 tab × 7 days
	100-mg vag tab	2 tab × 3 days
	500-mg vag tab	1 tab single dose
*Miconazole	2% cream	5 g × 7 days
	100-mg vag supp	1 supp × 7 days
	200-mg vag supp	1 supp × 3 days
	1,200-mg vag supp	1 supp once
Econazole	150-mg vag tab	1 tab × 3 days
Fenticonazole	2% cream	5 g × 7 days
*Tioconazole	2% cream	5 g × 3 days
	6.5% cream	5 g single dose
Terconazole	0.4% cream	5 g × 7 days
	0.8% cream	5 g × 3 days
	80-mg vag supp	80 mg × 3 days
Nystatin	100,000-U vag tab	1 tab × 14 days
Oral Agents		
Ketoconazole	400 mg bid	× 5 days
Itraconazole	200 mg bid	× 1 day
	200 mg	× 3 days
Fluconazole	150 mg	Single dose

* Over-the-counter medications.
vag = vaginal; tab = tablets; supp = suppository.

agents.[111-115] Oral agents cannot be expected to accomplish immediate local relief; hence, severe local symptoms may necessitate adjunct topical treatment for the first 48 hours.

Over the years, conventional use of vaginal antimycotics has been remarkably safe and free from untoward side effects. Certainly, no major morbidity or serious complications have been reported, although high-dose regimens of terconazole were associated with fever and flu-like symptoms that resulted in the withdrawal of this topical agent in these concentrations.[116] Mild to moderate vulvovaginal burning is an underestimated and not infrequent side effect of topical azoles. Accordingly, physicians should respect the preference of the patient when prescribing, in relation to choice of both the route of administration and the individual agent. Both itraconazole and fluconazole are extremely well tolerated, with good safety profiles, and are not comparable to ketoconazole with regard to risk of complications. Nevertheless, recently an untoward drug interaction was reported between intraconazole and astemizole or terfenadine (both commonly used antihistamines). Accordingly, the ideal antimycotic agent continues to evade us. Among the major shortcomings of the current agents is their efficacy in vaginitis caused by non-*albicans* species of *Candida* (see later section) as well as the potential for *C. albicans* strains to become resistant to fluconazole.

There has been a growing tendency to use shorter and shorter courses of both topical and oral agents.[106] Although justified on the basis of convenience and improved compliance, these new regimens have also been introduced to provide a marketing edge for one therapeutically equivalent agent over another. Testing of the efficacy of short, often single-dose courses has not been subject to the same careful and thorough scrutiny as has conventional 5- to 7-day regimens. Nevertheless, single-dose therapy by any route is effective in mild to moderate disease. Many of the single-dose drugs (e.g., vaginal clotrimazole, 500-mg suppository, and fluconazole, 150-mg oral tablet) possess pharmacokinetic properties such that following the single administration of these agents, concentrations of the antimycotic persist in the vagina for up to 5 days.[116, 117] Hence single-dose therapy may be more than "single-day" therapy. In a large multicenter study, severe vaginitis, particularly in women with recurrent CV, responded less well to treatment with single-dose antimycotic therapy.[21]

The aforementioned clinical observations have recently been incorporated into a new classification of CV[119] that forms the practical basis for treatment recommendations (Table 2-5). Uncomplicated CV occurs in normal hosts with mild to moderate severity of infection, is caused by *C. albicans*, and occurs in the absence of a history of recurrent CV. Uncomplicated infections, which constitute the majority of symptomatic episodes of CV, respond well to oral or topical therapy with all antimycotics, including short-course and single-dose regimens. Complicated CV refers to severe infections, including those caused by relatively resistant non-*albicans Candida* species, specifically in women with a history of physician-confirmed recurrent CV and those with underlying immunodeficiency. Complicated infections respond less well to short-course antimycotic regimens and require more prolonged antifungal regimens, of at least 7 days' duration.

TABLE 2-5 ▶ CLASSIFICATION OF VULVOVAGINAL CANDIDIASIS (VVC)	
Uncomplicated	**Complicated**
Sporadic/infrequent VVC	Recurrent VVC
and	*or*
Mild-to-moderate VVC	Severe VVC
and	*or*
Likely to be *Candida albicans*	Non-albicans candidiasis
and	*or*
Normal, nonpregnant host	Abnormal host e.g., Uncontrollable diabetes Debilitation Immunosuppression

Acute Vaginitis in Pregnancy

Management of CV during pregnancy has been poorly studied, but it is considered more difficult because clinical response tends to be slower and recurrences more frequent.[120-122] In general, most topical antifungal agents are effective, especially when prescribed for longer periods (i.e., 1 to 2 weeks). Longer duration of therapy may be necessary to eradicate yeast infection. However, single-application, high-dosage topical therapy with clotrimazole has been shown to be effective in pregnancy and may be considered for the initial therapeutic attempt.[123] In the past, nystatin was considered the drug of choice in the first trimester of pregnancy; however, all topical agents can be used throughout pregnancy. Oral azoles are, however, contraindicated.

RECURRENT *CANDIDA* VAGINITIS

Recurrent CV is a form of complicated vaginitis and is defined as four or more episodes of proven infection during a 12-month period. Most women with recurrent CV are normal hosts, otherwise healthy women without superficial candidiasis elsewhere. As with uncomplicated CV, vaginitis in women with recurrent CV is usually caused by azole-sensitive *C. albicans*. While a subpopulation of women exist with recurrent CV due to repeated courses of antibiotics, in the majority of patients repeated episodes occur in the absence of recognized precipitating factors. Current views regarding the pathogenesis of recurrent disease favor host factors as predisposing to infections. Hence, repeated episodes are thought to be due not to more frequent introduction of yeast into the lower genital tract (i.e., by sexual transmission) or a more virulent or resistant organism, but rather to host factors that result in frequent relapses.

The role of sexual transmission in women with recurrent CV is unclear. As mentioned previously, sexual transmission by vaginal intercourse and orogenital sex undoubtedly occurs, but it is not thought to be a cause in most women with recurrent CV. Moreover, most studies have failed to establish that treatment of the male partner puts an end to recurrent CV.[124–126] In one study,[127] Spinillo and colleagues were able, however, to reduce the recurrence of CV in women whose culture-positive partners were treated with antimycotics. Still, most practitioners do not recommend treatment of sexual partners.

Vaginal bacterial flora has not been shown to be altered or defective in lactobacilli in women with recurrent CV.[128] Thus, many view idiopathic recurrent CV due to C. albicans as an acquired breakdown in the local protective immunity in the vagina due to altered or impaired local cell-mediated immunity.[129] Whether similar factors apply to recurrent CV caused by more resistant C. glabrata is unknown.

Prior to initiation of treatment, diagnosis must be confirmed by culture. Thousands of women carry the label of "recurrent CV" when, in fact, their symptoms are due to noninfectious etiologies, such as allergic and hypersensitivity vulvitis. Following confirmation of CV, every effort should be made to eliminate factors predisposing to CV. However, in the majority of women, no reversible or correctable causal factors are present.

Initial antimycotic therapy requires an induction course of either oral or vaginal antimycotic therapy, which must be continued daily until the patient is completely asymptomatic and a culture-negative status has been achieved. In recurrent CV, failure to initiate a maintenance regimen results in a clinical relapse of vaginitis in 50% of patients within 3 months.[130] Maintenance suppressive regimens include ketoconazole, 100 mg daily, or once-weekly regimens of either clotrimazole, 500-mg suppositories, or fluconazole, 100 mg orally. All three maintenance regimens are effective in preventing breakthrough vaginitis.[124, 130–132] The superior safety profile of fluconazole and clotrimazole has resulted in the latter two agents largely replacing ketoconazole-suppressive prophylaxis. Whatever the maintenance regimen, cessation of therapy is accompanied by symptomatic relapse in half the women within a short time of stopping therapy.[124, 130]

Dennerstein[133] reported a reduced rate of recurrence in recurrent CV in 15 patients during a 3-month period of depot medroxy-progesterone acetate therapy.

In a small study using patients as their own controls, Hilton[134] reported fewer episodes of CV in women placed on oral yogurt. Given the small numbers and the lack of controls in this unblinded study, the role of yogurt in preventing CV remains unproven.

An alternative approach to long-term maintenance of antifungal therapy is the use of hyposensitization with Candida antigen preparation. Two small studies achieved encouraging results.[98, 135]

Resistant Yeast Infections

Vaginitis caused by azole-resistant strains of C. albicans is extremely rare. More recently, fluconazole-resistant strains of C. albicans have been isolated from the oral cavity of males and females with AIDS.[136] It should be emphasized that azole-resistant strains of C. albicans are rarely the cause of CV or recurrent CV. In contrast, not infrequently recurrent CV is due to non-albicans species, the majority of which show reduced susceptibility to all azoles. Particularly common is Candida (Torulopsis) glabrata, and approximately half the strains show reduced sensitivity to available azoles.[108, 137] Boric acid, 600 mg administered vaginally once daily in a gelatin capsule, has been shown to be highly effective in this clinically resistant infection.[19, 138] Therapy should be continued until cultures are negative (usually 10 to 14 days), and when the history suggests recurrent CV a maintenance regimen of alternate-day and then twice-weekly boric acid prescribed. Unfortunately, there is still not much experience published on the efficacy of this maintenance regimen; neither has the long-term safety of intravaginal boric acid been confirmed. An alternative to maintenance boric acid is daily nystatin vaginal suppositories.

The only alternative to vaginal boric acid in resistant infections is flucytosine cream. However, the latter agent is not available commercially and must be prepared by a pharmacist.[139] Flucytosine for vaginal use should be limited because of the potential for the acquisition of resistance.

Candida Vaginitis in HIV-Positive Women

From the onset of the AIDS epidemic, both the prevalence and the significance of oral and esophageal candidiasis have been recognized.[140] As the percentage and numbers of women with HIV grew in the 1980s, CV was increasingly reported.[141, 142]

The increased prevalence of oral candidiasis has been explained on the basis of the loss of oral mucosal cell-mediated immunity defense mechanisms, and the deficiency was thought also to apply to the vagina. Furthermore, given the enormous quantities of broad-spectrum antibiotics administered for prophylactic and therapeutic purposes to women with HIV, together with progressive debilitation, one might similarly predict the frequent occurrence of symptomatic CV, especially with severe immunodeficiency.

A 1987 report indicated that 24 HIV-infected women followed at the Walter Reed Army Medical Center had a history of unexplained chronic CV for at least 1 year.[141] All the patients described had oral thrush and severe helper T-cell depletion, and most were anergic. Within a 30-month follow-up, 80% developed other severe opportunistic infections. Recurrent CV was the presenting complaint, predating the recognition of oral thrush, and was frequently the only clinical indication of severe underlying immunodeficiency. HIV-associated recurrent CV was considered unique, with only temporary symptomatic improvement following the use of intravaginal antifungal agents and requiring constant therapy for control of symptoms. The authors concluded that HIV-positive women with recurrent CV are at serious risk for rapid progression to AIDS. Rhoads and colleagues[141] concluded that women with "chronic refractory" CV should be tested for HIV without defining either term.

A subsequent report described CV in 70% of a female cohort from Rhode Island.[142] In this study, CV responded well to appropriate therapy but had a tendency to recur. These authors also reported increased severity and duration of episodes of CV.[143] More than half the women with new onset of increased frequency or increased severity of CV described their symptoms as originating 6 months to 3 years before the diagnosis of HIV infection had been considered. More than 90% of the women presenting with oral candidiasis had experienced new onset of increased frequency of CV. The location and severity of Candida infections in these HIV-positive women were closely related to the degree of immunosuppression at the time the infection developed, as measured by CD4 counts. A total of 30% of HIV-positive women with only CV and no oral disease had CD4 counts identical to those of HIV-positive women without evidence of mucosal candidiasis. The authors concluded that mucosal infections by Candida organisms occur in a hierarchical (first vaginal, then oral, and later esophageal candidiasis) pattern in women with HIV infection, and that recurrent, often severe CV was common with little or no suppression of CD4 cells.[143]

A major limitation of the aforementioned studies is the lack of information concerning the diagnosis of CV. Any epidemiologic information based on the history only or on physical examination without KOH or culture confirmation is unreliable. A more definitive method of confirming the high prevalence of vulvovaginal candidiasis in women with HIV should emerge from a prospective longitudinal cohort study of HIV-positive women compared to a matched cohort of HIV-negative women with similar risk factors. Such studies have only recently been initiated. In the absence of an HIV-negative control group, it is possible that the CV and recurrent CV in HIV-positive women with high CD4 counts, as described by Imam and colleagues,[143] reflect background CV prevalence in a sexually active group of women still possessing a sense of well-being. Moreover, if progressive loss of mucosal immunity accompanies the decline in CD4 cells, one would anticipate a further increase in the frequency of recurrent CV accompanying advanced AIDS, but none of the published reports have described this occurrence. In contrast to the aforementioned studies, Duerr and coworkers[144] observed that the rate of vaginal carriage of Candida organisms did not increase until the CD4 count dropped below 200 cells/μL.

The issue of HIV testing in the presence of CV remains controversial. Most women experiencing a single episode of CV today are obviously not HIV infected and clearly do not require testing. Even in the case of women with recurrent CV, the issue is anything but clear, since most women with recurrent CV are HIV negative. Only women with recurrent CV who have risk factors for HIV infection should be tested, but high-risk women should be tested anyway, regardless of the presence of CV.

PREVENTION

Since the pathogenesis of CV and recurrent CV remains poorly understood, preventive measures are limited and directed largely at secondary prophylaxis in women known to be at risk for repeated episodes. Accordingly, patients with poorly controlled diabetes have fewer episodes when blood sugar levels are controlled. Similarly, women with a documented history of antibiotic-precipitated CV should avoid unnecessary use of systemic or vaginal antibiotics. If antibiotic use is essential, suppressive prophylaxis with fluconazole, 150 mg, once-weekly, for the duration of antibiotic use is highly effective. Discontinuing the use of oral contraceptives in women prone to recurrent CV has not been shown to reduce the repeated recurrences. A causal relationship between CV and IUDs and spermicidal sponges is more clear-cut, and discontinuing their use seems prudent. Much of prevention is anecdotal, with individuals reporting benefits from discontinuing orogenital sex, avoiding candy binges, and using yogurt either orally or by the vaginal route. The issue of probiotic therapy using FDA-approved Lactobacillus preparations via the vaginal route is similarly interesting but requires study after their release. There is no doubt that long-term suppressive therapy with systemic or topical azoles effectively prevents recurring infections, but most patients return to their original pattern of recurrence following discontinuation of maintenance antifungal therapy. Finally, the widespread abuse of OTC antimycotics requires attention, in order to prevent a further increase in non-albicans

Candida infections as well as resistant *C. albicans.* Responsibility for abuse also lies with practitioners, in situations where indiscriminate use of vaginal antimicrobials contributes to CV and especially resistant disease.

REFERENCES

1. Berg AO, Heidrich FE, Fihn SD, et al: Establishing the cause of symptoms in women in a family practice. JAMA 1984; 251:620.
2. Odds FC (ed): Candidosis of the genitalia. In: Candida and Candidosis. A Review and Bibliography, 2nd ed. Philadelphia, WB Saunders, 1988, p 124.
3. Geiger AM, Foxman B, Gillespie BW: Epidemiology of vulvovaginal candidiasis among university students. Am J Public Health 1995; 85:1146.
4. Hurley R, De Louvois J: *Candida* vaginitis. Postgrad Med J 1979; 55:645.
5. Geiger AM, Foxman B: Risk factors in vulvovaginal candidiasis: A case-control study among college students. Epidemiology 1996; 7:182.
6. Hurley R: Inveterate vaginal thrush. Practitioner 1975; 215:753.
7. Reed BD: Risk factors for *Candida* vulvovaginitis. Obstet Gynecol Surv 1992; 47:551.
8. Annual Reports of Chief Medical Officer, Department of Health and Social Security, 1976–1984 (England and Wales).
9. Centers for Disease Control: Non-reported sexually transmitted diseases. MMWR 1979; 38:61.
10. Fleury FJ: Adult vaginitis. Clin Obstet Gynecol 1981; 24:407.
11. Drake TE, Maibach HI: *Candida* and candidiasis: Culture conditions, epidemiology, and pathogenesis. Postgrad Med J 1973; 53:83.
12. Chow AW, Percival-Smith R, Bartlett KH, et al: Vaginal colonization with *Escherichia coli* in healthy women: Determination of relative risks by quantitative cultures and multivariate statistical analysis. Am J Obstet Gynecol 1986; 154:120.
13. Goldacre MJ, Watt B, Loudon N, et al: Vaginal microbial flora in normal young women. Br Med J 1979; 1:1450.
14. McCormack WM Jr, Zinner SH, McCormack WM: The incidence of genitourinary infections in a cohort of healthy women. Sex Trans Dis 1994; 21:64.
15. Sobel JD: Epidemiology and pathogenesis of recurrent vulvovaginal candidiasis. Am J Obstet Gynecol 1985; 152:924.
16. Morton RS, Rashid S: Candidal vaginitis: Natural history, predisposing factors and prevention. Proc R Soc Med 1977; 70(suppl 4):3.
17. Cauwenbergh G: Vaginal candidiasis: Evolving trends in the incidence and treatment of non–*Candida albicans* infection. Curr Probl Obstet Gynecol Fertil 1990; 8:241.
18. Horowitz BJ, Giaquinta D, Ito S: Evolving pathogens in vulvovaginal candidiasis: Implications for patient care. J Clin Pharmacol 1992; 32:248.
19. Sobel JD, Chaim W: Treatment of *Candida glabrata* vaginitis: A retrospective review of boric acid therapy. Clin Infect Dis 1997; 24:649.
20. Spinillo A, Capuzzo E, Egbe TO, et al: *Torulopsis glabrata* vaginitis. Obstet Gynecol 1995; 85:993.
21. Sobel JD, Brooker D, Stein G, et al: Single oral dose fluconazole compared with conventional topical therapy of *Candida* vaginitis. Am J Obstet Gynecol 1995; 172:1263.
22. Agatensi L, Franchi F, Mandello F, et al: Vaginopathic and proteolytic species of *Candida* among outpatients attending a gynecological center. J Clin Pathol 1991; 44:826.
23. O'Connor MI, Sobel JD: Epidemiology of recurrent vulvovaginal candidiasis, identification and strain differentiation of *Candida albicans.* J Infect Dis 1986; 154:358.
24. Soll DR, Galask R, Isley S, et al: Switching of *Candida albicans* during successive episodes of recurrent vaginitis. J Clin Microbiol 1989; 27:681.
25. King RD, Lee JC, Morris AL: Adherence of *Candida albicans*

and other *Candida* species to mucosal epithelial cells. Infect Immun 1980; 27:667.
26. Sobel JD, Myers P, Levison ME, Kaye D: *Candida albicans* adherence to vaginal epithelial cells. J Infect Dis 1981; 143:76.
27. Sobel JD, Muller G, Buckley H: Critical role of germination in the pathogenesis of experimental candidal vaginitis. Infect Immun 1984; 44:576.
28. Sobel JD, Muller G: Ketoconazole prophylaxis in experimental vaginal candidiasis. Antimicrob Agents Chemother 1984; 25:281.
29. DeBernardis F, Agatens L, Ross IK, et al: Evidence for a role for secreted aspartate proteinase of *Candida albicans* in vulvovaginal candidiasis. J Infect Dis 1990; 161:1276.
30. DeBernardis F, Cassone A, Sturtrant J, Calderone R: Expression of *Candida albicans* SAP 1 and SAP 2 in experimental vaginitis. Infect Immun 1995; 63:1887.
31. Shah DT, Glover DD, Larsen B: In situ mycotoxin production by *Candida albicans* in women with vaginitis. Gynecol Obstet Invest 1995; 39:67.
32. Slutsky B, Buffo J, Soll DR: High-frequency switching colony morphology in *Candida albicans.* Science 1985; 230:666.
33. Soll DR: High-frequency switching in *Candida albicans.* Clin Microbiol Rev 1992; 5:183.
34. Soll DR: High-frequency switching in *Candida albicans* and its relations to vaginal candidiasis. Am J Obstet Gyecol 1988; 158:997.
35. Soll DR, Galask R, Isley S, et al: Switching of *Candida albicans* during successive episodes of recurrent vaginitis. J Clin Microbiol 1989; 27:681.
36. Schroppel K, Rotman M, Galask R, et al: Evolution and replacement of *Candida albicans* strains during recurrent vaginitis demonstrated by DNA fingerprinting. J Clin Microbiol 1994; 32:2646.
37. Moors MA: A novel mechanism for the iron acquisition by *Candida albicans.* Presented at Symposium on *Candida,* American Society of Microbiology. Baltimore, MD, March 1993.
38. Bertholf ME, Stafford MJ: Colonization of *Candida albicans* in vagina, rectum, and mouth. J Family Pract 1983; 16:919.
39. Bland PB: Experimental vaginal and cutaneous moniliasis: Clinical and laboratory studies of certain monilias associated with vaginal oral and cutaneous thrush. Arch Dermatol Syphil 1937; 36:760.
40. McCourtie J, Douglas LG: Relationship between cell surface composition of *Candida albicans* and adherence to acrylic after-growth on different carbon sources. Infect Immun 1981; 32:1234.
41. Powell BL, Drutz DI: Identification of a 173-estradiol-binding protein in *Candida albicans* and *Candida (Torulopsis) glabrata.* Exp Mycol 1984; 8:304.
42. Madani ND: *Candida albicans* estrogen-binding protein gene encodes an oxidoreductase that is inhibited by estradiol. Proc Nat Acad Sci 1994; 91:922.
43. Spinillo A, Capuzzo F, Nicola S, et al: The impact of oral contraception on vulvovaginal candidiasis. Contraception 1995; 5:293.
44. Apisarnthanarax P: Oral contraceptives and candidiasis. Cutis 1974, p 77.
45. Davidson F, Oates JK: The pill does not cause "thrush." Br J Obstet Gynaecol 1985; 92:1265.
46. Foxman B: The epidemiology of vulvovaginal candidiasis: Risk factors. Am J Public Health 1990; 80:329.
47. Barbone F, Austin H, Louv WC, Alexander WJ: A follow-up study of methods of contraception, sexual activity and rates of trichomoniasis, candidiasis and bacterial vaginosis: Am J Obstet Gynecol 1990; 163:510.
48. Rahman KM, Chowdhury TA, Nahar N, Ashraful T: General yeast infection in Bangladesh women using contraceptives. Bangladesh Med Res Counc Bull 1984; 10:65.
49. Parewijck W: Candidiasis in women fitted with an intrauterine contraceptive device. Br J Obstet Gynaecol 1988; 95:408.
50. Spellacy WN, Zaias N, Buhi WC, Birk SA: Vaginal yeast growth and contraceptive practices. Obstet Gynecol 1971; 38:343.
51. Peddie BA, Bishop V, Baily RR, McGill H: Relationship between contraceptive method and vaginal flora. Aust NZ J Obstet Gynecol 1984; 24:217.

52. Hooton TM, Roberts PL, Stamm WE: Effects of recent sexual activity and use of the diaphragm on the vaginal microflora. Clin Infect 1994; 19:274.

53. Caruso LJ: Vaginal moniliasis after tetracycline therapy. Am J Obstet Gynecol 1964; 90:374.

54. Oriel JD, Waterworth PM: Effect of minocycline and tetracycline on the vaginal yeast flora. J Clin Pathol 1975; 28:403.

55. Liljemark WF, Gibbons RJ: Suppression of Candida albicans by human oral streptococci in gnotobiotic mice. Infect Immun 1973; 8:846.

56. Auger P, Joly J: Microbial flora associated with Candida albicans vulvovaginitis. Obstet Gynecol 1980; 55:397.

57. Hawes SE, Hillier SL, Beneditti J, et al: Hydrogen peroxide–producing lactobacilli and acquisition of vaginal infections. J Infect Dis 1996; 174:1058.

58. Bluestein D, Rutledge C, Lumsden L: Predicting the occurrence of antibiotic-induced candidal vaginitis. Family Pract Res J 1991; 11:319.

59. Rodin P, Kolator B: Carriage of yeasts on the penis. Br Med J 1976; 1:1123.

60. Thin RN, Leighton M, Dixon MJ: How often is genital yeast infection sexually transmitted? Br Med J 1977; 2:93.

61. Spinelli A: Recurrent vaginal candidiasis: Results of a cohort study of sexual transmission and intestinal reservoir. J Reprod Med 1992; 37:343.

62. Hellburg D, Zdolsek B, Nilsson S, Mardh PA: Sexual behavior in women with repeated bouts of vulvovaginal candidiasis. Eur J Epidemiol 1995; 11:575.

63. Markos AR, Wade AA, Walzman M: Oral sex and recurrent vulvovaginal candidiasis. Genitourin Med 1992; 68:61.

64. Elegbe IA, Elegbe I: Quantitative relationships of Candida albicans infections and dressing patterns in Nigerian women. Am J Public Health 1983; 73:450.

65. Davidson F, Hayes JP, Hussein S: Recurrent genital candidosis and iron metabolism. Br J Vener Dis 1977; 53:123.

66. De Sousa HM, Van Uden N: The mode of infection and infection in yeast vulvovaginitis. Am J Obstet Gynecol 1960; 80:1096.

67. Miles MR, Olsen L, Rogers A: Recurrent vaginal candidiasis: Importance of an intestinal reservoir. JAMA 1977; 238:1836.

68. Milne JD, Warnock DW: Effect of simultaneous oral and vaginal treatment on the rate of cure and relapse in vaginal candidosis. Br J Vener Dis 1979; 55:362.

69. Vellupillai S, Thin RN: Treatment of vulvovaginal yeast infection with nystatin. Practitioner 1977; 219:897.

70. Meinhof WL: Demonstration of typical features of individual Candida albicans strains as a means of studying sources of infection. Chemotherapy 1982; 28(suppl 1):51.

71. Odds FC: Genital candidosis. Clin Exp Dermatol 1982; 7:345.

72. Garcia-Tamayo J, Castello E, Martinez AJ: Human genital candidosis: Histochemistry, scanning and transmission electron microscopy. Acta Cytol (Balt) 1982; 26:7.

73. Waldman RH, Cruz JM, Rowe DS: Immunoglobulin levels and antibody to Candida albicans in human cervicovaginal secretions. Clin Exp Immunol 1972; 10:427.

74. Mathur S, Virella G, Koistinen J, et al: Humoral immunity in vaginal candidiasis. Infect Immun 1977; 15:287.

75. Cassone A, Boccarera M, Andreori DA, Santomi G, de Bernardes F: Rats clearing a vaginal infection by Candida albicans acquire specific antibody-mediated resistance to vaginal infection. Infect Immun 1995; 63:2619.

76. Gough PM, Warnock DW, Richardson MD, et al: IgA and IgG antibodies to Candida albicans in the genital tract secretions of women with or without vaginal candidosis. Sabouraudia 1984; 22:265.

77. Polonelli L, de Bernardis F, Conti S, et al: Idiotypic intravaginal vaccination to protect against candidal vaginitis by secretory, yeast killer toxin antiidiotypic antibodies. J Immunol 1994; 152:3175.

78. Mathur S, Goust JM, Horger EO III, et al: Immunoglobulin E anti-Candida antibodies and candidiasis. Infect Immun 1977; 18:257.

79. Witkin SS: IgE antibodies to Candida albicans in vaginal fluids of women with recurrent vaginitis. Abstract No. 9, American Society for Microbiology Meeting, Palm Springs, CA, 1987, p 10.

80. Witkin SS, Yu IR, Ledger WJ: Inhibition of Candida albicans–induced lymphocyte proliferation by lymphocytes and sera from women with recurrent vaginitis. Am J Obstet Gynecol 1983; 147:809.

81. Hobbs JR, Briden D, Davidson F, et al: Immunological aspects of candidal vaginitis. Proc Res Soc Med 1977; 70(suppl 4):1114.

82. Syverson RE, Buckley H, Gibian J, Ryan JR: Cellular and humoral immune status in women with chronic Candida vaginitis. Am J Obstet Gyneco 1979; 123:624.

83. Mathur S, Melcher JT, Ades EW, et al: Antiovarian and anti-lymphocyte antibodies in patients with chronic vaginal candidiasis. J Reprod Immunol 1980; 2:247.

84. Fidel PL Jr, Lynch ME, Rendondo-Lopez V, Sobel JD: Systemic cell-mediated immune reactivity in women with recurrent vulvovaginal candidiasis. J Infect Dis 1993; 168:1458.

85. Fidel PL Jr, Lyndh ME, Sobel JD: Effects of preinduced Candida-specific systemic cell-mediated immunity on experimental vaginal candidiasis. Infect Immun 1994; 62:1032.

86. Fidel PL Jr, Lynch ME, Sobel JD: Candida-specific Th-1 responsiveness in mice with experimental vaginal candidiasis. Infect Immun 1993; 61:4202.

87. Fidel PL Jr, Lynch ME, Sobel JD: Mice immunized by primary vaginal C. albicans infection develop acquired vaginal mucosal immunity. Infect Immun 1994; 63:547.

88. Fidel PL Jr, Wolf NA, Kukuruga MA: T lymphocytes in the murine vaginal mucosa are phenotypically distinct from those in the periphery. Infect Immun 1996; 64:3793.

89. Witkin SS: Inhibition of Candida-induced lymphocyte proliferation by antibody to Candida albicans. Obstet Gynecol 1986; 68:696.

90. Witkin SS, Hirsch J, Ledger WJ: A macrophage defect in women with recurrent Candida vaginitis and its reversal in vitro by prostaglandin inhibitors. Am J Obstet Gynecol 1986; 155:790.

91. Kalo-Klein A, Witkin SS: Prostaglandin E_2 enhances and interferon gamma inhibits germ-tube formation in Candida albicans. Infect Immun 1990; 58:260.

92. Witkin SS: Immunologic factors influencing susceptibility to recurrent Candida vaginitis. Clin Obstet Gynecol 1991; 34:662.

93. Savage DC: Microbial interference between indigenous yeast and lactobacilli in the rodent stomach. J Bacteriol 1969; 98:1278.

94. Pollack JJ, Denepitiya L, MacKay BJ, Iacono VJ: Fungistatic and fungicidal activity of human parotid salivary histidine-rich polypeptides on Candida albicans. Infect Immun 1984; 44:702.

95. Sobel JD, Muller G, McCormick R: Experimental chronic vaginal candidiasis in rats. Sabouraudia 1985; 23:199.

96. Kudelko NM: Allergy in chronic monilial vaginitis. Ann Allergy 1971; 29:266.

97. Palacios HJ: Hypersensitivity as a cause of dermatologic and vaginal moniliasis resistant to topical therapy. Ann Allergy 1976; 37:110.

98. Rigg D, Miller MM, Metzger WJ: Recurrent allergic vulvovaginitis treatment with Candida albicans allergen immunotherapy. Am J Obstet Gynecol 1990; 162:332.

99. Schaaf VKM, Perex-Stable EJ, Borehardt K: The limited value of symptoms and signs in the diagnosis of vaginal infections. Arch Intern Med 1990; 150:1929.

100. Bergman JJ, Berg AO, Schneeweiss R, Heidrich FE: Clinical comparison of microscopic and culture techniques in the diagnosis of Candida vaginitis. J Family Pract 1984; 18:549.

101. Ferris DG, Dekle C, Litaker MS: Women's use of over-the-counter antifungal pharmaceutical products for gynecologic symptoms. J Family Pract 1996; 42:595.

102. Rosenberg M: Vaginal candidiasis: Its diagnosis and relation of urinary tract infection. South Med J 1976; 69:1347.

103. Merson-Davies LA, Odds FC, Malet R, et al: Quantification of Candida albicans morphology in vaginal smears. Eur J Obstet Gynecol Reprod Biol 1991; 42:49.

104. Evans EGV, Lacey CJN, Carney JA: Criteria for the diagnosis of vaginal candidosis: Evaluation of a new latex agglutination test. Eur J Obstet Gynecol Reprod Biol 1986; 22:365.

105. Sobel JD, Schmitt CA, Meriwether C: A new slide latex agglutination for the diagnosis of acute *Candida* vaginitis. Am J Clin Pathol 1990; 94:323.

106. Sobel JD: Therapeutic considerations in fungal vaginitis. In: Ryley JF (ed): Chemotherapy of Fungal Diseases. 1990, Vol 14, pp 365–383.

107. Reef S, Levine W, McNeil M, et al: Treatment options for vulvovaginal candidiasis: Background paper for development of 1993 STD treatment recommendations. Clin Infect Dis 1995; 20:80.

108. Lynch ME, Sobel JD: Comparative in vitro activity of antimycotic against pathogenic vaginal yeast isolates. J Med Vet Mycol 1994; 32:267.

109. Tooley PJ: Patients and doctor preferences in the treatment of vaginal candidiasis. Practitioner 1985; 229:655.

110. Lewis JH, Zimmerman HJ, Benson GD, Ishak KG: Hepatic injury associated with ketoconazole therapy: Analysis of 33 cases. Gastroenterology 1984; 86:503.

111. Silva-Cruz A, Androle L, Sobral J, Francisca A: Itraconazole versus placebo in the management of vaginal candidiasis. J Gynecol Obstet 1991; 36:229.

112. Brammer KW: Treatment of vaginal candidiasis with a single oral dose of fluconazole. Eur J Clin Microbiol Infect Dis 1988; 7:364.

113. Kutzer E, Oittner R, Leodolter S, Brammer KW: A comparison of fluconazole and ketoconazole in the oral treatment of vaginal candidiasis: Report of a double-blind multicenter trial. Eur J Obstet Gynecol Reprod Biol 1988; 29:305.

114. Tobin JM, Loo P, Granger SE: Treatment of vaginal candidosis: A comparative study of the efficacy and acceptability of itraconazole and clotrimazole. Genitourin Med 1992; 68:36.

115. Osser S, Haglind A, Weström L: Treatment of *Candida* vaginitis: A prospective randomized multicenter study comparing econazole with oral fluconazole. Acta Obstet Gynecol Scan 1991; 70:73.

116. Moebius UM: Influenza-like syndrome after terconazole. Lancet 1988; 2:966.

117. Breuker G, Jurezok F, Lenaerts M, et al: Single-dose therapy of vaginal mycoses with clotrimazole vaginal cream 10%. Mykosen 1986; 29:427.

118. Ritter W: Pharmacokinetic fundamentals of vaginal treatment with clotrimazole. Am J Obstet Gynecol 1985; 152:945.

119. Sobel JD, Faro S, Force RW, et al: Vulvovaginal candidiasis: Epidemiologic, diagnostic and therapeutic considerations. Am J Obstet Gynecol 1998; 178:203.

120. Lang WR, Stella JG, Benchakan V: Nystatin vaginal tablets in treatment of candidal vulvovaginitis. Obstet Gynecol 1956; 8:364.

121. Wallenburg HCS, Wladimiroff JW: Recurrence of vaginal candidiasis during pregnancy: Comparison of miconazole and nystatin treatments. Obstet Gynecol 1976; 48:491.

122. McNellis D, McLeod M, Lawson J, Pasquale SA: Treatment of vulvovaginal candidiasis in pregnancy: A comparative study. Obstet Gynecol 1977; 50:674.

123. Lindeque BG, Van Niekerk WA: Treatment of vaginal candidiasis in pregnancy with a single clotrimazole 500-mg vaginal pessary. S Afr Med J 1984; 65:123.

124. Sobel JD: Recurrent vulvovaginal candidiasis: A prospective study of the efficacy of maintenance ketoconazole therapy. N Engl J Med 1986; 315:1455.

125. Fong IW: The value of treating the sexual partners of women with recurrent vaginal candidiasis with ketoconazole. Genitourin Med 1992; 68:174.

126. Bisschop MP, Merkus JM, Scheygrand H, et al: Co-treatment of the male partner in vaginal candidiasis: Double-blind randomized control study. Br J Obstet Gynecol 1986; 93:79.

127. Pizzoli G, Lombardi G, Cavanna C, et al: Recurrent vaginal candidiasis: Results of a cohort study of sexual transmission and intestinal reservoir. J Reprod Med 1992; 37:343.

128. Sobel JD, Chaim W: Vaginal microbiology of women with acute recurrent vulvovaginal candidiasis. J Clin Microbiol 1990; 34:2497.

129. Fidel PL Jr, Sobel JD: Immunopathogenesis of recurrent vulvovaginal candidiasis. Clin Microbiol Rev 1996; 9:335.

130. Sobel JD: Management of recurrent vulvovaginal candidiasis with intermittent ketoconazole prophylaxis. Obstet Gynecol 1985; 65:435.

131. Davidson F, Mould RF: Recurrent genital candidosis in women and the effect of intermittent prophylactic treatment. Br J Vener Dis 1978; 54:176.

132. Sobel JD: Fluconazole maintenance therapy in recurrent vulvovaginal candidiasis. Int J Gynecol Obstet 1992; 37:17.

133. Dennerstein GJ: Depot-Provera in the treatment of recurrent vulvovaginal candidiasis. J Reprod Med 1986; 31:801.

134. Hilton E, Isenberg HD, Alperstein P, et al: Ingestion of yogurt containing *Lactobacillus acidophilus* as prophylaxis for candidal vaginitis. Ann Intern Med 1992; 116:353.

135. Rosedale N, Brown MB: Hyposensitization in the management of recurring vaginal candidiasis. Ann Allergy 1979; 43:250.

136. Ng TT, Denning DW: Fluconazole resistance in *Candida* in patients with AIDS: A therapeutic approach. J Infect 1993; 26:117.

137. Redondo-Lopez V, Lynch ME, Schmitt CA, et al: *Torulopsis glabrata* vaginitis: Clinical aspects and susceptibility to antifungal agents. Obstet Gynecol 1990; 76:651.

138. Jovanovic R, Congema E, Ngujen HT: Antifungal agents versus boric acid for treating chronic mycotic vulvovaginitis. J Reprod Med 1991; 36:593.

139. Horowitz B: Topical flucytosine therapy for chronic recurrent *Candida tropicalis* infections. J Reprod Med 1986; 31:821.

140. Klein RS, Harris CA, Small CB, et al: Oral candidiasis in high-risk patients as the initial manifestation of the acquired immunodeficiency syndrome. N Engl J Med 1984; 311:354.

141. Rhoads JL, Wright C, Redfield RR, Burke DS: Chronic vaginal candidiasis in women with human immunodeficiency virus infection. JAMA 1987; 257:3105.

142. Carpenter CCJ, Mayer KH, Fisher A, et al: Natural history of acquired immunodeficiency syndrome in women in Rhode Island. Am J Med 1989; 86:771.

143. Imam N, Carpenter CCJ, Mayer KH, et al: Hierarchical pattern of mucosal *Candida* infections in HIV-seropositive women. Am J Med 1990; 89:142.

144. Duerr A: Gynecologic conditions in HIV-infected women in Brooklyn, New York. VIIIth International Conference on AIDS/IIIrd STD World Congress, July 19–24, 1992, Amsterdam, The Netherlands, vol 2, Abstr PB 3051, B95.

145. Schuman P, Sobel JD, Ohmit S, et al: Mucosal *Candida* colonization and candidiasis in women living with or at risk for HIV infection. Clin Infect Dis 1998; 27:1161.

Obstetric Infections

3

Toxoplasmosis

Oliver Liesenfeld ▶ Jack S. Remington

INTRODUCTION

Toxoplasma gondii infection acquired by the parturient during gestation places the fetus at risk for becoming infected with a parasite that can cause devastating damage to its central nervous system. Yet in the pregnant woman it most often goes unrecognized and is of little, if any, clinical consequence. Herein lies one of the most perplexing problems in the field of prevention, recognition, and management of infection in pregnant women. Whereas there is a heightened awareness of the untoward outcomes associated with infection acquired during gestation with a variety of bacterial and viral agents, *Toxoplasma* goes essentially unrecognized and unappreciated as a significant cause of disease in the newborn, older child, and adult who suffer the unfortunate sequelae of the congenital infection. This chapter focuses primarily on infection in the pregnant woman.

A fatal case of infantile granulomatous encephalitis—initially believed to be caused by an encephalitozoon[1]—was later correctly diagnosed as toxoplasmosis by Sabin and Olitski. *Toxoplasma* as a cause of prenatally transmitted human disease was established soon thereafter.[2, 3] Development of the dye test by Sabin and Feldman led to studies that revealed the high prevalence and broad (most often asymptomatic) spectrum of disease in humans.[4] In 1969, *Toxoplasma* was determined to be a coccidian and the definitive host was found to be the cat.

Transmission of *T. gondii* to the fetus occurs essentially only when the mother has been infected for the first time during gestation. Except for the rare exception, women infected prior to conception do not run the risk of passing the parasite on to their fetus unless they are severely immunocompromised during gestation. We do not have reliable data accumulated in recent years to permit an accurate estimate of the prevalence of *T. gondii* infection among different populations (including geographic locales and ethnic and economic groups) of women of childbearing age in the United States. Such data would allow for an estimate of the number of women actually at risk for acquiring the infection during gestation and, therefore, those whose infants potentially are at risk. Lacking also are data on the prevalence of congenitally infected babies born in the United States in recent years. It has been estimated that as many as 4,100 of the 4.1 million infants born annually in recent years in the United States have the congenital infection. The majority of infected infants do not have clinical signs at birth but suffer sequelae of the congenital infection later in life. All these events occur in the setting of a preventable infection and disease.

Diagnosis of the acute acquired infection is based largely on serologic methods. Since the infection most often goes unnoticed in pregnant women, only routine serologic screening of women during pregnancy (successfully performed in Austria and France) can detect acute acquired infection and thereby allow treatment intended to prevent infection of the fetus. However, such routine testing is not conducted in the United States. Since the vast majority of infected newborns have subclinical infection at birth, they go unnoticed and suffer the unfortunate sequelae of this congenital infection. Because of the lack of mandatory screening in the United States, a single serum sample—in most cases obtained either late in the first trimester or during the second or third trimester—is often the only source of information on whether the fetus is at risk.

Serologic screening and—perhaps more relevant and important in the era of managed care—the education of patients on how to prevent infection with this parasite have not been routinely or systematically undertaken. This situation, and the use of commercially available serologic test kits for detection of *T. gondii* antibodies that do not correctly distinguish acute and distant infection, have often done more harm than good to the individual patient. All these considerations highlight the importance of and problems associated with *T. gondii* infection in women.

MICROBIOLOGY

The Organism

Toxoplasma, an obligate intracellular protozoan in the subclass coccidia, exists in three forms: the oocyst that contains two sporozoites and is the product of the sexual cycle in members of the cat family; the asexual

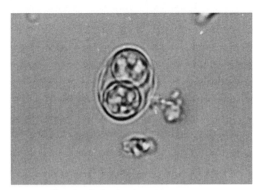

FIGURE 3-1 ▶ Sporulated oocyst.

invasive form, referred to as the tachyzoite; and the tissue cyst, which contains bradyzoites.

Oocyst

An enteroepithelial cycle occurs only in the intestines of members of the cat family (see section on transmission) and results in oocyst formation (Fig. 3–1).[5] Oocysts measure 10 x 12 μm, and as many as 10 million in a single day are shed in the feces for periods varying from 7 to 20 days. The sporulated oocyst is infective when ingested, giving rise to the extraintestinal forms in the cat and other mammals, including humans. Depending on temperature and availability of oxygen, sporulation occurs in 1 to 21 days.[6] Oocysts do not sporulate below 4°C or above 37°C.[6]

Tachyzoite

Tachyzoites are crescentic or oval, with one end attenuated (pointed) and the other rounded (Figs. 3–2 and 3–3); they are 2 to 4 μm wide and 4 to 8 μm long and

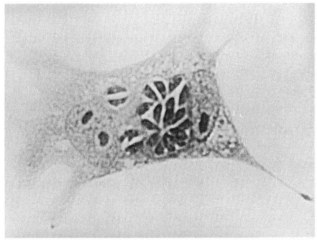

FIGURE 3-3 ▶ Tachyzoites in the cytoplasm of a fibroblast.

require an intracellular habitat to survive and multiply. They cannot survive desiccation or freezing and thawing.[7] Tachyzoites are destroyed within a few minutes in gastric juice and therefore usually do not survive passage through the stomach following oral infection. Tachyzoites enter both phagocytic and nonphagocytic cells by direct penetration as well as by being phagocytosed where they exist within cytoplasmic vacuoles.[8–10] Repeated replication results in disruption of the infected host cell, and released tachyzoites go on to invade contiguous cells or are phagocytosed. The tachyzoite form is seen during the acute stage of the infection. They can invade virtually every cell type and cause cell death, resulting in an inflammatory response and tissue destruction.

Cyst

Tissue cysts (Fig. 3–4) are formed within host cells and may vary in size from those that contain only a few bradyzoites to those that contain several thousand.[11] Cysts are demonstrable as early as the first week of

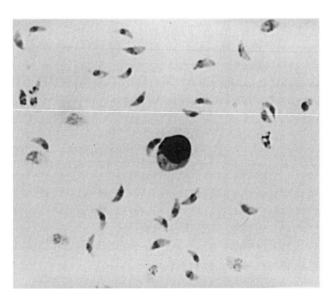

FIGURE 3-2 ▶ Tachyzoites in peritoneal fluid of a mouse infected 3 days previously.

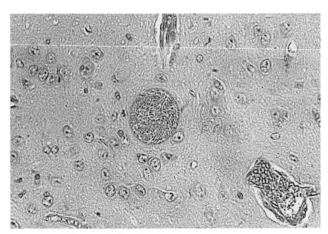

FIGURE 3-4 ▶ Cyst of *T. gondii* in brain.

infection and appear to persist throughout the life of many mammalian hosts. The brain (see Fig. 3–4), and skeletal and heart muscles appear to be the most common sites of latent infection. This form of the parasite is considered to be the cause of recrudescence of the infection in immunocompromised patients. When bradyzoites are released from cysts, they invade contiguous cells and differentiate into the tachyzoite form. Because of their persistence in tissues, demonstration of cysts in histologic sections does not necessarily mean that the infection was recently acquired. The cyst wall is disrupted by peptic or tryptic digestion. Liberated parasites can remain viable for at least 2 hours in pepsin-hydrochloric acid and for as long as 6 hours in trypsin,[7] thereby allowing them to survive the normal digestive period in the stomach and even longer in the duodenum. Development of immunity has been suggested as a factor in cyst formation. Using in vitro culture systems, the induction of bradyzoite-specific genes has been shown with pH shift, temperature, antimitochondrial drugs, and cytokines, including interferon gamma (IFN-gamma).[12]

Life Cycle

Ingestion of *T. gondii* cysts or oocysts (Fig. 3–5) is the most common means by which infection is acquired. Congenital transmission is much less common. After ingestion, cysts are disrupted and the bradyzoites are released into the intestinal lumen, where they rapidly enter cells and multiply as tachyzoites. Spread of tachyzoites occurs by disruption of infected cells and subsequent invasion of adjacent cells and via the blood stream. The sexual cycle occurs in the small intestine in members of the cat family, where the zygote (oocyst) is excreted into the environment. In secondary hosts and in extraintestinal tissues of the cat, development of specific immunity is paralleled by formation of cysts. Immunity in the host is lifelong, and reinfection does not appear to result in clinically apparent disease. In contrast, immunodeficiency may result in reactivation of latent infection and severe disease.

Different Strains of T. gondii

Virulence in laboratory mice, isoenzyme pattern analysis, and restriction fragment length polymorphism have been used to differentiate virulent and nonvirulent strains of *T. gondii*. More recently, genetic analysis has revealed that *T. gondii* consists of three clonal lineages designated types I, II, and III.[13, 14] Most strains isolated from patients with acquired immunodeficiency syndrome (AIDS) are type II, whereas type I strains are commonly found in cases of congenital disease. Identification of strain types for epidemiologic studies is now feasible.

EPIDEMIOLOGY

Transmission

Ingestion

In humans, *Toxoplasma* infection is most commonly acquired through ingestion of undercooked or raw meat containing tissue cysts; oocysts excreted in the feces of infected cats that have ingested contaminated

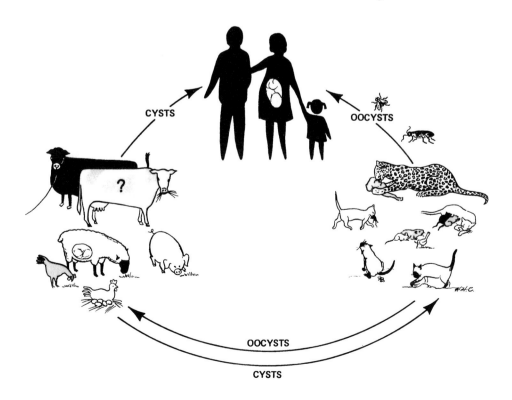

FIGURE **3–5** ▶ The life cycle of *T. gondii*. Members of the cat family are the definitive host.

water or food have also been reported as the source of infection. Thus, the natural route of transmission in nature proceeds from animals (and contaminated soil) to humans by way of ingestion.

The seroepidemiology of *T. gondii* infection in domestic animals used for human consumption and the ability of cysts to withstand the digestive process led to the hypothesis that meat may serve as a source of human *T. gondii* infection.[7] Humans consuming undercooked pork are more likely to have antibody titers,[15] and the parasite has been demonstrated in samples of meat from sheep, cattle, and swine.[7, 16]

In 1965, Desmonts and colleagues[17] proved the meat-man hypothesis of transmission when they found that consumption of undercooked meat resulted in development of antibodies to *T. gondii* at a rate five times that in the general population. Miniepidemics of toxoplasmosis and prevalence rates that vary depending on habits and customs of various populations have also strongly implicated ingestion of undercooked meat as the source of infection.[16, 18] The relative importance of oocysts and cysts in transmission has not been defined and probably varies among different populations and geographic locales. Epidemiologic studies in areas devoid of cats, and epidemics of toxoplasmosis in humans and sheep that have been attributed to exposure to infected cats, support the importance of the cat (oocyst) in transmission.[19, 20]

The organism has been transmitted successfully via milk directly to suckling young in experimental mouse models, but transmission during breast-feeding in humans has not been demonstrated. Whereas pasteurization of milk and cooking of other food products makes transmission by food products unlikely, the organism may be transmitted through unpasteurized milk (e.g., goat milk). Outbreaks within families and other groups are common[21]; however, there is no evidence of direct human-to-human transmission other than that from mother to fetus. Outbreaks caused by contamination of drinking water have been reported.[22]

Other Means of Transmission

Toxoplasma has been recovered from blood donated by an asymptomatic person for transfusion and was shown to survive in whole citrated blood stored at 4°C for up to 50 days.[23] *Toxoplasma* may remain viable in leukocytes, and development of overt toxoplasmosis in patients with acute leukemia following transfusion of leukocytes from donors with chronic myelogenous leukemia has been reported.[24] Laboratory-acquired cases of toxoplasmosis caused by handling of infected animals or contaminated needles and glassware have been reported.[25, 26] Transmission of *T. gondii* by organ transplantation from a seropositive donor to a seronegative recipient has proved to be a significant cause of infection.[27, 28]

Congenital Transmission

Congenital transmission of *T. gondii* from an infected woman to her fetus was the first form of transmission to be recognized.[1, 2] The current concept is that the parasite reaches the placenta via the blood stream during maternal parasitemia, invades and multiplies within cells of the placenta, and eventually gains access to the fetal circulation. Frequency of transmission to the fetus probably depends on a variety of factors, including maternal parasitemia, maturity of the placenta, and competency of the maternal immune response to *T. gondii* (see section on pathophysiology). Parasitemia and widespread infection most likely occur very early after infection in previously seronegative women. It is during the parasitemic phase of the infection in the mother that the placenta is infected. Isolation of *T. gondii* from placental tissues and infection of the fetus are very closely correlated. Congenital transmission has been shown to vary considerably, depending on the time during gestation that the mother acquired her infection (Table 3–1). Fetal infection is less frequent when the mother is treated during pregnancy (see sections on treatment and prevention). Maternal infection acquired around the time of conception and within the first 2 weeks of gestation usually does not result in transmission.[29] Maternal infection acquired during weeks or a few months prior to gestation rarely has been reported to result in fetal infection.[16]

Approximately 85% of infants with congenital infection appear normal at birth.[30, 31] This is the reason that such infants so frequently go undiagnosed in the newborn period. There is an inverse relationship of frequency of transmission and severity of disease. Infants who have been infected in the first and second trimester more frequently show severe congenital toxo-

---

TABLE 3–1 ▶ INCIDENCE OF CONGENITAL *T. GONDII* INFECTION ACCORDING TO GESTATIONAL AGE AT TIME OF INFECTION OF THE MOTHER

Weeks of Gestation*	No. of Infected Fetuses/ Total No. of Fetuses (%)
0–2	0/100 (0)
3–6	6/384 (1.6)
7–10	9/503 (1.8)
11–14	37/511 (7.2)
15–18	49/392 (13)
19–22	44/237 (19)
23–26	30/116 (26)
27–30	7/32 (22)
31–34	4/6 (67)
Unknown	8/351
Total	194/2632 (7.4)

*Patients were treated with spiramycin.

Adapted from Hohlfeld P, Daffos, F, Costa J-M, et al: Prenatal diagnosis of congenital toxoplasmosis with a polymerase-chain-reaction test on amniotic fluid. N Engl J Med 1994; 331:695–699.

TABLE 3-2 ▶ OUTCOME OF OFFSPRING AMONG WOMEN WHO ACQUIRED *T. GONDII* INFECTION DURING PREGNANCY

Outcome in Offspring	Infection Acquired During		
	First Trimester %	Second Trimester %	Third Trimester %
Congenital toxoplasmosis	9.0	27.0	59.0
Subclinical	22.2	74.4	89.8
Clinically apparent	77.8	15.6	10.2
Perinatal death or stillbirth	5.0	2.0	0

Adapted and modified from Desmonts G, Couvreur J: Congenital toxoplasmosis: A prospective study of the offspring of 542 women who acquired toxoplasmosis during pregnancy. Pathophysiology of congenital disease. In: Thalhammer O, Baumgarten K, Pollak A (eds): Perinatal Medicine, Sixth European Congress, Stuttgart: Georg Thieme Verlag, 1979, pp 51–60, with permission.

plasmosis (Table 3–2). In contrast, the majority of children, (e.g., those in whom maternal infection was acquired during the third trimester) are born with the subclinical form of the infection. However, if the condition goes untreated, as many as 85% of these children will develop signs and symptoms of the disease, in most cases chorioretinitis or delays in development.[16, 32, 33] Whereas placental blood flow appears to play a major role in the frequency of transmission of the parasite, the age of the fetus appears to be an important factor in determining clinical signs in the newborn. The period of highest risk of development of clinically apparent congenital infection was shown to be weeks 10 to 24; the low-risk period was weeks 26 to 40.[34]

Congenital Transmission in Immunocompromised Women

Whereas infection with *T. gondii* acquired before pregnancy poses little or no risk to the fetus when the mother is immunocompetent, immunocompromised patients with prior *Toxoplasma* infection may transmit *T. gondii* to their fetus. Pregnant women who are receiving corticosteroids or other immunosuppressive drugs for their underlying disease and those with human immunodeficiency virus (HIV) infection (e.g., AIDS) have an increased risk of transmitting the parasite to their offspring. HIV-infected women who are seropositive for *T. gondii* are at risk for reactivation of their infection and, thus, of congenital transmission. There are insufficient data for quantifying the risk of congenital transmission by HIV-infected mothers who have chronic *Toxoplasma* infection. Mitchell and colleagues[35] reported that the transmission rate of congenital infection was remarkably and significantly higher in HIV-infected *Toxoplasma*-seropositive women than in HIV-negatives ones.[35] In other studies, low rates of transmission have been reported.[36, 37] The differ-

ences in rates of transmission in these studies might be caused by differences in the stage of HIV infection in the mother.

Prevalence of *T. gondii* Infection and Toxoplasmosis

The prevalence of positive serologic test titers increases with age, indicating past exposure, and there is no significant difference in prevalence between men and women in the United States.[38] However, reports from other countries do indicate such differences.[39, 40] There are considerable geographic differences in prevalence rates possibly caused by differences in exposure to the tissue cyst and the oocyst and the habits of different populations at risk.

Prevalence of Toxoplasma Antibodies

Recent data on the prevalence of antibodies in pregnant women or women of childbearing age vary considerably in different geographic regions (Table 3–3). Reports from Europe and the United States suggest that there has been a decrease in the prevalence of *T. gondii* infection among women of childbearing age and the general population that may, in part, be attributed to preventive measures implemented by women during pregnancy and by differences in food processing and handling (see section on prevention).[41] The decrease in rates of prevalence of *Toxoplasma* antibodies among women of childbearing age results in a higher proportion of (seronegative) pregnant women at risk for acquisition of the infection during pregnancy and transmission of the microbe to their offspring. Thus, knowledge of the rate of seroprevalence among pregnant women is important in estimating the population at risk.

Incidence of Acquired Infection During Pregnancy and of Congenital Infection

Serologic screening of pregnant women, which is compulsory in France, has revealed rates of incidence of

TABLE 3-3 ▶ RATES OF PREVALENCE OF *T. GONDII* ANTIBODIES AMONG WOMEN OF CHILDBEARING AGE IN DIFFERENT LOCALES IN THE UNITED STATES

Geographic Locale	% Positive
Denver, Colorado	3
Palo Alto, California	10
Houston, Texas	12
Chicago, Illinois	12
Boston, Massachusetts	14
Los Angeles, California	30
Birmingham, Alabama	30

Adapted from Remington JS, McLeod R, Desmonts G: Toxoplasmosis. In: Remington JS, Klein JO (eds): Infectious Diseases of the Fetus and Newborn Infant. Philadelphia, WB Saunders, 1995, pp 140–267.

T. gondii infections acquired during pregnancy of 2.3% in French women and 1.6% in immigrant women living in France.[42] The frequency of acquired *Toxoplasma* infection during pregnancy and prevalence of congenital infection vary considerably in different geographic locales (Table 3–4). Similar investigations have not been performed in the United States, but the incidence of acute acquired infection among pregnant women in the United States has been estimated at 0.2% to 1%. The incidence of congenital infection in the United States has been estimated to range from 1 in 1,000 to 1 in 8,000 live births. Thus, among the approximately 4.2 million live births in the United States annually, approximately 500 to 4,100 infants are congenitally infected.[16] In France and Austria, there appears to have been a decrease in the incidence of congenital infection. Preventive measures, as well as improvements in diagnosis and subsequent abortion of infected fetuses, most likely caused this decrease.

Incidence of Toxoplasmic Encephalitis in the Immunocompromised Host

The incidence of toxoplasmic encephalitis directly correlates with the prevalence of *Toxoplasma* antibodies in a given population and the degree of immunosuppression in individuals in that population. *Toxoplasma* seroprevalence among patients with diseases that are associated with a higher risk of reactivated toxoplasmosis, including Hodgkin's disease or transplant recipients, has not been studied in detail. The prevalence of *Toxoplasma* antibodies among HIV-infected patients varies from 15% to 40% in the United States[43] and up to 96% in certain areas of Western Europe and Africa.[44] In areas of high seroprevalence, 25% to 50% of all AIDS patients may develop toxoplasmic encephalitis if they are not receiving appropriate prophylaxis. In the United States, toxoplasmic encephalitis has been observed in 1% to 5% of patients with AIDS.[44] The introduction of primary and secondary prophylaxis, as well as the recent introduction of new antiretroviral compounds including protease inhibitors, in HIV-infected *Toxoplasma*-seropositive patients probably has led to a decrease in the incidence of opportunistic infections, including toxoplasmic encephalitis.

PATHOPHYSIOLOGY

The course of the infection is influenced by a number of factors, including inoculum size and virulence of the organism and the genetic background and immunologic status of the individual. Following ingestion or inoculation, the organisms invade cells directly[45] or are phagocytosed.[8] Following host cell disruption, parasites are disseminated widely via the blood stream and infect multiple organs, including the central nervous system and eye, skeletal and heart muscle, and placenta, where they continue to multiply intracellularly, cause cell death, and go on to invade contiguous cells. Both cellular and humoral immunity appear to play major roles in control of the initial acute infection and to terminate continued tissue destruction by the parasite. Tachyzoites are cleared from the host by a variety of immune mechanisms resulting primarily from their activation of the cytokine system, especially the helper T-cell (T_H) 1 response. IFN-gamma is the major mediator of the immune response to the parasite. Antibodies act in concert with the cidal effect of activated macrophages and cytotoxic CD8[+] T cells (see later). Cyst formation occurs during the first week of infection, and this form of the parasite persists lifelong.[46] They do not cause clinical signs of the infection in the immunologically intact host. The immunologically pristine nature of the central nervous system likely is the reason for this site's being the most heavily infested with the cyst form. During acute infection in the immunocompromised host or fetus, the failure of limitation of tachyzoite replication may result in massive tissue destruction in multiple organs and tissues. Disruption of cysts in a setting of impaired host immunity is most probably the mechanism that leads to recrudescence of the infection and the subsequent severe clinical manifestations.[16]

Host Immune Response

In recent years, studies of the infection in humans and animal models have substantially increased our knowledge of the immune response against *T. gondii* and revealed the intricate balance of the cytokine network, lymphocytes, and the monocyte-macrophage system in host resistance to the parasite. In humans, the infection triggers production of IgG, IgM, IgA, and

| TABLE 3–4 ▶ | FREQUENCY OF ACQUIRED *TOXOPLASMA* INFECTION DURING PREGNANCY AND ESTIMATED PREVALENCE OF CONGENITAL INFECTION IN DIFFERENT GEOGRAPHIC LOCALES |

Geographic Locale	Frequency of Acquired *Toxoplasma* Infection During Pregnancy per 1000 Births	Estimated Prevalence of Congenital *Toxoplasma* Infection per 1000 Births
Birmingham, Alabama	0.6	0.12
Melbourne, Australia	5	2
Brussels, Belgium	14.3	2
Geneva, Switzerland	9	3.5
Karvina, Czechoslovakia	3.2	1.6
Paris, France	16	N.D.
London, U.K.	N.D.	0.07–0.25

N.D. = not determined.

Adapted from Remington JS, McLeod R, Desmonts G: Toxoplasmosis. In: Remington JS, Klein JO: Infectious Diseases of the Fetus and Newborn Infant. Philadelphia, WB Saunders, 1995, pp 140–267, with permission.

IgE antibodies against multiple *T. gondii* proteins. The activated macrophage inhibits or kills intracellular *T. gondii*, and sensitized CD4+ and CD8+ T lymphocytes are cytotoxic for *T. gondii*–infected cells.[48] Both upregulatory cytokines (e.g., IFN-gamma and TNF) and downregulatory cytokines (e.g., interleukin-10 [IL-10], TGF-beta) effect the response; IFN-gamma plays the pivotal role in this immunity.[49, 50] A relative increase in the percentages of γδ T cells has been observed in the acute stage of the infection.[51, 52] In vitro, these cells expand preferentially in response to *T. gondii*, are cytotoxic against *T. gondii*–infected cells, and produce IFN-gamma.[53] Expression of heat-shock proteins by γδ cells has been shown to closely correlate with protection against the infection.[54] Humoral and cellular immunity do not confer protection against reinfection. However, reinfections in immunologically intact animal models revealed that such reinfection does not result in disease or in congenital transmission of the parasite.

Pathology

Since the acute acquired infection in immunocompetent individuals most often goes unnoticed, knowledge regarding the pathology caused by *T. gondii* derives mainly from cases in immunocompromised individuals and in congenitally infected fetuses and newborns.

Acute Acquired Infection in Immunocompetent Individuals

During the acute infection, histologic changes in lymph nodes are characteristic and include reactive follicular hyperplasia, irregular clusters of epithelioid histiocytes encroaching on and blurring the margins of the germinal centers, and focal distention of sinuses with monocytoid cells (Fig. 3–6).[55] Langerhans giant

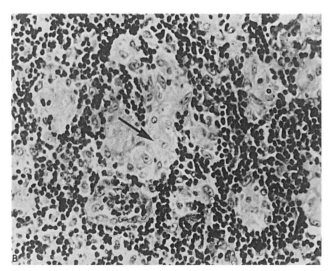

FIGURE 3–6 ▶ Histologic section of a lymph node from a *T. gondii*–infected patient. Arrow = cluster of epithelioid histiocytes.

cells, granulomas, microabscesses, and foci of necrosis are usually not found. Parasites are only rarely demonstrable in affected lymph nodes.[55] In rare cases in seemingly immunocompetent patients, clinical signs may reflect involvement of other organs, including the lungs, heart, and skeletal muscle. Tachyzoites surrounded either by areas of inflammation and necrosis or organisms without associated inflammation, as well as *T. gondii* cysts with or without associated inflammation, may be present.

Congenital Infection

Tachyzoites without significant histopathologic lesions in the placenta have been described,[56] as have *T. gondii* cysts and inflammatory reactions in the decidua capsularis and villi.[57] Although multiple organs and tissues are involved in the infected fetus, the major ones affected are the brain and eye, with resulting acute and chronic inflammation and destruction of vital tissue. Tachyzoites and cysts may be present in and around necrotic areas as well as in areas without obvious inflammation. Obstruction of the aqueduct of Sylvius or the foramen of Monro results in hydrocephalus. Infection in the eye causes inflammatory changes in the choroid and retina, with resulting impairment of vision if it involves the area of the macula (see later). For a more detailed discussion of the pathology observed in congenitally infected infants, the reader is referred to reference 16.

Infection in the Eye

The eyes may be involved as a result of the congenital or postnatally acquired infection. Primary lesions are in the retina and choroid and are accompanied by inflammation and necrosis associated with exudation into the vitreous.[58] Infiltrates contain mononuclear phagocytes, lymphocytes, and plasma cells. Single or multiple foci may occur. Adults with toxoplasmic chorioretinitis as a result of recrudescence of latent congenital infection more often have bilateral involvement, old scars, and involvement of the macula as hallmarks of retinal infection.[59] Patients with chorioretinitis in the setting of the acute acquired infection most often are older and have unilateral disease without old scars; less often, macular involvement is seen.[59] In most cases, toxoplasmic chorioretinitis following congenital infection runs the course of episodic flares without a systemic reaction. Glaucoma, iridocyclitis, and cataracts may develop as the result of chorioretinitis.[58]

Infection in Immunocompromised Patients

In the immunocompromised patient (e.g., the patient with AIDS or Hodgkin's disease, or the organ transplant recipient receiving high-dose immunosuppressive therapy), the dominant pathologic picture following reactivation of the infection is in the brain. Single, but more often, multiple brain abscesses are commonly found in patients with toxoplasmic encephalitis (Fig. 3–7). The abscesses are characterized by an avascular central zone with amorphous material and few organisms, an intermediate hyperemic zone with prominent inflammatory infiltrates, and an outer zone containing necrotic areas with numerous tachyzoites and often *T. gondii* cysts at the margins.[60] A "diffuse" form of toxoplasmic encephalitis with widespread microglial nodules without abscess formation has been observed in the gray matter.[60, 61] Lesions are most commonly found in the cerebral hemispheres and basal ganglia.[62, 63] Recently, Suzuki and colleagues[64] reported the first evidence of genetic regulation of susceptibility to toxoplasmic encephalitis in AIDS patients. HLA-DQ3 appeared to be a genetic marker of susceptibility, whereas HLA-DQ1 was found to be a genetic marker of resistance to the development of toxoplasmic encephalitis.[64] Involvement of the lungs presenting as interstitial or necrotizing pneumonitis is second in frequency and severity only to toxoplasmic encephalitis in AIDS patients and is associated with a high mortality.[65, 66] Involvement of other organs, including heart, skeletal muscle, and the intestinal tract, has frequently been observed in cases of AIDS and toxoplasmic encephalitis that come to autopsy.[44] Histologic changes vary from tissues that are parasitized but exhibit no other pathologic abnormality to those with marked inflammatory infiltrates with focal or widespread necrosis.

CLINICAL MANIFESTATIONS

Toxoplasmosis in immunologically normal patients can be broadly classified into three categories: acquired, congenital, or ocular (which may result from either the congenital or the acquired infection). Although the same categories can be applied to immunodeficient patients, the severity of the disease and its clinical manifestations in such patients deserve special consideration.

Acute Acquired Infection in Immunocompetent Individuals

Signs and symptoms of the acute infection most often go unrecognized by the pregnant woman. Yet the outcome of this infection may be an infant with congenital toxoplasmosis. The most commonly recognized clinical manifestation is lymphadenopathy. This may be accompanied by fatigue and is not usually associated with fever. The groups of nodes most commonly involved are the cervical, suboccipital, supraclavicular, axillary, and inguinal. The adenopathy is most often localized to one or a few lymph nodes in the neck but may

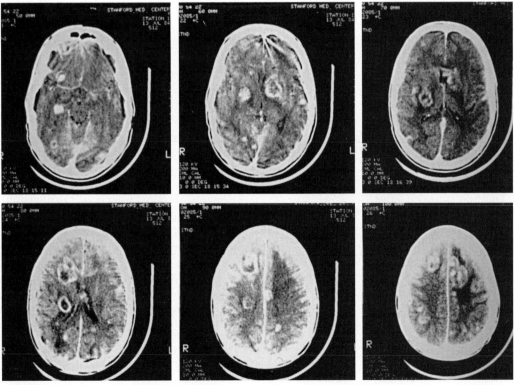

FIGURE 3–7 ▶ Computed tomography (CT) scan of the brain in a patient with toxoplasmic encephalitis. The patient had 12 abscesses in his brain at the time of diagnosis.

involve multiple areas. Involvement of nodes in the parapectoral region is often diagnosed clinically as suspect cancer of the breast in women. Enlarged nodes are usually discrete and nontender, do not suppurate, and vary in firmness.[67] The spleen and liver may also be involved.[16] Polymyositis, dermatomyositis, and exanthem have been described.[16] The clinical course of toxoplasmic lymphadenitis is benign and self-limited; clinically apparent symptoms usually resolve within 6 months but may persist for longer periods. The differential diagnosis of toxoplasmic lymphadenitis includes lymphoma, infectious mononucleosis, cytomegalovirus mononucleosis, cat scratch disease, sarcoidosis, tuberculosis, tularemia, metastatic carcinoma, and leukemia. The adenopathy is most often misdiagnosed as being due to Hodgkin's disease or other lymphoma. Chorioretinitis is an uncommon manifestation of the acute acquired infection (see later). An acute fulminant course with severe morbidity or even fatal outcome has been observed in rare cases in whom the acute acquired infection presented as myocarditis, pericarditis, hepatitis, polymyositis, pneumonitis, or encephalitis. Whether these latter cases were associated with an underlying condition that predisposed to the seriousness of the infection is unclear.

Congenital Toxoplasmosis

Depending on the stage of gestation when the infection is acquired by the mother, the clinical spectrum of congenitally infected infants may vary from normal appearance at birth to a newborn with hydrocephalus, chorioretinitis, and intracranial calcifications (see section on pathophysiology). The presence of clinical signs in the neonate usually indicates a high probability of severe sequelae, whereas infants without signs of disease at birth may experience mild or severe sequelae. Newborns without obvious signs of the infection at birth may suffer untoward sequelae of the infection months or even years later, including hydrocephalus, microcephaly, seizure disorders, psychomotor and mental retardation, strabismus, blindness, or deafness.[33, 69] Parameters suitable for predicting the outcome of the infection in a newborn with subclinical infection are unknown. Most signs and clinical presentations are nonspecific and may be indistinguishable from disease due to other pathogens, including *Treponema pallidum*, herpes simplex virus, cytomegalovirus, and rubella virus. When present, the most common signs are chorioretinitis, strabismus, blindness, epilepsy, psychomotor or mental retardation, encephalitis, pneumonitis, hydrocephalus, microcephaly, intracranial calcification, anemia, jaundice, rash, petechiae due to thrombocytopenia, diarrhea, hypothermia, and nonspecific illness.[16, 70] For a more detailed discussion of clinical manifestations in congenitally infected infants, the reader is referred to reference 16.

Congenital *Toxoplasma* Infection and HIV/AIDS

Congenital transmission of *T. gondii* from pregnant women co-infected with *T. gondii* and HIV is a tragic but, fortunately, uncommon occurrence. Such transmission has occurred from HIV-infected mothers who have clinical toxoplasmosis as a manifestation of their AIDS as well as HIV-infected mothers who have no clinical signs of toxoplasmosis. Congenital transmission has occurred from mothers who do not have demonstrable IgM *Toxoplasma* antibodies. The incidence of congenital transmission of *T. gondii* from these women remains unclear but may depend on the stage of HIV infection in the mother.[35-37] The clinical presentation of congenital toxoplasmosis appears to be similar to that in the non–HIV-infected infant but appears to run a more progressive course. Most dually infected newborns do not have clinical signs of either infection at birth but go on to develop severe signs of disseminated infection within the first weeks or months of life.[35, 71] Multiorgan involvement, including the central nervous system, heart, and lungs, is frequent.

Ocular Toxoplasmosis

Toxoplasmic chorioretinitis in adults appears most often to be the result of a congenital infection, rather than a manifestation of acquired toxoplasmosis. In the patient with congenital infection, toxoplasmic chorioretinitis most often presents clinically in the second or third decade. Lesions appear as yellowish-white, cotton-like patches in the fundus (Fig. 3–8). The more acute lesions are soft and cotton-like, with indistinct borders; the older lesions are whitish-gray, sharply outlined, and spotted by accumulations of choroidal pigment. Symptoms may range from blurred vision, scotoma, photophobia, and eye pain, to loss of vision. As inflammation resolves, vision improves; complete recovery of visual acuity may not be achieved. Periodic flare-ups of toxoplasmic chorioretinits months or years after the primary episode are common and may lead to destruction of retinal tissue and glaucoma.[72, 73]

Toxoplasmosis in the Immunocompromised Host

Toxoplasmosis in the immunocompromised patient most often is the result of reactivation of the latent infection. The highest frequency is in patients with Hodgkin's disease or other lymphoma, seronegative recipients of an organ transplant from a seropositive donor, patients with AIDS, and other patients who are on high-dose corticosteroids and/or other immunosuppressive drugs.[44, 74] Thirty to 50 percent of HIV-infected *Toxoplasma*-seropositive individuals develop toxoplasmic encephalitis if they are not receiving ap-

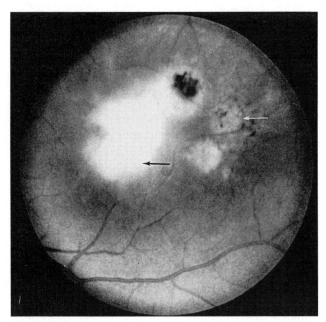

FIGURE 3–8 ▶ Chorioretinitis due to *Toxoplasma*. The characteristic lesion is a focal necrotizing retinitis with cotton-like patches in the fundus. Note that the acute lesions (*black arrow*) have indistinct borders and appear soft and white, while older lesions (*white arrow*) are whitish gray, sharply outlined, and spotted by accumulations of choroidal pigment. (Courtesy of Dr. G. Richard O'Connor.)

propriate prophylaxis. Multifocal involvement of the central nervous system leads to a wide variety of clinical findings, ranging from disturbances of consciousness to motor impairment, seizures, headache, and focal neurologic signs.[44, 75] A subacute onset with focal neurologic abnormalities can present as hemiparesis or speech impairment, but more abrupt clinical manifestations with seizures have also been reported. The differential diagnosis of toxoplasmic encephalitis includes central nervous system lymphoma, progressive multifocal leukoencephalopathy, and other infectious etiologies. Pulmonary disease due to toxoplasmosis in AIDS patients may present with prolonged fever, cough, and dyspnea—symptoms commonly found in patients with *Pneumocystis carinii* pneumonia. Disseminated toxoplasmosis has been reported to present with a picture of septic shock. In patients with AIDS, ocular disease due to toxoplasmosis is less common than cytomegalovirus retinitis and often does not differ from that seen in immunocompetent patients. Toxoplasmic chorioretinitis in these patients can often be differentiated from cytomegalovirus retinitis because of the marked hemorrhagic lesions in the latter. For a complete review of toxoplasmosis in AIDS patients, the reader is referred to reference 42. Toxoplasmosis in the non-AIDS immunocompromised host has recently been reviewed in detail.[74]

DIAGNOSIS

A variety of methods are available for the diagnosis of infection in the pregnant woman and fetus. These include serology, techniques for the isolation of the parasite, demonstration of the presence of the organism by polymerase chain reaction, and histologic demonstration of *T. gondii* in tissue sections.

Histology

Demonstration of tachyzoites in tissues (e.g., brain biopsy, bone marrow aspirate) or body fluids (e.g., cerebrospinal fluid,[76, 77] aqueous humor[78]) establishes the diagnosis of acute toxoplasmosis. Characteristic histologic criteria alone are probably sufficient for establishing the diagnosis of toxoplasmic lymphadenitis.[55] Histologic demonstration of the cyst form establishes that the patient is infected with *T. gondii* but does not warrant the conclusion that the infection is acute unless there is associated inflammation and necrosis. Since it is often difficult to demonstrate tachyzoites in tissue sections stained with conventional stains, an immunoperoxidase method has been developed and is highly successful for demonstration of the organism in tissues.[79] This method should be performed, whenever feasible, on placental tissue examined for suspect infection with *T. gondii*.

Isolation of the Parasite

Isolation of *T. gondii* from blood or other body fluids,[77, 80, 81] subretinal fluid,[82] aqueous humor,[83] or amniotic fluid[84-86] has been successfully used for the diagnosis of acute infection. Whereas isolation of the organism from the placenta usually means that the fetus has been infected, isolation from fetal tissues establishes the diagnosis. Isolation from the tissues (e.g., skeletal muscle, lung, brain, or eye) of adults does not necessarily prove active infection, since the isolation may be due to the presence of tissue cysts. Isolation studies are performed by injection of suspect material into laboratory mice or into mammalian cell tissue culture.[76, 87, 88] Tissue culture is less sensitive but yields results more rapidly than does mouse inoculation (usually 1 week or less, compared to 2 to 6 weeks, respectively).

In pregnant women who acquired the infection during pregnancy, cordocentesis has frequently been performed in the past to obtain fetal blood for isolation studies. The sensitivity of inoculation of mice with fetal blood ranges between 64% and 72% and was higher than that of inoculation of mice with amniotic fluid, which ranged between 52% and 64%.[29, 31] However, the hazards of cordocentesis appear to be higher than those of amniocentesis.

Polymerase Chain Reaction (PCR)

Molecular analysis of genes in *T. gondii* have allowed for development of molecular biologic detection methods for rapid diagnosis of the infection. PCR that detects the *B1* gene of *T. gondii* has been used with great success in amniotic fluid and is the preferred method for prenatal diagnosis of infection in the fetus.[29, 89–91] Performed at 18 weeks of gestation, sensitivity and negative predictive values, compared to conventional parasitologic methods, were 97.4% versus 89.5% and 99.7% versus 98.7%, respectively.[29] Combined with increased sensitivity, the earlier availability of results, compared with isolation methods, represents a major advancement in the prenatal diagnosis of infection. Furthermore, amniocentesis entails a substantially lower risk of fetal loss than does fetal-blood sampling using cordocentesis. We no longer recommend cordocentesis unless PCR testing is not available. PCR has also been successfully used on samples of cerebrospinal fluid, blood, bronchoalveolar lavage fluid, and formalin or fresh tissues.[90, 92, 93]

Serology

A major problem in serologic diagnosis of the acute infection in adults is the high prevalence of IgG antibody titers to *T. gondii* in most populations. In the United States, seroprevalence among pregnant women of childbearing age ranges from approximately 3% to 45%, depending on the geographic locale and the population being examined within that locale. For example, the prevalence of antibodies is much higher among Hispanic women in Los Angeles than among some groups of non-Hispanic women in the same locale. Knowledge of the percentage of women infected prior to pregnancy is critical to our understanding of the risk of a population for acquiring the infection during gestation (seronegative women) and therefore for giving birth to infected offspring. Such information is also pertinent to strategies for prevention of the infection. Since IgG antibody can persist at high titers for many years in healthy individuals, discrimination between a recently acquired infection and an infection acquired in the more distant past is often difficult. This is especially frustrating for the clinician trying to diagnose the infection in pregnant women, in whom it is so vital to establish whether their infection was acquired during or prior to gestation. Correct interpretation of serologic test results may be difficult not only because of persistence of IgG, IgM, and IgA antibodies, but also because commercial kits may be unreliable and may give false-negative or false-positive results, especially for IgM antibodies. At present, the serologic diagnosis of acute infection can be made only if a significant rise in antibody titers can be demonstrated. Using a panel of different methods[94, 95] helps discriminate between recent and more distant infection. We, as well as the U.S. Food and Drug Administration (FDA) and the Centers for Disease Control and Prevention have recommended that physicians consult with a reference serology laboratory whenever an IgM test result is positive in a pregnant woman or in a woman about to become pregnant. It is important to recognize that a positive IgM *Toxoplasma* antibody titer does not necessarily mean that the patient has recently been infected. A negative IgM antibody test result in a pregnant woman essentially means that she was not recently infected.

Tests for IgG Antibodies

The serologic tests most commonly used for measurement of IgG antibodies are the Sabin-Feldman dye test,[4] the immunofluorescent antibody (IFA) test,[96] the enzyme-linked immunosorbent assay (ELISA),[97] the IgG avidity test,[98] the agglutination test,[99] and the differential agglutination test.[100] IgG antibodies usually appear within 1 to 2 weeks of acquisition of infection, peak within 1 to 2 months, fall at variable rates, and likely persist for the life of the individual. High titers may persist for years. In contrast to commercial kits for measurement of IgM antibodies, in our experience most commercially available kits that test for IgG antibodies are reliable. The Sabin-Feldman dye test is based on the lysis of living organisms in the presence of antibody and complement. The titer reported is the dilution of serum at which half of the organisms are not killed (stained) and the other half are killed (unstained). The dye test is considered the reference serologic test against which other methods are evaluated.

Titers in the IgG-IFA essentially parallel those in the dye test[96]; however, reliable quantitative titers are frequently difficult to obtain. False-positive results may occur in sera that contain antinuclear antibodies,[101] and false-negative results in sera with low titers of IgG antibodies.

The most widely used method for the demonstration of IgG antibodies is the IgG ELISA. Information regarding the correlation between titers in IgG ELISA tests and those obtained in the dye test or other tests for IgG antibodies has been controversial.[102, 103]

Based on the observation that specific antibodies bind to *T. gondii* only weakly (low-avidity antibodies) during the acute phase of infection, whereas binding by antibodies in the chronic phase of infection is stronger (high-avidity antibodies), avidity tests have been designed to help discriminate between recently acquired infection and infections acquired in the more distant past. Important in their interpretation is that low-avidity antibodies can persist beyond 3 months of infection. High-avidity antibodies essentially rule out the infection as having been acquired in the previous 3 months. In addition, there is a wide range of equivocal results. As is true for IgM antibody tests, the avidity test is most useful when performed early in gestation, since a "chronic" pattern occurring late in pregnancy does not rule out the possibility that the acute infection may have occurred during the first months of gestation.[98, 104, 105] IgG avidity tests should be used to confirm positive results in tests for IgM antibodies performed in pregnant women during the first trimester. The presence of high-avidity antibodies essentially rules out recently acquired infection. Thus, the method is useful for identifying positive IgM antibody test results that are falsely positive or for detecting the presence of persisting IgM antibodies; the presence of low avidity antibodies or an equivocal result should result in further investigation by confirmatory testing in a reference laboratory. At the time of the writing of this chapter, no test for avidity had been released by the FDA for use in the United States.

The agglutination test[99] employs whole parasites that have been preserved in formalin. Since the method is very sensitive to IgM antibodies, nonspecific agglutination (related to "naturally" occurring IgM agglutinins) has been observed.[106] False-positive results are avoided by the addition of 2-mercaptoethanol to the sera.[107] The agglutination test is accurate, simple to perform, and inexpensive and has proved useful in the screening of pregnant women.[107]

The differential agglutination (AC/HS) test compares titers obtained with formalin-fixed tachyzoites (HS antigen) with those obtained with acetone- or methanol-fixed tachyzoites (AC antigen).[100] The different antigen preparations vary in their ability to recognize antibodies in sera from patients with recent or chronic infection. Essentially, this is also an avidity test. This test has proved helpful in differentiating between a probable acute or chronic infection in the pregnant patient[100, 108] and is best used in combination with a panel of other assays.

Tests for IgM Antibodies

The double-sandwich IgM ELISA and IgM immunosorbent assay are most frequently used for detection of IgM antibodies. IgM antibodies appear earlier and decline more rapidly than do IgG antibodies. They typically appear within the first week of infection, rapidly rise, and thereafter decrease at variable rates to disappear after a few months. IgM antibody tests have been widely used for the diagnosis of acute infection and to determine whether a pregnant woman has been infected during pregnancy or before conception. There has been a heightened awareness of the fact that titers in tests for IgM antibodies may persist for years after the acute infection and that the reliability of commercially available assays varies considerably.[95, 109] Both the laboratory performing the test and the physician requesting the test should be aware of this problem. The FDA has issued a health advisory to obstetricians, gynecologists, pediatricians, clinical pathologists, and infectious disease specialists warning about the use

of *Toxoplasma* IgM commercial test kits as the sole determinant of recent infection in pregnant women.[110]

The IgM-IFA has been successfully used to diagnose acute congenital and acquired infections.[70, 111, 112] High titers of IgG antibodies may inhibit or prevent the demonstration of IgM antibodies in the IFA test. The presence of rheumatoid factor and antinuclear factors may cause false-positive results.[113]

Naot and Remington and colleagues[114–116] developed a double-sandwich IgM ELISA for detection of IgM antibodies to *Toxoplasma*. The double-sandwich IgM ELISA is more sensitive than the IgM IFA test, and the presence of antinuclear antibodies or rheumatoid factor does not cause false-positive results. IgM-capture ELISA kits are most commonly used. Despite their wide distribution, commercially available tests for IgM antibodies often have low specificity, and results are frequently misinterpreted. False-positive results and the problems associated with the persistence of positive titers even years after initial infection remain major obstacles to correct interpretation of results obtained in these tests.

The IgM immunosorbent agglutination assay (ISAGA)[117] combines the advantages of both the direct agglutination test and the double-sandwich (capture) ELISA in its specificity and sensitivity for demonstration of IgM antibodies. It is easy to perform and more sensitive and specific than the IgM IFA test. It avoids false-positive results related to the presence of rheumatoid factor and/or antinuclear antibodies in serum samples. Due to its sensitivity, it is frequently used for the diagnosis of congenital infection in newborns.

Tests for IgA and IgE Antibodies

Methods for the detection of IgA and IgE antibodies have been used, along with those for the detection of IgG and IgM antibodies, in attempts to more accurately define whether the *Toxoplasma* infection is acute. The capture ELISA is the most common method used for detection of IgA *Toxoplasma* antibodies in the fetus, newborn, and pregnant patient.[118, 119] It appears to be more sensitive than the IgM ELISA or IgM ISAGA for diagnosis of the infection in the fetus and newborn.[119] The kinetics of IgA antibodies in adults with the early, acute acquired infection are similar to those of IgM antibodies, although IgA antibodies frequently disappear earlier than do IgM antibodies. However, as with the latter, they may remain positive for a year or longer. Very high titers of IgA antibodies correlate well with more recent onset of the infection. The usefulness of the IgE ISAGA in the diagnosis of acute acquired infection in the pregnant woman and in the congenitally infected newborn has been reported.[120, 121] IgE antibodies rise early, along with IgM and IgA antibodies, but disappear much earlier, often within 4 months. As is true of all other serologic tests for diagnosis of the acute infection, appropriate interpretation requires that it be used only in combination with other serologic methods.

Other Laboratory Measurements

Fetal *Toxoplasma* infection may be indicated by a variety of other laboratory abnormalities in cord blood obtained at cordocentesis, including elevation of gamma-glutamyltransferase, total IgM concentration, and leukocyte and eosinophil counts as well as thrombocytopenia. Abnormal results are not specific for *Toxoplasma* infection but have been used by clinicians to determine the need for initiation of treatment with pyrimethamine-sulfadiazine in the mother while awaiting results of isolation studies and to determine the need for repeat fetal blood sampling to establish infection.

Ultrasonography

Infection-related abnormalities in fetal biology can be found in as many as 45% of cases of the congenital infection.[31] Unilateral or, more often, bilateral and symmetrical dilatation of the ventricles is the most common finding. Other findings include hydrocephalus, intracranial calcifications, increased placental thickness, hepatic enlargement, and ascites. In pregnancies at risk for fetal infection (established or suspected maternal infection during pregnancy), ultrasound should be performed at least monthly until term, if the initial examination revealed no abnormalities. The presence of hydrocephalus in ultrasonographic examinations has been used as an indication for therapeutic abortion by researchers in France.

Diagnosis in Specific Clinical Settings

Diagnosis in the Immunocompetent Patient

Immunocompetent individuals who present with signs or symptoms suggestive of toxoplasmosis should be initially investigated with tests for IgG and IgM antibodies. Negative results virtually rule out the diagnosis of toxoplasmosis. Seroconversion or a significant rise in serologic test titers in serial specimens tested in parallel are supportive of the diagnosis of the acute infection. Montoya and colleagues[94] recently reported that a panel of serologic tests, the toxoplasma serologic profile, performed on the first serum specimen drawn after onset of the clinical syndrome of toxoplasmic lymphadenitis had a sensitivity of 100%. IgM antibodies were detected during the first 3 months after clinical onset of lymphadenopathy in all patients and persisted for as long as 12 months. A *Toxoplasma* serologic profile should be performed in cases of suspected toxoplasmic lymphadenitis to avoid an unnecessary biopsy procedure.

Diagnosis in the Pregnant Woman

Since routine screening is implemented only in France and Austria, maternal infection in the United States is most often diagnosed as a result of routine serologic testing by the patient's physician, or the presentation of a pregnant woman with clinical signs suggestive of acute toxoplasmosis, or as a request of concerned, informed patients. In the routine laboratory, tests for IgG and IgM antibodies are usually performed. The presence of a positive titer (except for the false-positive results mentioned earlier) in these tests establishes that the patient has been infected. The greatest value of detection of IgM antibodies is in determining that a pregnant woman has not been recently infected. Negative results in tests for IgM antibodies virtually rule out a recently acquired infection unless sera have been obtained so early that an IgM antibody response is not yet detectable. Because titers in any serologic test (e.g., in tests for IgM antibodies) may remain elevated for years, a single high titer does not indicate whether the infection is recently acquired or chronic.[122] In pregnant women in whom IgM antibodies are demonstrated during the first trimester, the presence of high-avidity IgG antibodies has proved helpful in ruling out recently acquired infection. In most cases, the diagnosis of acute *Toxoplasma* infection or toxoplasmosis requires demonstration of a rise in titers in serial specimens (either conversion from a negative to a positive titer or a significant rise from a low to a higher titer).[122] These specimens should be obtained at least 3 weeks apart and should be tested in parallel. Because the diagnosis is frequently considered relatively late in the course of the patient's illness, serologic test titers may have already reached their peak at the time the first serum specimen is obtained for testing. It therefore is often difficult to discriminate between infections acquired recently (possibly during pregnancy) and those acquired in the more distant past. Figure 3–9 presents guidelines for the interpretation of serologic tests for diagnosis of maternal *T. gondii* infection. The use of confirmatory testing with a panel of serologic tests in a reference laboratory has proved helpful in discriminating between recently and more distantly acquired infections.[95] Results of confirmatory testing in a reference laboratory suggested that recently acquired infections had occurred in only 40% of women who had positive results in tests for IgM antibodies in commercial laboratories; 17% of these women had their pregnancies terminated when informed of the results.[123] In that study, communication of the results and their correct interpretation by an expert in *Toxoplasma* serology decreased the rate of unnecessary abortions by 50% among the women with positive IgM *Toxoplasma* test results reported by commercial laboratories.[123]

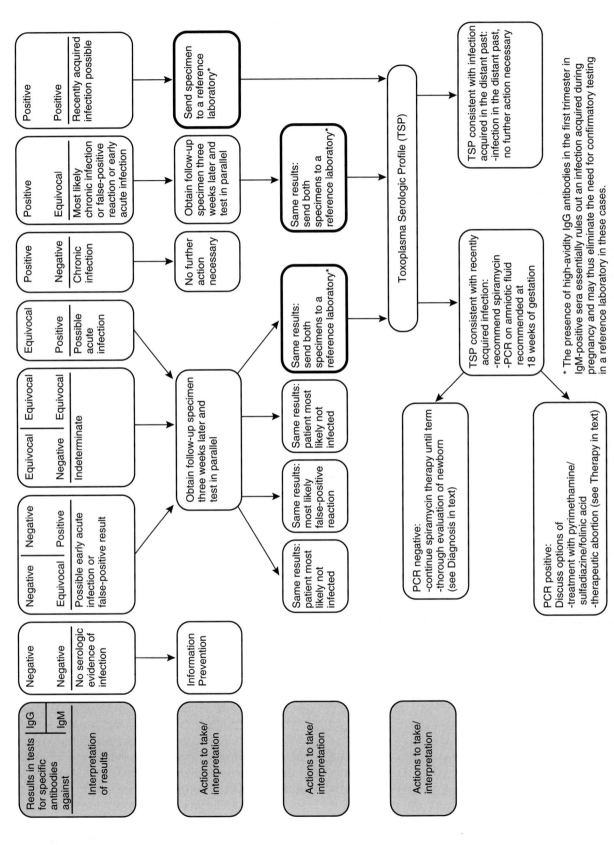

Results in tests for specific antibodies against	IgG	Negative	Negative	Equivocal	Equivocal	Equivocal	Positive	Positive	Positive
	IgM	Negative	Positive	Negative	Equivocal	Positive	Negative	Equivocal	Positive
Interpretation of results		No serologic evidence of infection	Possible early acute infection or false-positive result	Indeterminate		Possible acute infection	Chronic infection	Most likely chronic infection or false-positive reaction or early acute infection	Recently acquired infection possible

Actions to take/interpretation

Information
Prevention

Obtain follow-up specimen three weeks later and test in parallel

No further action necessary

Obtain follow-up specimen three weeks later and test in parallel

Send specimen to a reference laboratory*

Actions to take/interpretation

Same results: patient most likely not infected

Same results: most likely false-positive reaction

Same results: patient most likely not infected

Same results: send both specimens to a reference laboratory*

Same results: send both specimens to a reference laboratory*

Actions to take/interpretation

Toxoplasma Serologic Profile (TSP)

TSP consistent with recently acquired infection:
-recommend spiramycin
-PCR on amniotic fluid recommended at 18 weeks of gestation

TSP consistent with infection acquired in the distant past:
-infection in the distant past, no further action necessary

Actions to take/interpretation

PCR negative:
-continue spiramycin therapy until term
-thorough evaluation of newborn (see Diagnosis in text)

PCR positive:
Discuss options of
-treatment with pyrimethamine/sulfadiazine/folinic acid
-therapeutic abortion (see Therapy in text)

* The presence of high-avidity IgG antibodies in the first trimester in IgM-positive sera essentially rules out an infection acquired during pregnancy and may thus eliminate the need for confirmatory testing in a reference laboratory in these cases.

FIGURE 3-9 ▶ Guidelines for interpretation of serologic tests for IgG and IgM antibodies in pregnant women.

Diagnosis in the Fetus

Prenatal diagnosis of fetal infection is advised when a diagnosis of acute maternal toxoplasmosis is established or highly suspected in a pregnant woman, either based on clinical manifestations or as a result of serologic test results. Ultrasonography and amniocentesis are commonly used for this purpose.[29, 31, 124] Daffos and co-workers[31] reported that definitive diagnosis of fetal infection (based on isolation of the parasite from fetal blood or amniotic fluid obtained at 20 to 26 weeks of gestation and on serologic examination of the serum of the fetus for evidence of synthesis of IgM *Toxoplasma* antibodies) led to prenatal diagnosis in 92% of all cases of congenital infection. The complication rate related to the procedure in general was 0.3 fetal losses per 1000. More recently, development of PCR testing of amniotic fluid for the detection of *T. gondii*–specific DNA led to a major advancement in prenatal diagnosis. This technique, performed at 18 weeks of gestation, was shown to be more sensitive, more rapid, and safer than the conventional diagnostic procedures.[29, 93] PCR testing of amniotic fluid should be used in all cases of established maternal infection or cases with serologic test results highly suggestive of acute acquired infection during pregnancy. Such testing allows for the prompt initiation of specific therapy if the parents wish to continue the pregnancy. If PCR testing is not available, cordocentesis and fetal blood sampling may be used, with some success.

Diagnosis in the Newborn

Because the clinical picture of congenital toxoplasmosis may range from subclinical to nonspecific signs and symptoms, serologic tests are commonly performed for the diagnosis. Since maternal IgG antibodies present in the newborn may reflect merely past or recent infection in the mother, serologic tests for the detection of IgA and IgM antibodies are commonly employed. It is essential that maternal contamination of blood obtained at birth be excluded.[125] Detection of IgA antibodies appears to be more sensitive than IgM antibodies for the detection of infection in the newborn.[118] If IgG antibodies are detected but serologic tests for IgM and IgA antibodies are negative and *Toxoplasma* is not isolated, follow-up serologic testing is indicated in order to attempt to establish the diagnosis. Maternally transferred antibodies usually decline and disappear within 6 to 12 months. Additional diagnostic methods successfully used in infants are direct demonstration of the organism by inoculation in mice or cell culture or detection of *T. gondii* DNA from body fluid (e.g., cerebrospinal fluid, blood, and urine).[90, 92, 126] Evaluation of infants with suspected congenital toxoplasmosis should always include ophthalmologic testing, radiologic studies, and examination of cerebrospinal fluid.

For a more detailed discussion of diagnostic procedures in congenitally infected infants, the reader is referred to reference 16.

Diagnosis of Ocular Infection

Since retinal lesions in most cases are characteristic, most authorities consider that toxoplasmic chorioretinitis can be diagnosed with the use of eye examination.[127] In the adult with congenital infection, low levels of IgG antibodies are usually present, indicating past infection; IgM antibodies are only rarely detectable. A negative result in tests for IgG antibodies excludes the diagnosis in all but rare cases. In cases of atypical lesions, a positive result in tests for IgM antibodies may allow a presumptive diagnosis of acquired toxoplasmic chorioretinitis. Recently, PCR testing of aqueous humor and vitreous fluid has proved useful for diagnosis of toxoplasmic chorioretinitis in patients with atypical lesions.[128] Calculation of the immune load on aqueous fluid is commonly used in France and has proved to be an excellent method for diagnosis.[129]

Diagnosis in the Immunocompromised Patient

No single antibody test has proved useful for the definitive diagnosis of reactivated toxoplasmosis. However, by using the panel of serologic tests discussed previously, clinicians have been able to diagnose toxoplasmic encephalitis in up to 70% of AIDS patients.[44] In AIDS patients, higher IgG antibody titers are associated with increased risk of development of toxoplasmic encephalitis.[130] The definitive diagnosis of toxoplasmosis in most immunocompromised patients relies on histologic demonstration of the organism or demonstration of specific DNA in body fluids or tissue by PCR testing.

TREATMENT

The need for and the choice of appropriate antimicrobial therapy for infection with *T. gondii* depends on the clinical setting. Therefore, this section introduces drugs used for the treatment of the infection and thereafter comments on the use of these drugs in specific clinical settings.

Specific Therapy

Pyrimethamine-Sulfadiazine

Pyrimethamine and sulfadiazine act synergistically against *Toxoplasma*[131]; the simultaneous use of both drugs is indicated. Pyrimethamine-sulfadiazine therapy is the treatment of choice in patients with toxoplasmic chorioretinitis or toxoplasmic encephalitis and for the infection in the fetus and newborn. Combinations of pyrimethamine with most other sulfonamides are less effective and are not recommended. Although Fansidar (pyrimethamine-sulfadoxine) is widely used in parts of Europe, its associated severe untoward side effects have precluded its use for this purpose in the United States.[132] Both pyrimethamine and the sulfonamides are potentially toxic. Untoward reactions to sulfonamides include skin hypersensitivity, gastrointestinal discomfort, crystalluria, and hematuria. Pyrimethamine produces reversible, dose-dependent and usually gradual depression of the bone marrow.[133, 134] Thrombocytopenia associated with bleeding is the most serious consequence of toxicity, which also includes leukopenia, anemia, gastrointestinal distress, headaches, and an unpleasant taste in the mouth. All patients treated with pyrimethamine should have a peripheral blood cell and platelet count twice weekly. Folinic acid (in the form of leucovorin calcium) *but not folic acid* should be administered to prevent hematologic toxicity. Pyrimethamine is potentially teratogenic and should not be used during the first trimester of pregnancy.[135]

Spiramycin

Spiramycin is a macrolide antibiotic that is available to physicians in Canada and Europe. In the United States, it can be obtained through the U.S. Food and Drug Administration (FDA; telephone: 301-827-2335). Spiramycin reaches high titers in tissues (e.g., the placenta[136, 137]), which may explain its stated efficacy in reducing transmission of *T. gondii* to the fetus. It is administered for the express purpose of attempting to prevent transmission of the parasite to the fetus. Adverse effects of spiramycin include nausea, vomiting, diarrhea, and anorexia. Vertigo, nonvertiginous dizziness, flushing of the face, and a feeling of coolness have been reported less frequently.

Other Drugs

The high rate of untoward side effects associated with recommended regimens has been an impetus to search for new, less toxic, and more active drugs and therapeutic regimens. At present, there are insufficient clinical data to allow for recommendation of any of the drugs described later for treatment of the immunocompetent pregnant patient. These include trimethoprim-sulfamethoxazole; clindamycin, comparable in activity to pyrimethamine-sulfadiazine when used in combination with pyrimethamine in AIDS patients with toxoplasmic encephalitis[138, 139]; newer macrolides, including roxithromycin,[140] clarithromycin,[141] and azithromycin[142]; atovaquone[143]; and the newer quinolones.[144]

Treatment in Specific Clinical Settings

Treatment of the Acute Acquired Infection

Immunocompetent adults rarely require specific treatment unless persistent or severe disease develops. In such cases, treatment should be initiated with the combination pyrimethamine-sulfadiazine (Table 3–5) along with folinic acid. Treatment is usually for 2 to 4 weeks, followed by reevaluation of the patient's condition. Since infections acquired by laboratory accident or transfusion of blood may be more severe, these patients should always be treated.[145] For treatment of the special situation of the infection acquired following organ transplantation, the reader is referred to reference 74.

Treatment of the Pregnant Woman

Treatment of women with acute acquired infection may reduce but does not eliminate the incidence and severity of fetal infection. Spiramycin has been accepted by most investigators as being effective in reducing the frequency of maternal transmission of *T. gondii* to the fetus by approximately 60%.[146] Since there is a delay between the onset of maternal and fetal infection, therapy should be initiated as immediately as feasible after the diagnosis of recently acquired maternal infection is made. Treatment should be continued throughout the pregnancy. Dosage regimens for spiramycin are listed in Table 3–5. If spiramycin cannot be used or is not available, it may be replaced by sulfadiazine alone with appropriate precautions at term. However, there are no data on the efficacy of sulfonamides, including sulfadiazine, when these drugs are used for this purpose.

Treatment of the Fetus

Treatment with pyrimethamine-sulfadiazine is recommended when infection of the fetus is established or very highly probable.[16] Such treatment might be an alternative to termination of pregnancy when abortion is not allowed by law or for women who desire to continue the pregnancy. Therapy should be continued throughout pregnancy. Dosage regimens are listed in Table 3–5. Folinic acid should be administered to reduce the likelihood of bone marrow suppression, and the woman should be carefully monitored for development of hematologic toxicity. The occurrence of untoward toxic effects on the fetus is unknown. Routine use of pyrimethamine-sulfadiazine treatment is not recommended for every pregnant woman suspected or proven to have acquired the infection during pregnancy because of the real risk of serious adverse effects on mother and fetus. If fetal infection is demonstrated, pyrimethamine-sulfadiazine therapy should be initiated. Protocols that alternate pyrimethamine-sulfadia-

TABLE 3-5 ▶ GUIDELINES FOR THERAPY OF *TOXOPLASMA* INFECTION

	Therapy/Drug	Dosage	Duration
Acute acquired infection	Symptomatic[a]		
Acute toxoplasmosis in pregnant women	Spiramycin	3 g qd in 3 divided doses without food	Until term or until fetal infection is documented
Documented fetal infection (after 12 weeks of gestation)	Pyrimethamine	Loading dose: 100 mg qd in two divided doses for 2 days, then 50 mg qd	Until term
	plus		
	Sulfadiazine	Loading dose: 75 mg/kg qd in 2 divided doses (max 4 g qd) for 2 days, then 100 mg/kg qd in 2 divided doses (max 4 g qd)	Until term
	plus		
	Leucovorin (folinic acid)	5–20 mg qd	During and for 1 wk after pyrimethamine therapy
Congenital *Toxoplasma* infection in the infant	Pyrimethamine	Loading dose 2 mg/kg qd for 2 days, then 1 mg/kg qd for 2–6 mo, then this dose every Monday, Wednesday, Friday	1 y
	plus		
	Sulfadiazine	100 mg/kg qd in 2 divided doses	1 y
	plus		
	Leucovorin	10 mg 3 times weekly	During and for 1 wk after pyrimethamine therapy
	Corticosteroids[b] (prednisone)	1 mg/kg qd in 2 divided doses	Until resolution of signs and symptoms
Toxoplasmic chorioretinitis in adults	Pyrimethamine	Loading dose: 200 mg qd, then 50–75 mg qd	Usually 1–2 wk after resolution of symptoms
	plus		
	Sulfadiazine	Oral 1–1.5 g qd	Usually 1–2 wk after resolution of symptoms
	plus		
	Leucovorin	5–20 mg 3 times weekly	During and for 1 wk after pyrimethamine therapy
	Corticosteroids[b]	1 mg/kg qd in 2 divided doses	Until resolution of signs and symptoms
Acute/primary therapy for TE in patients with AIDS	Standard regimens: Pyrimethamine	Oral 200-mg loading dose, then 50–75 mg qd	At least 4–6 wk after resolution of signs and symptoms (see text)
	Leucovorin	Oral, IV, or IM 10–20 mg qd (up to 50 mg qd)	During and for 1 wk after pyrimethamine therapy
	plus		
	Sulfadiazine	Oral 0.5 to 1.0 g qid	[c]
	or		
	Clindamycin	Oral or IV 600 mg q6h (up to IV 1,200 mg q6h)	[c]
	Possible alternative regimens:		
	Trimethoprim-sulfamethoxazole	Oral or IV 5 mg (trimethoprim component)/kg q6h	[c]
	Pyrimethamine *plus* leucovorin plus one of the following:	As in standard regimens	[c]
	Clarithromycin	Oral 1 g q12h	[c]
	Atovaquone	Oral 750 mg q6h	[c]
	Azithromycin	Oral 1,200 to 1,500 mg qd	[c]
	Dapsone	Oral 100 mg qd	[c]

[a]Acute acquired infection in immunocompetent patients does not require specific treatment unless severe or persistent symptoms or evidence of damage to vital organs is present. If such signs or symptoms occur, treatment with pyrimethamine/sulfadiazine, and leucovorin should be initiated (for dosages, see section on toxoplasmic chorioretinitis in adults).

[b]When cerebrospinal protein is ≥1 g/dL and when active chorioretinitis threatens vision.

[c]Duration of treatment as for pyrimethamine in patients with TE.

Adapted from Remington JS, McLeod R, Desmonts G: Toxoplasmosis. In: Remington JS, Klein JO (eds): Infectious Diseases of the Fetus and Newborn Infant. Philadelphia, WB Saunders, 1995, pp 140–267; and Liesenfeld O, Wong S-Y, Remington JS: Toxoplasmosis in the setting of AIDS. In: Merigan TC, Bolognesi D (eds): Textbook of AIDS Medicine, 2nd ed. Baltimore, Williams & Wilkins, 1998.

zine and spiramycin have also been successfully used; in these cases, each regimen is alternated every 3 weeks.

Therapeutic Abortion

Therapeutic abortion is often considered by the physician and the patient when fetal infection is confirmed by prenatal testing (see section on diagnosis). Therapeutic abortion is offered to all women in France who have been infected during the first trimester and in whom ultrasonography reveals cerebral abnormalities in the fetus. Hohlfeld and colleagues[147] reported on termination of seven pregnancies in which infection was acquired during the first trimester. Ultrasound did not reveal obvious lesions: Severe brain damage was found in each of the fetuses at autopsy. Management of women who are suspected of having acquired the infection in the first trimester, although risk of fetal transmission is low, should include a recommendation for PCR testing of amniotic fluid before recommendations for abortions are made. Depending on the results, treatment options that consist of either spiramycin (in case of a negative PCR result) or pyrimethamine-sulfadiazine (in the case of a positive PCR result) or therapeutic abortion can be discussed with the patient, bringing into the discussion what the likelihood is of her giving birth to an infected child. In a recent study, we have shown that approximately 17% of pregnant women in whom recently acquired *T. gondii* infection was suggested by serologic test results chose therapeutic abortion.[123] Few of them had PCR testing performed on amniotic fluid, and the actual number of fetal infections remained unknown. However, since the frequency of transmission is low during the first trimester, the vast majority of these women will have aborted their pregnancies unnecessarily.

Treatment of Ocular Toxoplasmosis

Pyrimethamine-sulfadiazine combined with folinic acid is the therapy of choice for treatment of toxoplasmic chorioretinitis. Active chorioretinitis usually resolves within 1 to 2 weeks of specific treatment. Treatment is recommended to be administered for 1 to 2 weeks beyond resolution of signs and symptoms.[25, 148, 149] Dosage regimens are listed in Table 3–5. Clindamycin has been used with favorable clinical outcome.[150] In cases of accompanying inflammation that threatens the macula, optic disk, or optic nerve, the use of prednisone is recommended in conjunction with pyrimethamine-sulfadiazine. For an excellent review of toxoplasmic chorioretinitis and its management, the reader is referred to reference 149.

Treatment of Immunocompromised Patients

Acute *T. gondii* infection in immunocompromised patients is life-threatening and should always be treated. First-line treatment is pyrimethamine-sulfadiazine, along with folinic acid (see Table 3–5). Pyrimethamine-clindamycin has been shown to be comparable in efficacy to pyrimethamine-sulfadiazine in AIDS patients with toxoplasmic encephalitis.[138] Treatment should be administered for at least 4 to 6 weeks after resolution of all signs and symptoms, and in AIDS patients maintenance therapy is necessary for the lifetime of the patient.[44] Treatment guidelines are listed in Table 3–5. A variety of alternative therapies, usually used along with pyrimethamine, include dapsone, macrolides, and atovaquone. They have been used in patients in whom adverse side effects associated with pyrimethamine-sulfadiazine therapy occurred; however, because data on their use in sufficient numbers of patients are not available, they are to be considered second-line drugs. Pyrimethamine remains the mainstay of therapy. Unless there are circumstances that negate its use, pyrimethamine should always be included in the treatment regimen.

PREVENTION

As described earlier, the major route of infection is the oral route—primarily through ingestion of undercooked meat that contains *T. gondii* cysts or food contaminated with oocysts. Thus, infection with the parasite is preventable in almost all cases. Measures that can be taken to avoid the infection include education (primary prevention) and treatment of women who acquire the infection during pregnancy (secondary prevention). Whereas in the seronegative immunocompromised patient, acquisition of infection with *T. gondii* can be avoided, the seropositive immunocompromised patient is at risk for reactivation of the latent infection. In these patients (e.g., the patient with AIDS), prophylactic antimicrobial therapy has been highly successful (see later).

Primary Prevention

Education of patients by their physicians or other health care workers remains the main principle of primary prevention. Since the congenital infection is almost exclusively the result of acute infection during pregnancy, it is the responsibility of all physicians caring for pregnant women and women attempting to conceive (women at risk) to inform them appropriately of preventive measures that focus on the avoidance of ingestion of and contact with cysts or sporulated oocysts. Table 3–6 provides an overview of measures for preventing *Toxoplasma* infection. Measures of education include brochures (available from the National

TABLE 3-6 ▶	MEASURES TO PREVENT *T. GONDII* INFECTION

Wash fruits and vegetables prior to consumption.
Refrain from skinning animals.
Avoid mucous membrane contact when handling raw meat.
Wash hands thoroughly after contact with raw meat.
Kitchen surfaces and utensils that have come in contact with raw meat should be washed.
Cook meat to well done (meat that is smoked or cured in brine may be infectious).
Avoid ingestion of dried meat.
Avoid contact with materials potentially contaminated with cat feces, especially handling of cat litter and gardening. Gloves are advised when these activities are necessary.
Disinfect cat litter with near-boiling water for 5 minutes prior to handling.

Adapted from Remington JS, McLeod R, Desmonts G: Toxoplasmosis. In: Remington JS, Klein JO (eds): Infectious Diseases of the Fetus and Newborn Infant. Philadelphia, WB Saunders, 1995, pp 140–267.

Institutes of Health, Bethesda, MD; and Abbott Laboratories, Abbott Park, IL) and audiovisual programs.

In the seronegative immunocompromised patient (e.g., the patient with HIV or AIDS), the same educational measures should be used. In seronegative recipients of organ transplants (e.g., heart) from seropositive donors, primary prophylaxis using antimicrobial therapy (pyrimethamine) has been successful. Transfusion of whole blood from seropositive donors to seronegative immunosuppressed patients or pregnant women should be avoided whenever feasible.

In addition to primary prevention, secondary prevention is employed to prevent transmission from the acutely infected mother to her fetus by identifying and treating the mother or, if infection of the fetus has been diagnosed by prenatal testing, to discuss the options of antimicrobial therapy during gestation to treat the fetus, and therapeutic abortion.

Serologic Screening

Since acute infection with *T. gondii* most often goes unnoticed, systematic serologic screening of all pregnant women would detect those who acquired the infection during gestation. The usefulness of these programs has been shown in France and Austria.[16] In the United States, the role of a systematic screening program is controversial, mainly owing to the problems in weighing the costs of such a program (the screening at several times during gestation of the approximately four million pregnancies each year in the United States) against the costs to society of caring for children with congenital toxoplasmosis; accurate data on the incidence of congenital infection in the United States have not been determined in recent years.[16, 151] Furthermore, one must take into regard that serologic screening of all pregnant women would result in unfortunate psychological trauma and uncertainty for women who have abnormal results and who then have

to endure repeated serologic or even prenatal diagnostic testing. The significant problems with sensitivity and specificity of a number of serologic tests, discussed in the previous section on diagnosis, also have to be considered (e.g., an unacceptably high prevalence of false-positive IgM antibody test results in a setting of low incidence of the acute acquired infection, which is the situation in the United States at present). The success of mandatory serologic screening as performed in France (all women are tested early in pregnancy, and seronegative women are tested monthly thereafter) led to proposals for a screening program in the United States[151] that would consist of mandatory early serologic testing for IgG antibodies using the dye test (or a comparably sensitive, specific, and reproducible test); all seronegative women (approximately 85% of pregnant women in the United States) would be tested again at defined intervals. At the time that serologic screening began in France, as many as 75% of women were infected prior to gestation and thus were not at risk. This left a relatively small population of women (approximately 25%) who were at risk, compared to the approximately 85% at risk in the United States at present. If testing in seronegative women is chosen, the frequency of testing will depend on all the factors described previously. A commonly practiced method is to screen as early in gestation as feasible, at the beginning of each of the trimesters thereafter, and at the time of delivery. An initial positive IgG antibody test result would lead to testing for IgM antibodies; women with IgG antibodies who lack IgM antibodies in early pregnancy are very unlikely to have been recently infected. The current practice, in the United States, of sporadic serologic screening, especially with serologic tests that have ill-defined sensitivities and specificities, and incorrect interpretation of test results often lead to unnecessary concern on the part of the pregnant woman and unnecessary abortion.[123]

When acute infection acquired during pregnancy has been diagnosed, prophylactic treatment with spiramycin has been stated to reduce by 60% the frequency of transmission of *T. gondii* to the fetus, but it does not appear to modify the pattern of infection in the infected fetus.[146]

Because of the lack of feasibility of screening of all pregnant women, a secondary prevention program that consists of serologic testing of all newborns for IgM antibodies against *T. gondii* has been implemented in Massachusetts. Using routine screening of all newborns, 100 of 635,000 infants tested positive in the IgM ELISA; congenital infection was confirmed in 52, resulting in an incidence of approximately 1 in 12,000.[152] Fifty of these were identified only through neonatal screening, and not through initial clinical examination. Since testing for IgM antibodies in newborns is only 25% to 75% sensitive, this program will not detect a number of subclinically infected infants or those infected late in the third trimester (when the frequency of transmission is highest but antibody formation has not yet occurred).

A frequently asked question is, when is it safe for a woman to become pregnant following recently acquired infection with *T. gondii*. There is no definitive answer. The data reveal that *in very rare instances* women infected 4 to 6 months prior to their becoming pregnant have given birth to infected offspring. Most experts consider it advisable to wait at least 4 months and some suggest waiting 6 months from the calculated time of infection. The time of infection, if seroconversion was not demonstrated, is best estimated from the results of a serologic panel, as discussed under the previous section on diagnosis.

Antimicrobial Prophylaxis

Secondary prophylaxis in the immunocompromised patient focuses on prevention of recrudescence of the latent infection, primarily in the HIV-infected patient. Pyrimethamine-sulfadiazine is recommended for this purpose.[44] Information regarding the use of primary prophylaxis in the seropositive pregnant HIV-infected woman has been controversial.[35–37] At present, sufficient data are not available to quantify the risk of congenital transmission by HIV-infected mothers who are chronically infected with *T. gondii*. Whether antimicrobial prophylaxis is necessary and effective in preventing both recrudescence and congenital transmission is unknown. Until more data become available, we recommend prophylactic treatment of these women (e.g., those with CD4+ T cell counts below $200/mm^3$) with spiramycin. Trimethoprim-sulfamethoxazole is recommended for primary prophylaxis in these seropositive HIV-infected patients. For a detailed discussion of primary and secondary preventive measures in the HIV-infected patient and those with AIDS, the reader is referred to reference 44.

REFERENCES

1. Wolf A, Cohen D: Granulomatous encephalomyelitis due to an encephatitozoon (encephalitozoic encephalomyelitis): A new protozoon disease of man. Bull Neurol Inst N Y 1937; 7:306.
2. Wolf A, Cohen D, Paige B: Human toxoplasmosis. (Occurrence in infants as an encephalomyelitis. Verification by transmission to animals.) Science 1939; 89:226.
3. Wolf A, Cohen D, Paige B: Toxoplasmic encephalomyelitis. Trans Am Neurol Assoc 1939; 65:76.
4. Sabin AB, Feldman HA: Dyes as microchemical indicators of a new immunity phenomenon affecting a protozoon parasite (*Toxoplasma*). Science 1948; 108:660.
5. Frenkel JK: Toxoplasmosis: Parasite life cycle, pathology and immunology. In: Hammond DM (ed): The Coccidia. Baltimore: University Park Press, 1973, pp 343–410.
6. Dubey, JP, Miller NL, Frenkel JK: The *Toxoplasma gondii* oocyst from cat feces. J Exp Med 1970; 132:636.
7. Jacobs JK, Remington JS, Melton ML: The resistance of the encysted form of *Toxoplasma gondii*. J Parasitol 1960; 46:11.
8. Jones TC, Yeh S, Hirsch JG: The interaction between *Toxoplasma gondii* and mammalian cells. I. Mechanism of entry and intracelluar fate of the parasite. J Exp Med 1972; 136:1157.
9. Klainer AS, Krahenbuhl JL, Remington JS: Scanning electron microscopy of *Toxoplasma gondii*. J Gen Microbiol 1973; 75:111.
10. Zaman V, Colley FC: Ultrastructural study of penetration of macrophages by *Toxoplasma gondii*. Trans R Soc Trop Med Hyg 1972; 66:781.
11. Remington JS, in discussion, Lainson R: Observations on the nature and transmission of *Toxoplasma* in the light of its wide host and geographical range. Surv Ophthalmol 1961; 6:721.
12. Gross U: *Toxoplasma gondii* research in Europe. Parasitol Today 1996; 12:30.
13. Sibley LD, Boothroyd JC: Virulent strains of *Toxoplasma gondii* comprise a single clonal lineage. Nature 1992; 359:82.
14. Howe DK, Sibley LD: *Toxoplasma gondii* comprises three clonal lineages: Correlation of parasite genotype with human disease. J Infect Dis 1995; 172:1561.
15. Weinman D, Chandler AH: Toxoplasmosis in man and swine: An investigation of the possible relationship. JAMA 1956; 161:229.
16. Remington JS, McLeod R, Desmonts G: Toxoplasmosis. In: Remington JS, Klein JO (eds): Infections in the Fetus and Newborn Infant, 4th ed. Philadelphia, WB Saunders, 1995, pp 140–267.
17. Desmonts G, Couvreur J, Alison F, et al: Etude epidemiologique sur la toxoplasmose: De l'influence de la cuisson des viandes de boucherie sur la frequence de l'infection humaine. Rev Fr Etud Clin Biol 1965; 10:952.
18. Kean BH, Kimball AC, Christenson WC: An epidemic of acute toxoplasmosis. JAMA 1969; 208:1002.
19. Wallace GD: The role of the cat in the natural history of *Toxoplasma gondii*. Am J Trop Med Hyg 1973; 22:313.
20. Teutsch SM, Juranek DD, Sulzer A, et al: Epidemic toxoplasmosis associated with infected cats. N Engl J Med 1979; 300:695.
21. Luft BJ, Remington JS: Acute *Toxoplasma* infection among family members of patients with acute lymphadenopathic toxoplasmosis. Arch Intern Med 1984; 144:53.
22. Bowie WR, King AS, Werker DH, et al: Outbreak of toxoplasmosis associated with municipal drinking water. Lancet 1997; 350:173.
23. Ráisánen S: Toxoplasmosis transmitted by blood transfusions. Transfusion 1978; 18:329.
24. Siegel SE, Lunde MN, Geldermann AH, et al: Transmission of toxoplasmosis by leukocyte transfusion. Blood 1971; 37:388.
25. Kayhoe DE, Jacobs L, Beye HK, et al: Acquired toxoplasmosis: Observations on two parasitologically proved cases treated with pyrimethamine and triple sulfonamides. N Engl J Med 1957; 257:1247.
26. Remington JS, Gentry LO: Acquired toxoplasmosis: Infection vs. disease. Ann N Y Acad Sci 1970; 174:1006.
27. Brooks RG, Remington JS: Transplant-related infections. In: Bennet JV, Brachman PS (eds): Hospital Infections, 2nd ed. Boston, Little, Brown and Co., 1986, pp 581–618.
28. Israelski DM, Remington JS: Toxoplasmosis in the non-AIDS immunocompromised host. In: Remington JS, Swartz MN (eds): Current Clinical Topics in Infectious Diseases-13. Cambridge: Blackwell Scientific, 1993, pp 322–356.
29. Hohlfeld P, Daffos F, Costa J-M, et al: Prenatal diagnosis of congenital toxoplasmosis with a polymerase-chain-reaction test on amniotic fluid. N Engl J Med 1994; 331:695.
30. Hohlfeld P, Daffos F, Thulliez P, et al: Fetal toxoplasmosis: Outcome of pregnancy and infant follow-up after in utero treatment. J Pediatr 1990; 115:765.
31. Daffos F, Forestier F, Capella-Pavlovsky M, et al: Prenatal management of 746 pregnancies at risk for congenital toxoplasmosis. N Engl J Med 1988; 318:271.
32. Koppe JG, Loewer-Sieger DH, deRoever-Bonnet H: Results of 20-year follow-up of congenital toxoplasmosis. Lancet 1986; 101:254.
33. Wilson CB, Remington JS, Stagno S, et al: Development of adverse sequelae in children born with subclinical congenital *Toxoplasma* infection. Pediatrics 1980; 66:767.
34. Desmonts G: Toxoplasmose acquise de la femme enceinte:

Estimation du risque de transmission du parasite et de toxoplasmose congenitale. Lyon Med 1982; 248:115.

35. Mitchell CD, Lewis L, McLellan S, et al: Increased risk of congenital toxoplasmosis (Ct) among infants born to mothers infected with HIV-1 and *Toxoplasma gondii*. Abstract in Program and Abstracts of 3rd Conference on Retroviruses and Opportunistic Infections, Jan. 28–Feb. 1, 1996, Washington DC.

36. European Collaborative Study Group: Low incidence of congenital toxoplasmosis in children born to women infected with human immunodeficiency virus. Eur J Obstet Gynecol Reprod Biol 1996; 68:93.

37. Minkoff H, Remington JS, Holman S, et al: Vertical transmission of *Toxoplasma* by human immunodeficiency virus–infected women. Am J Obstet Gynecol 1997; 176:555.

38. Feldman HA, Miller LT: Serological study of toxoplasmosis prevalence. Am J Hyg 1956; 64:320.

39. Harboe A: *Toxoplasma* dye titres in 1600 blood donors in Oslo. Acta Pathol Microbiol Scand Suppl 1952; 93:325.

40. Remington JS, Efron B, Cavanaugh E, et al: Studies on toxoplasmosis in El Salvador: Prevalence and incidence of toxoplasmosis as measured by the Sabin-Feldman dye test. Trans R Soc Trop Med Hyg 1970; 64:252.

41. Smith KL, Wilson M, Hightower AW, et al: Prevalence of *Toxoplasma gondii* antibodies in U.S. military recruits in 1989: Comparison with data published in 1965. Clin Infect Dis 1996; 23:1182.

42. Jeannel D, Niel G, Costagliolat D, et al: Epidemiology of toxoplasmosis among pregnant women in the Paris area. Int J Epidemiol 1988; 17:595.

43. Luft B, Remington JS: Toxoplasmic encephalitis in AIDS. Clin Infect Dis 1992; 15:211.

44. Liesenfeld O, Wong S-Y, Remington JS: Toxoplasmosis in the setting of AIDS. In: Bolognesi D, Bartlett J, Merrigan B (eds): Textbook of AIDS Medicine, 2nd ed. Baltimore, Williams & Wilkins, 1998.

45. Lycke E, Carlberg K, Norrby R: Interactions between *Toxoplasma gondii* and its host cells: Function of the penetration-enhancing factor of *Toxoplasma*. Infect Immun 1975; 11:853.

46. Lainson R: Observations on the development and nature of pseudocysts and cysts of *Toxoplasma gondii*. Trans R Soc Trop Med Hyg 1958; 52:396.

47. Werner H, Pichl H: Vergleichende Untersuchungen an zystenbildenden Toxoplasma-Stämmen. II. Mitteilung: Zystenentwicklung und humorale Antikörperbildung. Zentralbl Bakterior 1969; 210:402.

48. Wong S-Y, Remington JS: Biology of *Toxoplasma gondii*. AIDS 1993; 7:299.

49. McCabe RE, Luft BJ, Remington JS: Effect of murine interferon gamma on murine toxoplasmosis. J Infect Dis 1984; 150:961.

50. Suzuki Y, Conley FK, Remington JS: Treatment of toxoplasmic encephalitis in mice with recombinant gamma interferon. Infect Immun 1990; 58:3050.

51. de Paoli P, Basaglia G, Gennari D, et al: Phenotypic profile and functional characteristics of human gamma and delta T cells during acute toxoplasmosis. J Clin Microbiol 1992; 30:729.

52. Scalise F, Gerli R, Castelluci G, et al: Lymphocytes bearing the γδ T-cell receptor in acute toxoplasmosis. Immunology 1992; 76:668.

53. Subauste CS, Hung JY, Do D, et al: Preferential activation and expansion of human peripheral blood γδ T cells in response to *Toxoplasma gondii* in vitro and their cytokine production and cytotoxic activity against *T. gondii*–infected cells. J Clin Invest 1995; 96:610.

54. Hiseada H, Nagasawa H, Maeda K, et al: γδ T cells play an important role in hsp65 expression and in acquiring protective immune responses against infection with *Toxoplasma gondii*. J Immunol 1995; 154:244.

55. Dorfman RF, Remington JS: Value of lymph-node biopsy in the diagnosis of acute acquired toxoplasmosis. N Engl J Med 1973; 289:878.

56. Beckett RS, Flynn FJ Jr: Toxoplasmosis: Report of two new cases, with a classification and with a demonstration of the organisms in the human placenta. N Engl J Med 1953; 249:345.

57. Bernischke K, Driscoll SG: The Pathology of the Human Placenta. New York, Springer-Verlag, 1967, p 512.

58. Hogan MJ: Ocular Toxoplasmosis. New York, Columbia University Press, 1951.

59. Montoya JG, Remington JS: Toxoplasmic chorioretinitis in the setting of acute acquired toxoplasmosis. Clin Infect Dis 1996; 23:277.

60. Post MJ, Chan JC, Hensley GT, et al: Toxoplasmic encephalitis in Haitian adults with acquired immunodeficiency syndrome: A clinical-pathologic-CT correlation. Am J Neuroradiol 1983; 4:155.

61. Gray F, Gheradi R, Wingate E, et al: Diffuse "encephalitic" cerebral toxoplasmosis in AIDS. J Neurol 1989; 236:273.

62. Levy RM, Bredesen DE, Rosenblum ML: Neurological manifestations of the acquired immunodeficiency syndrome (AIDS): Experience at UCSF and review of the literature. J Neurosurg 1985; 62:475.

63. Strittmatter C, Lang W, Wiestler OD, et al: The changing pattern of human immunodeficiency virus–associated cerebral toxoplasmosis: A study of 46 postmortem cases. Acta Neuropathol 1992; 83:475.

64. Suzuki Y, Wong S-Y, Grumet FC, et al: Evidence for genetic regulation of susceptibility to toxoplasmic encephalitis in AIDS patients. J Infect Dis 1996;173:265.

65. Oksenhendler E, Cadranel J, Sarfati C, et al: *Toxoplasma gondii* pneumonia in patients with the acquired immunodeficiency syndrome. Am J Med 1990; 88:5.

66. Schnapp L, Geaghan S, Campagna A, et al: *Toxoplasma gondii* pneumonitis in patients infected with the human immunodeficiency virus. Arch Intern Med 1992; 152:1073.

67. McCabe RE, Brooks RG, Dorfman RF, et al: Clinical spectrum in 107 cases of toxoplasmic lymphadenopathy. Rev Infect Dis 1987; 9:754.

68. Kean BH: Clinical toxoplasmosis—50 years. Trans R Soc Trop Med Hyg 1972; 66:549.

69. Rossier A, Blancher G, Designolle L, et al: Toxoplasmose congenitale a manifestation retardee: Effet du traitement. Semin Hop 1961; 37:1266.

70. Alford CA Jr, Stagno S, Reynolds DW: Congenital toxoplasmosis: Clinical, laboratory, and therapeutic considerations with special reference to subclinical disease. Bull N Y Acad Med 1974; 2:160.

71. Miller MJ, Remington JS: Toxoplasmosis in infants and children with HIV or AIDS. In: Pizzo PA, Wilfert CM (eds): Pediatric AIDS: The Challenge of HIV Infection in Infants, Children, and Adolescents. Baltimore, Wiliams & Wilkins, 1990, pp 279–307.

72. Canamucio C, Hallet J, Leopold I: Recurrence of treated toxoplasmic uveitis. Am J Ophthalmol 1963; 55:1035.

73. Lakhanpal V, Schocket SS, Nirankari VS: Clindamycin in the treatment of toxoplasmic retinochoroiditis. Am J Ophthalmol 1983; 95:605.

74. Israelski D, Remington JS: Toxoplasmosis in the non-AIDS immunocompromised host. In: Remington JS, Schwartz M (eds): Current Clinical Topics in Infectious Diseases-13. Boston, Blackwell Scientific, 1993, pp 322–356.

75. Porter SB, Sande M: Toxoplasmosis of the central nervous system in the acquired immunodeficiency syndrome. N Engl J Med 1992; 327:1643.

76. Hayes K, Billson FA, Jack I, et al: Cell culture isolation of *Toxoplasma gondii* from an infant with unusual ocular features. Med J Aust 1973; 1:1297.

77. Verlinde JD, Makstenieks O: Repeated isolation of *Toxoplasma* from the cerebrospinal fluid and from blood, and the antibody response in four cases of congenital toxoplasmosis. Antonie Van Leeuwenhoek 1950; 16:366.

78. Habegger H: Toxoplasmose humaine; mise en evidence des parasites dans les milieux intra-oculaires; humeur aqeuse, exudat retroretinien. Arch Ophthalmol (Paris) 1954; 14:470.

79. Conley FK, Jenkins KA, Remington JS: *Toxoplasma gondii* infection of the central nervous system: Use of the peroxidase-antiperoxidase method to demonstrate *Toxoplasma* in formalin-fixed, paraffin-embedded tissue sections. Hum Pathol 1981; 12:690.

80. Desmonts G, Couvreur J: L'isolement du parasite dans la toxoplasmose congenitale: Interet pratique e theorique. Arch Fr Pediatr 1974; 31:157.

81. Wolf A, Cowen D, Page BH: Toxoplasmic encephalomyelitis. VI. Clinical diagnosis of infantile or congenital toxoplasmosis: Survival beyond infancy. Arch Neurol Psych 1942; 48:689.

82. Matsubayashi H, Koike T, Uyemura M, et al: A case of ocular toxoplasmosis in an adult, the infection being confirmed by the isolation of the parasite from subretinal fluid. Keio J Med 1961; 10:209.

83. Frezotti R, Guerra R, Terragna A, et al: A case of congenital toxoplasmosis with active chorioretinitis. Ophthalmologica 1974; 169:321.

84. Schmidke L: Nachweis von Toxoplasma im Fruchtwasser; vorläufige wissenschaftliche Mitteilung. Dtsch Med Wochenschr 1957; 82:1342.

85. Teutsch SM, Sulzer AJ, Ramsey JE Jr, et al: *Toxoplasma gondii* isolated from amniotic fluid. Obstet Gynecol 1980; 55(suppl):2S.

86. Derouin F, Thulliez P, Candolfi E, et al: Early prenatal diagnosis of congenital toxoplasmosis using amniotic fluid samples and tissue culture. Eur J Clin Microbiol Infect Dis 1988; 7:423.

87. Chang CH, Stulberg C, Bollinger RO, et al: Isolation of *Toxoplasma gondii* in tissue culture. J Pediatr 1972; 81:790.

88. Derouin F, Mazeron MC, Garin YJF: Comparative study of tissue culture and mouse inoculation methods for demonstration of *Toxoplasma gondii*. J Clin Microbiol 1987; 25:1597.

89. Grover CM, Thulliez P, Remington JS, et al: Rapid prenatal diagnosis of congenital *Toxoplasma* infection by using polymerase chain reaction and amniotic fluid. J Clin Microbiol 1990; 28:2297.

90. Cazenave J, Forestier F, Bessieres M, et al: Contribution of a new PCR assay to the prenatal diagnosis of congenital toxoplasmosis. Prenat Diagn 1992; 12:119.

91. Pelloux H, Weiss J, Simon J, et al: A new set of primers for the detection of *Toxoplasma gondii* in amniotic fluid using polymerase chain reaction. FEMS Microbiol Lett 1996; 138:11.

92. van de Ven E, Melchers W, Galama J, et al: Identification of *Toxoplasma gondii* infections by B1 gene amplification. J Clin Microbiol 1991; 19:2120.

93. Dupouy-Camet J, Bougnoux ME, Lavreda de Souza S, et al: Comparative value of polymerase chain reaction and conventional biological tests for the prenatal diagnosis of congenital toxoplasmosis. Ann Biol Clin (Paris) 1992; 50:315.

94. Montoya JG, Remington JS: Studies on the serodiagnosis of toxoplasmic lymphadenitis. Clin Infect Dis 1995; 20:781.

95. Liesenfeld O, Press C, Montoya JG, et al: False-positive results in immunoglobulin M (IgM) toxoplasma antibody tests and importance of confirmatory testing: The Patelia Toxo IgM test. J Clin Microbiol 1997; 35:174.

96. Walton BC, Benchoff BM, Brooks WH: Comparison of indirect fluorescent antibody test and methylene blue dye test for detection of antibodies against *Toxoplasma gondii*. Am J Trop Med Hyg 1966; 15:149.

97. Balsari A, Poli G, Molina V, et al: ELISA for *Toxoplasma* antibody detection: A comparison with other serodiagnostic tests. J Clin Pathol 1980; 33:635.

98. Hedman K, Lappalainen M, Seppala I, et al: Recent primary *Toxoplasma* infection indicated by a low avidity of specific IgG. J Infect Dis 1989; 159:736.

99. Serologie de l'Infection Toxoplasmique en Particulier a Son Debut: Methodes et Interpretation des Resultats. Lyon, 11–12 Janvier, 1975. Lyon, Fondation Merieux, p 182.

100. Dannemann BR, Vaughan WC, Thulliez P, et al: Differential agglutination test for diagnosis of recently acquired infection with *Toxoplasma gondii*. J Clin Microbiol 1990; 28:1928.

101. Araujo FG, Barnett EV, Gentry LO, et al: False-positive anti-*Toxoplasma* fluorescent antibody tests in patients with antinuclear antibodies. Appl Microbiol 1971; 22:270.

102. Walls KW, Bullock SL, English DK: Use of the enzyme-linked immunosorbent assay (ELISA) and its microadaptation for the serodiagnosis of toxoplasmosis. J Clin Microbiol 1977; 5:273.

103. Voller A, Bidwell DE, Bartlett A: A microplate enzyme–immunoassay for *Toxoplasma* antibody. J Clin Pathol 1976; 29:150.

104. Lappalainen M, Koskela P, Koskiniemi M, et al: Toxoplasmosis acquired during pregnancy: Improved serodiagnosis based on avidity of immunoglobulin G. J Infect Dis 1993; 167:691.

105. Jenum PA, Stray-Pedersen B, Gundersen A-G: Improved diagnosis of primary *Toxoplasma gondii* infection in early pregnancy by determination of antitoxoplasma immunoglobulin G activity. J Clin Microbiol 1997; 35:1972.

106. Desmonts G, Baufine-Ducrocq H, Couzineau P, et al: Anticorps toxoplasmique naturels. Nouv Presse Med 1974; 3:1547.

107. Desmonts G, Remington JS: Direct agglutination test for diagnosis of *Toxoplasma* infection: Method for increased sensitivity and specificity. J Clin Microbiol 1980; 11:562.

108. Thulliez P, Remington JS, Santoro F, et al: A new agglutination test for the diagnosis of acute and chronic *Toxoplasma* infection. Pathol Biol 1986; 34:173.

109. Wilson MA, Remington JS, Clavet C, et al: Evaluation of six commercial kits for detection of human immunoglobulin M antibodies to *Toxoplasma gondii*. J Clin Microbiol 1997; 35:3112.

110. Public Health Service, Department of Health and Human Services, Food and Drug Administration. FDA Public Health Advisory: Limitations of Toxoplasma IgM Commercial Test Kits (letter). July 25, 1997.

111. Remington JS, Miller MJ, Brownlee I: IgM antibodies in acute toxoplasmosis. I. Diagnostic significance in congenital cases and a method for their rapid demonstration. Pediatrics 1968; 41:1082.

112. Remington JS, Miller MJ, Brownlee I: IgM antibodies in acute toxoplasmosis. II. Prevalence and significance in acquired cases. J Lab Clin Med 1968; 71:855.

113. Naot Y, Barnett EV, Remington JS: Method for avoiding false-positive results occurring in immunoglobulin M enzyme-linked immunosorbent assays due to presence of both rheumatoid factor and antinuclear antibodies. J Clin Microbiol 1981; 14:73.

114. Naot Y, Desmonts G, Remington JS: IgM enzyme-linked immunosorbent assay test for the diagnosis of congenital *Toxoplasma* infection. J Pediatr 1981; 98:32.

115. Naot Y, Remington JS: An enzyme-linked immunosorbent assay for detection of IgM antibodies of *Toxoplasma gondii*: Use for diagnosis of acute acquired toxoplasmosis. J Infect Dis 1980; 142:757.

116. Siegel JP, Remington JS: Comparison of methods for quantitative antigen-specific immunoglobulin M antibody with a reverse enzyme-linked immunosorbent assay. J Clin Microbiol 1983; 18:63.

117. Desmonts G, Naot Y, Remington JS: An IgM immunosorbent agglutination assay for diagnosis of infectious diseases: Diagnosis of acute congenital and acquired *Toxoplasma* infections. J Clin Microbiol 1981; 14:486.

118. Stepick-Biek P, Thulliez P, Araujo FG, et al: IgA antibodies for diagnosis of acute congenital and acquired toxoplasmosis. J Infect Dis 1990; 162:270.

119. Decoster A, Slizewicz B, Simon J, et al: Platelia-Toxo IgA, a new kit for early diagnosis of congenital toxoplasmosis by detection of anti-P30 immunoglobulin A antibodies. J Clin Microbiol 1991; 29:2291.

120. Pinon JM, Thoannes H, Pouletty PH, et al: Detection of specific immunoglobulin E in patients with toxoplasmosis. J Clin Microbiol 1990; 28:1739.

121. Wong S-Y, Hadju M-P, Ramirez R, et al: Role of specific immunoglobulin E in diagnosis of acute *Toxoplasma* infection and toxoplasmosis. J Clin Microbiol 1993; 31:2952.

122. Wong S-Y, Remington JS: Toxoplasmosis in pregnancy. Clin Infect Dis 1994; 18:853.

123. Liesenfeld O, Montoya JG, Tathieni NJ, et al: Confirmatory serological testing results in remarkable decrease in unnecessary abortion among pregnant women in the United States with positive *Toxoplasma* serology. Am J Obstet Gynecol 2000; in press.

124. Desmonts G, Daffos F, Forestier F, et al: Prenatal diagnosis of congenital toxoplasmosis. Lancet 1985; 1:500.

125. Forestier F, Cox W, Daffos F, et al: The assessment of fetal blood samples. Am J Obstet Gynecol 1988; 158:1184.

126. Fuentes I, Rodriguez M, Domingo CS, et al: Urine sample used for congenital toxoplasmosis diagnosed by PCR. J Clin Microbiol 1996; 34:2368.

127. O'Connor GR: Manifestations and management of ocular toxoplasmosis. Bull N Y Acad Med 1974; 50:192.

128. Montoya JG, Parmley S, Liesenfeld O, et al: Use of the polymerase chain reaction for diagnosis of ocular toxoplasmosis. Ophthalmology 1999; 106:1554.

129. Desmonts G: Definitive serological diagnosis of ocular toxoplasmosis. Arch Ophthalmol 1966; 76:839.

130. Derouin F, Leport C, Pueyo S, et al: Predictive value of *Toxoplasma gondii* antibody titres on the occurrence of toxoplasmic encephalitis in HIV-infected patients. AIDS 1996; 10:1521.

131. Eyles DE, Coleman M: Synergistic effect of sulfadiazine and Daraprim against experimental toxoplasmosis in the mouse. Antibiot Chemother 1953; 3:483.

132. Partisani M, De Mautort E, Hassari N, et al: Primary prophylaxis of cerebral toxoplasmosis with pyrimethamine–sulfadoxine in human immunodeficiency virus–infected individual seropositive for *Toxoplasma*. VIIIth International Conference on AIDS, Amsterdam, Netherlands, July 1991. Abstract PoB1216.

133. Ryan RW, Hart WM, Culligan JJ, et al: Diagnosis and treatment of toxoplasmic uveitis. Trans Am Acad Ophthalmol 1954; 58:867.

134. Perkins S, Smith CH, Schofield PB: Treatment of uveitis with pyrimethamine (Daraprim). Br J Ophthalmol 1956; 40:577.

135. Thiersch JB: Effect of certain 2,4-diaminopyrimidine antagonists of folic acid on pregnancy and rat fetus. Proc Soc Exp Biol Med 1954; 87:571.

136. MacFarlane JA, Mitchell AAB, Walsh JM, et al: Spiramycin in the prevention of postoperative staphylococcal infection. Lancet 1968; 1:1.

137. Garin J-P, Pellerat J, Maillard M, et al: Bases theoretiques de la prevention par la spiramycine de la toxoplasmose congenitale chez la femme enceinte. Presse Med 1968; 76:2266.

138. Dannemann BR, McCutchan JA, Israelski DA, et al: Treatment of toxoplasmic encephalitis in patients with AIDS: A randomized trial comparing pyrimethamine plus clindamycin to pyrimethamine plus sulfadiazine. Ann Intern Med 1992; 116:33.

139. Luft BJ, Hafner R, Korzun AH, et al: Toxoplasmic encephalitis in patients with the acquired immunodeficiency syndrome. N Engl J Med 1993; 329:995.

140. Luft BJ: In vivo and in vitro activity of roxithromycin against *Toxoplasma gondii* in mice. Eur J Clin Microbiol Infect Dis 1987; 6:479.

141. Fernandez-Martin J, Leport C, Morlat P, et al: Pyrimethamine-clarithromycin combination for therapy of acute *Toxoplasma* encephalitis in patients with AIDS. Antimicrob Agents Chemother 1991; 35:2049.

142. Araujo FG, Guptill DR, Remington JS: Azithromycin, a macrolide antibiotic with potent activity against *Toxoplasma gondii*. Antimicrob Agents Chemother 1988; 32:755.

143. Kovacs JA: Efficacy of atovaquone in treatment of toxoplasmosis in patients with AIDS. Lancet 1992; 340:637.

144. Khan AA, Slifer T, Araujo FG, et al: Activity of trovafloxacin in combination with other drugs for treatment of acute murine toxoplasmosis. J Clin Microbiol 1997; 41:893.

145. Haverkos HW: Assessment of therapy for toxoplasmic encephalitis. The TE Study Group. Am J Med 1987; 82:907.

146. Forestier F: Les foetopathies infectieuses—prevention, diagnostic prenatal, attitude pratique. Presse Med 1991; 20:1448.

147. Hohlfeld P, MacAleese J, Capella-Pavlovsky M, et al: Fetal toxoplasmosis: Ultrasonographic signs. Ultrasound Obstet Gynecol 1991; 1:241.

148. Gosh M, Levy P, Leopold IH: Therapy of toxoplasmic uveitis. Am J Ophthalmol 1965; 59:55.

149. Holland GN, O'Connor GR, Belfort R Jr, Remington JS: Toxoplasmosis. In: Pepose JS, Holland GN, Wilhelmus KR (eds): Ocular Infection and Immunity. St Louis, Mosby Yearbook, 1996, pp 1183–1223.

150. Tabbara KF, O'Connor GR: Treatment of ocular toxoplasmosis with clindamycin and sulfadiazine. Ophthalmology 1980; 87:129.

151. McCabe R, Remington JS: Toxoplasmosis: The time has come. N Engl J Med 1988; 318:313.

152. Guerina NG, Hsu H-W, Meissner HC, et al: Neonatal serologic screening and early treatment for congenital *Toxoplasma gondii* infection. N Engl J Med 1994; 330:1858.

4

Rubella

J. M. ERNEST

Prior to 1969, rubella was a universal disease in the United States. Its usually innocuous effects on children and young adults masked its potentially devastating course in the fetus, which had been recognized in 1941 by the Australian ophthalmologist Sir Norman McAllister Gregg. His association of cataracts in children with an epidemic of maternal rubella infection underscored the importance of the viral infection during pregnancy and the need for wide-scale prevention of the disease as well as an adequate understanding of the virus by health care providers, especially those who care for pregnant women.

EPIDEMIOLOGY

Before the advent of the rubella vaccine, epidemics usually occurred in the United States and around the world in varying cycles of 6 to 9 years. The last worldwide epidemic occurred in 1964. In 1969, three live attenuated rubella vaccines were licensed for use in the United States: the HPV-77 (DE-5 and DK-12) vaccines and the Cendehill vaccine. In that year, the incidence of rubella infection in the United States was 29 per 100,000 population, and the number of cases of congenital rubella syndrome (CRS) was 62.[1] Since the widespread availability of the vaccine and the development of the more immunogenic strain RA 27/3 (developed in human diploid cells and available since 1979), the numbers of cases of rubella and CRS have fallen dramatically. In 1982, the incidence of rubella had dropped to 1 per 100,000 population, and the number of cases of CRS to 13. In 1989, only one case of CRS was reported to the Centers for Disease Control and Prevention (CDC) National Congenital Rubella Syndrome Registry. However, in 1990, 25 cases were reported, and in 1991 a total of 31 indigenous cases of CRS were reported in the United States. Factors associated with this transient increase in cases of CRS include an increasing population in the United States of unvaccinated persons of Asian or Pacific Island background or Hispanic ethnicity (3% of cases in 1991, compared to 20% to 30% more recently) and a large number of cases in Pennsylvania in persons with religious objections to vaccination (20 of the 31 cases in the entire U.S. in 1991 were from that state).[2] Since

that rise, the number of cases of CRS has continued to fall, with only five cases reported in 1992 and none in 1993. In 1993, of the 190 persons in the U.S. with rubella (none of whom had CRS), only 6 of the 97 with known vaccination status (6%) over the age of 1 year reported receiving the recommended two doses of vaccine.[3]

These recent surges in the occurrence of CRS and the rarity of the disease in vaccinated individuals underscore the importance of widespread vaccination, since the likelihood of CRS in a vaccinated woman is extremely unlikely.

BIOLOGY OF THE MICROORGANISM

Named "rubella" by Henry Veale in 1866, the organism is a single-stranded RNA virus that belongs to the togavirus family. The illness caused by rubella is generally mild and rarely produces serious complications. The virus is highly communicable, and an infected person may shed virus in the upper respiratory tract from 1 week before to as long as 3 weeks after the acute illness.[4] Transmission to susceptible persons occurs by the respiratory route, the disease occurring 14 to 18 days after exposure. About one half of infected individuals have no symptoms, and in the remainder the simultaneous occurrence of a low-grade fever, mild upper respiratory tract symptoms, and rash signals the onset of the disease. The rash is typically a pink or salmon-colored, macular pruritic exanthem that begins on the face and neck, spreads to the trunk and proximal extremities, and fades within 1 to 3 days of onset. Posterior cervical and occipital adenopathy is a hallmark of the infection and may present as the only symptom. Node enlargement, which presents as early as 1 week before the rash, peaks with the onset of the rash. Occasionally, generalized adenopathy and splenomegaly lead to the mistaken diagnosis of infectious mononucleosis. Pharyngitis and conjunctivitis are common. Most persons recover uneventfully within 3 to 4 days. The major complication is acute polyarthralgia involving the proximal interphalangeal joints, metacarpal phalangeal joints, wrists, elbows, or knees, with tenosynovitis or the carpal tunnel syndrome. Joint symptoms usually are first noted during convalescence and persist for days to several weeks. Rare complications include thrombocytopenic purpura, pancytopenia, and postinfectious meningoencephalitis.[5]

CLINICAL MANIFESTATIONS IN PREGNANCY

Rubella infection during pregnancy has an appearance similar to that of infection in the nonpregnant adult, yet the potential sequelae are quite different. Infection is most likely to cause fetal damage when maternal infection occurs during the first 16 weeks of pregnancy. In a study of 61 women with confirmed rubella occurring from 5 weeks before to 6 weeks after the last menstrual period, no confirmed cases of fetal infection were seen if the rubella infection occurred 11 days or less after the last menstrual period. In contrast, all 10 of the pregnancies in which rubella occurred from 3 to 6 weeks after the last menstrual period had evidence of fetal infection.[6] In a study from 1982 in which all maternal cases were serologically confirmed and sensitive antibody assays were used to detect congenital infection, the risk of congenital defects was 90% when maternal infection occurred before 11 weeks of gestation, 33% for infection during the 11th to 12th week, 11% for the 13th to 14th week, 24% for the 15th to 16th week, and 0% after 16 weeks.[7]

DIAGNOSIS

Because of the transient nature of the rash, the occasional presence of only adenopathy to signal the presence of infection, and the similarity of skin rashes resembling rubella that are caused by adenovirus, enterovirus, or other respiratory virus infections, definitive diagnosis of rubella can be difficult. In September 1996, the CDC defined rubella as an illness that has all of the following characteristics:

Acute onset of generalized maculopapular rash

Temperature greater than 99.0°F (greater than 37.2°C), if measured

Arthralgia and/or arthritis, lymphadenopathy, or conjunctivitis

Laboratory criteria for diagnosis include the following:

Isolation of rubella virus, or

Significant rise between acute- and convalescent-phase titers in serum rubella immunoglobulin G (IgG) antibody level by any standard serologic assay, or

Positive serologic test for rubella immunoglobulin M (IgM) antibody

According to the CDC, rubella case classification includes *suspected*, *probable*, and *confirmed*. A suspected case involves any generalized rash illness of acute on-set. A probable case meets the clinical case definition, has no or noncontributory serologic or virologic testing, and is not epidemiologically linked to a laboratory-confirmed case. A *confirmed* case is laboratory confirmed or meets the clinical case definition and is epidemiologically linked to a laboratory-confirmed case. Serum rubella IgM test results that are false-positives have been reported in persons with other viral infections—for example, acute infection with Epstein-Barr virus (infectious mononucleosis), recent cytomegalovirus infection, and parvovirus infection—or in the presence of rheumatoid factor. Patients who have laboratory evidence of recent measles infection are excluded from the diagnosis of rubella.[8]

Congenital rubella syndrome is defined by the CDC as an illness usually manifesting in infancy, resulting from rubella infection in utero and characterized by signs or symptoms from the following categories:

1. Cataracts/congenital glaucoma, congenital heart disease (most commonly patent ductus arteriosus, or peripheral pulmonary artery stenosis), loss of hearing, pigmentary retinopathy
2. Purpura, splenomegaly, jaundice, microcephaly, mental retardation, meningoencephalitis, radiolucent bone disease

A clinical case is defined as the presence of any defects or laboratory data consistent with congenital rubella infection. Laboratory criteria for diagnosis include the presence of the following:

Isolation of rubella virus, or

Demonstration of rubella-specific IgM antibody, or

Infant rubella antibody level that persists at a higher level and for a longer period than expected from passive transfer of maternal antibody (i.e., rubella titer that does not drop at the expected rate of a twofold dilution per month)

Case classification includes the following categories:

Suspected: a case with some compatible clinical findings but not meeting the criteria for a probable case

Probable: a case that is not laboratory-confirmed and that has any two complications from paragraph a) of the clinical description or one complication from paragraph a) and one from paragraph b), and lacks evidence of any other etiology

Confirmed: a clinically compatible case that is laboratory-confirmed

Infection Only: a case that demonstrates laboratory evidence of infection, but without any clinical symptoms or signs

In probable cases, either or both of the eye-related findings (i.e., cataracts and congenital glaucoma) are interpreted as a single complication. In cases classified as infection only, if any compatible signs or symptoms (e.g., hearing loss) are identified later, the case is reclassified as confirmed.[9]

As is apparent from the CDC criteria, laboratory confirmation is critical for definitive diagnosis in the patient. Several methods are available for confirming the presence of rubella.

Viral Isolation. Rubella virus can be isolated from the blood stream and throat 7 to 10 days after exposure and continues to be shed from the throat for about a week. Few laboratory facilities provide this service, however, and rubella isolation usually takes 4 to 6 weeks to complete.

Serologic Tests. Although reinfection during pregnancy has been reported,[10] the presence of *any* detectable rubella antibody prior to or at the time of exposure usually indicates proof of immunity from subsequent systemic infections. The serologic diagnosis of *recent* rubella infection requires either detection in acute and convalescent sera of a significant (i.e., fourfold or higher) rise in rubella antibody levels, either total or IgG, or the presence of rubella IgM antibody.

In the United States today, the most commonly used assays for the diagnosis of acute rubella infection are hemagglutination inhibition (the "gold standard"), enzyme-linked immunosorbent assay (ELISA), and agglutination tests. Complement fixation tests are now used infrequently because they are less sensitive and because complement fixation antibodies appear later in the course of disease than do antibodies measured by other assays. Passive hemagglutination and passive latex agglutination tests are fast and convenient tests that are useful for detecting evidence of immunity but are not recommended for quantitating antibody or for confirming rubella illness. Neutralization tests are very sensitive but are not usually available in clinical laboratories.

Hemagglutination inhibition, ELISA, and indirect fluorescent immunoassays have been developed for detection of the serum rubella IgM fraction as well as for measurement of IgG antibody levels. Total rubella antibodies are rarely measured now by commercial laboratories, since most ELISA and indirect fluorescent immunoassays use conjugates specific for IgG.

Rubella IgM antibody can be detected from early after the onset of illness, reaching a peak at 7 to 10 days and persisting up to 4 weeks after the appearance of rash. Some sensitive assays may detect IgM antibody for more than 4 weeks. False-positive tests for IgM antibody can occur with any indirect assay, such as ELISA or indirect fluorescent immunoassay, if the laboratory technique used does not avoid nonspecific reactions due to complexes with rheumatoid antibody. A negative IgM test, unless supported by additional laboratory or other data, cannot definitively prove lack of

infection because of the potential for a false-negative result owing to early waning of IgM antibody in as little time as 4 or 5 weeks or less.[11] A particularly difficult diagnostic situation can occur in a pregnant woman who is vaccinated but who has a significant rise in total or IgG antibody level after recent exposure to rubella. If IgM is present, then acute infection or reinfection has occurred. If no IgM antibody is detected, the rise in IgG level probably represents a boosting of antibody due to reinfection, rather than a primary response to infection and generally is felt to represent no risk to the fetus.[12]

MATERNAL IMPLICATIONS

Pregnant women with confirmed rubella infection should receive recommendations for symptomatic relief of pharyngitis, fever, or generalized aches and pains typical of a viral infection. They should be reassured that the symptoms are self-limited, and should be cautioned to be aware of the potential for persistent joint aches and the rare but serious complications of thrombocytopenia or those involving the central nervous system. Counseling should be given to all pregnant women with rubella regarding the potential for serious consequences to the fetus, depending on the trimester of pregnancy.

FETAL IMPLICATIONS

The fetal risk from maternal rubella is determined by the nature of the virus (wild or attenuated) and the timing of the infection.

Rubella vaccine virus is known to cross the placenta and may infect the fetus during the early stages of development, but there is no evidence that it causes birth defects or illness. Between 1971 and 1988, the CDC collected data on 307 infants born to susceptible women who had received rubella vaccine up to 3 months before conception or during the first trimester of pregnancy. Ninety-four infants were born to mothers who had received the previously used Cendehill or HPV/77 vaccines, and 212 were born to mothers who had received the RA 27/3 vaccine. None of the infants had defects indicative of CRS. A total of three of the infants born to mothers receiving the Cendehill or the HPV/77 vaccine and three born to mothers receiving the RA 27/3 vaccine had laboratory evidence of subclinical fetal infection but no illness or defects. The observed risk of congenital malformations following rubella vaccination with the RA 27/3 vaccine therefore is 0; the theoretic risk may be up to 1.7%.[13]

Infection prior to the onset of the last menstrual period (LMP) does not appear to be associated with CRS. Infections occurring as early as 12 days after the LMP, however, have been seen to precede fetal infection, and the potential exists for neonatal or childhood complications. Because decreased cell replication is a direct effect of rubella infection, fetal growth retardation and failure of normal cellular differentiation during embryogenesis can be expected. Because of the body's inflammatory response to the infection and possibly because of autoimmune reactions, additional tissue damage and longer-term effects can also be predicted.

When maternal infection occurs prior to 16 weeks of gestation, the eyes, heart, and central nervous system are the most frequently affected systems noted at birth. Cataracts, glaucoma, microphthalmia, and chorioretinitis are common ophthalmologic problems. Cardiac defects include peripheral pulmonic stenosis, patent ductus arteriosus, and septal defects. Mental retardation, microcephaly, and encephalitis are neurologic effects of the virus. Sensorineural deafness is the most common consequence.

In approximately 20% of individuals, including those with intrauterine infections as late as the sixth gestational month, late manifestations of infection develop at 10 to 20 years of age. These include endocrinopathies, such as insulin-dependent diabetes, thyroid abnormalities, and hypoadrenalism; hearing loss or additional ocular damage; and, rarely, progressive rubella panencephalitis.[14] Since the absence of obvious defects at birth does not preclude the child from subclinical or subsequent damages discovered at a later date, careful follow-up is imperative.

TREATMENT IN PREGNANCY

There is no treatment to ameliorate maternal disease or reduce the risk to the fetus when maternal infection is present. Therefore, prevention of fetal infection requires prevention of maternal infection through widespread vaccination programs. The CDC has recommended the establishment of an additional routine visit for adolescents, 11 to 12 years of age, for the purposes of vaccinating adolescents who have not previously received varicella virus vaccine, hepatitis B vaccine, or the second dose of the measles, mumps, and rubella (MMR) vaccine and of providing a booster dose of tetanus and diphtheria toxoids.[15] Vaccination at this time should provide sufficient immunity for most women of childbearing age, since RA 27/3–induced antibody levels, which are present in at least 95% of vaccinees, have been shown to persist for at least 18 years in 92% of vaccinees who had originally seroconverted.[16] Women being seen for a preconceptional counseling visit are excellent candidates for rubella vaccination if they have a negative history of MMR vaccination. While they should be counseled to avoid pregnancy for at least 3 months after the vaccine, the risk of CRS, should pregnancy occur within those 3 months, is low and is not considered to be at a level for pregnancy termination to be recommended.[17] Postpartum women who are rubella antibody–negative are also ideal candidates for rubella vaccine at the time of discharge from the hospital after delivery. Viral shedding for several weeks can occur after receipt of the vaccine, but does not appear to pose a risk for pregnant women with whom they have contact or their breast-fed infant.

Pregnant women documented as having an acute rubella infection should be counseled about the significant risk to the fetus and the likelihood of the effects as determined by the trimester of infection. Pregnancy termination is considered by many affected women because of the likelihood and the potential severity of the infection in the developing fetus.

Rubella infection in pregnancy is fortunately becoming extremely rare because of the increasing number of women who have received adequate vaccination prior to pregnancy. As health care providers in the United States encounter more women from countries where rubella vaccination is not common, and as religious and other factors continue to prevent women from receiving vaccination, all providers of health care for women should be constantly searching for opportunities to educate and vaccinate rubella-susceptible women to continue to reduce this potentially preventable neonatal disease.

REFERENCES

1. MMWR. Rubella and Congenital Rubella Syndrome—United States, January 1, 1991–May 7, 1994. June 3, 1994. Vol 43/No 21, p 400.
2. MMWR. Rubella and Congenital Rubella Syndrome—United States, January 1, 1991–May 7, 1994. June 3, 1994. Vol 43/No 21, p 399.
3. MMWR. Rubella and Congenital Rubella Syndrome—United States, January 1, 1991–May 7, 1994. June 3, 1994. Vol 43/No 21, p 399.
4. Green RH, Balsamo MR, Giles JP, et al: Studies of the natural history and prevention of rubella. Am J Dis Child 1965; 110:348.
5. Modlin J: Systemic viral infections. In: Harvey A, Johns R, McKusick V, et al (eds): The Principles and Practice of Medicine, 23rd ed. Norwalk, CT, Appleton & Lange, 1988, p 647.
6. Enders G, Nickerl-Pacher U, Miller E, et al: Outcome of confirmed periconceptional maternal rubella. Lancet 1988; 1:1445.
7. Miller E, Cradock-Watson JE, Pollock TM: Consequences of confirmed maternal rubella at successive stages of pregnancy. Lancet 1982; 2:781.
8. Centers for Disease Control: Case definitions for infectious complications under public health surveillance. MMWR 1997; 46(No RR-10):29.
9. Centers for Disease Control: Case definitions for infectious complications under public health surveillance. MMWR 1997; 46(No RR-10):30.
10. Robinson J, Lemay M, Vaudry WL: Congenital rubella after anticipated maternal immunity: Two cases and a review of the literature. Pediatr Infect Dis J 1994; 13:812.
11. Rubella and pregnancy. ACOG Technical Bulletin 171, Aug 1992.
12. Rubella and pregnancy. ACOG Technical Bulletin 171, Aug 1992.

13. Centers for Disease Control: Rubella vaccination during pregnancy—United States 1971–1988. MMWR 1989; 38:289.

14. Grossman JH: Rubella in pregnancy. Contemp Ob/Gyn July 1997; July 29–36.

15. Centers for Disease Control: Immunization of Adolescents. MMWR 1996; 45:No RR-7.

16. O'Shea S, Best JM, Banatvala JE, et al: Persistence of rubella antibody 8–18 years after vaccination. Br Med J 1984; 288:1043.

17. Centers for Disease Control, Immunization Practices Advisory Committee: Increase in rubella and congenital rubella syndrome—United States, 1988–1990. MMWR 1991; 40:93.

5 Cytomegalovirus Infections in Women, Pregnancy, and the Neonate

Antonio V. Sison ▶ John L. Sever

INTRODUCTION

Cytomegalovirus (CMV) is one of the most ubiquitous viral infections in humans. Worldwide, infection rates range from 20% to 100%. The highest rates of infection occur in developing countries and in areas of low socioeconomic status within developed countries. Regions such as Southeast Asia, Africa, and the South Pacific have infection rates of more than 90%, compared to less than 50% in Europe and North America.

Transmission of virus among adults and children occurs primarily through contact with individuals who are actively shedding virus. Among infected individuals, CMV is commonly shed from, and hence detectable in, nasopharyngeal secretions, urine, saliva, tears, genital secretions (cervicovaginal fluid, semen), breast milk, and blood.[1, 2] Virus can also be easily acquired through transfusion of blood products or tissue transplantation and from an infected mother to her infant.

The high seroprevalence of CMV in humans, the ability of the virus to remain dormant in the infected host and cause latent infection, the extended period of viral-shedding in acute infection in children, and the majority of CMV infections being asymptomatic all have contributed to high transmission rates in humans. CMV is the most common viral cause of congenital infection. Approximately 35,000 infants are born with CMV annually in the United States, or about 1% of all live births.[3] Perinatal transmission occurs through exposure of the fetus in utero to virus from an acutely infected pregnant woman, although the majority of transmission has been documented in mothers with reactivated disease.[4] The most severe case of congenital infection, "cytomegalic inclusion disease," results primarily from intrauterine infection.

Developments in CMV infections in humans within the last decade have included the following: (1) the recent emergence of complications from CMV infection, such as CMV retinitis, specific only to immunocompromised hosts; for example, patients with ac- quired immunodeficiency syndrome (AIDS)[5]; (2) the altered clinical course and presentation of CMV due to other coinfecting viruses, such as human immunodeficiency virus (HIV)[6, 7]; and (3) the use of molecular biologic techniques, such as the polymerase chain reaction (PCR) in the diagnosis of adult, fetal, and neonatal infection.[8–10] Unfortunately, advances in therapy among infected individuals and neonates, as well as in developing vaccines against CMV, have been lacking. This chapter discusses the epidemiology, biology, clinical manifestations, diagnosis, and management of CMV infections in adults, pregnant women, and neonates.

EPIDEMIOLOGY AND MODES OF TRANSMISSION

CMV infections in humans follow three common patterns: (1) both adult seroprevalence and perinatal transmission rates are significantly higher in areas of low socioeconomic status and in nonindustrialized countries; (2) seroprevalence rates are inversely proportional to age; and (3) the incidence of perinatal infection directly correlates with seroprevalence rates within an infected population. The most common periods in life during which CMV infection is acquired are infancy and at the onset of sexual activity.[11, 12] The risk that a pregnant seronegative woman will convert while pregnant is approximately 1% to 4%, although the rate may be higher among women of low socioeconomic status.

The mode of horizontal transmission of virus, especially to women, is not clearly understood. Published studies have shown that both pregnant and nonpregnant women commonly acquire infection through exposure to infected children.[13–15] Yeager reported a seroconversion rate of 47% in 1 year among previously uninfected women whose infants had acquired primary CMV in nurseries.[15] Viral shedding is both common and prolonged especially among infected children, thus contributing to the persistent reservoir of virus in many communities. The average duration of viral shedding was approximately 13 months in one study of infants in an Iowa day care center.[16] Other methods by which virus is acquired by adults, children, and infants are summarized in Table 5–1.

Virus can also be spread through sexual transmission. In several studies, seropositivity to CMV among sexually active adults correlated with high numbers of sexual partners and with early age of intercourse.[11, 17] Virus has been detected in genital tract secretions. Assaying for a CMV-specific immediate early (IE) gene sequence by PCR, Shen and co-workers[18] demonstrated viral shedding in the cervix of infected pregnant women from 13% to 40% as pregnancy advanced. Semen has also been shown to harbor virus and hence can be infectious.[5, 19]

Among serosusceptible pregnant women, about 1% to 4% will acquire primary infection during pregnancy, and approximately half of these will transmit the virus to their children.[4, 20, 21] Infants also acquire CMV perinatally from chronic or reactivated infection in the mother, but transmission occurs in fewer than 1% of these cases. An additional 1% to 15% of seronegative, uninfected infants acquire CMV during the first 6 months of life through intimate contact with their mothers, the nursery, and other infected household members, and rarely through blood transfusion and organ transplantation.

Breast-feeding appears to be a significant factor in the postnatal transmission of virus.

Minamishima and co-workers[1] identified postnatal infection in 64.7% of breast-fed infants, in contrast to only 27.6% of bottle-fed infants from seropositive mothers.

TABLE 5–1 ▶ METHODS OF ACQUISITION AND TRANSMISSION OF CMV IN ADULTS AND NEONATES

Congenital
    In utero (transplacental)
    Passage through infected birth canal
Neonatal
    Breastfeeding
    Exposure to infected individual (other infectious neonates, mother, health care provider)
    Blood transfusion
    Tissue transplantation
Children
    Exposure to infected individual (other children, infected adults, household members)
    Blood transfusion
    Tissue transplantation
Adult/maternal
    Exposure to infected individual (infants, children, nurseries, day care centers, household members, sexual contacts)
    Blood transfusion
    Tissue transplantation

BIOLOGY AND PATHOGENESIS OF CMV DISEASE

Cytomegalovirus was first successfully described by Weller in 1953[22] and was subsequently isolated by Rowe and co-workers in 1956.[23] The term *cytomegalovirus* was first used by Weller to replace the term *cytomegalic inclusion disease virus*.[24] CMV is the largest member of the Herpesviridae family of viruses, measuring about 180 to 200 nm with an icosahedral capsid containing 162 capsomeres. The genomic material of CMV is double-stranded DNA, measuring about 240 kilobases. The phrase *cytomegalic inclusion disease* (CID), which has been used to describe severe cases of congenital infection, originated from the ability of the virus to induce cellular cytomegalia or "swelling" within the infected host cell. This cytopathic effect induced by viral infection generally gives the cell the classic "owl's-eye" appearance on histologic sections, in which cells contain large intranuclear or cytoplasmic inclusions (Fig. 5–1A and B). These cells, which have undergone cytopathologic change, were actually first described by Ribbert in 1881 in the kidney of a stillborn infected with congenital syphilis.[25] CMV has been isolated in many different organs in humans, including the lungs, liver, kidneys, and pancreas. CMV has been detected in the vitreous and aqueous humor from an AIDS patient with CMV retinitis.[26]

Spread of infection with CMV generally involves cell-to-cell transfer of virus. Muhlemann and associates[27] perfused human placental tissues with high titers of CMV, demonstrated failure of cell-free virus to traverse the placental barrier, and provided evidence that transplacental passage of cell-free virus is inefficient. There are specific cells, however, that are important in preserving the virus. Using immunohistochemical stains on various infected organs, Sinzger and colleagues[28] showed that macrophages play a major role in the hematogenous spread of virus within the infected host. These "reservoir sites" have been implicated in the pathogenesis of perinatal transmission of the virus as well. In pregnant guinea pigs, infectious virus was detected in fetal tissue not only at the time of initial maternal inoculation with virus but also after 3 to 4 weeks from inoculation, suggesting that primary infection may lead to development of reserved sites, such as placenta, where virus is present despite its clearance in the circulation.[29] Humoral immunity may therefore play a small role in the pathogenesis of infections with CMV.

Nevertheless, differences in humoral response alter the severity of clinical presentation with CMV. Britt and Vugler[30] demonstrated that clinically symptomatic infants were more likely to have higher levels of CMV IgG antibodies in cord blood than in those of infected infants who were asymptomatic.

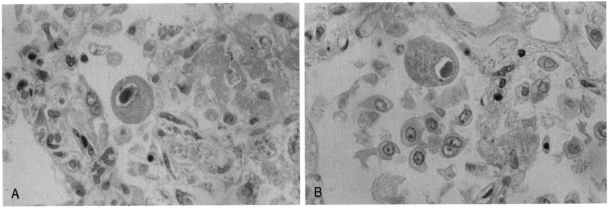

FIGURE 5-1 ▶ Photomicrograph of type II pneumocytes infected with CMV, showing the classic "owl's-eye" appearance of an infected cell transformed by CMV, taken at autopsy from a 35-year-old male with Hodgkin's lymphoma and CMV pneumonia. *A*, Intracytoplasmic inclusions. *B*, Intranuclear inclusions with CMV. Magnification ×10; H&E staining was used. (Courtesy of Fernando U. Garcia, Department of Pathology, Allegheny University Hospitals, Philadelphia, PA.)

CLINICAL MANIFESTATIONS OF ADULT, PEDIATRIC, AND CONGENITAL INFECTION WITH CMV

Women and Mothers. Table 5–2 summarizes the protean manifestations of CMV infection among adults and children. The vast majority of acute CMV infections in women are asymptomatic. Symptomatic infection typically presents with generalized malaise, fever, lassitude, lymphadenopathy, and pharyngitis, similar to a mononucleosis-like syndrome caused by Epstein-Barr virus (EBV). CMV mononucleosis is difficult to differentiate clinically from the one induced by EBV, although the heterophile-agglutinin test is typically negative in EBV infections. In the acute phase of CMV infection, virus is commonly excreted from the nasopharynx, throat, blood, saliva, and urine. Viremia is usually transient. CMV has also been detected in cervical secretions and semen. Severe complications, which include hepatitis, interstitial pneumonitis, and meningoencephalitis, and *Guillain-Barré syndrome* from CMV-induced mononucleosis are rare. Immunocompetent patients typically recover in a few weeks. Acute infection in children may present with a mononucleosis-like syndrome similar to adults. Of infants and children with this clinical presentation, Lajo and co-workers[31] showed that 16.1% of cases were attributable to CMV and 84% to EBV.

Acute CMV infection follows a more aggressive and protracted course in patients with HIV infection, with other immunocompromised states, or following organ transplantation. Among HIV-infected patients, CMV infection can cause pneumonitis, retinitis (Fig. 5–2), encephalopathy, and gastrointestinal ulcerations. In children with HIV, infants who had positive cultures to CMV had a statistically significant decrease in survival compared to the infants without CMV.[32]

Both CMV IgG and IgM are produced within days following infection. CMV IgM remains elevated for

TABLE 5-2 ▶ CLINICAL MANIFESTATIONS OF CMV INFECTION
ADULTS AND CHILDREN
Mostly asymptomatic
CMV-induced mononucleosis
Lymphadenopathy
Pharyngitis
Fever
Rare complications: petechiae, hepatitis, encephalitis, Guillain-Barré syndrome
IMMUNOCOMPROMISED HOST
Pneumonitis (most common)
Retinitis
Hepatitis
Gastrointestinal ulcerations

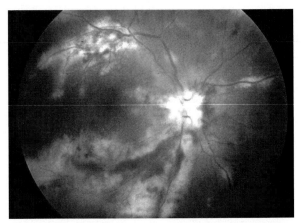

FIGURE 5-2 ▶ CMV retinitis from a 30-year-old, HIV-infected male, with a CD4 count of less than 50/mm³, complaining of decreased vision and floaters. Funduscopic examination showed full-thickness retinitis with hemorrhage in the posterior pole of the retina. (Courtesy of Todd Margolis, M.D., Ph.D., Dept. of Ophthalmology, U.C. San Francisco, F.I. Proctor Foundation.)

several months, and CMV IgG persists for life. Humoral immunity does not prevent transmission from a seropositive individual because the virus becomes latent and has the potential for reactivation in the future. With reactivation, virus is again shed from the nasopharynx, urine, and throat and patients are usually infectious. CMV IgM may be positive during periods of reactivation. Perinatal transmission from otherwise seropositive pregnant women is well documented from reactivation of latent CMV infection.[4, 33, 34] Most patients with recurrent infection are asymptomatic. The factors that control reactivation of virus are not clearly understood.

Infant. Table 5–3 summarizes the diverse clinical manifestations of CMV disease in newborns. Like adults, the vast majority of infected infants will be asymptomatic at birth. Severe cases of CMV infection with associated multiorgan damage and fetal anomalies result, in most cases, from acute infection in a pregnant woman, and not from reactivated disease. Since the incidence of primary infection is low in pregnancy (1% to 4%), the majority of infants born with CMV acquire the infection from recurrent disease.

When symptomatic, the most common clinical manifestations of congenital infection include hepatosplenomegaly, jaundice, and a generalized petechial rash. These findings are characteristic of infants with classic CID. The rash of congenital CMV is generalized and typically purpuric, appears within a few hours to days after birth, and is commonly associated with thrombocytopenia. Neonatal morbidity has been as high as 30% in severe cases of CID.[35] The most common cause of death is complications from liver involvement with CMV. Chorioretinitis is a relatively common complication of CID, affecting 14% of infants.[36] Sequelae from chorioretinitis with congenital CMV include blindness, strabismus, and retinal calcifications.

Approximately 10% of patients with symptomatic infections at birth will develop more serious sequelae, such as optic atrophy, learning disability, and psychomotor and mental retardation. Similarly, 10% of asymptomatic newborns will eventually develop late-onset findings which may include hearing loss, mental retardation, spastic diplegia, dental abnormalities, and learning disabilities. Hanshaw and co-workers[37] prospectively followed asymptomatic infants who had serologic evidence of congenital infection (i.e., presence of CMV IgM in cord blood) and found a lower mean IQ and a higher rate of hearing loss in these infants compared with matched control subjects.

Congenitally infected newborns shed virus for extended periods of time, typically pronounced in the first 6 months of life, but shedding may last up to a year. Virus is commonly shed and easily cultured from the nasopharynx and urine of these infants. Co-infec-

TABLE 5–3 ▶	CLINICAL MANIFESTATIONS OF CONGENITAL CMV INFECTION

PRENATAL DIAGNOSIS
  Fetal hydrops–intrauterine growth retardation, polyhydramnios, fetal ascites
CLINICALLY APPARENT FINDINGS AT BIRTH
Most Common Findings
  Hepatosplenomegaly, petechiae, purpura, microcephaly, jaundice, hemolytic anemia, hepatitis, thrombocytopenia
Less Common Findings
  Chorioretinitis, optic atrophy, microphthalmia, cerebral calcifications, seizures, cerebral/cerebellar atrophy, interstitial pneumonitis, dental abnormalities, lethargy, hypotonia, hyperbilirubinemia, inguinal hernias in males; prenatal findings: intrauterine growth retardation, fetal death in utero, prematurity
LATE ONSET FINDINGS
  Mental retardation, hearing loss, optic atrophy, spasticity, dental defects, neuromuscular defects, learning disability, psychomotor retardation

tion with other viruses, such as HIV, affects the clinical course of both CMV and the co-infecting virus.[6, 32] In HIV-infected children who also had acute CMV, Nigro and colleagues[6] demonstrated significantly shorter mean survival times among infants who had evidence by PCR testing of CMV DNA compared to infants who had no CMV DNA detectable.

Infants also acquire the infection postnatally through ingestion of infectious breast milk,[1, 38, 39] through intimate contact with an actively shedding mother, or nosocomially from other infectious neonates and hospital personnel in the nursery. These infants are generally asymptomatic. Premature infants who require extensive handling by neonatal nurses, stay for extended periods of time in the nursery, and receive multiple blood transfusions are at significant risk for acquiring the infection. Postnatally infected infants present with milder clinical findings compared to congenitally infected patients. Using in situ hybridization techniques, Maeda and associates[40] demonstrated that congenitally infected infants lacked intracellular CMV-specific IE gene sequence compared to postnatally infected newborns who harbored high levels of intracellular antigen, suggesting differences in the pathogenesis of infection between these two groups.

DIAGNOSIS OF CMV INFECTIONS

Clinical diagnosis of CMV is not useful, owing to the large percentage of asymptomatic infections. In addition, the clinical manifestations of symptomatic disease in adults and infants are generally nonspecific. Even newborns with CID present with symptoms similar to other infections, such as those caused by *Toxoplasma gondii*, herpes simplex virus, rubella, and syphilis. Table

TABLE 5-4 ▶	METHODS OF DIAGNOSING CMV INFECTIONS IN WOMEN AND INFANTS

PREGNANT WOMEN, ADULTS, AND CHILDREN
   CMV-Specific IgG and IgM
   Virus isolation
   Detection of CMV DNA (PCR)
      (Sources: nasopharynx, throat, cervical secretions, semen,
         blood, urine)
IN UTERO/CONGENITAL
   CMV-specific IgM
   Virus isolation
   Detection of viral antigen (monoclonal antibody, shell vial)
   Detection of CMV DNA (in situ hybridization, PCR)
      (Sources: fetal tissue, chorionic villus samples, amniotic fluid,
         cordocentesis sample, cord blood sample at delivery,
         placenta)
NEONATAL/POSTNATAL
   CMV-specific IgM
   Persistently elevated CMV-specific IgG
   Virus isolation
   Detection of viral antigen (monoclonal antibody, shell vial)
   Detection of CMV DNA (in situ hybridization, PCR)
      (Sources: nasopharyngeal/throat swabs, urine, saliva/sputum,
         blood, cerebrospinal fluid, tissue biopsies, postmortem
         autopsied tissue)

5–4 summarizes the different methods of diagnosis of CMV in adults, children, and infants.

Women and Mothers. Diagnosis of acute infection in adults is usually made serologically. CMV-specific IgM becomes positive within a few days following acute infection, implies recent infection, but develops in only 80% of cases.[41] Presence of CMV IgG confirms previous infection to CMV but does not preclude infected individuals from transmitting the virus, owing to reactivated disease. Despite the availability of serology, virus culture is still the gold standard for detection of virus. The most common sites of culture include the nasopharynx, throat, cervical secretions, semen, blood, and urine. Detection of virus does not differentiate between acute and reactivated disease.

The development of the PCR has led to a myriad of maternal, prenatal, and neonatal tests for CMV.[9, 10, 39, 42–45] PCR has been applied to test for CMV in cervical tissue,[10] breast milk,[39] cerebrospinal fluid,[44] and brain biopsy specimens.[45] Furukawa and co-workers,[10] for example, documented CMV DNA in glandular epithelial cells, leukocytes, and endothelial cells from cervical tissue of infected autopsied organs, using PCR and in situ hybridization techniques. Other less common methods of detecting virus have been reported by Wang and Adler,[46] using salivary IgG antibodies to CMV glycoprotein B.

Fetus/Prenatal Diagnosis. Prenatal ultrasound findings of fetal hydrops, intrauterine growth retardation, polyhydramnios, and fetal ascites have been associated with intrauterine CMV infection but generally remain nonspecific and nonpathognomic for CMV.[47] Differential diagnoses for fetal hydrops with an infectious etiology include infections caused by parvovirus B19, syphilis, *Toxoplasma gondii*, and herpes simplex virus. The earliest attempts at prenatal diagnosis of congenital infection have involved virus isolation of CMV in amniotic fluid,[48] and detection of CMV-specific IgG and IgM in fetal blood samples.[49] PCR techniques have again revolutionized the prenatal diagnosis of CMV. Revello and colleagues[50] successfully detected CMV DNA in 10 of 13 amniotic fluid samples from pregnant women who had developed acute CMV infection, resulting in a specificity for CMV by PCR in amniotic fluid of 100%. Hogge and co-workers[51] compared virus isolation techniques and CMV-specific IgM in fetal sera to PCR in chorionic villus samples and found good correlation between non-PCR techniques and those based on DNA amplification.

Neonatal Diagnosis. Clinical diagnosis of congenital infection relies on detection of classic manifestations of CID. In decreasing frequency, the three most common clinical signs in congenitally infected newborns are petechiae, hepatosplenomegaly, and jaundice.[36] Congenital infection with CMV is confirmed by serologic testing of cord blood for CMV IgM or persistently elevated levels of CMV IgG.[52] Because IgM does not cross the placenta, detection of CMV IgM is diagnostic of fetal infection. However, among infected newborns, CMV IgM is elevated in only 80% of cases. Other nonspecific laboratory abnormalities include hyperbilirubinemia, elevations of liver transaminases, and thrombocytopenia.

As with adult CMV infections, virus isolation is the most specific test for congenital infection. The most common sites for sampling the neonate include urine and nasopharynx. The samples are then inoculated into cultured human fibroblasts. A viral cytopathic effect is observed with regular light microscopy several days later. Recent techniques are able to detect viral antigen by monoclonal antibody using a shell-vial technique for rapid diagnosis.[53] In this system, samples are usually read within 24 hours and reports show a specifity of 100%.

Detection of CMV DNA by hybridization and PCR has proved very useful in the diagnosis of congenital infection. Borg and co-workers[54] detected viral DNA in nasopharyngeal aspirates and urine of congenitally infected newborns using nested PCR techniques. Daiminger and colleagues[8] compared virus isolation and early viral antigen (EA) assay to PCR in detecting CMV from urine samples. Sensitivity and specificity of the EA assay were 85.5% and 99%, respectively, compared with viral culture. Positive viral isolation results correlated with the PCR assay in 88% of cases using primers from the IE gene region.[8]

Finally, examination of the placenta in congenitally

infected cases provides useful, though nonspecific, evidence of intrauterine infection. The characteristic cytopathic effects of CMV infection can be seen in placental trophoblast, with villitis and plasma cell infiltration on histologic staining.[55] CMV DNA has also been detected in the same specimens by PCR and in situ hybridization techniques.[55]

TREATMENT AND PREVENTION

Women and Mothers. Universal screening for previous immunity to CMV in adults and pregnant women is currently not recommended. The reasons for this include the following: (1) seroprevalence rates in most communities are high; (2) risk of seroconverting while pregnant is low (1% to 4%); (3) effective ways of preventing fetal or neonatal infection are lacking; and (4) immunity is not protective against mother-to-child transmission of virus. Treatment of symptomatic infections in women and mothers is usually symptomatic. Among immunocompetent individuals, the acute phase of infection is self-limited, and adverse sequelae are rare. Seronegative adults with HIV or AIDS, or who are recent recipients of multiple and frequent blood products or organ transplants, are at significant risk for acquiring CMV and developing severe complications. These individuals may benefit from prenatal screening for CMV serology. Hospital personnel, especially those who work with neonates, in day care centers,[56] and in dialysis units are at substantial risk for developing acute infection. Pregnant women who have been identified as seronegative should either avoid these environments or minimize close contact with infectious patients. Frequent handwashing and appropriate handling of potentially infectious bodily fluids (e.g., universal use of gloves) have been shown to be effective in minimizing nosocomial transmission of the virus.[57]

DNA polymerase inhibitors, such as acyclovir, ganciclovir, and trisodium phosphonoformate (foscarnet), have been the principal chemotherapeutic agents used in the management of CMV and its complications.[58–60] Prophylactic acyclovir, for example, has been used to reduce the incidence of acute infection in renal allograft recipients.[59] Boeckh and co-workers[60] recently reported the successful use of ganciclovir in the treatment of acute CMV in bone marrow transplant recipients by using the presence of antigen in the host as a guide to when treatment should be initiated.[60] Ganciclovir has been effective in the control of CMV-induced retinitis, pneumonitis, and gastrointestinal complications in patients with AIDS.[61]

There are currently no recommended vaccines that prevent primary infection with CMV among seronegative individuals. Plotkin and co-workers[62] reported the use of a live attenuated CMV vaccine (Towne strain) to prevent infection among renal transplant patients. In a randomized protocol, Adler and co-workers[63] utilized this Towne vaccine to determine whether administration effectively prevented seronegative women from acquiring infection from their children. They reported similar mean lymphoproliferative responses to CMV antigens between wild-type and Towne vaccine–induced infections. Finally, Harrison and colleagues[64] reported the experimental use of guinea pig CMV glycoprotein vaccine and showed reduced congenital infection rates in litters of immunized dams (18%), compared to the unimmunized group (48%).

Infant. Treatment of congenitally infected infants is generally directed at management of symptoms. In severe cases such as CID, antiviral agents have been used to control viral replication. In most cases, however, discontinuation of the drug leads to resurgence of viral activity. Snydman and co-workers[65] undertook a randomized, placebo-controlled, double-blind study to use CMV immunoglobulin (CMVIG) to protect premature uninfected newborns against infection. Among infants born to CMV-seropositive mothers, the rate of acquisition of virus in the CMVIG-treated group was 3.2%, compared to 12.5% in the placebo-treated group.

There are no approved vaccines that prevent congenital or neonatal infection. Prevention of spread appears to be the most effective method of reducing cases of neonatal infection. Proper isolation of congenitally infected newborns who shed virus in high titers and for prolonged periods of time is therefore vital once they are identified.

CONCLUSIONS

Cytomegalovirus is the most common viral cause of congenital infection in the United States, affecting almost 35,000 infants annually. The majority of adults, children, and newborns with acute infection are asymptomatic, making close surveillance of the infection difficult. In general, women of low socioeconomic status and who reside in developing countries carry a substantially higher risk of being infected with CMV than do those of high economic status. Regardless of economic status, the incidence of acute infection is highest during the first few years of life and during the onset of sexual activity among individuals.

Mothers acquire the infection horizontally from their infants, from other neonates, from household contacts, or through sexual transmission. Rarely, virus is transmitted through blood transfusions or organ transplants. Infants acquire the infection in utero (congenital infection) or postnatally through exposure of the newborns to infectious maternal fluids (e.g., breast milk, cervical secretions) or to other infected individuals (in the nursery, household, day care centers). The most severe cases of congenital CMV develop from women who acquire acute infection while pregnant, with the most common symptoms presenting as hepatosplenomegaly, petechial rash, and jaundice. Approximately 10% of symptomatic newborns develop late-onset and multiorgan complications, such as mental retardation, hearing loss, or learning disability.

During acute infection, viremia is typical and virus is commonly shed in the nasopharynx, urine, and genital secretions. CMV IgG and IgM develop within days. CMV IgG persists for life. Because CMV remains latent and reactivation is possible, seropositivity to CMV actually increases, rather than eliminates, the risk of horizontal and subsequently perinatal infection. Molecular biologic techniques, such as PCR and in situ hybridization, have significantly improved the sensitivity and specificity of testing for virus in infants. The same techniques have also been applied to adult infections.

Treatment of acute CMV in immunocompetent adults and children and in congenitally infected newborns is directed toward the symptoms. The goals of therapy using antiviral agents (acyclovir, ganciclovir, foscarnet) have been to suppress the replication of virus, prevent the spread of infection, and minimize the development of severe complications (e.g., in patients with CID or patients co-infected with HIV). Currently, no vaccines have been universally effective in preventing infection or transmission, although experimental vaccines in both human and animal models have been reported to reduce infection.

REFERENCES

1. Minamishima I, Ueda K, Minematsu T, et al: Role of breastmilk in acquisition of cytomegalovirus infecton. Microbiol Immunol 1994; 38:549.
2. Lang DJ, Krummer JF: Cytomegalovirus in semen: Observations in selected populations. J Infect Dis 1975; 132:472.
3. Alford CA, Stagno S, Pass RF, et al: Congenital and perinatal cytomegalovirus infections. Rev Infect Dis 1990; 12:S745.
4. Stagno S, Pass RF, Dworsky ME, et al: Congenital cytomegalovirus infections: The relative importance of primary and recurrent maternal infections. N Engl J Med 1982; 306:945.
5. Collier AC, Meyers JD, Corey L, et al: Cytomegalovirus infection in homosexual men. Am J Med 1987; 82:493.
6. Nigro G, Krzysztofiak A, Gattinara GC, et al: Rapid progression of HIV disease in children with cytomegalovirus DNAemia. AIDS 1996; 10:1127.
7. Kilani RT, Chang LJ, Garcia-Lloret MI, et al: Placental trophoblasts resist infection by multiple human immunodeficiency virus (HIV) type 1 variants even with cytomegalovirus coinfection but support HIV replication after provirus transfection. J Virol 1997; 71:6359.
8. Daiminger A, Schalasta G, Betzl D, et al: Detection of human cytogemalovirus in urine samples by cell culture, early antigen assay and polymerase chain reaction. Infection 1994; 22:24.
9. Xu W, Sundqvist VA, Brytting M, et al: Diagnosis of cytomegalovirus infections using polymerase chain reaction, virus isolation and serology. Scand J Infect Dis 1993; 25:311.
10. Furukawa T, Jisajki F, Sakamuro D, et al: Detection of human cytomegalovirus genome in uterus tissue. Archiv Virol 1994; 135:265.
11. Chandler SJ, Holmes KK, Wentworth BB, et al: The epidemiology of cytomegaloviral infection in women attending a sexually transmitted disease clinic. J Infect Dis 1985; 152:597.
12. Schopfer K, Lauber E, Krech U: Congenital cytomegalovirus infection in newborn infants of mothers infected before pregnancy. Arch Dis Child 1978; 53:536.
13. Pass RF, Little EA, Stagno S, et al: Young children as a probable source of maternal and congenital cytomegalovirus infection. N Engl J Med 1978; 316:1366.
14. Adler SP: Molecular epidemiology of cytomegalovirus: Viral transmission among children attending a day care center, their parents, and caretakers. J Pediatr 1988; 112:366.
15. Yeager AS: Transmission of cytomegalovirus to mothers by infected infants: Another reason to prevent transfusion-acquired infections. Pediatr Infect Dis 1983; 2:295.
16. Murph JR, Bale JF: The natural history of acquired cytomegalovirus infection among children in group day-care. Am J Dis Child 1988; 142:843.
17. Drew WL, Mintz L, Miner RC, et al: Prevalence of cytomegalovirus infection in homosexual men. J Infect Dis 1981; 152:597.
18. Shen CY, Chang SF, Yen MS, et al: Cytomegalovirus excretion in pregnant and nonpregnant women. J Clin Microbiol 1993; 31:1635.
19. Lang DJ, Kummer JF: Demonstration of cytomegalovirus in semen. N Engl J Med 1972; 287:756.
20. Monif GRG, Egan EA, Held B, et al: The correlation of maternal cytomegalovirus infection during varying stages in gestation with neonatal involvement. J Pediatr 1972; 80:17.
21. Stern H, Tucker SM: Prospective study of cytomegalovirus infection in pregnancy. Br Med J 1973; 2:268.
22. Weller TH: Serial propagation of agents producing inclusion bodies derived from varicella and herpes zoster. Proc Soc Bxp Biol Med 1953; 83:340.
23. Rowe EWP, Hartley JW, Waterman S, et al: Cytopathogenic agent resembling human salivary gland virus recovered from tissue cultures of human adenoids. Proc Soc Exp Biol Med 1956; 92:418.
24. Weller TH, Hanshaw JB, Scott DE: Serologic differentiation of viruses responsible for cytomegalic inclusion disease. Virology 1960; 12:130.
25. Ribbert H: Ueber proozoanartige Zellen in der Niere eines syphilitischen Neugeborenen und in der Parotis von Kindern. Zentrabl Allg Pathol 1904; 15:945.
26. Friedman AH, Orellana J, Freeman WR, et al: Cytomegalovirus retinitis: A manifestation of the acquired immune deficiency syndrome (AIDS). Br J Ophthalmol 1981; 67:372.
27. Muhlemann K, Menegus MA, Miller RK: Cytomegalovirus in the perfused human term placenta in vitro. Placenta 1995; 16:367.
28. Sinzger C, Plachter B, Grefte A, et al: Tissue macrophages are infected by human cytomegalovirus in vivo. J Infect Dis 1996; 173:240.
29. Griffith BP, McCormick SR, Booss T, et al: Inbred guinea pig model of intrauterine infection with cytomegalovirus. Am J Pathol 1986; 122:112.
30. Britt WJ, Vugler LG: Antiviral antibody responses in mothers and their newborn infants with clinical and subclinical congenital cytomegalovirus infections. J Infect Dis 1990; 161:214.
31. Lajo A, Borque C, Del Castillo F, et al: Mononucleosis caused by Epstein-Barr virus and cytomegalovirus in children: A comparative study of 124 cases. Pediatr Infect Dis J 1994; 13:56.
32. Kitchen BJ, Engler HD, Gill VJ, et al: Cytomegalovirus infection in children with human immunodeficiency virus infection. Pediatr Infect Dis J 1997; 16:358.
33. Ahlfors K, Harris S, Ivarsson S, et al: Secondary maternal cytomegalovirus infection causing symptomatic congenital infection. N Engl J Med 1981; 305:284.
34. Morris DJ, Sims D, Chiswick M, et al: Symptomatic congenital cytomegalovirus infection after maternal recurrent infection. Pediatr Infect Dis J 1994; 13:61.
35. Stagno S, Pass RE, Dworsky ME, et al: Congenital and perinatal cytomegaloviral infections. Semin Perinatol 1983; 7:31.
36. Boppana SB, Pass RF, Britt WJ, et al: Symptomatic congenital cytomegalovirus infection: Neonatal morbidity and mortality. Pediatr Infect Dis J 1992; 11:93.
37. Hanshaw JB, Scheiner AP, Moxley AW, et al: School failure and

deafness after "silent" congenital cytomegalovirus infection. N Engl J Med 1976; 295:468.

38. Numazaki K: Human cytomegalovirus infection of breast milk. FEMS Immunol Med Microbiol 1997; 18:91.

39. Hotsubo T, Nagata N, Shimada M, et al: Detection of human cytomegalovirus DNA in breast milk by means of polymerase chain reaction. Microbiol Immunol 1994; 38:809.

40. Maeda A, Sata T, Sato Y, et al: A comparative study of congenital and postnatally acquired human cytomegalovirus infection in infants: Lack of expression of viral immediate early protein in congenital cases. Virchows Archiv 1994; 424:121.

41. Stago S, Tinker MK, Irod C, et al: Immunoglobulin M antibodies detected by enzyme-linked immunosorbent assay and radioimmunoassay in the diagnosis of cytomegalovirus infections in pregnant women and newborn infants. J Clin Microbiol 1985; 21:930.

42. Studahl M, Bergstrom T, Ekeland-Sjoberg K, et al: Detection of cytomegalovirus DNA in cerebrospinal fluid in iummunocompetent patients as a sign of active infection. J Med Virol 1995; 46:274.

43. Souza IE, Gregg A, Pfab D, et al: Cytomegalovirus infection in newborns and their family members: Polymerase chain reaction analysis of isolates. Infection 1997;25:144.

44. Kohyama J, Kajiwara M, Shimohira M, et al: Human cytomegalovirus DNA in cerebrospinal fluid. Arch Dis Child 1994; 71:414.

45. Darin N, Bergstrom T, Fast A, et al: Clinical, serological and PCR evidence of cytomegalovirus infection in the central nervous system in infancy and childhood. Neuropediatrics 1994; 25:316.

46. Wang JB, Adler SP: Salivary antibodies to cytomegalovirus (CMV) glycoprotein B accurately predict CMV infections among preschool children. J Clin Microbiol 1996; 34:2632.

47. Watt-Morse ML, Laife SA, Hill SA: The natural history of fetal cytomegalovirus infection as assessed by serial ultrasound and fetal blood sampling: A case report. Prenat Diagn 1995; 15:567.

48. Davis LE, Tweed GV, Chin TDY, et al: Intrauterine diagnosis of cytomegalovirus infection: Viral recovery from amniocentesis fluid. Am J Obstet Gynecol 1971; 109:1217.

49. Lynch L, Daffos F, Emanuel D, et al: Prenatal diagnosis of fetal cytomegalovirus infection. Am J Obstet Gynecol 1991; 165:714.

50. Revello MG, Baldanta F, Furione M, et al: Polymerase chain reaction for prenatal diagnosis of congenital human cytomegalovirus infection. J Med Virol 1995; 47:462.

51. Hogge WA, Buffone GJ, Hogge JS: Prenatal diagnosis of cytomegalovirus (CMV) infection: A preliminary report. Prenat Diagn 1993; 13:131.

52. Fung JC, Tilton RC: TORCH serologies and specific IgM antibody determination in acquired and congenital infections. Ann Clin Lab Science 1985; 15:204.

53. Stagno S, Pass RF, Reynolds DW, et al: Comparative study of diagnostic procedures for congenital cytomegalovirus infection. Pediatrics 1980; 65:251.

54. Borg KL, Nordbo SA, Winge P, et al: Detection of cytomegalovirus using 'boosted' nested PCR. Mol Cell Probes 1995; 9:251.

55. Ozono K, Mushiake S, Takeshima T, et al: Diagnosis of congenital cytomegalovirus infection by examination of placenta: Application of polymerase chain reaction and in situ hybridization. Pediatr Pathol Lab Med 1997; 17:249.

56. Hutto C, Little A, Ricks R, et al: Isolation of cytomegalovirus from toys and hands in a day care center. J Infect Dis 1986; 154:527.

57. Adler SP, Finney JW, Manganello AM, et al: Prevention of child-to-mother transmission of cytomegalovirus by changing behaviors: A randomized controlled trial. Pediatr Infect Dis J 1996; 15:240.

58. Canpolat C, Culbert S, Gardner M, et al: Ganciclovir prophylaxis for cytomegalovirus infection in pediatric allogenic bone marrow transplant recipients. Bone Marrow Transplant 1996; 17:589.

59. Balfour H, Chace BA, Stapleton JT, et al: A randomized placebo-controlled trial of oral acyclovir for the prevention of cytomegalovirus disease in recipients of renal allografts. N Engl J Med 1989; 320:1381.

60. Boeckh M, Gooley TA, Myerson D, et al: Cytomegalovirus pp65 antigenemia–guided early treatment with ganciclovir versus ganciclovir at engraftment after allogeneic marrow transplantation: A randomized double-blind study. Blood 1996; 88:4063.

61. Collaborative DHPG Treatment Study Group: Treatment of serious cytomegalovirus infections with 9-(1,3-dihydroxy-2-propoxylmethyl) guanine in patients with AIDS and other immmunodeficiencies. N Engl J Med 1986; 314:801.

62. Plotkin SA, Friedman HM, Fleischer GR, et al: Towne-vaccine–induced prevention of cytomegalovirus disease after renal transplants. Lancet 1984; 1:528.

63. Adler SP, Starr SE, Plotkin SA, et al: Immunity induced by primary human cytomegalovirus infection protects against secondary infection among women of childbearing age. J Infect Dis 1995; 171:26.

64. Harrison CJ, Britt WJ, Chapman NM, et al: Reduced congenital cytomegalovirus (CMV) infection after maternal immunization with a guinea pig CMV glycoprotein before gestational primary CMV infection in the guinea pig model. J Infect Dis 1995; 172:1212.

65. Snydman DR, Werner BG, Meissner HC, et al: Use of cytomegalovirus immunoglobulin in mutiply transfused premature neonates. Pediatr Infect Dis J 1995; 14:34.

6

Varicella-Zoster

Marvin S. Amstey ▶ Pamela Gilmore

INTRODUCTION

Varicella and herpes zoster infections are different manifestations of the same virus. The primary infection produces highly contagious varicella or chickenpox, usually during childhood. Like all members of the Herpesviridae family, the virus remains latent in sensory root ganglia for a number of years. The same infection, reactivated later in life, is manifested as herpes zoster or "shingles." Shingles is most commonly seen in an older population or in immunocompromised patients. However, it can appear in early childhood if the primary infection occurred in utero.[1]

Varicella is usually a childhood illness, with 98% of cases occurring before age 20. However, in tropical and subtropical countries, varicella is more frequently a disease of the reproductive age group.[2] When women born in subtropical countries were compared to women born in the United States, their immunity was 84% and 95%, respectively.[3] This finding has potential consequences, when one considers the large migrant population to the United States of reproductive-age women who are susceptible to varicella infection.

EPIDEMIOLOGY

Chickenpox is a highly contagious disease; humans are its only reservoir. Varicella-zoster virus (VZV) is transmitted from person to person by droplets or aerosols from vesicular fluid or from secretions from the upper respiratory tract, which is also the site of entry for the exposed individual. Most commonly, the virus is spread through household exposure, and most susceptible individuals become infected. Ross and colleagues[4] have demonstrated that 96% of susceptible household contacts will be infected after two incubation periods. Noscomial spread of infections is well known, as is transplacental spread of the virus.

Varicella-zoster infections have a worldwide distribution occurring at all times of the year. There is, however, a slight prevalence in winter and spring. The peak age incidence of chickenpox is 4 to 8 years. Approximately 7% of varicella cases occur between the ages of 14 and 45, or about 150,000 cases annually.[5] There are approximately 1 to 7 cases per 10,000 preg-

nancies, for an annual total of 3,000 to 10,000 pregnancies complicated by varicella.[6] While only 2% of varicella cases occur after the age of 20, approximately 25% of the deaths from complications occur in this older age group.[7] From 1985 through 1990, there were nearly 8,400 hospitalizations for varicella infection and its complications.[8] The mean number of persons dying as a result of complications of VZV infection decreased from 106 deaths, from 1973 to 1979, to 57 deaths during the period 1982 to 1986. However, during the period 1987 to 1991, the mean annual number of VZV-related deaths increased to 92 for unknown reasons. In persons older than 14 years, the risk of death increases with increasing age, from 2.7 per 100,000 at ages 15 to 19, to 25.2 per 100,000 at ages 30 to 49 (personal communication, CDC).

MICROBIOLOGY

Varicella-zoster virus is a member of the alpha Herpesviridae family of viruses and only infects humans. It contains a linear double-stranded DNA with a molecular weight of approximately 100×10^6 daltons. The icosahedral nucleocapsid is enveloped and measures approximately 180×250 nm. Varicella-zoster, like most human herpes group viruses, produces latent infections in sensory ganglia by mechanisms that are as yet unclear; it is reactivated as shingles also by unknown mechanisms.

Varicella-zoster virus is cytopathic for a number of tissue-cultured cells and produces type A intranuclear inclusions. These inclusions are large acidophilic bodies separated by a halo from marginated chromatin material (Table 6–1). The best source of material for virus isolation is vesicular fluid from the skin lesions of this infection. Cytologically, this VZV produces large multinucleated giant cells containing the eosinophilic intranuclear inclusions described previously. The Tzanck smear, which stains vesicle fluid with Giemsa or Wright's stain, will demonstrate these intranuclear inclusions.

Viral antigen can be demonstrated by direct fluorescent staining of cellular material from fresh vesicles. However, serologic assays are used most commonly to demonstrate both IgG and IgM antibodies to VZV. The

TABLE 6-1 ▶	CHARACTERISTICS OF VARICELLA-ZOSTER VIRUS

Family
　Alpha Herpesviridae
Nucleic Acid
　Linear double-stranded DNA MW 100×10^6
Size
　Enveloped virus, 180×250 nm
Inclusions
　Type A intranuclear (single, large acidophilic inclusion)

IgM antibodies remain present for several weeks, while the IgG antibodies are theoretically present for life. The IgM antibody level sometimes rises with the clinical onset of herpes zoster, even though this is a reactivation of the original VZV infection. Complement fixation (CF) antibodies are present within 1 week to 10 days and reach a peak in 2 to 3 weeks. These antibodies tend to disappear with time. A large percentage of individuals will not have detectable CF antibody within 1 year after infection; therefore, this serologic test is too insensitive for accurate demonstration of immunity.

The most commonly used techniques for estimating the presence of antibodies are the enzyme-linked immunosorbent assay (ELISA) and the fluorescent antibody against membrane antigen (FAMA). The ELISA test requires several hours for completion, while the FAMA test is more labor intensive. More recently, the U.S. Food and Drug Administration (FDA) approved a commercially available latex agglutination assay that produces results within 15 minutes with adequate sensitivity and specificity. While the latex agglutination assay is generally as sensitive as the FAMA and ELISA tests following natural infection, it is not as sensitive in detecting antibody after vaccination.[9] All of these antibodies are present by the time the initial chickenpox lesions are beginning to heal.

The level of protective antibody by any particular test is not clear. For example, four women developed chickenpox during pregnancy even though they had antibody as measured by FAMA, ELISA, and latex agglutination. These authors concluded that the criteria for protective VZV immunity remains ill defined.[10]

PATHOGENESIS

The initial site of viral entrance is thought to be the respiratory tract. However, once virus gains entrance into the body, dissemination occurs rapidly by viremia and it is difficult to distinguish virus in respiratory secretions from virus shed from lesions in the respiratory tract.

Skin lesions start as a macule that proceeds rapidly to a papule, vesicle, and crust. All of the stages of the disease are present at the same time, which distinguishes chickenpox from other viral exanthems such as smallpox, in which there is an orderly sequence of lesions.[11] It is believed that the various stages of the skin lesions (i.e., "crops" of vesicles) are the result of viremic "showers." Patients are infectious from a short prodromal stage of 1 or 2 days until the lesions are crusted. Immunocompromised individuals are contagious for a longer period of time.[12] Patients are generally not infectious 6 days after the onset of chickenpox.[13] As with chickenpox, virus can be isolated from the lesions of herpes zoster for 5 days after onset.[14]

After clinical infection, the virus continues in a latent phase, incorporating itself into the dorsal root ganglia. The reactivation of the latent virus infection is manifested as a localized skin eruption that is usually limited to the skin area (dermatomes) of the distribution of one to three sensory root ganglia. Pain and paresthesias occur in the involved dermatome several days prior to the outbreak of the vesicular lesions and may last for months.

CLINICAL PRESENTATION AND EVALUATION

After an incubation period that varies from 12 to 18 days, a low-grade fever is followed within 24 hours by rash that begins on the face and scalp. The rash spreads quickly to the trunk, with less effect on the extremities. New "crops" of lesions continue to appear for 5 days associated with intense pruritus. The total number of lesions varies from just a few pox to almost confluence. Antibody begins to appear on the fourth day after the appearance of the rash, after which the infection begins to subside (Fig. 6–1). Unlike smallpox, the crusts are not infectious. The virus is considered contagious prior to the onset of rash, but this is difficult to prove because virus has not been isolated from respiratory secretions prior to the development of rash.[3]

Varicella produces a mild infection in children, but adults infected with VZV have an increased risk of hospitalization.[15] Adults frequently have pronounced symptoms and have more frequent episodes of headache, arthralgia, myalgia, and malaise. Zoster, on the other hand, tends to be self-limited and targets an older or immunocompromised population, as described earlier. Potential complications of varicella infection include cellulitis secondary to superimposed bacterial infection and central nervous system complications, such as cerebellar ataxia, Guillain-Barré syndrome, and aseptic meningitis. Varicella encephalitis tends to be more serious and can produce severe headache, vomiting, and decreased consciousness. The frequency with which these complications occur is very low.

The most frequent cause of hospitalizations in adults

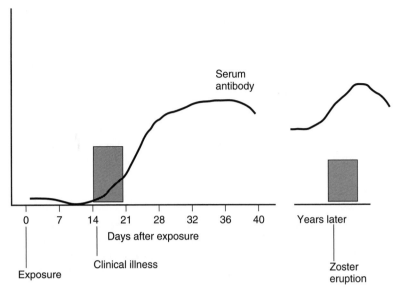

FIGURE 6-1 ▶ The clinical course of varicella-zoster virus infection.

with varicella is pneumonia. Mortality secondary to varicella pneumonia prior to adequate chemotherapy was reported to be as high as 40%. Pulmonary involvement usually occurs 2 to 6 days after rash appears and can progress to dyspnea, pleuritic chest pain, cyanosis, and hemoptysis. Chest radiograph often reveals a diffuse interstitial and peribronchiolar reaction with consolidation and hemorrhage. The intranuclear inclusions can be seen in the alveolar cells and endothelial cells, and elsewhere in the respiratory epithelium. A patient's pulmonary status may change drastically from an uncomplicated pneumonitis to that requiring mechanical ventilation. Antiviral therapy is necessary to reduce the pulmonary complications. A majority of immunocompetent adults recover from varicella with minimal sequelae.

VARICELLA AND PREGNANCY

Varicella occurring in pregnancy is significant because of the risk of more serious symptoms in adults. Varicella is considered more severe in pregnant women, but proof is lacking.[4] It appears that varicella in pregnancy is no more serious than that in the nonpregnant woman.[16] Approximately 14% of pregnant women will develop varicella pneumonitis, but pregnancy itself does not seem to increase this risk.

Maternal varicella infection can lead to fetal or neonatal infection by vertical transmission. The risk to the fetus depends on the timing of the infection. In most gestations complicated by varicella, the risk to the fetus is minimal and there are no reported abnormalities. Laforet and Lynch[17] were the first to describe a syndrome in newborns whose mothers acquired varicella in the first half of pregnancy. The latest gestational age of exposure in which the syndrome was docu-

mented was in the third trimester[16]; however, this is a single case, and most cases are from first trimester maternal infection. This syndrome, varicella embryopathy, is characterized by fetal growth retardation, hypoplasia of a limb, mandible, or chest wall, cicatrization of the skin, neurologic damage, and ocular damage[18]; some or all of these malformations may occur. It is estimated that 1% to 2% of infected mothers will deliver babies with varicella embryopathy.[15] A prospective study from the United Kingdom and Germany from 1980 to 1993 noted that when maternal infection occurred between 13 and 20 weeks, the embryopathy was seen in 0.4% of infected pregnancies, but in only 0.2% if the infection occurred between 0 and 12 weeks of gestation.[19] The virus has never been isolated from an affected neonate.

Ultrasonography may be useful in the detection of obvious structural abnormalities, but polyhdramnios may be the only finding. The use of cordocentesis to estimate fetal IgM antibody has been demonstrated,[20] and chorionic villus sampling has been used to diagnose congenital varicella infection by polymerase chain reaction. However, this technique may not truly distinguish maternal from fetal viral infection because of maternal blood contamination.[21]

A more common complication of maternal varicella for the newborn is related to the timing of the maternal infection relative to delivery. The newborn who develops varicella within 10 days of birth is considered to have acquired the infection in utero. This is deduced from the fact that the incubation period for varicella is almost always more than 12 days. Congenital varicella infection has been distinguished from neonatal varicella by this 10-day period and the fact that the most severe illness occurs in infants with congenital infection. However, there has been sufficient overlap between these two entities (congenital varicella and neonatal varicella) in severity and prognosis that one should think of them together simply as varicella of the newborn. The severity of the infection seems to be related to the amount of passively transferred antibody and therefore to the duration of the mother's infection. Thus, an infant born to a mother whose onset of disease is less than 5 days before delivery is at greatest risk for developing varicella of the newborn.[22]

The manifestations of congenital varicella include atrophy of an extremity, cicatrical skin lesions usually found on the affected extremity, cortical atrophy, and other neurological findings. Other prominent features include cataracts, microphthalmia, and Horner's syndrome. The largest series of cases was 4 found in 141 pregnancies followed prospectively.[23]

Varicella of the newborn acquired from nonimmune mothers occurs in approximately 50% to 60% of newborns.[24] Most of the infants had mild disease; however, 19 of 118 infants whose mothers had onset of varicella within 4 days before and 2 days after delivery had more severe illnesses, but no deaths. Interestingly, the severity did not relate to the treatment of these infants with VZIG. One of the explanations for this may be related to the amount of antibody in current lots of VZIG.[25]

ZOSTER IN PREGNANCY

This manifestation of VZV is less common and less serious for both the nonpregnant and the pregnant woman. It is estimated that about 6,000 cases of zoster infection occur in pregnancy annually.[26] Usually, the antibody to VZV is at a low level with the onset of "shingles" but rises rapidly owing to an anamnestic response. Therefore, babies born to women with zoster infection late in pregnancy or during delivery show no evidence of acute infection with VZV. On the other hand, zoster is highly contagious to a susceptible individual with chickenpox as the result of the transmitted infection.

Zoster occurs in young children who have never had chickenpox, but in almost every case varicella infection occurred in the mother during pregnancy. Presumably, the baby had its chickenpox in utero.[5]

TREATMENT

There is no need for treating uncomplicated varicella. It is almost always a self-limited disease; only in an immunocompromised host or when complications such as pneumonitis or encephalitis occur should antiviral therapy be considered.

Acyclovir is the prototypical drug that is effective against this and several other viruses of the herpesvirus group, such as herpes simplex 1 and 2. Acyclovir has less intrinsic activity in vitro against VZV than does herpes simplex, and generally larger doses are required for clinical varicella-zoster infections. The effectiveness of this drug is related to the availability of a specific (herpes simplex), viral-specified thymidine kinase. Human cellular thymidine kinases (or other viral-specified enzymes) are not nearly as good at activating acyclovir by a factor of several hundred.

Oral acyclovir for treating chickenpox in children was approved by the FDA in 1992 after placebo-controlled studies showed beneficial effects when acyclovir was given within 24 hours of the onset of rash. It reduced the duration and severity of the infection. Acyclovir did not reduce the transmission of the virus or the duration of school absences, nor did it reduce the complication rate; the same findings have occurred in clinical trials of adolescents and adults. Acyclovir is considered by the FDA as a class C drug for use in pregnancy, since the safety of this drug has not been established in pregnancy. Therefore, it is recommended that this drug not be used for uncomplicated varicella in pregnancy. To date, there have been no teratogenic effects in animal models.

On the other hand, the use of acyclovir is recommended for complicated varicella in pregnancy, that is, pneumonitis or encephalitis. Dosing recommendations are 10 to 15 mg/kg IV three times a day for 7 to 10 days. Dosing for infants with disseminated varicella syndrome can range from 500 to 700 mg/m^2 three times a day for 7 days. Intravenously, crystallization within the renal tubules occurs, which can lead to obstructive nephropathy, renal failure, and anuria. This renal insufficiency is completely reversible with discontinuation of the drug. The drug should be administered over a 1-hour period, and patients should be well hydrated and the volume of urine should be at least 500 mL/24 h; the blood urea nitrogen (BUN) and creatinine (Cr) levels should be monitored closely. Phlebitis at the site of injection can occur as a result of the drug's high pH; headaches, lethargy, tremor, seizure, and delirium have been reported. Drug concentrations, compared to maternal serum levels, are higher in cord serum, amniotic fluid, and placental tissue. In collections of cases and in anecdotal reports, acyclovir appears safe for the developing fetus; no substantial adverse effects have been reported.

Sorivudine is a new antiviral drug effective against VZV[24] with activity 1,000 times greater than that of acyclovir.[28] In a randomized, placebo-controlled trial, it was effective in shortening the mean time to lesion crusting and in shortening the duration of viral shedding. In contrast to acyclovir, which must be started within 24 hours of the onset of rash, sorivudine was effective even up to 96 hours after the onset of rash.[29] There is currently no experience with this drug in pregnancy.

PREVENTION

Passive Prevention with Varicella-Zoster Immune Globulin (VZIG)

VZIG is a 10% to 18% solution of the globulin fraction from human plasma. The processing of VZIG eliminates hepatitis B virus, human immunodeficiency virus (HIV), and other infectious agents. VZIG tests negative for hepatitis C RNA by the polymerase chain reaction.

Varicella-zoster immune globulin should be offered only to individuals who are seronegative for VZV. A positive history of chickenpox is a sensitive method of determining immunity. Without a history, serologic testing is necessary for determining the presence or absence of antibody. VZIG should be offered to the following individuals if they are susceptible: immunocompromised women, newborns born to mothers who developed the disease within 5 days before delivery or within 48 hours after delivery, and premature infants. Premature infants with birth weights less than 1,000 g or who are less than 28 weeks will require VZIG, whereas infants born after 28 weeks should have protective antibodies. Table 6-2 illustrates the exposure criteria for the use of VZIG.

Pregnant women who are susceptible and have significant exposure are also candidates for VZIG. This immune globulin has been used to modify the infection in pregnant women; however, there are no data demonstrating clearly that the maternal risk of complications from varicella is reduced by VZIG. There is no evidence that administration of VZIG will prevent viremia, fetal infection, varicella embryopathy, or congenital or neonatal varicella. The purpose of VZIG therapy is to prevent serious complications in seronegative pregnant women. Administration of VZIG extends the incubation period to 28 days; thus, if it is administered during the last month of pregnancy, neonates born to these mothers should receive VZIG also.

VZIG must be administered within 96 hours of exposure if it is to be effective.

VZIG is available through the American Red Cross. Adult dosages are 125 U/10 kg of body weight, to a maximum dose of 625 U (5 vials) by intramuscular injection. In the neonate, only one 125-U vial is required. The effectiveness of VZIG is greatest when it is given within 96 hours of exposure. The product is safe,

TABLE 6-2 ▶ EXPOSURE CRITERIA FOR USE OF VZIG
Continuous household contact
Playmate contact >1 hour indoors
Hospital contact—adjacent bed or infected staff member
Newborn of infected mother—from 5 days before to 2 days after delivery
AND
Time lapse from exposure is less than 96 hours

TABLE 6-3 ▶ INDICATIONS FOR USING VZIG
Susceptible to varicella-zoster virus
Significant exposure (see Table 6-2)
<15 years of age, or immunocompromised; e.g., leukemia or lymphoma, congenital or acquired immunodeficiency, immunosuppressive therapy
Newborn whose mother had onset of varicella 5 days before or 2 days after delivery
Premature, <28 weeks of gestation

but it can produce pain plus swelling at the injection site and, occasionally, constitutional symptoms. Table 6-3 summarizes the indications for the use of VZIG.

Active Prevention with Live Attenuated Varicella Virus Vaccine

Varivax, the live attenuated varicella vaccine, was approved for use in the United States in March 1995. A similar vaccine has been used for more than 10 years in Europe and Japan and has shown to be effective. In studies by the manufacturer involving healthy children, 98.8% had persistent antibodies at 1 year after one injection, and 99.5% had antibodies at a 4-year follow-up. In adolescents and adults who received two doses at scheduled intervals, 97% had persistence of antibody after 1 year. The question of duration of protection after vaccination in the absence of wild-type boosting is unknown at this time.[30] However, Gershon[31] has shown the persistence of antibody after 10 years in 95% of healthy children and 75% of vaccinated adults.

Varivax is recommended for individuals 12 months of age and older. It is administered subcutaneously as a single 0.5-mL dose in children. Adults and adolescents should receive two 0.5-mL subcutaneous doses 4 to 8 weeks apart. Following administration of Varivax, close contact with susceptible individuals should be avoided because there has been some suggestion that vaccine virus can be transmitted.

The risk of developing zoster after vaccination has also been examined. There appears to be no increased risk of developing zoster infection after the vaccine administration than after natural exposure to wild virus. Studies of children with leukemia show that the rate of developing herpes zoster is lower after vaccination.[32] The risk of developing herpes zoster was higher only if the vaccinated individual had a history of rash after vaccination, suggesting that virus may establish latency only if it has access to sensory nerves in skin. Since vaccination rarely produces skin infection, the virus is unable to establish itself in the dorsal root ganglia. Some researchers also suggest that because the virus is attenuated and not as virulent, it is unable to produce a dormant form that could reactivate.

Varivax is contraindicated in anyone who has a hypersensitivity to any of the components of the vaccine, such as neomycin or gelatin. It is contraindicated in individuals with hematologic malignancies or immunodeficiency states, and patients receiving immunosuppressive therapies. It is contraindicated in active infectious states and should not be administered to pregnant women, since fetal risks are unknown. Also, women should avoid pregnancy for 3 month after vaccination. Varivax should not be administered for approximately 5 months following receipt of blood, plasma, or immunoglobulin. Salicylates should be avoided for 6 weeks after vaccination because of the potential risks of Reye's syndrome.

Adverse effects have been reported following administration of Varivax; the most frequent symptoms include pain at the injection site, rashes, and fever. Rarely have severe complications been reported.

Routine use of this vaccine should reduce the number of susceptible pregnant women over time; however, the reality of our vaccination record suggests that we will not achieve universal vaccination. The immunity provided by wild virus infection in childhood will be diminished so that there will be a larger pool of susceptible childbearing women in the coming decades. This projection means that the future risk of seeing more varicella infections in adults—and particularly pregnant women—will be higher than it currently is.

REFERENCES

1. Dworsky M, Whitley RL, Alford CA: Herpes zoster in early infancy. Am J Dis Child 1982; 134:618.
2. Matetric Z, Couray MPM: Comparison between chickenpox in a tropical and a European country. J Trop Med Hyg 1963; 66:311.
3. Gershon AA, Raker R, Steinberg S, et al: Antibody to varicella-zoster virus in parturient women and their offspring during the first year of life. Pediatrics 1976; 58:692.
4. Ross AH, Lenchver E, Reitman G: Modification of chickenpox in family contacts by administration of gamma globulin. N Engl J Med 1962; 267:369.
5. Brunell PA: Varicella in pregnancy, the fetus, and the newborn: Problems in management. J Infect Dis 1992; 166(suppl 1):s42.
6. Freij BJ, Sever JL: Varicella. In: Queenan JT, Hobbins JC (eds): Protocols for High Risk Pregnancies, 3rd ed. Cambridge, MA, Blackwell Science, pp 387–397.
7. Centers for Disease Control: Varicella-zoster immune globulin for prevention of chickenpox. Ann Intern Med 1984; 100:859.
8. Personal communication, Merck Vaccine Division.
9. Steinberg SP, Gershon AA: Measurement of antibodies to varicella-zoster virus using the latex agglutination test. J Clin Microbiol 1991; 29:527.
10. Martin KA, Junker AK, Thomas EE, et al: Occurrence of chickenpox during pregnancy in women seropositive for varicella-zoster virus. J Infect Dis 1994; 170:991.
11. Gershon AA, LaRussa P: Varicella-zoster virus infections. In: S Krugman, et al (eds). Infectious Diseases of Children, 9th ed. St. Louis, Mosby, 1993, pp 586–614.
12. Gershon AA, Steinberg S, Brunell PA: Zoster immune globulin. N Engl J Med 1974; 290:243.
13. Thomson FH: Contact infection of chickenpox. Lancet 1991; 1:397.
14. Ribble JC: Chickenpox (varicella) and herpes zoster. In: Harrison's Principles of Internal Medicine, 7th ed. Wintrobe MM, et al (eds): New York, McGraw-Hill, 1974, pp 969–972.
15. Guess HA, Broughton DD, Melton CJ, et al: Population-based studies of varicella complications. Pediatrics 1986; 78:723.
16. Steiner G, Forsgren M, Erickson E, et al: Varicella-zoster infections in late pregnancy. Scand J Infect Dis Suppl. 1990; 71:30.
17. Laforet EG, Lynch CL: Multiple congenital defects following maternal varicella. N Engl J Med 1947; 236:534.
18. Brunell PA: Fetal and neonatal varicella-zoster infections. In: Amstey M (ed): Virus Infection in Pregnancy, New York, Harcourt Brace Jovanovich, 1984, pp 131–145.
19. Enders G, Miller E, Cradock-Wilson J, et al: Consequences of varicella and herpes zoster in pregnancy: Prospective study of 1739 cases. Lancet 1994; 343:1547.
20. Cuthhertson G, Weiner CP, Giller RH, et al: Prenatal diagnosis of 2nd trimester congenital varicella syndrome by virus specific immunoglobulin M. J Pediatr 1987; 111:592.
21. Amstey MS: Identification of varicella-zoster virus infection (letter). Am J Obstet Gynecol 1992; 167:1480.
22. Myers JD: Congenital varicella in term infants: Risk considered. J Infect Dis 1974; 129:215.
23. Enders G: Management of varicella-zoster contact and infection in pregnancy using a standardized varicella-zoster ELISA test. Postgrad Med J 1985; 61:23.
24. Miller E, Watson-Cradock JE, Ridehalgh MKS: Outcome in newborn babies given anti–varicella-zoster immunoglobulin after perinatal maternal infection with varicella-zoster virus. Lancet 1989; 2:371.
25. Lipton SV, Brunell PA: Management of varicella exposure in neonatal intensive care unit. JAMA 1989; 26:1782.
26. Brazan SA, Simkorrch JW, Johnson WT: Herpes zoster during pregnancy. Obstet Gynecol 1979; 53:175.
27. Gramm JW: New antivirals with activity against varicella-zoster virus. Ann Neurol 1994; 34:s69.
28. Machida H, Watanabe Y: Inhibition of DNA synthesis in varicella-zoster virus–infected cells by BV-araU. Microbiol Immunol 1991; 35:139.
29. Wallace MR, Chamberlin CJ, Sawyer MM, et al: Treatment of adult varicella with sorivudine: A randomized, placebo-controlled trial. J Infect Dis 1996; 174:249.
30. Merck and Co., Inc. Varivax product monograph, 1995.
31. Gershon AA: Varicella vaccine. Is J Med Sci 1994; 30:482.
32. Hardy IB, Gershon AA, Steinberg S, et al: The incidence of zoster after immunization with live attenuated varicella vaccine: A study in children with leukemia. N Engl J Med 1991; 325:1545.

7 Parvovirus

STUART P. ADLER ❯ JAMES H. HARGER ❯ WILLIAM C. KOCH

NATURE AND CHARACTERISTICS OF PARVOVIRUSES

The Parvoviridae family of viruses are the smallest known DNA-containing viruses and encode for only a few proteins. Within the Parvoviridae family is the genus Parvovirus. These viruses differ from other Parvoviridae mainly because their genome replicates without a helper virus. Parvoviruses infect many mammalian species, but there is no cross-infection among species. Thus, the canine parvovirus infects only dogs, and not humans, and the human parvovirus does not infect dogs. Each mammalian parvovirus also causes a different illness in its mammalian host. Thus, parvovirus disease in dogs is very different from that in humans. The human parvovirus, called human parvovirus B19, is the only known parvovirus to infect humans, but this single virus causes a wide spectrum of both acute and chronic human diseases.

It was understood that parvoviruses caused illness in small mammals long before it was discovered that a parvovirus infected humans. In 1975, Cossart and colleagues[1] discovered parvovirus B19 in human sera while testing sera for hepatitis B surface antigen. They found several sera (one of which was encoded B19) that had small, spherical viral particles with many disrupted fragments and empty shells. They showed that this virus was not hepatitis B virus and that 40% of adults had IgG antibodies to the new viral antigen.[1, 2] The virus was subsequently shown by genetic and biochemical analysis to be a parvovirus. At first, parvovirus B19 was not associated with any specific disease. However, the availability of serologic tests for parvovirus B19 infection allowed testing of sera from patients, and this eventually led to the discovery of human disease caused by this virus.

PATHOGENESIS

Parvovirus B19 requires a mitotically active host cell for its own replication.[3] Parvovirus B19 can propagate only in human erythroid progenitor cells from bone marrow,[4] fetal liver,[5] peripheral blood,[6] umbilical cord blood,[7] and a few leukemic cell lines.[8] The cellular receptor for parvovirus B19 is a globoside, a neutral glycosphingolipid found primarily on erythroid cells, which is called the P blood group antigen.[9] This receptor is necessary for parvovirus B19 infection. Bone marrow from patients who lack the P antigen (p phenotype) cannot be infected in vitro with parvovirus B19, and those without this antigen on their red cells are immune to parvovirus B19 infection.[10] The tissue distribution of the cellular receptor explains the predominance of hematologic effects in parvovirus B19 infection. P antigen is also found on vascular endothelial cells, megakaryocytes, placenta, fetal liver, and fetal myocardial cells, a tissue distribution that may have implications for the pathogenesis of other parvovirus B19 syndromes.[9]

Parvovirus B19 infection kills erythroid progenitor cells in the marrow, near the pronormoblast stage.[4] This leads to an arrest of erythropoiesis.[11] Susceptibility to infection increases with cellular differentiation, and the pluripotent stem cells are spared.[12] Infected bone marrow cultures contain giant pronormoblasts, or so-called "lantern cells."[13] These large, early erythroid cells are recognized by their cytoplasmic vacuolization, immature chromatin, and large eosinophilic nuclear inclusion bodies. These cells are also in the bone marrow of infected patients.[14, 15]

The arrest of erythropoiesis by parvovirus B19 occurs in vitro. The addition of virus to erythroid colony assays results in inhibition of erythroid colony-forming units (CFU-E) and variable inhibition of erythroid blast-forming units (BFU-E).[16] This suppression is reversed by IgG antibodies to parvovirus B19. The virus has no effect on the myeloid cell lines (granulocyte-macrophage colony-forming units [CFU-GM]) but causes inhibition of megakaryocytopoiesis in vitro without viral replication or cell lysis.[17] Infection of such cells that are nonpermissive for replication leads to the accumulation of a viral nonstructural protein, NS1, that may itself be toxic to the cell.[18]

Parvovirus B19 crosses the placenta after a primary maternal infection. Fetal viremia occurs, and there may be hematologic manifestations.[19] The fetus has a rapidly expanding red cell mass, a relatively short red cell half-life, and impaired humoral immunity. Intrauterine infection occasionally causes profound fetal anemia and consequent high-output cardiac failure.

Fetal hydrops ensues, and then fetal mortality is high. There may also be a direct effect of the virus on the fetal heart, as evidenced by the presence of parvovirus B19 DNA in myocardial tissue from abortuses and supported by the tissue distribution of the P antigen.[9, 20]

CLINICAL MANIFESTATIONS IN IMMUNOCOMPETENT ADULTS AND CHILDREN

Since its discovery, parvovirus B19 has been associated with several diverse clinical syndromes. Recent understanding of the molecular aspects of parvovirus B19 infection has shed light on the relationships between these syndromes. Asymptomatic infection with parvovirus B19 also occurs commonly in both children and adults. In studies of large outbreaks, asymptomatic infection occurs in approximately 20% of serologically proven cases.[21, 22]

Erythema infectiosum (EI) is the most common syndrome caused by parvovirus B19. This is a benign illness, also known as "fifth disease" because it was the fifth in a numeric classification scheme of common childhood exanthems.[23] Although the numbering scheme is obsolete, the name "fifth disease" for EI persists. Anderson first proposed parvovirus B19 as the cause of EI in 1983, and subsequent studies confirmed this.[22, 24, 25]

In children, EI begins with a mild prodromal phase consisting of low-grade fever, headache, malaise, and upper respiratory tract symptoms. This prodrome may be so mild that it goes unnoticed. The hallmark is the rash. The rash occurs in three phases, but these are not always distinguishable.[26] The initial stage is an erythematous facial flushing with a "slapped-cheek" appearance. In the second stage, the rash spreads quickly or concurrently to the trunk and proximal extremities as a diffuse, macular erythema. Central clearing of macular lesions occurs promptly, giving the rash a lacy, reticulated appearance. Palms and soles are usually spared, and the rash tends to be more prominent on the extensor surfaces. At this point, children are afebrile and feel well.

Adolescents and adult patients often complain of arthralgias concurrent with the rash. The rash resolves spontaneously, usually within 3 weeks, but typically may recur in response to a variety of environmental stimuli, such as sunlight, heat, exercise, and stress.[27] Lymphadenopathy may occur but is unusual. Atypical rashes not recognizable as classic EI have also been associated with acute parvovirus B19 infections, including morbilliform, vesiculopustular, desquamative, petechial, and purpuric.[27, 28]

Normal volunteers infected with parvovirus B19 develop a mild, biphasic illness, rather than an aplastic crisis.[29] Seven to eleven days after inoculation, volunteers develop viremia with fever, malaise, and mild upper respiratory tract symptoms. The reticulocyte counts drop to undetectable levels, but with a normal red cell half-life of 120 days there is only an insignificant dip in serum hemoglobin concentration. With the appearance of specific antibodies, symptoms resolve and the reticulocyte count returns to normal. Some volunteers develop a generalized rash 17 to 18 days after inoculation, and arthralgias coincident with the appearance of specific antibodies.

CLINICAL MANIFESTATIONS IN THOSE WITH ERYTHROID APLASIA

Transient aplastic crisis was the first syndrome to be definitively linked to parvovirus B19 infection. An infectious agent was suspected as the cause of the aplastic crisis of sickle cell disease because it occurs only once in a given patient, has a specific incubation period and duration, and occurs in clusters within families and communities.[27] Until 1981, attempts to find the infectious agent that caused the transient aplastic crisis repeatedly failed. Then, Pattison and colleagues[30] reported six positive tests for parvovirus B19 (seroconversion or antigenemia) among 600 admissions to a London hospital. All six patients were children with sickle cell anemia and aplastic crisis. This association was later confirmed by retrospective studies on the population with sickle cell disease in Jamaica.[31]

Unlike children with EI, those with an aplastic crisis are ill at presentation, with fever, malaise, and signs and symptoms of profound anemia (e.g., pallor, tachypnea, tachycardia). Rash is rarely present in these patients.[28, 32] The infection causes a transient arrest of erythropoiesis with a profound reticulocytopenia leading to a sudden and often life-threatening fall in serum hemoglobin. Children with sickle cell hemoglobinopathies may also develop a concurrent vaso-occlusive pain crisis that further complicates the diagnosis.

Any patient with disease causing a shortened red cell half-life and increased erythropoiesis can develop an aplastic crisis due to parvovirus B19. These diseases include hemoglobinopathies (e.g., thalassemia, sickle-C hemoglobin), red cell membrane defects (hereditary spherocytosis, stomatocytosis), enzyme deficiencies (e.g., pyruvate kinase deficiency, glucose-6-phosphate dehydrogenase deficiency), antibody-mediated red cell destruction (autoimmune hemolytic anemia), and decreased red cell production (e.g., iron deficiency, blood loss).[28] Parvovirus B19, however, is not a cause of transient erythroblastopenia of childhood (TEC), another condition of transient red cell hypoplasia that usually occurs in younger, hematologically normal children and follows a more indolent course.[13]

In addition to anemia, neutropenia and thrombocytopenia can also occur during an aplastic crisis, but the incidence varies. In a French study of 24 episodes of aplastic crisis (mostly hereditary spherocytosis), 35%

to 40% of patients were either leukopenic or thrombocytopenic, compared with 10% to 15% in a large American study (mainly sickle cell disease).[32, 33]

For patients with a transient aplastic crisis, the pathophysiology makes the syndrome understandable. In individuals with increased red cell turnover, infection with parvovirus B19 leads to a transient arrest in red cell production and a resultant precipitous fall in serum hemoglobin and hematocrit that usually requires transfusion. The reticulocyte count falls to nearly zero, reflecting the lysis of infected erythroblasts. Viral-specific IgM appears within 1 to 2 days of the peak of viremia, followed by IgG antibodies to parvovirus B19, and the infection is controlled. Control of the infection and the relative resistance of the pluripotent stem cells to infection contribute to bone marrow recovery, with a reactive reticulocytosis and a rise in serum hemoglobin.

A typical transient aplastic crisis may be the first symptom of an underlying hemolytic condition in certain patients. This is often the case for patients with hereditary spherocytosis.[33] The diagnosis of a typical transient aplastic crisis in an otherwise well patient should prompt a thorough hematologic investigation to exclude underlying hemolytic conditions.

CLINICAL MANIFESTATIONS IN THE IMMUNOCOMPROMISED/ IMMUNODEFICIENT HOST

Those with an impaired ability to produce antibodies can develop chronic and recurrent infections with parvovirus B19. Persistent anemia, sometimes profound, with reticulocytopenia is common and may be accompanied by neutropenia, thrombocytopenia, or complete bone marrow suppression. Chronic infections with parvovirus B19 occur in children with cancer who are receiving cytotoxic chemotherapy,[34, 15] children with congenital immunodeficiency states,[14] children and adults with acquired immunodeficiency syndrome (AIDS),[35, 36] transplant recipients,[37] and even patients with more subtle and specific defects in IgG class-switching who are able to produce measurable antibodies to parvovirus B19 but are unable to generate adequate neutralizing antibodies.[38]

Parvovirus B19 has also been associated with the viral-associated hemophagocytic syndrome (VAHS).[34, 39] This condition of histiocytic infiltration of bone marrow and associated cytopenias usually occurs in immunocompromised patients. Parvovirus B19 is only one of several viruses that have been implicated as causing VAHS. Thus, VAHS is generally considered a nonspecific response to a variety of viral insults, rather than a specific manifestation of a single pathogen.

EPIDEMIOLOGY AND TRANSMISSION

Parvovirus B19 is a highly contagious infection. In the United States, 60% or more of white adults are seropositive (have IgG antibodies to parvovirus B19 in their sera). This indicates a previous infection, usually acquired in childhood. Among black Americans, the rate of seropositivity is lower, about 30%. Transmission of parvovirus B19 from person to person is probably by droplets from oral or nasal secretions. This is suggested by the rapid transmission among those in close physical contact, such as schoolmates or family members, and by the fact that in a study of healthy volunteers, virus was found in blood and nasopharyngeal secretions for several days beginning a day or two before symptoms appeared.[29] In the volunteer study, no virus was detected in urine or stool.

Given the highly contagious nature of parvovirus B19 infections, it is not surprising that most outbreaks occur in elementary schools. Seronegative adult school personnel are at high risk for acquiring the infection from students.[40] Some outbreaks in schools may be seasonal (often late winter and spring) and epidemic, with many children and staff acquiring the infection and developing symptoms of EI. At other times the infection is often endemic, with transmission occurring slowly and only a few manifesting symptoms.

Other settings in which parvovirus B19 transmission is facilitated include the hospital and the family. Parvovirus B19 can be readily transmitted from infected patients to hospital workers.[41] Therefore, patients with erythrocyte aplasia should be presumed to have a parvovirus B19 infection until proved otherwise. These patients should receive respiratory and contact isolation while hospitalized. The family is another setting where transmission is rapid, although no intervention is generally necessary to interrupt transmission here.

RISK OF PARVOVIRUS B19 ACQUISITION FOR WOMEN OF CHILDBEARING AGE

The authors completed a large epidemiologic study to determine the relative risk of parvovirus B19 acquisition for women of childbearing age who are in daily contact with children, including nurses, day care employees, and teachers at all levels.[40] We identified risk factors for parvovirus B19 infections for hospital and school employees during an endemic period. Using serologic testing, we monitored 2,730 employees of 135 schools in three school systems and 751 employees of a hospital, all in Richmond, Virginia. A total of 60% were initially seropositive. After adjusting for age, race, and gender, risk factors for seropositivity (IgG antibodies to parvovirus B19) were contact with children 5 to 18 years of age at home (odds ratio = 1.2) or at work (odds ratio = 1.2), and employment in elementary schools (odds ratio = 1.4). Over 42 months (1988 to 1992), only 1 of 198 susceptible hospital employees seroconverted (0.42% annual rate), compared with 62 of 927 (2.93% annual rate) school employees (relative risk = 6.9). Four factors associated with seroconversion were employment at elementary schools (rate ratio = 2.2); contact with children 5 to 11 years of age at home (rate ratio = 2.3); contact with children 5 to 18 years of age at work (rate ratio = 4.8); and age less than 30 years (rate ratio = 1.9). Those in daily contact with school-aged children had a five-fold increased annual occupational risk for parvovirus B19 infection.[40]

The seropositivity rates the authors measured reflected parvovirus B19 infections among the study subjects prior to 1989. There was a marked association of age, race, and sex with seroprevalence. Age-related fluctuations in seroprevalence rates probably reflect prior epidemics of parvovirus B19 in the Richmond area. Assuming no racial effects on parvovirus B19 susceptibility or transmission, the fact that blacks had a lower infection rate than that of whites most likely reflects the racial segregation of children that has existed within the Richmond area schools and community for decades. The significantly higher infection rate for women, compared with men, may simply reflect that women, both at work and at home, spend more time with children. The 63% average seroprevalence rate for 2,730 school employees was similar to the 58% rate observed for 558 school employees in Connecticut before an outbreak in 1988.[42] For the Connecticut school employees, no association of age or sex with seroprevalence was detected.

Several observations indicate that parvovirus B19 infections were endemic—but not epidemic or pandemic—in the Richmond area during the 42-month prospective evaluation.[40] First, few cases of parvovirus B19 infection were reported by the school nurses, and no cluster of cases was observed at any single school or group of schools. Second, the seroconversion rates during each of three consecutive study periods were the same for all groups or subgroups. Third, for employees, parvovirus B19 infections were not clustered at individual or groups of schools. Fourth, the infection rates that the authors observed, even for those teaching elementary school, were less than those observed for the 1988 Connecticut epidemic in which 46 infections occurred among 236 susceptible individuals exposed in the schools, for a minimal annual infection rate of 19%.[42] Also, in a study of secondary parvovirus B19 infections among exposed household members, rates ranged from 30% to 50%.[43]

Parvovirus B19 infections are often asymptomatic or without a rash, and low-level endemics generally go unnoticed. The authors observed that 28 of 60 infected employees were asymptomatic, and only 20 knew of a specific exposure. In a study of 52 household contacts of patients with parvovirus B19 infections during an Ohio epidemic, infections without a rash occurred in 15 of 16 (94%) blacks and 17 of 35 (47%) whites, and completely asymptomatic infections occurred in 11 of 16 (69%) blacks and 6 of 30 (20%) whites.[43] During the Connecticut outbreak 5 of 65 (8%) teachers who were never exposed to a child with a rash became infected.[42] Thus, the observations of high rates of secondary attack during epidemics, and the high rates of rashless or asymptomatic infections, provide strong evidence that even during periods when EI is not apparent in the community, school or hospital personnel who come into contact with children have a significant occupational risk for parvovirus B19 infections.

Contact with elementary school–aged children, whether at home or at work, may be the most important risk factor for parvovirus B19 acquisition. When seropositivity for those patients with children at home was stratified by the child's age, the association between seropositivity and having children at home was significant ($P < .05$) when all children between 5 and 18 years of age were included, and for seroconversion the significant association was with elementary school–aged children at home.[40]

The low seroprevalence and seroconversion rates among hospital employees without known contact with children indicate that this group has a low occupational risk of acquiring parvovirus B19 infections. Parvovirus B19 is a known hazard for susceptible hospital employees exposed to patients with aplastic crisis, and secondary attack rates of 30% and 37% have been reported.[41, 44] Hospitalized patients with hemolytic anemias and fever or aplastic crisis should be in respiratory isolation, and pregnant women with unknown serologic status should not care for such patients.

In summary, the major conclusions from these studies are as follows:

1. When EI is inapparent in the community, school or hospital personnel in contact with children still have a significant occupational risk of parvovirus B19 infections.
2. Elementary school–aged children, whether at home or at work, are the most important risk factor for parvovirus B19 acquisition.[40]
3. Employees have an approximately two-fold greater risk of acquiring parvovirus B19 from children at work than from elementary school–aged children at home.
4. Hospital employees who do not have contact with children have a low risk of acquiring parvovirus B19.
5. Assuming that, on average, 50% of pregnant women are immune, that in endemic periods between 1% and 4% of susceptible women will become infected during pregnancy, and that the rate of fetal death following maternal infection may be as high as 5% to 10%, then the occupational risk of fetal death for a pregnant woman

with unknown serologic status will be between 1 in 500 and 1 in 4,000. These rates are so low that they do not justify intervention, such as serologic testing for pregnant women, and furloughing or temporary transfer of pregnant seronegative employees to administrative or other positions without child contact.

6. Knowing the parvovirus B19 infection rates during endemic periods may be more important than knowing the rates during epidemic periods. In the U.S., parvovirus B19 infections are endemic most of the time. Because more than 75% of parvovirus B19 infections are inapparent, the majority of women who acquire parvovirus B19 infection during pregnancy do so during endemic periods, not during epidemics. Therefore, for establishing public health policy and assessing the potential importance of immunizing against parvovirus B19, knowing that for seronegative women the endemic rate is between 1% and 4% is more important than knowing epidemic rates.

RISK OF PARVOVIRUS B19 ACQUISITION FOR PREGNANT WOMEN

The authors have also completed several studies to determine the incidence of human parvovirus B19 infections occurring during pregnancy. We used three strategies for estimating the incidence of parvovirus B19 infections during pregnancy:

1. Using the data from the study of school personnel, the authors are able to accurately estimate the average parvovirus B19 infection rate among pregnant school personnel.[40] Of the 60 individuals who seroconverted in that study, eight (13%) were pregnant. However, not all pregnant women in the school system participated in the study. Although we had data on the pregnancy rates for the female school personnel who participated, these volunteers may have been biased toward younger females, and therefore not representative of all school employees. Of the approximately 11,637 total school employees in Richmond, VA, the authors enrolled 2,730 (24%) in their study. Therefore, to determine whether the sample enrolled was representative of the entire school personnel population, we performed a survey (poll) of 733 school employees at schools studied. Schools were selected randomly by computer, and participants were selected randomly from the personnel working at each school. Compliance was more than 99%. The poststudy questionnaire, administered in person, included age, sex, race, number of pregnancies in the last 5 years, marital status, ages of

children at home, participation in the parvovirus B19 study, and job classification. The results (Table 7-1) show that volunteers were representative of the school personnel. Thus, we have strong evidence that the seroprevalence and annual infection rates observed among our study subjects are applicable to the entire school employee population. Assuming no seasonality to parvovirus B19 infections (none was observed) and that pregnancy does not affect susceptibility, we predicted that without regard to risk factors, seronegative pregnant personnel will have an average annual infection rate of 3%, or a 2.25% rate per pregnancy, and that 22% of all personnel will become pregnant in a 5-year period.

2. In Richmond, from 1989 to 1991, we collected sera from 1,650 pregnant women from a lower socioeconomic group who attended a high-risk pregnancy clinic for patients without medical insurance. Eighty percent of this group were black Americans, and the average maternal age was 24 years. We randomly selected a subset of 395 women for serotesting and monitoring, and 35% were seropositive. Of 256 seronegative women, 2 women seroconverted, for a 1.2% rate of seroconversion or an annual rate of 1.7%. This rate was similar to the rate observed among low-risk and black American school personnel in Richmond.[40]

3. We also collaborated with Dr. Sergio Stagno, who collected serial sera from a large number of private-practice obstetric patients. From this serum bank, we randomly selected 200 patients per year over 4 years (1987 to 1990) Of the 800 patients (average age 27 years and 88% white), there were no significant differences observed by year and, overall, 46% were seropositive (Table 7-2). Of 413 seronegative women serially tested, 5 seroconverted over 4 years. Overall,

TABLE 7-1 ▶	RESULTS OF A RANDOM POST-STUDY SURVEY OF SCHOOL PERSONNEL	
Characteristic	Study Population (n = 2730)	Post-Study Random Sample of all School Personnel (n = 733)
% female	90	83
% white	82	83
Average age	39 years	42 years
% married	74	75
% teachers	76	74
% pregnant in past 5 years	22.6	21.6
% participating in B19 study	100	27.5 (predicted = 24%)

From Adler SP, Manganello A-M, Koch WC, et al: Risk of human parvovirus B19 infections among school and hospital employees during endemic periods. J Infect Dis 1993; 168:361–368.

TABLE 7–2 ▶ PARVOVIRUS B19 INFECTIONS IN BIRMINGHAM, AL, FOR PREGNANT WOMEN BY YEAR OF FIRST SERUM SAMPLE*				
	1987	1988	1989	1990
No. of women tested	200	200	200	200
No. of seronegative women	85	103	113	112
No. seroconverting in pregnancy	0	1	2	2
Percentage of seroconversion	0	0.9	1.6	1.7
Annual seroconversion rate	0	1.60	2.75	2.80

*Authors' unpublished data.

1.2% of the women seroconverted. These women were observed for an average of 212 days, with an annual seroconversion rate of 2%, nearly identical to that observed in Richmond. Combining Richmond and Birmingham, we observed that 7 of 669 seronegative women seroconverted in pregnancy, for a rate of 1% per pregnancy with a 95% confidence interval (CI) of 0.3% to 21%. A recent South African study found that 64 (3.3%) of 1,967 pregnant women had acquired a parvovirus B19 infection during pregnancy, and another in Barcelona found that 60 (3.7%) of 1,610 pregnant women became infected with parvovirus B19 during pregnancy.[45, 46] Thus, our estimates may be low compared with other areas where parvovirus B19 may be more prevalent.

SYMPTOMS AND SIGNS OF PARVOVIRUS B19 INFECTIONS IN PREGNANT WOMEN

The symptoms reported by pregnant women in whom recent infection by parvovirus B19 has been serologically proved are typically vague and nonspecific, so there are no pathognomonic features that permit the diagnosis without serologic confirmation. It is important to realize that the signs and symptoms of classic EI in children are significantly different from those in adults: the classic sunburn-like "slapped-cheek" facial rash considered to be the hallmark of the exanthem in children rarely appears in adults. In contrast, malaise is a common feature of parvovirus B19 infection in children and in adults, but this symptom is so nonspecific in both groups that it is virtually useless in diagnosis, especially because pregnant women often report fatigue as a normal component of advancing pregnancy. In pregnant women, including pregnant adolescents, the most characteristic symptom is symmetrical arthralgias, occasionally with signs of arthritis, and usually affecting the small (distal) joints of the hands, wrists, and feet. We shall consider each of the reported symptoms and signs separately as clues to further serologic testing.

Asymptomatic Infection

First, the proportion of antiparvovirus B19-IgM-positive pregnant women who are entirely asymptomatic varies with the perspective provided by the inclusion criteria in the few studies that even address the issue. In a cohort of 1,610 pregnant women studied in Barcelona, 30 women were IgM-positive at initial prenatal screening and another 30 seroconverted during the pregnancy after being initially seronegative. Among this total of 60 women, only 18 (30%) reported any combination of fever, rash, and arthralgias, leaving fully 70% of the parvovirus B19–infected women asymptomatic. The authors did not report when questions about symptoms were asked in relation to the serologic results, and no comment was made about the distribution of symptoms, nor about which joints were affected by the arthralgias.[46] Similarly, during an epidemic of EI in Connecticut, fully 69% of nonpregnant antiparvovirus B19-IgM-positive adults were asymptomatic; but ascertainment of symptoms was by mailed questionnaires after the woman had been informed of her serologic results.[42, 47] In the British multicenter study, only 6 (3%) of 184 patients were asymptomatic, but the population was ascertained largely by recruiting women with typical symptoms, and thus is not comparable.[48] In contrast, we studied 618 pregnant women with known exposure to sources of parvovirus B19, and only 33% of the 52 antiparvovirus B19-IgM-positive women reported no symptoms of rash, fever, arthralgias, coryza, or malaise.[49] We questioned each exposed patient in our cohort about the symptoms before serologic testing, thereby minimizing recall bias; although the mere fact of known exposure could have increased their recall and led to over-representation of symptoms.

Malaise

Malaise, while a very vague and nonspecific finding, was reported by 27 (52%) of our 52 antiparvovirus B19-IgM-positive patients.[49] In contrast, only 5.5% of 307 exposed pregnant women with serologic evidence of previous parvovirus B19 infection (IgG-positive but IgM-negative) reported malaise; since they were essentially immune to parvovirus B19, some other illness or the pregnancy itself must be responsible for the complaint. Other reports of parvovirus B19 infections in adults rarely, if ever, mention such complaints from adults, although this symptom is often cited along with others in children with EI.

Arthralgias

Symmetrical arthralgias were the second most common symptom reported by our 52 parvovirus B19–infected patients, and other studies implicate distal arthralgias and arthritis as the most distinctive finding in adults with EI. The relative risk of arthralgias among nonpregnant adults in the Torrington, Connecticut, epidemic was 2.12 (P = .02) in the 11 of 46 (24%) IgM-positive subjects, compared with 61 of 512 (12%) of IgM-negative people.[42] Similarly, a parallel study in Connecticut revealed significantly more (P < .01) arthralgias in 5 of 19 (26%) IgM-positive adults but only 30 of 460 (7%) IgM-negative people.[48] In 618 known exposures to pregnant women, 24 (46%) of the 52 IgM-positive patients reported arthralgias, compared with 11 (3.6%) of 307 IgG-positive, IgM-negative women and 12 (4.6%) of 259 IgG- and IgM-negative women (P < .0001).[49]

The distribution of affected joints in pregnant women has not been reported before our recent paper.[49] Among the 24 IgM-positive women with arthralgias, the symmetrical joints most commonly affected by pain, swelling, and erythema were the knees (75%), followed by the wrists (71%), fingers (63%), ankles (42%), feet (29%), elbows (29%), shoulders (17%), hips (13%), and back and neck (8%). Only 2 of the 24 had only one set of joints involved, and very few other women reported monarticular pain or swelling. Arthralgias were almost always (N = 23) associated with malaise, and a rash occurred in 16 of the 24 women. Seven women had arthralgias with coryza, and seven had arthralgias with a fever. These arthralgias were easily controlled with anti-inflammatory drugs, and they usually lasted 1 to 5 days; but a few cases persisted for 10 to 14 days, and others were so painful that the woman was incapacitated for 2 to 3 days. Similarly, arthralgias were even more common among nonpregnant people during outbreaks in Ireland: they occurred in 79% of 47 anti-parvovirus B19-IgM-positive females and six IgM-positive males between 5 and 49 years of age, and 93% of those with arthralgias reported that their knees were involved.[50]

Rash

Maternal rash is less commonly observed in pregnant women than in children with EI, and the rash in pregnant women is not pathognomonic. We found a rash in 38% of 52 IgM-positive pregnant women compared (P < .0001) with 3.3% of 307 previously infected patients and 8.5% of 259 susceptible, uninfected patients.[49] In comparison, 91% of 184 women studied by the British Public Health Service Laboratory Working Party had a rash; but, again, this study found its patients predominantly through maternal symptoms.[48] In one report of the Connecticut epidemic, rashes were found in 6 (13%) of 46 IgM-positive cases, compared with 49 (10%) of 512 IgM-negative cases, whereas another report of the nonexposed community population there found rashes in 3 (16%) of 19 IgM-positive cases but only 33 (7%) of 460 IgM-negative cases

tested, a difference (P = 0.16) that seems appreciable but may represent random variation.[42] In contrast to the classic "lacy" truncal rash in children, the pregnant women often display a maculopapular (80%) pattern that rarely involves the face and may even be urticarial or morbilliform. In adults, these rashes are rarely pruritic and usually resolve within 1 to 5 days.

Coryza

Maternal coryza was reported by only 23% of our 52 IgM-positive patients but was seen in only 6.8% of the 307 previously infected women and 5.8% of the 259 seronegative cases.[49] This difference was significant at P < .0001, but the nonspecific nature of coryza in pregnant women afflicted with their typical upper respiratory tract congestion renders this symptom relatively useless as a guide to serologic testing unless it accompanies arthralgias and rash.

Fever

Maternal fever is also a relatively nonspecific symptom of dubious utility in the decision about serologic testing. We observed a maternal temperature ⩾ 38.0°C in 19% of 52 IgM-positive women exposed to parvovirus B19, compared (P < .0001) with 2.6% of 307 previously infected patients and 3.1% of 259 susceptible, noninfected patients.[49] In 9 of our 10 patients with fever, at least one other symptom was present; and none of the febrile pregnant women had temperatures exceeding 38.9°C. In the 16 IgM-negative patients with fever, all had at least one other symptom, but some of their fevers rose as high as 40.0°C, leading us to surmise that a higher fever (i.e., >39.0°C) in a pregnant woman should direct the clinician's attention to other infections. In a London outbreak of parvovirus B19 infection, 7 of the 10 IgM-positive adults had a fever.[44] In the Connecticut epidemic, fever was reported in 15% of the 46 IgM-positive cases but also in 16% of the 512 IgM-negative cases.[42] Clearly, pregnant women with fever are likely to be very concerned about the effect on their fetus of whatever caused the temperature elevation and thus will seek medical attention for diagnosis.

Fetal Signs

Occasionally, pregnant women infected with parvovirus B19 present with symptoms of rapidly increasing fundal height, preterm labor, or even symptoms and signs of preeclampsia. Such symptoms are rarely indicative of maternal parvovirus B19 infection and are too nonspecific to be good predictors of serologic testing, but these conditions are appropriate indications for fetal ultrasound assessment. If hydrops fetalis is discovered in that fashion, questioning about exposure to sources of EI or specific symptoms such as arthralgias is an essential part of the clinical evaluation. Further, serologic testing for anti-parvovirus B19-IgM should be an integral part of the evaluation of nonimmune hydrops fetalis.

INTRAUTERINE TRANSMISSION RATES AND FETAL OUTCOMES

Primary maternal infection with parvovirus B19 during gestation has been associated with adverse outcomes, such as nonimmune hydrops fetalis and intrauterine fetal death, asymptomatic neonatal infection, and normal delivery at term.[51, 52] Initial reports of fetal hydrops related to maternal parvovirus B19 infection were anecdotal and retrospective, suggesting rates of adverse outcomes as high as 26% and generating concern that parvovirus B19 may be more fetotropic than rubella or CMV.[54, 55] Subsequent reports of normal births following documented maternal parvovirus B19 infection made clear the need for better estimates of the rate of intrauterine transmission and the risk of adverse outcomes.[56, 57]

Fetal Outcomes

Prospective studies report rates of intrauterine viral transmission ranging from 25% to 33%.[48, 58, 59] These studies indicate that the risk of an adverse fetal outcome is less than 10% (probably much less) and greatest during the first 20 weeks of pregnancy.[28] A large prospective study in Great Britain identified 186 pregnant women with confirmed parvovirus B19 infections during an epidemic and followed them to term.[48] There were 30 (16%) fetal deaths in all, with as many as 17 (9%) estimated to be due to parvovirus B19 on the basis of DNA studies of a sample of the abortuses. Most of the fetal deaths occurred in the first 20 weeks, with an excessive fetal loss in the second trimester.[48] The intrauterine transmission rate was estimated at 33%, based on analysis of the abortuses, fetal IgM in cord blood, and persistence of parvovirus B19 IgG at 1 year follow-up of the infants. A smaller study of 39 pregnancies complicated by maternal parvovirus B19 infection and followed to term found 2 fetal deaths (fetal loss rate of 5%), one (3%) of which was attributable to parvovirus B19 and occurred at 10 weeks of gestation.[58] A prospective study conducted by the Centers for Disease Control and Prevention (CDC) identified 187 pregnant women with parvovirus B19 infection and compared their outcomes to 753 matched control subjects.[59] The overall fetal loss rate in the infected group was 5.9%, with 10 of 11 occurring before the 18th week of gestation, compared to a 3.5% fetal loss rate in the control group, suggesting a fetal loss rate of 2.5% attributable to parvovirus B19. In a prospective Spanish study during an endemic period,

1,610 pregnant women were screened for parvovirus B19 infection and 60 (3.7%) were identified.[46] There were five abortions among this group, but only one (1.7%) was caused by parvovirus B19 based on histologic and virologic analyses of fetal samples. The incidence of vertical transmission was estimated at 25%, based on serologic evaluation of the infants at delivery and at 1 year of age. In a similar prospective study of an obstetric population, 1,967 pregnant women were screened and 64 (3.3%) were identified as recently infected.[45] Among this group, no adverse effects were seen by serial ultrasound examinations and no fetal hydrops was noted; one abortion occurred, but the fetus was not examined for evidence of parvovirus B19 infection (maximal fetal loss attributable = 1.6%).

While the published prospective studies of parvovirus B19 infection in pregnancy have varied in their estimates of adverse fetal outcome and rates of vertical transmission, it is clear that the majority of women infected during pregnancy deliver normal-appearing infants at term. Among these infants, some will have asymptomatic infection.[60] A more recent prospective study that combined serologic with virologic markers of infection suggests that intrauterine transmission may be even higher.[61] In this study, 43 pregnant women with a confirmed parvovirus B19 infection were followed to delivery. The infants were tested at birth and at intervals throughout the first year of life for IgM and IgG to parvovirus B19 and also by polymerase chain reaction (PCR) for viral DNA in serum, urine, or saliva. No fetal losses or fetal hydrops were observed in this study; however, the rate of intrauterine viral transmission was 51%.

Other outcomes related to parvovirus B19 infection in pregnancy have been described rarely. There has been one case of congenital malformation due to parvovirus B19: an abortus with eye anomalies and histologic evidence of parvovirus B19 infection in other tissues.[62] However, from the studies to date, there is no evidence that B19 infection in utero causes an increase in the risk of birth defects among liveborne infants.[28, 57] Meconium ileus and peritonitis have been associated with maternal parvovirus B19 infection in a few reports.[51, 63] One case of fatal hepatic disease associated with in utero parvovirus B19 infection has also been reported.[64] Three infants with congenital anemia following maternal infection and intrauterine hydrops have also been reported.[51] All three had abnormalities on bone marrow examination and parvovirus B19 DNA detected in bone marrow by PCR.

While parvovirus B19 infection in utero may cause nonimmune hydrops fetalis, it is one of the many causes of this syndrome and probably accounts for only 10% to 15% of fetal hydrops.[65] Hydrops fetalis is rare, occurring in only 1 in 3,000 births, and in 50% of cases the etiology is unknown. In a study of 50 cases, parvovirus B19 DNA was detected by in situ hybridization in the tissues of four fetuses, while the majority of the cases were due to chromosomal or cardiovascular abnormalities.[66] In a more recent study, parvovirus B19 DNA was demonstrated in 4 of 42 cases of nonimmune hydrops fetalis.[67]

Data regarding the long-term outcomes of liveborn children infected in utero are very limited. Only one study has addressed this issue.[68] Several years after delivery, 113 pregnant women with parvovirus B19 infection during pregnancy and a control group of immune women were questioned about the health and development of their children when the median age of the children was 4 years for both groups. The incidences of developmental delays in speech, language, information processing, and attention were similar between the study group and the control subjects (7.3% vs. 7.5%). Of note, two cases of cerebral palsy were found in the study group, compared to none in the control subjects. Although not statistically significant, this 2% incidence of cerebral palsy in the infected group is 10-fold higher than the reported national incidence.[68] Large long-term, prospective studies are needed to further define the outcomes of children exposed to B19 in utero.

Fetal Immune Responses to Parvovirus B19

In studies in which both serologic and virologic markers of infection have been sought, fetal immune responses to parvovirus B19 were variable.[28, 61, 69] Parvovirus B19–specific IgM in cord blood is a recognized marker of fetal infection, but sensitivity can be increased by adding other markers, such as IgA, PCR positivity, and persistence of parvovirus B19 IgG at 1 year.[48, 61, 69] Infants exposed to parvovirus B19 earlier in gestation may be less likely to demonstrate a positive IgM response because of either immaturity of the fetal immune system or interference by passively acquired maternal antibodies. In one study, only 2 of 9 infected infants whose exposure occurred in the first 14 weeks of pregnancy were IgM-positive at delivery, whereas all 4 infected infants who were exposed in the last trimester had parvovirus B19 IgM in cord blood.[61] Serum IgA, like IgM, does not cross the placenta, so for some congenital viral infections (e.g., rubella and human immunodeficiency virus [HIV]) viral-specific IgA responses in cord blood are associated with intrauterine infection.[70] In the only study where this was examined, parvovirus B19 IgA in cord blood was associated with maternal B19 infection, and for a few infants this was the only marker of intrauterine infection.[61]

CURRENT DIAGNOSTIC TESTS

The diagnosis of EI in children is usually based on the clinical recognition of the typical exanthem and exclusion of other similar conditions. A presumptive diagnosis of a parvovirus B19–induced transient aplastic crisis in a patient with hemoglobinopathy is likewise based on compatible clinical findings, a severe fall in serum hemoglobin with an absolute reticulocytopenia. Specific laboratory diagnosis is often not necessary. This may pose a problem when the index case is a child whose mother is pregnant, as a specific diagnosis is needed to fully assess the mother's risk (see later).

Antibodies

Specific laboratory diagnosis depends on identification of parvovirus B19 antibodies, viral antigens, or viral DNA in clinical samples. In the immunologically normal patient, determination of antiparvovirus B19-IgM is the best marker of recent or acute infection on a single serum sample. Specific IgM antibodies develop rapidly after infection and are detectable for up to 6 to 8 weeks.[71] IgG antibodies become detectable within a few days after IgM do, and persist for years and probably for life. Seroconversion from IgG-negative to IgG-positive status on paired sera can also confirm a recent infection. Anti-parvovirus B19-IgG, however, serves primarily as a marker of past infection or immunity. Patients with parvovirus-B19-related rash illness or acute arthropathy are almost always IgM-positive, so a diagnosis can generally be made from a single serum sample. Patients with parvovirus B19–induced transient red cell aplasia may present before specific antibodies are detectable; however, IgM will be detectable within 1 to 2 days, and IgG will follow soon thereafter.

Seroconversion is the hallmark of asymptomatic infections with parvovirus B19 and, as noted earlier, many cases of maternal infection during pregnancy are totally asymptomatic following exposure to an infected contact. Still, the pattern described earlier will be observed in the immunologically normal patient; IgM will appear first, followed by IgG. The IgG response may continue to increase over a period of weeks and may reach very high titers, especially during pregnancy.[60] Persistence of low titers of IgM beyond the typical 6 to 8 weeks has also been observed in this patient group.[61]

The availability of serologic assays for parvovirus B19 has been limited by the lack of a reliable and renewable source of antigens for diagnostic use. The recent development of recombinant cell lines that express parvovirus B19 capsid proteins has begun to provide antigens suitable for use in commercial test kits.[72] There currently are a few commercial kits available for the detection of parvovirus B19 antibodies, but they employ a variety of different antigens (e.g., recombinant capsid proteins, fusion proteins, synthetic peptides). And their performance in large studies has been variable.[73] Until serologic tests are more standardized and results more consistent, some knowledge of the methods used and the antigens employed will be necessary for proper interpretation of specific test results.

Diagnosis in Immunodeficient Patients

In immunocompromised or immunodeficient patients, serologic diagnosis is unreliable because humoral responses are impaired, so methods of detecting viral particles or viral DNA are necessary for diagnosis. As noted, the virus cannot be isolated on routine cell cultures, so viral culture is not useful. Detection of viral DNA by hybridization techniques or by PCR is useful methods in these patients.[74–76] Both techniques can be applied to a variety of clinical specimens including serum, amniotic fluid, fresh tissues, bone marrow, and paraffin-embedded tissues.[28]

Histology

Histologic examination can also be helpful in establishing a diagnosis of parvovirus B19 infection in certain situations. Examination of bone marrow aspirates in anemic patients with parvovirus B19–induced red cell aplasia typically reveals giant pronormoblasts with a general erythroid hypoplasia. However, the absence of such cells does not exclude B19 infection.[77] Electron microscopy may reveal viral particles in the serum of some infected patients and cord blood or serum of hydropic infants. Pathologic studies of infected fetuses report leukoerythroblastic reactions in the liver and large pale cells with eosinophilic inclusion bodies and peripheral condensation or margination of the nuclear chromatin.[65] Parvovirus B19 DNA has been detected by DNA dot blot and in situ hybridization in fetal remains, and parvovirus B19 viral particles have been visualized in electron microscopic studies.[78–80]

Diagnosis in Liveborn Infants

Diagnosis of parvovirus B19 infection in infants should include serologic and virologic tests. Demonstration of parvovirus B19 IgM or IgA in cord blood is an indication of intrauterine infection, but false-positive IgM reactions to rheumatoid factor and to rubella can occur and should be excluded if the clinical picture is ambiguous. As noted earlier, since the fetal immune response can be variable, tests for viral DNA should also be included (e.g., PCR, hybridization). Reliance on serologic diagnosis alone may miss some infected infants.[61, 61, 69] Prenatal diagnosis of parvovirus B19–related hydrops fetalis is possible by testing fetal blood obtained via cordocentesis or amniotic fluid.[81–83] However, the decision to administer intrauterine treatment for hydrops fetalis should be based on clinical parameters, rather than on a viral diagnosis (see section on treatment).

MANAGEMENT OF THE WOMAN AND FETUS EXPOSED TO OR INFECTED BY PARVOVIRUS B19 DURING PREGNANCY

Since EI may be seasonal, occurring in the spring in temperate climates, physicians may be consulted about the exposure of pregnant women to parvovirus B19 from March through July; but sporadic cases of exposure and infection may occur at any time of the year. To manage these exposures and potential fetal parvovirus B19 infections, the clinician must follow a logical and complete algorithm for preventing fetal morbidity while minimizing the emotional and financial toll for the patient. This algorithm should include (1) knowledge of the prevailing status of EI in the community, (2) a detailed history of the exposure, (3) characteristic symptoms and signs of maternal EI and signs of parvovirus B19 infection in the fetus, (4) appropriate laboratory tests for confirming maternal and fetal infection, (5) methods of monitoring the fetus at risk for nonimmune hydrops fetalis, (6) therapeutic approaches for treating the hydropic fetus, and (7) the prognosis of maternal and fetal infection and the expected outcomes for the therapeutic interventions. In this section, we discuss these topics in that order.

Prevalence of EI

The public health department in the area may have knowledge of outbreaks of EI, but often it is the school systems where such outbreaks or epidemics are first noticed by school nurses or elementary school teachers. Health care professionals should maintain an increased level of suspicion for symptoms and signs of EI from March until July.[49] We have also observed that the increasing use of day care by working parents may lead to the persistence of outbreaks of EI throughout the summer months, as many family members of preschoolers are kept in close proximity with elementary school–aged siblings. This mechanism may prevent the subsidence of outbreaks that normally accompanies the end of school in June.

History of Exposure

Pregnant women who are suspected of having been exposed to EI should be questioned in detail about their exposure. The identity of the source contact and the duration and location of the exposure are important because brief outdoor contact is less likely to result in maternal parvovirus B19 infection than is prolonged, close indoor contact.[49] Face-to-face exposures with a source or handling of fomites contaminated with the respiratory secretions of preschool– or elementary school–aged children represent the closest contact and are the highest risk factor for susceptible pregnant women. The single greatest risk for a pregnant woman comes from children living in her own household, where 29.4% of susceptible pregnant women were probably infected.[49] On the other hand, brief contact not involving touching the potential source carries less risk, as does car pooling with other related or unrelated children. However, the duration of time spent in an enclosed automobile may affect the risk of parvovirus B19 transmission.

Since young children may develop a variety of upper respiratory tract symptoms with or without an exanthem, the nature of the illness in the source contact must be characterized carefully. Were typical symptoms of EI observed, including a low-grade fever and a typical slapped-cheek rash that soon spread to the trunk or limbs in a lacy pattern? Did the rash disappear and then re-appear when the child was warm from exercise or bathing? Had the child been exposed to any known source of EI, such as an outbreak in his or her school, preschool, or day care center, a family gathering, a play group, or a church nursery? Most important, was the child seen by a health care professional familiar with viral exanthems and dermatologic manifestations of allergic reactions? In our studies, we did not require serologic confirmation of a child's rash illness because experienced pediatricians can identify EI and other exanthems by sight, avoiding the trauma of drawing a blood sample from an uncomprehending child. The most difficult task faced by mothers of the source contact has been convincing their clinician that the child with a typical rash and mild symptoms must be seen at all; yet if the exposure can be determined to be insignificant, further testing can be obviated and pregnant women reassured and educated about avoiding future high-risk exposures through the remainder of the outbreak.

Similarly, exposure of pregnant hospital personnel to an adult source of parvovirus B19, such as another employee, or to a neonate presenting with idiopathic hydrops fetalis seems to carry a very small risk of parvovirus B19 infection.[49] Exposures from one adult to another do not usually result in maternal parvovirus B19 infection because of the greater care and cleanliness shown by adults with respiratory tract illnesses compared with young children.

Signs and Symptoms of Parvovirus B19 Infection

When the reason for concern on the part of the pregnant woman is derived from her own symptoms and signs, the physician must attempt to distinguish the relatively nonspecific signs of adult parvovirus B19 infection. In our prospective study of 618 pregnant women exposed to sources of parvovirus B19, we found that 67% of the 52 IgM-positive, parvovirus-infected women reported at least one symptom of malaise (52%), arthralgia (46%), rash (38%), coryza

(23%), or fever ≥38.0°C (19%).[49] In a serologic survey of 1,610 consecutive, unselected women in Barcelona, however, Gratecos and co-workers[46] found that only 30% of the 60 IgM-positive women recalled any such symptoms. The difference may be due to recall bias in the Barcelona patients, not remembering mild symptoms after the serologic results were available. Pregnant women expressing such symptoms, especially malaise with symmetrical arthralgias in the hands, wrists, knees, or feet, should be considered at high risk and good candidates for serologic testing.

Similarly, women lacking such systemic symptoms but presenting with signs of a rapidly enlarging uterus (fundal height exceeding dates by more than 3 centimeters), an elevated level of serum alpha-fetoprotein (MSAFP), preterm labor, or decreased fetal movement should be questioned about exposure to parvovirus B19 sources. They should be considered for diagnostic testing if ultrasound reveals evidence of hydrops fetalis. Further, women whose fetus is found to have any evidence of hydrops fetalis, such as ascites, pleural or pericardial effusion, skin thickening, polyhydramnios, or placentomegaly at any period of gestation, should be questioned about parvovirus B19 exposure and tested serologically for recent parvovirus B19 infection.

Laboratory Diagnosis in the Pregnant Woman

When there is any evidence of a significant maternal exposure to parvovirus B19, of maternal symptoms or signs of parvovirus B19 infection, or of fetal signs of hydrops fetalis, the diagnostic algorithm should be initiated. First, a maternal blood sample should be drawn for IgG and IgM antibodies against parvovirus B19. If the only indication is maternal exposure to a definite source of parvovirus B19, the first sample should be drawn at least 10 days after the exposure, to allow development of a sufficient titer of IgG and IgM antibodies to be detected. Fetal morbidity rarely occurs within 2 weeks of exposure, so immediate serologic testing should be reserved for a woman or a fetus already displaying symptoms or signs of actual parvovirus B19 infection. This strategy reduces both the financial cost and the need for multiple maternal blood samples. This sample should be sent to a reliable laboratory that keeps an aliquot of the serum sample for later testing, if it becomes necessary.

If a first sample is IgG-positive but IgM-negative (indicating previous maternal infection by parvovirus B19), there is no need for another sample to measure the IgG titer and detect a possible rise. The IgM assay is sufficiently sensitive that very few false-negative results occur in high-quality laboratories. If the serologic result is negative for IgM and IgG (indicating no previous maternal infection, remote or recent), the clinician can conclude that parvovirus B19 is not responsible for maternal symptoms and signs, nor for hydrops fetalis.

A negative IgM and positive IgG result suggests previous maternal parvovirus B19 infection remote in time, so the patient can be reassured that her risk of another significant parvovirus B19 infection is near zero. If the negative IgM result is accompanied by a negative IgG result, the finding suggests no recent parvovirus B19 infection; but the patient remains susceptible to parvovirus infection and should be counseled appropriately regarding further exposures (see later).

If the IgM result is positive, parvovirus B19 infection should be strongly considered regardless of the IgG titer. A concomitant negative IgG titer should be interpreted as early parvovirus B19 infection, with insufficient time for the later-appearing IgG to develop, but the same clinical management should be followed.[58, 84, 85] A second blood sample could be sent to another laboratory or even a reference laboratory, since commercial laboratories seem to have a high rate of false-positive IgM test results; but even if a negative IgM result is reported, it leaves open the question of which laboratory result to believe.[87]

With a positive IgM, then, the fetus must be assessed for signs of hydrops fetalis by ultrasound within 24 to 48 hours. If the gestational age is less than 18 weeks, the absence of hydrops may be reassuring; but hydrops could appear later and yet the only intervention possible before 18 to 20 weeks of pregnancy would be termination of pregnancy. Several case reports have indicated, however, that even severe hydrops fetalis may spontaneously revert to normal over a period of 3 to 6 weeks, so pregnancy termination depends on the wishes of the affected mother.[63, 85–88]

Fetal Monitoring

If the gestational age of the fetus exceeds 20 weeks, an initial negative ultrasound should be repeated each week to detect the onset of hydrops fetalis. The number of weekly ultrasound scans, however, remains controversial: Rodis and colleagues[84] originally suggested continuing weekly scans for 6 to 8 weeks after exposure. In that same paper, they reported a fetal death at 23 weeks of gestation after maternal fever and arthralgias "in first trimester," leaving an uncertain interval between maternal parvovirus B19 infection and fetal morbidity.[84] Based on this case, then, Sheikh and co-workers recommended continuing the weekly ultrasound scans for 14 weeks after maternal parvovirus B19 infection.[85] While the latter recommendation usually appeals to pregnant women fearful of fetal death, this approach requires many office visits, financial expense, and expert time to detect each case of hydrops fetalis due to parvovirus B19. While the first ultrasound scan to assess the fetus requires a complete fetal survey for anatomic anomalies and fetal measurements, subse-

quent weekly scans could be brief evaluations looking only for ascites, pleural or pericardial effusions, skin and placental thickening, and polyhydramnios. Such scans would require less time and, therefore, reduce financial cost while reassuring the patient.

The duration of monitoring for hydrops fetalis might be best determined by examination of the interval between maternal exposure or symptoms of parvovirus B19 infection and the appearance of hydrops fetalis or fetal death. Table 7–3 summarizes those reports with adequate information to evaluate the interval. Table 7–3 shows 14 intervals between maternal parvovirus B19 exposure/infection and fetal death and 7 intervals between maternal exposure/infection and the first diagnosis of hydrops fetalis. Taken together, the range is 1 to 19 weeks with a median of 6 weeks and 17/21 (81%) cases developed between 3 and 11 weeks. Eleven of the 21 cases developed between 4 and 8 weeks after maternal exposure/infection, so this range is the most common time for fetal hydrops to appear. On this basis, we continue to recommend weekly ultrasound monitoring of the fetus for 12 weeks after maternal exposure, realizing that such a protocol will not detect all unusually delayed cases and may be more expensive than some would advocate.

Depending on the incidence of hydrops fetalis in women with IgM-positive evidence of recent parvovirus B19 infection, such extensive scanning may not be considered reasonable or cost-effective by some. For example, our recent study found that none of the 52 IgM-positive women developed hydrops fetalis; and the 95% confidence interval based on that sample suggested a 0 to 8.6% risk for hydrops fetalis.[49] Yet other studies, using presence of maternal symptoms as the most common ascertainment criteria for maternal parvovirus B19 infection, have suggested a 9% incidence of fetal death due to parvovirus B19 in IgM-positive women.[48]

Serial maternal serum alpha-fetoprotein measurements have been suggested as a way to monitor the fetus in parvovirus B19-infected women.[89] Carrington and co-workers reported that elevated MSAFP was associated with fetal death (in utero) in five cases but that 11 IgM-positive women with parvovirus B19 infection but normal MSAFP values had no fetal deaths.[90] Anand and co-workers have described a fatal case discovered due to an elevated MSAFP at 16 weeks in a routine test on an asymptomatic woman.[53] In adding a seventh case of fetal death associated with elevated MSAFP in parvovirus B19-IgM-positive women, Bernstein and Capeless suggested using the MSAFP values to indicate a good fetal prognosis.[89] Currently there is insufficient experience using the MSAFP, however, and MSAFP measurements at any gestational age are relatively nonspecific indicators of fetal well-being. Since ultrasound scans are as readily available, equally as expensive, and

TABLE 7-3 ▶ REPORTED FETAL DEATHS DUE TO PARVOVIRUS B19 INFECTION

Reference Number (year published)	Infection–Death Interval (weeks)	Gestational Age at Fetal Death (weeks)	Fetal Weight at Death (grams)	Gender
51 (1984)	NR	19	320	M
52 (1984)	1	39	3,840	F
55 (1986)	NR	NR	NR	NR
	NR	NR	NR	NR
94 (1986)	10	25	NR	NR
90 (1987)	13	22	409	M
	4	20	161	M
95 (1987)	4	24	420	M
96 (1988)	NR	22	230	NR
97 (1988)	NR	23	600	NR
98 (1988)	4	26	695	M
	9	24	580	F
99 (1989)	7	18	300	M
89 (1989)	8	19	236	F
100 (1985)	1	4	NR	NR
	3	NR	NR	NR
	6	17	NR	NR
101 (1988)	NR	27	920	M
91 (1988)	NR	13	NR	NR
	NR	18	NR	NR
	NR	18	NR	NR
	NR	18	NR	NR
	NR	18	NR	NR
	NR	27	NR	NR
	NR	27	NR	NR
85 (1988)	10–19	23	NR	NR
	5	16	NR	NR
82 (1990)	(10)*	(11)†	Hydrops fetalis	NR
86 (1991)	(4)	(25)	Hydrops, 3,320	M
87 (1991)	(11)	(21)	Hydrops, 3,111	M
88 (1992)	(7)	(13)	Hydrops fetalis	NR
	(4)	(24)	Hydrops, 1,495	F
85 (1992)	(3)	(30)	Hydrops, 3,550	M
63 (1993)	(8)	(25)	Hydrops fetalis	Twins, one affected

*Number in parentheses refers to intervals between exposure or onset of symptoms and diagnosis of hydrops fetalis.
†Numbers in parentheses refer to gestational age at time of diagnosis of hydrops fetalis.
NR = not reported.

give instant, specific information about the presence or absence of hydrops fetalis, ultrasound remains the preferred method to monitor the fetus under these circumstances.

Electronic fetal monitoring (EFM) has not been shown effective in detecting hydrops fetalis nor in predicting the outcome of pregnancy in parvovirus B19-IgM-positive women. Contraction stress tests and "non-stress" tests are not accurate predictors of fetal well-being in cases of fetal anemia and/or hydrops fetalis, whereas ultrasound scans provide specific information about fetal status in these cases. Similarly, fetal assessment with estriol measurements or other biochemical markers have no documented role in cases of hydrops fetalis.

Fetal Therapy

If hydrops fetalis is detected before 18 weeks, there is no effective intervention available currently. Naturally, the mother should be assessed for other causes such as chromosomal disorders and the fetus for anatomic abnormalities responsible for hydrops. The fetus should be scanned again by ultrasound at 18 weeks and, if it is still viable, consideration given to percutaneous umbilical blood sampling (PUBS), also termed cordocentesis. At 18 weeks the umbilical vein diameter is about 4 millimeters, the minimum size required for successful PUBS. Fetal blood should be obtained for hematocrit, Kleihauer-Betke test, reticulocyte count, platelet count, leukocyte count, antiparvovirus B19-IgM, karyotype, and perhaps tests for parvovirus B19-DNA by polymerase chain reaction. The hematocrit must be determined immediately and, if fetal anemia is present, an intrauterine intravascular fetal transfusion performed with the same needle puncture. If anemia is not confirmed, another cause of hydrops fetalis other than parvovirus B19 considered in lieu of fetal transfusion.

If the fetus is already between 18 and 32 weeks of gestation at the diagnosis of hydrops fetalis, fetal transfusion should be considered and presented as an option to the parents immediately. There are at least seven successful reported cases of fetal transfusion for parvovirus B19–induced hydrops fetalis, but the infant follow-up is limited to a few months.[82, 91–93] In addition, unsuccessful attempts at fetal transfusion are not reported, so the success rate of the procedure remains unknown. Finally, reported cases usually required two or three separate transfusions to resolve the fetal anemia and hydrops fetalis, increasing the 1% to 2% risk of each single PUBS procedure; and resolution of the hydrops has required 3 to 6 weeks after the first transfusion. While several cases of spontaneous resolution have been reported in the literature, it seems difficult to advise parents prospectively that they should wait for such an uncertain outcome since the longer the fetal transfusion attempt is delayed, the less likely it is to be successful and the worse the potential harm to the fetus caused by continued fetal hypoxia.[63, 82, 85–88] More data are needed to clarify the risk factors for fetal death versus spontaneous resolution of the hydrops fetalis, but in the meantime an active effort to transfuse the fetus in utero seems most prudent.

If the fetus is ≥32 weeks when hydrops is discovered, immediate delivery with neonatal exchange transfusion, thoracentesis, and paracentesis as indicated is usually the safest management for the baby. If amniotic fluid has been obtained during a PUBS procedure to investigate the cause of hydrops fetalis, it could be tested for the level of fetal lung maturity; or maternal corticosteroid therapy could be employed to accelerate fetal lung maturation. In view of the critical condition of the hydropic fetus and the usual uncertainty about the progression of the condition, however, immediate delivery usually is the best alternative. The most likely exception would be a hydropic fetus ≥32 weeks found in a medical facility lacking a level III nursery: immediate corticosteroid therapy and maternal transfer to a level III neonatal intensive care unit would be essential.

Fetal Outcomes

From the beginning of any consultation with a pregnant woman, the clinician can reassure the patient about the relatively low risk of fetal morbidity resulting from exposure to a source of parvovirus B19 infection. Since approximately 50% (1/2) of women between 20 and 40 years of age will already be seropositive, the maternal parvovirus B19 infection rate ranges from 29% (3/10) for exposures by the woman's own children to 10% to 18% (1/40–1/6) for other exposures, and the expected fetal morbidity/mortality risk is around 2% (1/50), the overall risk of fetal death varies between a high of only 0.3% ($1/2 \times 3/10 \times 1/50 = 3/1000$) to a mere 0.1% ($1/2 \times 1/10 \times 1/50 = 1/1000$).[49] Discussing the risks using simple multiplication models has proved very reassuring in our hands, though many pregnant women naturally conclude that

they will fall into the unfavorable group. Most, however, respond positively to such low risks and feel much better knowing that these risk calculations have been prepared from individualized figures for their age, exposure source, and later serologic results. Those few women who are IgM-positive have proven to be very compliant with serial ultrasound scanning and grow more assured with each normal scan.

Prevention

In counseling seronegative women about avoiding future exposures, we emphasize that they should not disrupt their own children by sending them away since the value of a parent's care exceeds the small risk of parvovirus B19 to the pregnancy. Schools and day care centers cannot stop parvovirus B19 outbreaks by excluding children with rash illnesses because parvovirus B19 is transmissible before the rash gives the first sign of infection. We have not advocated removing pregnant day care workers or school teachers from their workplace even during outbreaks in the school, but some very concerned teachers have chosen to do so because of great individual concern. Clinicians should work closely with public health officials, school district administrations, and even the media to educate the public about parvovirus B19 epidemics and appropriate, measured responses.

FUTURE APPROACHES

With the exception of intravenous gamma globulin for the immunocompromised patient who develops a chronic parvovirus B19 infection and intrauterine transfusion for the fetus with hydrops fetalis, both of which are highly experimental, no other specific therapy exists for parvovirus B19 infections. Work is in progress on developing a parvovirus vaccine. Given the broad spectrum of disease caused by parvovirus B19, the large number of persons infected annually, the high rate of parvovirus B19 infection during pregnancy with high rates of intrauterine transmission, and the unknown effects on the live-born fetus, it is likely that an effective parvovirus B19 vaccine will be routinely administered in early childhood. Because specific therapy or other interventions are unlikely soon, a vaccine remains the best immediate hope for control of this ubiquitous infection. Finally, before it can be assumed that a parvovirus B19 vaccine is unnecessary for pregnant women, it will be necessary to demonstrate by careful prospective evaluation that parvovirus B19 infection of the fetus does not cause postnatal neurologic, hematologic, or other adverse sequelae.

REFERENCES

1. Cossart YE, Cant B, Field AM, et al: Parvovirus-like particles in human sera. Lancet 1975; 1:72.

2. Paver WK, Clarke SKR: Comparison of human fecal and serum parvo-like viruses. J Clin Microbiol 1976; 4:67.

3. Hauswirth WW: Autonomous parvovirus DNA structure and replication. In: Berns KI (ed): The Parvoviruses. London, Plenum Press, 1984, pp 129–152.

4. Ozawa K, Kurtzman G, Young N: Productive infection by B19 parvovirus of human erythroid bone marrow cells in vitro. Blood 1987; 70:384.

5. Yaegashi N, Shiraishi H, Takeshita T, et al: Propagation of human parvovirus B19 in primary culture of erythroid lineage cells derived from fetal liver. J Virol 1989; 63:2422.

6. Schwarz TF, Serke S, Hottentrager B, et al: Replication of parvovirus B19 in hematopoietic progenitor cells generated in vitro from normal human peripheral blood. J Virol 1992; 66:1273.

7. Sosa CE, Mahoney JB, Luinstra KE, et al: Replication and cytopathology of human parvovirus B19 in human umbilical cord blood erythroid progenitor cells. J Med Virol 1992; 36:125.

8. Shimomura S, Komatsu N, Frickhofen N, et al: First continuous propagation of B19 parvovirus in a cell line. Blood 1992; 79:18.

9. Brown KE, Anderson SM, Young NS: Erythrocyte P antigen: Cellular receptor for B19 parvovirus. Science 1993; 262:114.

10. Brown KE, Hibbs JR, Gallinella G, et al: Resistance to parvovirus B19 infection due to lack of virus receptor (erythrocyte P antigen). N Engl J Med 1994; 330:1192.

11. Young N: Hematologic and hematopoietic consequences of B19 parvovirus infection. Semin Hematol 1988; 25:159.

12. Takahashi T, Ozawa K, Takahashi K, et al: Susceptibility of human erythropoietic cells to B19 parvovirus in vitro increases with differentiation. Blood 1990; 75:603.

13. Brown KE, Young NS: Parvovirus B19 infection and hematopoiesis. Blood Rev 1995; 9:176.

14. Kurtzman GJ, Ozawa K, Cohen B, et al: Chronic bone marrow failure due to persistent B19 parvovirus infection. N Engl J Med 1987; 317:287.

15. Van Horn DK, Mortimer PP, Young N, et al: Human parvovirus–associated red cell aplasia in the absence of underlying hemolytic anemia. Am J Pediatr Hematol Oncol 1986; 8:235.

16. Mortimer PP, Humphries RK, Moore JG, et al: A human parvovirus–like virus inhibits haematopoietic colony formation in vitro. Nature 1983; 302:426.

17. Srivastava A, Bruno E, Briddell R, et al: Parvovirus B19–induced perturbation of human megakaryocytopoiesis in vitro. Blood 1990; 76:1997.

18. Ozawa K, Ayub J, Kajigaya S, et al: The gene encoding the nonstructural protein of B19 (human) parvovirus may be lethal in transfected cells. J Virol 1988; 62:2884.

19. Anderson LJ: Human parvoviruses. J Infect Dis 1990; 161:603.

20. Porter HJ, Quantrill AM, Fleming KA: B19 parvovirus infection of myocardial cells. [Letter.] Lancet 1988; 1:535.

21. Chorba T, Coccia P, Holman RC, et al: The role of parvovirus B19 in aplastic crisis and erythema infectiosum (fifth disease). J Infect Dis 1986; 154:383.

22. Plummer FA, Hammond GW, Forward K, et al: An erythema infectiosum–like illness caused by human parvovirus infection. N Engl J Med 1985; 313:74.

23. Thurn J: Human parvovirus B19: Historical and clinical review. Rev Infect Dis 1988; 10:1005.

24. Anderson MJ, Jones SE, Fisher-Hoch SP, et al: Human parvovirus, the cause of erythema infectiosum (fifth disease)? [Letter.] Lancet 1983; 1:1378.

25. Anderson MJ, Lewis E, Kidd IM, et al: An outbreak of erythema infectiosum associated with human parvovirus infection. Epidemiol Infect 1984; 93:83.

26. Cherry JD: Parvoviruses. In: Feigin RD, Cherry JD (eds): Textbook of Pediatric Infectious Diseases. Philadelphia; WB Saunders Co; 1992, pp 1626–1633.

27. Anderson LJ: Role of parvovirus B19 in human disease. Pediatr Infect Dis J 1987; 6:711.

28. Török TJ: Parvovirus B19 and human disease. Adv Intern Med 1992; 37:431.

29. Anderson MJ, Higgins PG, Davis LR, et al: Experimental parvoviral infection in humans. J Infect Dis 1985; 152:257.

30. Pattison JR, Jones SE, Hodgson J: Parvovirus infections and hypoplastic crisis in sickle-cell anaemia. [Letter.] Lancet 1981; 1:664.

31. Serjeant GR, Topley JM, Mason K, et al: Outbreak of aplastic crises in sickle cell anaemia associated with parvovirus-like agent. Lancet 1981; 2:595-97.

32. Saarinen UM, Chorba TL, Tattersall P, et al: Human parvovirus B19–induced epidemic acute red cell aplasia in patients with hereditary hemolytic anemia. Blood 1986; 67:1411.

33. Lefrere J-J, Courouce A-M, Bertrand Y, et al: Human parvovirus and aplastic crisis in chronic hemolytic anemias: A study of 24 observations. Am J Hematol 1986; 23:271.

34. Koch WC, Massey G, Russell CE, et al: Manifestations and treatment of human parvovirus B19 infection in immunocompromised patients. J Pediatr 1990; 116:355.

35. Frickhofen N, Abkowitz JL, Safford M, et al: Persistent B19 parvovirus infection in patients infected with human immunodeficiency virus Type 1 (HIV-1): A treatable cause of anemia in AIDS. Ann Intern Med 1990; 113:926.

36. Naides SJ, Field EH: Transient rheumatoid factor positivity in acute human parvovirus B19 infection. Arch Intern Med 1988; 148:2587.

37. Weiland HT, Salimans MMM, Fibbe WE, et al: Prolonged parvovirus B19 infection with severe anaemia in a bone marrow transplant recipient. [Letter.] Br J Haematol 1989; 71:300.

38. Kurtzman G, Frickhofen N, Kimball J, et al: Pure red-cell aplasia of ten years' duration due to persistent parvovirus B19 infection and its cure with immunoglobulin therapy. N Engl J Med 1989; 321:519.

39. Muir K, Todd WTA, Watson WH, et al: Viral-associated haemophagocytosis with parvovirus B19–related pancytopenia. Lancet 1992; 339: 1139.

40. Adler SP, Manganello A-M, Koch WC, et al: Risk of human parvovirus B19 infections among school and hospital employees during endemic periods. J Infect Dis 1993; 168:361.

41. Bell LM, Naides SJ, Stoffman P, et al: Human parvovirus B19 infection among hospital staff members after contact with infected patients. N Engl J Med 1989; 321:485.

42. Gillespie SM, Cartter ML, Sachs S, et al: Occupational risk of human parvovirus B19 infection for school and day-care personnel during an outbreak of erythema infectiosum. JAMA 1990; 263:2061.

43. Chorba T, Coccia P, Holman RC, et al: The role of parvovirus B19 in aplastic crisis and erythema infectiosum (fifth disease). J Infect Dis 1986; 154:383.

44. Pillay D, Patou G, Hurt S, et al: Parvovirus B19 outbreak in a children's ward. Lancet 1992; 339:107.

45. Schoub BD, Blackburn NK, Johnson S, et al: Primary and secondary infection with human parvovirus B19 in pregnant women in South Africa. S Afr Med J 1993; 83:505.

46. Gratecos E, Torres PJ, Vidal J, et al: The incidence of parvovirus B19 infection during pregnancy and its impact on perinatal outcome. J Infect Dis 1995; 171:1360.

47. Cartter ML, Farley TA, Rosengren SS, et al: Occupational risk factors for infection with parvovirus B19 among pregnant women. J Infect Dis 1991; 163:282.

48. Public Health Laboratory Service Working Pary on Fifth Disease: Prospective study of human parvovirus (B19) in pregnancy. Br Med J 1990; 300:1166.

49. Harger JH, Adler SP, Koch WC, et al: Prospective evaluation of 618 pregnant women exposed to parvovirus B19: Risks and symptoms. Obstet Gynecol 1998 (in press).

50. Kerr JR, Curran MD, Moore JE: Parvovirus B19 infection—persistence and genetic variation. Scand J Infect Dis 1995; 27:551.

51. Brown T, Anand A, Ritchie LD, et al: Intrauterine parvovirus infection associated with hydrops fetalis. [Letter.] Lancet 1984; 2:1033.

52. Knott PD, Welply GAC, Anderson MJ: Serologically proved intrauterine infection with parvovirus. Br Med J 1984; 289:1660.

53. Anand A, Gray ES, Brown T, et al: Human parvovirus

infection in pregnancy and hydrops fetalis. N Engl J Med 1987; 316:183.

54. Schwarz TF, Roggendorf M, Hottentrager B, et al: Human parvovirus B19 infection in pregnancy. [Letter.] Lancet 1988; 2:566.

55. Gray ES, Anand A, Brown T: Parvovirus infections in pregnancy. [Letter.] Lancet 1986; 1:208.

56. Brown T, Ritchie LD: Infection with parvovirus during pregnancy. Br Med J 1985; 290:559.

57. Kinney JS, Anderson LJ, Farrar J, et al: Risk of adverse outcomes of pregnancy after human parvovirus B19 infection. J Infect Dis 1988; 157:663.

58. Rodis JF, Quinn DL, Gary GW, et al: Management and outcomes of pregnancies complicated by human parvovirus B19 infection: A prospective study. Am J Obstet Gynecol 1990; 163:1168.

59. Torok TJ, Anderson LJ, Gary GW, et al: Reproductive outcomes following human parvovirus B19 infection in pregnancy. [Abstract 1374.] In: Program and Abstracts of 31st ICAAC (Chicago). Washington, DC, American Society for Microbiology, 1991, p 328.

60. Koch WC, Adler SP, Harger J: Intrauterine parvovirus B19 infection may cause an asymptomatic or recurrent postnatal infection. Pediatr Infect Dis J 1993; 12:747.

61. Koch WC, Harger JH, Barnstein B, et al: Serologic and virologic evidence for frequent intrauterine transmission of human parvovirus B19 following a primary maternal infection during pregnancy. Pediatr Infect Dis J 1998; 17:489.

62. Hartwig NG, Vermeij-Keers C, Van Elsacker-Niele AMW, et al: Embryonic malformations in a case of intrauterine parvovirus B19 infection. Teratology 1989; 39:295.

63. Zerbini M, Musiani M, Gentilomi G, et al: Symptomatic parvovirus B19 infection of one fetus in a twin pregnancy. Clin Infect Dis 1993; 17:262.

64. Metzman R, Anand A, DeGuilio PA, et al: Hepatic disease associated with intrauterine parvovirus B19 infection in a newborn premature infant. J Pediatr Gastroenterol Nutr 1989; 9:112.

65. Brown KE: Human parvovirus epidemiology and clinical manifestations. In: Anderson LJ, Young NS (eds): Human Parvovirus B19. Monographs in Virology, vol 20, Basel, Karger, 1997.

66. Porter HJ, Khong TY, Evans MF, et al: Parvovirus as a cause of hydrops fetalis: Detection by in situ DNA hybridisation. J Clin Pathol 1988; 41:381.

67. Yaegashi N, Okamura K, Yajima A, et al: The frequency of human parvovirus B19 infection in nonimmune hydrops fetalis. J Perinatol Med 1994; 22:159.

68. Rodis JF, Rodner C, Hansen AA, et al: Long-term outcome of children following maternal human parvovirus B19 infection. Obstet Gynecol 1998; 91:125.

69. Zerbini M, Musiani M, Gentilomi G, et al: Comparative evaluation of virological and serological methods in prenatal diagnosis of parvovirus B19 fetal hydrops. J Clin Microbiol 1996; 34:603.

70. Lewis DB, Wilson CB: Developmental immunology and role of host defenses in neonatal susceptibility to infection. In: Remington JS, Klein JO (eds): Infectious Diseases of the Fetus and Newborn Infant, 4th ed. Philadelphia, WB Saunders, 1995, pp 20–98.

71. Anderson LJ, Tsou C, Parker RA, et al: Detection of antibodies and antigens of human parvovirus B19 by enzyme-linked immunosorbent assay. J Clin Microbiol 1986; 24:522

72. Brown CS, van Bussel MJ, Wassenaar AL, et al: An immunofluorescence assay for the detection of parvovirus B19 IgG and IgM antibodies based on recombinant viral antigen. J Virol Methods 1990; 29:53.

73. Cohen BJ, Bates CM: Evaluation of 4 commercial test kits for parvovirus B19–specific IgM. J Virol Methods 1995; 55:11.

74. Clewly JP: Detection of human parvovirus using a molecularly cloned probe. J Med Virol 1985; 15:173.

75. Clewly JP: Polymerase chain reaction assay of parvovirus B19 DNA in clinical specimens. J Clin Microbiol 1989; 27:2647.

76. Koch WC, Adler SP: Detection of human parvovirus B19 DNA using the polymerase chain reaction. J Clin Microbiol 1990; 28:65.

77. Brown KE, Young NS: Parvovirus B19 infection and hematopoiesis. Blood Rev 1995; 9:176.

78. Clewly JP, Cohen BJ, Field AM: Detection of parvovirus B19 DNA, antigen, and particles in the human fetus. J Med Virol 1987; 23:367.

79. Salimans MM, van de Rijke FM, Raap AK, et al: Detection of parvovirus B19 DNA in fetal tissues by in situ hybridisation and polymerase chain reaction. J Clin Pathol 1989; 42:525.

80. Field AM, Cohen BJ, Brown KE, et al: Detection of B19 parvovirus in human fetal tissues by electron microscopy. J Med Virol 1991; 35:85.

81. Peters MT, Nicolaides KH: Cordocentesis for the diagnosis and treatment of human fetal parvovirus infection. Obstet Gynecol 1990; 75:501.

82. Kovacs BW, Carlson DE, Shahbahrami B, et al: Prenatal diagnosis of human parvovirus B19 in nonimmune hydrops fetalis by polymerase chain reaction. Am J Obstet Gynecol 1992; 167:461.

83. Török TJ, Wang Q-Y, Gary GW, et al: Prenatal diagnosis of intrauterine infection with parvovirus B19 by the polymerase chain reaction technique. Clin Infect Dis 1992; 14:149.

84. Rodis JF, Hovick TJ, Quinn DL, et al: Human parvovirus infection in pregnancy. Obstet Gynecol 1988; 72:733.

85. Sheikh AU, Ernest JM, O'Shea M: Long-term outcome from fetal hydrops from parvovirus B19 infection. Am J Obstet Gynecol 1992; 167:337.

86. Humphrey W, Magoon M, O'Shaughnessy R: Severe nonimmune hydrops secondary to parvovirus B-19 infection: Spontaneous reversal in utero and survival of a term infant. Obstet Gynecol 1991; 78:900.

87. Morey AL, Nicolini U, Welch CR, et al: Parvovirus B19 infection and transient fetal ascites. Lancet 1991; 337:496.

88. Pryde PG, Nugent CF, Pridjian G, et al: Spontaneous resolution of nonimmune hydrops fetalis secondary to human parvovirus B19 infection. Obstet Gynecol 1992; 79:859.

89. Bernstein IA, Capeless EL: Elevated maternal serum alpha-fetoprotein and hydrops fetalis in association with fetal parvovirus B19 infection. Obstet Gynecol 1989; 774:456.

90. Carrington D, Whittle MJ, Gibson AAM, et al: Maternal serum alpha feto-protein: A marker of fetal aplastic crisis during uterine human parvovirus infection. Lancet 1987; 1:433.

91. Schwartz TF, Roggendorf M, Hottentrager B, et al: Human parvovirus B19 infection in pregnancy. Lancet 1988; 2:566.

92. Soothill P: Intrauterine blood transfusion for non-immune hydrops fetalis due to parvovirus B19 infection. Lancet 1990; 356:121.

93. Sahakian V, Weiner CP, Naides SJ, et al: Intrauterine transfusion treatment of nonimmune hydrops fetalis secondary to human parvovirus B19 infection. Am J Obstet Gynecol 1991; 164:1090.

94. Bond PR, Caul EO, Usher I, et al: Intrauterine infection with human parvovirus. [Letter.] Lancet 1986; 1:448.

95. Woernle CH, Anderson LJ, Tattersall P, et al: Human parvovirus B19 infection during pregnancy. J Infect Dis 1987; 156:17.

96. Anderson MJ, Kousman MN, Maxwell DJ, et al: Human parvovirus and hydrops fetalis. [Letter.] Lancet 1988; 1:535.

97. Porter JH, Khong TY, Evans MF, et al: Parvovirus as a cause of hydrops fetalis: Detection by in situ hybridization. J Clin Pathol 1988; 41:381.

98. Maeda H, Shimokawa H, Satoh S, et al: Nonimmunologic hydrops fetalis resulting from intrauterine human parvovirus B19 infection: Report of 2 cases. Obstet Gynecol 1988; 71:482.

99. Samra JS, Obhrai MS, Constantine G: Parvovirus infection in pregnancy. Obstet Gynecol 1989; 73:832.

100. Mortimer PP, Cohen BJ, Buckley MM, et al: Human parvovirus and the fetus. Lancet 1985; 2:1012.

101. Franciosi R, Tattersall P: Fetal infection with human parvovirus B19. Human Pathol 1988; 19:489.

8

Hepatitis A to E

Joseph G. Pastorek, II ▶ Raul Yordan-Jovet

The causes of hepatic inflammation are numerous (Table 8–1). Many common medications and chemicals (e.g., acetaminophen and chloroform) may cause hepatic necrosis. Historically, viruses have been major causes of liver disease (e.g., yellow fever). Today, especially in developed countries, a variety of viruses are perhaps the most common causes of clinical hepatitis. The liver may be directly affected by cytomegalovirus (CMV), Epstein-Barr virus (EBV), herpes simplex virus (HSV), coxsackievirus type-B, and even mumps virus. Nonetheless, the usual cause of viral hepatitis is one of the specific viral hepatitis viruses, now generally denoted by the letters of the Roman alphabet.

The Centers for Disease Control and Prevention (CDC) has been tracking hepatitis since the 1950s (Fig. 8–1).[1] However, only since the mid-1960s has it been possible in the laboratory to differentiate hepatitis A virus (HAV) and hepatitis B virus (HBV), thus allowing separate epidemiologic data.[2, 3] Today, it is clear that the epidemiology of viral hepatitis, at least in the United States and other industrialized countries, has shifted from fecal-oral transmission to exposure to blood products, sexual activity, both heterosexual and homosexual, and illicit drug use.

Current medical knowledge described delta hepatitis, also called hepatitis D virus (HDV), as a small, incomplete virus that needs coinfection with HBV to replicate.[4, 5] The obstetrician caring for pregnant women with hepatitis must therefore look to their lifestyles as more dangerous than the infection itself.

The observations of Krugman and Blumberg had given the clinician access for the serologic diagnosis of viral hepatitis. The number of distinct forms of viral hepatitis has expanded from hepatitis A (originally termed *infectious hepatitis*) and hepatitis B (*serum hepatitis*) to the recognition of several types, and maybe more agents yet to come.[6] The medical practitioner faces a changing scientific understanding of the viruses that cause hepatitis. The insight provided by molecular techniques should lead to further improvements and effective treatment.

Disclaimer: The opinions contained herein are the private opinions of the authors and are not to be construed as official or as reflecting the views of the Department of the Air Force or the United States Department of Defense.

HEPATITIS A

The agent that causes the clinical illness of HAV is in the hepatavirus group of picornaviruses transmitted primarily by the fecal-oral route. Only one serotype exists as a small RNA virus, similar to other enteroviruses. Previously called *short incubation hepatitis,* it is also referred to as *infectious hepatitis* because it is often related to poor hygienic conditions. After 15 to 35 days of incubation, the usual acute onset of illness resembles a gastroenteritis syndrome, with low-grade fever, nausea, vomiting, malaise, and fatigue. HAV infection may also manifest as a classic case of hepatitis, with liver pain and tenderness, and clinical jaundice, even though it rarely results in relapsing disease or fulminant, fatal hepatitis. Most cases of HAV go unrecognized because of subclinical or anicteric disease, but as many as 70% of all adults and health care workers are seropositive.

No chronic HAV infections have been recognized after the normal immunologic response.[7] Recently, an increased prevalence of HAV among male homosexuals has given an indication of a "new" sexually transmitted disease.[8] Infection may be transmitted through blood products from asymptomatic blood donors during a short viremic phase of the prodromal phase of the illness.[9] In 1997, the CDC reported 30,021 cases of HAV infection in the United States. However, this is probably a gross underestimate, considering the percentage of cases that are subclinical or unrecognized, and therefore unreported.

The CDC reported the first documented transmission of HAV through clotting factor concentrates

TABLE 8–1 ▶	MAJOR CAUSES OF LIVER DISEASE IN PREGNANCY
	Viral hepatitis
	Cholestasis of pregnancy
	Gallbladder disease/stone
	Pre-eclampsia/HELLP syndrome
	"Acute fatty liver"
	Drug toxicity (e.g., acetaminophen)
	Cirrhosis
	Pyelonephritis
	Hyperemesis gravidarum

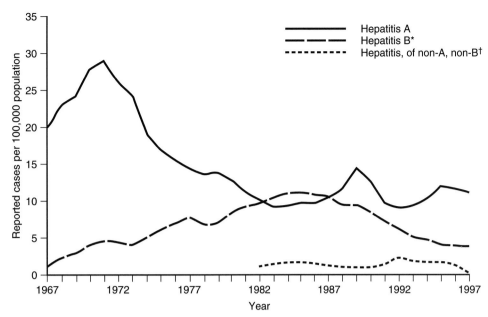

FIGURE 8-1 ▶ Hepatitis, by year, United States, 1967–1997. (From MMWR 46[54]:1–88, 1998.)

* The first hepatitis B vaccine was licensed in June 1982.
† Anti-HCV antibody test was available as of May 1990.

among persons with hemophilia in the U.S.[10] Spreading of HAV may occur whether or not the index case is symptomatic. Peak infectivity occurs about 1 week prior to illness and may be minimal at the onset of symptoms. Recent findings support the existence of a carrier state, although this is apparently uncommon and generally confined to patients with compromised immunity.[11]

Serologic Testing

The two antibody tests for HAV are IgM anti-HAV and total (IgM and IgG) anti-HAV. No commercially available tests exist for HAV antigen or RNA. The IgM anti-HAV implies acute or recent infection; the IgG anti-HAV implies immunity status.

Hepatitis A and Pregnancy

The course of HAV infection seems to vary according to the patient's health status and the reporting source. The world literature suggests possibly a more severe course and sequelae when HAV is contracted during pregnancy by women from developing countries. This fact might reflect their deprived nutritional states, deteriorated medical conditions, and inadequate medical care. However, recent studies suggest that pregnant patients from industrialized countries do not appear to experience a more dangerous course or more severe clinical manifestations than do nonpregnant women.

Nonetheless, careful attention is warranted with regard to the potential adverse effects of HAV infection on the gravid patient. Premature contractions and possibly preterm delivery or spontaneous abortion could

be the consequence from dehydration, fever, and hypovolemia. Immunologic mediators may cause myometrial irritability, mainly in severe cases.

The major threats to the fetus are premature birth and inadequate placental perfusion. Neonates exposed to acutely ill cases may develop HAV owing to an insufficient humoral immunity from the lack of transplacentally acquired maternal antibody. One case of intrauterine infection with HAV has been reported,[12] but there has been no evidence of teratogenicity associated with the virus.

Diagnosis

Serologic testing remains the main diagnostic tool, since HAV is not routinely cultured. According to the degree of suspicion, anti-HAV IgM antibodies may be detected in the early acute phase.[13] The presence of IgG alone suggests prior infection or immunity from previous administration of immune serum globulin (ISG) prophylaxis (or now vaccination).

Management

The lack of curative modalities of HAV infection calls for supportive and palliative measures instead. Fortunately, the illness is rarely fatal (<0.1%) and nearly always self-limited. Fluid replacement, bed rest, and preventive hygienic precautions are all that is recommended. Antiemetics and nutritional support depend on the severity of the illness. Intramuscular administration of 0.02 mL/kg of ISG is recommended by the CDC within 2 weeks of exposure regardless of pregnancy, and is said to be more than 85% efficacious in

TABLE 8–2 ▶	RECOMMENDED VACCINATION SCHEDULE FOR HAVRIX*			
Age group (Years)	Dose (EL-U†)	Volume (mL)	No. Doses	Schedule (Months)‡
2–18 and >18	720–1440	0.5–1.0	3 doses twice	0, 1, 6–12 0, 6–12

*Distributed by SmithKline Beecham Pharmaceuticals (Philadelphia, PA); used for identification only.
†Enzyme-linked immunosorbent assay units.
‡Zero months if the initial dose: Subsequent numbers are the months after the initial dose.

preventing HAV infection after exposure, the benefits lasting from 3 to 6 months.[14] Newborns of infected mothers may receive 0.5 mL ISG also. There is no known risk to the fetus from passive immunization of pregnant women with ISG.[15] Since 1995, the U.S. Food and Drug Administration (FDA) has approved two inactivated HAV vaccines (Table 8–2). Used in a two-dose series, 6 to 12 months apart, these vaccines are 99% to 100% immunogenic, and 94% to 100% effective in preventing HAV disease. Candidates for vaccination include travelers to endemic areas, children living in high-prevalence areas, homosexual males, illicit intravenous drug users, patients older than 30 years of age with chronic liver disease, persons having (or planning to have) a liver transplant, and persons working directly with HAV in medical or veterinary situations.[16]

HEPATITIS B

Ever since the description of the Australia antigen,[5] specific tests for the HBV have been aggressively developed. Of course, HAA was shown to be the viral surface envelope glycoprotein, now called HBV surface antigen (HBsAg). The agent that causes HBV infection is in the human hepadnavirus family transmitted through blood and body fluids. A DNA hepadnavirus, HBV was formerly known as "long incubation" hepatitis because incubation lasted months (average 100 days), regardless of an acute phase similar to that of HAV. Also called "serum hepatitis" because of its connection with tainted blood transfusions or serum obtained from a human "plasma pool."[17] Lately, routine screening of banked blood has decreased the transmission of HBV by transfusion, so most cases still occur by parenteral drug abuse.[18, 19] Official records underestimate the actual incidence as much as five-fold, but report 5,000 deaths annually in the U.S. In 1997, the CDC reported 10,416 cases of HBV infection,[1] again, probably a significant underestimate.

In addition to self-limited, asymptomatic, anicteric, and icteric disease as well as the uncommon fulminant case (<1%), chronic infection (antigenemia persisting for more than 6 months) occurs in as many as 10% of acute cases. The chronic asymptomatic carrier shows serologic evidence for HBsAg but normal liver transaminase levels. Chronic persistent infection may be histologically mild (asymptomatic but with abnormal

liver transaminases) or aggressive chronic active hepatitis with abnormal liver profile and systemic symptoms indistinguishable from those of acute hepatitis. The latter can progress to cirrhosis and hepatocellular carcinoma.[20] Most normal patients (90%) clear the antigen and develop antibody within an arbitrary time period of 6 months. The prevalence for chronic carriers ranges from 0.1% to 0.2%, in many industrialized countries, to 10% to 30%, in the developing world. In the U.S., about 5% of the population show evidence of previous infection.

Neonates are less resilient than the normal adult, with as many as 85% to 90% developing chronic sequelae of HBV after acquisition by vertical transmission from the mother; and a 50% chance for cirrhosis or primary hepatocellular carcinoma. Intimate sexual contact can primarily transmit HBV, even though casual transmission in the house or hospital is unusual owing to a great variability in HBV infectivity from patient to patient. Although about 1% of surgeons are infected with HBV, uncommonly outbreak transmissions to patients have been reported despite apparent compliance with recommended infection-control practices.[21, 22] It is unknown what role blood-feeding insects play in transmissibility.

Serologic Testing

HBsAg is routinely measured in the serum as an indicator of carrier status or infectivity. Several subtypes exist, and the HBV genome encodes four other antigens: the nucleocapsid (core) antigen (HBcAg); a post-translationally modified form of high-infectivity core antigen e (HBeAg); a DNA polymerase; and the x-antigen (HBxAg). HBcAg does not circulate freely in the blood, and HBxAg and DNA polymerase assays are not generally available. Measuring antibody against HBsAg for immunity or recovery, against HBcAg (IgG and IgM) for partial convalescence, and against HBeAg for greater infectivity (or conversely, against anti-HBe for lesser infectivity) can be done. Growing the virus in tissue culture cannot be done. Measurements of serum levels of HBV DNA reflect the circulating HBV.[6] Recently, problematic point mutations in the core gene have been described which no longer allow expression of immunologically detectable HBeAg while the patient has very high levels of HBV.[24, 25]

Hepatitis B and Pregnancy

The acute febrile onset and vomiting in severe HBV infection can be associated with premature labor and insufficient placental perfusion. Nonetheless, acute or chronic HBV disease does not represent teratogenic or any specific untoward direct effects on the fetus or neonate. The outcomes of pregnancies complicated by HBsAg carriage are no different from or worse than those of other women in the same population.[26] However, vertical transmission to the fetus or neonate predisposes to more than a 90% chance of developing chronic HBV infection and possible long-term hepatic dysfunction.[20] The intrauterine infection appears to be caused by microscopic leakage through the aged-porous placenta during maternal viremia.[27] Perinatal exposure or infection seems to be the contagious source for siblings and the rest of the population.[28] Among inner-city pregnant women not registered for prenatal care, a positive result of urine drug screening is a rapidly available marker for increased risk of HBsAg positivity.[29]

Diagnosis

The clinical manifestations of acute and chronic HBV infection resemble those of viral hepatitis of other etiologies. Modern clinical medicine allows diagnostic accuracy through interpretation of the available serologic testing. A usual "hepatitis B panel" consists of HBsAg, HBeAg, anti-HBs, anti-HBe, and anti-HBc. Interpretation of these data leads the medical practitioner to deduce the patient's stage of disease (Table 8–3).

Diagnosis of HBV infection in a suspected patient is made by evaluating the serologic presence of HBsAg and HBeAg. HBsAg appears in the blood before clinical symptoms arise, implying contagiousness before diagnosis is made. HBeAg is found in the serum as the infection progresses, indicating high infectivity until it disappears. The appearance of anti-HBe signals a decrease in infectivity. Other antibodies develop during the course of the disease, that is, anti-HBc and anti-HBs. Anti-HBc rises, initially as IgM and later as IgG, as an immunologic response to the illness but not as a sign of resolution, as it is seen in chronic HBV infection. Recovery is signaled by the disappearance of associated antigens, and the development of anti-HBs. Patients in the "window" test negative to both HBsAg and anti-HBs, but have high levels of anti-HBc (IgM) and variable findings concerning HBeAg and anti-HBe. Arbitrarily, the persistence of HBsAg over 6 months is defined as "chronic" illness, although in fewer patients it might take longer for resolution to occur. At such times, liver transaminase and symptoms characterize the chronicity status.

Seroconversion to anti-HBe precedes clearance of HBsAg, predicting recovery. HBeAg and HBV DNA, markers of viral replication, remain detectable in active hepatitis, progression to chronicity or reactivation of asymptomatic carriers.[30] HBeAg is a nonstructural protein (16 kD) of HBV with an amino acid sequence essentially identical to the protein that makes the HBcAg particle (27 nm). Its function or pathogenesis in liver disease is unknown; however, it has been used as an index of infectiousness and severity of the disease. The level of liver transaminase (alanine transaminase [ALT]) does not correlate well with histologic activity.

Management

Safe and effective disease prevention is the primary strategy for the treatment of HBV infection. Large-scale preventive technology applies immunization strategies to reach those at high risk, that is, children,[31] adolescents,[32] and illicit intravenous drug users. Outreach programs offer innovative and cost-effective approaches to facilitate adherence to long-term prophylaxis regimens and to provide protection to all others in the population.[33] Patients with HBV infection may require physiologic and pharmacologic support, with hydration and antinauseants as the basic form of treatment. HBV infection could be prevented by both passive and active immunization. Hepatitis B immunoglobulin (HBIG) is used for postexposure prophylaxis, in an adult dose of 0.06 mL/kg IM, as soon as possible after exposure, that is, needle sticks or sexual encoun-

TABLE 8–3 ▶ CLASSIFICATION OF HEPATITIS B CLINICAL COURSE					
Clinical Stage	HBsAg	HBeAg	Anti-HBs	Anti-HBe	Anti-HBc
Susceptible	− −	− −	− −	− −	− −
Acute HBV (highly infectious; less infectious)	+ +	+ − −	− − − −	− − +	Variable Variable
Chronic infection (highly infectious; less infectious)	+ +	+ − −	− − − −	− − +	High High
Recovering	− −	− −	+	+	High
Old natural infection	− −	− −	+	+	+
Postvaccination	− −	− −	+	− −	− −
HBsAg "window"	− −	±	− −	±	+

ters. Simultaneous initiation of the purified, surface-antigen-particles vaccine series is recommended for persons at high risk for HBV infection.[13] This regimen is equally applicable to health care professionals owing to continuous and potential exposure, and vaccination should be accomplished early in their careers. Immunization is also recommended for all infants and children, especially in high-risk population,[34] travelers to endemic areas, and inmates of long-term correctional facilities.

Neonatal vaccination with 0.5 mL HBIG within 12 hours of birth, and 0.5 mL HBV vaccine (separate site) prevents nearly 90% of cases of vertical transmission. The CDC has recommended the screening of high-risk gravidae in an effort to identify neonates for vaccination (Table 8–4).[35] High-risk women are re-tested in the third trimester. Additional recommendations for prenatal hepatitis B virus screening were amended in 1988 to include universal screening of pregnant women for HBsAg (Table 8–5).[36] This strategy has been equally reinforced by the Committee on Obstetrics of the American College of Obstetricians and Gynecologists.[37] Neither HBIG nor HBV vaccine appears to have adverse reactions, either maternal or fetal, when given to pregnant women.

HBV infection results in more than 10,000 hospitalizations per year and 5,000 deaths due to cirrhosis and liver cancer. The current vaccines offer a protective efficacy in healthy adults of 85% to 95%, once the primary series is completed. The duration of effect is at least 7 years. Recommendations on revaccination are still under study. Booster doses that appear to last around 9 years are offered to elderly persons or high-risk persons with declining or low antibody status. Some persons fail to seroconvert after three additional doses.

Prevention of HBV infection is much more important with HBV than with HAV, since HBV has an associated chronic infection state in a significant proportion of patients. The treatment of this chronic infection is problematic. There may be clinical remission of as much as 25% to 50% after treatment of chronic

TABLE 8–4 ▶ PERSONS AT HIGH RISK FOR HEPATITIS B INFECTION

Women of Asian, Pacific, or Eskimo descent (whether or not born in the United States)
Women born in Haiti or sub-Saharan Africa
Women in any of the following categories:
    Acute or chronic liver disease
    Work or treatment in a hemodialysis unit
    Work or residence in an institution for the mentally retarded
    Previous rejection as a blood donor
    Multiple blood transfusions
    Professionals' exposure to blood and blood products
    Household contact with a known carrier or dialysis patient
    Multiple sexually transmitted diseases
    Parenteral drug use

TABLE 8–5 ▶ PRENATAL HEPATITIS B VIRUS SCREENING RECOMMENDATIONS

All pregnant women screened for HBsAg
Additional testing later for high risk or symptoms
If no test done, test at delivery (hospital should have 24-hour turnaround)
Infants born to positive mothers receive active and passive immunizations
Household members and sexual partners of positive women addressed
Endemic populations can be universally vaccinated
Enforced education of patients and health professionals

HBV infection with interferon alpha. The clearance of HBeAg after treatment with interferon alpha is associated with improved clinical outcome.[38] Preliminary short trials with lamivudine therapy reduced HBV-DNA to undetectable levels in a few patients.[39] Discontinuation of either therapy resulted in relapse in most of these patients. Therefore, prevention remains the prime strategy for the treatment of HBV infection.

HEPATITIS C

For many years, patients with clinical hepatitis who tested negative for HAV and HBV were considered to have "non-A, non-B hepatitis" (NANB). However, molecular biology techniques developed in the 1980s elucidated the presumed viral causes of NANB hepatitis.[40, 41] Studies of NANB hepatitis of human origin demonstrated that it could be transmitted to primates and mammals by intravenous or percutaneous inoculation of infected plasma, serum, factor VIII concentrates, factor IX preparations, or commercially prepared fibrinogen. Cases of multiple episodes of NANB hepatitis, and variance-length incubation period, offered presumptive evidence of the existence of two or more etiologic agents.[42] Also known as post-transfusion NANB hepatitis, the cause of most cases was isolated and was named hepatitis C virus (HCV).[43] Routine screening of blood donors for HCV began shortly after its discovery.[44, 45] However, despite the intensive screening of blood products that has been performed in recent years, HCV remains the most common blood-borne pathogen in the U.S. today, with a rate of approximately 180,000 new cases per year during the decade of the 1980s.[1]

HCV is a distinct, blood-borne, single-stranded RNA virus similar in structure and function to the flaviviruses and pestiviruses, members of the Flaviviridae family.[46] It is a small virus, approximately 30 to 60 nm in diameter, is coated by a lipid envelope, and comprises 9,500 to 10,000 nucleotide bases encoding for 3,000 amino acids that code for three structural proteins and four to six nonstructural proteins. These proteins replicate through a negative-stranded RNA intermediate without integration into the host's cellular DNA.[47]

Through a collaborative effort between the CDC and the Chiron Corporation, HCV was the first virus isolated and cloned by molecular methods prior to identification by direct visualization (electron microscopy) or growth from culture media. In 1989, HCV was isolated and cloned from pooled plasma extracted from chronically infected chimpanzees.[43] Phylogenetically, HCV is classified into 6 main genotypes and 11 subtypes through molecular analysis of the nonstructural protein NS-5. HCV types 1a and 1b are the predominant types of HCV in the U.S. and Japan.[48]

HCV has been thought to be transmittable parenterally, sexually, occupationally, and vertically from mother to infant during pregnancy. However, the prevalence of HCV has been found to be constant worldwide in a pattern that suggests that socioeconomic status, age, climate, insect vectors, or sexual practices do not significantly influence the spread of the virus. Parenteral transmission via blood transfusions, intravenous drug usage, or hemodialysis is the most identifiable risks for the spread of HCV to date. The prevalence of HCV is 70% to 90% in intravenous drug users, and 70% to 90% of severe hemophiliacs have HCV secondary to their frequent requirement of factor VIII collected from various donors. Nevertheless, about half of the patients have no identifiable risk factor for the spread of the HCV.

Transfusions currently account for approximately 5% of cases of HCV; hemodialysis and occupational hazards account for fewer than 7% of cases, and sexual transmission of HCV infection, unlike HBV infection, is relatively rare but definitely possible.[49] Recent findings provide evidence that HCV may have been transmitted from surgeons to patients.[50]

Serologic Testing

Enzyme immunoassays (EIA) based on recombinant-technology–produced antigens are available initially for a single antigen (C-100, a nonstructural HCV component) and subsequently with a combination of three antigens. The confirmatory immunoblot assays are more antibody-specific. No antigen or anti-HCV IgM assay exists. Serum RNA assays, reflecting levels of circulating HCV, seem to represent the "gold standard" for determining the degree of active HCV infection.

Hepatitis C and Pregnancy

HCV can be transmitted directly across the placenta to infect the fetus, but transmission rarely occurs in acute maternal HCV infections prior to the third trimester of pregnancy.[51] The underlying etiology for such a fact has not been elicited, and the exact time for maternal-to-fetal transmission (antepartum versus intrapartum) is not exactly clear.[52, 53]

The most recent study suggests that vertical transmission and the risk of transmission of HCV from mother to infant correlates with the HCV RNA titer in the mother.[54] Seroconversion was observed in infants of parturient women who were positive for anti-HCV antibody by recombinant immunoblot assay (RIBA-2) and were positive for HCV RNA by polymerase chain reaction (PCR) testing. It is difficult to assess the vertical transmission of HCV owing to inadequate sampling size and post-partum follow-up of infants born to women positive for the HCV antibody. Transmission to the fetus appears to be rare after acute maternal infections before the third trimester. Hepatitis C can directly cross the placenta to infect the fetus; however, precisely when it occurs is not exactly clear. While no teratogenic effects are known, there probably is no effect on pregnancy outcome.

Diagnosis

Currently, a highly sensitive enzyme immunoassay (EIA) is utilized to detect the presence of HCV antibodies in serum. The EIA are composed of multiple HCV-specific antigen proteins; as opposed to the first-generation EIA, which were specific for only the C-100 antigen. The sensitivities of available methods for antibody detection range from 94% to 100% with greater than 97% specificities. False-negative results with the second-generation immunoassays are thought to be secondary to variation among HCV genotypes. Whereas false-positive test results with the second-generation immunoassays are thought to be secondary to connective tissue diseases and hypergammaglobulinemia.

Confirmation of EIA results are performed by one of two possible tests, the RIBA-2 or the PCR. The RIBA test is similar to the Western blot test and is a highly specific confirmatory test for HCV. It involves the attachment of HCV antibodies in serum to at least two of four HCV-specific antigen bands on a nitrocellulose strip. It is thought that the variations in the HCV genotypes allow for less reactivity between serum antibodies and the four viral antigens contained on the nitrocellulose strips in the RIBA-2. However, this problem is thought to be nonexistent with the PCR test.

The PCR test for HCV is a direct RNA detection method that also allows for quantification of HCV RNA. The serum of infected blood is rapidly separated from the cellular components of blood, and HCV RNA is isolated. The RNA then undergoes conversion to cDNA by reverse transcriptase and is then replicated by PCR. It is a highly sensitive and specific test for confirming HCV infection.

Management

In view of the recent understanding of HCV, therapeutic modalities are still evolving. Screening all banked blood in the U.S. for anti-HCV has shown to be reasonable for prevention. However, no universal prenatal screening for HCV is recommended, as for HBV. Screening for high-risk groups may be reasonable. The most recent recommendations by the CDC for routine testing for HCV include persons who have a history, no matter how remote, of illicit drug use, persons with selected medical histories (e.g., those who received clotting factor concentrate before 1987, were on long-term hemodialysis, or had persistently abnormal ALT levels), persons who received blood, blood components, or tissue donation before 1992 or from a known HCV-positive donor, and persons who have ongoing occupational or family exposure to HCV (e.g., neonates of HCV-positive mothers).[55]

Patients found to be HCV positive should be evaluated at intervals for evidence of chronic hepatitis, primarily by serial testing for alanine aminotransferase. Antiviral therapy is suggested for patients with chronic HCV who have persistently elevated ALT levels in the setting of positive anti-HCV testing, with detectable HCV RNA, and in whom liver biopsy indicates portal or bridging fibrosis and moderate inflammation and necrosis.[55]

The treatment of chronic/active HCV infection is still problematic. The only drug that has withstood the test of time, but at the same time is only passably adequate, is interferon alpha. Currently, the combination of interferon alpha plus ribavirin, a nucleoside analogue previously used to treat influenza, is approved by the FDA for the treatment of chronic HCV infection.[55, 56] Patients being considered for such therapy are best advised to seek care within a formal clinical trial, on account of the costs of therapy, the side effects of the drugs, and the rapidly changing nature of the knowledge and expertise in this area of hepatology and infectious disease. It should also be stated that ribavirin is teratogenic and thus contraindicated in pregnancy, and that interferon has, at least theoretically, the possibility of causing adverse pregnancy outcome (primarily prematurity) by virtue of its systemic effects.

No vaccine against HCV exists. Passive immunization with ISG has been used in an attempt to prevent transmission. The recommended neonatal dose for an infant born to an HCV-infected mother has been 0.5 mL IM at birth and again at 28 days of life. However, the CDC does not recommend ISG prophylaxis anymore, because of its lack of efficacy. On the other hand, the CDC does *not* recommend *against* breastfeeding in this situation, as breast-fed and bottle-fed infants apparently have the same rate of HCV infection from positive mothers.[55]

HEPATITIS D

Hepatitis D virus (HDV), previously called the "delta agent," is the smallest virus (37 mm, 1,700 base)

known to infect humans. Since identified in Italy in 1977,[4] this single-stranded circular RNA virus remains unclassified, because its genome seems unrelated to other mammalian virus families. HDV requires an obligatory helper function from HBV, which supplies HBsAg as a coat, for successful infection. Inextricably intertwined with HBV, HDV infection occurs only in the presence of HBV infection. However, the replication of the "defective virus" can occur without HBV sequences enclosed in an envelope of HBsAg as a Trojan horse.[57] The epidemiology of HDV is closely linked to HBV, including transmission through intravenous drug abuse and sexual activity.

HDV infection develops in two clinical patterns: (1) endemic, with high prevalence of both HDV and HBV (Mediterranean, Amazon basin, Middle East), and (2) epidemic, with low prevalence of HDV (U.S., Northern Europe, Australia) but high prevalence of HBV carriers (China, Taiwan, and Japan). Clinically, HDV can cause both acute and chronic hepatitis, in either case mimicking the hepatitis caused by other viruses except that it can be more severe. The clinical illness can be separated into coinfection or superinfection, or considered a superimposition on preexisting HBV infection. Compared to HBV infection alone, HDV infection (together with HBV) has higher rates of morbidity and mortality: 5% to 20% mortality, 75% chronicity, and 70% to 80% development of cirrhosis and portal hypertension.[5]

Serologic Testing

Commercial assays for IgM and total (IgM and IgG) anti-HDV are available, and delta antigen (HDVAg) can be measured in the blood. Serum HDV RNA can be measured as a function of circulating virus, but such testing is not clinically available.[6]

Hepatitis D and Pregnancy

Theoretically, HDV should affect a pregnant woman in the same relatively low-rate, vertical transmission of HBV.[58] Patients with active HBV/HDV are likely to be "sicker" and may be less likely to conceive, so concomitant pregnancy is relatively rare. Overall, the impact on pregnancy and neonatal statistics is minimal compared to all other viral hepatitis. Ultimately, if one assumes there are more severe manifestations in pregnancy than HBV alone, as in the nonpregnant patient, more cases of perinatal transmission will happen, even though such a finding remains to be elucidated.

Diagnosis

Key serologic markers are needed for the diagnosis of acute HDV infection. Tests for both the early-phase

(IgM anti-HDV) and the late-phase (IgG anti-HDV) antibody, and/or documentation of anti-HDV antibody, in a patient with an unusually severe HBV infection or relapses of apparent HBV infection, are ordered for laboratory documentation of HDV infection. Anti-HDV IgM, usually high in the acute phase, can remain in low titers in cases of persistent HDV infection. Anti-HDV IgG, which appears late in the illness, does not imply resolution or lack of infectivity as does anti-HBs. Western blot identification of HDVAg is a more sensitive test for HDV, and molecular hybridization techniques enable research laboratories to identify HDV RNA. Isolation of HDVAg in hepatic tissue is the gold standard for comparison. PCR techniques improve diagnostic sensitivities.

Patients should be tested with one or more modalities, and concurrent documentation of HBV infection should be performed in cases that are particularly severe, have become chronic, or have seemed to resolve but have now "relapsed." Documentation of concurrent HBV infection may be difficult because HDVAg suppresses replication of HBV and disappearance of HBV markers. Patients from endemic areas or intravenous drug abusers are reasonable candidates for HDV testing.

Management

Mainstay preventive therapy is the avoidance of HBV infection. Therefore, vaccination against HBV is the "treatment of choice" for the prevention of HDV infection. Physiologic support, for acute or chronic HDV infection, is best, since no effective treatments are available. Immunosuppression with prednisone and azathioprine is ineffective. Treatment with interferon alpha has had a poor success rate, the main difficulty being relapse, regardless of an initial normalization of ALT levels, a decrease in hepatic inflammation, and lessened viremia.[56] Recurrence after liver transplantation has been reported regardless of suppression of HDVAg expression in liver tissue after recombinant interferon-alpha therapy.

HEPATITIS E

An RNA virus, closely related to the calicivirus family, hepatitis E virus (HEV) was isolated from the stool of patients during the acute phase of enterically transmitted NANB hepatitis.[59] HEV causes a sporadic or an epidemic, often water-borne infection in developing countries, as well as occasional cases in international travelers or immigrants returning to the U.S.[60, 61]

The epidemiology of HEV differs from HCV, as it is transmitted primarily enterally, in a manner very similar to that of HAV; that is, through oral-fecal contamination. Not limited to contaminated water, food-borne transmission has been seen after a short incubation of

about 6 weeks (20 to 40 days). HEV infection affects young to middle-aged adults (15 to 39 years of age), with males infected more frequently (2.8%), although pregnant women have the highest incidence (5.3%). The clinical course is characterized by jaundice, anorexia, malaise, abdominal pain, arthralgia, and fever. The low household incidence (2.5%) contrasts with the high rate of attack in contacts of HAV (10% to 20%).

HEV can present as acute fulminating hepatitis, especially in pregnant women, in whom reported fatality rates range between 20% and 40%,[62] varying directly with the duration of pregnancy. Nonetheless, pregnancy is not the major predisposing factor, since the mortality seen in HAV- and HBV-infected pregnant women is as low as 3% to 8%. There are no long-term sequelae after recovery from the acute infection, and no carrier state has been described.[63]

Serologic Testing

No commercial assays for HEV are available in the U.S., regardless of the viral genome's having been cloned. Testing, however, is available through the CDC: Tel. (404) 639-3048.

Hepatitis E and Pregnancy

Since HEV has only recently been described, the literature documenting the clinical course during pregnancy is scarce.[64] Extrapolating from reports of NANB hepatitis transmitted enterically, pregnant women showed a higher rate of disease and a worsening prognosis as pregnancy advanced into the third trimester.[62] It is unclear whether the clinical correlation is with the pregnancy itself and the patient's previous nutritional or medical status, since malnutrition, malaria, and other illnesses common to developing countries could have contributed to a more severe course during pregnancy. Some studies reported preterm labor accompanying the illness, even when no maternal deaths were reported.[65] No perinatal (transplacental) transmission has yet been described, even though neonatal infection appears reasonable, as is the case with HAV.[63, 65]

Diagnosis

One type of viral particle associated with HEV has been isolated in the laboratory from infected cynomolgus monkeys and other primates, including marmosets.[66] An antigen denoting HEVAg (and associated antibodies) was identified, leading to the development of tests for anti-HEV, by both fluorescent antibody blocking assay and Western blot assay, as an experimental tool for investigating epidemics.[66, 67]

The diagnosis of HEV is suggested by supportive

epidemiologic circumstances and by exclusion of other possible etiologic agents of infectious hepatitis. In the setting of the lack of available routine clinical testing, HEV might be suspected in the patient with acute hepatic symptoms after probable enteric transmission from exposure to foreign travel *and* after excluding seroconversion to HAV, HBV, and HCV. (Thus, HEV becomes "non-A, non-B, non-C hepatitis," or "NANBNC.") After a report is received by the local health department, the CDC's Hepatitis Branch may request further testing.[60]

Management

The lack of definitive knowledge of HEV makes it impossible to reach satisfactory recommendations regarding treatment. Support of the acutely ill patient is indicated. No guidelines can be followed concerning prevention (i.e., prophylactic ISG), since previous failure has been reported.[63] Prevention of infection after exposure (including at the time of birth of an infant to a mother who is acutely ill with HEV) can be attempted with ISG, as is used for HAV. However, ISG prepared from pooled donors in nonendemic countries may lack sufficient anti-HEV for any significant efficacy.[60] Ultimately, prevention is best achieved by improving hygienic conditions or avoiding exposure of HEV from fecal contamination, or simply by avoidance of travel to endemic areas. If a vaccine is not available, prevention of exposure remains the best way of "treating" HEV infection.

HEPATITIS F

With modern electron microscopic and recombinant DNA techniques, another parenteral NANB agent, hepatitis F virus (HFV), has been isolated from HCV-negative patients. However, it is uncertain whether HFV is an important cause of NANB since it was described; that is, is it simply a viral particle looking for a disease?[68] It may be possible that multiple attacks of NANB in intravenous drug abusers and hemophiliacs are due to serologic variants of HCV, rather than to distinct new alphabet viruses.[69]

Serologic and epidemiologic data suggest that a novel agent, a togavirus-like particle (60 to 70 nm), was detected from patients with fulminant hepatitis. Electron microscopy demonstrated the presence of cytoplasmic tubular structures in the liver cells of infected chimpanzees.[70]

Serologic Testing

No serologic test is yet available for HFV, if indeed this microbe exists as a distinct viral agent.

Hepatitis F and Pregnancy

No cases of HFV infection have been described in pregnancy.

Diagnosis

There are no commercially available tests for the diagnosis of HFV infection. Suspicious cases, in which all other known viruses have been excluded, may be evaluated by the CDC or research laboratories on a case-by-case basis.

Management

Physiologic support and pharmacologic palliative measures are the only recommended treatments for the various rare, poorly understood NANBNC hepatitis viruses. The development of an effective vaccine is hindered by the extensive genetic and antigenic diversity among these viruses.[71]

HEPATITIS G

Plasma from patients with chronic hepatitis yielded the entire genome (9,392 nucleotides) from an immunoreactive cDNA clone. Hepatitis G virus (HGV) was identified as an RNA virus with amino acid sequences similar to others of the Flaviviridae family, including HCV.[72] Preliminary reports have linked this virus to syncytial giant-cell hepatitis (hepatitis G) due to virus-like particles resembling the measles virus (paramyxoviruses).

The clinical characteristics in patients with acute HGV hepatitis are similar to those in patients infected with HCV. The risk factors are not different between the two groups, and include transfusion, intravenous drug use, and multiple sexual partners. Preliminary data might support the sexual transmission of HGV, owing to a significantly higher prevalence among heterosexual partners.[73]

Serologic Testing

The detection of HGV RNA is possible from serum samples of index cases by immunoassays and PCR. No commercial serologic testing for anti-HGV is yet available.

Hepatitis G and Pregnancy

No data are yet available about perinatal transmission, regardless of presumptive transmission among heterosexual partners.[74] Further studies are required for determining the natural history of HGV infection and for establishing its full clinical significance. Again, perhaps a virus searching for its disease.

Diagnosis and Management

Serum specimens from patients with community-acquired non-A–E hepatitis can be tested by immunoassays and PCR. Initially, molecular cloning was performed from suspected plasma through the CDC Sentinel Counties Study of Viral Hepatitis. Demonstration of replication of the virus, animal transmission studies, and characterization of changes in viral genome will be helpful in understanding the full pathogenesis of HGV infection. Exclusion of conventional measles virus is necessary because this microbe can also cause hepatitis. Effective vaccines or immunization regimens are not available yet because of the unavailability of cell culture or animal models.

HEPATITIS GB

The agent of hepatitis GB (HGBV), originally found in marmosets, has been found to be different by neutralization and cross-challenge experiments.[75] The virus was so named in 1967, because it was isolated from the serum of a 34-year-old Chicago surgeon with acute hepatitis whose initials were GB. The true origin of the GB agent remained questionable until the recent application of modern molecular virologic techniques on stored blood samples.

Morphologic characteristics suggest that the virus is about 20 nm in diameter, resembling a parvovirus in both infectious and convalescent serum. The genomic organization designates it as belonging to the Flaviviridae family.[76]

GB viral particles do not appear to be shed in the feces, unlike the enteroviruses or other enterically transmitted NANB hepatitis virus.[77] Infection has been achieved by intravenous, intramuscular, and even oral inoculation of serum, suggesting some similarities to human parenterally transmitted NANB hepatitis.

Serologic Testing

Reverse transcription-PCR (RT-PCR) and EIA detected the RNA and antibodies associated with the three flavivirus-like genomes, GB virus-A, GB virus-B, and GB virus-C.[78, 79] No commercial testing is yet available.

Hepatitis GB and Pregnancy

Little is known about the transmission, epidemiology, and disease-inducing capacity of HGBV, except that it sometimes produces a fulminant non-A–E hepatitis. In general, disease occurring after transfusion or community-acquired infection has a benign course. HGBV accounts for a minority of all cases of unexplained liver disease, and there is no documentation of histologic progression from acute to chronic hepatitis, cirrhosis, hepatocellular carcinoma, or end-stage liver disease, unlike the case with HCV infection.[80]

No cases of HGBV infection have been reported or documented in pregnant women, but the search is still on.

Diagnosis and Management

A high degree of suspicion, and exclusion of non-A–G hepatitis, is the mainstay of clinical diagnosis of HGBV infection. Supportive management of the acutely ill patient is reasonable. Antiviral modalities are equally speculative at this time, as is the case with chronic NANB hepatitis.[56]

HEPATITIS H

Hepatitis H virus (HFV) is transmitted in a manner similar to that for the NANB F strains, but HFV is morphologically different owing to hepatic nuclear ultrastructural particles.[70] Otherwise, little is known about this (so far) last alphabet hepatitis virus, with regard to both diagnosis and management.

CONCLUSION

The field of viral hepatitis has become much more complex than could have been foreseen a few years ago. Screening for HCV with second-generation antibody tests should extend beyond transfusion practice to include nonparenterally transmitted cases and any underlying liver disease. Testing for HEV is currently cumbersome, but enzyme-linked immunoassays are being developed to help determine its worldwide importance.

Epidemiology and cross-challenge studies support the presence of more than one non-A–E agent, as well as help to establish the overall prevalence and clinical significance of the various HCV-like viruses. Cloning and nucleic acid sequencing of the viral genome bring insight into the genetic heterogeneity of hepatotropic viruses.

Effective treatment will be possible when the immune processes are better understood and through improved culture media and animal models. The search continues for the development of new immunomodulators and antiviral drugs for these new agents, and any of their as-yet-unknown fellows just around the molecular laboratory "corner."[25]

REFERENCES

1. Centers for Disease Control and Prevention: Summary of notifiable diseases, United States, 1997. MMWR 1998; 46:1.
2. Krugman S, Ward R, Giles JP: The natural history of infectious hepatitis. Am J Med 1962; 32:717.
3. Blumberg BS, Alter HJ, Vinich S: A "new" antigen in leukemia sera. JAMA 1965; 191:541.
4. Rizzeto M: The delta agent. Hepatology 1984; 3:729.
5. Hoofnagle JH: Type D (Delta) hepatitis. JAMA 1989; 261:1321.

6. Lutwick LI: Serodiagnosis of viral hepatitis. Infect Dis Pract Clinician 1994; 18:65.
7. Hollinger FB, Glombicki AP: Hepatitis A virus. In: Mandell GB, Douglas RG, Bennett JE (eds): Principles and Practice of Infectious Disease, 3rd ed. New York, Churchill Livingstone, 1990, pp 1383–1399.
8. Centers for Disease Control: Hepatitis A among homosexual men—United States, Canada and Australia. MMWR 1992; 41:155.
9. Lemon SM: The natural history of hepatitis A: The potential for transmission by transfusion of blood or blood products. Vox Sang 1994; 67:19.
10. Centers for Disease Control: Hepatitis A among persons with hemophilia who received clotting factor concentrate—United States, September–December 1995. MMWR 1996; 45:29.
11. Fagan EA, Yousef G, Brahm J, et al: Persistence of hepatitis A virus in fulminant hepatitis and after transplantation. J Med Virol 1990; 30:131.
12. Leiken E, Lyhsikiewicz A, Garry D, Tejani N: Intrauterine transmission of hepatitis A virus. Obstet Gynecol 1996; 88:690.
13. Snydman DR, Dienstag JL, Stedt BL, et al: Use of IgM–hepatitis A antibody testing: Investigating a common source, food-borne outbreak. JAMA 1981; 245:827.
14. Centers for Disease Control and Prevention: 1998 Guidelines for treatment of sexually transmitted diseases. MMWR 1998; 47(No. RR-1):99.
15. Centers for Disease Control: General recommendations on immunization: Recommendations of the Advisory Committee on Immunization Practices (ACIP). MMWR 1994; 43(RR-1):1.
16. Duff B, Duff P: Hepatitis A vaccine: Ready for prime time. Obstet Gynecol 1998; 91:468.
17. Barker LF, Shulman NR, Murray R, et al: Transmission of serum hepatitis. JAMA 1970; 211:1509 (quoted in JAMA 1996; 276:841).
18. Centers for Disease Control: Protection against viral hepatitis: Recommendations of the Immunization Practices Advisory Committee (ACIP). MMWR 1990; 39(RR-2):1.
19. Schreiber GB, Busch MP, Kleinman SH, et al: The risk of transfusion-transmitted viral infections. N Engl J Med 1996; 334:1685.
20. Beasley RP, Hwang L-Y: Epidemiology of hepatocellular carcinoma. In: Vyas GN, Dienstag JL, Hoofnagle JH (eds): Viral Hepatitis and Liver Disease. New York, Grune & Stratton, 1984, pp 209–224.
21. Harpaz R, Von Seidlein L, Averhoff FM, et al: Transmission of hepatitis B virus to multiple patients from a surgeon without evidence of inadequate infection control. N Engl J Med 1996; 334:549.
22. Heptonstall J and The Incident Investigation Teams: Transmission of hepatitis B to patients from four infected surgeons without hepatitis B e antigen. N Engl J Med 1997; 336:178.
23. Alter MJ: The birth of serological testing for hepatitis B virus infection. JAMA 1996; 276:845.
24. Liang TJ, Hasegawa K, Rimon N, et al: A hepatitis B virus mutant associated with an epidemic of fulminant hepatitis. N Engl J Med 1991; 324:1705.
25. Fagan EA: Hepatitis A to G and beyond. Br J Hosp Med 1992; 47:127.
26. Pastorek JG, Miller JM, Summers PR: The effect of hepatitis B antigenemia on pregnancy outcome. Am J Obstet Gynecol 1988; 158:486.
27. Ohto H, Lin H-H, Kawana T, et al: Intrauterine transmission of hepatitis B virus is closely related to placental leakage. J Med Virol 1987; 21:1.
28. Franks AL, Berg CJ, Kane MA, et al: Hepatitis B virus infection among children born in the United States to Southeast Asian refugees. N Engl J Med 1989; 321:1301.
29. Silverman NS, Darby MJ, Ronkin SL, Wapner RJ: Hepatitis B prevalence in an unregistered prenatal population. JAMA 1991; 266:2582.
30. Decker RH: Diagnosis: Hepatitis B virus. In: Zuckerman AJ, Thomas HC (eds): Viral Hepatitis: Scientific Basis and

Clinical Management. New York, Churchill Livingstone, 1993, pp 165–184.
31. Chen HL, Chang MH, Ni YH, et al: Seroepidemiology of hepatitis B virus infection in children: Ten years of mass vaccination in Taiwan. JAMA 1996; 276:906.
32. Centers for Disease Control: Hepatitis B vaccination of adolescents—California, Louisiana, and Oregon, 1992–1994. MMWR 1994; 43:605.
33. Margolis HS, Coleman PJ, Brown RE, et al: Prevention of hepatitis B virus transmission by immunization: An economic analysis of current recommendations. JAMA 1995; 274:1201.
34. Centers for Disease Control: Update: Recommendations to prevent hepatitis B virus transmission—United States. MMWR 1995; 44:574.
35. Immunization Practices Advisory Committee: Postexposure prophylaxis of hepatitis B. MMWR 1984; 33:285.
36. Immunization Practices Advisory Committee: Prevention of perinatal transmission of hepatitis B virus: Prenatal screening of all pregnant women for hepatitis B surface antigen. MMWR 1988; 37:341.
37. Committee on Obstetrics: Maternal and Fetal Medicine: Guidelines for Hepatitis B virus screening and vaccination during pregnancy. ACOG Committee Opinion No. 111. American College of Obstetricians and Gynecologists, Washington, DC, May 1992.
38. Niederau C, Heintges T, Lange S, et al: Long-term follow-up of HBeAg-positive patients treated with interferon alpha for chronic hepatitis B. N Engl J Med 1996; 334:1422.
39. Dienstag JL, Perrillo RP, Schiff ER, et al: A preliminary trial of lamivudine for chronic hepatitis B infection. N Engl J Med 1995; 333:1657.
40. Prince AM, Brotman B, Grady GF, et al: Long-incubation post-transfusion hepatitis without serological evidence of exposure to hepatitis B virus. Lancet 1974; 2:241.
41. Anonymous: Non-A, non-B? Lancet 1975; 2:64.
42. Bradley DW, Maynard JE, Popper J, et al: Post-transfusion non-A, non-B hepatitis: Physicochemical properties of two distinct agents. J Infect Dis 1983; 148:254.
43. Choo QL, Kuo G, Weiner AJ, et al: Isolation of a cDNA clone derived from a blood-borne non-A, non-B viral hepatitis genome. Science 244:359.
44. Stevens CE, Aach RD, Hollinger FB, et al: Hepatitis B virus antibody in blood-donors and the occurrence of non-A, non-B hepatitis in transfusion recipients: An analysis of the Transfusion-Transmitted Viruses Study. Ann Intern Med 1984; 101:733.
45. Alter MJ, Hadler SC, Judson FN, et al: Risk factors for acute non-A, non-B hepatitis in the United States and association with hepatitis C virus infection. JAMA 1990; 264:2231.
46. Miller RH, Purcell RH: Hepatitis C virus shares amino acid sequence similarity with pestiviruses and flaviviruses as well as members of two plant virus supergroups. Proc Natl Acad Sci USA 1990; 87:2057.
47. Gross JB, Persing DH: Hepatitis C: Advances in diagnosis. Mayo Clin Proc 1995; 70:296.
48. Farci P, Purcell RH: Hepatitis C virus: Natural history and experimental models. In: Zuckerman AJ, Thomas HC (eds): Viral Hepatitis: Scientific Basis and Clinical Management. New York, Churchill Livingstone, 1993, pp 241–267.
49. Kumar RM: Interspousal and intrafamilial transmission of hepatitis C virus: A myth or a concern? Obstet Gynecol 1998; 91:426.
50. Esteban JI, Gomez J, Martell M, et al: Transmission of hepatitis C virus by a cardiac surgeon. N Engl J Med 1996; 334:555.
51. Thaler MM, Park CK, Landers DV, et al: Vertical transmission of hepatitis C virus. Lancet 1991; 388:17.
52. Lynch-Salamon DI, Combs CA: Hepatitis C in obstetrics and gynecology. Obstet Gynecol 1992; 79:621.
53. Joffe GM: Hepatitis C virus in pregnancy: Case reports and literature review. Infect Dis Obstet Gynecol 1995; 3:248.
54. Ohto H, Terazawa S, Sasaki N, et al: Transmission of hepatitis C virus from mothers to infants. N Engl J Med 1994; 330:744.
55. Centers for Disease Control and Prevention:

Recommendations for prevention and control of hepatitis C virus (HCV) infection and HCV-related chronic diseases. MMWR 1998; 47(No. RR-19):1.

56. Hoofnagle JH, DiBisceglie AM: The treatment of chronic viral hepatitis. N Engl J Med 1997; 336:347.

57. Nowicki MJ, Balisteri WF: Three important new hepatitis viruses: C, D, and E. Contemp Ob/Gyn 1993; 33:71.

58. American College of Obstetricians and Gynecologists: Hepatitis in pregnancy. ACOG Technical Bulletin Number 174, American College of Obstetricians and Gynecologists, Washington, DC, November 1992.

59. Reyes GR, Purdy MA, Kim JP, et al: Isolation of a cDNA from the virus responsible for enterically transmitted non-A hepatitis. Science 1990; 247:1335.

60. Centers for Disease Control: Hepatitis E among U.S. travelers, 1989–1992. MMWR 1993; 42:1.

61. Smalley DL, Brewer SC, Dawson GJ, et al: Hepatitis E virus infection in an immigrant to the United States. South Med J 1996; 89:994.

62. Christie AB, Allan AA, Aref MKK, et al: Pregnancy hepatitis in Libya. Lancet 1976; 2:827.

63. Velazquez O, Stetler HC, Avila C, et al: Epidemic transmission of enterically-transmitted non-A, non-B hepatitis in Mexico, 1986–1987. JAMA 1990; 263:3281.

64. Khurdo S, Teli MR, Skidmore S, et al: Incidence and severity of viral hepatitis in pregnancy. Am J Med 1981; 70:252.

65. Bradley W, Maynard JE: Etiology and natural history of post-transfusion and enterically-transmitted non-A, non-B hepatitis. Semin Liver Dis 1986; 6:56.

66. Krawczynski K, Bradley DW: Enterically-transmitted non-A, non-B hepatitis: Identification of virus-associated antigen in experimentally infected cynomolgus macaques. J Infect Dis 1989; 159:1042.

67. Favorov MO, Fields HA, Purdy MA, et al: Serologic identification of hepatitis E virus infections in epidemic and endemic settings. J Med Virol 1992; 36:246.

68. Bradley DW, Maynard JE, Popper J, et al: Post-transfusion non-A, non-B hepatitis: Physicochemical properties of two distinct agents. J Infect Dis 1983; 148:254.

69. Craske J, Spooner RJD, Vandervelde EM: Evidence for the existence of at least two types of factor VIII–associated non-B transfusion hepatitis. Lancet 1978; 2:1051.

70. Shimizu YK, Feinstone SM, Purcell RH: Non-A, non-B hepatitis: Ultrastructural evidence for two agents in experimentally infected chimpanzees. Science 1979; 205:197.

71. Lemon SM, Thomas DL: Vaccines to prevent viral hepatitis. N Engl J Med 1997; 336:196.

72. Linnen J, Wages J, Zhang-Keck ZY, et al: Molecular cloning and disease: Association of hepatitis G virus: A transmission-transmissible agent. Science 1996; 271:505.

73. Rubio A, Rey C, Sanchez-Quijano, et al: Is hepatitis G virus transmitted sexually? N Engl J Med 1997; 277:532.

74. Alter HJ: The cloning and clinical implications of HGV and HGBV-C. N Engl J Med 1996; 334:1536.

75. Deinhardt F, Holmes AW, Capps RB, Popper H: Studies on the transmission of human viral hepatitis to marmoset monkeys. J Exp Med 1967; 125:673.

76. Muerhoff AS, Leary TP, Simons JN, et al: Genomic organization of GB viruses A and B: Two new members of the Flaviviridae associated with GB agent hepatitis. J Virol 1995; 69:5621.

77. Karayiannis P, Petrovic LM, Fry M, et al: Studies of GB hepatitis agent in tamarins. Hepatology 1989; 9:186.

78. Schlauder GG, Dawson GJ, Simons JN, et al: Molecular and serologic analysis in the transmission of the GB hepatitis agent. J Med Virol 1995; 46:81.

79. Simons JN, Leary TP, Dawson GJ, et al: Isolation of novel virus-like sequences associated with human hepatitis. Nat Med 1995; 1:564.

80. Masuko K, Mitsui T, Iwano K, et al: Infection with hepatitis GB virus C in patients on maintenance hemodialysis. N Engl J Med 1996; 334:1485.

9

Lyme Disease

SEBASTIAN FARO

Lyme disease is the most common vector-borne disease in the United States.[1] The disease was first described in 1977, and since then there have been an estimated 10,000 cases annually in the United States.[1] The bacterium that causes Lyme disease is the spirochete *Borrelia burgdorferi*, which is transmitted through the bite of the tick *Ixodes dammini*. The disease was named after the town in Connecticut where the first cluster of arthritis cases caused by Lyme disease occurred.[2]

EPIDEMIOLOGY

Lyme disease was first reported as a new disease in 39 children and 12 adults.[1] Although the disease affected the joints, it differed from juvenile rheumatoid arthritis. Lyme disease was not persistently chronic, but it manifested acute episodes laced with intermittent symptom-free periods. Since the initial report of 51 cases in 1975, thousands of cases have been documented in 24 states, 3 continents, and 18 countries.[3] The largest number of cases reported was from Connecticut, Massachusetts, Minnesota, New Jersey, New York, Oregon, Wisconsin, and Washington. The disease was reported in 47 states through 1996, and in 1996 there were 16,000 cases reported.[4] In Europe, there are approximately 50,000 cases each year.[5]

The tick *Ixodes dammini* (now known as *Ixodes scapularis*) was first found in the United States in 1926, and it was believed to have originated in Europe and to have been brought to the United States on sea birds.[6] The tick has been recovered from a variety of birds and animals, including deer. The birds and mammals are the primary and maintenance hosts, whereas humans are incidental hosts. White-footed mice also play an important role in the life cycle of *I. scapularis* and the transmission of *B. burgdorferi*. Nymphs carrying the spirochete *B. burgdorferi* infect the white-footed mice, and larvae become infected by feeding on them during the summer.[7, 8] The adult *I. scapularis* mates and remains on the deer throughout the winter.[8, 9] *Borrelia burgdorferi* was first isolated from *I. scapularis* by Burgdorfer and co-workers in 1982.[10]

Infection occurs most frequently during the summer months, when people tend to be outdoors and spend time in wooded areas.[11-13] Once an individual receives a bite from an infected tick, the rash (erythema migrans) appears in 9 to 10 days.[9]

CLINICAL MANIFESTATIONS

The clinical appearance of Lyme disease begins within 3 to 30 days (average 9 to 10 days) following infection with *B. burgdorferi*. Initially, a red papule forms at the site of the bite from *I. scapularis* and infection with *B. burgdorferi*. The area of erythema expands centrifugally, with clearing in the center. The annular rash may expand to a diameter of 20 cm (Fig. 9–1). This rash is referred to as erythema chronicum migrans (ECM). This manifestation of the disease is referred to as stage 1 and occurs in 50% of infected children and 30% of infected adults.[14] During this stage, patients frequently develop headache, malaise, fever, chills, stiff neck, arthralgia, and myalgia.[15] These symptoms may persist for several weeks. However, some patients can remain totally asymptomatic during this stage.

Stage 2 occurs within weeks to months of the onset of disease. Approximately 8% of infected patients develop cardiac dysfunction and 15% neurologic sequelae.[15] These individuals develop lymphocytic meningitis, motor or sensory radiculoneuritis, cranial neuropathy, and, most commonly, facial palsy.[16-18] Lyme borreliosis can result in chronic neurologic disease affecting either the central nervous system or the peripheral nervous system.

In Germany, Ackermann and associates[18] described 44 cases of progressive borreliosis whose clinical manifestations were spastic paraparesis or tetraparesis, ataxia, cognitive impairment, bladder dysfunction, and cranial neuropathy involving the seventh or eighth cranial nerve. In all of these cases the diagnosis was confirmed by the presence of intrathecal IgG antibody to *B. burgdorferi*. Other investigators in Europe have described a skin condition associated with Lyme disease known as acrodermatitis chronica atrophicans that is associated with sensory polyneuropathy and mental dysfunction.[19-21]

In the United States, Halperin and colleagues[22] described two chronic neurologic syndromes caused by

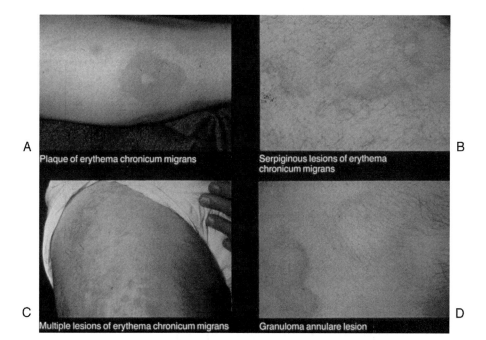

A — Plaque of erythema chronicum migrans

B — Serpiginous lesions of erythema chronicum migrans

C — Multiple lesions of erythema chronicum migrans

D — Granuloma annulare lesion

FIGURE 9-1 ▶ *A*, The enlarging of erythema centrifugally with clearing in the center. *B*, Serpiginous lesions of erythema chronicum migrans. *C*, Multiple lesions of erythema chronicum migrans. *D*, Granuloma annulare lesion. (Images courtesy of Pharmacia and Upjohn. Special thanks to Dr. Marvin Amstey for providing the slide.)

Lyme disease. One syndrome involved the peripheral nervous system and is characterized by paresthesias and axonal polyneuropathy, and the other is charaterized by encephalopathy.[22, 23] Logigian and co-workers[24] reported on 27 patients with Lyme disease with chronic neurologic manifestations; 8 of the patients were followed for 8 to 12 years (Table 9–1). Logigian and colleagues also described three neurologic conditions associated with Lyme disease; chronic encephalopathy, polyneuropathy, and leukoencephalopathy (Table 9–2). Antibiotic therapy results in improvement of these neurologic conditions associated with Lyme disease.

Logigian and co-workers[24] treated all patients with ceftriaxone, 2 g, as a single intravenous dose for 14 days. Patients did not respond immediately but a positive response occurred, in most patients, within several months of completing therapy. Six months after the completion of therapy, 17 patients (63%) were considered significantly improved, 6 patients (22%) were improved but experienced a relapse, and 4 (15%) did not show any response.[24]

Individuals can also develop cardiac disease in association with Lyme disease. This has been demonstrated in patients in both the United States and Europe.[25–27] The incidence in studies conducted in 1989 revealed a rate of 4% to 10% in the United States and 0.5% to 4% in Europe.[28, 29] However, recent studies have demonstrated a decrease in the incidence of carditis.[30, 31] Clinical manifestations of carditis are fluctuating degrees of atrioventricular block, myopericarditis, and left ventricular dysfunction. Typically, the clinical appearance of cardiac abnormalities associated with Lyme disease occurs within 5 weeks of the tick bite.[32] The clinical appearance of carditis is transient and rarely results in sustained damage.

Stage 3 Lyme disease is characterized by oligoarthritis and can occur within months to years after the tick bite. Approximately 69% of infected, untreated individuals with Lyme disease develop arthritis, with the knee the most frequently affected joint.[33] Other joints affected are the shoulder, the elbow, the wrist, the ankle, and the hip. The affected joint becomes swollen and warm and is painful. The inflammation can last for several months. The patient is likely to experience recurrences, and usually several joints, in addition to the initial one, are involved. The stages of Lyme disease are summarized in Table 9–3.

Acrodermatitis chronica atrophicans (ACA) is an associated condition that is a late manifestation of Lyme disease. ACA is characterized by chronic and long-lasting progressive erythematous and bluish-red lesions that develop on the extensor surface of the extremities.[34] This condition is apparently common in Europe but relatively rare in the United States. Molecular analysis of the bacteria isolated from patients with ACA revealed that the etiologic agent is primarily *Borrellia afzelii*. In a recent study of 22 patients, 17 isolates were identified as *B. afzelii*, 4 were *Borrellia garinii*, and 1 was *B. burgdorferi*.[35]

DIAGNOSIS

Initially, the disease should be strongly suspected in the patient who complains of a flu-like syndrome and the development of a rash, ECM. This rash, although considered to be pathognomonic of Lyme disease, is not seen in approximately 50% of infected children and 30% of infected adults. The diagnosis of Lyme disease is based on clinical findings, a history of a tick bite, and serologic data.

TABLE 9-1 ▶ COURSE OF LYME DISEASE IN THE 27 STUDY PATIENTS

Mean age—yr (range)	49	(25–72)
Male/Female	14/13	(52%/48%)
Early Infection	**25**	**(92%)**
Tick bite	10	(37%)
Erythema migrans	23	(85%)
Influenza-like summer illness without rash	2	(7%)
Headache and neck stiffness or spinal pain	11	(41%)
Oral antibiotics for early symptoms		
Doxycycline or tetracycline	4	(15%)
Penicillin	2	(7%)
Erythromycin	1	(4%)
Early Neurologic Abnormalities	**8**	**(30%)**
Mean time from erythema migrans to early neurologic involvement—mo. (range)	1	(0.5–2)
Facial palsy	8	(30%)
Meningitis	2	(7%)
Radiculoneuritis	1	(4%)
Doxycycline for facial palsy	1	(4%)
Oligoarticular Arthritis	**19**	**(70%)**
Median time from erythema migrans to early neurologic involvement—mo. (range)	6	(1–57)
Antibiotics		
Oral tetracycline	1	(4%)
Intramuscular penicillin V benzathine	1	(4%)
Chronic Neurologic Abnormalities	**27**	**(100%)**
Median time from erythema migrans to chronic peripheral nervous system involvement—mo. (range)	16	(1–156)
Median time from erythema migrans to chronic central nervous system involvement—mo. (range)	26	(1–168)
Duration of chronic neurologic involvement at time of evaluation—mo. (range)	12	(3–168)
Intravenous antibiotics for arthritis and neurologic abnormalities		
Penicillin	3	(11%)
Ceftriaxone	3	(11%)

From Logigian EL, Kaplan RF, Steere AC: Chronic neurologic manifestations of Lyme disease. N Engl J Med 1990; 323:1438–1444.

The serologic tests most often used to detect antibodies to *B. burgdorferi* are enzyme-linked immunosorbent assay (ELISA), immunofluorescence assays, and Western blotting. The ELISA and immunofluorescence assays are the most frequently used, but both have a low specificity because of cross-reactivity with other antibodies produced by a variety of illnesses (Table 9–4).[36–39] Serologic testing in stage 1 of the disease is confirmatory, since the clinical findings are fairly distinctive. During the first few weeks of the disease, the specificity of serologic testing is 40% to 60%.[40, 41] All individuals who progress beyond stage 1 will have antibodies to *B. burgdorferi*. The two most commonly employed tests are the indirect immunofluorescence and ELISA, the latter being more sensitive and specific. Detection of IgM occurs within 2 to 4 weeks of infection, after the appearance of EM. IgM peaks within 6 to 8 weeks, remains elevated for 4 to 6 months, and then declines. If the IgM remains elevated or rises, recurrent illness should be suspected. IgG appears within 6 to 8 weeks of the initial infection, peaks at 4 to 6 months, and remains elevated indefinitely. Confirmation of Lyme disease can be achieved by Western blot analysis and polymerase chain reaction (PCR).[42, 43]

TREATMENT

Once the diagnosis is suspected, treatment should be instituted without delay. The following antibiotics can be used to treat Lyme disease:

1. Tetracycline, 500 mg qid, *or*
2. Doxycycline, 100 mg bid, *or*
3. Amoxicillin, 500 mg tid, *or*
4. Erythromycin, 250 mg qid

PREGNANCY

Borrelia burgdorferi can cross the placenta; thus, pregnant women need to prevent exposure to *I. scapularis* by avoiding the areas known to be infested with the tick. Once an infected tick has bitten the host, the microorganism enters the blood stream and gains access to the fetal circulation across the placenta. In 1985, Schlesinger and co-workers[44] reported the case of a pregnant women who acquired Lyme disease in the first trimester. The mother delivered an infant at 35 weeks with a poorly contractile left ventricle, aortic stenosis, patent ductus arteriosus, and coarctation of the aorta. The infant expired 39 hours after birth. An autopsy was performed, and spirochetes were identi-

---

TABLE 9–2 ▶ CLINICAL MANIFESTATION OF NEUROLOGIC SEQUELAE ASSOCIATED WITH LYME DISEASE

Subacute Encephalopathy (24 Patients)
Memory loss
Depression
Excessive daytime sleepiness
Extreme irritability
Language disturbance

Laboratory studies:
Serum IgG—elevated in 21 patients
Three remaining patients, all received antibiotics:
   1 patient was positive for IgM (1:3200)
   1 patient was positive for IgG (1:200)
   1 patient had a cellular immune response to *Borrelia* antigens
Cerebrospinal fluid analysis:
8 patients had only IgG antibody to *B. burgdorferi*
1 patient had IgG and IgA antibodies
1 patient had only IgA antibody
1 patient had only IgM antibody
11 patients had increased protein levels
1 patient had 7 lymphocytes/mm³ of spinal fluid

Axonal Polyneuropathy (19 Patients)
17 patients had encephalopathy
11 had cervical, thoracic, and lumbosacral pain with tingling, burning, spasms, or shooting pain of the limbs or trunk
7 patients had only distal paresthesia
12 had diminished sensation to light and sharp touch
2 had ankle hyporeflexia
2 had mild limb weakness
13 patients had symmetric sensory findings
6 patients had asymmetric sensory findings

Laboratory findings:
16/19 patients had electrophysiologic evidence of axonal polyneuropathy
9/11 patients had denervation in proximal paraspinal nerves and distal limb muscles
3/11 patients with spinal pain
4/7 patients with distal paresthesia had reduced conduction velocity of motor or sensory peroneal and tibial nerves

Leukoencephalitis
1/24 patients developed progressive stiffness, weakness, and increased tone in the muscles of the right arm and legs. Gait was reduced, with a swing on the right. There were diffuse and brisk tendon jerks as well as bilateral ankle clonus and Babinski signs. The patient had episodic urinary incontinence, and urinary urgency and frequency.

---

fied in the spleen, renal tubules, and bone marrow, but not in the heart.[44]

Markowitz and colleagues[45] reported 19 pregnancies affected by Lyme disease. Fourteen pregnancies had uneventful outcomes. Among these pregnancies, infection occurred in the first trimester in 7 patients, in the second trimester in 4 patients, and in the third trimester in 2 patients; 1 patient did not know when the

---

TABLE 9–3 ▶ CHARACTERISTIC FINDINGS IN VARIOUS CLINICAL STAGES OF LYME DISEASE

Stage	Findings
1	Lasts a median of 4 weeks
	Erythema migrans
	Influenza-like illness
	Severe fatigue
	Musculoskeletal pains
	Headache
	Stiff neck
2	Lasts days to months
	Central nervous system disease with meningitis, encephalitis, Bell's palsy
	Peripheral nervous system involvement with radiculopathy or neuropathy or both
	Cardiac involvement with variable heart block, myopericarditis, congestive heart failure
	Ophthalmitis
3	Lasts months to years
	Asymmetric, pauciarticular arthritis—often intermittent but chronic in 10% of cases
	Severe, chronic, late central nervous system disease with encephalitis, demyelinating syndromes, and psychiatric disorders

From Duffy J, Mertz LE, Wobig GH, Katzmann JA: Diagnosing Lyme disease: The contribution of serologic testing. Mayo Clin Proc 1988; 63:1116–1121.

infection occurred.[45] Five patients experienced abnormal pregnancy outcomes: syndactyly, cortical blindness, spontaneous abortion, prematurity, and rash.[45] Although the spirochete could not be directly implicated in these adverse outcomes, the incidence is too high; Lyme disease in pregnancy should be treated aggressively.

Successful treatment of Lyme disease in the pregnant patient is probably dependent on early diagnosis and institution of therapy. Mikkelsen and Palle[46] reported on the successful treatment of a pregnant patient diagnosed with Lyme disease. A tick bit the patient in the 24th week of gestation, and 12 weeks later she developed ECM. The patient was treated with penicillin and gave birth to a normal infant.[46] Weber and co-workers[47] reported the case of a mother who acquired Lyme disease in the first trimester. She developed ECM within 2 weeks and was treated with penicillin. She delivered a term infant who appeared normal, but within 23 hours of birth the infant expired. Postmortem examination revealed a well-developed newborn, 51 cm in length and weighing 3,400 g. Spirochetes, believed to be *B. burgdorferi,* were identified in the brain and liver. Although the available data do not link Lyme disease to an increase in teratogenicity, there is a potential for poor fetal outcome; thus, all suspected cases of exposure should be treated aggressively.[48]

PREVENTION

Preventing Lyme disease can best be achieved by avoiding areas known to be endemic to *I. scapularis* (*I. dammini*). In the event that this is not possible, when one enters wooded areas the neck, arms, and legs should be covered. On returning home, the individual should check all areas of the skin, including the scalp, for the presence of ticks. Any tick found should be removed and saved for identification.[49] Ticks should not be discarded but brought to the physician, so that they can be sent to the laboratory for identification.

Treatment with ceftriaxone (Table 9–5) resulted in a patient developing the Jarisch-Herxheimer reaction.[50] This is especially important in pregnant women, since treatment of spirochete infection resulting in the Jarisch-Herxheimer reaction can result in intrauterine fetal death.[51] Therefore, a pregnant woman treated

TABLE 9–4 ▶	CONDITIONS THAT CAN PRODUCE A FALSE-POSITIVE SEROLOGIC TEST FOR LYME DISEASE

Spirochete infections
Nonspirochetal bacterial endocarditis
Epstein-Barr virus infection
Rheumatoid arthritis
Systemic lupus erythematosus

TABLE 9–5 ▶	TREATMENT REGIMENS

Erythema migrans—20 days
First-degree heart block—30 days
Arthritis—30 days
Acrodermatitis chronica atrophicans—30 days
Bell's palsy—30 days
Ceftriaxone, 2 g IV daily, or penicillin G, 20 million units IV in 6 doses for 14 days for the treatment of:
Neurologic disease
High-degree atrioventricular block
Persistent arthritis

with intravenous antibiotics should be monitored for 12 hours. This includes monitoring her temperature, blood pressure, pulse rate, and respiratory rate, and the fetal heart rate.

A vaccine has been developed that was shown, in 1990, to induce high titers to the outer surface protein A (OspA) of *B. burgdorferi* and prevented infection in mice.[52, 53] The vaccine, which contained 30 μg of purified L-OspA (L = lipid moiety), was absorbed to aluminum hydroxide in phosphate buffer.[54] Steere and colleagues[47] conducted a multicenter, randomized, double-blind vaccine trial involving 10,936 individuals. Participants received an injection at enrollment, 1 month, and 12 months later. During the first year, 22 patients in the vaccine group and 43 in the placebo group contracted Lyme disease ($P = .009$).[54] Vaccine efficacy went from 49% in the first year to 76% in the second, following the third injection. The efficacy of the vaccine for preventing asymptomatic disease was 83% in the first year and 100% in the second year. Steere and colleagues[54] concluded that three doses of the L-OspA vaccine prevented both symptomatic and asymptomatic Lyme disease.

Sigal and co-workers[55] performed a double-blind study administering 30 μg of OspA vaccine to 10,305 patients in 14 states. The individuals (5156) were randomly assigned to receive either 30 μg of OspA vaccine or placebo (5149). The first two injections were administered at enrollment and 1 month later. The efficacy of the vaccine in the first year was 68%. Then, 3,745 individuals were selected to receive a booster dose, and 3,770 received a placebo. The vaccine was 92% effective in the group receiving the booster.[55] Sigal followed the group for 4 years after vaccination and has not found any late cases of Lyme disease. This indicates that the vaccine is safe and did not mask any subclinical infection.

REFERENCES

1. Anonymous: Lyme disease—United States, 1995. MMWR 1996; 45:481.
2. Steere AC, Malawista SE, Snydman DR, et al: Lyme arthritis: An epidemic of oligoarticular arthritis in children and adults in three Connecticut communities. Arthritis Rheum 1977; 20:7.
3. Steere AC, Green J, Schoen RT, et al: Successful parenteral

penicillin therapy of established Lyme arthritis. N Engl J Med 1985; 312:869.

4. Centers for Disease Control and Prevention: Lyme Disease—United States, 1996. MMWR 1997; 46:531.

5. O'Connell S, Granstrom M, Gray JS, Stanek G: Epidemiology of European Lyme borreliosis. Zentralbl Bakteriol 1998; 287:229.

6. Oliver JHJ, Owsley MR, Hutcheson HJ, et al: Conspecificity of the ticks *Ixodes dammini* and *Ixodes scapularis* [Acari: Ixodidae]. J Med Entomol 1993; 30:54.

7. Spielman A, Wilson ML, Levine JF, Piesman J: Ecology of *Ixodes dammini*–borne babesiosis and Lyme disease. Annu Rev Entomol 1985; 30:439.

8. Main AJ, Carey AB, Carey MG, Goodwin RH: Immature *Ixodes dammini* (Acari: Ixodidae) on small animals in Connecticut, USA. J Med Entomol 1982; 19:655.

9. Wilson ML, Telford SR 3d, Piesman J, Spielman A: Reduced abundance of immature *Ixodes dammini* (Acari: Ixodidae) following elimination of deer. J Med Entomol 1988; 25:224.

10. Burgdorfer W, Barbour AG, Hayes SF, et al: Lyme disease—a tick-borne spirochetosis? Science 1982; 216:1317.

11. Hanrahan JP, Benach JL, Coleman JL, et al: Incidence and cumulative frequency of endemic Lyme disease in a community. J Infect Dis 1984; 150:489.

12. Williams CL, Curran AS, Lee AC, Sousa VO: Lyme disease: Epidemiologic characteristics of an outbreak in Westchester County, NY. Am J Public Health 1986; 76:62.

13. Steere AC, Taylor E, Wilson ML, et al: Longitudinal assessment of the clinical and epidemiological features of Lyme disease in a defined population. J Infect Dis 1986; 154:295.

14. Johnson RC: Lyme borreliosis: A disease that has come into its own. Lab Manag 1988; 26:34.

15. Hamilton DR: Lyme disease: The hidden pandemic. Postgrad Med 1989; 85:303–308, 313–314.

16. Reik L, Steere AC, Bartenhagen NH, et al: Neurologic abnormalities of Lyme disease. Medicine (Baltimore) 1979; 58:281.

17. Pachner AR, Steere AC: The triad of neurologic manifestations of Lyme disease: Meningitis, cranial neuritis, and radiculoneuritis. Neurology 1985; 35:47.

18. Ackermann R, Rehse-Kupper B, Gollmer E, Schmidt R: Chronic neurologic manifestations of erythema migrans borreliosis. Ann NY Acad Sci 1988; 539:16.

19. Asbrink E, Hovmark A: Early and late cutaneous manifestations in *Ixodes*-borne borreliosis (erythema migrans borreliosis, Lyme borreliosis). Ann NY Acad Sci 1988; 539:4.

20. Hopf HC: Peripheral neuropathy in acrodermatitis chronica atrophicans (Herxheimer). J Neurol Neurosurg Psychiatry 1975; 38:452.

21. Gans O, Landes E: Acrodermatitis atrophicans atrophica. Hautarzt 1952; 3:151.

22. Halperin JJ, Little BW, Coyle PK, Dattwyler RJ: Lyme disease: Cause of treatable peripheral neuropathy. Neurology 1987; 37:1700.

23. Halperin JJ, Luft BJ, Anand AK, et al: Lyme neuroborreliosis: Central nervous system manifestations. Neurology 1989; 39:753.

24. Logigian EL, Kaplan RF, Steere AC: Chronic neurologic manifestations of Lyme disease. N Engl J Med 1990; 323:1438.

25. Cimmino MA: Relative frequency of Lyme borreliosis and of its clinical manifestations in Europe. Infection 1998; 26:298.

26. Steere AC, Batsford WP, Weinberg M, et al: Lyme carditis: Cardiac abnormalities of Lyme disease. Ann Intern Med 1980; 93:8.

27. van der Linde MR: Lyme carditis: Clinical characteristics of 105 cases. Scand J Infect Dis Suppl 1991; 77:81.

28. Ciesieiski CA, Markowitz LE, Horsley R, et al: Lyme disease surveillance in the United States, 1983–1986. Rev Infect Dis 1989; 11(suppl 6):S1435.

29. Steere AC: Lyme Disease. N Engl J Med 1989; 321:586.

30. Gerber MA, Shapiro ED, Burke GS, et al: Lyme disease in children in southeastern Connecticut. N Engl J Med 1996; 335:1270.

31. Berglund J, Eiterm R, Ornstein K, et al: An epidemiologic study of Lyme disease in southern Sweden. N Engl J Med 1995; 333:1319.

32. Stechenberg BW: Lyme disease: The latest great imitator. Pediatr Infec Dis J 1988; 7:402.

33. Wang G, van Dam AP, Schwartz I, Dankert J: Molecular typing of *Borrelia burgdorferi* sensu lato: Taxonomic, epidemiologic and clinical implications. Clin Microbiol Rev 1999; 12:633.

34. Stanek G, O'Connell S, Cimmino M, et al: European Union concerted action on risk assessment in Lyme borreliosis: Clinical case definitions for Lyme borreliosis. Wien Klin Wochenschr 1996; 108:741.

35. Picken RN, Strle F, Picken MM, et al: Identification of three species of *Borrelia burgdorferi* sensu lato (*B. burgdorferi* sensu stricto, *B. garnii*, and *B. afzelii*) among isolates from acrodermatitis chronica atrophicans lesions. J Invest Dermatol 1998; 110:211.

36. Magnarelli LA: Current status of laboratory diagnosis for Lyme disease. Am J Med 1995; 98:10S.

37. Magnarelli LA, Miller JN, Anderson JF, Riviere GR: Cross-reactivity of nonspecific treponemal antibody in serologic tests for Lyme disease. J Clin Microbiol 1990; 28:1276.

38. Hofmann H: Lyme borreliosis—problems of serological diagnosis. Infection 1996; 24:470.

39. Tugwell P, Dennis DT, Weinstein A, et al: Laboratory evaluation in the diagnosis of Lyme disease. Ann Intern Med 1997; 127:1109.

40. Mertz LE, Wobig GH, Duffy J, Katzmann JA: Improved sensitivity in a Lyme disease enzyme-linked immunosorbent assay using *Treponema reiteri* adsorbent (abstract). Arthritis Rheum 1987; 30(suppl):S17.

41. Shrestha M, Grodzicki RL, Steere AC: Diagnosing early Lyme disease. Am J Med 1985; 78:235.

42. Anonymous: Recommendations for test performance and interpretation from the Second International Conference on Serologic Diagnosis of Lyme disease. MMWR 1995; 44:590.

43. Nocton JJ, Bloom BJ, Rutledge BJ, et al: Detection of *Borrelia burgdorferi* DNA by polymerase chain reaction in cerebrospinal fluid in Lyme neuroborreliosis. J Infect Dis 1996; 174:623.

44. Schlesinger PA, Duray PH, Burke BA, et al: Maternal-fetal transmission of the Lyme disease spirochete, *Borrelia burgdorferi*. Ann Intern Med 1985; 103:67.

45. Markowitz LE, Steere AC, Benach JL, et al: Lyme disease during pregnancy. JAMA 1986; 255:3394.

46. Mikkelsen AL, Palle C: Lyme disease during pregnancy. Acta Obstet Gynecol Scand 1987; 66:477.

47. Weber K, Bratzke HJ, Neubert U, et al: *Borrelia burgdorferi* in a newborn despite oral penicillin for Lyme borreliosis during pregnancy. Pediatr Infect Dis J 1988; 7:286.

48. Smith LG Jr, Pearlman M, Smith LG, Faro S: Lyme disease: A review with emphasis on the pregnant woman. Obstet Gynecol Surv 1991; 46:125.

49. Stafford KC 3d: Lyme disease prevention: Personal protection and prospects for tick control. Conn Med 1989; 53:347.

50. Steere AC, Hutchinson GJ, Rahn DW, et al: Treatment of the early manifestations of Lyme disease. Ann Intern Med 1983; 99:22.

51. Wendel GD Jr, Stark HS, Jamison RB, et al: Penicillin allergy and desensitization in serious infections during pregnancy. N Engl J Med 1985; 312:1229.

52. Fikrig E, Barthold SW, Kantor FS, Flavell RA: Protection of mice against the Lyme disease agent by immunizing with recombinant OspA. Science 1990; 250:553.

53. Schaible UE, Kramer MD, Eichmann K, et al: Monoclonal antibodies specific for the outer surface protein A (OspA) of *Borrelia burgdorferi* prevent Lyme borreliosis in severe combined immunodeficiency (scid) mice. Proc Natl Acad Sci USA 1990; 87:3768.

54. Steere AC, Sikand VK, Meurice F, et al: Vaccination against Lyme disease with recombinant *Borrelia burgdorferi* outer-surface lipoprotein A with adjuvant. N Engl J Med 1998; 339:209.

55. Sigal LH, Zahradnik JM, Lavin P, et al: A vaccine consisting of recombinant *Borrelia burgdorferi* outer–surface protein A to prevent Lyme disease. N Engl J Med 1998; 339:216.

10 Group B Streptococcal Infections in Pregnancy

JOHN W. LARSEN ▸ SUSANNE L. BATHGATE

Group B *Streptococcus* (GBS) is the leading cause of bacterial sepsis in newborns. Vertical transmission of the bacteria from mother to baby can occur during parturition. Clinical management strategies are directed at efficient detection, treatment, and prevention.

EPIDEMIOLOGY

GBS colonization has been found in every ethnic group and geographic location for which studies have been carried out. While colonization rates have been reported to vary from 5% to 40%,[1-4] it is difficult to separate the true biologic variance from variance due to study methods. In general, studies that have cultured only the cervix and have used neither selective nor enriched culture medium have reported isolation rates less than 10%, while studies that have cultured both the vagina and the rectum and have used enriched and selective broth medium report isolation rates of 15% to 30%.[5, 6]

The Centers for Disease Control and Prevention (CDC) has reported that both black race and maternal age less than 20 years may increase the risk of GBS carriage twofold.[7] Also, diabetes may be an independent risk factor for increased GBS colonization during pregnancy.[8, 9] While the scientific basis for these observations has not been worked out, it is speculated that younger pregnant women may be more susceptible to genital tract infections in general than older women. On the other hand, young black women may have been subject to ascertainment bias in the process of being more aggressively studied for genital tract pathogens. While it is tempting to presume that diabetic women have more GBS colonization because of increased glucose levels, there is no proof that this simple reasoning is in fact valid. In the authors' clinical experience, GBS colonization has appeared among every group with sufficient frequency that testing and/or prevention programs should be applied to all pregnant women. Further, no epidemiologic factor has eliminated the possibility of GBS colonization.

Longitudinal studies of GBS carriage during pregnancy have suggested that genital colonization may change spontaneously from positive to negative, and vice versa, from trimester to trimester.[10] However, we believe that this apparent change in colonization is largely a sampling phenomenon in which colonization is chronic while the number of GBS bacteria present varies. At a moment of heavy colonization, it is relatively easy to find abundant GBS colonies on culture plates, whereas a sample taken during light colonization may be more easily reported as negative. If an individual patient's management depends on one screening culture, it is currently recommended by the CDC guidelines that the specimen be collected as a swab of the lower vagina and rectum taken at 35 to 37 weeks of gestation.[5, 6] We believe that if a patient has had one positive sample for GBS it is preferable to regard her as chronically positive, and that repeat cultures are unnecessary. Nonetheless, in clinical obstetrics, there are patients who have had multiple cultures done over time, often by different doctors using different laboratories. When both positive and negative GBS cultures have been reported, it is safest to consider the patient truly a GBS carrier and to treat her accordingly during parturition.

BIOLOGY OF THE MICROORGANISM

Streptococci are gram-positive cocci that characteristically grow in chains or as diplococci. They are classified serologically or on the basis of their hemolytic reactions on blood agar plates. The beta-hemolytic streptococci cause complete destruction of red blood cells on the agar plates, and colonies have a clear zone surrounding them. The reaction of carbohydrate antigens on their cell walls with antisera forms a basis for serologic classifications. The Lancefield classification scheme was begun in the 1930s, based in part on studies of human puerperal sepsis.[11, 12] Colonies of streptococci cultured from fatal cases usually showed large beta-hemolytic rings (and were called group A). Colonies of streptococci cultured from women who had fever but did not die usually showed small beta-hemolytic rings (and were called group B).

Lancefield's group B *Streptococcus* is also known as *Streptococcus agalactiae*. *Streptococcus agalactiae* was historically associated with bovine mastitis. Although Fry[13] reported fatal cases of human puerperal sepsis due to GBS in 1938, GBS was only widely appreciated as a human pathogen beginning in the 1960s.[14, 15] There is no evidence for cattle as a reservoir for transmission of GBS disease to humans. Many differences exist between human and bovine isolates,[4] and indeed the current epidemic of neonatal disease has occurred in an era in which most humans have little contact with dairy cattle, and pasteurization is the rule.

GBS is suspected of causing disease through production of several enzymes and metabolic products. Some strains of type III GBS make quantities of neuraminidase, and these strains are found more often in conjunction with invasive GBS disease in neonates than strains that produce less neuraminidase, suggesting a role for this enzyme in pathogenesis.[16] These same strains produce large amounts of extracellular protease and type-specific polysaccharide, which also may contribute to virulence.[17] Acylated and deacylated glycerol teichoic acids may promote attachment to human cells.[18]

Eight serotypes of *Streptococcus agalactiae* are currently recognized (Ia, Ib, Ia/c, II, III, IV, V, and VI) on the basis of carbohydrate antigens. Most neonatal disease is caused by serotype III, although all serotypes have been found to cause clinical disease. The first carbohydrate cell wall antigens were identified by Lancefield, including the group-B specific, "C" substance common to all strains of this species, and the type-specific, or "S", substance that permitted classification into four serotypes: Ia, Ib, II, and III.[12, 19–22] Initially, the GBS strains were classified as I, II, and III, but type I was later found to be made up of two antigenically separate strains, while having a shared polysaccharide antigen common to all type I strains, the Iabc antigen.[22, 23] Type Ic was characterized by Wilkinson and co-workers,[24, 25] who found that it shares a polysaccharide antigen with type Ia strains (the type Ia antigen)[26–28] as well as a protein antigen common to all type Ib, up to 60% of type II,[29] and an occasional type III strain.[30, 31] This protein antigen, the c protein, historically called the type Ibc antigen, is never found in type Ia strains.

In 1983, Jelínková introduced a nomenclature system designed to simplify classification of GBS[32] in which the polysaccharide antigens are designated as type antigens and the protein antigens as additional markers for supplementary characterization of serotypes. Roman numerals, sometimes followed by a lowercase letter, designate the capsular polysaccharide type antigens. Protein antigen Ibc was simplified to "c" to avoid confusion with polysaccharide antigens. In this system, type Ic becomes type Ia/c because all have the Ia polysaccharide antigen and the c protein antigen. Perch and colleagues[33] introduced type IV in 1979, and types V and VI have been more recently characterized.[34–36]

DIAGNOSIS

Since current culture-based strategies for prevention of early-onset neonatal GBS disease depend on screening pregnant women who are GBS carriers, it is important for clinicians and laboratories to use the methods that will maximize carrier detection.[5, 6, 37] The use of selective broth enhances the recovery of GBS greatly compared with nonselective or selective solid agar. Media that inhibit the growth of gram-negative bacilli as well as other normal flora, such as Todd-Hewitt broth with gentamicin or colistin and nalidixic acid, are preferred. The initial incubation in broth media enhances the recovery of low numbers of organisms compared to methods that rely on standard transport medium or initial inoculation of swabs onto agar.[38]

Recovery of GBS from clinical specimens depends on both the site of culture and the culture media. Obtaining specimens from the anorectum and vaginal introitus increases the likelihood of isolation of GBS by 5% to 37% over obtaining specimens from the vagina alone.[6, 39, 40] Appreciation of this point is critically important to the development and effective implementation of clinical screening protocols. While many obstetricians have been trained to carefully sample the endocervix when attempting to diagnose gonorrhea or chlamydia, this is not the best way of screening for GBS. In the case of GBS infection, a positive endocervical sample may have up to 50% positive predictive value for the mother or baby developing a symptomatic perinatal infection; however, the incidence of positive endocervical cultures is very low (<5%).[41] It is important to ascertain the largest number of asymptomatic carriers if positive carrier status is to be effective as the main clinical trigger for intrapartum antibiotic prophylaxis.

Performing cultures at more than one point in time increases the cumulative likelihood that GBS will be found in at least one specimen. While repeated cultures are *not* recommended as a screening protocol, the authors recommend that clinicians interpret any GBS-positive genitourinary culture during pregnancy as evidence of chronic colonization. The most common example of this scenario might be a urine culture taken early in pregnancy that grows GBS. The urinary tract infection should be treated, and the patient also should be given antibiotic prophylaxis intravenously during labor. These patients do not require additional screening cultures for GBS.[6]

Women with heavier colonization may be more likely to transmit GBS to their newborns, and those infants may be more likely to have resulting disease.[42, 43] The risks of chorioamnionitis[44] and neonatal GBS disease increase with the duration of amniorrhexis.[45–47] In women with light GBS colonization of the vagina and rectum, the risk for early-onset neonatal disease should increase with the duration of amniorrhexis, since the GBS can multiply rapidly in the amniotic fluid. As the amount of GBS present in the amniotic fluid increases, the concentration of antibiotic necessary for preventing neonatal disease may also increase.[48, 49]

Several types of nonculture rapid assays have been tested for use in diagnosing GBS colonization in labor, ultimately with disappointing results.[50, 51] Initially, it was hoped that a rapid (less than 1 hour) result from a vaginal swab would identify the patients at clinically significant risk, thereby selecting the patients who would receive antibiotics.[41–43] Several latex particle agglutination and enzyme-linked immunosorbent assay (ELISA) tests have been shown to have fair sensitivity for heavy colonization, but poor sensitivity for light colonization.[47, 48] An optical immunoassay has been shown to be very sensitive (near 100%) for heavily colonized women; however, the sensitivity falls to 31% with only light colonization.[51] Incubating specimens in enriched media prior to assaying increases sensitivity but also increases the time to obtain results.[52, 53] The occurrence of early-onset neonatal disease in babies born to mothers with light vaginal and rectal colonization has minimized the clinical usefulness of currently available rapid tests for screening pregnant women. Rapid assays may yet be shown to be clinically useful if sensitivity can be increased to compete with selective enriched cultures.

Communication between clinician and laboratorian may be particularly important when one starts a clinical screening program for GBS. Many laboratories have been in the practice of using nonselective media,[6, 54] and they may not have emphasized the importance of identifying a few GBS colonies on a culture plate of mixed growth. Laboratory emphasis on GBS identification may lead to a process that may include the following:

▶ Coding for GBS on the order forms sent to the laboratory
▶ Not freezing the specimen prior to processing
▶ Inoculation of the swab onto selective medium (to prevent overgrowth) and into broth (to increase the yield from lightly colonized women)
▶ Prompt double reporting of results to physicians' offices and the proposed labor and delivery unit

IMPLICATIONS FOR THE MOTHER

While GBS is usually present as asymptomatic colonization, GBS also can cause symptomatic infection of the urinary tract or cervix ante partum, plus intrauterine and myometrial infection during or immediately after parturition. These symptomatic infections due to GBS are clinically indistinguishable from infection of the

same anatomic sites due to other bacteria. The GBS may act as the sole or predominant bacteria causing symptomatic maternal infection, or the GBS may act in combination with other aerobes and anaerobes (particularly in the instance of puerperal endomyometritis and sepsis).[55] Since pelvic soft tissue infections are known to be frequently polymicrobial in origin, treatment with broad-spectrum antibiotics is recommended for symptomatic chorioamnionitis, in contrast to the recommended use of penicillin for intrapartum GBS chemoprophylaxis in the absence of symptoms.

The GBS-colonized woman who remains afebrile during labor is unlikely to develop puerperal endometritis if there has been an atraumatic vaginal delivery. However, the GBS-positive woman who delivers by cesarean section after amniorrhexis and/or labor has a high probability of developing endomyometritis once there is amniotic fluid infection even if antibiotics are given as prophylaxis or early treatment.[56] In general, antibiotic prophylaxis continued as treatment if fever persists should decrease the overall duration and extent of morbidity by at least 50% (see Chapter 14).

Other scenarios of symptomatology that may require treatment of the mother for GBS include

▶ Urinary tract infections: These should be treated as often as symptoms recur and when a GBS culture is positive.
▶ Cervicitis: A copious yellow, purulent discharge due to GBS may be seen more often in the presence of a cerclage suture.
▶ Preterm amniorrhexis or labor: There is some evidence that GBS colonization is a minor risk factor for these conditions.[57, 58] There is stronger evidence that once these clinical conditions are present there is an increased risk for early-onset infection in the baby.[6, 45, 46]

IMPLICATIONS FOR THE BABY

While the baby has about a 50% chance of being colonized from its GBS-positive mother during birth,[59] the baby is most likely to remain asymptomatic and unharmed if born at term. However, in the absence of antibiotic prophylaxis, approximately 2% of colonized babies will develop early-onset disease.[4–6] This syndrome of sepsis, pneumonia, and meningitis affects about 8,000 babies in the United States each year.[6] The attack rate among babies born before 37 completed weeks of gestation increases as gestational age decreases.[46] While antibiotic treatment has decreased the fatality rate for infected babies, there is still considerable risk for short-term morbidity and residual neurologic damage.

Current strategies for minimizing early-onset GBS infection in babies begin with intravenous antibiotic chemoprophylaxis given to the mother during labor.[6] It is possible to achieve therapeutic levels of penicillin and ampicillin in the baby's blood and amniotic fluid if prophylaxis is given to the mother in a timely manner[42, 60, 61] (see section on treatment). This approach is estimated to be capable of decreasing the incidence of early-onset GBS disease in newborns by 70% to 90%.[6, 43, 46] Some newborns, but not all, will need further antibiotics after birth to follow up the prophylaxis or treatment given during labor.[6] In general, healthy-appearing term babies will not need further antibiotics. Conversely, babies with sepsis, pneumonia, or meningitis will require full treatment. The CDC guidelines[6] include recommendations pertinent to the management of GBS colonization and disease in different subcategories of newborns.

There is also a late-onset GBS neonatal sepsis syndrome that manifests at after 1 week of age. The majority of these infants have meningitis, but there may be localized infection of the eyes, sinuses, joints, bones, skin, ears, or lungs. About half of these infections are due to mother-baby transmission at birth.[4]

Treatment in Pregnancy

Intravenous penicillin is the drug of choice for prophylaxis and for symptomatic infections due to GBS. Nonetheless, the clinician often cannot be sure that GBS or another penicillin-sensitive microbe is the exclusive cause of disease in symptomatic women. Therefore, it has been customary to begin empirical therapy for pelvic infections with a broader spectrum antibiotic, such as ampicillin. For penicillin-allergic patients, erythromycin or clindamycin may be used, even though randomized clinical trials are still needed to measure the degree of clinical efficacy.[6] While GBS resistance to clindamycin and erythromycin has been expected in about 2% to 3% of cases, Pearlman and associates[62] have now reported an increase of up to 15% in the incidence of resistant strains.

Urinary Tract Infections

Treatment of culture-proven GBS cystourethritis with oral penicillin alone has been shown to reduce the frequency of preterm labor and premature amniorrhexis by Thomsen and associates,[63] who were studying a high-risk population. Multiple courses of oral penicillin treatment may be given during the course of pregnancy, repeating treatment each time a positive urine culture is obtained. This approach has not been rigorously studied to determine the optimal frequency of repeat cultures and treatment, or to compare to asymptomatic gravidas with positive rectovaginal cultures given the same course of antibiotics. Since GBS is a much less frequent cause of urinary tract infections than is *Escherichia coli*, it has been customary to begin oral outpatient treatment that focuses on gram-negative coverage unless GBS has been shown to be present (see Chapter 32).

Pyelonephritis during pregnancy usually requires hospitalization for effective treatment and monitoring of fetal well-being. A cephalosporin is usually given intravenously (with gentamicin added for more severely ill patients). Either agent may be discontinued on receipt of culture and sensitivity results that show the other antibiotic to be inappropriate. In the instance of isolation of a bacteria sensitive to both ampicillin and gentamicin, the more toxic drug, gentamicin, is discontinued. Hydration and lateral positioning have been recognized as an important part of the treatment regimen that is continued until the patient is afebrile and free from pain. Some clinicians[64, 65] recommend long-term antibiotics taken orally for suppression of bacterial growth in the urine of a patient who has recovered from pyelonephritis during pregnancy. We prefer to monitor the remainder of pregnancy with monthly urine cultures. Repeated courses of oral antibiotics are given for recurrent asymptomatic bacteriuria.

Amniotic Fluid Infection

Amniotic fluid infections and puerperal endometritis have a polymicrobial etiology in the majority of cases. Anaerobic bacteria are highly likely to be present, even though they are unlikely to be identified through routine cultures. If GBS is the predominant bacteria present, and if symptoms of intrauterine infection are minimal in a mother with an intact immune system, penicillin alone may produce satisfactory results, provided that the patient is delivered. Although individual cases of successful eradication of GBS from the amniotic fluid without immediate delivery of the baby have been reported, the general safety and efficacy of this approach are not known and so it is not recommended.[66, 67]

When selecting the route and timing of delivery of a pregnancy with amniotic fluid infection due to GBS, the obstetrician must consider various factors bearing on the well-being of both the mother and the baby:

▶ Maternal puerperal endometritis and the risks of wound infection or sepsis are less if there is a prompt vaginal delivery. If symptomatic amniotic fluid infection has occurred prior to cesarean delivery, symptomatic puerperal endometritis almost always occurs.
▶ The attack rate for early-onset neonatal sepsis due to GBS increases with the duration of exposure of the fetus to the colonizing bacteria. This relationship has been shown best in studies of the relationship between the duration of amniorrhexis and neonatal sepsis.[45]

▶ Uterine contractions may be weaker or less effective in the presence of myometrial infection.
▶ Intravenous penicillin or ampicillin given to the mother reaches standard therapeutic levels rapidly in the fetus. Levels in the amniotic fluid increase over a few hours to achieve a concentration that will have some therapeutic effect against GBS.[42] However, since the concentration of GBS in the amniotic fluid can reach 10^9 CFU/mL, an inoculum effect may be operative such that standard dosing and standard antibiotic levels may be ineffective for eliminating the infection.[4, 48, 49]
▶ The preterm baby seems to be at a substantially increased risk for developing symptomatic infection in utero or in the early neonatal period.[6, 45]
▶ A fetus who has become infected with GBS in utero may have heart rate decelerations that convey a more ominous prognosis than the same patterns in the absence of infection.
▶ Empirical antibiotics given to the mother may invalidate negative results from cultures taken later from mother or baby. While this argument has been used for years as a reason to delay maternal antibiotics until after delivery of the baby, the documentation of infectious risk to the baby can be obtained by the obstetrician via cultures of maternal vagina, cervix, rectum, blood, and urine prior to starting intrapartum antibiotics.

ANTIBIOTIC PROPHYLAXIS

A History of GBS Prophylaxis

Although mortality due to early-onset GBS sepsis has decreased with efforts to achieve early detection and treatment, GBS remains the leading cause of bacterial sepsis in neonates.[4, 6] Treated infants, particularly those with meningitis, may have residual neurologic damage. Since early-onset GBS sepsis in neonates is a vertically transmitted infection due to a bacteria that is susceptible to penicillin, there has been considerable interest in developing effective strategies for prevention.

Initial efforts involved oral or parenteral antibiotics given ante partum with an intent to eradicate GBS from the mother. In general, these efforts did not succeed. Transient decreases in colonization were noted, with return of colonization after antibiotics were stopped.[68–70] The exact mechanism for this is unclear, but it is reasonable to assume that the GBS remain within the genital tract or gastrointestinal tract in sites not reached by antibiotics. In many instances, the apparent variation in colonization may just have been a phenomenon related to the low sensitivity of culture methods.

Although antepartum antibiotic regimens have not succeeded in eradicating GBS colonization, intrapartum intravenous regimens have succeeded in inter-

rupting vertical transmission of GBS from mother to baby. This was first demonstrated by Yow and colleagues[59] in 1979, using a dose of 500 mg of ampicillin given intravenously to the laboring woman at the time of admission. Subsequent studies have shown that both penicillin and ampicillin are effective during labor in reducing both the transmission of colonization and the incidence of newborn infection. In 1986, Boyer and Gotoff[46] reported a successful prospective randomized trial in which ampicillin was given both to the mother during labor and to the baby after birth. GBS colonization was established by vaginal and rectal cultures done at 26 to 28 weeks of gestation. Maternal treatment (ampicillin 2 g IV, followed by 1 g IV every 4 hours) was begun for a culture-positive woman if there was

▶ preterm labor (less than 37 completed weeks)
▶ amniorrhexis for more than 12 hours
▶ maternal fever defined as a temperature $>37.5°C$

This regimen significantly reduced, but did not eliminate, surface colonization of mother and baby, and reduced maternal postpartum febrile morbidity. Most important was the elimination of GBS bacteremia in the newborns whose mothers received ampicillin, compared to a 6.3% bacteremia rate in untreated control subjects. Additional studies showing the efficacy of intrapartum intravenous ampicillin for reducing early-onset GBS neonatal septicemia were reported in 1986 and 1987 by Morales and co-workers.[42, 52]

The effectiveness of intrapartum penicillin was shown in 1989 by Tuppurainen and Hallman,[43] who had a study design that identified heavy vaginal colonization with GBS by a latex rapid test administered to parturients at the time of admission in labor. Study patients were given 5 million units of penicillin G intravenously every 6 hours during labor. Babies born to penicillin-treated parturients had a 1.1% incidence of early-onset GBS sepsis compared to 9.0% among control subjects. While this study showed that penicillin would work, it also showed that 50% of the cases in Helsinki, Finland, occurred without clinical risk factors other than heavy GBS colonization.

In 1991, Garland and Fliegner[71] reported an 8-year protocol management study from Royal Women's Hospital in Melbourne in which all public patients had their GBS colonization status checked at 32 weeks of gestation by a low vaginal culture. Carriers were treated with an intrapartum regimen of 1 million units of intravenous penicillin, repeated every 6 hours. No cases of early-onset neonatal infection due to GBS were reported in the babies born to treated carriers in a total public patient group of 30,197 livebirths. Over the same period of time, there were 27 neonatal GBS infections with 8 deaths among an unscreened control group of 26,915 private patients. Since these authors did detect some cases of early-onset newborn sepsis among public patients delivered prior to 32 weeks, they recommended moving the time for screening back to 28 weeks.

Other authors have approached the GBS problem by emphasizing clinical risk factors. In 1986, the same year Boyer and Gotoff published their study based on 26- to 28-week cultures plus clinical risk factors, Minkoff and Mead[72] published an essay suggesting an approach that advised prompt empirical intravenous ampicillin for patients in preterm labor if GBS was shown to be present or if the GBS status was unknown. Minkoff and Mead recommended that cultures for GBS be performed at the time of evaluation of the patient with preterm labor and/or amniorrhexis at less than 37 weeks of gestation, and that ampicillin be given before the results of the cultures are known if labor is not inhibited by tocolytics. They recognized that their protocol emphasized the management of patients at very high risk without suggesting a solution for the patients at term. While Minkoff and Mead advised starting prophylaxis without bacterial test results, they incorporated test results by stopping prophylaxis if a GBS culture came back negative a few days after antibiotics were started.

In devising protocols for GBS, many attempts have been made to avoid the need to perform cultures. GBS cultures have been criticized as

- unnecessary, if antibiotics will be given anyway
- costly, particularly if considered as a universally performed test
- cumbersome, when all administrative efforts to process specimens and report results are considered
- inaccurate (up to 50% false-negative results), if done as "routine" genital cultures, rather than using selective medium and using optimal sampling technique (vaginal plus rectal swab)

Manufacturers of rapid nonculture tests for GBS have offered kits that can produce results in about 1 hour; however, none to date have had sufficient sensitivity to equal or come close to equaling the performance of a culture that is done with enriched and selective medium.[73] Yet, the rapid tests are useful if positive. The clinician can treat or give prophylaxis when a positive rapid test result is reported. If a rapid test result is negative, the clinician must remain concerned about the low test sensitivity (16% to 53%) and possible failure to detect light colonization. While heavy maternal GBS colonization is an accepted risk factor for early-onset GBS disease in the neonate,[5, 43] infants born to lightly colonized mothers still have some risk, particularly since the vagaries of sampling and specimen handling can cause a truly heavily colonized patient to seem (falsely) to be only carrying a light colonization.[74]

In attempts to give clinical guidance and education

regarding GBS and methods of prophylaxis both the American College of Obstetricians and Gynecologists (ACOG)[75] and the American Academy of Pediatrics (AAP)[76] published bulletins for their members in 1992. Both groups consulted extensively with each other to find common ground for their recommendations. Ultimately, the two groups produced documents with small but significant differences. The ACOG Technical Bulletin on GBS described what action could be advised for OB/GYNs based on the current literature. This was basically an endorsement of the Minkoff-Mead protocol[72] for patients who had no culture results and advised intrapartum prophylaxis for asymptomatic patients with clinical risk factors known to have positive cultures. The AAP document took a more activist position and suggested that universal screening for GBS at 26 to 28 weeks of gestation was a method on which antibiotic prophylaxis given during labor could be based.[76]

Subsequent surveys of clinical practices showed a small change in clinical practice, but nothing suggesting a thorough national change.[77, 78] In a continued effort to find a protocol that would have efficacy plus political acceptability to physicians and patients, the CDC convened a series of meetings that led to guidelines published in 1996.[6]

Current Guidelines for GBS Prophylaxis

The CDC guidelines urge obstetricians to screen patients by vaginal plus rectal cultures, but now suggest doing the cultures just before term, at 35 to 37 weeks of gestation (Fig. 10–1).[6] It is presumed that this timing allows accurate reporting of results for the vast majority of patients. All positive gravidas then get antibiotic prophylaxis during labor, regardless of the clinical risk factors (Table 10–1). Antibiotics are recommended for preterm patients in labor. While the CDC guidelines suggest that patients with preterm amniorrhexis without labor may either begin antibiotics while awaiting

TABLE 10–1 ▶	RECOMMENDED REGIMENS FOR INTRAPARTUM ANTIMICROBIAL PROPHYLAXIS FOR PERINATAL GROUP B STREPTOCOCCAL DISEASE
Recommended	Penicillin G, 5 mU IV load, then 2.5 mU IV q4h until delivery
Alternative	Ampicillin, 2 g IV load, then 1 g IV q4h until delivery
If penicillin-allergic	
Recommended	Clindamycin, 900 mg IV q8h until delivery
Alternative	Erythromycin, 500 mg IV q6h until delivery

*Note: If the patient is receiving treatment for amnionitis with an antimicrobial agent active against group B streptococci (e.g., ampicillin, penicillin, clindamycin, or erythromycin), additional prophylactic antibiotics are not needed.
Data from CDC.[6]

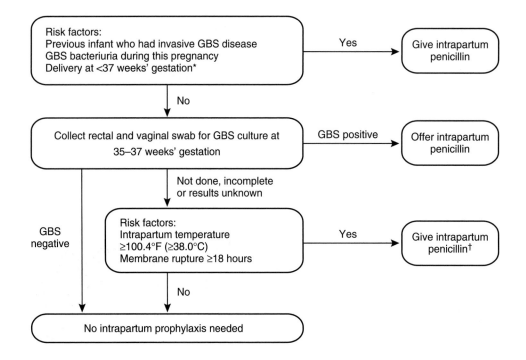

* If membranes ruptured at <37 weeks' gestation, and the mother has not begun labor, collect
group B streptococcal culture and either a) administer antibiotics until cultures are completed
and the results are negative or b) begin antibiotics only when positive cultures are available.
No prophylaxis is needed if culture obtained at 35–37 weeks' gestation was negative.
† Broader spectrum antibiotics may be considered at the physician's discretion, based on clinical
indications.

FIGURE 10-1 ▶ Algorithm for the prevention of early-onset group B streptococcal (GBS) disease in neonates, using prenatal screening at 35 to 37 weeks of gestation. (Data from CDC.[6])

culture results or may begin antibiotics only after the GBS culture has been shown to be positive, more recent evidence suggests that prompt use of empirical antibiotics may produce better results in the management of premature amniorrhexis.[79]

For practitioners who do not obtain screening cultures for GBS, the CDC urges initiation of intravenous penicillin prophylaxis (or broader spectrum antibiotics at the physician's discretion based on clinical indications) if one or more of the following clinical risk factors are present:

▶ amniorrhexis greater than or equal to 12 hours
▶ onset of labor at <37 completed weeks of gestation
▶ maternal temperature >100.4°F (38°C)
▶ History of prior GBS-infected child[6]

The CDC recommendations have a logical basis and reasonably broad support among the obstetric and pediatric communities. However, since the CDC recommendations were devised without waiting for scientific proof that the protocols recommended are the best course of action, clinicians should expect changes as data from clinical trials become available. The following issues seem particularly likely for clarification and revision:

I. Timing of Testing: Although the recommended time for culture collection is currently 35 to 37 weeks, other gestational timing may be shown to be equivalent or superior. It is possible that a culture done at the time of the first obstetric visit, when other cultures and a Papanicolaou (Pap) smear are conventionally done, will be more efficient and clinically equivalent. Earlier studies that showed maternal cultures shifting from positive to negative, and vice versa, during the course of pregnancy[5, 10, 39] may not hold up against studies done with current sampling methods and improved laboratory medium.[38] The authors believe that it is highly likely that vaginal or rectal colonization is chronic, with some fluctuation in the quantity of bacteria present.

II. Testing Method: While a culture with enriched/selective medium is the current "gold standard,"[6] a rapid test may yet be developed that will replace most GBS culture applications. The currently marketed tests only had to have performance comparable to a nonselective "standard" culture method in order to receive approval of the U. S. Food and Drug Administration (FDA). Since the current CDC recommendations include universal screening, there is a strong market incentive to develop an exquisitely sensitive rapid test for GBS. If this test is available, it would be logical to use the test on hospital admission in many instances to avoid difficulties in antenatal transmission of information among the physician's office, the laboratory, and the hospital.

III. Choice of Clinical Risk Factors

A. Maternal Temperature: While there is a consensus that fever is a sign of maternal infection and thus a risk factor for transmission of infection to the baby, there is no database that will allow the physician to say exactly how much risk is conveyed by each increment of temperature increase. The prospective study of early-onset GBS sepsis by Boyer and Gotoff[46] used maternal temperature above 37.5°C as the point at which antibiotics were started. Other studies of the clinical impact of chorioamnionitis on the baby have used 37.8°C[80, 81] and 38.0°C[82] as thresholds. The current CDC recommendations advise beginning antibiotic chemoprophylaxis at the onset of labor and continuing it every 4 hours until delivery, for women who are known to be GBS positive. If the GBS status is unknown, a maternal temperature of 38°C or higher is used to trigger the same antibiotic regimen. The higher temperature threshold was chosen (38.0°C vs. 37.5°C) to gain acceptance from skeptical clinicians, and may well be equivalent to the action point of 37.5°C used by Boyer and Gotoff.[46] Prospective clinical reports should contribute directly to clarification of this point.

B. Duration of amniorrhexis: For mothers known to be GBS positive, an issue is, "Should I begin antibiotics at home if I rupture membranes prior to hospitalization?" If the answer is "yes," the obstetrician needs a practical method for obtaining a therapeutic level. Oral antibiotics may convey some benefit, but given the expected decrease in gastrointestinal mobility related to labor, absorption of oral antibiotics may not be sufficient for efficacy. This question may be moot if the patient is within a short travel distance from her intended labor and delivery area. On the other hand, homebirths occur, sometimes inadvertently, and a prophylaxis option that did not *require* hospitalization would be attractive. One option may be to give benzathine penicillin, 4.8 million units IM at 36 weeks of gestation. This regimen has been reported by Weeks and colleagues[83] to achieve therapeutic penicillin levels in cord blood for up to 4 weeks and to reduce maternal GBS colonization at the time of delivery. However, this promising method has not yet been used in a clinical trial sufficient to demonstrate effectiveness compared with the method recommended by the CDC.[6]

For mothers whose GBS status is unknown, the question is, "What duration of amniorrhexis should trigger antibiotic chemoprophylaxis?" According to the current CDC guidelines, all preterm women whose GBS status is unknown should be treated if delivery is expected before 37 weeks. In the absence of labor, the clinician has had the option either to wait for a positive culture prior to starting antibiotics[10] or to follow the Minkoff-Mead protocol and begin antibiotics empirically, with the alternative of stopping if the culture is negative.[72] Information published since the CDC guidelines were released favors the use of empirical antibiotics for all women with preterm amniorrhexis.[79] The CDC guidelines recommend that intrapartum antibiotic chemoprophylaxis be given to women at term when the duration of amniorrhexis is 18 hours or more.[6] Boyer and Gotoff[46] gave ampicillin after 12 hours of ruptured membranes in women in their 1986 study who were known to be GBS positive. Earlier data reported by Boyer and associates[45] showed that the attack rate of neonatal infection increased more than 10-fold as the duration of amniorrhexis increased from ≤6 hours to >48 hours. Further studies might produce data that would permit the time threshold for starting intrapartum antibiotic prophylaxis in the "risk factors only" approach to be reduced to as little as a few minutes prior to delivery.

IV. Choice of Antibiotic Regimen: The CDC currently recommends intravenous penicillin for GBS carriers.[6] Ampicillin could also be expected to be efficacious. The recommendation favoring penicillin is based on the belief that penicillin's narrower spectrum of activity against GBS will minimize the risk of darwinian selection of resistant strains of bacteria in the population.[84] On the other hand, ampicillin may be the preferred drug for use in patients whose GBS status is unknown. In this instance, the broader spectrum of activity against other bacterial species that also cause amniotic fluid infection may override the "use penicillin for a narrow spectrum" strategy. Likewise clinical trials could show that an antibiotic with an even wider spectrum of activity, such as ampicillin-sulbactam, is preferable in all patients with clinical risk factors. It should be remembered that GBS is commonly one of several pathogens producing clinical illness in chorioamnionitis. Furthermore, the currently recommended antibiotics for penicillin-allergic patients (clindamycin and erythromycin) have not had their clinical effectiveness measured for GBS prophylaxis.[6] Both resistant strains of GBS (reported to be as frequent as 15% to 16% of clinical isolates by Pearlman and associates[62]) and limited placental transfer may decrease efficacy.

Vaccine

Ideally, prevention of GBS disease in the newborn would involve provision of type-specific immunity to the newborn. Theoretically, this could occur by passive immunization of the mother or the newborn with type-specific immune globulin. Unfortunately, currently available human immune globulins for intravenous use contain only low levels of group B streptococcal type-specific antibodies. Limited studies providing immune globulin to neonates at risk have been disappointing and impractical.[85]

Active immunization of the mother holds more promise. Protective levels of maternal serum antibodies may prevent neonatal infection,[86–88] although they do not prevent maternal colonization.[89] Unfortunately, about 80% to 90% of the population does not have protective antibodies.[90] Sera containing type III specific antibody at levels consistent with immunity in humans shows at least a partial protective benefit against lethal challenge in animal models of infection.[91–95] This is true of other serotypes also.[96–101]

Capsular polysaccharides from serotypes Ia, II, and III have been isolated, purified, and immunochemically characterized and have been tested as immunogens in adults.[102–107] Vaccination of adults with low levels of antibodies in their sera resulted in an immune response in 48%, 88%, and 60% of adults given type Ia, II, or III vaccine, respectively, within 2 weeks of subcutaneous immunization.[106] Serum antibody levels among vaccine responders remain at presumably protective levels for 5 to 7 years after immunization.

One study of immunization of pregnant women with type III polysaccharide showed a rise in type-specific antibody levels in the sera in 35 of 40 who had low levels of type III antibody before immunization.[108] There was evidence of transplacental passage of the antibody. Among infants born to vaccine responders, 83% and 75% had protective levels of antibody in their sera at 1 and 2 months after birth, respectively. Although this vaccine was not optimally immunogenic (overall immune response rate was 54%), it is apparent that active vaccination of mothers during pregnancy can provide passive immunity against invasive infection of many of their infants during the critical period of

susceptibility.[108] The GBS capsular polysaccharide is poorly immunogenic in nonimmune adults, and several studies have investigated a protein-polysaccharide conjugate as a better antigen.[109–111] The first GBS conjugate vaccines were composed of type III GBS antigen conjugated to tetanus toxoid and used random activation of polysaccharide fragments before conjugation.[111–113] These vaccines are immunogenic and produce functional antibody in rabbits and mice. Safety and immunogenicity of these vaccines in humans await human trials.

Another approach involves choosing the optimal oligosaccharide by selective activation of the polysaccharide before conjugation. Theoretically, oligosaccharides may be better than full-length polysaccharides when conjugated to a protein antigen because they elicit better T-cell help. However, smaller saccharides may be conformationally altered in a way that adversely affects immunogenicity. Paoletti and co-workers[114] conjugated a type III oligosaccharide to tetanus toxoid and found the conjugate to be immunogenic in rabbits, with intermediate-sized oligosaccharide conjugates producing the best response.[115] Although type III GBS produces most neonatal disease, some research activity has also been directed against type II. Serum from rabbits vaccinated with type II polysaccharide conjugated to tetanus toxoid provided 100% protection in a mouse model of GBS infection.[116]

An alternative to tetanus toxoid protein conjugate is the protein c of GBS. This protein is common to several serotypes, and 2 of its 4 antigens have been shown to elicit protective antibodies in an animal model.[117, 118] A type III polysaccharide–c protein conjugate vaccine theoretically could prevent an estimated 85% of neonatal systemic infections.[4] Protein c is composed of an alpha and a beta polypeptide,[119] which can be expressed independently,[120] can elicit protective immunity,[121, 122] but are usually not expressed by type III strains. Another protein, protein Rib (resistance to proteases, immunity, group B) is expressed by type III strains, and immunity to protein Rib has been shown to be protective against GBS disease in a mouse model.[123]

Because most women do not have type-specific antibody, the most logical strategy for immunoprophylaxis is active immunization of all women of childbearing age, either before pregnancy or later in gestation. One approach would be to vaccinate all pregnant women. However, successfully vaccinated women could deliver so early in gestation that placental transfer of antibody had not yet reached protective levels. This group has been estimated to represent fewer than 2% of all early-onset infections.[4] If immunogenic vaccines were given to all pregnant women early in the third trimester, 95% of late- and early-onset disease of infants born at term would theoretically be prevented. Another approach would be vaccination of all women prior to pregnancy; however, this approach might be difficult to implement. While the cost of developing and implementing protective vaccines is substantial, it ultimately may be less than the cost of treating these infections and their lifelong sequelae.[124, 125] Immunizing pregnant women would provide the greatest benefit to full-term infants, who are the majority of infants affected. It is likely that premature infants would still need antibiotics as well.

REFERENCES

1. Franciosi RA, Knostman JD, Zimmerman RA: Group B streptococcal neonatal and infant infections. J Pediatr 1973; 82:707.
2. Joshi AK, Chen CI, Turnell RW: Prevalence and significance of group B streptococcus in a large obstetric population. Can Med Assoc J 1987; 137:209.
3. Aber RC, Allen N, Howell JT, et al: Nosocomial transmission of group B streptococci. Pediatrics 1976; 58:346.
4. Baker CJ, Edwards MS: Group B streptococcal infections. In: Remington J, Klein JO, (eds): Infectious Diseases of the Fetus and Newborn Infant, 4th ed. Philadelphia, WB Saunders, 1995, pp 980–1054.
5. Boyer KM, Gadzala CA, Kelly PD, et al: Selective intrapartum chemoprophylaxis of neonatal group B streptococcal early-onset disease. II. Predictive value of prenatal cultures. J Infect Dis 1983; 148:802.
6. Centers for Disease Control: Prevention of perinatal group B streptococcal disease: A public health perspective. MMWR 1996; 45(RR-7):1.
7. Schuchat A, Oxtoby M, Cochi S, et al: Population-based risk factors for neonatal group B streptococcal disease: Results of a cohort study in metropolitan Atlanta. J Infect Dis 1990; 162:672.
8. Matorras R, Garcia-Perea A, Usandizaga JA, et al: Rectovaginal colonization and urinary tract infection by group B Streptococcus in the pregnant diabetic patient. Acta Obstet Gynecol Scand 1988; 67:617.
9. Ramos E, Gaudier FL, Hearing LR, et al: Group B streptococcus colonization in pregnant diabetic women. Obstet Gynecol 1997; 89:257.
10. Yow MD, Leeds LJ, Mason EO, et al: The natural history of group B streptococcal colonization in the pregnant woman and her offspring. I. Colonization studies. Am J Obstet Gynecol 1980; 137:34.
11. Lancefield RC: A serological differentiation of human and other groups of hemolytic streptococci. J Exp Med 1933; 57:571.
12. Lancefield RC, Hare R: The serological differentiation of pathogenic and nonpathogenic strains of hemolytic streptococci from parturient women. J Exp Med 1935; 61:335.
13. Fry RM: Fatal infections by haemolytic streptococcus group B. Lancet 1938; 1:199.
14. Hood M, Janney A, Dameron G: Beta-hemolytic streptococcus group B associated with problems of perinatal period. Am J Obstet Gynecol 1961; 82:809.
15. Eickhoff TC, Klein JO, Daly AL, et al: Neonatal sepsis and other infections due to group B beta-hemolytic streptococci. N Engl J Med 1964; 271:1221.
16. Milligan TW, Baker CJ, Straus DC, et al: Association of elevated levels of extracellular neuraminidase with clinical isolates of type III group B streptococci. Infect Immun 1978; 21:738.
17. Straus DC, Mattingly SJ, Milligan TW, et al: Protease production by clinical isolates of type III group B streptococci. J Clin Microbiol 1980; 12:421.
18. Neallon TJ, Mattingly SJ: Role of cellular lipoteichoic acids in mediating adherence of serotype III strains of group B streptococci to human embryonic, fetal, and adult epithelial cell. Infect Immun 1984; 43:523.
19. Lancefield RC: A serological differentiation of specific types

20. Lancefield RC, Freimer EH: Type-specific polysaccharide antigens of group B streptococci. J Hyg (Camb) 1966; 64:191.
21. Freimer EH: Type-specific polysaccharide antigens of group B streptococci. II. The chemical basis for serological specificity of the type II HCl antigen. J Exp Med 1967; 125:381.
22. Lancefield RC, McCarty M, Everly WN: Multiple mouse-protective antibodies directed against group B streptococci. J Exp Med 1975; 142:165.
23. Kubin V, Frank J, Prochazka O: Use of fluorescent antibodies for identification of streptococci. II. Determination of Streptococcus agalactiae (group B). J Hyg Epidemiol Microbiol Immun 1968; 12:330.
24. Wilkinson HW, Moody MD: Serological relationships of type I antigens of group B streptococci. J Bacteriol 1969; 97:629.
25. Wilkinson HW, Eagon RG: Type-specific antigens of group B type Ic streptococci. Infect Immun 1971; 4:596.
26. Wilkinson HW: Immunochemistry of purified polysaccharide type antigens of group B streptococcal types Ia, Ib, and Ic. Infect Immun 1975; 11:845.
27. Kane JA, Karakwa WW: Multiple polysaccharide antigens of group B Streptococcus, type Ia: Emphasis on a sialic acid type–specific polysaccharide. J Immunol 1977; 118:2155.
28. Kane JA, Karakawa WW: Existence of multiple immunodeterminants in the type-specific capsular substance of group B streptococci. Infect Immun 1978; 19:983.
29. Johnson DR, Ferrieri P: Group B streptococcal Ibc protein antigen: Distribution of two determinants in wild-type strains of common serotypes. J Clin Microbiol 1984; 19:506.
30. Anthony BF, Okada DM: The emergence of group B streptococci in infections of the newborn infant. Annu Rev Med 1977; 28:355.
31. Wilkinson HW: Analysis of group B streptococcal types associated with disease in human infants and adults. J Clin Microbiol 1978; 7:176.
32. Henrichsen J, Ferrieri P, Jelínková J, et al: Nomenclature of antigens of group B streptococci. Int J Systematic Bacteriol 1984; 34:500.
33. Perch B, Kjems E, Henrichsen J: New stereotypes of group B streptococci isolated from human sources. J Clin Microbiol 1979; 10:109.
34. Jelínková J, Motlová J: Worldwide distribution of two new serotypes of group B streptococci: Type IV and provisional type V. J Clin Microbiol 1985; 21:361.
35. Wessels MR, DiFabio JL, Benedí V-J, et al: Structural determination and immunochemical characterization of type V group B Streptococcus capsular polysaccharide. J Biol Chem 1991; 266:6714.
36. Von Hunolstein C, D'Ascenzi S, Wagner B, et al: Immunochemistry of capsular type polysaccharide and virulence properties of type VI Streptococcus agalactiae (group B streptococci). Infect Immun 1993; 61:1280.
37. Baker CJ, Goroff DK, Alpert SL, et al: Comparison of bacteriological methods for the isolation of group B streptococcus from vaginal cultures. J Clin Microbiol 1976; 4:46.
38. Silver HM, Struminsky J: A comparison of the yield of positive antenatal group B Streptococcus cultures with direct inoculation in selective growth medium versus primary inoculation in transport medium followed by delayed inoculation in selective growth medium. Am J Obstet Gynecol 1996; 175:155.
39. Dillon HC, Gray E, Pass MA, et al: Anorectal and vaginal carriage of group B streptococci during pregnancy. J Infect Dis 1982; 145:794.
40. Badri MS, Zawnaeh S, Cruz AC, et al: Rectal colonization with group B streptococcus: Relation to vaginal colonization of pregnant women. J Infect Dis 1977; 135:308.
41. Grossman JH, Kaye MF, Isada NB, et al: Rapid test plus ampicillin protocol for reduction of preterm group B streptococcal perinatal morbidity. J Matern Fetal Med 1995; 4:1.
42. Morales WJ, Lim DV, Walsh AF: Prevention of neonatal group B streptococcal sepsis by the use of a rapid screening test and selective intrapartum chemoprophylaxis. Am J Obstet Gynecol 1986; 155:979.
43. Lancefield RC: A serological differentiation of specific types of bovine hemolytic streptococci (group B). J Exp Med 1934; 59:441.

43. Tuppurainen N, Hallman M: Prevention of neonatal group B streptococcal disease: Intrapartum detection and chemoprophylaxis of heavily colonized parturients. Obstet Gynecol 1989; 73:583.

44. Soper DE, Mayhall CG, Froggatt JW: Characterization and control of intra-amniotic infection in an urban teaching hospital. Am J Obstet Gynecol 1996; 175:304.

45. Boyer KM, Gadsala CA, Burd LI, et al: Selective intrapartum chemoprophylaxis of neonatal group B streptococcal early-onset disease. I. Epidemiologic rationale. J Infect Dis 1983; 148:795.

46. Boyer KM, Gotoff SP: Prevention of early-onset group B streptococcal disease with selective intrapartum chemoprophylaxis. N Engl J Med 1986; 314:1665.

47. McLaren RA, Chauhan SP, Gross TL: Intrapartum factors in early-onset group B streptococcal sepsis in term neonates: A case-control study. Am J Obstet Gynecol 1996; 174:1934.

48. Weeks JL, Mason EO Jr, Baker CJ: Antagonism of ampicillin and chloramphenicol for meningeal isolates of group B streptococci. Antimicrob Agents Chemother 1981; 20:281.

49. Feldman WE: Concentrations of bacteria in cerebrospinal fluid of patients with bacterial meningitis. J Pediatr 1976; 88:549.

50. Yancey MK, Armer T, Clark P, Duff P: Assessment of rapid identification tests for genital carriage of group B streptococci. Obstet Gynecol 1992; 80:1038.

51. Baker CJ: Inadequacy of rapid immunoassays for intrapartum detection of group B streptococcal carriers. Obstet Gynecol 1996; 88:51.

52. Morales WJ, Lim D: Reduction of group B streptococcal maternal and neonatal infections in preterm pregnancies with premature rupture of the membranes through a rapid identification test. Am J Obstet Gynecol 1987; 157:13.

53. Altaie SS, Bridges F, Loghamanee D, et al: Preincubation of cervical swabs in Lim broth improves performance of ICON rapid test for detection of group B streptococci. Infect Dis Obstet Gynecol 1996; 4:20.

54. Whitney CG, Plikaytis BD, Gozansky WS, et al: Prevention practices for perinatal group B streptococcal disease: A multistate surveillance analysis. Obstet Gynecol 1997; 89:28.

55. Faro S: Group B beta-hemolytic streptococci and puerperal infections. Am J Obstet Gynecol 1981; 139:686.

56. Watts H, Hillier S, Eschenbach D: Upper genital tract isolates at cesarean section predict postpartum endomyometritis despite antibiotic prophylaxis. Obstet Gynecol 1991; 77:287.

57. Alger LS, Lovchik JC, Hebel JR, et al: The association of *Chlamydia trachomatis, Neisseria gonorrhoeae,* and group B streptococci with preterm rupture of the membranes and pregnancy outcome. Am J Obstet Gynecol 1988; 149:397.

58. Gibbs RS, Romero R, Hillier SL, et al: A review of premature birth and subclinical infection. Am J Obstet Gynecol 1992; 166:1515.

59. Yow MD, Mason EO, Leeds LJ, et al: Ampicillin prevents intrapartum transmission of group B streptococcus. JAMA 1979; 241:1245.

60. Bray RE, Boe RW, Johnson WL: Transfer of ampicillin into fetus and amniotic fluid from maternal plasma in late pregnancy. Am J Obstet Gynecol 1966; 96:938.

61. MacAulay MA, Abou-Sabe M, Charles D: Placental transfer of ampicillin. Am J Obstet Gynecol 1966; 96:943.

62. Pearlman MD, Pierson CL, Faix RG: Frequent resistance of clinical group B streptococci isolates to clindamycin and erythromycin. Obstet Gynecol 1998; 92:258.

63. Thomsen AC, Morup L, Hansen KB: Antibiotic elimination of group B streptococcus in urine in prevention of preterm labor. Lancet 1987; 1:591.

64. Harris R, Gilstrap L: Prevention of recurrent pyelonephritis during pregnancy. Obstet Gynecol 1974; 44:637.

65. Whalley P, Cunningham FG: Short-term versus continuous antimicrobial therapy for asymptomatic bacteriuria in pregnancy. Obstet Gynecol 1977; 49:262.

66. Haesslein HC, Goodlin RC: Delivery of the tiny newborn. Am J Obstet Gynecol 1979; 134:192.

67. Goodlin RC: Intra-amniotic antibiotic infusion. [Letter.] Am J Obstet Gynecol 1981; 139:975.

68. Gardner SE, Yow MD, Leeds LJ, et al: Failure of penicillin to eradicate group B streptococcal colonization in the pregnant woman. Am J Obstet Gynecol 1979; 135:1062.

69. Hall RT, Barnes W, Krishnan L, et al: Antibiotic treatment of parturient women colonized with group B streptococci. Am J Obstet Gynecol 1976; 124:630.

70. Lewin EB, Amstey MS: Natural history of group B *Streptococcus* colonization and its therapy during pregnancy. Am J Obstet Gynecol 1981; 139:512.

71. Garland SM, Fliegner JR: Group B *Streptococcus* (GBS) and neonatal infections: The case for intrapartum chemoprophylaxis. Aust N Z J Obstet Gynaecol 1991; 31:119.

72. Minkoff H, Mead P: An obstetric approach to the prevention of early-onset group B beta-hemolytic streptococcal sepsis. Am J Obstet Gynecol 1986; 154:973.

73. Baker CJ: Inadequacy of rapid immunoassays for intrapartum detection of group B streptococcal carriers. Obstet Gynecol 1996; 88:51.

74. Ostroff RM, Steaffens JW: Effect of specimen storage, antibiotics, and feminine hygiene products on the detection of group B *Streptococcus* by culture and the STREP B OIA test. Diagn Microbiol Infect Dis 1995; 22:253.

75. American College of Obstetricians and Gynecologists: Group B streptococcal infections in pregnancy. ACOG technical bulletin No. 170. Washington, DC, American College of Obstetricians and Gynecologists, 1992.

76. American Academy of Pediatrics: Guidelines for prevention of group B streptococcal infection by chemoprophylaxis. Pediatrics 1992; 90:775.

77. Gigante J, Hickson GB, Entman SS, Oquist NL: Universal screening for group B *Streptococcus:* Recommendations and obstetricians' practice decisions. Obstet Gynecol 1995; 85:440.

78. Whitney CG, Plikaytis BD, Gozansky WS, et al: Prevention practices for perinatal group B streptococcal disease: A multi-state surveillance analysis. Obstet Gynecol 1997; 89:28.

79. Mercer BM, Miodovnik M, Thurnau GR, et al: Antibiotic therapy for reduction of infant mortality after preterm premature rupture of the membranes: A randomized controlled trial. JAMA 1997; 278:989.

80. Sperling RS, Ramamurthy RS, Gibbs RS: A comparison of intrapartum versus immediate postpartum treatment of intra-amniotic infection. Obstet Gynecol 1987; 70:861.

81. Soper DE, Mayhall G, Froggatt JW: Characterization and control of intra-amniotic infection in an urban teaching hospital. Am J Obstet Gynecol 1996; 175:304.

82. Gilstrap LC, Leveno KJ, Cox SM, et al: Intrapartum treatment of acute chorioamnionitis: Impact on neonatal sepsis. Am J Obstet Gynecol 1988; 159:579.

83. Weeks JW, Myers SR, Lasher L, et al: Persistence of penicillin G benzathine in pregnant group B *Streptococcus* carriers. Obstet Gynecol 1997; 90:240.

84. Amstey MS, Gibbs RS: Is penicillin G a better choice than ampicillin for prophylaxis of neonatal group B streptococcal infections? Obstet Gynecol 1994; 84:1058.

85. Noya FJD: Intravenously administered immune globulin for premature infants: A time to wait. J Pediatr 1989; 115:969.

86. Baker CJ, Kasper DL: Group B streptococcal vaccines. Rev Infect Dis 1985; 7:458.

87. Baker CJ, Edwards MS, Kasper DL: Immunogenicity of polysaccharides from type III, group B streptococcus. J Clin Invest 1978; 61:1107.

88. Baker CJ, Edwards MS, Kasper DL: Role of antibody to native type III polysaccharide of group B streptococcus in infant infection. Pediatrics 1981; 68:544.

89. Baker CJ, Rench MA, Edwards MS, et al: Immunization of pregnant women with a polysaccharide vaccine of group B streptococcus. N Engl J Med 1988; 319:1180.

90. Baker CJ: Immunization to prevent group B streptococcal disease: Victories and vexations. J Infect Dis 1990; 161:917.

91. Baltimore RS, Baker CJ, Kasper DL: Antibody to group B *Streptococcus* type III in human sera are measured by a mouse protection test. Infect Immun 1981; 32:56.

92. Larsen JW Jr, Harper JS III, London WT, et al: Antibody to type III group B *Streptococcus* in the rhesus monkey. Am J Obstet Gynecol 1983; 146:958.

93. Santos JI, Shigeoka AO, Rote NS, et al: Protective efficacy of a

modified immune serum globulin in experimental group B streptococcal infection. J Pediatr 1981; 99:873.

94. Hemming VG, London WT, Fischer GW, et al: Immunoprophylaxis of postnatally acquired group B streptococcal sepsis in neonatal rhesus monkeys. J Infect Dis 1987; 156:655.

95. Rodewald AK, Onderdonk AB, Warren HB, et al: Neonatal mouse model of group B streptococcal infection. J Infect Dis 1992; 166:635.

96. Klegerman ME, Boyer KM, Papierniak CK, et al: Estimation of the protective level of human IgG antibody to the type-specific polysaccharide of group B *Streptococcus* type Ia. J Infect Dis 1983; 148:648.

97. Boyer KM, Kendall LS, Papierniak CK, et al: Protective levels of human immunoglobulin G antibody to group B *Streptococcus* type Ib. Infect Immun 1984; 45:618.

98. Gotoff SP, Odell C, Papierniak CK, et al: Human IgG antibody to group B streptococcus type III: Comparison of protective levels in a murine model with levels in infected human neonates. J Infect Dis 1986; 153:511.

99. Gotoff SP, Papierniak CK, Klegerman ME, et al: Quantitation of IgG antibody to the type-specific polysaccharide of group B streptococcus type 1b in pregnant women and infected infants. J Pediatr 1984; 105:628.

100. Gray BM, Pritchard DG, Dillon HC Jr: Seroepidemiological studies of group B Streptococcus type II. J Infect Dis 1985; 151:1073.

101. Madoff LC, Michell JL, Gong EW, et al: Protection of neonatal mice from group B streptococcal infection by maternal immunization with beta C protein. Infect Immun 1992; 60:4989.

102. Baker CJ, Kasper DL, Davis CE: Immunochemical characterization of the native type III polysaccharide of group B *Streptococcus*. J Exp Med 1976; 143:258.

103. Kasper DL, Baker CJ, Glades B, et al: Immunochemical analysis and immunogenicity of the type II group B streptococcal capsular polysaccharide. J Clin Invest 1983; 72:260.

104. Jennings HJ, Katzenellenbogen E, Lugowski C, et al: Structure of the native polysaccharide antigens of type Ia and type Ib group B *Streptococcus*. Biochemistry 1983; 22:1258.

105. Baker CJ, Edwards MS, Kasper DL: Immunogenicity of polysaccharides from type III group B *Streptococcus*. J Clin Invest 1978; 61:1107.

106. Baker CJ, Kasper DL: Group B streptococcal vaccines. Rev Infect Dis 1985; 7:458.

107. Wessels MR, Paoletti LC, Kasper DL, et al: Immunogenicity in animals of a polysaccharide-protein conjugate vaccine against type III group B *Streptococcus*. J Clin Invest 1990; 58:687.

108. Baker CJ, Rench MA, Edwards MS, et al: Immunization of pregnant women with a polysaccharide vaccine of group B *Streptococcus*. N Engl J Med 1988; 319:1180.

109. Baker CJ: Immunization to prevent group B streptococcal disease: Victories and vexations. J Infect Dis 1990; 161:917.

110. Baker CJ: Group B streptococcal infection in newborns: Prevention at last? N Engl J Med 1986; 314:1702.

111. Jennings H: Further approaches for optimizing polysaccharide-protein conjugate vaccines for prevention of invasive bacterial disease. J Infect Dis 1992; 165(suppl 1): S156.

112. Wessels MR, Paoletti LC, Kasper DL, et al: Immunogenicity in animals of a polysaccharide-protein conjugate vaccine against type III group B *Streptococcus*. J Clin Invest 1990; 86:1428.

113. Lagergard T, Shiloach J, Robbins JB, et al: Synthesis and immunological properties of conjugate composed of group B streptococcus capsular polysaccharide covalently bound to tetanus toxoid. Infect Immun 1990; 58:687.

114. Paoletti LC, Kasper DL, Michon F, et al: An oligosaccharide–tetanus toxoid conjugate vaccine against type III group B *Streptococcus*. J Biol Chem 1990; 265:18278.

115. Paoletti LC, Kasper DL, Michon F, et al: Effects of chain length on the immunogenicity in rabbits of group B *Streptococcus* type III oligosaccharide–tetanus toxoid conjugate. J Clin Invest 1992; 89:203.

116. Paoletti LC, Wessels MR, Michon F, et al: Group B *Streptococcus* type II polysaccharide–tetanus toxoid conjugate vaccine. Infect Immun 1992; 60:4009.

117. Madoff LC, Michel JL, Gong EW, et al: Protection of neonatal mice from group B streptococcal infection by maternal immunization with beta C protein. Infect Immun 1992; 60:4989.

118. Michel JL, Madoff LC, Kling DE, et al: Cloned alpha and beta C-protein antigens of group B streptococci elicit protective immunity. Infect Immun 1991; 59:2023.

119. Wilkerson HW, Eagon RG: Type-specific antigens of groups B type Ic streptococci. Infect Immun 1971; 4:596.

120. Johnson DR, Ferrieri P: Group B streptococcal Ibc protein antigen: Distribution of two determinants in wild-type strains of common serotypes. J Clin Microbiol 1984; 19:506.

121. Bevanger L, Naess AI: Mouse-protective antibodies against the Ibc proteins of group B streptococci. Acta Pathol Microbiol Scand 1985; Sect B 93:121.

122. Michel JL, Madoff LC, Kling DE, et al: Cloned alpha and beta c-protein antigens of group B streptococci elicit protective immunity. Infect Immun 1991; 59:2023.

123. Stalhammar-Carlemalm M, Stenberg L, Lindahl G: Protein Rib: A novel group B streptococcal cell surface protein that confers protective immunity and is expressed by most strains causing invasive infections. J Exp Med 1993; 177:1593.

124. Institute of Medicine, National Academy of Sciences. Appendix P. New vaccine development: Establishing priorities. In: Diseases of Importance in the United States, Vol 1. Washington, DC, National Academy Press, 1985, pp 242–439.

125. Mohle-Boetani JC, Schuchat A, Plikaytis BD, et al: Comparison of prevention strategies for neonatal group B streptococcal infection: A population-based economic analysis. JAMA 1993; 270:1442.

Clinical Syndromes

11

Premature Labor and Infection

SEBASTIAN FARO

The exact role of the presence of bacteria in amniotic fluid is not very well understood. Bacteria are found in the amniotic cavity in approximately 10% of patients with premature rupture of amniotic membranes (PROM).[1-4] Bacteria ascend into the intrauterine cavity in both the presence and the absence of intact membranes.[5, 6] The bacteria most commonly found invading the intra-amniotic fluid and the amniotic membranes have their origin in the endogenous vaginal microflora. Preterm PROM occurs in approximately 5% of all pregnancies and accounts for 30% to 40% of all premature deliveries. Thus, it is important to understand the conditions and factors that contribute to this event because of the significant short- and long-term neonatal morbidity, mortality, and extreme cost associated with PROM and delivery.

MICROBIOLOGY

There is little doubt that the vaginal microflora make a significant contribution to the bacteriology of preterm PROM. However, it is not understood how these bacteria actually initiate infection or colonize the amniotic membranes. The differences that exist between pregnant women that result in some (5%) having PROM is also not understood. The incidence of PROM ranges from a high of 18% to a low of 2%.[7-9]

Bacteria migrate from the vagina up the endocervical canal to reach the membranes that overlay the internal cervical os. The bacteria follow one of two courses or simultaneously take advantage of both opportunities; that is, they adhere to the amniotic membranes or travel and adhere to the basal lining of the uterus, resulting in a deciduitis. A progesterone-dominant mucus plug blocks bacteria from entering the endocervical canal during much of the pregnancy. This prohibits bacteria from ascending the canal and reaching the amniotic membranes and decidua of the uterus.

The bacteriology of the vagina is complex and consists of a great variety of gram-positive, gram-negative, aerobic, facultative, and obligate anaerobic bacteria. The bacterial make-up of the endogenous vaginal microflora can be altered by a variety of factors, especially the sexual practices of the patient and her partner. Consideration should also be given to the possibility of an oral-hand-vagina route as well as an oral-hematogenous-vaginal route. *Fusobacterium nucleatum*, *F. nucleatum* subspecies *vincentii*, *Capnocytophaga*, and other typically dominant oral bacteria have been isolated from amniotic fluid.[10, 11] This indicates and raises the concern that potentially virulent bacteria can be added to the complex vaginal microflora, thus increasing the risk for amnionitis, chorioamnionitis, and deciduitis. In addition to the bacteria that consistently make up the endogenous vaginal flora, other microorganisms that play a significant role are *Streptococcus agalactiae* (group B streptococci [GBS]), *Trichomonas vaginalis*, and *Candida* (Table 11–1). In addition to the organisms listed in Table 11–1, other bacteria have been isolated in association with preterm labor and PROM, including *Neisseria gonorrhoeae*, *Chlamydia trachomatis*, *Mycoplasma hominis*, and *Ureaplasma urealyticum*.

Many different bacteria have been isolated from pregnant women in premature labor with and without rupture of amniotic membranes. Bacteria of particular interest are the mycoplasmas and ureaplasmas.[12] Several investigators have studied the relationship between *U. urealyticum* and *M. hominis* and premature labor. Abele-Horn and colleagues[13] prospectively studied the relationship between *U. urealyticum* colonization of the genital tract and pregnancy and neonatal outcome. These authors found 170 pregnant women were colonized and 83 women were not colonized by

TABLE 11–1 ▶	BACTERIA ISOLATED FROM AMNIOTIC FLUID	
Gram-Positive	**Gram-Negative**
Streptococcus agalactiae	Escherichia coli
Streptococcus pneumoniae	Enterobacter aerogenes
Streptococcus viridans	Enterobacter cloacae
Enterococcus faecalis	Gardnerella vaginalis
Streptobacillus moniliformis	Klebsiella pneumoniae
Staphylococcus aureus	Morganella morganii
Staphylococcus epidermidis	Salmonella
Peptococcus	Fusobacterium nucleatum
Peptostreptococcus	Prevotella
	Bacteroides

U. urealyticum. Both groups of women included those with an impending or premature delivery. Compared with uncolonized women, women colonized by *U. urealyticum* had a significantly increased risk of amnionitis (2% vs. 35%; $P < .001$), chorioamnionitis (0% vs. 10%; $P < .05$), PROM (12% vs. 35%; $P < .001$), and delivery of a premature infant (10% vs. 41%; $P < .001$).[13] Several investigators have found a statistically significant relationship between *U. urealyticum* colonization, preterm delivery, and poor perinatal outcome.[14–18] Bashri and co-workers[19] demonstrated that an increase in intra-amniotic fluid levels of interleukin-6 (IL-6) was indicative of intra-amniotic infection with *U. urealyticum* and adverse pregnancy outcome.

Antsaklis and colleagues[20] treated 18 pregnant women between 26 and 34 weeks' gestation who were in premature labor and had intact amniotic membranes with erythromycin and ritodrine. Their control group consisted of 17 matched pregnant women who did not receive antibiotics. The patients in the treated group received erythromycin, 500 mg PO every 8 hours for 10 days. These investigators reported that the treated group had a statistically significant greater mean delay of delivery (36.4 days) than the control group (23.1 days).[20] Ogasawara and Goodwin[21] found that a single dose of azithromycin, 1 g, did not affect colonization of the lower genital tract by *U. urealyticum.*

Candida is gaining recognition as a primary pathogen causing infection in healthy women. Sfameni and associates[22] reported two cases of chorioamnionitis secondary to infection with *Candida glabrata.*

EPIDEMIOLOGY

Approximately 10% of all perinatal deaths are associated with PROM.[23] The risk to the mother may also be significant because prolonged PROM (>48 hours) increases the risk of postpartum endometritis, especially if cesarean delivery is necessary. Duration of PROM for longer than 48 hours is associated with an increase in antepartum, intrapartum, and postpartum infectious and febrile morbidity.[24] Thus, infection does appear to be a main factor leading to PROM. Minkoff and co-workers[25] found that women with PROM had a higher incidence of vaginal *T. vaginalis* and *Staphylococcus* infection. Although there has been a great deal of investigation and discussion regarding bacterial vaginosis and the occurrence of PROM, a statistical association between the two has not been established. McDonald and colleagues[26] performed a double-blind, placebo-controlled study on 879 pregnant women comparing oral metronidazole, 400 mg twice daily, with placebo for 2 days administered at 24 and 29 weeks' gestation if *Gardnerella vaginalis* was found at the 4-week evaluation. In the group with bacterial vaginosis (480 patients) treated with metronidazole versus placebo, metronidazole treatment had no effect on the spontaneous preterm birth rate (11/242 [4.5%] vs. 15/238 [6.3%]).[26] However, they did find that in women who had experienced a previous preterm birth, 46 patients treated with metronidazole exhibited a significant reduction in the spontaneous preterm birth rate (2/22 [9/1%] vs. 10/24 [41.7%], odds ratio 0.14, 95% confidence interval 0.01 to 0.84).[26] Thus, in women with bacterial vaginosis and no previous history of spontaneous preterm birth, treatment with metronidazole did not reduce the risk of preterm delivery. However, pregnant women with bacterial vaginosis and a previous history of preterm delivery do benefit from treatment with metronidazole. Treatment of pregnant women with a history of previous preterm birth with intravaginal clindamycin 2% cream does not reduce their risk of a spontaneous preterm birth.[27]

Colonization of the lower genital tract with GBS has been identified as a risk factor for preterm delivery. GBS colonization is twice as common among women who deliver prematurely than those who deliver at term.[28] The acquisition of GBS and subsequent colonization of the vagina is a perplexing problem. How does a person acquire GBS and initially become colonized? The answer to this question is not known. However, there are data to suggest that if either partner becomes colonized, transmission to the other partner by sexual intercourse is possible. Yamamoto and associates[29] studied married couples and found that GBS could be recovered from 18.5% of pregnant women and from 18% of their husbands' urine.

Group B streptococci continue to be a significant problem for both the obstetrician and the neonatologist. They are the most common cause of systemic infection in neonates younger than 7 days of age. Mortality rates are 4% to 6% of term infants and up to 20% in preterm infants.[30–32] However, early-onset disease is not a common event, with approximately 1% of neonates having early-onset disease after birth from a colonized woman. In view of the fact that vertical transmission from mother to neonate is common, rates of 29% to 72% have been reported.[33–36] The most frequent strains colonizing pregnant women and healthy neonates were equally divided between serotypes I, II, and III.[33–36] Since the late 1980s, new serotypes, IV, V, VI, and VIII, have been described.[37–40] Hickman and colleagues[41] reported a GBS colonization rate of 28% for 546 pregnant women, with the highest rate, 40.6%, in black women, 20.3% in whites, and 26.9% in Hispanics. Vertical transmission was significantly reduced in mothers receiving intrapartum antibiotic prophylaxis (0% vs. 54%), in those with time from rupture of the amniotic membranes to delivery less than 12 hours (38.4% vs. 73.3%), or in those whose delivery was accomplished by cesarean section (4% vs. 20%).[41] The common serotypes reported were Ia (32%), II (25%), III (22.4%), and V (11.8%).[41]

Group B streptococci, like other bacteria that inhabit the lower genital tract, have the potential to ascend through the endocervical canal and colonize the amniotic membranes. The mechanism by which bacteria are able to penetrate the mucus barrier that occludes the endocervical canal appears to reside in the ability of endogenous bacteria to produce enzymes such as mucinase and sialidase that can degrade the endocervical mucus.[42] Because GBS typically exist alongside other bacteria, it is likely that these organisms act in concert to effect colonization of the amniotic membranes, amniotic fluid, or decidua, resulting in infection and preterm labor.

Several other factors have been linked to PROM and preterm labor. Although these may not be associated with infection, they are presented in Table 11–2 for comprehensiveness.

MICROBIAL PATHOPHYSIOLOGY

The interaction between bacterial invasion and infection of the uterus, whether the membranes are intact or ruptured, depends on the bacteria or microorganisms initiating an action. This action may in turn create synergistic effects with the host, uterus, amniotic membranes, or fetus, initiating a secondary or even tertiary action. The end result is usually an adverse one— premature delivery and an infected infant. Infection is a common precursor to premature labor and PROM. The difficulty is that the mother often does not exhibit signs of infection, and therefore, even though the amniotic membranes have ruptured spontaneously and labor may ensue, there may not be any clinical sign or symptom of an associated infection.

Many investigators have reported on the results of transabdominal amniocentesis of women presenting in premature labor. The mean rate of positive amniotic fluid cultures obtained from 1,866 amniocenteses was 12.7%, reported by Gomez and colleagues[48] in a review of 22 studies. Although women with bacteria isolated from their amniotic fluid typically did not have clinical

TABLE 11-2 ▸ FACTORS ASSOCIATED WITH PREMATURE RUPTURE OF AMNIOTIC MEMBRANES AND PREMATURE LABOR

1. Amniocentesis, when performed in the second or third trimester, is associated with a 1.2% risk of rupture of the amniotic membranes.[43]
2. Cigarette smoking is associated with PROM.[44]
3. Zinc deficiency in amniotic fluid was found in 70% of women with PROM. Zinc is a component of the antibacterial peptide found in amniotic fluid.[45]
4. Coitus associated with inflammation of the amniotic membranes is associated with PROM.[46, 47]
5. Spontaneous premature delivery places the pregnant patient at risk for a recurrence of premature delivery. The approximate recurrence rate is 21%, compared with a rate of 14% to 17% for the general obstetric population.[48, 49]

PROM = premature rupture of amniotic membranes.

findings suggestive of infection, they were nevertheless more likely to acquire chorioamnionitis than women whose amniotic fluid was sterile (37.5% vs. 9%).[49–51] Women with bacteria isolated from their amniotic fluid were more likely to be refractory to tocolytic agents for inhibition of labor (85.6% vs. 16.3%).[52–55] In addition, women with intact membranes, in preterm labor, and positive amniotic fluid cultures were more likely to experience spontaneous rupture of amniotic membranes than women with negative amniotic fluid cultures (40% vs. 3.8%).[56–59]

Data on positive amniotic fluid cultures obtained by transabdominal amniocentesis from women with PROM are similar to those obtained from women with intact amniotic membranes. The mean rate of positive amniotic fluid cultures was reported to be 36.1%, based on analysis of 14 studies.[48] In all likelihood, this is a low estimate because in many instances specimens cannot be obtained because of a lack of amniotic fluid, or there is significant oligohydramnios and amniocentesis was not attempted.

Romero and co-workers[60] reported that 51.5% of women presenting with cervical dilatation of at least 2 cm and intact amniotic membranes, between 14 to 24 weeks' gestation, had positive amniotic fluid culture. Regardless of whether the membranes are intact, the eventual outcome of intra-amniotic infection or chorioamnionitis is PROM, premature delivery, fetal or neonatal infection, and possible postpartum endometritis. The mortality rate of neonates who acquire the infection in utero is 25% to 90%.[36, 61] Fetal bacteremia occurs in 33% of fetuses if bathed in infected amniotic fluid, compared with 4% of fetuses surrounded by sterile amniotic fluid.[51] This finding supports the position that the amniotic fluid of women in preterm labor is likely to be infected.

Infection may also be a direct link to the induction of prostaglandins from the amnion and chorion. Bacteria can produce phospholipase A_2 and C, which cleave and release arachidonic acid from membrane phospholipids.[55, 62–64] Infecting bacteria cause an increase in production of prostaglandins in the amnion, chorion and, probably, decidua through the activity of inflammatory agents such as cytokines, growth products, bacterial products, and other inflammatory substances.[65, 66] Once arachidonic acid is released, it can be metabolized further by different pathways (Fig. 11–1), including the cyclooxygenase pathway, which leads to the formation of prostaglandins, prostacyclin (prostaglandin I_2 [PGI_2]), and thromboxanes. It can also be metabolized by the lipoxygenase pathway to synthesize leukotrienes, hydroxyeicosatetraenoic acids, and lipoxins; or the epoxygenase pathway, leading to the formation of epoxide.[48] Women with preterm labor and intra-amniotic infection have significantly elevated concentrations of PGE_2 and $PGF_{2\alpha}$ compared with women in preterm labor without infection[56] (Fig. 11–

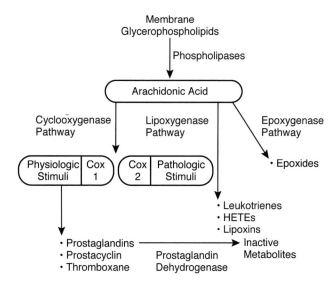

FIGURE 11-1 ▶ Metabolism of arachidonic acid. (From Gomez R, Romero R, Edwin SS, David C: Pathogenesis of preterm labor and premature rupture of membranes associated with intra-amniotic infection. Infect Dis Clin North Am. 1997; p 144.

2). Additional evidence supporting the role of bacteria and infection in causing an increase in prostaglandin synthesis comes from the demonstration of a similar association in those patients with preterm labor and high concentrations of proinflammatory agents in the amniotic fluid, such as IL-1β, tumor necrosis factor (TNF), and IL-6.[67, 68] Lopez-Bernal and co-workers[69] demonstrated that prostaglandin production was higher in amnion cells derived from patients with chorioamnionitis compared with those from women who did not have chorioamnionitis.

Several bacterial products are capable of stimulating

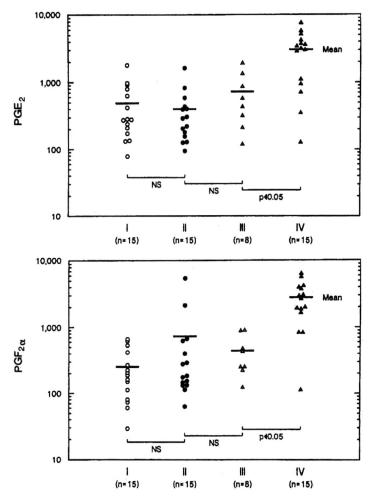

FIGURE 11-2 ▶ Amniotic fluid concentrations of PGE_2, and $PGF_{2\alpha}$ in women with labor and intra-amniotic infection (Group IV) are significantly higher than in women without these conditions (Group I: no infection, no labor; Group II: no infection, labor; Group III: infection, no labor). (From Romero R, Emamian M, Wan M, et al: Prostaglandin concentrations in amniotic fluid of women with intra-amniotic infection and preterm labor. Am J Obstet Gynecol 1987; 157:1461, with permission.)

prostaglandin production from the amnion, chorion, and decidua. Gram-negative bacterial infection of amniotic fluid releases endotoxin and lipopolysaccharide into the amniotic fluid. Endotoxin can stimulate the production of prostaglandins from the amnion and decidua. Endotoxin levels are higher in women with PROM and labor than in women with PROM and no labor.[70] That both groups of patients have amniotic fluid infected with gram-negative bacteria producing endotoxin, but in different concentrations, suggests that endotoxin alone is not sufficient to initiate labor or that a critical threshold of endotoxin must be achieved (Fig. 11–3). In addition, endotoxin may not be necessary, but may serve as an enhancing agent because preterm labor also develops in pregnant women with intra-amniotic infection caused by gram-positive bacteria.

Bacteria produce a variety of proteolytic enzymes and collagenases. These agents can weaken amniotic membranes and cause them to rupture under the pressure exerted by the weight of the amniotic fluid and fetus. McGregor and associates[71] demonstrated in vitro that bacterial collagenase causes a dose-dependent reduction in membrane strength, elasticity, work-to-rupture of membranes.

Preterm and term labor are associated with an increase in the platelet-activating factor (PAF) in amniotic fluid.[72] PAF has been associated with stimulation of PGE_2 synthesis by the amnion.[73] The enzyme responsible for activation of PAF, PAF-acetylhydrolase, is se-creted by decidual macrophages and is regulated by bacterial endotoxin and cytokines. Secretion of PAF-acetylhydrolase from decidual macrophages is inhibited by endotoxin, IL-1α, IL-1β, and TNF.[48] Endotoxin can be partially blocked by the natural IL-1 receptor antagonist, and this cytokine can also block the action of IL-1α and IL-1β on secretion of PAF-acetylhydrolase by the decidua.[74] Thus, PAF appears to play a role in the mechanism of both term and premature labor.

The macrophages in the decidua and fetal and maternal tissues can be stimulated by bacterial products (endotoxin) to secrete a variety of proinflammatory cytokines (e.g., IL-1, IL-6, IL-8, and TNF). Endotoxin and cytokines can act synergistically to create septic shock. The effects of deciduitis, chorioamnionitis, and intra-amniotic infection on the fetus can be equated with those of septic shock. Thus, the proinflammatory response initiated in the maternal compartment in response to infection can also be seen in the fetus.

Interleukin-1 is produced by monocytes and macrophages in response to bacterial infection and liberation of endotoxin. IL-1 has multiple effects because it is a pleiotropic cytokine. When IL-1 acts with IL-6 and TNF, it mediates host responses to infection and tissue injury. IL-1 exists in two forms, IL-1α and IL-1β, which are derived from two distinct genes. IL-1 is responsible for mediating febrile response to infection as well as hypotension, activation of B and T lymphocytes, stimulation of collagenase activity, and prostaglandin synthesis.

Romero and co-workers[48, 75, 76] postulated that IL-1 produced by the mother or fetus serves as the signal for the initiation of labor. Support for this hypothesis includes the facts that IL-1 stimulates prostaglandin synthesis from the amnion, decidua, and myometrium; decidual cells produce IL-1 in response to bacterial infection; women in preterm labor with intra-amniotic infection or chorioamnionitis have been demonstrated to have elevated levels of IL-1 in the amniotic fluid; and women with PROM, labor, and infection have higher levels of IL-1 than women with PROM, infection, and no labor (Figs. 11–4 and 11–5).[77, 78] Plasma levels of IL-1β from fetuses born prematurely to women with intra-amniotic infection are markedly elevated.[48] Placental tissue derived from women in labor with and without infection was analyzed and found to have higher levels of IL-1 than placental tissue obtained from women not in labor.[79] Additional supporting data come from animal experiments. IL-1 administered to pregnant mice and guinea pigs, with the latter also receiving TNF, induces preterm labor.[80, 81] IL-1β gene expression is increased in fetal membranes and decidua from patients with clinical and histologic chorioamnionitis.[48] This expression has been localized to macrophages found in the chorion and decidua, and, at a lower level, to neutrophils.[48] Thus, the increase in IL-1β concentrations found in patients with

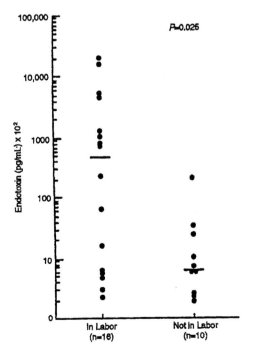

FIGURE 11–3 ▶ Endotoxin concentrations in amniotic fluid of women with premature rupture of membranes with and without labor. (From Romero R: Labor and infection II: Bacterial endotoxin in amniotic fluid and its relationship to the onset of preterm labor. Am J Obstet Gynecol 1988; 158:1044, with permission.)

chorioamnionitis appears to be derived from infiltrating inflammatory cells.[82, 83] The evidence is therefore mounting that premature labor and intra-amniotic infection, chorioamnionitis, and deciduitis cause the release of IL-1, which, in turn, activates the prostaglandin cascade to facilitate the initiation of labor.

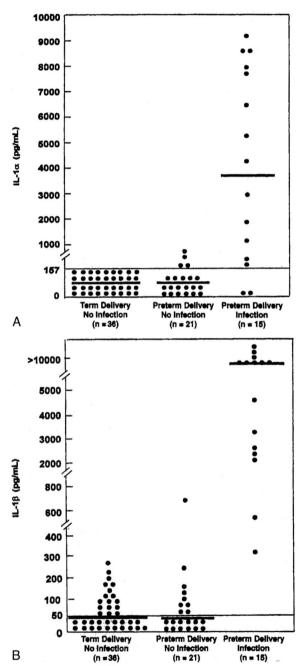

FIGURE 11-4 ▶ Amniotic fluid IL-1 concentrations in patients with preterm labor and intact membranes. *A* and *B* show that amniotic fluid concentrations of both IL-1α and IL-1β are significantly higher in women with intra-amniotic infection than in women with negative amniotic fluid cultures, respectively. (From Romero R, Mazor M, Brandt F, et al: Interleukin-1α and interleukin-1β in preterm and term parturition. Am J Reprod Immunol 1992; 27:117, © 1992 Munksgaard International Publishers Ltd., Copenhagen, Denmark, with permission.)

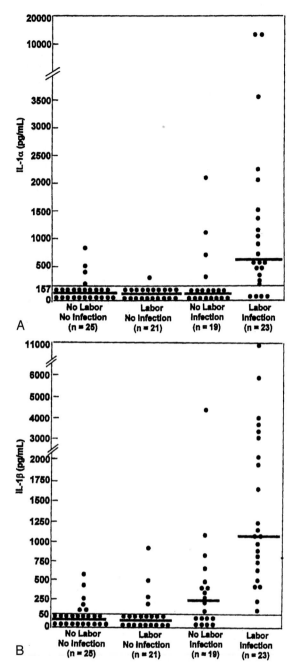

FIGURE 11-5 ▶ Amniotic fluid IL-1 concentrations in patients with preterm PROM. *A* and *B* show that amniotic fluid concentrations of both IL-1α and IL-1β are significantly higher in women with intra-amniotic infection and labor than in women of the other three groups, respectively. (From Romero R, Mazor M, Brandt F, et al: Interleukin-1α and interleukin-1β in preterm and term parturition. Am J Reprod Immunol 1992; 27:119, © 1992 Munksgaard International Publishers Ltd., Copenhagen, Denmark, with permission.)

Tumor necrosis factor is produced and secreted by macrophages, and its properties are similar to those of IL-1. It appears that TNF also has a role in premature parturition because, like IL-1, it can stimulate the amnion, chorion, and decidual cells to produce prostaglandin.[84] TNF is produced in decidual cells in the presence of infection.[85, 86] It is markedly elevated in patients with preterm labor and infection compared with those patients with preterm labor without infection[87, 88] (Fig. 11–6). TNF and IL-1 appear to have a synergistic effect on decidua, amnion, and chorion to produce prostaglandin.[89]

Interleukin-6 is produced by fibroblasts, monocytes, macrophages, endothelial cells, keratinocytes, and endometrial stromal cells. IL-6 expression is induced by IL-1, TNF, bacterial products, viruses, and second messenger agonists (diacylglycerol, cyclic adenosine monophosphate, and Ca^{2+}) that activate any of three major signal transduction pathways.[48] IL-6 can stimulate the acute-phase plasma protein response, activate T cells and natural killer cells, stimulate B cells, and stimulate the liver to produce C-reactive protein.[48] The latter is probably significant because C-reactive protein levels are elevated in the presence of infection. Early detection of a rise in the C-reactive protein can be a signal that a woman in preterm labor with or without rupture of the amniotic membranes may have an infection. Several investigators have demonstrated that the C-reactive protein level can be elevated even though clinical signs of maternal infection have not materialized.[90–92] IL-6 is similar in profile to IL-1 and TNF: it stimulates the production and release of prostaglandins from the amnion and decidua; its production by the decidua is stimulated by IL-1 and TNF; it is elevated in women with preterm labor and infection; plasma levels are elevated in those fetuses likely to deliver compared with those that remain in utero; and fetal red blood cells can produce IL-6 before and after stimulation.[93–97]

Other factors have been implicated in preterm labor and infection, including colony-stimulating factors, IL-8, macrophage inflammatory proteins 1-α and 1-β, and monocyte chemotactant protein-1. However, the role of these agents is less clear than that of IL-1, IL-6, and TNF.

The role of inhibitory agents, such as IL-1 receptor antagonist and transforming growth factor-β, has yet to be elucidated. However, the role of these agents in premature labor and their interaction with other cytokines is not understood.

DIAGNOSIS AND MANAGEMENT

The most difficult aspect of diagnosing premature labor with or without ruptured membranes is establishing that the patient is actually in labor. The second most difficult aspect is determining if an infection is present. Frequently, the patient presents with uterine contractions with or without spontaneous rupture of the amniotic membranes, and it is extremely difficult to determine if an infection is present. Patients with clinical intra-amniotic infection of chorioamnionitis can be diagnosed easily. These patients typically present with fever, elevated white blood cell count, uterine tenderness, and labor, and the amniotic fluid can be purulent.

The history is extremely important in evaluating the patient with premature labor, ruptured amniotic membranes, and possible infection. Initially, the history should establish if there has been any exposure

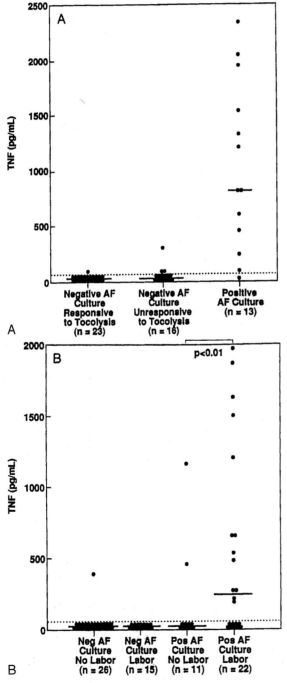

FIGURE 11–6 ▶ Amniotic fluid concentrations of TNF in patients with preterm labor and intact membranes (A) and women with preterm PROM (B). Amniotic fluid concentrations of TNF are significantly higher in patients with positive amniotic fluid cultures than in the other groups. (From Romero R, Mazor M, Sepulveda W, et al: Tumor necrosis factor in preterm and term labor. Am J Obstet Gynecol 1992; 166:1580, with permission.)

to people with a known infectious disease. The viral illnesses are common and often easily transmitted. Next, the patient should be questioned regarding oral intake (e.g., consumption of dairy products, such as cheese, salads that have a dairy base, ice cream, creamed cakes, and pies). The patient should be asked if there have been any signs of illness, general aches and pains, gastrointestinal discomfort, low-grade fever, or urinary frequency, pain, or burning.

The physical examination should begin with an assessment of the patient's skin, searching for a rash or other lesions. The pelvis should be addressed last. The pregnancy should be evaluated by measuring the fundal height and determining if this is consistent with the gestational age according to the patient's menstrual history. The patient should be asked if she has had any abdominal pain, and if so, its location, whether the pain radiated in any direction, if the pain is rhythmic, and if it can be palpated.

Once the general physical examination has been concluded, an ultrasonogram of the fetus should be obtained. This examination is very important because the fetal age must be accurately determined. Subsequent decisions are influenced by the fetal age. The amniotic fluid volume should be determined, and fetal assessment should be performed using a biophysical profile. This gives an impression of the wellness of the fetus. Fetal weight, heart rate, position, presenting part, and placental location, as well as general condition of the placenta should be assessed. If amniotic fluid is present, a transabdominal amniocentesis should be performed. Amniotic fluid should be analyzed as follows: Gram stain; glucose concentration; culture for aerobic, facultative and obligate anaerobic bacteria, and *Mycoplasma* and *Ureaplasma*; and fetal maturation studies.

The pelvic examination should begin with a close inspection of the external genitalia, searching for lesions and erythema. Skene's and Bartholin's glands should be palpated and compressed to elicit discharge, which should be clear. If it is not, a specimen should be Gram stained and cultured for the previously specified bacteria. However, specific tests for *N. gonorrhoeae* and *C. trachomatis* should also be performed. The vagina should be inspected for lesions and the discharge analyzed for infection as well as for an alteration in the natural or healthy vaginal ecosystem. This can be easily accomplished by noting the pH of the vagina, with a pH of 4.5 or more considered abnormal. A drop or two of vaginal fluid should be mixed with a drop of concentrated potassium hydroxide. If a fish-like odor is emitted, this indicates the presence of a large number of anaerobic bacteria, which is indicative of bacterial vaginosis. The absence of bacterial vaginosis and lactobacilli suggests that the patient's vagina may be colonized by a large number of *Escherichia coli*, GBS, or other bacteria. A drop or two of vaginal discharge

should be mixed with 1 to 2 mL of saline to dilute it and examined microscopically under $40\times$ magnification. This permits the dominant bacterial morphotype to be established and can determine whether any other pathogens are present (e.g., *T. vaginalis* or *Candida albicans*).

The cervix should be closely inspected for lesions or necrosis, which is indicative of infection (e.g., human papilloma virus, herpes simplex virus). The endocervix should be gently sampled with a Dacron- or cotton-tipped applicator. The color of the endocervical discharge retrieved on the applicator should be noted. Yellow endocervical discharge or the presence of mucopus is indicative of cervical infection (e.g., *N. gonorrhoeae*, *C. trachomatis*).

Inspection of the vagina for pooling of amniotic fluid can be done during the assessment of the lower genital tract. If no pooling is noted, the patient should be asked to cough and gentle pressure can be exerted by the patient or the examiner on the uterine fundus to determine if fluid exits the cervical os. If fluid is observed, or there is a collection of fluid in the posterior cul de sac, a sample of this fluid can be streaked on a glass slide and allowed to air dry. The specimen is then examined microscopically to detect if ferning of the amniotic fluid has occurred because of the formation of sodium chloride crystals on protein as the amniotic fluid dries. The presence of ferning is highly indicative of the leakage of amniotic fluid. The difficulty in relying on the patient's historical account of possible spontaneous rupture of amniotic membranes is that the loss of fluid may represent a transient episode of urinary incontinence. Another test to confirm the presence of ruptured amniotic membranes is staining the vaginal fluid with Nile blue for the presence of fetal cells. Also, indigo carmine dye can be instilled into the amniotic sac at the time of amniocentesis. A tampon is then placed in the vagina and the patient is permitted to ambulate for at least 1 hour. The tampon is removed and examined for the presence of blue dye, indicating that the amniotic membranes is not intact.

Once a diagnosis of ruptured amniotic membranes is established, the patient should be closely monitored for uterine contractions. Evaluation for the presence of infection should continue because further aggressive management—whether to maintain the fetus in utero or expedite delivery—will be based on whether infection is present. The amniotic glucose concentration may be helpful, especially in those instances where the patient is completely asymptomatic. Dildy and colleagues[98] and Kirshon and associates[99] have demonstrated the usefulness of the amniotic fluid glucose concentration in establishing the presence of infection. Dildy and colleagues[98] found that an amniotic fluid glucose concentration of less than 15 mg/dL was indicative of infection. Gauthier and Meyer[100] found that positive leukocyte esterase activity and a glucose concentration less than 16 mg/dL was indicative of intra-amniotic infection. Kirshon and associates[99] also found that a low glucose concentration (5 vs. 39.8 mg/dL, $P < .0005$) was indicative of intrauterine infection. Coultrip and Grossman[101] examined amniotic fluid for glucose concentration, leukocyte esterase activity, Gram staining, and Limulus amebocyte assay. They found that a glucose concentration no greater than 10 mg/dL had a specificity of 88%, a sensitivity of 90%, and a negative predictive value of 98% for the prediction of clinical infection in patients with PROM.[101]

Management of the patient with PROM and labor depends on the presence or absence of infection. The patient with infection requires antibiotic therapy and, most likely, expedient delivery. The antibiotic regimen should include coverage against gram-positive and gram-negative facultative and obligate anaerobic bacteria. Coverage should include *S. agalactiae* because this is a common bacterium found in the lower genital tract of up to 30% of pregnant women. Women with PROM who are not infected should be given penicillin for prophylaxis against *S. agalactiae* until culture data are available establishing the patient's status with regard to GBS. Penicillin should be used instead of ampicillin because it has a narrower spectrum of activity and it is less likely to select for *E. coli.*

The benefit of antibiotics in increasing the latency period (i.e., time to delivery) is somewhat unsettled. Some studies have reported a benefit, but others have not been able to confirm this observation. McGregor and associates[102] reported a significant mean increase in latency in patients receiving erythromycin compared with those receiving a placebo (32.5 vs. 22.4 days, $P = .027$). However, they were unable to demonstrate any benefit in patients administered clindamycin in a similar setting.[103] Morales and colleagues[104] administered ampicillin, erythromycin, or no antibiotics and also found an increased period of latency in those subjects receiving antibiotics. They found that there was a significant decrease in preterm delivery among those women receiving ampicillin, but not erythromycin.[104] Winkler and co-workers[105] found that women culture positive for *U. urealyticum* and treated with erythromycin had a prolonged latency period compared with untreated women (43 vs. 20 days, $P < .05$). Newton and colleagues[106] reported that administration of ampicillin followed by erythromycin did not have any beneficial effect on women with preterm labor. In a second study, Newton and colleagues[107] administered ampicillin with sulbactam but found no difference compared with the group receiving a placebo. Romero and associates,[108] in a multicenter study on 275 women in preterm labor randomized to ampicillin and erythromycin, or placebo, reported no difference with regard to increased latency period. Cox and colleagues[109] compared ampicillin plus sulbactam to placebo in 78 women in preterm labor and found no benefit from antibiotic therapy.

Management of the patient with documented intra-amniotic infection or chorioamnionitis is straightforward, especially if the patient is febrile or septic. These patients should be given broad-spectrum antibiotics and vaginal delivery should be attempted. Infected patients should undergo a trial of labor as long as their condition does not deteriorate. Delivering an infected patient by cesarean section increases her morbidity. Failure to recognize that the patient's uterus is converting to anaerobic metabolism and therefore cannot contract efficiently results in a prolonged labor that terminates in cesarean section. This can result in serious morbidity and mortality in infected patients with or without ruptured membranes. Therefore, it is important to determine if the amniotic membranes are ruptured or intact, and whether infection is present.

Many investigators have reported on antibiotic treatment in patients with PROM and prolongation of the latency phase. These studies have shown an increase in the latency period, but 61% of the women treated with antibiotics still deliver within 1 week.[110] The goal of expectant management is to achieve a gestation that lasts beyond 32 weeks because significant neonatal morbidity associated with long-term sequelae is thereby greatly reduced.[111, 112] Mercer and colleagues[113] conducted a placebo-controlled trial of erythromycin and found that pregnancy could be delayed, but the incidence of chorioamnionitis was not reduced.

Several trials have addressed the effect of intrapartum antibiotics on the incidence of chorioamnionitis and postpartum endometritis and neonatal outcome in patients with PROM. An improvement in the rate of chorioamnionitis, postpartum endometritis, or neonatal complications has not been demonstrated.[114–117]

REFERENCES

1. Arias F, Rodriquez L, Rayne SC, Kraus FT: Maternal placental vasculopathy and injection: Two distinct subgroups among patients with preterm labor and preterm ruptured membranes. Am J Obstet Gynecol 1993; 168:585.
2. Duff P, Kopelman JN: Subclinical intra-amniotic infection in asymptomatic patients with refractory preterm labor. Obstet Gynecol 1987; 69:756.
3. Romero R, Sirtori M, Oyarzun E, et al: Infection and labor. V: Prevalence, microbiology, and clinical significance of intraamniotic infection in women with preterm labor and intact membranes. Am J Obstet Gynecol 1989; 161:817.
4. Romero R, Yoon BH, Mazor M, et al: The diagnostic and prognostic value of amniotic fluid white blood cell count, glucose, interleukin-6, and Gram-stain in patients with preterm labor and intact membranes. Am J Obstet Gynecol 1993; 169:805.
5. Romero R, Avila C, Brekus CA, Morotti R: The role of systemic and intrauterine infection in preterm parturition. Ann NY Acad Sci 1991; 622:355.
6. Faro S, Walker C, Pierson RL: Amnionitis with intact amniotic membranes involving *Streptobacillus moniliformis*. Obstet Gynecol 1980; 55(suppl 3):9s.
7. Gunn GC, Mishell DR Jr, Morton DG: Premature rupture of the fetal membranes: A review. Am J Obstet Gynecol 1970; 106:469.

8. Polansky GH, Varner MW, O'Gorman T: Premature rupture of the membranes and barometric pressure changes. J Reprod Med 1985; 30:189.

9. Trap R, Helm P, Lidegaard O, Helm E: Premature rupture of the fetal membranes, the phases of the moon and barometer readings. Gynecol Obstet Invest 1989; 28:14.

10. Hill GB: Preterm birth: Associations with genital and possibly oral microflora. Ann Periodontol 1998; 3:222.

11. Davenport ES, Williams CE, Sterne JA, et al: East London study of maternal chronic periodontal disease and preterm low birth weight infants: Study design and prevalence data. Ann Periodontol 1998; 3:213.

12. Hillier SL, Martius J, Krohn M, et al: A case-control study of chorioamnionitic infection and histologic chorioamnionitis in prematurity. N Engl J Med 1988; 319:972.

13. Abele-Horn M, Peters J, Genzel-Boroviczeny O, et al: Vaginal *Ureaplasma urealyticum* colonization: Influence on pregnancy outcome and neonatal morbidity. Infection 1997; 25:286.

14. Yoon BH, Chang JW, Romero R: Isolation of *Ureaplasma urealyticum* from the amniotic cavity and adverse outcome in preterm labor. Obstet Gynecol 1998; 92:77.

15. Paul VK, Gupta U, Singh M, et al: Association of genital mycoplasma colonization with low birth weight. Int J Gynaecol Obstet 1998; 63:109.

16. Wang EE, Matlow AG, Ohlsson A, Nelson SC: *Ureaplasma urealyticum* infections in the perinatal period. Clin Perinatol 1997; 24:91.

17. Knox CL, Cave DG, Farrell DJ, et al: The role of *Ureaplasma urealyticum* in adverse pregnancy outcome. Aust N Z J Obstet Gynecol 1997; 37:45.

18. Knudsin RB, Leviton A, Allred EN, Poulin SA: *Ureaplasma urealyticum* infection of the placenta in pregnancies that ended prematurely. Obstet Gynecol 1996; 87:122.

19. Bashiri A, Horowitz S, Huleihel M, et al: Elevated concentrations of interleukin-6 in intra-amniotic infection with *Ureaplasma urealyticum* in asymptomatic women during genetic amniocentesis. Acta Obstet Gynecol Scand 1999; 78:379.

20. Antsaklis A, Daskalakis G, Michalas S, Aravantinos D: Erythromycin treatment for subclinical *Ureaplasma urealyticum* infection in preterm labor. Fetal Diagn Ther 1997; 12:89.

21. Ogasawara KK, Goodwin TM: Efficacy of azithromycin in reducing lower genital *Ureaplasma urealyticum* colonization in women at risk for preterm delivery. J Matern Fetal Med 1999; 8:12.

22. Sfameni SF, Talbot JM, Chow SL, et al: *Candida glabrata* chorioamnionitis following in vitro fertilization and embryo transfer. Aust N Z J Obstet Gynaecol 1997; 37:88.

23. Naeye RL: Causes of perinatal mortality in the US Collaborative Perinatal Project. JAMA 1977; 238:228.

24. Burchell RC. Premature spontaneous rupture of the membranes. Am J Obstet Gynecol 1964; 88:251.

25. Minkoff H, Grunebaum AN, Schwarz RH, et al: Risk factors for prematurity and premature rupture of membranes: A prospective study of the vaginal flora in pregnancy. Am J Obstet Gynecol 1984; 150:965.

26. McDonald HM, O'Loughlin JA, Vigneswaran R, et al: Impact of metronidazole therapy on preterm birth in women with bacterial vaginosis flora (*Gardnerella vaginalis*): A randomized, placebo-controlled trial. Br J Obstet Gynaecol 1997; 104:1391.

27. Vermeulen GM, Bruinse HW: Prophylactic administration of clindamycin 2% vaginal cream to reduce the incidence of spontaneous preterm birth in women with an increased recurrence risk: A randomized placebo-controlled double-blind trial. Br J Obstet Gynaecol 1999; 106:652.

28. Regan JA, Chao S, James LS: Premature rupture of membranes, preterm delivery, and group B streptococcal colonization of mothers. Am J Obstet Gynecol 1981; 141:184.

29. Yamamoto T, Nagasawa I, Nojima M, et al: Sexual transmission and reinfection of group B streptococci between spouses. J Obstet Gynaecol Res 1999; 25:215.

30. Schuchat A: Epidemiology of group B streptococcal disease in the United States: Shifting paradigms. Clin Microbiol Rev 1998; 11:497.

31. Schuchat A, Deaver-Robinson K, Plikaytis BD, et al: Multistate case-control study of maternal risk factors for neonatal group B streptococcal disease. Pediatr Infect Dis J 1994; 13:623.

32. Baker CJ: Group B streptococcal infections. Clin Perinatol 1997; 24:59.

33. Baker CJ, Barrett FF: Transmission of group B streptococci among parturient women and their neonates. J Pediatr 1973; 83:919.

34. Anthony BF, Okada DM, Hobel CJ: Epidemiology of the group B streptococcus: Maternal and nosocomial sources for infant acquisitions. J Pediatr 1979; 95:431.

35. Ancona RJ, Ferrieri P, Williams PP: Maternal factors that enhance the acquisition of group B streptococci by newborn infants. J Med Microbiol 1980; 13:273.

36. Boyer KM, Gotoff SP: Prevention of early-onset neonatal group B streptococcal disease with selective intrapartum chemoprophylaxis. N Engl J Med 1986; 314:1665.

37. Jelinkova J, Motlova J: Worldwide distribution of two new serotypes of group B streptococci: Type IV and provisional type V. J Clin Microbiol 1985; 21:361.

38. Rench MA, Baker CJ: Neonatal sepsis caused by a new group B streptococcal serotype. J Pediatr 1993; 122:638.

39. Lin FY, Clemens JD, Azimi PH, et al: Capsular polysaccharide types of group B streptococcal isolates from neonates with early-onset systemic infection. J Infect Dis 1998; 177:790.

40. Lachenauer CS, Kasper DL, Shimada J, et al: Serotypes VI and VII predominate among group B streptococcal isolates from pregnant Japanese women. [Abstract.] In: Program and Abstracts of the 37th Interscience Conference on Antimicrobial Agents and Chemotherapy 1997; 318:K80.

41. Hickman ME, Rench MA, Ferrieri P, Baker CJ: Changing epidemiology of group B streptococcal colonization. Pediatrics 1999; 104:203.

42. Howe L, Wiggins R, Soothill PW, et al: Mucinase and sialidase activity of the vaginal microflora: Implications for the pathogenesis of preterm labor. Int J STD AIDS 1999; 10:442.

43. Gold RB, Goyert GL, Schwarz DB, et al: Conservative management of second trimester post-amniocentesis fluid leakage. Obstet Gynecol 1989; 74:745.

44. Harger JH, Hsing AW, Tuomala RE, et al: Risk factors for preterm premature rupture of fetal membranes: A multicenter case-controlled study. Am J Obstet Gynecol 1990; 163:130.

45. Blanco JD, Gibbs RS, Krebs LF, Castaneda YS: The association between the absence of amniotic fluid bacterial inhibitory activity and intra-amniotic infection. Am J Obstet Gynecol 1982; 143:749.

46. Naeye RL, Ross S: Coitus and chorioamnionitis: A prospective study. Early Hum Dev 1982; 6:91.

47. Naeye RL: Factors that predispose to premature rupture of fetal membranes. Obstet Gynecol 1982; 60:93.

48. Gomez R, Romero R, Edwin SS, David C: Pathogenesis of preterm labor and premature rupture of membranes associated with intraamniotic infection. Infect Dis Clin North Am 1997; 11:135.

49. Galask RP, Varner MW, Petzold CR, Wilbur SL: Bacterial attachment to the chorioamniotic membranes. Am J Obstet Gynecol 1984; 148:915.

50. Romero R, Manogue KR, Murray MD, et al: Infection and labor. IV: Cachectin tumor necrosis factor in the amniotic fluid of women with intraamniotic infection and preterm labor. Am J Obstet Gynecol 1989; 161:336.

51. Carroll SG, Papaioannou S, Nitumazah IL, et al: Lower genital tract swabs in the prediction of intrauterine infection in preterm prelabour rupture of the membranes. Br J Obstet Gynaecol 1996; 103:54.

52. Bejar R, Curbelo V, Davis C, Gluck L: Premature labor. II: Bacterial sources of phospholipase. Obstet Gynecol 1981; 57:479.

53. Keirse MJ, Flint AP, Turnbull AC: F prostaglandins in amniotic fluid during pregnancy and labour. J Obstet Gynecol Br Commonw 1974; 81:131.

54. Matsuzaki N, Saji F, Kameda T, et al: In vitro and in vivo production of interleukin-6 by fetal mononuclear cells. Clin Immunol Immunopathol 1990; 55:305.

55. Embrey MP: Induction of abortion by prostaglandins E_1 and E_2. BMJ 1970; 1:258.

56. Balavoine JF, de Rochemonteix B, Williamson K, et al: Prostaglandin E_2 and collagenase production by fibroblasts and synovial cells is regulated by urine-derived human interleukin-1 and inhibitor(s). J Clin Invest 1986; 78:1120.

57. Bobitt J, Hayslip CC, Damato JD: Amniotic fluid infection as determined by transabdominal amniocentesis in patients with intact membranes in premature labor. Am J Obstet Gynecol 1981; 140:947.

58. Arend WP: Interleukin 1 receptor antagonist: A new member of the interleukin family. J Clin Invest 1991; 88:1445.

59. Feinstein SJ, Vintzileos AM, Lodeiro JG, et al: Amniocentesis with premature rupture of membranes. Obstet Gynecol 1986; 68:147.

60. Romero R, Gonzalez R, Sepulveda W, et al: Infection and labor. VIII: Microbial invasion of the amniotic cavity in patients with suspected cervical incompetence: Prevalence and clinical significance. Am J Obstet Gynecol 1992; 167:1086.

61. Gerdes JS: Clinicopathologic approach to the diagnosis of neonatal sepsis. Clin Perinatol 1991; 18:361.

62. Bennet PR, Rose MP, Myatt L, Elder MG: Preterm labor: Stimulation of arachidonic acid metabolism in human amnion cells by bacterial products. Am J Obstet Gynecol 1987; 156:649.

63. Lamont RF, Anthony F, Myatt L, et al: Production of prostaglandin E2 by human amnion in vitro in response to addition of media conditioned by microorganisms associated with chorioamnionitis and preterm labor. Am J Obstet Gynecol 1990; 162:819.

64. McGregor JA, French JI, Jones W, et al: Association of cervicovaginal infections with increased vaginal fluid phospholipase A2 activity. Am J Obstet Gynecol 1992; 167:1588.

65. Gomez R, Ghezzi F, Romero R, et al: Premature labor and intra-amniotic infection: Clinical aspects and role of the cytokines in diagnosis and pathophysiology. Clin Perinatol 1995; 22:281.

66. Kelly RW: Pregnancy maintenance and parturition: The role of prostaglandin in manipulating the immune and inflammatory response. Endocr Rev 1994; 15:684.

67. Romero R, Wu YK, Mazor M, et al: Amniotic fluid concentration of 5-hydroxyeicosatetraenoic acid is increased in human parturition at term. Prostaglandins Leukot Essent Fatty Acids 1989; 35:81.

68. Cox SM, King MR, Casey ML, MacDonald PC: Interleukin-1β, 1α, and 6 and prostaglandins in vaginal/cervical fluids of pregnant women before and during labor. J Clin Endocrinol Metab 1993; 77:805.

69. Lopez-Bernal A, Hansell DJ, Canete Soler R, et al: Prostaglandins, chorioamnionitis and preterm labour. Br J Obstet Gynaecol 1987; 94:1156.

70. Romero R, Roslansky P, Oyarzun E, et al: Labor and infection. II: Bacterial endotoxin in amniotic fluid and its relationship to the onset of preterm labor. Am J Obstet Gynecol 1988; 158:1044.

71. McGregor JA, French JI, Lawellin D, et al: Bacterial protease-induced reduction of chorioamniotic membrane strength and elasticity. Obstet Gynecol 1987; 69:167.

72. Hoffman DR, Romero R, Johnston JM: Detection of platelet-activating factor in amniotic fluid of complicated pregnancies. Am J Obstet Gynecol 1990; 162:525.

73. Morris C, Khan H, Sullivan M, Elder MG: Effects of platelet-activating factor on prostaglandin E2 production by intact fetal membranes. Am J Obstet Gynecol 1992; 166:1228.

74. Narahara H, Johnston JM: Effects of endotoxins and cytokines on the secretion of platelet-activating factor acetylhydrolase by human decidual macrophages. Am J Obstet Gynecol 1993; 169:531.

75. Romero R, Durum S, Dinerallo C, et al: Interleukin-1: A signal for the initiation of labor in chorioamnionitis. Presented at the 33rd Annual Meeting for the Society for Gynecologic Investigation, Toronto, Canada, March 19–22, 1986.

76. Romero R. LaFreniere D, Duff G, et al: Human decidua: A potent source of interleukin-1 like activity. Presented at the 32nd Annual Meeting of the Society of Gynecologic Investigation, Phoenix, Arizona, March 20–23, 1985.

77. Romero R, Brody DT, Oyarzun E, et al: Infection and labor. III: Interleukin-1: a signal for the onset of parturition. Am J Obstet Gynecol 1989; 160:1117.

78. Romero R, Mazor M, Brandt F, et al: Interleukin-1α and interleukin-1β in preterm and term human parturition. Am J Reprod Immunol 1992; 27:117.

79. Romero R, Mazor M, Tartakovsky B: Systemic administration of interleukin-1 induces preterm parturition in mice. Am J Obstet Gynecol 1991; 165:969.

80. Bukowski R, Scholz P, Hasan S, et al: Induction of preterm parturition with interleukin-1β (IL-1β), tumor necrosis factor (factor-α [TNF-α]) and LPS in guinea pigs. Presented at the 40th Annual Meeting of the Society for Gynecological Investigation, Toronto, Canada, March 31–April 3, 1993.

81. Taniguchi T, Matsuzaki N, Kameda T, et al: The enhanced production of placental interleukin-1 during labor and intrauterine infection. Am J Obstet Gynecol 1991; 165:131.

82. Kauma SW, Walsh SW, Nestler JE, Turner TT: Interleukin-1 is induced in human placenta by endotoxin and isolation procedures for trophoblasts. J Clin Endocrinol Metab 1992; 75:951.

83. Kauma SW: HLA-DR and interlukin-1β (IL-1β) mRNA expression in human decidua. Presented at the 36th Annual Meeting for the Society of Gynecologic Investigation, San Diego, California, March 15–18, 1989.

84. Romero R, Mazor M, Manogue K, et al: Human decidua: A source of cachectin-tumor necrosis factor. Eur J Obstet Gynecol Reprod Biol 1991; 41:123.

85. Gauldie J, Richards C, Harnish D, et al: Interferon 2/B-cell stimulatory factor type 2 shares identity with monocyte-derived hepatocyte-stimulating factor and regulates the major acute phase protein response in liver cells. Proc Natl Acad Sci U S A 1987; 84:7251.

86. Casey ML, Cox SM, Beutler B, et al: Cachectin/tumor necrosis factor-alpha formation in human decidua: Potential role of cytokines in infection-induced preterm labor. J Clin Invest 1989; 83:430.

87. Romero R, Manogue KR, Mitchell MD, et al: Infection and labor. IV: Cachectin-tumor necrosis factor in amniotic fluid of women with intra-amniotic infection and preterm labor. Am J Obstet Gynecol 1989; 161:336.

88. Romero R, Mazor M, Munoz H, et al: The preterm labor syndrome. Ann NY Acad Sci 1994; 734:414.

89. Bry K, Hallman M: Synergistic stimulation of amnion cell prostaglandin E2 synthesis by interleukin-1, tumor necrosis factor and products from activated human granulocytes. Prostaglandins Leukot Essent Fatty Acids 1991; 44:241.

90. Evans MI, Hajj SN, Devoe LD, et al: C-reactive protein as a predictor of infectious morbidity with premature rupture of membranes. Am J Obstet Gynecol 1980; 138:648.

91. Farb HF, Arnesen M, Geistler P, Knox GE: C-reactive protein with premature rupture of membranes and premature labor. Obstet Gynecol 1983; 62:49.

92. Hawrylyshyn P, Bernstein P, Milligan JE, et al: Premature rupture of membranes: The role of C-reactive protein in the prediction of chorioamnionitis. Am J Obstet Gynecol 1983; 147:240.

93. Mitchell MD, Dudley DJ, Edwin SS, Schiller SL: Interleukin-6 stimulates prostaglandin production by human amnion and decidual cells. Eur J Pharmacol 1991; 192:189.

94. Dudley DJ, Trautman MS, Araneo BD, et al: Decidual cell biosynthesis of interleukin-6: Regulation by inflammatory cytokines. J Clin Endocrinol Metab 1992; 74:884.

95. Saito S, Kasahara T, Kato, et al: Elevation of amniotic fluid interleukin 6 (IL-6), IL-8 and granulocyte colony stimulating factor (G-CSF) in term and preterm parturition. Cytokine 1993; 5:81.

96. Salmon JA, Amy JJ: Levels of prostaglandin F2a, in amniotic fluid during pregnancy and labor. Prostaglandins 1973; 4:523.

97. Matsuzaki N, Saji F, Kameda T, et al: In vitro and in vivo production of interleukin-6 by fetal mononuclear cells. Clin Immunol Immunopath 1990; 11:205.

98. Dildy GA, Pearlman MD, Smith LG, et al: Amniotic fluid glucose concentration: A marker for infection in preterm labor and preterm premature rupture of membranes. Infect Dis Obstet Gynecol 1993; 1:166.

99. Kirshon B, Rosenfeld B, Mari G, Belfort M: Amniotic fluid glucose and intraamniotic infection. Am J Obstet Gynecol 1991; 164:818.

100. Gauthier DW, Meyer WJ: Comparison of Gram stain, leukocyte esterase activity, and amniotic fluid glucose concentration in predicting amniotic fluid culture results in preterm prema-

ture rupture of membranes. Am J Obstet Gynecol 1992; 167:1092.

101. Coultrip LL, Grossman JH: Evaluation of rapid diagnostic tests in the detection of microbial invasion of amniotic cavity. Am J Obstet Gynecol 1992; 167:1231.

102. McGregor JA, French JI, Reller LB, et al: Adjunctive erythromycin treatment for idiopathic preterm labor: Results of a randomized, double-blinded, placebo controlled trial. Am J Obstet Gynecol 1986; 154:98.

103. McGregor JA, French JI, Seo K: Adjunctive clindamycin therapy for preterm labor: Results of a double-blind, placebo-controlled trial. Am J Obstet Gynecol 1991; 165:867.

104. Morales WJ, Angel JL, O'Brien WF, et al: A randomized study of antibiotic therapy in idiopathic preterm labor. Obstet Gynecol 1988; 72:829.

105. Winkler M, Baumann L, Ruckhäberle KE, Schiller EM: Erythromycin therapy for subclinical intrauterine infections in threatened preterm delivery: A preliminary report. J Perinat Med 1988; 16:253.

106. Newton ER, Dinsmoor MJ, Gibbs RS: A randomized, blinded, placebo-controlled trial of antibiotics in idiopathic preterm labor. Obstet Gynecol 1989; 74:562.

107. Newton ER, Shields L, Ridgway LE III, et al: Combination antibiotics and indomethacin in idiopathic preterm labor: A randomized double-blind clinical trial. Am J Obstet Gynecol 1991; 165:1753.

108. Romero R, Sibai B, Caritis S, et al: Antibiotic treatment of preterm labor with intact membranes: A multicenter, randomized, double-blinded, placebo-controlled trial. Am J Obstet Gynecol 1993; 169:764.

109. Cox SM, Bohman VR, Sherman ML, Leveno KJ: Randomized investigation of antimicrobials for the prevention of preterm birth. Am J Obstet Gynecol 1996; 174:206.

110. Mercer BM, Lewis R: Premature labor and preterm premature rupture of the membranes: Diagnosis and management. Infect Dis Clin North Am 1997; 11:177.

111. Copper RL, Goldenberg RL, Creasy RK, et al: A multicenter study of preterm birth weight and gestational age-specific neonatal mortality. Am J Obstet Gynecol 1993; 168:78.

112. Johnston MM, Sanchez-Ramos L, Vaughn AJ, et al: Antibiotic therapy in preterm premature rupture of the membranes: A randomized prospective, double-blind trial. Am J Obstet Gynecol 1990; 163:743.

113. Mercer BM, Moretti ML, Prebost RR, Sibai BM: Erythromycin therapy in preterm premature rupture of the membranes: A prospective, randomized trial of 220 patients. Am J Obstet Gynecol 1992; 166:794.

114. Amon E, Lewis SV, Sibai BM, et al: Ampicillin prophylaxis in preterm premature rupture of the membranes: A prospective randomized study. Am J Obstet Gynecol 1988; 159:539.

115. Christmas JT, Cox SM, Andrews W, et al: Expectant management of preterm ruptured membranes: effects of antimicrobial therapy. Obstet Gynecol 1992; 80:759.

116. Lockwood CJ, Costigan K, Ghidini A, et al: Double-blind placebo-controlled trial of piperacillin prophylaxis in preterm membrane rupture. Am J Obstet Gynecol 1993; 169:970.

117. Owen J, Groome LJ, Hauth JC: Randomized trial of prophylactic antibiotic therapy after preterm amnion rupture. Am J Obstet Gynecol 1993; 169:976.

12

Chorioamnionitis

SEBASTIAN FARO

Chorioamnionitis is a term that is commonly used to mean infection of the amniotic membranes and amniotic fluid. However, the term *chorioamnionitis* can be defined as the microorganisms and polymorphonuclear leukocytes that reside in the layers between the chorion and the amnion. Infection of the amniotic fluid is termed *intra-amniotic infection* and is described as the infiltration of microorganisms and polymorphonuclear leukocytes. The two conditions can coexist, or the patient can have either infection. A third condition—deciduitis infection of the innermost surface layer of the uterus—can also exist, but it has not been documented. *Chorioamnionitis* is used here to encompass all three entities, chorioamnionitis, intra-amniotic infection, and deciduitis. These infections can be overt and present with classic signs and symptoms of infection: fever, maternal tachycardia, uterine tenderness, premature labor, premature rupture of amniotic membranes, and elevated white blood cell count.

Chorioamnionitis and associated conditions may be subtle, with the patient presenting with premature labor or premature rupture of amniotic membranes with or without labor. Thus, chorioamnionitis can present with a wide spectrum of clinical signs and symptoms. This infection affects approximately 10% of all pregnancies. The term *chorioamnionitis*, however, is not applied to pregnancies in which the fetus has not reached viability; i.e., less than 500 g. Typically, a spontaneous termination of a pregnancy associated with infection is referred to as *septic abortion*. Thus, the term *chorioamnionitis* is applied only to pregnancies in which the fetus has achieved viability; i.e., weight exceeding 500 g.

Chorioamnionitis is a serious infection. The end result of unrecognized chorioamnionitis is septic shock for both the fetus and the mother. Thus, this infection must be recognized early in its course and treated aggressively. It must be pointed out that the pathologist often reports that the chorion and amnion reflect chorioamnionitis, but that the mother and the fetus are not infected.

EPIDEMIOLOGY

The actual incidence of chorioamnionitis is not known, but it has been estimated to occur in as many as 2% of all pregnancies.[1–4] When one considers this and the risk factors, the estimated incidence of acute chorioamnionitis is approximately 10%.[5] Various factors have been associated with an increased risk of chorioamnionitis (Table 12–1). Individuals with a preterm gestation who experience rupture of the amniotic membranes, and labor, have approximately a 10-fold increased risk of developing chorioamnionitis.[5] In two large studies with a total of 3,416 pregnant patients, the risk factors that were significantly predictive of who was at risk for developing chorioamnionitis were as follows: nulliparity, length of time the amniotic membranes were ruptured, use of internal fetal monitoring, and the number of digital vaginal examinations.[6, 7] Other investigators have reported an increased risk of chorioamnionitis among women younger than 21 years of age, nonwhite, and unmarried.[8] The presence of meconium was a factor in a study by Wen and colleagues.[9] These investigators found that there was an 8% incidence of infection in women with meconium-stained amniotic fluid, compared to 2% in women with meconium.[9]

The patients who are at greatest risk for chorioamnionitis are those who have an abnormal vaginal microflora. There is little doubt that the individuals colonized with large inoculum bacteria (e.g., *Streptococcus agalactiae* or *Escherichia coli*) are more likely to develop chorioamnionitis. Individuals who have a low inoculum but have prolonged rupture of the amniotic membranes are placed at risk because these bacteria gain entrance to the amniotic cavity and fluid. These bacteria can then multiply in this amniotic fluid and achieve numbers that serve as a suitable inoculum. Pinell and co-workers[10] demonstrated that bacterial reproduction does occur in either the uterine cavity or the amniotic fluid over the course of 12 hours. The bacterial counts for nonobligate anaerobes rose from 10^2 to more than 10^6 bacteria/mL of amniotic fluid.

MICROBIOLOGY

Most patients who develop chorioamnionitis usually have one or more risk factors. The nonmicrobiologic risk factors are lack of prenatal care, promiscuity, poor nourishment, and smoking. Microbiologic risk factors

TABLE 12-1 ▶	RISK FACTORS ASSOCIATED WITH CHORIOAMNIONITIS

First pregnancy
Preterm labor
Premature rupture of amniotic membranes
Ruptured membranes for a prolonged period
Prolonged labor
Use of intrauterine monitors (scalp electrode, pressure catheter)
Frequent and numerous vaginal examinations
Presence of meconium in the amniotic fluid
Presence of *Streptococcus agalactiae, Neisseria gonorrhoeae, Chlamydia trachomatis, Escherichia coli*, etc.

are an altered vaginal microflora, the acquisition of a sexually transmitted microorganism, and, possibly, the presence of chronic gingivitis. The main factor causing chorioamnionitis is the status of the endogenous microflora of the vaginal ecosystem.

The endogenous vaginal microflora is complex and consists of gram-negative and gram-positive aerobic, facultative, and obligate anaerobic bacteria (Table 12–2). These bacteria exist in a harmony that may be considered a synergistic relationship of coexistence without influencing one another or having an antagonistic relationship. The vaginal ecosystem is either in a healthy or an altered state. The altered state may be an infection or a disruption in the ecosystem resulting in a vaginal ecosystem that supports an abnormal or skewed microbiology. A healthy vaginal ecosystem is dominated by *Lactobacillus,* and the status of the ecosystem can be established very easily. The characteristics of the vaginal ecosystem can be established by determining the pH, and whether or not *Lactobacillus* is dominant by microscopically examining the vaginal discharge. Table 12–3 lists the characteristics of various conditions.

The important concept in the initiation of infection (chorioamnionitis) is that the number of bacteria, or inoculum size, plays an important role in causing infection. If the numbers of bacteria, or inoculum of virulent bacteria, is at least 10^5/mL of vaginal fluid, infection is more likely to occur. In addition to the

TABLE 12-2 ▶	BACTERIOLOGIC MAKE-UP OF THE VAGINAL ECOSYSTEM

Lactobacillus acidophilus	*Morganella morgagnii*
Corynebacterium	*Proteus vulgaris*
Diphtheroids	*Bacteroides fragilis*
Staphylococcus epidermidis	*Eubacterium*
Streptococcus agalactiae	*Fusobacterium*
Streptococcus viridans	*Prevotella*
Enterococcus faecalis	
Enterobacter aerogenes	
Enterobacter agglomerans	
Enterobacter cloacae	
Escherichia coli	

inoculum size, other criteria of importance include the ability of the bacteria to adhere to epithelial cells, penetrate into the deeper epithelium, reproduce, and overcome the host defenses.

Therefore, amnionitis can be unimicrobial (e.g., *S. agalactiae, E. coli*), or it can be polymicrobial. The polymicrobial infection can involve combinations of bacteria; for example, facultative and/or obligate anaerobic bacteria. In one study of 52 pregnant women found to have chorioamnionitis, an average of 2 organisms per patient was found.[11] The three most common organisms found were *S. agalactiae, E. coli*, and *Prevotella bivia*.[11, 13] This concept of a polymicrobial etiology of chorioamnionitis is interesting but raises significant questions. The fact that two of the three most common organisms are nonobligate anaerobic bacteria, *S. agalactiae* and *E. coli*, raises concern over the role or significance of obligate anaerobic bacteria in chorioamnionitis. These two bacteria are the most common causes of neonatal sepsis. Obligate anaerobic bacteria rarely cause neonatal sepsis.[14]

Additional supporting evidence for the lack of obligate anaerobic involvement in chorioamnionitis comes from the use of antibiotic regimens that do not provide adequate antibacterial activity against obligate anaerobic bacteria. These regimens include doses of ampicillin, or ampicillin plus gentamicin. In a study of 400 amniotic fluid cultures obtained from pregnant women with chorioamnionitis, *Ureaplasma urealyticum* was isolated in 76% and *Mycoplasma hominis* in 30%.[13] However, the role of these two organisms in chorioamnionitis is not fully understood. Several bacteria that are relatively uncommon have also been isolated via amniocentesis from women with acute chorioamnionitis, *Listeria monocytogenes, Lactobacillus, Haemophilus influenzae, Fusobacterium, Chlamydia trachomatis, Salmonella*, and *Candida*.[15-20]

MICROBIAL PATHOPHYSIOLOGY

The significance of chorioamnionitis resides in the realization that two patients may be infected. If only the maternal compartment is infected, the consequence of infection may have a deleterious effect on the fetus. Once the infection becomes established in the mother, a proinflammatory syndrome is initiated with the release of various cytokines that can cross the placenta and enter the fetal compartment. The maternal proinflammatory response can result in septic shock in the mother, causing adult respiratory distress syndrome coexisting with sepsis. Transplacental migration of maternal cytokines can also initiate a septic shock–like syndrome in the fetus.

Chorioamnionitis begins when the bacteria ascend the endocervical canal and colonize the amniotic membranes and decidua. The bacteria must adhere

TABLE 12-3 ▶ CHARACTERISTICS OF VARIOUS CONDITIONS AFFECTING THE VAGINA					
Character	Discharge	pH	Odor	Clue Cells	Lactobacillus
Healthy	White	3.8–4.2	None	None	Dominant
BV	Gray	≥5	Fishy	+	None*
Yeast	White	<5	None	None	Dominant
Trichomoniasis	Gray to purulent	≥5	Foul	±	None*
Unimicrobial	Gray	≥5	None	None	None*

*The counts of lactobacilli are usually extremely low; ≤10^3/mL of vaginal fluid.

to the tissue and reproduce. Bacterial growth on the amniotic membranes results in a decrease in the tensile strength of the membranes, causing them to rupture under the weight of the amniotic fluid. Once the membranes have ruptured, bacteria ascend into the uterine cavity and can infect the fetus. Intra-amniotic infection can also occur via transmigration across intact amniotic membranes.

Patients who develop chorioamnionitis are at risk for postpartum endometritis. This is especially true if they are delivered by cesarean section. During the course of labor, the bacteria that enter the uterine cavity and colonize amniotic fluid reproduce. Over a 12-hour labor, the gram-positive aerobes (e.g., *S. agalactiae,* facultative gram-negative anaerobes, and *E. coli*) increase from 10^2 to 10^6 bacteria/mL of amniotic fluid.[10] Thus, the bacteria that colonize the amniotic fluid can increase in number significantly and migrate across the amniotic membranes, colonizing and invading the uterus. Infection of the uterus can result in chorioamnionitis and maternal bacteremia. Chorioamnionitis can result in intra-amniotic infection, which in turn can cause fetal infection. Intra-amniotic infection may be asymptomatic or symptomatic. However, when the infection reaches the amniotic membranes, the bacteria can traverse the membranes invading and infecting the decidual layer of the uterus. Infection of the amniotic membranes can result in their premature rupture.

DIAGNOSIS

The classic presentations of chorioamnionitis are fever, maternal tachycardia, uterine tenderness, uterine contractions, and, possibly, fetal tachycardia. The increase in the fetal heart rate can be caused by maternal fever or fetal anemia, or both. It is important to determine the site of infection, and not to assume that it is intrauterine because the usual management of chorioamnionitis is to deliver the fetus, regardless of age. However, this action is also dependent on the significance or degree of infection. This may be difficult to accomplish, but the patient should be thoroughly evaluated and infection of the urinary tract (e.g., pyelonephritis) must be ruled out. With improperly treated pyelonephritis, not only can the patient deliver maturely, but also there is a significant risk of gram-negative sepsis and septic shock. Once other sites of infection have been ruled out, attention can be turned to determining whether the patient has chorioamnionitis. Amniocentesis should be performed under ultrasound guidance, if possible, and the amniotic fluid should be processed as outlined in Table 12–4.

The absence of bacteria on the Gram stain should not be interpreted as infection not being present. It may only mean that there are fewer than 10^3 bacteria/mL of amniotic fluid present at the time of amniocentesis. An amniotic fluid glucose level of more than 15 mg/dL and the fact that bacteria have not been seen are indicative of the absence of infection. A glucose

TABLE 12-4 ▶ EVALUATION OF AMNIOTIC FLUID FOR ESTABLISHING A DIAGNOSIS OF CHORIOAMNIONITIS
Gram-stain—a positive Gram stain establishes that there are ≥10^3 bacterial/mL of amniotic fluid present.
The Gram-stain characteristics may be helpful in guiding antibiotic therapy; e.g., gram-positive cocci suggest *S. agalactiae,* gram-positive bacilli suggest *Listeria monocytogenes*
Homogeneous morphologic gram-negative bacilli suggest *E. coli*
Pleomorphic gram-negative rods suggest *Prevotella*
Fusiform gram-negative rods suggest *Fusobacterium*
Large gram-positive cocci suggest anaerobic streptococci
White blood cells suggest an inflammatory response, e.g., infection
Glucose concentration <15 mg/dL suggests phagocytic activity and infection
The fluid should be cultured for aerobic, facultative, and obligate anaerobic bacteria as well as *C. trachomatis, Mycoplasma,* and *Ureaplasma*
Fetal lung maturation studies should also be performed

level of more than 15 mg/dL indicates that phagocytosis is not occurring.

The vaginal ecosystem should be evaluated to determine whether bacterial vaginosis is present. I would recommend the following assays:

1. pH determination—greater than 5 definitely indicates an alteration of the endogenous vaginal microflora.
2. A wet prep and a Gram stain should be performed. The presence of clue cells, the absence of a single dominant morphotype, and the presence of a variety of bacterial morphotypes is consistent with bacterial vaginitis (BV).
3. A positive whiff test strongly suggests the presence of BV.
4. The lower third of the vagina and rectum should be cultured for the presence of *S. agalactiae*.
5. Endocervical specimens should be obtained for the detection of *Neisseria gonorrhoeae* and *C. trachomatis*.

If the bacterial morphotype, on wet mount or Gram stain, is predominantly small coccal forms, this should be interpreted as the patient being colonized by *S. agalactiae*. If there is a noticeable absence of other bacteria, the diagnosis of *S. agalactiae* chorioamnionitis can be made with a relatively high degree of confidence. If the Gram stain of the amniotic fluid also reveals the presence of Gram-positive cocci, this finding will strengthen the diagnosis of *S. agalactiae* chorioamnionitis. If there are a variety of bacterial morphotypes detected on examination of the vaginal wet prep or Gram stain, one should strongly consider that the patient has bacterial vaginosis. Thus, the evaluation of the vagina and amniotic fluid via the microscope can be quite helpful in establishing a diagnosis and guiding antibiotic therapy.

The vaginal ecosystem should also be evaluated for the presence of yeast and *Trichomonas vaginalis*. Yeast has been reported to cause chorioamnionitis as well as neonatal infection. *Trichomonas vaginalis* is associated with an altered vaginal flora, and the presence of gram-negative bacteria is of concern.

In addition to evaluating the patient's amniotic fluid and vaginal ecosystem, the following laboratory tests should be performed: a complete blood count (CBC) with white blood cell (WBC) differential, C-reactive protein, and urine specimen for culture of uropathogens. If the patient has clinically apparent chorioamnionitis, venous blood should also be cultured to rule out bacteremia.

A WBC differential may or may not reveal a leukocytosis. Leukocytosis can be found in a healthy pregnant woman without infection, especially if she is in labor. Approximately 3% to 86% of pregnant women with chorioamnionitis demonstrate leukocytosis.[11, 21] Gibbs and co-workers[11] demonstrated a leukocytosis in 63% of women with acute chorioamnionitis and found 21% of uninfected healthy pregnant women with a leukocytosis. When one analyzes the WBC differential, the number of immature polymorphonuclear leukocytes or band forms should be evaluated. If more than 10% of the WBC are immature polymorphonuclear leukocytes, this is indicative of acute infection.

Amniotic fluid should also be gram-stained. The absence of bacteria does not concretely establish that the patient does not have an infection. If bacteria are present but not detectable by Gram stain, this implies that there are fewer than 10^3 bacteria/mL of amniotic fluid. The Gram stain also detects the presence of WBC, which may or may not be indicative of infection. Supporting evidence for chorioamnionitis can be obtained by the measurement of glucose concentration in amniotic fluid.[22-24] Amniotic glucose concentration less than 15 mg/dL is indicative of phagocytosis. The overall specificity and sensitivity ranges from 75% to 98%, to 100%, respectively.

Thus, patients not presenting with the classic clinical signs and symptoms of chorioamnionitis should be evaluated as follows:

1. CBC with WBC differential
2. C-reactive protein
3. Urine culture
4. Amniocentesis—culture, Gram stain, glucose concentration

C-reactive protein is a nonspecific measure of inflammation. It is a protein that is produced in the liver in response to infection or inflammation. This test has been used to assist in establishing the diagnosis of acute chorioamnionitis, but its reliability has been questioned. In one study, the C-reactive protein test was reported to have a sensitivity of 8% and a specificity of 96%.[25] In another study, the sensitivity was 8% and the specificity 29%. A total of 18% of the patients with chorioamnionitis had a C-reactive protein value that was in the normal range.[26]

MANAGEMENT

Once the diagnosis is suspected or has been established, there does not appear to be any reason to delay institution of antibiotic therapy and aggressive management, leading to delivery of the fetus. The dilemma always arises when the fetus is premature. However, one must weigh the risk to the mother and the fetus when attempting to delay delivery in order to achieve some degree of fetal enhancement and to prevent the sequelae that are associated with preterm delivery.

One common problem associated with true chorioamnionitis is dysfunctional labor. There appears to be a significant degree of dysfunctional labor associated with true chorioamnionitis, and this can lead to an increase in cesarean deliveries.[27] In one study of patients with acute chorioamnionitis and the use of oxytocin, it was observed that if infection occurred prior to the administration of oxytocin there was no increase in the cesarean section rate (15%). The control group had an incidence of 14%. This was in contrast to the group that received oxytocin after chorioamnionitis developed, in which 44% of the patients required delivery by cesarean section.[28]

Thus, in patients with fever (at least 101°F), maternal and fetal tachycardia, uterine tenderness, and, perhaps, purulent amniotic fluid, the diagnosis is easily made. However, the combination in a patient of a low-grade fever, less than or equal to 100.4°F but greater than or equal to 99.6°F, a slight elevation in maternal pulse rate, a normal fetal heart rate, the absence of uterine tenderness, or confusion over whether or not there is uterine tenderness (cannot distinguish the pain associated with uterine contractions and tenderness of another etiology) may represent a subtle presentation of chorioamnionitis, but may often be overlooked. The WBC does not aid in determining infection because it is less than or equal to 16,000. In the scenario previously presented, it is not uncommon to attribute these conditions to dehydration. However, if there is an increase in immature polymorphonuclear leukocytes and the labor is dysfunctional, it is likely that the patient is developing chorioamnionitis. If the patient has ruptured membranes for 6 hours or longer, the index of suspicion should be greater.

A delay in the administration of antibiotic therapy can lead to dysfunctional labor. Persistent dysfunctional labor is caused by the uterine muscle shifting to an anaerobic metabolism and lactic acid accumulating in the muscle, thus creating more fatigue. This results in inefficient uterine contractions that lead to the inability of the uterus to accomplish work; a cesarean section will be needed to accomplish delivery of the fetus. In addition, as time progresses, the mother is at risk for developing sepsis, septic shock, adult respiratory distress syndrome, and death. Once the proinflammatory response is initiated, cytokines can cross the placenta and induce a septic shock–like state in the fetus. This will result in significant hypoxia and likely produce long-term sequelae in the fetus (e.g., cerebral palsy).

Patients who show signs of dysfunctional labor should be managed aggressively. Oxytocin should not be withheld, but administration of oxytocin should be instituted early, when the initial signs of dysfunctional labor are first noted. Patients with chorioamnionitis delivered by cesarean section are at greater risk for developing postpartum endometritis. These patients are also at risk for developing necrotizing myositis of the uterus. This is most likely caused by the development of thrombosis of the uterine vascular bed and the inability of antibiotics to reach an effective level in the uterine tissue. Necrosis initially develops along the uterine incision. A significant degree of necrosis necessitates hysterectomy.[29]

Once the diagnosis of chorioamnionitis is established, antibiotic therapy should be initiated. There has been much discussion on the microbiology of chorioamnionitis; however, the approach can be simplified by assuming that the offending organism or organisms originated from the patient's own endogenous microflora. Therefore, the most likely organisms are *S. agalactiae* (group B streptococci [GBS]), *E. coli*, and an obligate anaerobe, most likely *Peptostreptococcus*, *Peptococcus*, or *Prevotella*. Antibiotic therapy requires an agent that can provide broad coverage against the organisms just listed. In Table 12–5, antibiotic recommendations are given for the treatment of acute chorioamnionitis.

Although there are no randomized, double-blind studies to support one antibiotic regimen over another, it would appear that any of the beta-lactamase–inhibiting agents, combined with piperacillin or ampicillin, would be a logical first choice. The combination of ampicillin plus gentamicin, although effective and possibly less expensive than piperacillin-tazobactam or ampicillin-sulbactam, does carry the potential of nephrotoxicity and ototoxicity. Perhaps metronidazole is not an ideal choice, since the combination of metronidazole and gentamicin does not provide antibacterial activity against GBS.

Oxytocin should be administered immediately on

TABLE 12–5 ▶ ANTIBIOTIC REGIMENS FOR THE TREATMENT OF ACUTE CHORIOAMNIONITIS

I. Patient not allergic to penicillin:
   A. Piperacillin-tazobactam (Zosyn), 3.375 g IV q6h, *or*
   B. Ampicillin-sulbactam (Unasyn), 3 g IV q6h, *or alternatives are*
   C. Cefoxitin (Mefoxin), 2 g q6h
   D. Cefotetan (Cefotan), 2 g q12h
II. Combination therapy:
   A. Ampicillin + gentamicin
   B. Clindamycin + gentamicin
III. Patients allergic to penicillin:
   A. Clindamycin, 900 mg IV q8h + gentamicin, 2 mg/kg body weight as a loading dose followed by 1.5
     mg IV q8h or metronidazole, 500 mg IV q12h, + gentamicin

recognizing that the labor has become ineffective or is beginning to show signs of ineffectiveness. Delaying the initiation of Pitocin to enhance the labor mechanism can only result in failure, and a cesarean section will have to be performed. This step is often delayed but should not be, since chorioamnionitis is not an indication for cesarean section and this route of delivery can often be avoided.

NEONATAL OUTCOME

Acute chorioamnionitis can result in significant neonatal morbidity, with a significant increase in morbidity and mortality among preterm infants. Gilstrap and colleagues[3] reported four intrauterine deaths and no neonatal deaths among 273 term pregnancies. This represents a perinatal mortality rate of 15:1,000. In 39 preterm deliveries, there were 9 neonatal deaths and no intrauterine deaths, yielding a perinatal mortality rate of 230:1,000. These neonatal deaths could not be attributed to sepsis.[3] Chorioamnionitis is not a common cause of fetal acidemia, hypoxia, or hypoxic ischemic injury.[3, 30, 31] Wendel and co-workers[4] reported that 35% of 197 infants born to mothers diagnosed with chorioamnionitis had cord arterial pH measurements of less than 7.20. In addition, none of the infants had evidence of fetal acidemia, that is, an umbilical artery pH of less than 7.20.[4] In a comparative study of preterm infants born to women with and without chorioamnionitis, Hankins and co-workers[32] reported a lower mean arterial pH (7.26) in infants born to women with chorioamnionitis than in control subjects (7.28). There was no fetal acidemia; however, Apgar scores were lower in the former group.

SUMMARY

Chorioamnionitis occurs in approximately 1% of all pregnancies and is more likely to occur in association with premature labor and premature rupture of amniotic membranes. Prolonged rupture of amniotic membranes is a significant risk factor in both preterm and term pregnancies. *Streptococcus agalactiae* and *E. coli* are the two most common bacteria to cause acute chorioamnionitis. Early indicators of chorioamnionitis are maternal fever that usually begins as low-grade, a slow increase in maternal pulse rate, maternal and fetal tachycardia, uterine tenderness, purulent amniotic fluid, dysfunctional labor, and an elevated number of immature polymorphonuclear leukocytes typically associated with an established chorioamnionitis. A decrease in the sequelae of chorioamnionitis (e.g., dysfunctional labor, cesarean section, postpartum endometritis, maternal sepsis) can be achieved by early and aggressive management. Broad-spectrum antibiotics and oxytocin should be instituted, to enhance labor

early in its course, in an attempt to effect a vaginal delivery.

REFERENCES

1. Gibbs RS, Castillo MS, Rogers PJ: Management of acute chorioamnionitis. Am J Obstet Gynecol 1980; 136:709.
2. Hauth JC, Gilstrap LC 3d, Hankins GD, Connor KD: Term maternal and neonatal complications of acute chorioamnionitis. Obstet Gynecol 1985; 66:59.
3. Gilstrap LC 3d, Leveno KJ, Cox SM, et al: Intrapartum treatment of acute chorioamnionitis: Impact on neonatal sepsis. Am J Obstet Gynecol 1988; 159:579.
4. Wendal PJ, Cox SM, Roberts SW, et al: Chorioamnionitis: Association of nonreassuring fetal heart-rate patterns and interval from diagnosis to delivery on neonatal outcome. Infect Dis Obstet Gynecol 1994; 2:162.
5. Newton ER: Chorioamnionitis and intraamniotic infection. Clin Obstet Gynecol 1993; 36:795.
6. Newton ER, Pirhoda TJ, Gibbs RS: Logistic regression analysis of risk factors for intra-amniotic infection. Obstet Gynecol 1989; 73:571.
7. Soper DE, Mayhall CG, Dalton HP: Risk factors for intra-amniotic infection: A prospective epidemiologic study. Am J Obstet Gynecol 1989; 161:562.
8. Sturchler D, Menegoz F, Daling J: Reproductive history and intrapartum fever. Gynecol Obstet Invest 1986; 21:182.
9. Wen TS, Eriksen NL, Blanco JD, et al: Association of clinical intra-amniotic infection and meconium. Am J Perinatol 1993; 10:438.
10. Pinell P, Faro S, Roberts S, et al: Intrauterine pressure catheter in labor: Associated microbiology. Infect Dis Obstet Gynecol 1993; 1:60.
11. Gibbs RS, Blanco JD, St Clair PJ, Castaneda YS: Quantitative bacteriology of amniotic fluid from women with clinical intraamniotic infection at term. J Infect Dis 1982; 145:1.
12. Yoder PR, Gibbs RS, Blanco JD, et al: A prospective, controlled study of maternal and perinatal outcome after intra-amniotic infection at term. Am J Obstet Gynecol 1983; 145:695.
13. Sperling RS, Newton E, Gibbs RS: Intraamniotic infection in low-birth-weight infants. J Infect Dis 1988; 157:113.
14. Yancy MK, Duff P, Clark P, et al: Peripartum infection associated with vaginal group B streptococcal colonization. Obstet Gynecol 1994; 84:816.
15. Petrilli ES, D'Ablaing G, Ledger WJ: *Listeria monocytogenes* chorioamnionitis: Diagnosis of transabdominal amniocentesis. Obstet Gynecol 1980; 55(3 suppl):5s.
16. Lorenz RP, Appelbaum PC, Ward RM, Botti JJ: Chorioamnionitis and possible neonatal infection associated with *Lactobacillus* species. J Clin Microbiol 1982; 16:558.
17. Cox SM, Phillips LE, Mercer LJ, et al: Lactobacillemia of amniotic fluid origin. Obstet Gynecol 1986; 68:134.
18. Winn HN, Egley CC: Acute *Haemophilus influenzae* chorioamnionitis associated with intact amniotic membranes. Am J Obstet Gynecol 1987; 156:458.
19. Altshuler G, Hyde S: Fusobacteria: An important cause of chorioamnionitis. Arch Pathol Lab Med 1985; 109:739.
20. Ault KA, Kennedy M, Seoud MAF, Reiss R: Maternal and neonatal infection with *Salmonella* Heidelberg: A case report. Infect Dis Obstet Gynecol 1993; 1:46.
21. Hoolander D: Diagnosis of acute chorioamnionitis. Clin Obstet Gynecol 1986; 29:816.
22. Kirshon B, Rosenfeld B, Mari G, Belfort M: Amniotic fluid glucose and intraamniotic infection. Am J Obstet Gynecol 1991; 164:818.
23. Romero R, Jimenez C, Lohda AK, et al: Amniotic fluid glucose concentration: A rapid and simple method for the detection of intraamniotic infection in preterm labor. Am J Obstet Gynecol 1990; 163:968.
24. Dildy GA, Pearlman MD, Smith LG, et al: Amniotic fluid glucose concentration: A marker for infection in preterm labor and preterm premature rupture of membranes. Infect Dis Obstet Gynecol 1993/1994; 1:166.

25. Romem Y, Artal R: C-reactive protein as a predictor for chorio-amnionitis in cases of premature rupture of the membranes. Am J Obstet Gynecol 1984; 150(5 pt, 1):546.

26. Ernest JM, Swain M, Block SM, et al: C-reactive protein: A limited test for managing patients with preterm labor or premature rupture of membranes? Am J Obstet Gynecol 1987; 156:449.

27. Duff P, Sanders R, Gibbs RS: The course of labor in term patients with chorioamnionitis. Am J Obstet Gynecol 1983; 147:391.

28. Satin AJ, Maberry MC, Leveno KJ, et al: Chorioamnionitis: A harbinger of dystocia. Obstet Gynecol 1992; 79:913.

29. Gilstrap LC 3d, Faro S: Infections in Pregnancy. New York, Wiley-Liss, 1997, pp 65–77.

30. Peevy KJ, Chalhub EG: Occult group B streptococcal infection: An important cause of intrauterine asphyxia. Am J Obstet Gynecol 1983; 146:989.

31. Maberry MC, Ramin SM, Gilstrap LC 3d, et al: Intrapartum asphyxia in pregnancies complicated by intra-amniotic infection. Obstet Gynecol 1990; 76(3 pt,1):351.

32. Hankins GD, Snyder RR, Yeomans ER: Umbilical arterial and venous acid-base and blood gas values and the effect of chorio-amnionitis on those values in a cohort of preterm infants. Am J Obstet Gynecol 1991; 164(5 pt, 1):1261.

13 Intra-Amniotic Infection

LISA M. HOLLIER ▶ SUSAN M. COX

Although intra-amniotic infection (IAI) is more common with preterm labor and delivery, as many as 0.5% to 2% of term pregnancies may be complicated by overt infection. IAI is associated with increased maternal and perinatal morbidity and mortality. There is an increased incidence of serious maternal pelvic infections and substantively increased maternal sepsis and deaths. Neonatal morbidity includes septicemia and pneumonia as well as increases in adverse neurologic outcomes, even in term infants. The purpose of this chapter is to review clinical and research aspects of intra-amniotic infection.

DEFINITION OF INTRA-AMNIOTIC INFECTION

The sheer volume of terminology for this type of infection underscores the difficulty in defining the term. *Intra-amniotic infection* is the term most commonly used to describe the clinical syndrome of intrapartum infection of the placenta and membranes accompanied by signs and symptoms in the mother and fetus. Other terms used include *chorioamnionitis, amnionitis, intrapartum infection, amniotic fluid infection,* and *amniotic sac infection syndrome.* The term *intrauterine infection* is no longer used because it does not distinguish intra-amniotic infection from postpartum uterine infections. *Intra-amniotic infection* is preferred because it distinguishes this clinical entity from chorioamnionitis—a histologic inflammation of the placenta and membranes. *Intra-amniotic infection (IAI)* is used throughout this chapter to indicate clinical infection, whereas *chorioamnionitis* is used to denote histologic infection.

PATHOPHYSIOLOGY

Intra-amniotic infection has traditionally been thought to occur in 0.5% to 2% of term pregnancies. As shown in Table 13–1, the frequency of infection varies from medical center to medical center and is based on whether clinical or histologic criteria are used to make the diagnosis. These differences may also reflect variations in both patient populations and obstetric management.

The incidence of intra-amniotic infection is also increased in the preterm gestation. The reported incidence of clinical disease varied from 1% to 4% in several recent series.

Pathogenesis

Prior to the onset of labor or rupture of the membranes, the amniotic cavity is virtually always sterile. There are several potential routes of infection of the amniotic cavity. First and most common is ascending infection involving flora from the vagina and cervix. Second, hematogenous or transplacental infection is possible. Third, infection can occur as a complication of invasive procedures, such as chorionic villous sampling, cordocentesis, amniocentesis, or cervical cerclage (Table 13–2).

Romero and Mazor[1] have proposed a four-stage process leading to intrauterine infection. The first stage consists of an overgrowth of facultative organisms or the presence of pathologic organisms in the vagina and cervix. With interruption of the chorioamniotic membrane or with cervical dilation, microorganisms from the lower genital tract can ascend to invade the uterine cavity, residing in the decidua (stage II). The infection may invade fetal vessels or proceed through the amnion into the amniotic cavity and lead to IAI (stage III). Once in the amniotic cavity, the organisms can gain access to the fetus by aspiration (pneumonia) or by direct contact (conjunctivitis), which represents

TABLE 13–1 ▶ INCIDENCE OF INTRA-AMNIOTIC INFECTION	
Study	Percentage
Gibbs et al[82]	0.8
Koh et al[79]	0.5
Yoder et al[87]	1.0
Hauth et al[19]	1.3
Ferguson et al[89]	0.9
Gilstrap et al[20]	1.5
Soper et al[17]	10.5
Newton et al[16]	4.3
Satin et al[81]	1.8
Wendel et al[36]	2.3

Adapted from Williams Supplement No. 12, 1995.

TABLE 13-2 ▶	RISK OF INTRA-AMNIOTIC INFECTION AFTER INVASIVE PROCEDURES	
Procedure		**Risk**
Early amniocentesis		1:1000
Intrauterine transfusion		5–10:100
Cervical cerclage		1–2:100
Cerclage after prolapsed membranes and cervical dilatation		1:4
Percutaneous blood sampling		0.7:100

Adapted from Williams Supplement No. 12, 1995.

stage IV. Organisms can also gain access to the fetus by spread of an infection from the decidua parietalis to the decidua basalis, and directly into the fetal villous circulation.

The initial histologic findings of chorioamnionitis include an inflammatory and exudative reaction involving the chorionic plate. As the infection progresses, the inflammatory process spreads to the amnion, decidua, and eventually the amniotic fluid (Fig. 13–1).

Microbiology

Bacteria indigenous to the lower genital tract are the most frequent amniotic fluid isolates in women with IAI (Table 13–3). In a case-controlled study of the microbiologic features of chorioamnionitis, 70% of infected women had more than 10^2 CFU/mL of virulent organisms compared with only 8% in an uninfected control group ($P < .001$).[2] In this same study, a mean

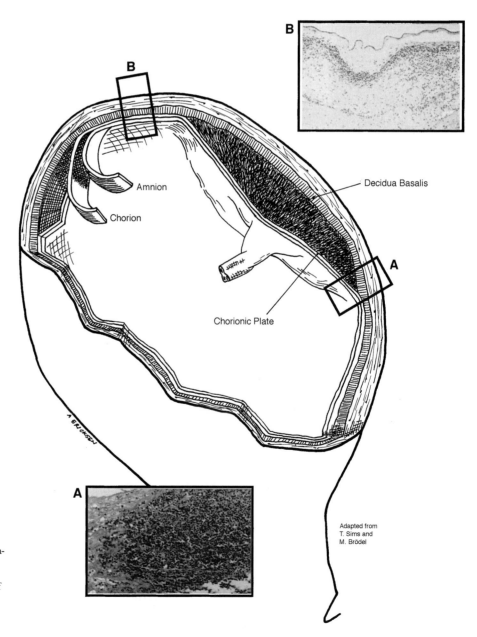

FIGURE 13-1 ▶ Cutaway view of gravid uterus showing acute and chronic deciduitis in the immature placenta *(A)* and inflammation of the chorion and amnion *(B)*. (From Benirschke K, Kaufmann P: Pathology of the Human Placenta, 3rd ed. New York, Springer-Verlag, 1995 pp 545, 549, with permission.)

TABLE 13–3 ▶ **AMNIOTIC FLUID ISOLATES FROM WOMEN WITH INTRA-AMNIOTIC INFECTION**

	Percentage
Aerobic	
Gram-Negative	
Escherichia coli	8.5
Other gram-negative bacilli	5.8
Gram-Positive	
Staphylococcus aureus	2.9
Streptococcus agalactiae	15.4
Enterococcus faecalis	5.3
Anaerobic	
Gram-Negative	
Gardnerella vaginalis	28.2
Bacteroides fragilis	3.0
Bacteroides bivius	30.8
Fusobacterium species	5.3
Gram-Positive	
Peptococcus species	11.9
Peptostreptococcus species	8.8
Clostridium species	10.0
Other	
Mycoplasma hominis	32.8
Ureaplasma urealyticum	47.3

Adapted from Gibbs et al,[75] Yoder et al,[87] and Sperling et al.[88]

of 2.2 organisms per patient was isolated and this included both aerobes and anaerobes. Listwa and colleagues[3] found similar results, with 2 to 3 organisms isolated per specimen; about 20% of those identified were anaerobes. Pankuch and associates[4] attempted isolation of bacterial and chlamydial organisms from 75 placentas. They found bacteria in 82% of placentas from patients with intra-amniotic infection. Nearly 50% of the organisms were anaerobes.

While anaerobic bacteria can be isolated, their role in the clinical syndrome is unclear. *Streptococcus agalactiae* and *Escherichia coli* are the two species of bacteria most commonly isolated in infected newborns delivered of mothers with IAI. Another important observation is that most women with chorioamnionitis respond favorably to simple antimicrobial regimens that do not provide specific anaerobic coverage. Finally, neonatal anaerobic bacteremia is uncommon.

A role for *Ureaplasma urealyticum* and *Mycoplasma hominis* has been suggested. Sperling and colleagues[5] studied 408 pregnancies complicated by chorioamnionitis and reported that these two organisms were isolated in 47% and 31% of amniotic fluid samples, respectively. In some of the placentas evaluated in this study, *Ureaplasma* was the only organism isolated.

The role of *Chlamydia trachomatis*, if any, in the etiology or pathogenesis of acute intra-amniotic infection is unclear. From sparsely available data, it appears that chlamydial infection is an unlikely cause of IAI.[6]

Newton and colleagues recently reported that there was a twofold increased incidence of chorioamnionitis if bacterial vaginosis (BV) was present intrapartum.[7] There is also a significant relationship between prenatal infection with BV and subsequent development of

IAI. Women with BV in the second or third trimester were twice as likely to have IAI.[8]

The influence of group B streptococcus on the frequency of IAI is somewhat unclear. Yancey and co-workers[9] showed a twofold increased incidence of chorioamnionitis in 216 women colonized with group B streptococci compared with 607 uncolonized women. Whereas the presence of rectovaginal group B streptococci was not helpful in predicting chorioamnionitis in women evaluated by Newton.[7]

As already mentioned, in some circumstances, organisms gain access to the amniotic space by hematogenous spread. The best example of this is infection with *Listeria monocytogenes*, which may occur as an epidemic or in isolated cases.[10] A California outbreak was found to be due to consumption of unprocessed Mexican cheese.[11] Other organisms capable of hematogenous spread include group A streptococci, *Campylobacter* species, *Fusobacterium* species, and *Treponema pallidum. Escherichia coli* may also be spread hematogenously. IAI following acute appendicitis has also been reported.[12]

Other rare causes of intra-amniotic infection include *Candida tropicalis*[13] infecting a woman who had an intrauterine device (IUD) in situ. IAI due to *Pseudomonas aeruginosa*[14] occurred after prolonged antimicrobial therapy in the setting of preterm ruptured membranes. A case of IAI due to *Salmonella typhi* was reported in a patient positive for human immunodeficiency virus (HIV) who presented with ruptured membranes.[15]

Risk Factors

Some reported risk factors for intra-amniotic infection are shown in Table 13–4. Ruptured membranes is the single most common risk factor. In two prospective studies, a positive association between obstetric manipulations and intra-amniotic infection was identified. Newton and colleagues[16] prospectively screened 2,908 women, of whom 705 (24%) were found to meet previously identified risk criteria. Of the 124 women with

TABLE 13–4 ▶ **RISK FACTORS FOR INTRA-AMNIOTIC INFECTION**

Ruptured membranes prior to labor
Labor duration
Preterm labor
Internal fetal monitoring
Cervical examinations during labor
Nulliparity
Young age
Meconium-stained amniotic fluid
Cervical colonization (with *Neisseria gonorrhoeae* or group B *Streptococcus*)
Bacterial vaginosis

Adapted from Cox SM, Gilstrap LC III: Chorioamnionitis. In: Williams Obstetrics, 19th ed. Supplement No. 12. Norwalk, CT, Appleton & Lange, April/May, 1995.

chorioamnionitis, 86% met the risk criteria. Logistic regression analysis showed that parity, duration of membrane rupture, and internal monitoring were significant risk factors. Likewise, Soper and colleagues[17] identified the duration of internal monitoring and membrane rupture, the number of cervical examinations, and the duration of labor as predictors of chorioamnionitis in 408 consecutive women.

In a population-based study, Sturchler and associates[18] investigated epidemiologic predictors of intrapartum fever and infection. The risk factors with the strongest association were preterm delivery and nulliparity. A history of amnionitis in a previous pregnancy did not increase the risk for subsequent intrapartum infection. These investigators found that socioeconomic factors such as being unmarried and nonwhite were important. Others, however, have not reported such an association. For example, the reported frequency of chorioamnionitis in a military population was 1.3%,[19] while an inner-city indigent population had an incidence of 1.5%.[20] Similarly, Looff and Hager[21] reported a 0.7% incidence of chorioamnionitis in women of predominately lower socioeconomic status. Other risk factors include BV and both preterm labor and preterm prematurely ruptured membranes. These latter two factors are associated with a tenfold-increased risk of chorioamnionitis.[22]

Meconium-stained amniotic fluid is associated with intra-amniotic infection and is presumed to be a marker for microbial invasion. A fourfold increase in the incidence of chorioamnionitis has been reported in women with meconium-stained fluid when compared with control subjects (8% versus 2%; $P = .05$).[23] These findings agree with earlier clinical studies,[24] as well as in vitro work.[25] The increased prevalence of infection in patients with meconium in the amniotic fluid may be explained in part by the ability of meconium to interfere with the antibacterial properties of amniotic fluid. Both light and very light meconium have been shown to inhibit the oxidative burst of neutrophils in vitro. Moderate meconium, in similar experiments, inhibited phagocytosis.[26]

Host Defense

Because ascending spread after ruptured membranes is the major route of infection, it is amazing that most laboring women do not develop IAI. There are a number of host defense mechanisms that probably prevent this. Some of these include amniotic fluid immunoglobulins, transferrin, inhibitory factors, lysozymes, and polymorphonuclear leukocytes.

Cattaneo[27] was the first to report that amniotic fluid produced zones inhibitory to bacterial growth. The specific inhibitor or inhibitors have not been identified and the precise mechanism of bacterial inhibition is unclear, although amniotic fluid may alter bacterial properties, such as virulence or attachment.

Amniotic fluid contains immunoglobulins specifically of the IgG class. There is little known of their actual role, although amniotic fluid IgG concentrations are higher in women with chorioamnionitis. While it is doubtful that these immunoglobulins are microorganism specific, they may provide some inhibitory activity.

Other substances, namely, polymorphonuclear leukocytes, lysozymes, and transferrin, all have been found in amniotic fluid from women in labor with ruptured membranes. Their exact role has not been clearly delineated. Leukocytes are commonly found in amniotic fluid in women with preterm labor but without evidence of infection. In contrast, in fulminant chorioamnionitis caused by group B streptococci, there may be very few or no white cells in the fluid. While Larsen[28, 29] and Schlievert[30] and their colleagues have isolated a low-molecular-weight peptide-zinc complex that inhibits bacterial replication, Gibbs and associates[2] were unable to duplicate their results.

There is an increasing body of evidence regarding the association of cytokines and intra-amniotic infection. IL-1β, IL-6, IL-8, IL-10, and TNF-α have all been found in elevated concentrations in women with IAI. IL-8 is a chemotactic and activating cytokine for neutrophils, which may eliminate invading bacteria by releasing bactericidal metabolites.[31]

The contribution of the fetus to the defense mechanisms is unknown, however, the fetal immune system clearly responds to the infection. Taniguchi and colleagues evaluated the ability of neonatal mononuclear cells to produce IL-8 and found rates comparable with that of maternal mononuclear cells.[32] Additionally, mononuclear cells obtained from cord blood in pregnancies complicated by IAI produced significantly higher amounts of IL-8 than those of neonates without chorioamnionitis, suggesting that the mononuclear cells of fetuses with IAI had been activated in utero. Recently it has been determined that polymorphonuclear leukocytes found in amniotic fluid in cases of IAI are of fetal origin.[33] Further investigation of this finding is important to delineate the contribution of the two immune systems.

DIAGNOSIS

There are no universally accepted criteria to diagnose IAI. While chorioamnionitis is a histological diagnosis, from a practical standpoint, the diagnosis of IAI is a clinical one based on maternal manifestations that include fever, tachycardia, and uterine tenderness (Table 13–5). Other reported diagnostic criteria include foul-smelling amniotic fluid and maternal leukocytosis.[6, 34] Fetal manifestations may include a nonreassur-

TABLE 13-5 ▶	CLINICAL FINDINGS REPORTED IN FIVE STUDIES OF WOMEN WITH INTRA-AMNIOTIC INFECTION				
Findings	Koh 1979 (n = 140)	Gibbs 1980 (n = 171)	Gibbs 1982 (n = 167)	Hauth 1985 (n = 103)	Wendel 1994 (n = 197)
Maternal fever (%)	96	85	100	99	100
Maternal tachycardia (%)	70	33	84	19	28
Uterine tenderness (%)	—	12	25	17	6
Fetal tachycardia (%)	70	37	58	82	73

Adapted from Cox SM, Gilstrap LC III: Chorioamnionitis. In: Williams Obstetrics, 19th ed. Supplement No. 12. Norwalk, CT, Appleton & Lange, April/May, 1995.

ing fetal heart rate pattern such as tachycardia and decreased variability.[35, 36]

Although some combination of these criteria is present in women with IAI, they are somewhat variable and certainly are not diagnostic. Maternal fever is the most significant and constant finding, and most consider it the hallmark for diagnosis. In fact, intrapartum fever in a woman with ruptured membranes and in the absence of other obvious causes almost always signifies intra-amniotic infection. The threshold for fever varies, but Gibbs and Duff[37] define it as an oral temperature of 37.8°C (100.0°F) or greater. If the importance of an isolated fever spike is questioned, the temperature should be monitored frequently.

Maternal Tests

Although many women with amnionitis have leukocytosis, so do many laboring women without obvious clinical infection. The criteria for diagnosing leukocytosis vary by study. In the case-control study by Gibbs and colleagues,[2] 63% of women with amniotic infection had a leukocyte count of greater than 15,000 per mL, while only 21% of uninfected controls exceeded this threshold. Defining leukocytosis as greater than 12,000 per mL was 67% sensitive and 86% specific, with negative and positive predictive values of 72% and 82%, respectively compared with clinical diagnosis of IAI.[34]

C-reactive protein is an acute-phase reactant that is generally increased in conjunction with an inflammatory response.[38] This protein is produced by the liver and levels are unaffected by pregnancy.[39] Elevated C-reactive protein was found to be sensitive yet not specific in identifying IAI.[40, 41] In a study of 100 women with prematurely ruptured membranes, amnionitis was identified in 18. Using a C-reactive protein level of more than 20 mg per L as a marker for IAI, this test was 82% sensitive and 55% specific, with low positive and negative predictive values of 36% and 9% respectively.[41] Practically speaking, this test adds little to the clinical diagnosis of IAI.

Amniotic Fluid Testing

IAI is frequently diagnosed in the term gravida with ruptured membranes whose only symptom is fever in

labor without another source of infection. Therefore, the vast majority of studies evaluating the ability of various biochemical markers to predict intra-amniotic infection are conducted in the setting of preterm labor, preterm premature rupture of membranes, or both. It is often difficult to compare their accuracy as testing methods because of the different endpoints (clinical disease, positive amniotic fluid culture, and chorioamnionitis) that have been selected by the various authors. Tests used for the diagnosis of intra-amniotic infection are found in Table 13-6.

During the past two decades, the diagnosis of IAI using inexpensive rapid techniques to assess amniotic fluid has been promoted. Larsen and associates[42, 43] found increased leukocyte concentrations in amniotic fluid taken from women with chorioamnionitis. In their population, the presence of white blood cells was associated with a 100% infection rate. This has not been confirmed by other investigators.[2, 3, 44] Thus, for women with suspected IAI, quantification of amniotic fluid leukocytes is considered to be of little predictive or diagnostic value.

Amniotic fluid leukocyte esterase has also been studied in intra-amniotic infection. This leukocyte enzyme may be present in the absence of intact cells, and its assay is a simple chemical test. Hoskins and associates evaluated 21 women with IAI at term and a control group of 21 matched uninfected laboring women.[34] Using IAI diagnosed clinically as the standard for com-

TABLE 13-6 ▶	TESTS USED IN THE DIAGNOSIS OF INTRA-AMNIOTIC INFECTION
Maternal	Cytokines
Leukocytosis	Interleukin-1β
C-reactive protein	Interleukin-6
Amniotic fluid analysis	Interleukin-8
Leukocytes	Interleukin-10
Leukocyte esterase	Tumor necrosis factor α
Gram stain	Gas liquid chromatography
Bacterial culture	Fetal evaluation
Glucose	Biophysical profile
Nitric oxide metabolites	Placenta and membranes
	Histologic evaluation

Adapted from Cox SM, Gilstrap LC III: Chorioamnionitis. In: Williams Obstetrics, 19th ed. Supplement No. 12. Norwalk, CT, Appleton & Lange, April/May, 1995.

parison, the leukocyte esterase test was sensitive as well as specific: 91% and 95% respectively. Similarly, they found a positive predictive value (PPV) of 95% and a negative predictive value (NPV) of 91%. In a subsequent study including 57 women, the sensitivity and specificity were 94% and 95% respectively. The PPV was 97% and NPV was 90%.[45]

Gram staining of amniotic fluid has been used as an adjunctive diagnostic test for IAI; however, the results to date are contradictory. A positive Gram stain is defined as the presence of any microorganism seen on high power field of unspun amniotic fluid. Miller and colleagues reported that a positive Gram stain correlated with subsequent culture growth, but not with the clinical diagnosis of IAI.[46] In a case-controlled study of amniotic fluid obtained via an intrauterine pressure catheter, organisms were found in 67% of women with chorioamnionitis, compared with only 12% of uninfected controls.[2] Similarly, Garite and associates reported a positive Gram stain of amniotic fluid obtained by amniocentesis, to be 78% specific and 81% sensitive for predicting infections.[47] In contrast, Listwa and coworkers reported a positive predictive value of only 7%. The sensitivity and positive predictive values range from 0 to 85% and 0 to 100%, respectively.[3] Thus, while the Gram stain is a frequently used rapid diagnostic test, there are no data to suggest that intervention based on a positive Gram stain alters perinatal morbidity.

Bacterial cultures are frequently obtained on amniotic fluid, however the inherent 48 hour delay limits their clinical application. Additionally, culture results do not correlate well with clinical disease. Romero and colleagues performed amniocentesis on 90 women in labor presenting at term.[48] Seventeen of the 90 samples (18.8%) obtained by amniocentesis had positive cultures. Clinical signs of IAI were present in only 3 women and only one of these three had a positive amniotic fluid culture. Others have also reported high culture-positive rates in women without chorioamnionitis.[2] To the contrary, one half of women with negative cultures had evidence of overt IAI in a study by Douvas and colleagues.[49]

Amniotic fluid glucose concentration has been studied as an aid to diagnose IAI. Amniotic fluid glucose levels of less than 10 to 20 mg per dL have been reported to be associated with positive cultures, but they are less strongly associated with clinical symptoms. Greig and associates evaluated the ability of low amniotic fluid glucose levels to predict subclinical intrauterine infection in women with preterm labor and intact membranes.[50] The sensitivity of low amniotic fluid glucose to predict either positive amniotic fluid cultures or histologic evidence of infection ranged from 41% to 55% depending on the threshold used. The specificity in detecting those cases with positive amniotic fluid cultures ranged from 94% to 100%. Coultrip and

Grossman reported that glucose concentration correlated most closely with semi-quantitative amniotic fluid leukocyte counts.[51] Women with many or moderate numbers of leukocytes were more likely to have glucose concentrations of less than 10 mg per dL, compared with women with few or no leukocytes seen on Gram-stained fluid.

The detection of cytokines, especially interleukin-1 (IL-1), IL-6, and tumor necrosis factor, has been used in research studies to diagnose subclinical intra-amniotic infection. To date, however, none of these cytokines has proved useful clinically. Most observations have been in women with preterm labor and intact fetal membranes.[31, 52–56] Yoon and colleagues[57] found that IL-6 concentrations greater than 17 pg/mL had a sensitivity of 79% and a specificity of 100% in the diagnosis of acute histologic chorioamnionitis. Amniotic fluid IL-8 concentrations have been reported to be significantly increased in women at term with chorioamnionitis.[31] Puchner and associates[58] documented chorioamnionitis in eight term women with intact membranes in whom amniotic fluid IL-8 concentrations ranged from 10,000 to 900,000 pg/mL, whereas IL-8 levels in women without chorioamnionitis were less than 10,000 pg/mL. IAI was associated with significantly increased concentrations of IL-10, with very high levels found in premature gestations.[59] Recently, amniotic fluid granulocyte colony stimulating factor (G-CSF) has been shown to be increased by a factor of 10 in women with chorioamnionitis, compared with control women.[60]

Amniotic fluid nitric oxide metabolites and cyclic guanosine 3',5'-monophosphate may play an important role in pregnant women with intra-amniotic infection. Hsu and colleagues[61] evaluated fluid obtained by amniocentesis from 72 pregnant women with preterm contractions, labor, or rupture of membranes. Levels of nitric oxide metabolites, endogenous nitrite, nitrate, and cyclic guanosine monophosphate were significantly higher in women with a positive amniotic fluid culture. Further studies are needed to confirm their findings.

Gas liquid chromatography has also been used to diagnose chorioamnionitis. This test is based on the identification of short-chain organic acids that are byproducts of bacterial metabolism. Gravett and colleagues studied 16 women with intra-amniotic infection along with 22 asymptomatic control subjects.[62] While 15 of 16 "infected" samples contained short-chain organic acids, such as acetate, butyrate, and propionate, only one of the control samples was positive. This abnormal chromatographic pattern was 94% sensitive and 95% specific for diagnosing infection. Other investigators have used this method to predict amniotic fluid culture results in women at risk for IAI because of preterm labor and preterm premature rupture of the membranes.[56, 63] Chromatography was

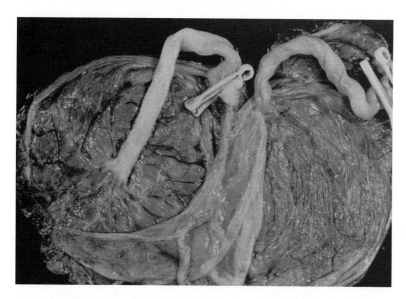

FIGURE 13-2 ▶ Diamniotic, dichorionic twin placenta from a cesarean section. Twin A (*left*, one cord clamp) was located higher in the uterus; twin B (*right*), with a marginally inserted cord, was near the lower uterine segment and had significant chorioamnionitis. Compare the luster of the normal placenta (*left*) with the indistinct features of the abnormal placenta (*right*), which are due to inflammation. (From Benirschke K, Kaufmann P: Pathology of the Human Placenta, 3rd ed. New York, Springer-Verlag, 1995, p 538, with permission.)

found to be only 29% sensitive and 55% specific in predicting a positive amniotic fluid culture. This technique is not used clinically because the instruments are not readily available and the cost is prohibitive.

Ultrasound

Ultrasonographic evaluation of the fetus could potentially provide a noninvasive method for the diagnosis of intrauterine infection. Early studies performed primarily in pregnancies at less than 34 weeks of gestation with prolonged membrane rupture had encouraging results. Vintzileos and colleagues[64] performed serial biophysical profiles in 75 pregnancies with prematurely ruptured membranes. A biophysical profile of less than 7 was associated with a 93% incidence of intra-amniotic infection. The most sensitive individual parameter was fetal breathing. Similar results were reported by Roussis and associates,[65] who found a biophysical profile of less than 5 had a 75% sensitivity in predicting amnionitis, with an accuracy of 92%. These observations were not confirmed in recent studies.[66–68]

Current data do not support the use of Doppler velocimetry to predict intra-amniotic infection. Leo and co-workers[69] prospectively performed Doppler flow studies of the umbilical artery in 51 pregnancies complicated by prematurely ruptured membranes. In the 10 women who developed chorioamnionitis, none of these fetuses had an abnormal systolic to diastolic (S/D) ratio.

Histology

Histologic examination of the placenta, membranes, and umbilical cord provide a retrospective diagnosis of chorioamnionitis. Grossly, the infected membranes may appear opaque and friable. The fetal surface appears to have lost its normal luster. The surface may

become yellow when much leukocytic exudate has accumulated and when the process has been of long duration (Fig. 13–2). In addition, the placenta is not uncommonly malodorous. Microscopic evaluation finds an acute inflammatory reaction in which polymorphonuclear leukocytes predominate. Macrophages and eosinophils may occasionally be present. Plasma cells are generally absent. In the third trimester, these leukocytes are of both maternal and fetal origin. The maternal cells migrate from the intervillous space, and the fetal cells from the fetal vessels on the surface of the placenta. The emigration of leukocytes appears to be toward the amniotic cavity. Tropism of leukocytes is a better indicator of infection than is Gram stain, culture, or chromatography.[70] Placental examination may help to differentiate hematogenous from ascending infection because the former characteristically involves the placental villi, but not the membranes. In contrast, with ascending infection, polymorphonuclear leukocytes infiltrate the extraplacental membranes adjacent to the cervical os. The infiltrate later involves the chorionic plate and adjacent intervillous space.

Unfortunately, histologic evaluation is nonspecific and insensitive for the identification of the clinical syndrome—IAI. For example, chorioamnionitis based on leukocyte infiltration is found in 11% to 16% of all full-term fetal membranes examined, while clinically evident chorioamnionitis was reported in only 1% of pregnancies.[71] Importantly, pathologic chorioamnionitis is found in greater than one half of low-birth-weight pregnancies.[72] To assess the time course of histologic chorioamnionitis and to correlate pathologic findings with the clinical syndrome, Dashe and colleagues[73] evaluated consecutive placentas from full-term deliveries in women whose membranes had been ruptured for more than 6 hours. Histologic evidence of infection was found to increase over time and was present in more than 70% of placentas with membranes that had been ruptured for more than 18 hours. Interestingly, between 6 and 18 hours after membrane rupture, only half of the women with histologic infection had fever.

TREATMENT

Antimicrobial Therapy

Appropriate management of IAI consists of parenteral antimicrobial agents and subsequent delivery. In this era of evidence-based medicine, it is surprising how few data exist regarding specific antimicrobial selection. In the absence of randomized clinical trials comparing antibiotic efficacy, several agents have been used empirically, as shown in Table 13–7. Penicillin or ampicillin, given in combination with an aminoglycoside such as gentamicin, has proven efficacy. Because approximately 20% of women with IAI may be colonized with anaerobic organisms, the addition of an agent with good anaerobic coverage may be appropriate. In contrast, Gibbs and Duff[37] recommend limiting empirical anaerobic coverage to women undergoing operative delivery. In one preliminary study, dual therapy for IAI with ampicillin plus gentamicin was compared with triple therapy composed of ampicillin-gentamicin-clindamycin.[74] They were unable to show significant differences in the frequency of pelvic infection following cesarean delivery. Surprisingly, there appeared to be a significant benefit to using the triple-antibiotic regimen to prevent postpartum metritis in women who delivered vaginally. Neonatal morbidity and mortality were similar in both groups.

Antimicrobial therapy should be given when IAI is diagnosed either before or during delivery. At least three studies have shown benefit from intrapartum therapy compared with therapy begun post partum (Table 13–8). Sperling and colleagues[5] reported significantly decreased neonatal bacteremia (20% vs. 3%) as well as neonatal deaths from sepsis (4.3% vs. 0.9%) in women in whom therapy was begun intra partum.

TABLE 13–7 ▶ EMPIRICAL ANTIMICROBIAL REGIMENS FOR TREATMENT OF INTRA-AMNIOTIC INFECTION

Combination therapy
  Ampicillin or penicillin plus gentamicin with/without clindamycin
Single-agent therapy
  Cefoxitin
  Third-generation cephalosporins
  Mezlocillin
  Piperacillin
  Ticarcillin-clavulanate
  Ampicillin-sulbactam
  Piperacillin-tazobactam

Adapted from Gilstrap LC, Faro S: Infections in Pregnancy: New York, Wiley-Liss, 1993, pp 37–44.

TABLE 13–8 ▶ OUTCOMES OF PREGNANCIES WITH INTRA-AMNIOTIC INFECTION BY TIMING OF THERAPY

	Treatment Before Delivery (%)	Treatment After Delivery (%)
Cesarean delivery	39.8	41.3
Maternal bacteremia	5.9	12.3
Endometritis	3.9	5.5
Early neonatal sepsis	2.2	10.2
Perinatal deaths	6.5	3.1
deaths from sepsis	0.9	4.3

Data from Sperling et al,[5] Gilstrap et al,[20] and Gibbs.[75]

Gilstrap and co-workers[20] reported significantly reduced neonatal sepsis. This was especially prominent with sepsis due to group B streptococci: 4.7% with postpartum therapy versus zero with intrapartum therapy. In the only randomized clinical trial to date, Gibbs and associates[75] reported that intrapartum therapy was of benefit to the neonate as well as the mother when compared with antimicrobial therapy begun post partum. They observed decreased rates of sepsis and decreased duration of hospitalization for the infants and decreased hospital stay for the mothers.

Delivery

The timing of delivery after IAI is diagnosed may be problematic. In women with IAI, the mean interval from diagnosis to delivery is generally 3 to 7 hours, and the critical interval after which neonatal or maternal complications increase has not been identified.[19, 75] Wendel and colleagues[36] reported that a diagnosis-to-delivery interval of 12 hours, and possibly even 18 hours, did not herald an unfavorable neonatal outcome, compared with intervals of 0 to 2 hours (Table 13–9). It is unclear whether intervals longer than 12 hours have a significant impact on fetal morbidity. There is little evidence to suggest that cesarean delivery offers advantages to the fetus over vaginal birth, and maternal morbidity may be increased by cesarean (see section on sequelae). Therefore, the route of delivery should be chosen according to standard obstetric indications. However, as discussed subsequently, the cesarean delivery rate is significantly increased in women with chorioamnionitis because of dysfunctional labor. When cesarean delivery is indicated, the standard transperitoneal low transverse incision is appropriate. Cesarean hysterectomy is reserved for women with refractory uterine atony or other indications.

In the past, some have recommended extraperitoneal cesarean delivery to decrease maternal infection-related complications.[76, 77] Others, however, found no benefit of such operations.[78] Twenty-six women undergoing extraperitoneal cesarean delivery were com-

TABLE 13-9 ▶ **NEONATAL OUTCOMES IN PREGNANCIES WITH IAI ACCORDING TO THE INTERVAL FROM DIAGNOSIS TO DELIVERY**

Outcome	Interval in Hours (percent)					
	0–2	2–4	4–6	6–12	12–18	P Value
Number of infants	80	57	39	18	3	—
Apgar score at 5 min						
≤6	2(3)	3(5)	1(3)	1(6)	0	0.72
≥3	0	1(2)	0	1(6)	0	0.17
Cord gas						
pH < 7.20	25(31)	19(33)	17(44)	6(33)	1(33)	0.76
pH < 7.00	0	0	0	0	0	—
Sepsis	2(3)	0	0	0	0	0.76
Oxygen requirement	7(9)	6(11)	2(9)	2(11)	0	0.85
Admission to special-care nursery	10(13)	10(18)	2(5)	2(11)	1(3)	0.26

From Wendel PJ, Cox SM, Roberts SW, et al: Chorioamnionitis: The association of nonreassuring fetal heart rate patterns and interval from diagnosis to delivery on neonatal outcome. Infect Dis Obstet Gynecol 1994; 2:162–166.

pared with 65 undergoing transperitoneal low transverse incisions. A similar incidence of wound infection, 12% versus 14%, and postoperative stay, 5.3 versus 4.8 days, were found in the two groups. Importantly, about 10% of the extraperitoneal procedures were associated with bladder injury or entry into the peritoneum. Practically speaking, the extraperitoneal technique is rarely taught.

Fetal Monitoring

Continuous fetal monitoring is preferable in pregnancies complicated by IAI because of the high frequency of abnormal tracings. Monitoring may be accomplished either externally or directly by using a fetal scalp electrode. The most common abnormal findings are tachycardia and decreased variability.[37] In this clinical setting, these findings do not necessarily indicate fetal acidosis.[36, 37] Gibbs and Duff[37] reported diminished or absent short-term variability in almost 80%, tachycardia in 67%, and bradycardia in about 10%. Sinusoidal patterns were documented in approximately 15% of these pregnancies complicated by chorioamnionitis.[37]

Wendel and colleagues[36] also evaluated the effects of intra-amniotic infection on fetal heart rate tracings. Tachycardia was found in 73%; it was mild (160 to 180 BPM) in 56% and severe (>180) in 17%. In 28%, there were absent accelerations, absent variability in 5%, and late decelerations in 4%. No sinusoidal fetal heart rate patterns were seen. Despite these findings, there were no intrapartum findings associated with poor neonatal outcomes, nor were any cases of pathologic fetal acidemia (pH < 7.00) identified.

SEQUELAE

Maternal

Women with IAI commonly have dysfunctional labor (Table 13–10). At least two possibilities exist: Clinical infection can result in dystocia and prolonged labor; alternatively, labor may be desultory because of infection. In several series, 50% to 70% of women required oxytocin augmentation of labor either before or after the diagnosis of IAI was made.[20, 79]

In 1983, Duff and co-workers[35] found an increased cesarean delivery rate for dystocia in women with IAI. They suggested that infection may have inhibitory effects on labor. Additionally, women with subclinical intra-amniotic infection require higher doses of oxytocin to achieve adequate uterine contractions.[80] Importantly, despite adequate uterine activity, labor progression was slow. In contrast, other investigators have implicated IAI in the stimulation of labor. Satin and colleagues[81] studied the impact of IAI on the course of labor and reported two clinical presentations. In the first, diagnosis of IAI before labor stimulation was not associated with an increased incidence of cesarean delivery. In the second, diagnosis of IAI after oxytocin stimulation was begun was a harbinger of dystocia and was associated with significantly increased cesarean delivery (40% vs. 9%). They, too, found that higher doses of oxytocin were required in women with IAI diagnosed after augmentation of labor was begun.

IAI may result in significant maternal infection–related morbidity. Bacteremia is occasionally associated with IAI. Reported prevalence ranges from 6.4% to 2.3% of women with IAI.[79, 82] The frequency of postpartum pelvic infection is related primarily to the route of

TABLE 13-10 ▶ **POTENTIAL COMPLICATIONS ASSOCIATED WITH IAI**

Maternal	Neonatal
Dysfunctional labor	Stillbirth
Cesarean delivery	Sepsis
Bacteremia	Pneumonia
Sepsis	Intraventricular hemorrhage
Endometritis	Periventricular leukomalacia
Wound infection	Cerebral palsy

delivery, and infection is especially common following cesarean delivery. This finding is magnified by the markedly increased incidence of cesarean delivery in women with IAI. Koh and colleagues[79] reported that nearly one third of women with IAI developed postpartum infection. When stratified by route of delivery, 11% had infection following vaginal delivery compared to 48% following cesarean delivery. Similarly, Hauth and co-workers[19] observed that approximately 10% of women with IAI who gave birth by cesarean required additional therapy or changes in empirical antimicrobial therapy because of persistent serious pelvic infection. In their report, two women required débridement and drainage of subcutaneous wound infections.[19] In this same study, only 1 of 59 women with chorioamnionitis whose infants were delivered vaginally required additional treatment.

IAI had been associated with maternal mortality. In several series, maternal deaths have resulted from IAI.[83, 84] In Gogoi's report,[83] 93% of deaths that occurred following cesarean delivery were attributed to sepsis and shock. In more recent studies, chorioamnionitis has become a rare cause of maternal mortality.[5, 20, 36, 75] No maternal deaths were reported in these series, which studied a total of more than 700 women.

Neonatal

Immediate Morbidity and Mortality

Certainly, in the past, there were abundant data to show that poor perinatal outcome was associated with chorioamnionitis.[85] One of the most devastating adverse fetal effects is death (see Table 13–10). Hauth and associates[19] reported 1 fetal death in 103 pregnancies complicated by IAI, while Gilstrap and co-workers[20] reported 2% stillbirths among 273 pregnancies of more than 34 weeks' gestation complicated by IAI. Unfortunately, fetal deaths still occur even with the most modern and aggressive therapy.

Although the neonatal death rate is increased as the result of IAI, it is difficult to separate deaths due to infection from those due to complications of preterm delivery. Gilstrap and associates[20] found that 9 of 39 newborns (23%) of less than 35 weeks' gestation succumbed, compared with none of the 269 newborns of more than 35 weeks' gestation born to mothers with IAI. In this study, none of the preterm infants died as a result of presumed sepsis. Similarly, Looff and Hager[21] reported a perinatal mortality rate of 123 per 1,000, with all excess mortality attributed to preterm delivery and none to sepsis.

Immediate infection-related neonatal morbidity is primarily from sepsis and pneumonia. Whether maternally administered antimicrobial therapy decreases this morbidity is unclear. For example, some studies have shown a benefit,[5, 20, 74, 75] while others have reported no

such advantages.[19, 79, 86, 87] The incidence of bacteremia overall is 3% to 4% but ranges from 0 to 21% in infants given intrapartum antimicrobial therapy. This rate was not significantly higher in infants who were treated only during the neonatal period.[20] Pneumonia is documented in 7% to 8% of those treated with intrapartum antibiotic medication, but ranges from 0 to 23%.

The preterm infant may be a more susceptible host to infection. A significantly increased rate of sepsis was found in infants weighing less than 2,500 g compared to infants weighing more than 2,500 g (16.2% vs. 4.1%).[88] Other investigators have found similar results.[89]

Hankins and associates[90] quantified the effects of IAI in 86 preterm infants (<37 weeks) by studying cord gases at birth. In these infants, there were no significant differences in the umbilical artery pH.[90] No differences in the frequency of acidemia were found in fullterm infants with and without intra-amniotic infection.[20, 36, 73]

The association of cytokines to immediate adverse neonatal outcome was investigated by Weeks and colleagues.[91] Umbilical cord IL-6 levels are elevated in neonates who subsequently develop sepsis, congenital pneumonia, necrotizing enterocolitis, or grade II to IV intraventricular hemorrhage.[91]

Long-Term Morbidity

Over the last several years, there is increasing evidence regarding the role of intra-amniotic infection in the development periventricular leukomalacia and ultimately cerebral palsy (CP).[92–97] In a case-control study of very preterm babies, any maternal infection, including IAI, was associated with a fourfold increased risk of cerebral palsy.[97] Intra-amniotic infection was associated with a doubling in the incidence of periventricular leukomalacia and more frequent intraventricular hemorrhage and seizures in infants with birthweights less than 1,500 g.[96]

Cytokines produced in the process of infection are associated with periventricular leukomalacia in preterm infants. Yoon and colleagues[98] quantified tumor necrosis factor and IL-1β levels in cord blood of 172 consecutive preterm births. Plasma concentrations of IL-6, but not of tumor necrosis factor-α, IL-1β, and IL-1 receptor antagonist were significantly higher in neonates with periventricular leukomalacia-associated lesions than in those without these lesions.

Exposure to maternal infection has also been associated with a marked increase in the risk of cerebral palsy in infants of normal birth weight.[93] In fact, Grether and Nelson[93] estimate that infection might account for 12% (95% confidence interval [CI], 4% to 20%) of total spastic CP in children of normal birth weight, 19% (95% CI, 7% to 31%) of unexplained spastic CP, and 35% (95% CI, 13% to 57%) of unexplained spastic quadriplegia.

In a recent report, experimentally induced intrauterine infection was associated with fetal white-matter brain lesions in rabbits. Yoon and associates[99] established ascending intrauterine infection with *E. coli* and found white matter lesions in 36% of living fetuses compared to no lesions in the control group inoculated with saline. This randomized study provides convincing evidence of a causal role of infection in the development of neurologic injury.

REFERENCES

1. Romero R, Mazor M: Infection and preterm labor. Clin Obstet Gynecol 1988; 31:553.
2. Gibbs RS, Blanco JD, St Clair PJ, et al: Quantitative bacteriology of amnionic fluid from women with clinical intra-amnionic infection at term. J Infect Dis 1982; 145:1.
3. Listwa HM, Dobek AS, Carpenter J, et al: The predictability of intrauterine infection by analysis of amnionic fluid. Obstet Gynecol 1976; 49:31.
4. Pankuch GA, Appelbaum PC, Lorenz RP, et al: Placental microbiology and histology and the pathogenesis of chorioamnionitis. Obstet Gynecol 1984; 64:802.
5. Sperling RS, Ramamurthy RS, Gibbs RS: A comparison of intrapartum versus immediate postpartum treatment of intraamnionic infection. Obstet Gynecol 1987; 70:861.
6. Gibbs RS, Schachter J: Chlamydial serology in patients with intra-amnionic infection and controls. Sex Transm Dis 1987; 14:213.
7. Newton ER, Piper J, Peairs W: Does the presence of bacterial vaginosis intrapartum increase the likelihood of intra-amniotic infection? Society of Perinatal Obstetricians annual meeting, abstract 147. Am J Obstet Gynecol 1995; 172:302.
8. Gravett MG, Nelson HP, DeRouen T, et al: Independent associations of bacterial vaginosis and *Chlamydia trachomatis* infection with adverse pregnancy outcome. JAMA 1986; 256:1899.
9. Yancey MK, Duff P, Clark P, et al: Peripartum infection associated with vaginal group B streptococcal colonization. Obstet Gynecol 1994; 84:816.
10. Halliday HL, Kirata T: Perinatal listeriosis: A review of twelve patients. Am J Obstet Gynecol 1979; 133:405.
11. Linnan MJ, Mascola L, Lou XD, et al: Epidemic listeriosis associated with Mexican-style cheese. N Engl J Med 1988; 319:823.
12. Bard JL, O'Leary JA: Chorioamnionitis and appendiceal abscess: A case report. J Reprod Med 1994; 39:321.
13. Nichols A, Khong TY, Crowther GA: *Candida tropicalis* chorioamnionitis. Am J Obstet Gynecol 1995; 172:1045.
14. Kyle P, Turner DPJ: Chorioamnionitis due to *Pseudomonas aeruginosa*: A complication of prolonged antibiotic therapy for premature rupture of membranes. Br J Obstet Gynaecol 1996; 103:181.
15. Hedriana HL, Mitchell JL, Williams SB: *Salmonella typhi* chorioamnionitis in a human immunodeficiency virus–infected pregnant woman: A case report. J Reprod Med 1995; 40P:157.
16. Newton ER, Prihoda TJ, Gibbs RS: Logistic regression analysis of risk factors for intra-amnionic infection. Obstet Gynecol 1989; 73:571.
17. Soper DE, Mayhall CG, Dalton HP: Risk factors for intraamnionic infection: A prospective epidemiologic study. Am J Obstet Gynecol 1989; 161:562.
18. Sturchler D, Menegoy F, Daling T: Reproductive history and intrapartum fever. Gynecol Obstet Invest 1986; 21:182.
19. Hauth JC, Gilstrap LC, Hankins GDV, et al: Term maternal and neonatal complications of acute chorioamnionitis. Obstet Gynecol 1985; 66:59.
20. Gilstrap LC, Leveno KJ, Cox SM, et al: Intrapartum treatment of acute chorioamnionitis: Impact on neonatal sepsis. Am J Obstet Gynecol 1988; 159:579.
21. Looff JD, Hager WD: Management of chorioamnionitis. Surg Gynecol Obstet 1984; 158:161.
22. Cox SM, Williams ML, Leveno KJ: The natural history of preterm ruptured membranes: What to expect of expectant management. Obstet Gynecol 1988; 71:558.
23. Wen TS, Eriksen NL, Blanco JD, et al: Association of clinical intra-amniotic infection and meconium. Am J Perinatol 1993; 10:438.
24. Meis PJ, Hall M, Marshall JR, et al: Meconium passage: A new classification for risk assessment during labor. Am J Obstet Gynecol 1978; 131:509.
25. Bryan CS: Enhancement of bacterial infection by meconium. Johns Hopkins Med J 1967; 121:9.
26. Clark P, Duff P: Inhibition of neutrophil oxidative burst and phagocytosis by meconium. Am J Obstet Gynecol 1995; 173:1301.
27. Cattaneo P: Portere lisizimico del liquido amnionico postere antilisizimico del meconio, recherche sperimentoli. La Clin Obstet 1949; 51:60.
28. Larsen B, Snyder I, Galask R: Bacterial growth inhibition by amnionic fluid. I. In vitro evidence for bacterial growth inhibiting activity. Am J Obstet Gynecol 1974; 119:492.
29. Larsen B, Snyder I, Galask R: Bacterial growth inhibition by amnionic fluid. II. Reversal of amnionic fluid bacterial growth inhibition by addition of a chemically defined medium. Am J Obstet Gynecol 1974; 119:497.
30. Schlievert P, Johnson W, Galask RP: Isolation of a low molecular weight antibacterial system from human amniotic fluid. Infect Immunol 1976; 14:1156.
31. Romero R, Ceska M, Avila C, et al: Neutrophil attractant/activating peptide-1/interleukin-8 in term and preterm parturition. Am J Obstet Gynecol 1991; 165:813.
32. Taniguchi T, Matsuzaki N, Shimoya K, et al: Fetal mononuclear cells show a comparable capacity with maternal mononuclear cells to produce IL-8 in response to lipopolysaccharide in chorioamnionitis. J Reprod Immunol 1993; 23:1.
33. Sampson JE, Theve RP, Blatman RN, et al: Fetal origin of amniotic fluid polymorphonuclear leukocytes. Am J Obstet Gynecol 1997; 176:77.
34. Hoskins IA, Johnson TRB, Winkel CA: Leukocyte esterase activity in human amnionic fluid for the rapid detection of chorioamnionitis. Am J Obstet Gynecol 1987; 157:730.
35. Duff P, Sanders R, Gibbs RS: The course of labor in term pregnancies with chorioamnionitis. Am J Obstet Gynecol 1983; 147:391.
36. Wendel PJ, Cox SM, Roberts SW, et al: Chorioamnionitis: The association of nonreassuring fetal heart rate patterns and interval from diagnosis to delivery on neonatal outcome. Infect Dis Obstet Gynecol 1994; 2:162.
37. Gibbs RS, Duff P: Progress in pathogenesis and management of clinical intraamnionic infection. Am J Obstet Gynecol 1991; 164:1317.
38. Morley JJ, Kushner I: Serum C-reactive protein levels in disease. Ann N Y Acad Sci 1982; 389:406.
39. Haran K, Augensen K, Elsayed S: Serum protein patterns in normal pregnancy with specific reference to acute-phase reactants. Br J Obstet Gynaecol 1983; 90:139.
40. Hawrylyshyn P, Bernstein P, Milligan J: Premature rupture of the membranes: The role of C-reactive protein in the prediction of chorioamnionitis. Am J Obstet Gynecol 1983; 147:240.
41. Ismail M, Zinaman M, Lowensohn R, et al: The significance of C-reactive protein levels in women with premature rupture of membranes. Am J Obstet Gynecol 1985; 151:541.
42. Larsen J, Goldkrand J, Hanson T, et al: Intrauterine infection on an obstetric service. Obstet Gynecol 1974; 43:838.
43. Larsen J, Weis K, Unihan J, et al: Significance of neutrophils and bacteria in the amnionic fluid of patients in labor. Obstet Gynecol 1976; 47:143.
44. Bobitt JR, Hayslip CC, Damato JD: Amniotic fluid infection as determined by transabdominal amniocentesis in patients with intact membranes in premature labor. Am J Obstet Gynecol 1981; 140:947.
45. Hoskins IA, Katz J, Ordorica SA, et al: Esterase activity in second- and third-trimester amniotic fluid: An indicator of chorioamnionitis. Am J Obstet Gynecol 1989; 161:1543.
46. Miller JM, Hiu GB, Welt SI, et al: Bacterial colonization of amnionic fluid in the presence of ruptured membranes. Am J Obstet Gynecol 1980; 137:451.

47. Garite TJ, Freeman RK: Chorioamnionitis in the preterm gestation. Obstet Gynecol 1982; 59:539.
48. Romero R, Nores J, Mazor M, et al: Microbial invasion of the amniotic cavity during term labor: Prevalence and clinical significance. J Reprod Med 1993; 38:543.
49. Douvas SG, Brewer MJ, McKay ML, et al: Treatment of premature rupture of the membranes. J Reprod Med 1984; 29:741.
50. Greig PC, Ernest JM, Teot L: Low amniotic fluid glucose levels are a specific but not sensitive marker for subclinical intrauterine infections in patients in preterm labor with intact membranes. Am J Obstet Gynecol 1994; 171:365.
51. Coultrip LL, Grossman JH: Evaluation of rapid diagnostic tests in the detection of microbial invasion of the amnionic cavity. Am J Obstet Gynecol 1992; 167:1231.
52. Casey ML, Cox SM, Beutler B, et al: Cachectin/tumor necrosis factor formation in human decidua. J Clin Invest 1989; 83:430.
53. Romero R, Brody DT, Oyarzun E, et al: Infection and labor III. Interleukin-1. A signal for the onset of parturition. Am J Obstet Gynecol 1989; 160:1117.
54. Romero R, Manogue KR, Mitchell MD, et al: Infection and labor. IV. Cachectin-tumor necrosis factor in the amnionic fluid of women with intraamnionic infection and preterm labor. Am J Obstet Gynecol 1989; 161:336.
55. Romero R, Avila C, Santhanam U, et al: Amnionic fluid interleukin-6 in preterm labor. J Clin Invest 1990; 85:1392.
56. Romero R, Scharf K, Mazor M, et al: The clinical value of gas-liquid chromatography in the detection of intra-amnionic microbial invasion. Obstet Gynecol 1988; 72:44.
57. Yoon BH, Romero R, Kim CJ, et al: Amniotic fluid interleukin-6: A sensitive test for antenatal diagnosis of acute inflammatory lesions of preterm placenta and prediction of perinatal morbidity. Am J Obstet Gynecol 1995; 172:960.
58. Puchner T, Egarter C, Wimmer C, et al: Amniotic fluid interleukin-8 as a marker for intra-amniotic infection. Arch Gynecol Obstet 1993; 253:9.
59. Greig PC, Herbert WNP, Robinette BL, et al: Amniotic fluid interleukin-10 concentrations increase through pregnancy and are elevated in patients with preterm labor associated with intrauterine infection. Am J Obstet Gynecol 1995; 173:1223.
60. Raynor D, Clark P, Duff P: Granulocyte colony stimulating factor (GCSF) in amniotic fluid. Society of Perinatal Obstetricians annual meeting, abstract 70. Am J Obstet Gynecol 1995; 172:280.
61. Hsu CD, Aversa K, Meaddough E, et al: Elevated amniotic fluid nitric oxide metabolites and cyclic guanosine 3',5'-monophosphate in pregnant women with intra-amniotic infection. Am J Obstet Gynecol 1997; 177:793.
62. Gravett MG, Eschenbach DA, Speigel-Brown CA, et al: Rapid diagnosis of amnionic fluid infection by gas-liquid chromatography. N Engl J Med 1982; 306:725.
63. Wager GP, Hanley LS, Farb HF, et al: Evaluation of gas-liquid chromatography for the rapid diagnosis of amniotic fluid infection: A preliminary report. Am J Obstet Gynecol 1985; 152:51.
64. Vintzileos AM, Campbell WA, Nochimson DJ, et al: The fetal biophysical profile in patients with premature rupture of membranes—an early prediction of fetal infection. Am J Obstet Gynecol 1985; 152:510.
65. Roussis P, Rosemond RL, Glass C, et al: Preterm premature rupture of membranes: Detection of infection. Am J Obstet Gynecol 1991; 165:1099.
66. Cox SM, Roberts S, Roussis P, et al: Prematurity, subclinical intra-amniotic infection, and biophysical parameters: Is there a correlation? Infect Dis Obstet Gynecol 1993; 1:76.
67. Del Valle GD, Joffe GM, Izquierdo LA, et al: The biophysical profile and the nonstress test: Poor predictors of chorioamnionitis and fetal infection in prolonged preterm premature rupture of membranes. Obstet Gynecol 1992; 80:106.
68. Miller JM, Kho MS, Brown HL, et al: Clinical chorioamnionitis is not predicted by an ultrasonic biophysical profile in patients with preterm premature rupture of membranes. Obstet Gynecol 1990; 76:1051.
69. Leo MV, Skurnick JH, Ganesh VV, et al: Clinical chorioamnionitis is not predicted by umbilical artery Doppler velocimetry in patients with premature rupture of membranes. Obstet Gynecol 1992; 79:916.
70. Pankuch GA, Cherouny PH, Botti JJ, et al: Amniotic fluid leukotaxis assay as an early indicator of chorioamnionitis. Am J Obstet Gynecol 1989; 161:802.
71. Driscoll SG: The placenta and membranes. In: Charles D, Finland M (eds): Obstetric and Perinatal Infections. Philadelphia: Lea & Febiger, 1973, p 532.
72. Hillier SL, Martius J, Krohn M, et al: A case-control study of chorioamnionic infection and histologic chorioamnionitis in prematurity. N Engl J Med 1988; 319:972.
73. Dashe JS, Rogers BB, McIntire DD, et al: Time course of clinical and histologic intrauterine infection at term. Am J Obstet Gynecol 1998; 178:S204.
74. Maberry MC, Gilstrap LC, Bawdon R: Anaerobic coverage for intra-amniotic infection: Maternal and perinatal impact. Am J Perinatol 1991; 8:338.
75. Gibbs RS, Dinsmoor MJ, Newton ER, et al: A randomized trial of intrapartum versus postpartum treatment of women with intraamnionic infection. Obstet Gynecol 1988; 72:823.
76. Hanson H: Revival of the extraperitoneal cesarean section. Am J Obstet Gynecol 1978; 130:102.
77. Imig JR, Perkins RP: Extraperitoneal cesarean section: A new need for old skills. A preliminary report. Am J Obstet Gynecol 1976; 125:51.
78. Yonekura ML, Wallace R, Eglinton G: Amnionitis—optimal operative management: Extraperitoneal cesarean section vs low cervical transperitoneal cesarean section. Abstract 24A. Proceedings of the Third Annual Meeting of the Society of Perinatal Obstetricians, San Antonio, TX, January 1983.
79. Koh KS, Chan FH, Monfared AH, et al: The changing perinatal and maternal outcome in chorioamnionitis. Obstet Gynecol 1979; 53:730.
80. Silver RK, Gibbs RS, Castillo M: Effect of amnionic fluid bacteria on the course of labor in nulliparous women at term. Obstet Gynecol 1986; 68:587.
81. Satin AJ, Maberry MC, Leveno KJ, et al: Chorioamnionitis: A harbinger of dystocia. Obstet Gynecol 1992; 79:913.
82. Gibbs RS, Castillo MS, Rodgers PJ: Management of acute chorioamnionitis. Am J Obstet Gynecol 1980; 136:709.
83. Gogoi MP: Maternal mortality from cesarean section in infected cases. Br J Obstet Gynaecol 1971; 78:373.
84. Gibbs CE, Locke WE: Maternal deaths in Texas, 1969 to 1973: A report of 501 consecutive maternal deaths from the Texas Medical Association's Committee on Maternal Health. Am J Obstet Gynecol 1976; 126:687.
85. Clark DM, Anderson GV: Perinatal mortality and amnionitis in a general hospital population. Obstet Gynecol 1968; 31:714.
86. Wiswell TE, Stou BJ, Tuggle JM: Management of asymptomatic, term gestation neonates born to mothers treated with intrapartum antibiotics. Pediatr Infect Dis J 1990; 9:826.
87. Yoder PR, Gibbs RS, Blanco JD, et al: A prospective controlled study of maternal and perinatal outcome after intra-amniotic infection at term. Am J Obstet Gynecol 1983; 145:695.
88. Sperling RS, Newton E, Gibbs RS: Intraamniotic infection in low birthweight infants. J Infect Dis 1988; 158:113.
89. Ferguson MG, Rhodes PG, Morrison JC, et al: Clinical amniotic fluid infection and its effects on the neonate. Am J Obstet Gynecol 1985; 151:1058.
90. Hankins GDV, Snyder RR, Yeomans ER: Umbilical arterial and venous acid-base and blood gas values and the effect of chorioamnionitis on those values in a cohort of preterm infants. Am J Obstet Gynecol 1991; 164:1261.
91. Weeks JW, Reynolds L, Taylor D, et al: Umbilical cord blood interleukin-6 levels and neonatal morbidity. Obstet Gynecol 1997; 90:815.
92. Murphy DJ, Sellers S, MacKenzie IZ, et al: Case control study of antenatal and intrapartum risk factors for cerebral palsy in very preterm singleton babies. Lancet 1995; 346:1449.
93. Grether JK, Nelson KB: Maternal infection and cerebral palsy in infants of normal birth weight. JAMA 1997; 278:207.
94. Verma U, Tejani N, Klein S, et al: Obstetrical antecedents of neonatal periventricular leukomalacia (PVL). Am J Obstet Gynecol 1994; 170:264.
95. Bejar R, Wozniak P, Allard M, et al: Antenatal origin of neurologic damage in newborn infants. I. Preterm infants. Am J Obstet Gynecol 1988; 159:357.
96. Alexander JA, Gilstrap LC, Cox SM, et al: Effects of acute mo-

noamnionitis in the premature infant. Obstet Gynecol 1998; 91:725.

97. Murphy DJ, Hope PL, Johnson A: Neonatal risk factors for cerebral palsy in very preterm babies: A case-control study. BMJ 1997; 314:404.

98. Yoon BH, Romero R, Yang SH, et al: Interleukin-6 concentrations in umbilical cord plasma are elevated in neonates with white matter lesions associated with periventricular leukomalacia. Am J Obstet Gynecol 1996; 174:1433.

99. Yoon BH, Kim CJ, Romero R, et al: Experimentally induced intrauterine infection causes fetal brain white matter lesions in rabbits. Am J Obstet Gynecol 1997; 177:797.

14 Postpartum Endometritis

SEBASTIAN FARO

Postpartum endometritis continues to be a major complication of pregnancy, resulting in significant morbidity and hospital costs. It is more likely to occur in patients delivering by cesarean section, but does occur following vaginal delivery. Patients at risk for developing postpartum endometritis are typically those who experience a prolonged labor with ruptured amniotic membranes and are delivered by cesarean section. However, there are patients who have a relatively uncomplicated labor and go on to develop postpartum endometritis. It appears that a major factor contributing to postpartum endometritis is the status of the lower genital tract. The bacteria commonly found to inhabit and make up the microflora of the vaginal ecosystem can cause significant infection. The morbidity associated with postpartum endometritis is related to the type of sequelae that can develop; for example, pelvic abscess, myonecrosis of the uterus, suppurative endometritis, ligneous cellulitis, and septic pelvic vein thrombosis. In order to prevent postpartum endometritis and its associated sequelae, the obstetrician must possess a working knowledge of the complexities of the vaginal ecosystem and microbial pathophysiology of postpartum endometritis.

EPIDEMIOLOGY

Postpartum endometritis can occur early or late in the postpartum period, up to 6 weeks following delivery. It is an infection that results, in more than 90% of the cases, from bacteria ascending from the lower genital tract into the uterus.[1, 2] Therefore, it is the status of the lower genital tract that is a significant predictor of the risk of postpartum endometritis (Table 14–1).

All pregnant patients are potentially at risk for developing postpartum endometritis. The individuals at greatest risk are those with little or no prenatal care as well as other factors (see Table 14–1). The incidence of postpartum endometritis is related to the mode of delivery; approximately 5% of patients delivering vaginally develop postpartum endometritis, whereas as many as 85% of those delivering by cesarean section develop this infection.[1, 3] However, among patients who consistently keep their prenatal appointments and ad-

here to the principles of prenatal care, approximately 10% of those delivered by cesarean section develop postpartum endometritis.

A small number of cases of postpartum endometritis, probably fewer than 1%, are caused by bacteria that are introduced from the exogenous environment, including the common sexually transmitted diseases (STDs), that is, *Neisseria gonorrhoeae* and *Chlamydia trachomatis*. Therefore, screening patients during the antepartum period for STDs, especially for gonococcus and chlamydia, can prevent not only neonatal infection but also maternal infection. It should be remembered that disseminated gonococcal infection occurs more frequently in the pregnant state than in the nonpregnant state.[4]

Obviously, intangible factors can contribute to placing the patient at risk for developing postpartum endometritis. The factors that can place the patient at risk for postpartum infection are chronic medical illness, immunosuppression, gingivitis, and malignancy. Chronic medical illness may result in decreased circulation, immunosuppression, and poor healing (Table 14–2). A relationship has been suggested between the presence of chronic gingivitis and postoperative infection.[5] The pathophysiology of this relationship has not been elucidated. Immunosuppression may result from a direct assault on the patient's immune systems (e.g., acquired immunodeficiency syndrome [AIDS]) or from treatment of a chronic disease (e.g., lupus) that requires the use of immunosuppressive agents.

MICROBIOLOGY

The lower genital tract is inhabited by a variety of bacteria that constitute the endogenous microflora of

TABLE 14–1 ▸ RISK FACTORS FOR DEVELOPING POSTPARTUM ENDOMETRITIS

Lack of prenatal care
Bacterial vaginosis
Colonization with *Streptococcus agalactiae*
Prolonged rupture of amniotic membranes
Prolonged labor
Use of internal fetal monitoring devices

181

TABLE 14-2 ▶	CHRONIC ILLNESSES THAT MAY PREDISPOSE THE PATIENT TO INFECTIONS
Diabetes	Sarcoidosis
Hypertension	Cardiac disease
Lupus	Pulmonary disease

TABLE 14-4 ▶	CHARACTERISTICS OF A HEALTHY VAGINAL ECOSYSTEM	
Characteristic	**Description**	
Discharge	Homogenous, liquid to pasty	
Color	White to slate-gray	
Odor	None	
pH	3.8 to 4.2	
Squamous cells	Well estrogenized, cell membrane and nucleus easily seen	
	Microscopically 10× and 40× magnification	
WBCs	Rare	
Bacteriology	One dominant morphotype, large bacillary rods	

the vaginal ecosystems (Table 14–3). These bacteria can exist independently of one another, in a commensal relationship, synergistically, or as antagonists. When the vaginal ecosystem is in a healthy state, the microflora is dominated by *Lactobacillus acidophilus*. Although other bacteria including pathogenic gram-negative and gram-positive bacteria are present, their numbers are usually less than 10^3 organisms/mL of vaginal fluid. The growth of these bacteria is held in check and suppressed by *L. acidophilus* through the production of lactic acid, hydrogen peroxide (H_2O_2), and bacteriocin.[6-8] A healthy vaginal flora is characterized by the presence of estrogen, dominance of *L. acidophilus* (at least 10^5 bacteria/mL of vaginal fluid) and odorless white discharge (Table 14–4).

Lactobacillus acidophilus favors a pH of 5 to 6 to achieve optimal growth, which also favors the growth of other bacteria (e.g., *Gardnerella vaginalis*, *Prevotella bivia*, *Escherichia coli*, *Streptococcus agalactiae*) as well as others. However, as *L. acidophilus* grows, it produces significant quantities of lactic acid, up to 26 moles/L of medium, H_2O_2, and bacteriocins.[9] The production of lactic acid results in a significant increase in the hydrogenous concentration, with the pH becoming 4 or less. The pH of a healthy vaginal ecosystem ranges between 3.8 and 4.2, which is unfavorable to other bacteria in the vaginal ecosystem. *Lactobacillus acidophilus* does not favor a pH less than or equal to 4 but is able to grow, although extremely slowly. Thus, *L. acidophilus* has adapted to this pH, 3.8 to 4.0, and is able to maintain itself and not have to compete with other bacteria.

Other factors that enable *L. acidophilus* to maintain dominance are H_2O_2 and bacteriocin. H_2O_2 is toxic to anaerobic bacteria because these organisms lack the enzyme catalase. Therefore, obligate anaerobic bacteria cannot degrade H_2O_2 to water and oxygen. Bacteriocin, also referred to as lactocin, is a protein that

inhibits the growth of bacteria.[10-12] This protein is capable of inhibiting a variety of bacteria, including bacteria that make up the endogenous microflora of the vaginal ecosystem.

When the vaginal ecosystem is altered, e.g., by organisms introduced into the ecosystem such as *Trichomonas vaginalis*, *N. gonorrhoeae*, *C. trachomatis*, and other factors such as frequent sexual intercourse, use of antibiotics, and unknown factors, the growth of *L. acidophilus* is inhibited. This results in an increase in pH, which allows bacteria other than *L. acidophilus* to grow. *L. acidophilus* is apparently not a good competitor and becomes suppressed. If the dominant organism becomes *G. vaginalis*, its growth continues to promote an increasing pH as well as depletes the oxygen concentration in the environment. These changes favor the growth of obligate anaerobes and eventually they, along with *G. vaginalis*, become the dominant organisms of the vaginal ecosystem. This state of the vaginal ecosystem has been termed *bacterial vaginosis* (BV), vaginal bacteriosis, or bacterial anaerobiosis syndrome.

This condition, BV, is not an infection and is not associated with inflammation. Treatment of BV should not be directed at achieving a cure but at returning the vaginal ecosystem to a healthy state. The overuse of antibiotics will only result in further alteration of the ecosystem.

Shifts in the vaginal ecosystem can result in dominance by other bacteria, such as *E. coli* and *S. agalactiae*. These two bacteria have particular importance because they can result in significant infectious morbidity. *Escherichia coli* is the most common cause of urinary tract infections in women and is the most common cause of pyelonephritis in pregnancy. *Escherichia coli* appears to be evolving into an organism that is being selected via the use of ampicillin prophylaxis against *S. agalactiae* (group B streptococcus [GBS]) colonization of pregnant women during labor.[13] *Streptococcus agalactiae* can also assume a role of dominance, causing vaginitis and postoperative infection, specifically postpartum endometritis.

Patients who acquire *T. vaginalis* vaginitis also develop a shift in the type of or abnormal microflora of the vaginal ecosystem. Typically, the microflora is not

TABLE 14-3 ▶	ENDOGENOUS BACTERIA OF THE VAGINA	
Lactobacillus acidophilus	*Klebsiella pneumoniae*	
Corynebacterium	*Proteus vulgaris*	
Diphtheroids	*Prevotella bivia*	
Nondescript streptococci	*P. melaninogenica*	
Staphylococcus epidermidis	*Bacteroides fragilis*	
Enterococcus faecalis	*Fusobacterium nucleatum*	
Escherichia coli	*F. necrophorum*	
Enterobacter cloacae	*Peptostreptococcus anaerobius*	

dominated by a single bacterial species, but there are numerous genera and species. Growth of *T. vaginalis* is associated with a pH of at least 5, and therefore *L. acidophilus* loses its role as a dominant organism and stabilizer of the microflora of the vaginal ecosystem.

The alteration of the vaginal flora has significance because it can result in or serve as a possible etiology of premature labor, premature rupture of amniotic membranes, and postoperative infection. There is general agreement that BV places the pregnant patient at risk for the development of postpartum endometritis, especially if delivered by cesarean section.[14–16]

PREVENTION OF POSTPARTUM ENDOMETRITIS

Prevention of postpartum endometritis begins with an understanding of the microbial pathophysiology and associated risk factors. It appears that an initial predisposing factor is an altered vaginal microflora in association with labor, especially if prolonged. An additional significant factor is the duration of ruptured amniotic membranes. These three conditions appear to function synergistically in establishing a myometrial infection that actually begins during labor.[17–19]

There is a general agreement among investigators that the vaginal microflora does have a central role in postpartum endometritis. Therefore, it is logical to screen all pregnant women, perhaps between 34 and 37 weeks, for the presence of an altered vaginal flora. In most instances, this would correlate with screening for *Streptococcus agalactiae*. Screening at this gestational age would permit adequate time prior to delivery, therefore permitting time for treatment to be completed. Determining the state of the microflora of the lower genital tract can be easily accomplished (see section on diagnosis). The goal is to determine the specific abnormality present; for example, BV, GBS, gram-negative or gram-positive bacilli, or *Trichomonas*. Screening for these conditions at the first prenatal visit may indicate a patient at risk for interruption of the pregnancy. Diagnosis of an altered vaginal ecosystem early in pregnancy should be an indication for sequential screening throughout the pregnancy.

Finding an altered vaginal microflora should initiate treatment in an attempt to restore the lower genital tract to a healthy state, if possible. One hypothetical consideration is the possibility that patients known to have recurrent vaginitis may have a low grade or "subclinical" endometritis. Coincident endometritis has been reported in 20% of women with BV.[20] This implies that bacteria have established an infection in the endometrium and perhaps the myometrium. Therefore, once a patient, especially if pregnant, is diagnosed with BV, treatment with oral antibiotics should be initiated. The agent should have a spectrum of

TABLE 14-5 ▶	ANTIBIOTICS EFFECTIVE IN THE TREATMENT OF BV

Metronidazole, 250 mg tid, 500 mg bid, 750 mg qd × 7 days
Clindamycin, 300 mg tid × 7 days
Amoxicillin-clavulanic acid, 500 mg tid × 7 days

activity that is effective against obligate anaerobes (Table 14–5).

Although none of these antibiotics have approval for use in pregnancy, they have been used and have not been found to adversely affect the fetus. Metronidazole, the agent that receives the most attention, has been given to approximately 4,000 pregnant women in various stages of pregnancy. Intravaginal preparations would not be indicated, since topical agents do not provide adequate tissue levels.

Individuals found to have vaginal trichomoniasis also have an altered vaginal microflora. The bacteria tend to be mainly obligate anaerobes, a situation that can resemble BV; or BV and trichomoniasis can coexist. These individuals should be treated with metronidazole, since no other antimicrobial is effective against *T. vaginalis*.

Patients colonized by GBS pose a significant problem, and antepartum management has not been established. Although it is not recommended to treat GBS-colonized patients in the antepartum period, individuals who have experienced a previous GBS event do not accept this recommendation. It may be prudent to determine the inoculum size, even in a semiquantitative manner. Treatment may reduce the inoculum to a low level. A complete discussion of GBS and pregnancy can be found in Chapter 10.

Individuals whose vaginal microflora is altered—but not by one of the specific conditions discussed earlier—may have unimicrobial vaginitis (e.g., *E. coli*), or a nonspecific vaginitis, and are at risk for the development of postpartum endometritis. Numerous investigators have demonstrated a beneficial effect by administering antibiotics prophylactically.[21–24] However, these studies did not address the status of the vaginal ecosystem with regard to the risk of developing postpartum endometritis. Although there are benefits to administering antibiotics prophylactically, there are also disadvantages. Administration of antibiotics can result in selection of resistant bacteria. Studies have demonstrated that administration of a single dose of a cephalosporin, cefazolin, or cefoxitin prophylactically resulted in a sixfold increase in enterococcal (*Enterococcus faecalis*) colonization of the lower genital tract.[18, 25] There has also been a selection of resistant strains from a population of a species that is typically sensitive to the antibiotic. An example of this is selection of *E. coli* resistant to cefoxitin in patient's receiving it for prophylaxis. Patients cultured prior to receiving cefoxitin for prophylaxis did not reveal any *E. coli* resistant to cefoxitin. Reculturing the patients 24 hours after receiving a single dose of cefoxitin did yield, in one patient, *E. coli* resistant to cefoxitin.[26]

Although antibiotic prophylaxis has reduced the incidence of postoperative infection, approximately 10% of surgical patients continue to experience infection; that is, postpartum endometritis. An important precursor of or risk factor for the development of postpartum endometritis is the presence of BV. Therefore, it would be beneficial to screen patients in the latter weeks of pregnancy for BV and treat them with oral metronidazole in an attempt to facilitate the restoration of the vaginal ecosystem to a healthy state.

Patients known to be colonized with GBS, who receive ampicillin or penicillin for prophylaxis to prevent perinatal transmission of GBS to the neonate, and subsequently are delivered by cesarean section are considered at risk for the development of postpartum endometritis. It is important to understand that other bacteria (e.g., *E. coli* or *P. bivia*) can increase in number during the labor process. They can achieve numbers exceeding 10^5 bacteria/mL of 5% amniotic fluid.[27] Therefore, these patients should receive a broader spectrum antibiotic (e.g., piperacillin/tazobactam, ampicillin/sulbactam, cefoxitin, or clindamycin plus gentamicin). However, it may be prudent to administer an antibiotic therapeutically until the patient is afebrile and demonstrates complete resolution of clinical and laboratory signs of infection.

DIAGNOSIS

The diagnosis of postpartum endometritis can, at times, be difficult to establish. Patients will frequently develop febrile morbidity without localizing signs of infection. Patients who develop fever within 24 to 48 hours following delivery may or may not have postpartum endometritis. Individuals who develop fever this early in the postpartum period must be evaluated for GBS endometritis as well as potentially other bacterial etiologies versus viral infection. The physical examination is extremely important in establishing a diagnosis of postpartum endometritis.

Postpartum endometritis that occurs within the first 48 hours following delivery most likely originates during labor. It is during labor that bacteria gain entrance to the myometrium, and if conditions are appropriate the organisms will become established within the myometrium. The infection process is initiated by the bacteria adhering to the myometrium, thus allowing them to reproduce and infiltrate deeper in the myometrium. If myometritis is established, once the patient manifests clinical signs of infection a common physical finding is a sub-involuted uterus and a dilated cervix (Table 14–6).

The lochia may or may not be purulent. It is often

TABLE 14-6 ▶ CLINICAL SIGNS OF POSTPARTUM ENDOMETRITIS

Fever ≥101°F or ≥100°F on two occasions is measured at least 6 h apart.
A tachycardia that parallels the patient's temperature course.
A WBC count ≥14,000/mm³ or ≥10% band forms.
Marked uterine tenderness.
Sub-involution of the uterus.
Significant cervical dilation is present.
Lochia may be purulent.
An adynamic ileus may be present.

difficult to determine whether the lochia is purulent because it is usually bloody. However, frequently when purulence is present, it forms streaks in the lochia. When it is thoroughly mixed with the lochia, the color tends to be dark and brownish.

Patients meeting the criteria for postpartum endometritis should have an endometrial specimen obtained via the use of an endometrial-sampling device. The lochia retained within the uterine cavity should be evacuated to facilitate obtaining tissue. This will produce a higher yield of organisms representative of the infected tissue. Utilizing an endometrial sampling device (e.g., the Pipelle) will produce a smaller number of genera of bacteria.[16] The specimen should immediately be placed in anaerobic transport medium and processed for the isolation of aerobic, facultative, and obligate anaerobic bacteria.

The value of obtaining specimens from the suspected site of infection will facilitate management of the patient who fails initial empirical antibiotic therapy. It is true that most studies have shown that as many as 90% of patients with postpartum endometritis will respond to initial empirical therapy.[28–32] However, the patients who do not respond often fall victim to "revolving" antibiotic therapy. Frequently, the change in antibiotic therapy offers an advantage over the previous antibiotics. Since most patients respond within 48 hours of administering antibiotics, those that do not are considered failures. The aerobically cultured specimens, if bacteria are present, should have colonies present on the agar surface. Failure to respond to initial antibiotic therapy can be due to a variety of causes (Table 14–7). When failure to respond can be attributed to the presence of a bacterium that is resis-

TABLE 14-7 ▶ ANTIBIOTIC THERAPEUTIC FAILURES

Presence of a resistant bacterium
Viral infection
Infected hematoma
Pelvic abscess
Myometrial abscess
Necrotizing myositis
Septic pelvic vein thrombosis
Drug fever

tant to the currently administered antibiotic regimens, it is most frequently because of the presence of a gram-positive aerobic or gram-negative facultative anaerobic bacterium. Rarely is antibiotic failure caused by the presence of an obligate anaerobic bacterium. Therefore, if an initial culture is obtained, growth will usually appear within 48 hours. Bacterial colony morphology may be helpful because if it varies, this would indicate the presence of more than bacterial species or genus. Bacterial specimens should be obtained from the various colony morphotypes for Gram staining. If blood cultures were performed, the bottles should be shaken vigorously and an aliquot obtained for Gram staining. A negative Gram stain, from an aliquot obtained from the blood culture, would be highly suggestive of the absence of bacteremia. The blood cultures will be monitored daily for the appearance of growth.

The results of the Gram stain of the bacteria growing on the agar cultures can be of significant assistance in determining which modifications to the current antibiotics should be made. For example, most patients delivered by cesarean section receive antibiotic prophylaxis. The most frequently administered antibiotics for prophylaxis are cephalosporins. Other antibiotics (e.g., penicillin and clindamycin) have also been used for prophylaxis. Antibiotics administered prophylactically, even when given as a single dose, have been demonstrated to select for resistant strains, such as *E. faecalis* and gram-negative facultative anaerobic bacteria. Therefore, if a patient who received a cephalosporin for prophylaxis subsequently develops postpartum endometritis and fails to respond to initial therapy, the possibility of selection of resistant bacteria should be considered. The management of this clinical dilemma can be conducted as outlined in Figures 14–1 to 14–3.

If the patient is being treated with a cephalosporin or cephamycin and the endometrial cultures reveal the presence of gram-positive cocci, the most likely bacterium is *E. faecalis*. The reason for this assumption is that the cephalosporins and cephamycin have good activity against the streptococci, specifically *S. agalactiae, Staphylococcus epidermidis*, and community-acquired *Staphylococcus aureus*. Changing to an expanded spectrum penicillin, such as piperacillin-tazobactam, provides coverage against gram-positive aerobic bacteria as well as gram-negative facultative anaerobic bacteria. The presence of the beta-lactamase inhibitor, tazobactam, expands the spectrum of piperacillin against gram-negative facultative anaerobic bacteria, especially the Enterobacteriaceae. This includes organisms that are resistant to piperacillin. If the patient has gram-positive bacteremia as well as endometritis, an aminoglycoside should be added to the expanded-spectrum penicillin to provide coverage against *Enterococcus*.

Patients who are treated with an expanded-spectrum penicillin and fail are likely to have a resistant member of the Enterobacteriaceae. All that is required in these cases is the addition of an aminoglycoside, which will expand the antibiotic activity against gram-negative facultative anaerobic bacteria. The initial choice should be gentamicin, as most gram-negative facultative anaerobic bacteria will be sensitive. A specific identification of the bacterium and antibiotic sensitivities should be available within the next 24 hours. The combination of an expanded spectrum penicillin (piperacillin-tazobactam or ampicillin-sulbactam) plus gentamicin is synergistic against *E. faecalis*. These penicillins have activity against a wide spectrum of anaerobic bacteria, including *Bacteroides fragilis* and members of the *B. fragilis* group, as well as the anaerobes commonly found in pelvic infections. The use of gentamicin is also cost-effective, and once-a-day dosing is as effective as multiple-dosing regimens.

Patients begun on the combination of clindamycin plus gentamicin lack coverage for approximately 15% to 20% of GBS, and this combination has no activity against enterococci. Therefore, it would be prudent to add ampicillin to provide coverage against both GBS and enterococci. The combination of ampicillin plus an aminoglycoside is synergistic against both GBS and the enterococci. If a gram-negative bacillus is isolated, gentamicin should be discontinued and amikacin begun. Once the identification and antibiotic sensitivities are known, adjustments can be made. Tobramycin should not be substituted for gentamicin because there is cross-resistance. An organism resistant to gentamicin will be resistant to tobramycin.

Patients treated with metronidazole pose a problem different from those receiving clindamycin; namely, metronidazole is active strictly against obligate anaerobes. Therefore, when these patients fail to respond to therapy, consideration must be given to discontinuing the metronidazole and instituting therapy with an antibiotic that not only provides similar antimicrobial coverage but also exceeds that provided by metronidazole (Fig. 14–4). Therefore, substituting clindamycin for metronidazole does not meet these criteria. The expanded-spectrum penicillins, piperacillin-tazobactam or ampicillin-sulbactam, do provide the spectrum of activity required and are synergistic with aminoglycosides against both GBS and enterococci.

Patients who are allergic to penicillin pose an interesting challenge. This group of patients may be treated with the fluoroquinolone levofloxacin; however, if these patients are breast-feeding their infants, they must stop breast-feeding during their treatment. The patient should pump her breast and discard the milk up to 24 hours after completely discontinuing the levofloxacin. Quinolones are contraindicated in parturients and breast-feeding mothers.

Imipenem-cilastatin is a carbapenem with a broad spectrum of activity, including obligate anaerobic bacteria. This agent is rarely used as initial enzyme therapy and is commonly the back-up antibiotic. It is suitable

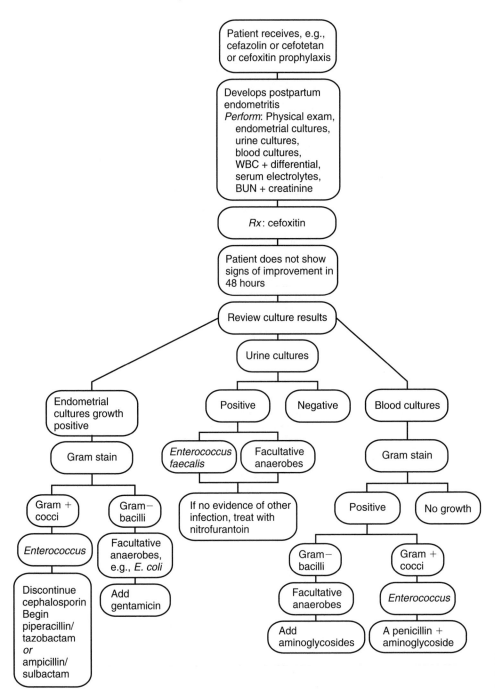

FIGURE 14–1 ▶ Management of therapeutic antibiotic failures: cephalosporins.

for treatment of postpartum endometritis but does not offer any significant advantage over the beta-lactam penicillin.

Since postpartum endometritis typically is an infection localized to the uterus and occurs in a population that is relatively healthy, patients respond to therapy quickly. Therefore, the antibiotic armamentarium can be kept simple and cost-effective. Newer antibiotics are not always better; in fact, there have not been any clinical studies demonstrating the superiority of one appropriate antibiotic over another. Therefore, the more traditional antibiotics continue to be effective and cost-effective (Table 14–8).

Comparative studies have demonstrated that the beta-lactam antibiotics, the expanded-spectrum cephalosporins, and penicillin are as efficacious as the combinations; that is, clindamycin or metronidazole plus an aminoglycoside and ampicillin (Table 14–9).[29–32] There has been very limited investigation regarding the use of quinolones. Ciprofloxacin has been used in combination with clindamycin and has not been shown to be very effective in the treatment of postpartum endometritis.[33] The quinolones, at this time, do not appear to be well suited for the treatment of postpartum endometritis because they are contraindicated in pregnancy and breast feeding women.

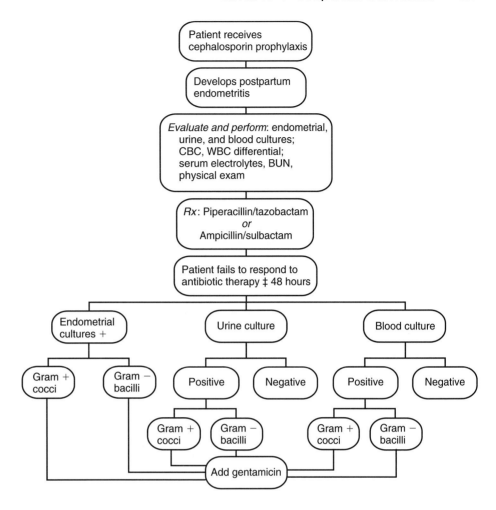

FIGURE 14-2 ▶ Management of therapeutic antibiotic failure: penicillin.

Treatment of postpartum endometritis should be instituted early, since delay can result in complications that lead not only to increased costs as well as increased hospital stay but also, often, conditions that place the patient at significant risk for other associated complications. The most serious of these complications are the following: necrotizing myositis of the uterus, pelvic abscess, septic pelvic vein thrombosis, and ligneous cellulitis.

Thus, patients who fail initial antibiotic therapy should be re-evaluated to determine whether the reason for not responding favorably is because of the presence of a resistant bacterium or another reason

(Table 14–10). A viral infection is characterized by the presence of a rapidly rising temperature, usually 103°F or greater, a white blood cell count of 13,000 to 15,000/mm³, and the absence of any physical findings

TABLE 14-9 ▶ ANTIBIOTICS SUITABLE FOR PROPHYLAXIS AND TREATMENT OF POSTPARTUM ENDOMETRITIS

Prophylaxis

First-generation cephalosporin
Keflin (cephalothin)
Cefazolin
Second-generation cephalosporin
Cefotetan
Cefoxitin
Ceftizoxime

Treatment of Postpartum Endometritis

Single Agents	Beta-Lactamase Inhibitor
Cefoxitin	Piperacillin-tazobactam
Cefotetan	Ampicillin-sulbactam
Ceftizoxime	

Combinations
Clindamycin + aminoglycoside
Clindamycin + aminoglycoside + ampicillin
Metronidazole + aminoglycoside
Metronidazole + aminoglycoside + ampicillin

TABLE 14-8 ▶ ANTIBIOTIC CHOICES FOR THE TREATMENT OF POSTPARTUM ENDOMETRITIS

Cephalosporins	Penicillins	Carbapenems
Cefoxitin	Ampicillin-sulbactam	Imipenem-cefazolin
Cefotetan	Piperacillin-tazobactam	Meropenem
Ceftizoxime	Ticarcillin-clavulanic acid	

Combinations
Clindamycin + aminoglycoside
Clindamycin + aminoglycoside + ampicillin
Metronidazole + aminoglycoside
Metronidazole + aminoglycoside + ampicillin

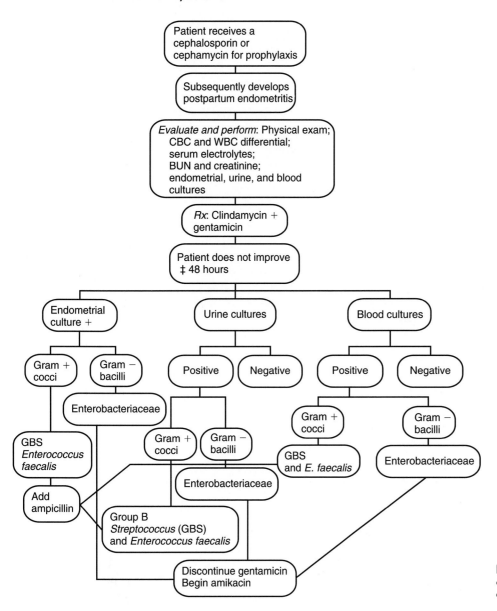

FIGURE 14-3 ▶ Management of therapeutic antibiotic failures: clindamycin and gentamicin.

of localized infection. The patient will usually relate the presence of nonspecific complaints of myalgias and malaise. In some instances, the physical examinations may reveal labial lesions or ulcers indicative of oral herpes. Typically, these patients will experience sponta-

neous resolution of symptoms within 48 to 72 hours. If they are started on antibiotic therapy and spontaneous resolution of all signs and symptoms of infection occurs, and they then remain afebrile for 24 hours, therapy can be discontinued.

The presence of an infected hematoma and abscess can be documented by ultrasonography. Localization of a collection of fluid should be approached aggressively. The fluid collection should be aspirated under ultrasound guidance. The fluid should be immediately placed into an anaerobic transport medium. An aliquot of the fluid should be gram-stained. The characteristics of the gram-stained bacteria can assist in choosing appropriate modifications to the currently administered antibiotic therapy. It would be prudent to obtain venous blood for culture, since there is a 10% to 20% risk of bacteremia in these patients. Aspiration of the fluid should be accompanied by the placement of a drain (percutaneous drainage) to allow

TABLE 14-10 ▶	DIFFERENTIAL DIAGNOSIS FOR ANTIBIOTIC TREATMENT FAILURES

Wrong diagnosis; example, viral and not bacterial infection
Presence of a resistant bacterium
Presence of an infected hematoma
Presence of an abscess
Presence of a wound infection
Necrotizing myositis of the uterus
Septic pelvic vein thrombosis
Ligneous cellulitis of the pelvis
Infection outside the pelvis
Drug fever

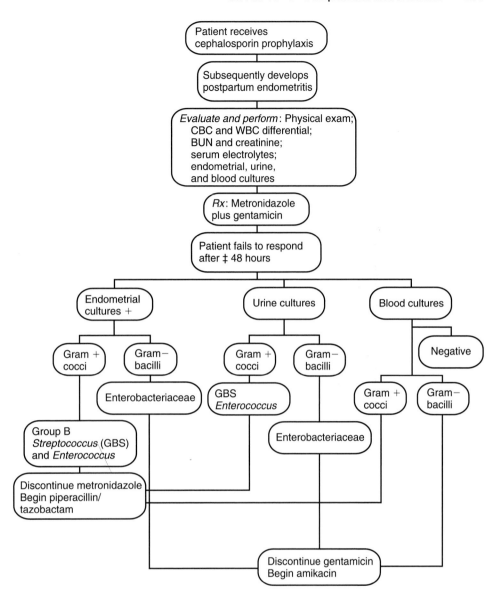

FIGURE 14-4 ▶ Management of antibiotic failures: metronidazole and gentamicin.

for complete drainage of the abscess or infected hematoma. The abscess cavity or infected hematoma should be completely evacuated. This is followed with copious irrigation of the cavity. Irrigation should be carried out until the fluid returns clear. Intravenous antibiotics are administered until the patient remains afebrile for 72 hours, all laboratory tests have returned to normal, and all physical signs and symptoms of infection have resolved. The drain should be removed when there is less than 30 mL of fluid collected over a 24-hour period.

Wound infections following cesarean section or vaginal delivery (episiotomy) should be managed aggressively, since they can be polymicrobial and there is a possibility that the bacteria can act synergistically to cause necrotizing fasciitis. The clinical manifestations usually begin on the second and third postoperative days, but they can occur later. One indication that the patient is developing a wound infection is the presence

of a persistent low-grade fever (e.g., fever peaks at 100.2°F and does not return to baseline; the lowest may be 99°F). Inspection of the wound may reveal one or more of the characteristics listed in Table 14–11. A logical approach to the management of a suspected infected wound is to truly determine whether an infection is present. This can be accomplished with the aid of ultrasonography and aspiration of fluid, if present.

TABLE 14-11 ▶	CHARACTERISTICS OF WOUND INFECTION

Induration of the surrounding tissue
Erythema of the tissue on either or both sides of the incision
The skin around the incision develops a sheen
Edema of the wound
Drainage from the incision
Pain to pressure
The skin overlying and adjacent to the incision appears tense.

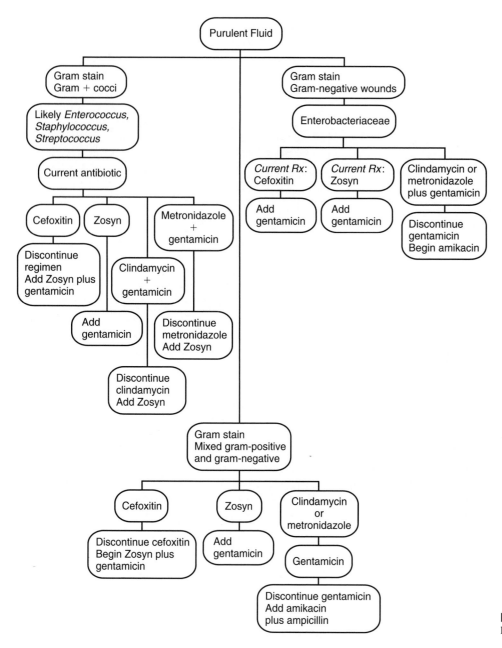

FIGURE 14–5 ▶ Aspirate purulent fluid from wound.

Ultrasonographic examination can locate a fluid collection, and aspiration can be easily and painlessly performed. Inserting the needle, an 18-gauge, through the incision line does not cause pain. The ultrasound can guide the placement of the needle into the fluid collection. The characteristics and Gram stain of the fluid can facilitate in establishing that an infection is present and the type of bacteria that are involved (Fig. 14–5). The key to management is to open and cleanse the wound. All necrotic tissue should be débrided. The wound should be patched with moistened gauze, and the dressing should be changed at least three times a day. Antibiotic therapy is definitely necessary if there is an area of advancing cellulitis. However, all patients should be administered antibiotics until the infection is under control.

If the patient has necrotic tissue and the area is not painful, the diagnosis of necrotizing fasciitis must be considered. Typically, the tissue will liquefy and the skin is not involved early in the course of infection. The patient also appears septic. In case of fasciitis or necrotizing myositis, the tissue must be excised and the débridement must be carried to healthy tissue. This can be determined by noting the contrast between necrotic tissue that does not bleed and the healthy tissue that bleeds. Healthy subcutaneous tissue is yellow compared to the white, blanched–appearing avascular color of necrotic tissue. Advanced infection of the tissue results in liquefaction. The bacteria involved result in liberation of endotoxin and exotoxin, and therefore these patients are at significant risk for developing septic shock. Following surgical excision of the infected tissue, the patient should be examined every 4 hours for signs of sepsis and shock. The wound should also be examined, and if there is evidence of necrosis the patient should be taken back to surgery and further débridement performed.

Patients with necrotizing fasciitis are best served with broad-spectrum agents; for example, metronidazole for anaerobes, gentamicin for gram-negative facultative bacteria, and ampicillin for gram-positive bacteria as well as synergy with gentamicin. When one administers an aminoglycoside, it is prudent to obtain several peak and trough levels. There have been suggestions and recommendations that it is not necessary to obtain gentamicin serum levels, but these are not sound because (1) subtherapeutic levels enhance the selection of resistant bacteria; (2) levels of antibiotic in postpartum patients are unpredictable because the patient goes through a phase of diuresis and oliguria; (3) obtaining levels is useful in preventing toxicity, since it is not dose dependent; and (4) if levels are subtherapeutic and the patient responds to therapy, the aminoglycoside was not needed.

Infrequently, patients will develop high spiking temperatures with a tachycardia that rises in conjunction with, and parallels, the patient's temperature. The oral temperature can rise to 103°F or higher. Physical examination, typically, does not reveal a focus of infection. However, on occasion, the patient may complain of pelvic pain that may be localized to the right or left lower quadrant, or both. The patient's white blood cell count is usually markedly elevated to at least 20,000/mm³. These findings are consistent with a diagnosis of septic pelvic vein thrombosis. A computed tomography scan can be of assistance in establishing the diagnosis. The patient is best treated with the administration of antibiotics and heparin. The antibiotic administered should have a broad spectrum of activity, including coverage of gram-negative facultative and obligate anaerobic bacteria. Heparin is typically administered intravenously, 10,000 units as a loading dose followed by 1,000 units per hour. The patient's prothrombin time should be monitored to ensure that a hypercoagulopathy is not created. The therapeutic regimen should be continued for at least 72 hours beyond the time that the patient defervesces, the white blood cell count returns to normal (normal is defined as that range of white blood cell count noted in her first prenatal visit), and any signs and symptoms of infection have resolved.

There is no need for prolonged anticoagulation therapy unless the patient was found to have persistence of a mass. This is best illustrated by a case:

The patient is a 16 y/o delivered vaginally after a labor of approximately 10 hours. The labor was uncomplicated, as was the delivery, which was spontaneous without an episiotomy and the absence of lacerations. On postpartum day 2, approximately 8 P.M., the patient complained of right lower quadrant pain. Evaluation revealed that the patient had a temperature of 102°F, pulse rate of 110, respiratory rate of 18, BP 110/70. Physical examination was remarkable for right lower quadrant pain, without rebound, and fullness that was asymmetrical and firm. The uterus was estimated at 12-week size, the os was closed, and the lochia was dark and without odor. The diagnosis was infected hematoma, abscess, endometritis, and appendicitis. The patient did not have the rebound tenderness that is typically seen in association with appendicitis. Ultrasonography of the pelvis revealed a nondescript mass in the right adnexal area. The patient was begun on piperacillin-tazobactam intravenously, 3.375 g every 6 hours. After receiving 12 doses of the antibiotic there was no improvement—in fact her pain was increasing and there was no pain with ambulation. Examination revealed that this mass appeared to be enlarging.

The patient was taken to surgery because of a suspected enlarging abscess from an infected hematoma. Exploratory laparotomy revealed the uterus to be involuting and firm. The left parametrial and adnexal areas were normal. The right parametrial area and lateral wall were significantly indurated. This finding is similar to what is seen with a phlegmon or ligneous cellulitis. No further exploration was performed. The patient was begun on heparin, and within 48 hours the patient's condition improved. After approximately 5 days of therapy she became asymptomatic. Therapy was continued for an additional 72 hours, at which time all parameters returned to normal. She was discharged with instructions to be seen in 1 week. The patient did well for approximately 4 weeks post partum and then was seen for recurrent pain in the right lower quadrant. Computed tomography scan of the pelvis revealed venous thrombosis of the venous plexus in the right parametrial area. Doppler flow studies of the lower extremities were normal. The patient was admitted, and anticoagulation therapy was begun. After 48 hours of therapy, her pain began to resolve. Coumadin (warfarin sodium) was started and heparin was discontinued after the Pitocin (oxytocin) resulted in anticoagulation being achieved. Coumadin therapy was continued for 6 months.

Ligneous cellulitis or phlegmon usually is not associated with pelvic vein thrombosis. These conditions do not require surgical intervention and should be managed medically. Affected patients usually develop signs and symptoms of pelvic infections. Pelvic examination in the case of a phlegmon reveals a unilateral asymmetrical solid mass, whereas the presence of ligneous cellulitis involves the entire pelvis. The latter condition resembles the "frozen pelvis" that is seen with extensive pelvic carcinoma. The patient usually responds to antibiotic therapy with initial defervescence but slow resolution of the pelvic floor induration. Therefore, these patients are usually continued on oral antibiotics on discharge until the mass resolves.

Drug fever is characterized by an elevated oral body temperature and a normal pulse rate. The white blood cell count may be slightly elevated, and in approximately 50% of the cases there is an eosinophilia. The physical examination is unremarkable. The approach is to discontinue all medications, especially antibiotics. The patient's signs and symptoms will resolve within 48 hours of discontinuing all medications.

When evaluating patients for postpartum infection prior to performing the pelvic examination, physicians should look for infection outside the pelvis. As stated earlier, the patient should be assessed for conditions such as possible viral infections, pneumonia, and tooth abscess. Although the antibiotic therapy used to treat postpartum infection will also be adequate for treating most other bacterial infections, in the case of pneumonia the therapy should include an antibiotic effective against *Mycoplasma pneumoniae.*

A common infection that is seen in the late postpartum period, but may also be seen within the first week, is mastitis. This condition can be accompanied with fever (e.g., 103°F) and should not be overlooked. The failure to recognize mastitis or a delay on the patient's part in seeking treatment can result in the formation of a breast abscess that requires surgical intervention. This results in increased morbidity and cost and can also result in disfigurement of the breast.

Antibiotic usage for the treatment of postpartum endometritis should be directed against three groups of bacteria: the streptococci, primarily *S. agalactiae* and the infrequently encountered *S. pyogenes;* Enterobacteriaceae, for example, *E. coli* and *Klebsiella, Proteus,* and *Enterobacter;* and obligate anaerobes—both gram-positive and gram-negative microbes. This concept has initiated the use of combinations such as clindamycin or metronidazole plus gentamicin plus ampicillin. Over the years, ampicillin has been held in reserve and added when the patient did not respond to the initial combination. Routine monitoring of peak and trough levels of gentamicin has been debated; however, the use of subtherapeutic levels of antibiotics should be avoided, since such dosing can contribute to the selection of resistant bacteria. In addition, since subtherapeutic levels do not affect bacteria in an adverse manner, and if the patient on such doses is cured, then gentamicin or another aminoglycoside is not necessary. This was demonstrated in two studies in which patients were treated with clindamycin alone: 88% of the patients were cured of postpartum endometritis.[20] The reason for this is that patients with early postpartum endometritis have a unimicrobial infection primarily and the most frequent bacterium that is isolated is *S. agalactiae.* Clindamycin is active against approximately 85% of the strains of *S. agalactiae.*

Single agents such as cefoxitin, piperacillin-tazobactam, cefotetan, ampicillin-sulbactam, and Primaxin (imipenem–cilastin sodium) all have been demonstrated to be as effective as the combinations. Even though clindamycin, gentamicin, ampicillin, and metronidazole are inexpensive, they require multiple dosing, which requires multiple tasks by pharmacy and nursing. Consideration should also be given to the increased risk of adverse effects because multiple agents are being administered multiple times.

The newer antibiotics may not offer a broader spectrum of activity compared with the agents already available. However, if less frequent dosing is an option, this could translate into a reduction in overall cost to the patient. To be factored into the cost analysis is the interruption of other nursing activity that results from the administration of these agents as well as the time spent in the actual administration of the agents; for example, when the nurse ascertains that the delivery system is functioning correctly.

REFERENCES

1. Phillips LE, Faro S, Martens MG, et al: Postcesarean microbiology of high risk patient treated for endometritis. Curr Ther Res 1987; 42:1157.
2. Gilstrap LC III, Cunningham FG: The bacterial pathogenesis of infection following cesarean section. Obstet Gynecol 1979; 53:545.
3. Amstey MT, Sheldon GW, Blyth JF: Infectious morbidity after cesarean section in private institution. Am J Obstet Gynecol 1980; 136:205.
4. Garcia-Kutzbach A, Dismuke S, Musi A: Gonococcal arthritis: Clinical features and results of penicillin therapy. J Rheumatol 1974; 1:210.
5. Faro S, Sanders CV, Aldridge KE: Use of single agent antimicrobial therapy in the treatment of polymicrobial female pelvic infections. Obstet Gynecol 1982; 60:232.
6. Whittenbury R: Hydrogen-peroxide formation and catalase activity in the lactic acid bacteria. J Gen Microbiol 1964; 35:13.
7. Eschenbach DA, Davich PR, Williams BL, et al: Prevalence of hydrogen peroxide producing *Lactobacillus* species in normal women and women with bacterial vaginosis. J Clin Microbiol 1989; 27:251.
8. Klebanoff SJ, Hillier SL, Eschenbach DA, Waltersdorph AM: Control of the microbial flora of the vagina by H_2O_2—generating lactobacilli. J Infect Dis 1991; 164:94.
9. Lin L, Song J, Kimber N, et al: The role of bacterial vaginosis in infection after major gynecologic surgery. Infect Dis Obstet Gynecol 1999; 7:169.
10. Skarin A, Sylwan J: Vaginal lactobacilli inhibiting growth of *Gardnerella vaginalis, Mobiluncus* and other bacterial species cultured from vaginal content of women with bacterial vaginosis. Acta Pathol Microbiol Immunol Scand, Sect B 1986; 94:399.
11. Tahara T, Kanatani K: Isolation and partial amino acid sequence of bacteriocins produced by *Lactobacillus acidophilus.* Biosci Biotech Biochem 1997; 61:884.
12. McGroarty JA, Reid G: Detection of a *Lactobacillus* substance that inhibits *Escherichia coli.* Can J Microbiol 1988; 34:974.
13. McDuffie RS Jr, McGregor JA, Gibbs RS: Adverse perinatal outcome and resistant Enterobacteriaceae after antibiotic usage for premature rupture of the membranes and group B streptococcus carriage. Obstet Gynecol 1993; 82(4 Pt 1):487.
14. Watts DH, Krohn MA, Hillier SL, Eschenbach DA: Bacterial vaginosis as a risk factor for post-cesarean endometritis. Obstet Gynecol 1990; 75:52.
15. Faro S, Phillips LE, Martens MG: Perspectives on the bacteriology of postoperative obstetric-gynecologic infections. Am J Obstet Gynecol 1988; 158:694.
16. Martens MG, Faro S, Hammill HA, et al: Transcervical uterine cultures with a new endometrial suction curette: A comparison of three sampling methods in postpartum endometritis. Obstet Gynecol 1989; 74:273.
17. Yonekura ML: Risk factors for postcesarean endomyometritis. Am J Med 1985; 78:177.
18. Stiver HG, Forward KR, Tyrrell DL, et al: Comparative cervical microflora shifts after cefoxitin or cefazolin prophylaxis against infection following cesarean section. Am J Obstet Gynecol 1984; 149:718.
19. Polk BF, Kruche W, Phillippe M, et al: Randomized clinical trial of preoperative cefoxitin in preventing maternal infection after primary cesarean section. Am J Obstet Gynecol 1982; 142:983.
20. Korn AP, Bolan G, Padian N, et al: Plasma cell endometritis in

women with symptomatic bacterial vaginosis. Obstet Gynecol 1995; 85:387.

21. McGregor JA, Gordon SF, Krotec J, Poindexter AN: Results of a randomized, multicenter comparative trial of a single dose of cefotetan versus multiple dose of cefoxitin as prophylaxis on cesarean section. Am J Obstet Gynecol 1988; 158:701.

22. Apuzzio JJ, Reyelt C, Pelosi M, et al: Prophylactic antibiotics for cesarean section: A comparison of high- and low-risk patients for endometritis. Obstet Gynecol 1982; 59:693.

23. Gonik B: Single- versus three-dose cefotaxime prophylaxis for cesarean section. Obstet Gynecol 1985; 65:189.

24. Petersen EE: Disturbed vaginal floor as a risk-factor in pregnancy. J Obstet Gynecol 1986; 45:1808.

25. Faro S, Martens MG, Hammill HA, et al: Antibiotic prophylaxis: Is there a difference? Am J Obstet Gynecol 1990; 162:900.

26. Martens MG, Faro S, Maccato M, et al: Prevalence of β-lactamase enzyme production in bacteria isolated from women with postpartum endometritis. J Reprod Med 1993; 38:794.

27. Pinell P, Faro S, Roberts S, et al: Intrauterine pressure catheter in labor: Associated microbiology. Infect Dis Obstet Gynecol 1993; 1:60.

28. Faro S, Martens M, Hammill H, et al: Ticarcillin/clavulanic acid versus clindamycin and gentamicin in the treatment of postcesarean endometritis following antibiotic prophylaxis. Obstet Gynecol 1989; 73:808.

29. Hemsell DC, Martens MG, Faro S, et al: A multi-center study comparing intravenous menopenem with clindamycin plus gentamicin for the treatment of acute gynecologic and obstetric pelvic infections in hospitalized women. Clin Infect Dis 1997; 24(suppl 2):S222.

30. Sweet RL, Roy S, Faro S, et al: Piperacillin and tazobactam versus clindamycin and gentamicin in the treatment of hospitalized women with pelvic infection: The Piperacillin/tazobactam Study Group. Obstet Gynecol 1994; 83:280.

31. Martens MG, Faro S, Hammill H, et al: Ampicillin/sulbactam versus clindamycin/gentamicin in the treatment of postpartum endometritis. Am J Gynecol Health 1990; 4:11.

32. Martens MG, Faro S, Phillips LE: Metronidazole-gentamicin vs. sulbactam-ampicillin in the treatment of postpartum endometritis. Diagn Microbiol Infect Dis 1989; 12(suppl 4):181s.

33. Maccato ML, Faro S, Martens MG, Hammill H: Ciprofloxacin versus gentamicin/clindamycin for postpartum endometritis. J Reprod Med 1991; 36:857.

15

Septic Pelvic Thrombophlebitis

JOHN W. RIGGS ▶ JORGE D. BLANCO

INTRODUCTION AND DEFINITION OF SYNDROME

Thrombosis in the veins of the pelvis may present in a variety of ways. Historically, subsets of potentially confusing syndromes can be found in the literature. The key difference lies in the presenting symptoms. This chapter focuses on the diagnosis and management of the thrombotic syndromes that present after pelvic infection.

It is possible for the ovarian vein to become greatly distended and/or thrombosed without a concurrent or preceding pelvic infection; however, this is rare. This condition, right ovarian vein syndrome, presents with ureteral obstruction above the point where it crosses the ovarian vein and presents clinically with urologic complaints.[1] Syndromes that do present in association with pelvic infections are acute ovarian vein thrombosis syndrome and enigmatic fever syndrome. While there is some overlap between these three syndromes, this chapter examines the latter two as they present clinically with pelvic infection. It is recognized that in some medical centers the term *septic pelvic thrombophlebitis* (SPT) is used only for the third syndrome; for the purposes of this discussion we use this term to describe the spectrum of disease including acute ovarian vein thrombosis syndrome and enigmatic fever syndrome (Fig. 15–1).

EPIDEMIOLOGY

Septic pelvic thrombophlebitis is an uncommon complication. It is typically found in the puerperium or following pelvic surgery when febrile morbidity does not respond to antibiotics. Also, it can be discovered incidentally when surgery is performed for appendicitis or another infection. These syndromes are presumed to be the result of infected thrombi of the ovarian, iliac, or uterine veins. The precise incidence of this condition is elusive because of the variety of ways in which it can present. The overall incidence of puerperal SPT has been estimated to be 1:500 to 2,000.[2] Witlin and Sibai[3] have reported 11 cases of ovarian vein thrombosis following vaginal delivery diagnosed by computed tomography (CT) scan or sur-

gery among 64,000 vaginal deliveries (1:5,000).[3] Two patients have been reported to have ovarian vein thrombophlebitis ante partum.[4] A presumptive diagnosis of SPT was made in some patients who defervesced after the addition of heparin to their treatment. This complication was equally found in patients treated with double-agent and single-agent antibiotics.[5] Not all cases of SPT occur following birth, however. In a series of 46 cases of SPT, 30% were preceded by vaginal delivery, 30% by cesarean section, 17% by abortion, 13% by vaginal hysterectomy, and 8% by a different operation.[6] In addition, the type of cesarean section seems to influence the frequency of SPT. Two percent of patients undergoing classic cesarean section may experience SPT.[7, 8] Approximately 80% of ovarian vein thromboses occur on the right, 14% occur bilaterally, and 6% are unilateral, on the left.[9] Septic pelvic thrombophlebitis is also typically considered as either a primary infectious process or an extension of one.[5, 9–11]

PATHOPHYSIOLOGY

The central step in the coagulation cascade is the formation of fibrin from fibrinogen and the cross-linking of these molecules to form clots or thrombi. Thrombin, the protein that produces the fibrinogen conversion, is produced through different pathways. Thrombin formation occurs through the activation of precursor proteins, which is appropriately triggered by injury to a vessel wall. This injury exposes the blood to foreign surfaces, allowing platelet adherence and the release of platelet granules. Stasis of blood flow, alteration of the vein wall, and an increase in the circulating coagulation factors, known as Virchow's triad, have been considered for years as predisposing factors in the development of venous thrombosis. All three of these factors may be present in women who are pregnant, are puerperal, have undergone surgery, or are suffering from severe pelvic infections. Microbes and tissue factors from infections or malignancies may contribute to the development of pelvic vein thrombosis.

The ovarian veins are responsible for most of the uterine venous drainage immediately following deliv-

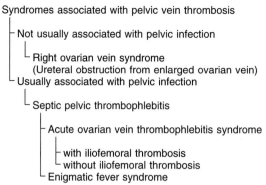

Syndromes associated with pelvic vein thrombosis

├ Not usually associated with pelvic infection

│ └ Right ovarian vein syndrome
│   (Ureteral obstruction from enlarged ovarian vein)
└ Usually associated with pelvic infection

   └ Septic pelvic thrombophlebitis

      ├ Acute ovarian vein thrombophlebitis syndrome
      │ ├ with iliofemoral thrombosis
      │ └ without iliofemoral thrombosis
      └ Enigmatic fever syndrome

FIGURE 15-1 ▶ The relationship of various syndromes associated with pelvic vein thrombosis.

ery. Near the end of a full-term gestation, the veins of the pelvis increase their diameter by threefold, but without a significant change in venous pressure. The veins have this capacity because there is little fibrous support in their surrounding sheaths. The increased capacity serves as a dynamic reservoir and a baffle between the central venous pressure and the pressures transmitted from the contracting uterus.[12] However, this capacity also means that the ovarian veins are more susceptible to extrinsic compression from the pregnant or puerperal uterus or from pelvic masses. Also, the ovarian veins enter the central circulation remote from their origin and hence follow a long and vulnerable course. The ovarian veins are particularly susceptible to compression as they emerge from the pelvis over its bony brim. Valves in the veins help to produce the cephalad flow of blood, but they are also the sites of pooling and stasis.

Munsick and Gillanders[9] performed uterine vein phlebography in four women 8 to 19 hours post partum by injecting contrast material into the uterus. Serial radiographs were taken, and in two women it showed retrograde flow of the left ovarian vein.[9] This study demonstrated that it is possible for bacteria and tissue thromboplastin to flow preferentially into the right ovarian vein. Since SPT is found more often on the right and is often preceded by infection, retrograde flow seems a logical explanation. The uterus is also more frequently rotated to the right, which may predispose the right ovarian vein to greater compression or alterations in its flow.

Some clues concerning vein wall alteration come from patients with nonpuerperal, right ovarian vein syndrome. As mentioned earlier, these patients often present to urologists with pyelonephritis or recurrent urinary tract infection due to compression of the ureter by the distended right ovarian vein. Dykhuizen and Roberts[1] found that ureteral obstruction could be provoked by pregnancy or administration of high-dose oral contraceptive pills owing to hormonally induced distention of the adjacent ovarian veins. Resected veins

from these patients showed muscle hypertrophy within the vein walls.[1]

Damage to the vessel intima triggers platelet adhesion and aggregation. Trauma to the vessels that could disrupt the intima is likely to take place during surgery or from the compression by the uterus and bony pelvis. Also, bacteria that enter the veins from the reproductive tract may injure the vascular endothelium.[2]

During pregnancy, there is a substantial increase in fibrinogen and vitamin K–dependent coagulation factors, coupled with a decrease in fibrinolytic activity.[13] The overall bleeding time during pregnancy, however, does not change.[14] In normal coagulation, proteins C and S are necessary to break down factors Va and VIIIa and therefore limit thrombosis. Protein S appears to be decreased in pregnancy.[13] The factor V Leiden mutation limits the ability of proteins C and S to break down factor V and is thought to be the most common genetic factor predisposing women to thrombosis. It has received great attention recently but its association with SPT, if any, has not yet been described.[15]

Knowledge about the contribution of different bacteria to these syndromes is limited. Most of the information about the microbiologic aspects of this condition comes from cases treated with ovarian vein excision. By the 1970s this treatment was replaced largely by medical management; therefore, few thrombi have been cultured recently. The organisms that have been isolated from the thrombi of SPT include *Escherichia coli,* anaerobic streptococci and staphylococci, microaerophilic streptococci, and coagulase-negative staphylococci. The presence of anaerobic organisms isolated from these thrombi contrasts with the absence of such organisms in intravenous catheter-related thrombophlebitis.[16] Both marked depression of ovarian vein oxygen saturation and the ovarian vein drainage of the potentially infected uterine cavity may support anaerobic bacterial growth.[9, 12]

While it is believed that febrile ovarian vein thrombosis typically represents a primary infection or an extension of an infectious process, a sterile thrombus that contained fetal squames and lanugo hair has also been reported.[17] Also, oncology patients undergoing chemotherapy have been identified to be at risk for SPT, possibly owing to thrombogenic factors released from dying tumor cells.[18]

DIAGNOSIS

Septic pelvic thrombophlebitis can present as a prominent, isolated ovarian vein thrombophlebitis or in a more obscure fashion, known as enigmatic fever.[2, 19, 20] Septic ovarian vein thrombophlebitis typically begins acutely as fever within 72 hours of surgery, but its occurrence has been described as late as 70 days postoperatively and has been described in many nonsurgical patients.[3, 9, 18] The average time to diagnosis of ovarian vein thrombosis following vaginal delivery was found to be 7.6 days post partum in one study.[3] Patients with iliofemoral involvement have the onset of their symptoms later than do women with only ovarian vein thrombosis.[21] Fever is not always present. The afflicted patient often has lower abdominal and pelvic pain that steadily worsens on the side of the thrombosis.

The diagnosis of ovarian vein thrombosis should be considered in women who have the diagnoses of endometritis *and* pyelonephritis following vaginal delivery. Iliofemoral thrombosis produces upper thigh pain, tenderness, and leg edema and usually becomes symptomatic later than does ovarian thromboses. Adynamic ileus and severe abdominal tenderness is common. A mass may be palpated along the course of the vein on the affected side, and the patient usually appears ill. Since most ovarian thromboses occur on the right, this diagnosis is often appropriately confused with appendicitis.[22] Other conditions that one should consider in the differential diagnosis are hematoma of the broad ligament, ovarian torsion, pyelonephritis, and abscess. Clinicians should be vigilant for signs and symptoms of septic emboli and evaluate pulmonary complaints expeditiously. The chest x-ray findings may be negative, since the emboli tend to be numerous but small.

Enigmatic fever is considered when patients have refractory febrile morbidity following delivery or pelvic surgery. Often, the patient is treated initially with broad-spectrum antibiotics for endometritis or cuff cellulitis, but the patient has persistent febrile morbidity. The temperature pattern commonly shows marked elevations, with tachycardia and malaise, followed by afebrile periods when the patient appears well. The examination of the patient is otherwise unremarkable, and the diagnosis is achieved when other sources of fever have been excluded and the patient shows defervescence with heparin treatment. The following conditions should also be carefully excluded in women with persistent febrile morbidity before the physician confidently makes the diagnosis of enigmatic fever: resistant bacterial infection, infected retained products of conception, viral infection, abscess, drug fever, and collagen vascular diseases.[19] Rapid defervescence after initiation of heparin therapy is often the only confirmatory finding.

While the diagnosis of SPT is based on the judgment of the clinician who has thoroughly evaluated the patient, until recently a confident diagnosis could be made only on the operating table or by observing the patient's response to heparin.[23] Numerous observational reports of diagnostic tests have described this condition over the last 20 years.[21, 24–40] Intravenous pyelography can give indirect proof of ovarian vein thrombosis when there is compression of the ureter on the affected side, but this is not often useful.[24] Imaging methods that can give direct evidence of an ovarian vein thrombus are CT scan, magnetic resonance imaging (MRI), and ultrasonography. Savader and coworkers[31] compared these three methods retrospectively in five patients who were referred for evaluation with the diagnosis of puerperal ovarian vein thrombosis. Bowel gas often obscured evaluation by ultrasound, whereas the diagnosis could be made in most patients with CT.[31] Diagnostic laparoscopy has been used in a puerperal patient with symptoms consistent with appendicitis. It revealed a 4×2 cm band of induration along the right lateral aspect of the uterus and upper broad ligament.[39] While it is helpful to be aware of the in situ appearance of SPT, laparoscopy is rarely necessary for making the diagnosis. CT scanning and the response to heparin are the preferred methods for diagnosis. An example of the CT findings of SPT is given in Figure 15–2.

As stated previously, the most common manner in which SPT presents is in the patient who does not respond to antibiotics for a pelvic infection. Gibbs and colleagues[41] sought to determine which patients are likely to fail to respond to antibiotic therapy for endometritis. A total of 35 of 160 patients with clinical postpartum endometritis failed treatment with penicillin and kanamycin. After more extensive anaerobic coverage was added, only 7 more failed, of whom 4 had either a hematoma or an abscess. The remaining 3 were presumed to have SPT.[41] Therefore, a more practical concern is the diagnostic evaluation of the patient with refractory postpartum or postoperative febrile morbidity.

Brown and colleagues[35] used CT to evaluate 74 women who had persistent puerperal infections despite the administration of appropriate antibiotics. Twenty-one per cent had SPT demonstrated by CT, of whom 75% were not suspected of having the condition by clinical evaluation. The disparity between the physical examination and the findings on CT scan is under-

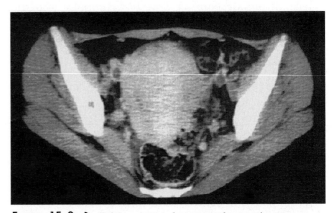

Figure 15–2 ▶ Pelvic computed tomography scan in postpartum woman demonstrating bilateral occlusion of the ovarian veins. The bilaterally occluded veins may be seen as circles with two different tissue densities on either side of the puerperal uterus, which is midline.

standable given the discomfort inherent in puerperal examinations. These findings support the use of CT scanning in women with refractory fever.[35] Although there remain some patients who have refractory fever and normal CT scans, heparin therapy may still be efficacious if other causes can be excluded. It is the condition of this subset of patients that we call enigmatic fever syndrome.

A serum test found to predict the clinical response to heparin in patients with refractory febrile morbidity is fibrinopeptide A. This peptide is the first peptide cleaved from fibrinogen during the process of fibrin formation. Fibrinopeptide A has been found to be elevated in patients with persistent fever who subsequently respond to heparin. However, it is not advised to delay heparin therapy when there is a reasonable clinical suspicion that SPT already exists, even if this laboratory test is highly accurate.[27] Therefore, the diagnostic evaluation of a patient with persistent febrile morbidity should include a thorough review of the patient's history, a detailed physical examination, and a CT scan of the abdomen and pelvis if no obvious source is found or if a pelvic mass is palpated. Any previously attained cultures should be reviewed. Treatment is guided by the results of these evaluations. One of the most useful tests is the patient's response to the addition of heparin.

TREATMENT

Although there are few scientifically designed studies of this condition, therapy for SPT has changed from predominantly surgical to medical over the last century.[11, 42] During the 1960s, treatment of SPT began to shift, owing to case series reporting efficacy with medical management, broad-spectrum antibiotics and heparin. This diagnosis had been considered an emergent indication for surgical ligation or excision of the affected veins to avoid pulmonary embolism.[43] Several doubts about medical management existed: (1) Can therapeutic efficacy be claimed for heparin if a definitive, i.e., surgical, diagnosis has not been made? (2) Does heparin obscure the clinical response in heparinized patients who are misdiagnosed with SPT? (3) Will anticoagulation resolve large thrombi? Despite these doubts, surgical excision was associated with a high mortality rate owing to embolization, and so certain case reports arose to answer these questions.

In 1965, O'Lane and Lebherz[44] reported on two patients in whom ovarian vein thrombosis was diagnosed surgically, followed by successful medical therapy without excision of the infected veins. Ledger and Peterson[45] described another surgically diagnosed patient who responded to heparin and antibiotics even though her ovarian vein thrombus extended into the vena cava above the renal vein. Later, Magee and colleagues[11] demonstrated the resolution of a thrombus

that filled the ovarian vein, femoral vein, and inferior vena cava to the diaphragm. CT scan and ultrasonography documented the SPT and its resolution. Ledger's report also described two patients in whom the true site of infection became apparent after treatment with heparin, showing that heparin is unlikely to mask an infection that lies elsewhere.[45] While these anecdotes leave many unanswered questions, they were indications of the increasing comfort with medical management of SPT. Larger series have given this therapy further credence.

In 1981, Brown and Munsick[9] summarized their experience with 36 patients with SPT. They found that pulmonary embolism was a rare event, and so they preferred medical therapy to venous ligation or excision. Josey and Staggers[6] presented a series of 46 patients of whom 42 responded to antibiotics and heparin. Defervescence occurred in 1 to 7 days. No complications of the heparin were identified in these patients. Four patients required laparotomy, of whom three had additional infectious processes (abscess in two and severe myometritis in the third). The fourth died from complications of anaerobic septicemia despite vena caval ligation and hysterectomy.[6]

These case series suggest that heparin and antibiotics are safe in most cases of SPT.[2] Surgical ligation or excision is now reserved for patients whose conditions are refractory to medical therapy with either persistent febrile morbidity or embolization. Like most pelvic infections, SPT should be considered a polymicrobial infection; therefore, broad-spectrum antibiotics should be used, including coverage of anaerobes. Since bacterial injury of the vascular endothelium is considered one of the important mechanisms of SPT, heparin alone is not believed to be sufficient. An example of a typical medical regimen would be ampicillin, gentamicin, and clindamycin plus heparin in a dose that achieves an activated partial thromboplastin time 1½ to 2 times normal.

The optimal duration of heparin therapy has not been established; however, anticoagulant therapy beyond 7 to 10 days is probably indicated only in selected patients. It is best to individualize the treatment based on the extent of documented thrombosis.[2] CT scan may be helpful in determining the endpoint of treatment when thrombi are large.[11] Broadspectrum, single-agent antibiotic therapy may also be effective, but it has not been widely described. Likewise, there are no studies of low-molecular-weight heparin therapy for the treatment of SPT; however, it may have a more predictable dose-response pattern and a longer half-life. These properties may afford it greater therapeutic acceptability.

Once antibiotics and heparin have been instituted, rapid improvement is typical.[21] The mean time until the patient is again afebrile ranges from 2.5 to 6 days.[6, 21] A recent study has drawn into question the need for heparin. Fourteen women with CT scan evidence of SPT were randomly assigned to receive antibiotics alone or with heparin. Their clinical courses were similar.[48] In the absence of a clinical response to medical therapy or for persistent embolization, a surgical approach may be indicated. No experience with thrombolytic therapy or vena cava filtering in SPT has been reported, and a concurrent infectious process is often found if surgery is performed at this point. When medical therapy fails, most often an abscess or myonecrosis of the uterus is found. The surgical procedure chosen depends on the anatomic location of the thrombus, the occurrence of repetitive emboli after heparinization, the presence of other pathologic conditions, and the experience of the surgeon.

Surgical procedures that have been described include unilateral or bilateral ovarian vein ligation or resection, and vena cava interruption.[46] For renal vein extension of the thrombus, thrombectomy may be necessary. Ligation of the infected vein with continued antibiotic and anticoagulant coverage is probably sufficient in most other cases. These procedures can be extremely difficult, owing to the degree of induration and inflammation surrounding the vessel.[2]

SEQUELAE

Perhaps the most serious complication of SPT is pulmonary embolism. Once heparin has been initiated, the probability of embolization is low. Most patients treated medically for SPT recover fully. Early reports of medical therapy failures are best explained by the relative lack of sophisticated antibiotics and diagnostic tests available today.

No long-term follow-up studies are available for patients following medical therapy. Nevertheless, the risk of SPT or pulmonary embolism in future pregnancies or with the use of hormonal contraception is probably small, since severe local infection is believed to play an essential role in the pathogenesis of SPT. On the other hand, surgical ligation of the infected veins may predispose the patient to edema and poor pregnancy outcomes. However, this finding may be the result of recall bias, since there was no follow-up available for 80% of the patients.[47]

CONCLUSION

Septic pelvic thrombophlebitis is an uncommon condition found most often following pregnancy or pelvic surgery. It can be subclassified as ovarian vein thrombophlebitis syndrome or enigmatic fever syndrome. Ovarian vein thrombophlebitis syndrome often presents with pain, a tender pelvic mass, fever, and an ileus, although it is often recognized only with a CT scan or surgery. Enigmatic fever syndrome is best illustrated in patients with fever refractory to antibiotics.

Both groups of patients typically respond rapidly to the addition of heparin. Patients with pelvic infections, who do not respond to broad-spectrum antibiotics, should be evaluated thoroughly to rule out the multiple other causes of persistent febrile morbidity. A CT scan should be used to evaluate patients with refractory fever to exclude abscesses and hematomas. In the absence of another explanation for the patient's persistent fever or if a frank thrombosis is found, heparin therapy should be started. Heparin plus continued broad-spectrum antibiotics results in the resolution of most cases of SPT, but surgical ligation may rarely be necessary. This medical regimen is typically continued for a total of 10 days, but it may be used for a longer period, depending on the size of the thrombus and the preferences of the physician. The need for long-term oral anticoagulants is rare, but such treatment should be individualized, based on the size of the thrombus and the occurrence of recurrent embolization. Since a local infectious process is necessary in the initiation of this type of thrombophlebitis, anticoagulation during future pregnancies or the avoidance of hormonal contraception is probably not justified.

REFERENCES

1. Dykhuizen RF, Roberts JA: The ovarian vein syndrome. Surg Gynecol Obstet 1970; 130:443.
2. Duff P, Gibbs RS: Pelvic vein thrombophlebitis: Diagnostic dilemma and therapeutic challenge. Obstet Gynecol Surv 1983; 38:365.
3. Witlin AG, Sibai BM: Postpartum ovarian vein thrombosis after vaginal delivery: A report of 11 cases. Obstet Gynecol 1995; 85:775.
4. Simons GR, Piwnica-Worms DR, Goldhaber SZ: Ovarian vein thrombosis. Am Heart J 1993; 126:641.
5. Stovall TG, Thorpe EM Jr, Ling FW: Treatment of post-cesarean section endometritis with ampicillin and sulbactam or clindamycin and gentamicin. J Reprod Med 1993; 38:843.
6. Josey WE, Staggers SR Jr: Heparin therapy in septic pelvic thrombophlebitis: A study of 46 cases. Am J Obstet Gynecol 1974; 120:228.
7. Blanco JD, Gibbs RS: Infections following classical cesarean section. Obstet Gynecol 1980; 55:167.
8. Rehu M, Nilsson CG: Risk factors for febrile morbidity associated with cesarean section. Obstet Gynecol 1980; 56:269.
9. Munsick RA, Gillanders LA: A review of the syndrome of puerperal ovarian vein thrombophlebitis. Obstet Gynecol Surv 1981; 36:57.
10. Duff P: Pathophysiology and management of postcesarean endomyometritis. Obstet Gynecol 1986; 67:269.
11. Magee KP, Blanco JD, Graham JM: Massive septic pelvic thrombophlebitis. Obstet Gynecol 1993; 82:662.
12. Hodgkinson CP: Physiology of the ovarian veins during pregnancy. Obstet Gynecol 1953; 1:26.
13. Barbour LA, Pickard J: Controversies in thromboembolic disease during pregnancy: A critical review. Obstet Gynecol 1995; 86:621.
14. Berge LN, Lyngmo V, Svensson B, et al: The bleeding time in women: An influence of the sex hormones? Acta Obstet Gynecol Scand 1993; 72:423.
15. Dizon-Townson DS, Nelson LM, Jang H, et al: The incidence of the factor V Leiden mutation in an obstetric population and its relationship to deep vein thrombosis. Am J Obstet Gynecol 1997; 176:883.
16. Collignon P, Sorrell T, Garret P: Are anaerobic bacteria involved in peripheral vein catheter-associated thrombophlebitis? Biomed Pharmacother 1988; 42:213.

17. Kern SB, Duff P: Localized amniotic fluid embolism presenting as ovarian vein thrombosis and refractory postoperative fever. Am J Clin Pathol 1981; 76:476.
18. Jacoby WT, Cohan RH, Baker ME, et al: Ovarian vein thrombosis in oncology patients: CT detection and clinical significance. Am J Roentgenol 1990; 155:291.
19. Dunn LJ, Van Voorhis LW: Enigmatic fever and pelvic thrombophlebitis: Response to anticoagulants. N Engl J Med 1967; 276:265.
20. Lamki H: Enigmatic puerperal pyrexia. J Irish Med Assoc 1973; 66:386.
21. Brown CE, Lowe TW, Cunningham FG, et al: Puerperal pelvic thrombophlebitis: Impact on diagnosis and treatment using x-ray computed tomography and magnetic resonance imaging. Obstet Gynecol 1986; 68:789.
22. Brown TK, Munsick RA: Puerperal ovarian vein thrombophlebitis: A syndrome. Am J Obstet Gynecol 1971; 109:263.
23. Lotze EC, Kaufman RH, Kaplan AL: Postpartum ovarian vein thrombophlebitis. Obstet Gynecol Surv 1966; 21:853.
24. Darney PD, Wilson EA: Intravenous pyelography in the diagnosis and management of postpartum ovarian vein thrombophlebitis: A case report. Am J Obstet Gynecol 1977; 127:439.
25. De Schepper A, Van Rompaey W: Computed tomographic diagnosis of dilated ovarian veins in a case of "ovarian vein syndrome." Eur J Radiol 1983; 3:324.
26. Ross M, Mintz M, Toumala R: The diagnosis of puerperal ovarian vein thrombophlebitis by computed tomography scan. Obstet Gynecol 1983; 62:131.
27. Weiner CP, Kwaan H, Duboe F: Diagnosis of septic pelvic thrombophlebitis by measurement of fibrinopeptide A. Am J Perinatol 1985; 2:93.
28. Mintz MC, Levy DW, Axel L, et al: Puerperal ovarian vein thrombosis: MR diagnosis. Am J Roentgenol 1987; 149:1273.
29. Baran GW, Frisch KM: Duplex Doppler evaluation of puerperal ovarian vein thrombosis. Am J Roentgenol 1987; 149:321.
30. Khurana BK, Rao J, Friedman SA, et al: Computed tomographic features of puerperal ovarian vein thrombosis. Am J Obstet Gynecol 1988; 159:905.
31. Savader SJ, Otero RR, Savader BL: Puerperal ovarian vein thrombosis: Evaluation with CT, US, and MR imaging. Radiology 1988; 167:637.
32. Rudoff JM, Astrauskas LJ, Rudoff JC, et al: Ultrasonographic diagnosis of septic pelvic thrombophlebitis. J Ultrasound Med 1988; 7:287.
33. Baka JJ, Lev-Toaff AS, Friedman AC, et al: Ovarian vein thrombosis with atypical presentation: Role of sonography and duplex Doppler. Obstet Gynecol 1989; 73:887.
34. Lev-Toaff AS, Baka JJ, Toaff ME, et al: Diagnostic imaging in puerperal febrile morbidty. Obstet Gynecol 1991; 78:50.
35. Brown CE, Dunn DH, Harrell R, et al: Computed tomography for evaluation of puerperal infections. Surg Gynecol Obstet 1991; 172:285.
36. Apter S, Shmamann S, Ben-Baruch G, et al: CT of pelvic infection after cesarean section. Clin Exp Obstet Gynecol 1992; 19:156.
37. Rooholamini SA, Au AH, Hansen GC, et al: Imaging of pregnancy-related complications. Radiographics 1993; 13:753.
38. Grant TH, Schoettle BW, Buchsbaum MS: Postpartum ovarian vein thrombosis: Diagnosis by clot protrusion into the inferior vena cava at sonography. Am J Roentgenol 1993; 160:551.
39. Silva PD, Glasser KE, Landercasper J: Laparoscopic diagnosis of puerperal ovarian vein thrombophlebitis: A case report. J Reprod Med 1993; 38:309.
40. Cranston PE, Hamrick-Turner J, Morano JU: Pseudothrombosis of the right ovarian vein: Pitfall of abdominal spiral CT. Clin Imaging 1995; 19:176.
41. Gibbs RS, Jones PM, Wilder CJ: Antibiotic therapy of endometritis following cesarean section: Treatment successes and failures. Obstet Gynecol 1978; 52:31.
42. Miller CJ: Ligation or excision of the pelvic veins in the treatment of puerperal pyaemia. Surg Gynecol Obstet 1917; 25:431.
43. Sanders JG, Malinak LR, Gready TG: Ovarian-vein thrombosis: A postpartum surgical emergency. Obstet Gynecol 1964; 24:903.
44. O'Lane JM, Lebherz TB: Puerperal ovarian thrombophlebitis. Obstet Gynecol 1965; 26:676.
45. Ledger WJ, Peterson EP: The use of heparin in the management of pelvic thrombophlebitis. Surg Gynecol Obstet 1970; 131:1115.
46. Collins CG: Suppurative pelvic thrombophlebitis: A study of 202 cases in which the disease was treated by ligation of the vena cava and ovarian vein. Am J Obstet Gynecol 1970; 108:681.
47. Collins JH, Bosco JAS, Cohen CJ: Pregnancy subsequent to ligation of the inferior vena cava and ovarian vessels. Am J Obstet Gynecol 1959; 77:760.
48. Brown CE, Stettler RW, Twickler D, Cunningham FG: Puerperal septic pelvic thrombophlebitis: incidence and response to heparin therapy. Am J Obstet Gynecol 1999; 181:143.

16

Septic Abortion

Mark D. Pearlman

DEFINITIONS

Abortion is usually defined as the termination of a pregnancy prior to the time of fetal viability. Beyond the time of fetal viability, and before birth, loss of pregnancy is termed *stillbirth* or *fetal death.* The time at which a fetus becomes viable is usually a legal definition and varies from state to state.[1]

Abortion can be either spontaneous or induced. Spontaneous abortions can result from an infectious process (e.g., due to *Neisseria gonorrhoeae, Campylobacter fetus*), or infection can complicate a spontaneous abortion that resulted from another cause. Induced abortion, whether surgical or medical, can also be complicated by infection. Certain risk factors increase the likelihood of postabortal infection, and are listed in Table 16–1.

PATHOPHYSIOLOGY

Because of the high frequency of induced and spontaneous abortion (>2 million each year in the United States), infectious morbidity is a common occurrence despite the fact that febrile morbidity complicates fewer than 1% of all induced abortions.[2, 3] The definition of pelvic infection following abortion constitutes a spectrum of disease. Some studies have attempted to characterize the frequency of these infections with the use of standard or modified definitions of febrile morbidity. However, pelvic infections that complicate abortion encompass a wide variety of anatomic involvement and associated systemic derangement, ranging from infection confined to the endometrium, to pelvic abscesses and septic shock. These infections can have both acute and chronic sequelae (Table 16–2). Fever following medical termination of pregnancy without evidence of infection can also occur, and has been recently reported with the use of mifepristone and misoprostol.[4] In this study of 2,121 women, the incidence of fever was 4%, and 19 women were diagnosed with endometritis (0.8%), one case of which was considered "severe."

Infection following abortion is a general progression of disease, beginning locally (in the endometrium) and, in some cases, either ascending to the fallopian tubes or spreading laterally via the lymphatics. This spread can result in soft tissue infection with or without suppuration. Certain bacteria can cause microabscess formation within the uterus, resulting in a necrotizing myonecrosis (e.g., *Clostridium perfringens*).[5] This progression of disease is summarized in a classification scheme first proposed in 1992 (Table 16–3), and is described in greater detail in the text that follows.[6]

Endometritis

If an infection develops and is confined to the endometrium and myometrium, the clinical presentation tends to be local. Abnormal uterine bleeding, fever, uterine tenderness, or foul-smelling discharge, or any combination of these, can occur. Because standard criteria has not been established for diagnosing endometriosis in this setting, the incidence of this complication is uncertain. However, in a study of 170,000 surgically induced abortions, "mild (uterine) infection" was identified in fewer than 1 in 200 of all cases.[3]

Parametritis

When the endometrial infection has extended beyond the uterus, the parametrial structures are usually involved (i.e., fallopian tubes, round ligament, uterosacral ligament, and the pelvic peritoneum that covers these structures). More serious sequelae, such as pelvic abscess, ligneous cellulitis, septic pelvic thrombophlebitis, and septic shock, occur more frequently follow-

TABLE 16–1 ▶ RISK FACTORS FOR POSTABORTAL INFECTION
Use of nonsterile equipment
Preexisting cervical infection (e.g., chlamydiosis, gonorrhea)
Illicit abortions
Procedure performed (e.g., risk higher with hysterotomy or hypertonic saline injection)
Failure to use antibiotic prophylaxis in high-risk patients
History of gonorrhea infection or pelvic inflammatory disease
More than two sexual partners
Nulliparity
Cervical infection with *Chlamydia trachomatis* or *Neisseria gonorrhoeae*

TABLE 16-2 ▶ IMPORTANT COMPLICATION SEQUELAE RESULTING FROM SEPTIC ABORTION

Acute Complications	Chronic Sequelae
Adult respiratory distress syndrome	Infertility
Septic shock	Ectopic pregnancy
Renal failure	Pelvic adhesions
Abscess formation	Pelvic pain
Septic emboli	

Adapted from Faro S, Pearlman MD: Infections and Abortion. New York, Elsevier, 1992, p 42, with permission.

---

ing parametritis than with endometritis alone. Accurate diagnosis and prompt treatment of parametritis is critically important in averting these more serious sequelae.

Uterine injury is one mechanism that can lead to the development of parametritis. There are a number of reasons for this:

▶ Injury to the uterus allows direct access of bacteria to the peritoneum
▶ Injury may cause local vascular injury, impairing perfusion and interfering with the host's immune response and with antibiotic delivery
▶ Possible injury to the bowel may result in fecal contamination
▶ Retained products of conception

Retained products serve as an excellent nidus of infection because they are poorly vascularized, provide a good culture media, and may obstruct the outflow tract, facilitating an ascending infection via the fallopian tubes, or the uterine lymphatics.

Suppuration of the infection results in an abscess that can be confined to the fallopian tubes (pyosal-pinx) or tube and ovary (tubo-ovarian abscess) or may extend beyond those pelvic structures (cul-de-sac abscess, small bowel interloop abscess). Contiguous structures, including the small and large bowel, and ometum may be involved in the inflammatory process because of their location. Large bowel involvement can be important from a microbiologic standpoint, because organisms such as *Bacteroides fragilis* can migrate across an inflamed colon and can contribute to the microbiologic composition of the abscess. In advanced infection, concomitant bacteremia occurs more frequently than the usual 5% seen in all women with septic abortion.[6] Fortunately, these serious infections are uncommon in the United States today, but they are occasionally seen following illicit abortions, abortion complicated by unrecognized bowel injury, incomplete abortion, or uterine perforation. Systemic illness, including adult respiratory distress syndrome (ARDS), hypotension, septic shock, and renal failure, and death may occur, and these sequelae are more common if there is a delay in presentation, a misdiagnosis, or inappropriate treatment.[7]

DIAGNOSIS

The ability to successfully treat the patient with septic abortion depends on the physician recognizing not only the presence of infection but also the severity and extent of disease. Because many of the symptoms of septic abortion are nonspecific (e.g., fever, lower abdominal pain, general malaise, myalgia, and nausea and vomiting), appropriate and judicious use of adjunctive testing is instrumental in establishing the extent of disease. The severity of infection depends on numerous factors, including duration from the time

---

TABLE 16-3 ▶ CLASSIFICATION OF SEPTIC ABORTION

Class	Anatomic Location	Signs and Symptoms	Incidence of Bacteremia	Treatment*
I	Endomyometrium	Abnormal uterine bleeding Uterine tenderness Abdominal pain (not always present) Fever (uncommon)	<5%	Antibiotics D&C if retained products
II	Endomyometrium Parametrium	Adnexal and uterine tenderness Cervical motion tenderness Fever	5–10%	Parenteral antibiotics D&C
III	Endometritis Parametrium Abscess formation (pyosalpinx, TOA, pelvic abscess)	High fever Tachycardia Leukocytosis Marked abdominal tenderness Abscess on physical exam and/or imaging	25%+	Resuscitation and stabilization Parenteral antibiotics Surgical drainage and/or removal of pelvic organs
IV	Rupture of pelvic abscess	Hypotension Tachycardia Tachypnea Signs of peritoneal inflammation High fever	25%+	Resuscitation and stabilization Parenteral antibiotics Surgical exploration and removal of infected tissue

*See treatment section for agents and doses.
D&C = dilatation and curettage; TOA = tubo-ovarian abscess.
Modified from Pearlman MD: In: Faro S, Pearlman MD. Infections and Abortion. New York, Elsevier, 1992, pp 46–49.

of the procedure; delay in seeking medical attention; presence of uterine perforation; and pre-existing infections.

A critical component of effective management of septic abortion involves prompt diagnosis. The diagnosis of septic abortion must be considered when there is vaginal bleeding, lower abdominal pain, and fever in a woman of reproductive age. Delayed treatment is one of the most common features of septic abortion resulting in death. Often, the patient is reluctant to share with caregivers the circumstances or even the presence of an induced abortion. The widespread availability of sensitive pregnancy tests is helpful, as these tests typically remain positive for 4 to 6 weeks following complete evacuation of the uterus.[8]

Contact with the health provider who performed the procedure can be helpful in determining the results of the bacteriologic evaluation, pathologic examination, ultrasound examination (if performed), and possible complication of the procedure. The type of procedure performed is also important because the use of rigid instruments increases the likelihood of uterine perforation. Hypertonic saline installation is associated with disseminated intravascular coagulation, and the use of pharmacologic agents such as misoprostol can result in retained products of conception.[8] Illicit abortion with installation of foreign materials (e.g., phenols or soaps) into the uterus to induce abortion can also cause uterine necrosis, central nervous system toxicity, renal failure, respiratory arrest, and cardiac depression.[9, 10]

Differentiating between mild and severe disease is critically important in appropriately prioritizing therapeutic interventions. Milder clinical presentations, such as fever, uterine tenderness, lower abdominal pain, and uterine-vaginal bleeding, are consistent with endometritis but may also represent incomplete or failed abortion (continuing pregnancy), or hematometra. Re-evacuation of the uterus is a critical component of successful therapy, and accurate diagnosis is an important first step in management. In a series of 170,000 cases by Hakim-Elahi and colleagues[3] re-evacuation was performed in 0.35% of cases. This was responsible in part for the very low rate of septic abortion in this series (0.02%).

The microbial etiology of sepsis associated with abortion is derived from two sources: primarily, it is derived from the endogenous vaginal bacterial flora, but may result from exogenous bacteria, mainly sexually transmitted organisms (*Chlamydia trachomatis, N. gonorrhoeae*). The setting in which the original procedure was performed can sometimes help predict the organisms encountered in the infectious sequelae. For example, genetic amniocentesis or chorionic villus sampling associated with subsequent septic abortion is rare, but is usually associated with endogenous flora (Table 16–4). Septic abortion is usually a polymicrobial infection.

TABLE 16–4 ▶	**BACTERIAL FLORA OF THE LOWER FEMALE GENITAL TRACT**
Aerobes and Facultative Anaerobes	**Obligate Anaerobes**
Gram-positive	Gram-positive
Bacillus spp.	*Peptostreptococcus* spp.
Diphtheroids	*Peptostreptococcus micros*
Corynebacterium spp.	*Peptostreptococcus tetradius*
Lactobacillus spp.	(*Gaffkya anaerobia*)
Enterococcus faecalis	*Clostridium* spp.
Staphylococcus aureus	Gram-negative
Staphylococcus epidermidis	*Bacteroides* spp.
Streptococcus spp.	*Prevotella bivia*
Streptococcus agalactiae	*Bacteroides disiens*
Gram-negative	*Bacteroides fragilis*
Acinetobacter calcoaceticus	*Prevotella melaninogenica*
Acinetobacter lwoffi	*Fusobacterium necrophorum*
Citrobacter freundii	*F. nucleatum*
Enterobacter aerogenes	*Veillonella* spp.
Enterobacter agglomerans	
Enterobacter cloacae	
Escherichia coli	
Klebsiella pneumoniae	
Proteus mirabilis	
P. vulgaris	
Pseudomonas aeruginosa	

Yeasts and viruses have rarely been associated with these infections.[6] An important species that is uncommonly isolated from septic abortions is *C. perfringens*, which has been associated with uterine myonecrosis.[5] *Haemophilus influenzae, C. fetus, Salmonella enteritis, Mycoplasma hominis*, and a variety of viruses have also been isolated from patients with septic abortion.[6]

Organisms associated with sexual transmission colonize the endocervical epithelium, and can readily access the upper genital tract through instrumentation at the time of abortion. In addition to *N. gonorrhoeae* and *C. trachomatis, Trichomonas vaginalis* and herpes simplex virus have been associated with septic abortion, in part because they can cause tissue destruction or alteration in the vaginal bacterial environment.[6] These organisms may provide a thoroughfare for endogenous lower genital tract organisms to access the upper genital tract. Because the endogenous flora of the lower genital tract contains many virulent factors, including endotoxins and exotoxins, significant tissue destruction or systemic derangement can occur. The most common organisms found to be responsible for bacteremia in patients with septic abortion are streptococcus and *Escherichia coli*.[11] In this study, Smith and colleagues found that 27% of patients with septic abortion were bacteremic, with 63% of these harboring anaerobic bacteria and 23% with gram-negative facultative bacteria, principally *E. coli*. Ascending infections are much more common prior to 10 weeks of gestation, after which time there is a mechanical obliteration of the uterine cavity by the amniotic membranes. In addition, the thick and tenacious cervical mucus provides an additional barrier to ascending infection.

The aseptic technique used in appropriately performed abortions results in an extremely low infectious complication rate, particularly if the myometrium is not damaged.[3] This low risk of subsequent infection is also true when mechanical evacuation of the uterus is used in the setting of spontaneous abortion infection. Appropriate management of an infected spontaneous abortion is the institution of parenteral antibiotics and evacuation of the uterus with the use of aseptic technique. The infection generally does not progress beyond the uterus if the infection is recognized and early aggressive antibiotic therapy is instituted.

DIAGNOSIS

The severity of the illness is first determined by a rapid initial assessment of the patient, including vital signs. Physical examination should elicit evidence of abdominal tenderness and the presence of peritoneal signs (e.g., guarding and rebound). Tenderness limited to the lower abdomen is suggestive of localized disease, whereas tenderness that extends to the upper abdomen suggests generalized peritonitis. Peritonitis is serious because the systemic response to the potentially higher bacterial burden is more likely to manifest as septic shock. Careful inspection for evidence of injury to the lower genital tract, including the cervix and the vagina, should be performed. Bimanual examination should be performed to detect the presence of uterine tenderness, uterine enlargement, and adnexal or cul-de-sac masses suggesting abscess or hematoma.

Radiologic studies can be useful in determining the presence of radiopaque foreign bodies or free air in the abdomen, suggesting uterine perforation. Ultrasound examination can be helpful in ascertaining the presence of a pelvic mass, and should be obtained particularly if pelvic tenderness on examination prohibits the performance of an adequate examination.

A specimen for culture isolation and identification of the bacterium responsible for the infection is very helpful in managing complicated infections following abortion. A disposable endometrial sampling instrument (e.g., Pipelle) has been demonstrated to be safe and practical for obtaining specimens from patients with endometritis.[12] The biopsy specimen should be placed in aerobic and anaerobic transport media and taken to the laboratory for processing. The specimen should be plated out on appropriate media for aerobes and facultative and obligate anaerobes. *Chlamydia trachomatis* and *N. gonorrhoeae* should be cultured by swabbing the endocervix. A complete blood count with white blood cell differential should be obtained. Liver and kidney function should be monitored, especially if there is evidence of systemic deterioration. Urine output should be monitored hourly to help evaluate the patient's hemodynamic status. Because many of the antibiotics are excreted by the kidneys, and are

TABLE 16-5 ▶	FREQUENTLY ORDERED LABORATORY TESTS FOR SEPTIC ABORTION

Complete blood count, including leukocyte differential and platelet count
Electrolytes
Arterial blood gases
Blood urea nitrogen and creatinine
Urinalysis
Prothrombin time, partial thromboplastin time, fibrinogen
Serum lactate
Cultures with antibiotic sensitivities
   Blood
   Urine
   Endometrium
Chest x-ray film
Adjunctive imaging studies as necessary; e.g., computed tomography, magnetic resonance imaging, abdominal radiograph

Modified from Pearlman MD, Faro S: Obstetric septic shock: A pathophysiologic basis for management. Clin Obstet Gynecol 1990; 33:488.

potentially nephrotoxic (e.g., aminoglycosides, vancomycin, and beta-lactams), early evaluation of renal function is important. This can be performed by checking blood urea nitrogen (BUN) and creatinine. If there is impaired kidney function, the dosages of these antibiotics will need to be adjusted. Commonly used laboratory tests in patients with septic abortion are included in Table 16–5.

Although uncommon, septic shock can occur in women with septic abortion. The hallmark of septic shock is peripheral circulatory failure, inadequate tissue perfusion, and ultimately cell dysfunction or death. The cell wall components of both gram-negative and gram-positive bacteria can activate at least three separate pathways in the host if bacteremia is present: (1) the complement pathway, (2) the coagulation cascade, and (3) cytokine production by macrophages. Cytokines are particularly important in the development of septic shock. Of the various cytokines, tumor necrosis factor (TNF) plays an important role. In animal studies, direct injection of TNF results in the changes typical of septic shock, including ARDS, acute tubular necrosis, bowel changes typical of endotoxic shock, and adrenal hemorrhage.[13, 14] The development of septic shock tends to be a physiologic continuum: simple sepsis (fever, tachycardia, tachypnea, leukocytosis), severe sepsis (sepsis associated with organ dysfunction, hypoperfusion, or hypotension), and septic shock, which is defined as sepsis with hypotension despite adequate fluid resuscitation, resulting in a variety of physiologic dysfunctions.[15] The common clinical manifestations of septic shock are shown in Table 16–6.

After diagnosis, imaging is also potentially extremely useful in evaluating and managing the patient with septic abortion. Ultrasound is useful in determining both the presence of uterine enlargement and whether there is any fluid or tissue within the uterine cavity. It can assist in evaluating whether there has been disrup-

TABLE 16–6 ▶ CLINICAL MANIFESTATIONS OF SEPTIC SHOCK

Organ System	Clinical Findings	Mechanism
Cardiovascular Hypotension	Systolic BP <60 mm Hg	Vasodilatation Decreased circulating volume due to increased vascular permeability
Cardiac dysfunction	Increase in cardiac index (early) Decrease in cardiac index (late) Decrease in ejection fraction	Myocardial depressant factor Decreased myocardial blood flow
Pulmonary (ARDS)	Bilateral diffuse infiltrates on CXR Hypoxemia Normal PCWP (<18 mm Hg)	Increased vascular permeability Direct endothelial damage

Renal
  Oliguria
  ATN
 	
  Intestinal nephritis
	<30 mL/h	Hypotension and renal vasoconstriction
		Prolonged cortical hypoxia secondary to decreased renal blood flow
		Immune mechanism

Hematologic
  DIC
 	
  Leukocytosis
	Elevated FDP, FT, PTT
	Decreased platelets and fibrinogen
	Spontaneous bleeding (uncommon)
	>20,000 cells/mm³
		Endotoxin activation of Hageman's factor
		
		Demargination
		Neutrophil-releasing substance

Neurologic (mental status changes)	Somnolence, coma, combativeness (uncommon, usually due to hypoxia)	Decreased cerebral blood flow Hypoxia
Fever	Temperature >38°C	Direct endotoxin/TNF effect on hypothalamus

Septic shock BP indicates blood pressure; ARDS = adult respiratory distress syndrome; CXR = chest x-ray films; PCWP = pulmonary capillary wedge pressure; ATN = acute tubular necrosis; DIC = disseminated intravascular coagulation; FDP = fibrin degradation products; PT = prothrombin time; PTT = partial thromboplastin time; TNF = tumor necrosis factor.

From Am Coll of Obstet Gynecol to use table 2 from ACOG Tech Bulletin, #204, Apr 1995.

tion of the myometrium or the presence of gas within the myometrium. A computed tomography (CT) scan is particularly useful because it can assess the entire abdomen and pelvis, searching for the presence of abscesses in the abdominal cavity (subdiaphragmatic, subhepatic, subsplenic, and interloop bowel abscess). The CT scan may also be used to allow percutaneous drainage under direct visualization. Fluid removed should be gram-stained and cultured for isolation of both aerobic and anaerobic bacteria. Both CT scans and plain radiography of the abdomen can detect the presence of gas in the uterus, or other pelvic tissues, an indication of anaerobic infection (e.g., *Clostridium* spp.). Clostridial myometritis can result in gas production, which will be apparent by an "onionskin" appearance of the myometrium. This is caused by *Clostridium* or other bacteria invading and growing within the myometrium, producing gas that dissects between the fibers of the myometrium. A thickened bowel wall can be an indication that inflammatory material has caused edema of the bowel.

MANAGEMENT

In the presence of sepsis, the initial steps taken to resuscitate and stabilize the patient are the most im-

portant in reducing both morbidity and mortality. The prioritization of management is as follows:

1. Maintain adequate oxygenation and circulating volume.
2. Transfer the patient to an appropriate care unit (e.g., intensive care unit).
3. Obtain appropriate laboratory data (see Table 16–5).
4. If the patient is hemodynamically unstable, despite crystalloid resuscitation, institute inotropic or vasopressin therapy.
5. Administer appropriate antimicrobial agents.
6. Surgically remove infected tissue or drain abscesses, or both, if indicated.[6]
7. Lee and colleagues[16] demonstrated that simply ignoring or delaying the removal of infected tissue in the obstetric patient with sepsis can substantially increase morbidity or even result in death.

Adequate oxygenation can be determined by pulse oximetry. Pulse oximetry saturation correlates predictably with arterial oxygen saturation, although it is less accurate in circumstances of low hemoglobin or impaired local perfusion. Oxygen therapy should be initiated to maintain oxygen saturation above 92% to 94% in the otherwise healthy patient. In the septic patient,

TABLE 16-7 ▶	ANTIBIOTICS SUITABLE FOR TREATMENT OF UNCOMPLICATED POSTABORTAL ENDOMETRITIS	

| Parenteral Therapy | | |
Penicillins	Cephalosporins	Oral Therapy
Timentin (ticarcillin/clavulanic acid), 3.1 g q4–6h	Cefotan (cefotetan), 2 g q12h	Augmentin (amoxicillin/clavulanic acid), 500 mg q8hr *or* 875 mg q12h
Unasyn (ampicillin/sulbactam), 3 g q6h	Mefoxin (cefoxitin), 2 g q6–8h	Floxin (ofloxacin), 400 mg q12h *plus*
Zosyn (piperacillin/tazobactam), 3.375 g q6h	Cefizox (ceftizoxime), 2 g q8–12h	Flagyl (metronidazole), 500 mg q8h *or* Clindamycin, 300 mg q6h

fluid resuscitation should begin with installation of 1 to 2 L of crystalloid (normal saline or lactated Ringer's solution) over 15 to 20 minutes. This can be performed without invasive monitoring initially; however, because of the frequent need for large volumes of crystalloid resuscitation, continued high-volume crystalloid resuscitation typically requires invasive hemodynamic monitoring (e.g., pulmonary artery catheter) to reduce the risk of, or to manage, pulmonary edema, ARDS, and myocardial dysfunction. Both patients with mild septic abortion and those with severe cases require antimicrobial therapy, but the degree of severity of the infection dictates the type of coverage. Antibiotics that are suitable for the treatment of uncomplicated postabortal endometritis are listed in Table 16–7.

For more serious infections, multiple-antibiotic combinations are sometimes necessary. For example, ampicillin, 2 g every 6 hours, and gentamicin, 4.5 mg/kg daily, plus metronidazole, 500 mg every 8 hours, has good efficacy over a wide antimicrobial spectrum for virtually all potential bacteria involved in septic abortion.

Determining whether infected tissue remains within the uterus or whether there has been injury to the uterus is critically important in continuing the management of patients. The use of imaging, as described earlier in this chapter, is important in attempting to evaluate these conditions. The reason for retained products is often uterine perforation; thus, attempts at removing the remainder of the tissue are best accomplished in combination with direct visualization by laparoscopy at the time of dilatation and curettage (D&C), if perforation is suspected. In addition, if several hours have transpired between the occurrence of uterine perforation and the time of diagnosis, significant myometrial infection can develop, which may require hysterectomy. The need for hysterectomy is often a difficult clinical decision, and is particularly challenging in young patients of low parity. At operation, if the area surrounding the perforation is bleeding and appears pink, and is not necrotic, simple closure or achieving hemostasis with cautery is all that is necessary. If the area is not bleeding and the tissue appears

viable, no further intervention other than evacuation of the uterine contents under direct laparoscopic visualization is necessary. However, if the tissue surrounding the traumatic area is black and easily falls apart, and the tissue immediately adjacent to the traumatized tissue is pale, this suggests the presence of a necrotizing infection. Attempting to salvage the uterus in these circumstances can potentially be disastrous, given the absence of adequate blood supply to the tissue edges. This lack of adequate blood flow interrupts antibiotic delivery to the infected tissue, and in general the uterus should be removed in this clinical setting. Fortunately, these circumstances are uncommon.

If abdominal contents are noted to be trapped in the uterine perforation, they should not be reduced through the perforation at the time of pelvic examination. The patient requires exploratory laparotomy and direct visualization of the bowel to determine whether bowel resection is necessary. In this circumstance, the involvement of a surgeon familiar with bowel resection is imperative.

In the seriously infected patient, activation of the coagulation cascade can result in consumption of clotting factors, leading to disseminated intravascular coagulation (DIC). The potential need for blood and coagulation factors should be anticipated in this setting. Typing and cross-matching should be performed for 4 units of packed red blood cells plus replacement of clotting factors and fibrinogen through the use of cryoprecipitate, or platelet transfusion may be necessary, depending on the results of laboratory values (fibrinogen, prothrombin time [PT], partial thromboplastin time [PTT], platelet count) and the patient's clinical status.

Patients seen early in the course of infection can be treated with single-agent antimicrobial therapy (see Table 16–7), and the uterus can be evacuated if necessary. Patients who have mild to moderate endometritis who have no evidence of disseminated infection and no products of conception within the uterus can be treated with oral antibiotics alone. Patients treated in an ambulatory setting should be advised to take their temperature at home at least three times daily and to report the onset of chills, nausea, vomiting, or increasing lower abdominal pain. Patient must be re-evaluated within 72 hours of the initiation of medication to ensure a prompt response to therapy. If there is no significant improvement, the patient requires hospitalization for parenteral antibiotic therapy and re-evaluation for potential retained products or uterine perforation. In the setting of failed ambulatory treatment and the presence of severe infection, combination antibiotic therapy should be administered. Appropriate bacteriologic cultures should be obtained from the endometrium by endometrial sampling. Laboratory tests including complete blood count, electrolytes, liver function studies, and renal function evaluation should be obtained so that changes in antibiotic dosage can be instituted if necessary.

The septic patient should be prepared for hysterectomy and possible removal of both ovaries and fallopian tubes. Even if the initial procedure is planned to be D&C, the finding of uterine perforation at that time will require laparoscopic visualization. Extensive injury to the bowel or uterus may require exploratory laparotomy and removal or resection of involved tissue. Potential complications should be discussed, such as damage to the bladder, ureters, and small and large bowel. If there has been a delay prior to presentation, dense adherence of the bowel to the uterus can be anticipated, and injury to the bowel is distinctly possible. The use of nasogastric suctions and pelvic drains are necessary if extensive bowel adhesions are detected at the time of surgery.

SUMMARY

The management of septic abortion depends on accurate assessment of the degree and severity of infection, with particular emphasis on the possibility of retained products of conception and uterine perforation. The need for surgical intervention in addition to antibiotic therapy is high. Because the potential for serious sequelae is significant, antibiotic therapy should not be delayed and strong consideration should be given to parenterally administered antimicrobial agents. The need for laparoscopy to evaluate the possibility of uterine perforation and to complete the abortion procedure is uncommon, and the patient must be prepared for the real but uncommon possibility of hysterectomy and oophorectomy.

REFERENCES

1. Standard terminology for reporting of reproduction health statistics in the US. In: Guidelines for Perinatal care, 4th ed. Washington, DC, American Academy of Pediatrics and American College of Obstetricians and Gynecologists 1997, pp 328–329.
2. Grimes DA, Schultz KF, Cates W Jr, et al: Midtrimester abortion by dilatation and evacuation: A safe and practical alternative. N Engl J Med 1971; 296:1141.
3. Hakim-Elaki E, Tovel HMM, Burnhill MS: Complications of the first trimester abortion: A report of 170,000 cases. Obstet Gynecol 1990; 76:129.
4. Spitz IM, Bardin CW, Benton L, Robbins A: Early pregnancy termination with mifepristone and misoprostol in the United States. N Engl J Med 1998; 338:1241.
5. Kowen DE, Hanslo DH, Botha PL, Davey DA: Incidence of aerobic and anaerobic infection in patients with incomplete abortion. S Afr Med J 1979; 55:129.
6. Faro S, Pearlman M: Infections in Abortion. New York, Elsevier, 1992, pp 41–50.
7. Cates W Jr, Rochat RW, Grimes DA, et al: Legalized abortion: Effect on national trends of maternal and abortion-related mortality, 1940–1976. Am J Obstet Gynecol 1978; 132:211.
8. Stubblefield PG, Grimes DA: Current concepts: Septic abortion. N Engl J Med 1994; 331:310.
9. Jain JK, Mishell DR Jr: A comparison of intravaginal misoprostol with prostaglandin E₂ for termination of second-trimester pregnancy. N Engl J Med 1994; 331:290.
10. Burnhill MS: Treatment of women who have undergone chemically induced abortion. J Reprod Med 1985; 30:610.
11. Smith JW, Southern PM, Lehman JD: Bacteremia and septic abortion: Complications and treatment. Obstet Gynecol 1970; 35:704.
12. Martens MG, Faro S, Hammed HA, et al: Transcervical uterine cultures with a new endometrial section curette: A comparison of three sampling methods in postpartum endometritis. Obstet Gynecol 1989; 74:273.
13. Remick DG, Kunkel RG, Larrick JW, Kunkel SL: Acute in vivo effects of human recombinant tumor necrosis factor. Lab Invest 1987; 56:583.
14. Tracey KJ, Beutler B, Lowrey SF, et al: Shock and tissue injury induced by recombinant human cachectin. Science 1986; 234:470.
15. Bone RC, Balk RA, Cerra FR, et al: ACCP/SCCM consensus conference: Definitions for sepsis and organ failure and guidelines for the use of innovative therapies in sepsis. Chest 1992; 101:1646.
16. Lee W, Clark SL, Cotton DB, et al: Septic shock during pregnancy. Am J Obstet Gynecol 1988; 159:410.

17 Episiotomy Infections

LARRY C. GILSTRAP, III

Until recently, episiotomy was one of the most common obstetric operations performed. However, it is now generally accepted that the routine performance of this procedure for vaginal deliveries can no longer be justified.[1-4] Moreover, episiotomies may be associated with significant morbidity and complications such as third- and fourth-degree extensions, dehiscence, rectal incontinence, fistula formation, infection, and death. This chapter deals primarily with the diagnosis and management of episiotomy infection and dehiscence.

INFECTION

Incidence

Fortunately, episiotomy infections are relatively uncommon, especially considering that episiotomy is not routinely performed in every woman in modern obstetrics. In one review by Owen and Hauth,[5] episiotomy infections occurred in only 0.05% of more than 20,000 women. One of the greatest risk factors for episiotomy infection is the presence of third- and fourth-degree episiotomy lacerations or extensions. Although the exact incidence of episiotomy infections is unknown, the incidence of infection associated with these lacerations has been reported to be from 0.1% to as high as 3.6%.[6, 7] These types of infections are not always reported in hospital infection control statistics.

Complications

The most serious sequelae of episiotomy infection include dehiscence, fistula formation, sepsis, necrotizing fasciitis, and even death. In addition, these infections

increase patient morbidity (i.e., pain and discomfort), hospital stay, costs, and the risk of "litigation" (Table 17–1).

In one review of 390 women with fourth-degree lacerations, Goldaber and associates[7] reported that 11 (2.8%) women experienced infection and dehiscence. Another three (0.8%) women experienced infection without dehiscence, and seven (1.8%) women had episiotomy dehiscence without apparent infection (Fig. 17–1). In another report by Ramin and colleagues,[8] 27 (79%) of 34 women experienced dehiscence secondary to infection—86% of women with midline and 69% of women with mediolateral episiotomy dehiscence. Hankins and colleagues,[9] in a review of 22 women with episiotomy dehiscence, reported that dehiscense was associated with infection in only eight (38%) women (Table 17–2). Fortunately, the occurrence of the other serious complications of episiotomy infection, such as sepsis, necrotizing fasciitis, and death, are extremely rare.

Signs and Symptoms

The signs and symptoms of "uncomplicated" infection of the episiotomy site include fever, pain, swelling,

TABLE 17-1 ▶	SEQUELAE OF EPISIOTOMY INFECTION
	Dehiscence
	Sepsis
	Necrotizing fasciitis
	Death
	Increased hospital days
	Increased cost
	Increased litigation

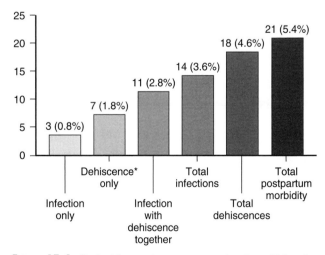

FIGURE 17–1 ▶ Incidence of postpartum perineal morbidity: dehiscence, infection, and rectovaginal fistula after fourth-degree perineal repair in 390 women. * Includes two rectovaginal fistulas. (From Goldaber KG, Wendel PJ, McIntire D, Wendel GD Jr: Postpartum perineal morbidity after fourth-degree perineal repair. Am J Obstet Gynecol 1993; 168:489, with permission of the publisher.)

TABLE 17-2 ▶ ASSOCIATION OF EPISIOTOMY INFECTION AND DEHISCENCE		
	No. with Dehiscence	Percent (%) Infected
Hankins et al.[9] (1990)	22	38
Ramin et al.[8] (1992)	34	79
Goldaber et al.[7] (1993)	18	61

tenderness, redness, purulent discharge, and dehiscence (Table 17–3). If the infection is associated with an episiotomy hematoma, the woman may also complain of difficulty in voiding or inability to void. If infection is further complicated by dehiscence, the woman may also complain of incontinence of flatus and stool.

Women with the more serious form of infection, necrotizing fasciitis, are much more likely to be immunocompromised or have insulin-dependent diabetes. In its earliest stages, necrotizing fasciitis is often manifested by intense pain, erythema, and cellulitis. However, the rapid progression of this infection may result in necrosis and anesthesia of the skin and underlying tissue. The skin may become "dusky" in appearance with dark ecchymotic areas. The area may also appear crepitant to the touch. The woman usually appears acutely ill, and sepsis, shock, and death can follow rapidly—even if treatment is timely and appropriate. A woman with necrotizing fasciitis 8 days post partum is shown in Figures 17–2 and 17–3. Her episiotomy had become infected, and she failed to respond to the usual therapy.[10]

Women may also have infection beneath the deep fascia.[10] Such infections may involve the underlying muscle, resulting in myonecrosis. These women may present with signs and symptoms similar to those with necrotizing fasciitis, although the severity of pain may be out of proportion to the physical findings.[10] Of special concern is the fact that such serious infection may have a very rapid onset and progression.

Treatment

Treatment is based on the extent or degree of infection and on the presence or absence of complications. Obviously, treatment is radically different for necrotiz-

TABLE 17-3 ▶ SIGNS AND SYMPTOMS OF EPISIOTOMY INFECTIONS
Pain
Erythema
Tenderness
Swelling
Purulent discharge
Dehiscence

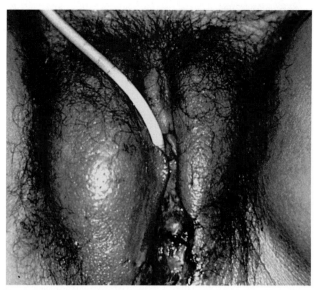

FIGURE 17-2 ▶ Woman with necrotizing fasciitis. (Courtesy of Dr. Gary D. V. Hankins, University of Texas Medical Branch at Galveston, Texas.)

ing fasciitis compared with uncomplicated infection with dehiscence.

Management of Uncomplicated Infection

The episiotomy is often "broken down," or dehisced, with infection. If not, it should be opened and drained. All suture material should be removed, and the wound should be débrided of all necrotic tissue. Copious irrigation with a dilute povidone–iodine solution should be used until the area appears clean and free from exudate. Initial therapy can usually be accomplished with intravenous sedation, although spinal analgesia

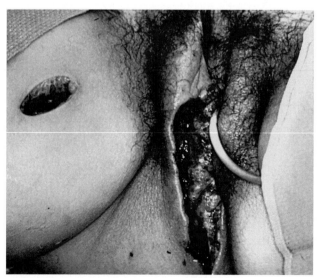

FIGURE 17-3 ▶ Necrotizing fasciitis. Opening in thigh was exploration to help determine extent of lesion. (Courtesy of Dr. Gary D. V. Hankins, University of Texas Medical Branch at Galveston, Texas.)

may be necessary in some women when extensive exploration is indicated. After initial treatment, the site should be cleaned at least twice daily, and the woman should be instructed on daily sitz baths. Before the wound is scrubbed and cleaned, it may be necessary to use intravenous sedation with meperidine, at least for the first day. Lidocaine gel (1%) applied to wound edges usually decreases patient discomfort. Wound care can often be accomplished as an outpatient process if the wound is clean and the woman is afebrile after initial therapy.

A wide variety of bacteria may be isolated from episiotomy infections, similar to those isolated from women with postcesarean infection. Although organisms such as *Staphylococcus aureus*, *Streptococcus faecalis*, and *Escherichia coli* may be isolated, it is not uncommon to recover a mixed aerobic-anaerobic flora (i.e., polymicrobial), similar to that found in women with postcesarean endometritis. Because of these bacteria, the author prefers to use one of the broad-spectrum beta-lactam antibiotics in women with an episiotomy infection. Antibiotics such as cefoxitin, cefotetan, or one of the penicillins combined with a beta-lactamase inhibitor usually prove satisfactory. The oral antibiotic, amoxicillin plus clavulanic acid, is especially useful for women being managed as outpatients. Antibiotics are not required in all women with episiotomy infection. For example, infection in the absence of abscess formation or significant cellulitis usually responds satisfactorily to the opening of the wound, copious irrigation, and simple débridement. However, if there is any question as to the extent of the process, it is prudent to use antibiotics for a minimum of 48 to 72 hours.

Necrotizing Fasciitis

Because the infection is life-threatening, with a mortality rate of 50% or higher, early diagnosis and treatment is of paramount importance.[11] The bacteriology of this infection is often polymicrobial, although it may also result from a clostridial cellulitis. Thus, a combination of antibiotics such as penicillin (or ampicillin), gentamicin, and clindamycin (or metronidazole) should be used after blood and tissue cultures have been obtained. Next, the woman should be taken to the operating room for thorough examination under adequate anesthesia (i.e., either regional or general). Extensive débridement of all necrotic and involved tissue must be accomplished in a timely fashion if the patient is to survive. Surgical débridement must be carried out until "healthy," bleeding tissue is encountered (see Fig. 17–3). The woman must be closely observed for signs and symptoms of septic shock and the wound should be inspected, cleaned, and débrided (if necessary) several times a day.

Myonecrosis

The most common organism associated with myonecrosis is *Clostridium perfringens*.[10] The treatment of myonecrosis includes high-dose penicillin and clindamycin. Because the bacteriology may not be known at the time of therapy, the author also adds an aminoglycoside to the aforementioned regimen. The patient should be taken to the operating room and, under adequate anesthesia, undergo extensive surgical débridement until the margins are free from nonviable tissue. As pointed out by Fisher and colleagues,[12] deep tissue necrosis usually extends farther than the obvious skin involvement. Hyperbaric oxygen therapy may also prove beneficial in some women with this life-threatening infection.

EPISIOTOMY DEHISCENCE

Infection most often results in dehiscence of the episiotomy site. Moreover, if spontaneous opening of the wound does not occur, it is necessary to open the episiotomy to explore and clean the wound adequately. Until recently, there was significant controversy over when to repair such dehiscences (i.e., early vs. late repair).

Initial Therapy

Antibiotics should be used in women with episiotomy dehiscence secondary to infection, especially in the presence of cellulitis, purulent discharge, a frank abscess, or an infected hematoma. As previously mentioned, either one of the newer penicillins with a beta-lactamase inhibitor or a broad-spectrum cephalosporin such as cefoxitin or cefotetan usually proves satisfactory. After initiation of antibiotic, the patient should be taken to a procedure or operating room and given adequate sedation (i.e., intravenous meperidine) or anesthesia (i.e., spinal). If not a total dehiscence, the wound should be opened completely and all suture material removed. The wound should be irrigated with a dilute povidone-iodine solution. We use a Betadine-impregnated scrub brush for débridement. Unless extensive cellulitis or fasciitis is present, plans are made for early repair of the episiotomy dehiscence.

Early versus Late Repair

Classically, it was taught that episiotomy breakdown or dehiscence should be managed by delayed closure in 2 to 3 months to allow for partial healing and revascularization of tissue. However, this approach was not based on scientific data and was associated with significant morbidity and cost.[1] Moreover, such an approach may lead to litigation.

More recently, it has been shown that early repair

after dehiscence can be accomplished with satisfactory results. Hauth and colleagues,[13] in a review of eight women with dehiscences of fourth-degree lacerations, reported successful early repair in seven (88%). In one woman, a pinpoint fistula developed, which was subsequently repaired with a small rectal flap. Follow-up of this patient revealed complete healing.

Hankins and colleagues,[9] in a review of 31 women with episiotomy dehiscence (including the 8 women initially reported by Hauth and colleagues[13]), reported successful early repair in 29 (94%). In the 22 women with fourth-degree lacerations in this series, the mean time from dehiscence to repair was 6.5 days. The mean time from repair to discharge was 9.7 days. In a 12-month follow-up of 17 of these 22 women, all were well, with the exception of 2 women who still had complaints of dyspareunia. None of these 17 women, however, had complaints of incontinence of flatus or stool.

In another review of early repair of episiotomy dehiscence, Ramin and colleagues[8] reported successful repair in 32 (94%) of 34 women. The women in this series were from a predominantly medically indigent population. In the 27 women with infection from this series, the mean time from vaginal delivery to dehiscence was 4.4 days, and from complication to repair was 6.7 days. The mean time from repair to discharge was 4.5 days.

Advantages of Early Repair

There are numerous, obvious advantages to early repair of an episiotomy dehiscence, especially one resulting from a fourth-degree extension or laceration. Early repair is convenient and is associated with decreased hospital stay, decreased costs, and decreased litigation. Moreover, the woman has fewer risks of dyspareunia and fecal incontinence and, most important, she is not sent home with a "cloaca."[1, 14, 15]

Preoperative Protocol for Early Repair

After the initial management of an infected episiotomy, as described previously, the open wound should be cleaned at least twice daily by scrubbing the site with a Betadine-impregnated brush (Fig. 17–4). Satisfactory pain relief can usually be provided with parenteral meperidine and 1% lidocaine jelly applied to the wound[14, 15] (Table 17–4). Repair should be scheduled only after the wound is pink or red with healthy granulation tissue. A mechanical bowel preparation should be done the night before surgery in women with dehiscence of an infected fourth-degree episiotomy.

Technique of Repair

Regional analgesia (e.g., epidural or spinal) usually provides satisfactory pain relief for repair of episiotomy

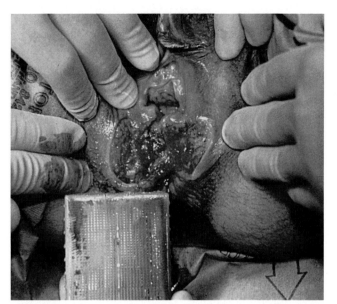

FIGURE 17–4 ▶ Wound has been scrubbed. Repair is done when wound surface is free from exudate and covered by granulation tissue.

dehiscence. After adequate analgesia, the episiotomy site can be further débrided as necessary (Fig. 17–5). Dissection should be carried out to ensure good tissue mobility, especially around the sphincter ani muscle.

Although a variety of suture material can be used for the repair, the author prefers to use chromic. The rectal mucosa is first sutured with a 4–0 chromic suture in a running submucosal closure, followed by reinforcement of the rectovaginal septal tissue with an interrupted 2–0 or 3–0 chromic suture. The sphincter muscle is approximated with several interrupted 2–0 chromic sutures.[8–10, 13–15] The remainder of the episiotomy is closed in the usual fashion of a second-degree episiotomy[10] (Fig. 17–6).

Postoperative Care

After closure of an episiotomy dehiscence secondary to infection, the author prefers to observe the woman in the hospital for at least 24 hours. After this initial observation period, she can usually be managed as an outpatient for the remainder of her postoperative care. She should be started on a low-residue diet, which can

TABLE 17–4 ▶	PREOPERATIVE WOUND CARE FOR EARLY REPAIR OF EPISIOTOMY DEHISCENCE

Continue antibiotics
Twice-daily cleaning
Removal of necrotic tissue
Sitz baths
Mechanical bowel preparation for fourth-degree tears

Adapted from Ramin SM, Gilstrap LC III: Episiotomy and early repair in dehiscence. Clin Obstet Gynecol 1994; 37:316, with permission.

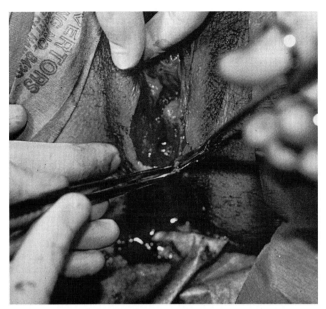

FIGURE 17-5 ▶ Débridement of wound at time of closure.

be advanced to a regular diet over the first week. The woman should be encouraged to have sitz baths three to four times per day for the first week. A heat lamp should be directed at the perineum for the first 24 to 48 hours, and nothing should be used per rectum or vagina until the wound is healed. The author also prefers to examine the wound in the office 48 to 72 hours post discharge (Table 17–5).

It is of paramount importance to avoid excessive use of stool softeners to prevent the development of watery stools or diarrhea. The presence of watery stools may

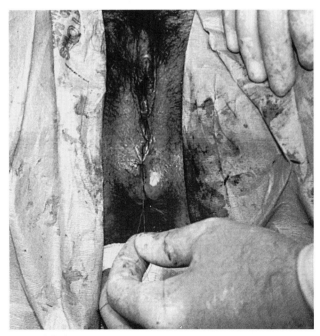

FIGURE 17-6 ▶ Secondary repair of dehiscence is almost complete.

TABLE 17-5 ▶	POSTOPERATIVE WOUND CARE AFTER EARLY REPAIR OF EPISIOTOMY DEHISCENCE

24-h minimal observation in hospital
Low-residue diet
Avoid diarrhea
Heat lamp for 24 to 48 h
Avoid anything per rectum/vagina until healed
Follow-up in office at 24–72 h and at 10 d to 2 wk

Adapted in part from Ramin SM, Gilstrap LC III: Episiotomy and early repair in dehiscence. Clin Obstet Gynecol 1994; 37:816, with permission.

interfere with the healing process or lead to breakdown because they may easily pass through the suture line. A low-residue diet without the addition of stool softeners usually provides satisfactory results.

Prevention

Not all cases of infection and dehiscence can be prevented. Because one of the greatest risk factors for episiotomy infection (and hence dehiscence) is a third- or fourth-degree laceration, it seems reasonable to use prophylactic antibiotics in these cases, especially with extension into the rectum. However, this recommendation is not based on firm scientific data.

Although it is of paramount importance to use good surgical technique in repairing episiotomies, it is doubtful that poor technique contributes significantly to episiotomy infection or dehiscence.

SUMMARY

The routine performance of episiotomies in all women undergoing vaginal delivery cannot be justified from available data.[1] Fortunately, episiotomy infections are relatively uncommon, and the most significant risk factor appears to be the presence of a fourth-degree laceration. Serious, life-threatening infection, such as necrotizing fasciitis and myonecrosis, may also develop. General principles in the management of episiotomy infection include antibiotics, opening of the wound if necessary, removal of all foreign material, and débridement of all nonviable or necrotic tissue, especially in the presence of fasciitis or myonecrosis.

Dehiscence is often due to episiotomy infection. Early repair can often be accomplished after débridement and antibiotics and has a success rate of up to 94%.[1] There are obvious advantages to early repair of episiotomy dehiscences associated with fourth-degree lacerations, including less hospitalization, lower cost, and less litigation.

REFERENCES

1. Owen J, Hauth JC: Episiotomy infection and dehiscence. In: Gilstrap LC III, Faro S (eds): Infections in Pregnancy, 2nd ed. New York, John Wiley & Sons, 1997, pp 87–94.

2. Thorp JM Jr, Bowes WA Jr, Brame RG, Cefalo R: Selected use of midline episiotomy: Effect on perineal trauma. Obstet Gynecol 1987; 70:260.

3. Thorp JM Jr, Bowes WA Jr: Episiotomy: Can its routine use be defined? Am J Obstet Gynecol 1989; 160:1027.

4. Shiono P, Klebanoff MA, Carey JC: Midline episiotomies: More harm than good? Obstet Gynecol 1990; 75:765.

5. Owen J, Hauth JC: Episiotomy infection and dehiscence. In: Gilstrap LC III, Faro S (eds): Infections in Pregnancy. New York, Liss, 1990, pp 61–74.

6. Harris RE: An evaluation of the median episiotomy. Am J Obstet Gynecol 1970; 106:660.

7. Goldaber KG, Wendel PJ, McIntire D, Wendel GD Jr: Postpartum perineal morbidity after fourth-degree perineal repair. Am J Obstet Gynecol 1993; 168:489.

8. Ramin SM, Ramus RM, Little BB, Gilstrap LC III: Early repair of episiotomy dehiscence associated with infection. Am J Obstet Gynecol 1992; 167:1104.

9. Hankins GDV, Hauth JC, Gilstrap LC III, et al: Early repair of episiotomy dehiscence. Obstet Gynecol 1990; 75:48.

10. Hankins GDV: Episiotomy. In: Hankins GDV, Clark SL, Cunningham G, Gilstrap LC III (eds): Operative Obstetrics. Norwalk, CT, Appleton & Lange, 1995, pp 93–127.

11. Patino JF, Castro D: Necrotizing lesions of the soft tissue: review. World J Surg 1991; 15:235.

12. Fisher JR, Conway MJ, Takeshita RT, Sandoval MR: Necrotizing fasciitis: Importance of roentgenographic studies for soft-tissue gas. JAMA 1979; 241:803.

13. Hauth JC, Gilstrap LC III, Ward SC, Hankins GDV: Early repair of an external sphincter ani muscle and rectal mucosal dehiscence. Obstet Gynecol 1986; 67:806.

14. Ramin SM, Gilstrap LC III: Episiotomy and early repair in dehiscence. Clin Obstet Gynecol 1994; 37:816.

15. Ramin SM: Early repair of episiotomy dehiscence: Association with infection. Contemp Obstet Gynecol 1996; 41:25.

18 Mastitis

W. David Hager ▸ Kate Pierce

BACKGROUND

Mastitis is a clinical term describing an inflammatory process of the breast tissue. Although the term indicates inflammation, it is usually considered to be synonymous with infection. Breast infections have been recognized as long as women have given birth and nursed infants. It is unfortunate, therefore, that there are few well-designed, randomized, prospective studies that have evaluated the etiology and treatment of this condition. There have been numerous reports on the epidemiologic aspects of mastitis.

Although the most frequent categorization of the disease is puerperal or nonpuerperal, others include epidemic or nonepidemic, sporadic or nonsporadic, and acute or chronic. Since epidemic outbreaks are unusual now, this discussion focuses on acute or chronic puerperal and nonpuerperal mastitis. In the past, epidemic occurrences were thought to be associated with longer maternal and neonatal hospital stays, staphylococcal infections in nurseries, and unavailability of antibiotics. The correction of these underlying risk factors has resulted in most cases being acute and nonepidemic.

INCIDENCE

The incidence of acute puerperal mastitis varies widely with the patient population studied. Rates of 2.9%,[1] 4.8%,[2] and 24%[3] have been reported. Infection usually occurs within the first 2 weeks of delivery, related to engorgement and milk stasis; at 5 to 6 weeks post partum; or late, in association with weaning or teething. If a mother has mastitis with one pregnancy, she has a threefold increased risk with a subsequent pregnancy.[3]

PATHOPHYSIOLOGY

Acute puerperal mastitis (nonepidemic, sporadic) is defined as an acute puerperal cellulitis with extension to the periglandular connective tissue. The connective tissue infection results in a V-shaped area of involvement between lobes along the lactiferous apparatus. Some disagreement exists as to whether the process is primarily the result of milk statis and engorgement, cracking and fissuring of nipples allowing ascension of bacteria, migration of the mother's skin flora into susceptible breast tissue, or an overwhelming inoculum of bacteria from the infant's oral flora. Actually, the infection probably results from a combination of these events. To be effectively managed, each of these factors must be addressed.

In a detailed study on the classification of lactation mastitis, Thomsen and co-workers[4] subdivided the infection into three categories—milk stasis, noninfectious inflammation, and acute mastitis—based on progression of disease (Table 18–1). They described milk stasis as an area of the breast where swelling and knots occur as the result of engorgement from the slowing of milk flow. The patient may feel warmth in the breast, the leukocyte count of the milk is less than 10^6/mL the bacterial count is less than 10^3 CFU/mL and the symptoms usually last only a few days.

When stasis of milk is persistent and marked, noninfectious inflammation may result. This process is characterized by edema, erythema, heat, pain, tenderness,

TABLE 18–1 ▸ STAGES OF BREAST INFLAMMATION

	Milk Stasis	Noninfectious Inflammation	Infectious Mastitis
Fever	Low grade	Low grade	High grade
Breast	Engorged, nodular	Tender, swollen, red, hot	Tender, swollen, red, hot
Milk			
Leukocytes	$<10^6$/mL	$>10^6$/mL	$>10^6$/mL
Bacteria	$<10^3$ CFU/mL	$<10^3$ CFU/mL	$>10^3$ CFU/mL

Modified from Thomsen AC, Espersen T, Maigaard S: Course and treatment of milk stasis, noninfectious inflammation of the breast, and infectious mastitis in nursing women. Am J Obstet Gynecol 1984; 149:492.

and low-grade fever. The number of leukocytes in the milk are more than 10^6/mL and the bacterial level is less than 10^3 CFU/mL. When self-limited, the condition usually lasts for 5 to 6 days.

If the stasis and inflammation do not resolve, acute infectious mastitis may occur. This stage is divided into two classes by Thomsen:

1. *Cellulitis*, which involves infection of interlobular connective tissues as the result of the introduction of bacteria through cracked or fissured nipples. The symptoms and signs include edema, erythema, pain, myalgias, chills, fever, and tenderness.[5]
2. *Adenitis*, which occurs when one or more ducts of the breast are plugged and then infected. The clinical signs and symptoms are usually less severe, but suppuration is more common. Abscesses usually do not occur if nursing is continued. Pathogens may ascend through the lactiferous sinuses from a nipple fissure, with spread to the periductal lymphatics. Hematogenous spread may also occur.[5]

Although this classification is helpful, in a practical sense the diagnostician must differentiate between stasis with or without inflammation that will respond to conservative treatment measures, and infection that requires these measures plus antibiotic therapy.

RISK FACTORS FOR DISEASE

Several investigators have reported that a combination of risk factors may be involved in predisposing the mother to mastitis. Women who have had mastitis with a previous pregnancy are three times more likely than women who never had mastitis to have the infection during the index pregnancy.[6] Cracking of nipples is a significant factor in allowing an avenue for ascension of potential pathogens. Engorgement and milk stasis, which may result from incomplete emptying or decreased frequency of feeding, present bacteria with an ideal medium for growth. Fatigue and stress have been associated with mastitis, as they indirectly predispose the woman to infection. When tired, the mother may not hold and/or position the baby properly, and nipple trauma may occur. Fatigue and stress may affect the immune system and decrease resistance to infection. Plugging of the ducts with keratinous debris may also result in stasis and infection. If other family members, especially the infant, are ill, the mother may be exposed to pathogens in an inoculum that overwhelms normal defense mechanisms.

Basically, anything that causes poor drainage of the duct, a segment of a duct itself or the alveolus, has the potential for causation. Cracked or fissured nipples caused by improper latch, candidal infections, teething, a tight or shortened frenulum, or a high palatal arch increase the potential for infection. A sudden change in the number of breast-feedings, breast trauma, engorgement, or insufficient emptying of obstructions in the duct caused by wearing tight clothing (brassiere, baby slings or carriers) may increase the risk. Breast shells used for flat or inverted nipples, although beneficial, can increase the risk of milk stasis if they are worn while sleeping or with a brassiere that is too small.

ETIOLOGY

Many different bacteria have been isolated from the infected milk of women with acute puerperal mastitis. Niebyl and co-workers[7] isolated pathogenic bacteria from 53% of their patients with this diagnosis. Among these women, 37% harbored *Staphylococcus aureus* alone or in combination with other bacteria. In specimens obtained by expressing milk from the infected breast, Carrol and colleagues[8] found that only 6% of the specimens contained *S. aureus*, and 7% Enterobacteriaceae. A total of 97% of isolates were similar to skin or mouth flora. Aerobes are the principal isolates in puerperal infection, as opposed to nonpuerperal mastitis, in which anaerobes are frequently isolated from purulent material.[9] In our recent analysis, we isolated staphylococci from 60% of women with acute infection.[2] All of these isolates were resistant to penicillin and sensitive to cephalosporins. We did not isolate anaerobes other than propionibacteria.

In other reports, *S. aureus*, staphylococcal species (coagulase-negative), group B streptococci, Enterobacteriaceae, *S. pneumoniae*, and various anaerobes have been isolated from infected breasts.[7, 8, 10] *Mycobacterium tuberculosis* and atypical mycobacteria have been recovered from patients with nonpuerperal mastitis.

It is difficult to obtain cultures in a sterile fashion from the breast. The nipple and areola should be prepared with povidone-iodine (Betadine). The patient should place the breast in a dependent position and have milk expressed from the inflamed area. After 3 to 5 drops are expressed, several drops should be collected in a sterile flushed tube to allow for aerobic and anaerobic culturing in a quantitative manner colony-forming units per milliliter (CFU/mL). It is not essential that cultures be obtained outside of a research setting unless the infection is persistent or epidemic or there is an abscess present.

When quantitative cultures of human milk from patients with clinical mastitis have been performed, 10^8 to 10^9 CFU/mL of milk have been found excreted. These cultures included organisms such as *S. aureus*, and yet neither mother nor baby were ill.[11] This observation has led most experts in the field to allow continued breast-feeding despite infection, since the infants do not appear adversely affected. They may tend to reject the breast in severe infection, and should not be allowed to nurse when an abscess, with quantitatively more bacteria, is present.

CLINICAL COURSE

The diagnosis of puerperal mastitis is made on clinical grounds with no asymptomatic state reported. The most frequent symptoms are malaise, myalgias, fever, chills, and pain in the breast and axilla. At the time of examination, the breast is usually edematous, erythematous, and tender to palpation. The erythema is in a V-shaped pattern, which corresponds to the lactiferous apparatus. As mentioned, milk stasis is often bilateral and is not associated with fever or erythema. Noninfectious inflammation and mastitis are more frequently unilateral and associated with fever and erythema.

In a recent report of 25 women,[2] the clinical parameters included days from delivery to onset of symptoms, 55.4, and duration of symptoms before the diagnosis was made, 47.4 hours. Cracking of nipples was found in 64% of patients. The mean temperature at diagnosis was 100.7°F (38.17°C), and the mean white blood cell count was 11,400/mL. A total of 2 of 25 women had bilateral involvement, and 1 developed an abscess. Abscesses have been reported in as many as 11% of women with mastitis.[12]

If patients are not diagnosed readily, they may become extremely ill. Malaise, lethargy, and marked debility may occur, and the mother may lose interest in breast-feeding.

DIAGNOSIS

The diagnosis of postpartum fever includes a careful history and a comprehensive physical examination that includes the breasts. The mother usually has complaints of throbbing pain and warmth in a particular segment of the breast. Complaints of fever, chills, myalgias, fatigue, and headache are common. She may complain that the baby is rejecting or pulling away from the breast. Although this can be a finding among women who have breast cancer and are attempting to nurse, it is usually due to the increase in sodium and chloride in the milk, which gives it a salty taste.

Examination usually reveals an anxious patient who is very uncomfortable. The breast or breasts are usually engorged and found to be erythematous and tender in the segment of involvement. The nipple often has a crack or fissure. The skin of the involved breast is often taut and shiny. The lactiferous area infected may be firm, lumpy, or indurated and is usually in the upper outer quadrant. Oral temperature is usually at least 100°F, and the pulse is elevated. The peripheral white blood cell count is greater than 10,000/mL.

TREATMENT

The basics of treatment for puerperal mastitis are conservative: continued nursing, the use of warm, moist

TABLE 18-2 ▶ MANAGEMENT OF ACUTE PUERPERAL MASTITIS

1. The patient should continue breast-feeding, starting on the affected side.
2. If the infant does not feed well or will not feed on the affected breast, empty the breast using a piston-type breast pump (hospital-grade breast pump).
3. Bed rest, if possible, for the first 48 h.
4. Increased intake of fluids.
5. Decreased intake of sodium chloride.
6. The patient should take acetaminophen or ibuprofen to reduce fever and decrease discomfort so letdown will occur and the breast can be emptied.
7. Moist heat should be used to facilitate letdown and decrease soreness; cool-packs may be used initially to decrease swelling.
8. Gentle massage should be employed to move the milk forward and increase drainage from the infected area.
9. The patient should avoid breast shells and tight-fitting brassieres.
10. The patient should avoid tight clothing and underwire brassieres.
11. Careful hand washing should be done before handling the breast.
12. Lanolin creams should be used to treat nipples. Treat fungal infections of the nipple.
13. Reinforce appropriate nursing position, use a lactation consultant to evaluate suck and technique.
14. The patient should take vitamin C (500 mg) and vitamin E (400 IU) once or twice a day.
15. If the patient is febrile, prescribe antibiotics for 7 to 10 days.
16. Schedule patient follow-up in 7 days to evaluate for abscess formation. If there is no clinical response within 48 hours of antibiotic treatment, the patient should notify the physician.

compresses, fluid intake, rest, and the use of antipyretics (acetaminophen) (Table 18-2).

Antibiotics may hasten the response to therapy and should be used in the febrile patient. No single antibiotic has been found to be preferred. Those studied have included beta-lactamase–susceptible penicillins, penicillinase-resistant penicillins, cephalosporins, erythromycin, trimethoprim-sulfamethoxazole, and metronidazole.[2, 4, 5] Although evaluation of the etiologic agents would indicate that the antibiotic used must cover staphylococci, our data[2] and that of others[7, 12] indicate that other antibiotics may be used successfully as well. In a comparison of amoxicillin versus cephradine, both treatment failures (15.6%) and the only abscess (1 of 13) occurred in the amoxicillin-treated group, but the difference was not significant.[2]

If a woman with mastitis is found to have a fluctuant area in the breast consistent with an abscess, drainage is indicated. Meguid[14] compared treatment of subareolar abscesses in 24 women using antibiotics alone (n = 4), antibiotics plus incision and drainage of the abscess only (n = 16), and excision of the abscess and plugged lactiferous duct (n = 4). All patients in the first two groups had recurrences, whereas none in the latter group did.

Women who have multiple recurrences or persistence of mastitis with no evidence of an abscess, should be treated with either erythromycin (250 to 500 mg q6h) or trimethoprim-sulfamethoxazole (160 mg/800 mg) twice daily for several weeks.[13] The best prevention for recurrences is to appropriately treat the initial infection with effective antibiotics and adequately instruct the mother in preventive techniques.

CONSEQUENCES OF INFECTION

The most frequent consequence of puerperal mastitis is persistent infection and/or development of an abscess. This complication has been reported in 4.0%,[2] 4.6%,[11] and 11.1%[12] of women with acute mastitis. When an abscess is diagnosed, the infant should not be allowed to nurse on the involved breast, but the breast should be emptied by pumping. Parenteral antibiotics should be used that are effective against staphylococci and anaerobes. If improvement is not noted within 48 hours, incision and drainage or excision should be performed.[15]

Inflammatory carcinoma of the breast may be very difficult to differentiate from mastitis with or without an abscess. Carcinoma is usually found in older, nonlactating women, but this is not always the case. The failure of a patient to respond to initial antibiotic therapy should result in a change to parenteral antibiotics, evaluation for an abscess, and consideration of breast biopsy.[16]

NONPUERPERAL MASTITIS

Infection of the breast in nonpregnant women is an uncommon clinical problem but can result in serious consequences if not treated appropriately. The signs and symptoms of disease are similar to those of puerperal mastitis but may not be detected as readily because the patient is not pregnant.

The disease is characterized by keratotic debris and squamous metaplasia of the epithelium lining the milk sinus, which partially blocks the lactiferous ducts and results in inflammation and pain. Staphylococci and anaerobic cocci and bacilli are the most frequent isolates from breast secretions and from abscesses.[17] Other causes of nonpuerperal mastitis include tuberculous and atypical mycobacterial infections, insect bites, silicone implants, lupus mastitis, lymphocytic mastitis in diabetes, and idiopathic granulomatous mastitis.[18–21] Oral stimulation of the breast is another possible inciting factor.

Nonpuerperal mastitis presents as acute, subacute, or chronic infection. Acute disease presents in a manner similar to that of acute puerperal infection, along with a firm, tender subareolar mass. Subacute disease presents in a similar manner but is associated with a tender, fluctuant mass. The chronic process presents with a history of multiple, recurrent infections that lead to sinus tract formation, suppuration, and possibly a fluctuant mass.

The treatment of nonpuerperal mastitis involves the use of a penicillinase-resistant penicillin in combination with an agent effective against anaerobes. Treatment should continue for 10 to 14 days. The presence of an abscess requires incision and drainage or excision. Treating skin lesions aggressively and avoiding oral stimulation to the breast may help prevent infection.

REFERENCES

1. Kaufmann J, Foxman B: Mastitis among lactating women: Occurrence and risk factors. Soc Sci Med 1991; 33:701.
2. Hager WD, Barton JR: Treatment of sporadic acute puerperal mastitis. Infect Dis Obstet Gynecol 1996; 4:97.
3. Jonsson S, Pulkkinen MO: Mastitis today: Incidence, prevention and treatment. Ann Chir Gynaecol 1994; 208:84.
4. Thomsen AC, Espersen T, Maigaard S: Course and treatment of milk stasis, noninfectious inflammation of the breast, and infectious mastitis in nursing women. Am J Obstet Gynecol 1984; 149:492.
5. McGregor JA, Neifert MR: Maternal problems in lactation. In: Neville MC, Neifert MR (eds): Lactation Physiology, Nutrition and Breastfeeding. Plenum Publishers, 1983, pp 333–348.
6. Riordan JM, Nichols FH: A descriptive study of lactation mastitis in long-term breastfeeding women. J Hum Lact 1990; 6:53.
7. Niebyl JR, Spence MR, Parmley TH: Sporadic (non-epidemic) puerperal mastitis. J Reprod Med 1978; 20:97.
8. Carrol L, Davies DP, Osman M, McNeigh AS: Bacteriologic criteria for feeding raw breast milk to babies on neonatal units. Lancet 1979; 2:732.
9. Leach RD, Eykyn SJ, Phillips I: Anaerobic subareolar breast abscess. Lancet 1979; 1:35.
10. Wust J, Rutsch M, Stocker S: Streptococcus pneumoniae as an agent of mastitis. Eur J Clin Microbiol Infect Dis 1995; 14:156.
11. Marshall BR, Heppler JK, Zirbel CC: Sporadic puerperal mastitis, an infection that need not interrupt lactation. JAMA 1975; 233:1377.
12. Devereux WP: Acute puerperal mastitis: Evaluation of its management. Am J Obstet Gynecol 1970; 108:78.
13. Cantlie HB: Treatment of acute puerperal mastitis and breast abscess. Can Fam Physician 1988; 34:2221.
14. Meguid MM: Pathogenesis-based treatment of recurring subareolar breast abscesses. Surgery 1995; 118:775.
15. Newton M, Newton NT: Breast abscess: A result of lactation failure. Surg Gynecol Obstet 1950; 91:651.
16. Dahlbeck SW, Donnelly JF, Theriault RL: Differentiating inflammatory breast cancer from acute mastitis. Am Fam Physician 1995; 52:929.
17. Admiston CE, Walker AP, Krepel CJ, et al: The nonpuerperal breast infection: Aerobic and anaerobic microbial recovery from acute and chronic disease. J Infect Dis 1990; 162:695.
18. Shinde SR, Chandawarkar RY, Deshmulch SP: Tuberculosis of the breast masquerading as carcinoma: A study of 100 patients. World J Surg 1995; 19:379.
19. Salam IM, Alhomsi MF, Daniel MF, et al: Diagnosis and treatment of granulomatous mastitis. Br J Surg 1995; 82:214.
20. Lee D, Goldstein EJ, Zarem HA: Localized Mycobacterium avium intracellulare mastitis in an immunocompetent woman with silicone breast implants. Plast Reconstr Surg 1995; 95:142.
21. DeBrandt M, Meyer O, Grossin M, et al: Lupus mastitis heralding systemic lupus erythematosus with antiphospholipid syndrome. J Rheumatol 1993; 20:1217.

Gynecologic Infections

19

Bacterial Vaginosis

JANICE I. FRENCH ▶ JAMES A. MCGREGOR

Bacterial vaginosis is a leading cause of abnormal vaginal discharge and odor. This condition is increasingly recognized as causing common and costly obstetric and gynecologic infectious complications worldwide.[1-21] Bacterial vaginosis constitutes a massive microecologic alteration of vaginal flora, which is similar to the "bloom," or "red tide," of microorganisms that can occur in large bodies of water. Complications related to bacterial vaginosis include preterm birth, chorioamnionitis, postpartum endometritis, postcesarean infection, and nonchlamydial nongonococcal endometritis and salpingitis, as well as post-termination and posthysterectomy infections.[4-21] The risks of sequelae have been shown to be partially preventable by identification and treatment of bacterial vaginosis.[22-26] Recognition of the morbidity, costs, and liabilities engendered by bacterial vaginosis has led some experts to recommend routine screening and treatment of bacterial vaginosis (1) during pregnancy, (2) prior to invasive upper reproductive tract procedures and surgeries, (3) subsequent to sexual assault, and (4) as part of routine gynecologic health maintenance.

HISTORY

The clinical signs consistent with bacterial vaginosis have long been recognized as abnormal.[27, 28] As early as 1894, findings consistent with bacterial vaginosis were described and termed *"nonspecific" vaginitis.*[28] Classic work by Gardner and Dukes,[29] published in 1955, described the characteristic "clue" cell, as well as the homogeneous "milky" discharge and amine odor that, along with increased pH, constitute the definition of bacterial vaginosis. Additionally, Gardner and Dukes proposed *Haemophilus vaginalis* as the causative agent and the name *"Haemophilus vaginalis vaginitis."*[29] Subsequently, this gram-variable aerobic bacteria was placed in its own classification and eponymously named *Gardnerella vaginalis.*[30] The synergistic roles of both *Gardnerella vaginalis* and vaginal anaerobic bacteria in the pathobiology of bacterial vaginosis was described in the early 1980s.[31] Subsequently, the term *bacterial vaginosis* or *"BV"* superseded other terms, including, *anaerobic colpitis* and *vaginal bacteriosis.*[31-33] The

suffix *osis* means discharge; therefore, *bacterial vaginosis* means vaginal discharge caused by bacteria.

MICROBIOLOGY AND PATHOGENESIS

Bacterial vaginosis consists of a massive polymicrobial overgrowth in which microbes act synergistically and cause local genital symptoms (i.e., amine odor and discharge) as well as upper reproductive tract abnormalities.[3, 31, 34] Bacterial vaginosis is best understood as a massive change in the vaginal ecosystem, rather than an infection caused by a single microorganism.[35, 36] During a woman's reproductive years, the acidophilic facultative, hydrogen peroxide (H_2O_2)–producing *Lactobacillus crispatus, L. jensenii, L. fermentum,* and *L. gasseri* constitute the predominant vaginal species.[37, 38] These "healthy" lactobacilli are found in concentrations of 10^5 to 10^6 colony-forming units (CFU)/g of vaginal fluid.[36-38] Other bacteria occur in much lower concentrations (10^2 to 10^5 CFU/g of vaginal fluid) and account for 10% of the bacterial species recovered from the healthy vagina.[37] These species include facultative aerobes such as *Staphylococcus epidermidis, Streptococcus* spp., and *Gardnerella vaginalis,* and anaerobic organisms including *Bacteroides* spp., *Prevotella* spp., and *Peptostreptococcus* spp., as well as *Mycoplasma hominis* and *Ureaplasma urealyticum.*[31, 34, 37, 39-41] Bacterial vaginosis is characterized by (1) decreased or absent *Lactobacillus* spp., (2) logarithmically increased concentrations ($\geq 10^8$ to 10^{11} CFU/g of fluid) of *G. vaginalis,* and (3) logarithmically increased concentrations of a set of potentially pathogenic bacteria. These bacterial vaginosis–associated microorganisms include *Prevotella* spp. (formerly *Bacteroides* spp.), *Peptostreptococcus* spp., *Porphomonas* spp., and *Mobiluncus* spp., along with *Ureaplasma urealyticum* and *Mycoplasma hominis.*[31, 37, 39-42]

Commensurate with shifts in microbial flora, characteristic vaginal fluid biochemical changes also occur with bacterial vaginosis. Bacterial vaginosis–associated biochemical factors include elevated pH, as well as increased vaginal fluid concentrations of diamines, polyamines, and organic acids.[34, 41, 43, 44] A number of established bacterial virulence factors occur in high concentrations in the vaginal fluid of women with

221

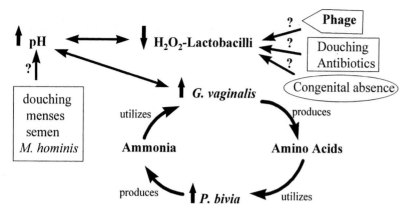

FIGURE 19-1 ▶ Pathophysiology of bacterial vaginosis.

bacterial vaginosis, such as endotoxin (lipopolysaccharide), mucinases, sialidase, IgA protease, collagenase, nonspecific proteases, and phospholipase A_2 and C.[31, 34, 45-51] Similarly, host inflammatory molecules including the cytokine interleukin-1α, and the prostaglandins E_2 and $F_{2α}$ occur in increased concentrations in the vaginal fluid of women with bacterial vaginosis.[51, 52] The potential roles of functions of these factors remain to be determined.

The importance of vaginal pH in maintaining normal vaginal microecology is increasingly recognized.[53] Attachment and growth of lactobacilli are favored in the acidic (pH range, 3.8 to 4.2) vaginal environment.[53-56] Conversely, this acidic environment limits attachment of *G. vaginalis* and other bacterial vaginosis–associated microorganisms.[55, 56] Increased pH tends to displace lactobacilli from vaginal epithelial cell receptor sites and to maximize adherence of *G. vaginalis*.[36, 53, 56] H_2O_2-producing lactobacilli also appear to play important roles in maintaining the healthy vaginal microecology.[53, 57, 58] In vitro studies demonstrate that H_2O_2-producing lactobacilli are toxic to *G. vaginalis* and *Prevotella bivia*.[58] Studies from Seattle show that women with bacterial vaginosis have low concentrations of H_2O_2-producing lactobacilli or none at all, and women without H_2O_2-producing lactobacilli who are followed prospectively are significantly more likely to acquire bacterial vaginosis.[54, 58-61] Separate studies by Rosenstein[62] and Boris[63] in Europe found no differences in the prevalence or concentration of H_2O_2-producing lactobacilli between women with or without bacterial vaginosis, and they suggest that other factors, such as lactobacillus-produced bacteriocins, play roles in suppressing *G. vaginalis* and other potentially pathogenic vaginal flora.

Synergistic relationships between *G. vaginalis* and bacterial vaginosis–associated anaerobic bacteria were postulated in 1979 by Chen.[43] Chen's early in vitro work demonstrated increased production of amino acids during the growth of *G. vaginalis* and increased metabolism of these amino acids into the amines, putrescine, cadaverine, and trimethylamine when grown with mixed anaerobic flora from women with bacterial vaginosis.[43] Recent, in vitro work by Pybus and Onderdonk[44] clearly demonstrates a commensal relationship between two of the predominant organisms in bacterial vaginosis, *G. vaginalis,* and *P. bivia.* Amino acids produced by *G. vaginalis* are utilized by *P. bivia* to produce ammonia and short-chain fatty acids, such as succinate and isovalerate. The growth of *G. vaginalis* is further enhanced by the presence of ammonia, which is produced during growth by *P. bivia* (Fig. 19–1).[44]

In addition to providing support for the growth of bacterial vaginosis–constituent bacteria, changes in vaginal fluid may serve to impair host defense mechanisms and facilitate passage of microorganisms and their products into the upper reproductive tract.[46, 47] Among the virulence factors present in bacterial vaginosis–associated vaginal fluid, mucinases and sialidases promote bacterial attachment by effectively lysing components of protective mucin in epithelial cell layers.[45, 46] Mucinase and sialidase may disrupt cervical mucus and promote bacterial attachment.[46] During pregnancy, phospholipase A_2 and C as well as nonspecific proteases may act on cervical and amniochorion connective tissue and promote cervical ripening and focal amniochorion weakening.[48, 49] In addition, phospholipase A_2 and C may promote the release of arachidonic acid and other molecules that promote intrauterine inflammation.

EPIDEMIOLOGY

Current understanding of the epidemiology of bacterial vaginosis is limited by several research methodologic problems. Bacterial vaginosis has been studied largely among self-selected women attending a variety of clinics. Since more than 50% of women with bacterial vaginosis are asymptomatic, large numbers of women with the condition are not included in studies of this type. An additional problem for epidemiologic study arises from the subjective nature of the clinical diagnosis of bacterial vaginosis. Variation in the diagnosis due to either the use of subjective clinical criteria or the use of different laboratory-based methods leads to misclassification of women as having or not having bacterial vaginosis. Thus, very different numbers of women may be deemed to have bacterial vaginosis, depending on which diagnostic criteria are used.[65] Despite these and other methodologic limitations, studies from various parts of the world in similar clinic populations tend to show surprisingly similar prevalences (Table 19–1).[3, 9, 12, 14–18, 24, 34, 35, 64–84] Among unselected women attending sexually transmitted disease (STD) clinics in the United States, Nova Scotia, Canada, and Sweden, the prevalence of bacterial vaginosis ranged from 26% to 37% of women.[3, 41, 66–73, 75] Among symptomatic women attending family planning clinics, bacterial vaginosis has been reported among 23% of Scandinavian women, 27% of French women, and 29% of U.S. women.[34, 77, 78] Among unselected gynecologic patients in the United Kingdom, the prevalence of bacterial vaginosis is 11%.[77, 78] This prevalence is similar to reports from Bump[81] and Gardner[82] of the findings of 5.6% and 12% of women with bacterial vaginosis in private gynecologic practices.

The prevalence of bacterial vaginosis in parturients is similar to that found among nonpregnant women with similar demographic characteristics. Bacterial vaginosis is found among 6% to 32% of pregnant women (see Table 19–1).[9, 12, 14–18, 85–91] The prevalence of bacterial vaginosis in the U.S. is highest among African American women and lowest among Asian American women; highest among women with multiple sexual partners and lowest among women with no history of heterosexual contact.[9, 24, 41, 81, 82, 92–94] Bacterial vaginosis is detected more often among women who report douching, those not using contraception, and those using an intrauterine contraceptive device.[34, 61, 95, 96]

Bacterial vaginosis is unrelated to oral contraceptive use. One study suggests that the use of the spermicide nonoxynol 9 may decrease the incidence of bacterial vaginosis (relative risk [RR], 0.86; 95% confidence interval [CI], 0.69 to 1.12).[97]

Multiple observations link the acquisition of bacterial vaginosis to sexual activity.[41, 61] Bacterial vaginosis most often occurs among sexually active women. Among sexually active women, bacterial vaginosis is found more frequently among women who have initiated sexual activity at an early age, among those reporting more sexual partners, and among women with concurrent or prior STDs.[34, 75, 97] Bacterial vaginosis is noted among sexually abused children and more commonly among lesbian partners of women with bacterial vaginosis.[98, 99] Among heterosexual women, acquisition of bacterial vaginosis can often be related to the introduction of a new male sexual partner, and male partners of women with bacterial vaginosis are five times more likely to have nongonococcal urethritis.[61, 97, 100] Bacterial vaginosis–associated microorganisms, including *M. hominis*, *G. vaginalis*, *Peptostreptococcus* spp., *Mobiluncus* spp., and *Prevotella* spp., are recovered from 17% to 52% of urethral cultures from male partners of women with bacterial vaginosis.[41, 101] Furthermore, the same *G. vaginalis* biotypes are isolated from heterosexual couples.[102] Conversely, detection of bacterial vaginosis among virginal women and children, even though the occurrence is low, militates against sexual transmission as the exclusive means for acquisition of bacterial vaginosis.[93, 98] Further evidence against exclusive sexual transmission arises from the consistent finding that the treatment of male partners does not prevent recurrence of bacterial vaginosis in their partners.[103, 104]

Natural History

Bacterial vaginosis may occur acutely or episodically, may become a persistent condition, or may resolve spontaneously.[90, 105] The natural history of bacterial vaginosis is best studied during pregnancy. Studies from various parts of the world show remarkably similar findings: (1) among initially negative women, fewer than 10% become positive between the first and third trimesters; (2) among positive women, 30% to 50% show resolution of signs of bacterial vaginosis without treatment; and (3) 10% to 30% of women have recurrent bacterial vaginosis approximately 4 to 16 weeks following treatment.[17, 46, 90, 92, 106]

Bacterial vaginosis is less well studied in nonpregnant women and children. Longitudinal studies among children and nonpregnant women demonstrate development of bacterial vaginosis among (1) 7% of adolescents followed for 3 months, (2) 13.6% and 25% of women attending STD clinics who are followed for 5 to 6 months, and (3) 50% of Scandinavian women

TABLE 19–1 ▶ PREVALENCE OF BACTERIAL VAGINOSIS IN SELECTED CLINIC POPULATIONS	
Population	**Prevalence (%)**
STD clinics	12.3–37*
	10.7–64†
Commercial sex workers	23*
Juvenile detention center	26*
Adolescents	15.5*
Abortion clinics	29*
	26.9‡
Family planning clinics	23*
	26.8–27.2†
	11–22.6‡
	5.6§
	9.5*
Gynecology clinics	5.6–13*
	12.2–32.2‡
	41†
Antenatal clinics	6–32‡

*Symptoms not described.
†Symptomatic.
‡Both symptomatic and asymptomatic.
§Asymptomatic.

followed for 4 to 9 years after successful treatment.[61, 63, 93, 97] Bacterial vaginosis also may appear to resolve spontaneously; Bump and colleagues[81] reported that only 36% of untreated women continued to have clue cells on examination at a 6-month follow-up visit.

Follow-up among nonpregnant women who were treated successfully demonstrates recurrent episodes of bacterial vaginosis among 30% to 40% of women within 3 months of oral metronidazole therapy.[105, 107] Prolonged follow-up of 44 Swedish women, followed continuously from 4.7 to 9 years after initial successful treatment for bacterial vaginosis, demonstrated recurrent bacterial vaginosis among 50% of patients.[63] Most recurrences (73% to 94%) occurred within the first year of follow-up.[63] Women who did not relapse within the first year following treatment were less likely to have subsequent episodes of bacterial vaginosis over the follow-up period.[63]

Individual factors that predispose to acquisition, persistence, resolution, and/or recurrence of bacterial vaginosis, continue to be studied. As noted, Eschenbach, Hillier, and their colleagues[59, 60] determined that the absence of H_2O_2-producing lactobacilli increased the likelihood of developing bacterial vaginosis in pregnancy. Among nonpregnant women, the absence of H_2O_2-producing lactobacilli, douching, and a new sexual partner all are independent risk factors for the acquisition of bacterial vaginosis.[58, 61] However, Boris and co-workers[63] found no association between recovery of H_2O_2-producing lactobacilli and recurrence of bacterial vaginosis. H_2O_2-producing lactobacilli were recovered from approximately 40% of women with and without relapsing bacterial vaginosis. Recurrent episodes of bacterial vaginosis were most often associated with the introduction of a new sexual partner.[63] Cook and colleagues[105] suggest that a number of individuals with bacterial vaginosis appear to be unable to reestablish a normal vaginal ecosystem following treatment. Cook and Sobel[105, 108] further suggest that the persistence of at least one abnormal microbiologic or vaginal fluid biochemical factor predicts the likelihood of frequent recurrence of bacterial vaginosis among nonpregnant women.

Tao and Pavlova and Mou and co-workers[109-111] introduced the idea of, and preliminary evidence supporting, a role for Lactobacillus-specific lytic bacteriophages causing the microbial shift that characterizes bacterial vaginosis. They demonstrated increased recovery of bacteriophages from women with bacterial vaginosis compared with women with normal vaginal flora.[109] In vitro studies demonstrate lysis of vaginal lactobacilli by these bacteriophages. They also showed that tobacco-associated chemicals, antibiotics, and nonoxynol 9 can increase concentrations of lytic phages in culture and therefore may lead to increased killing of protective vaginal lactobacilli.[110, 111] The acquisition and persistence of lytic bacteriophages is an intriguing explanation for how bacterial vaginosis becomes established and one that can also account for recurrent episodes. The absence of "healthy" lactobacilli due to persistence of lytic Lactobacillus bacteriophages may account for some cases of persistent and recurrent bacterial vaginosis. New treatment regimens may include probiotic treatment with "healthy" lactobacilli after completion of antimicrobial therapy, in order to foster reestablishment of a self-generating protective vaginal microecology.

GYNECOLOGIC COMPLICATIONS

Rapidly increasing knowledge shows that bacterial vaginosis is related to considerable, and possibly preventable, infectious morbidity in nonpregnant women. The sequelae of bacterial vaginosis now include endometritis, pelvic inflammatory disease, post–surgical abortion infections, posthysterectomy infection, increased risk of human immunodeficiency virus (HIV) acquisition, and, possibly, cervical intraepithelial neoplasia (Table 19–2).[4-8, 112-117]

Pelvic Inflammatory Disease

Constituents of bacterial vaginosis including anaerobic bacteria (i.e., *Bacteroides* spp., *Prevotella* spp., and *Pepto-*

TABLE 19–2 ▶ GYNECOLOGIC COMPLICATIONS ASSOCIATED WITH PRESENCE OF BACTERIAL VAGINOSIS

Gynecologic Complications	Risk Ratio	95% Confidence Intervals	Reference
Pelvic inflammatory disease	7.5	ND	Paavonen et al[4]
	19.6*	ND	Eschenbach et al[3]
Postabortion PID	3.7	(1.1–12.1)	Larsson et al[6]
Posthysterectomy cuff cellulitis	3.2		Soper et al[5]
	6.2	(1.5–6.7)	Larsson et al[129]
	3.0	(1.3–30.7)	Persson et al[129a]
Histologic endometritis	15	(2–686)	Korn et al[128]
Abnormal uterine bleeding	3.8	(1.8–8.2)	Wolner-Hanssen et al[123]
Cervical intraepithelial neoplasia	7.2	(3.7–14.0)	Platz-Christensen et al[117]

*Case Control Study: Bacterial vaginosis was present among 25.5% of cases and one of the control subjects.

streptococcus spp.) and *M. hominis* are associated with laparoscopically confirmed nonchlamydial, nongonococcal pelvic inflammatory disease (endometritis, salpingitis, peritonitis).[4, 112–115] In a uniquely detailed cross-sectional study of the microbiology of acute salpingitis, Soper and colleagues[114] identified vaginal fluid Gram stain findings of bacterial vaginosis among 61.8% of women with laparoscopically confirmed pelvic inflammatory disease. Paavonen and co-workers[4] examined vaginal wash specimens for volatile fatty acids and identified a profile consistent with bacterial vaginosis among 9 of 35 (25.5%) women with acute salpingitis or histologic endometritis. Importantly, women with pelvic inflammatory disease were 7.5 times more likely to have bacterial vaginosis compared with women who did not have pelvic inflammatory disease. Subsequently, in a cross-sectional study of 661 women attending a Seattle STD clinic, clinical signs of upper genital tract infection were present among approximately 4% of women with Gram stain findings of bacterial vaginosis and 1% of women without bacterial vaginosis.[3] Controlling for co-infection with *N. gonorrhoeae,* and *C. trachomatis,* women with bacterial vaginosis were 9.2 times more likely to have adnexal tenderness compared with women who did not have bacterial vaginosis.[3]

Conversely, Faro and colleagues[118] studied 41 women with clinical pelvic inflammatory disease and concluded that bacterial vaginosis could not be assigned a role in the development of pelvic inflammatory disease. Most of the subjects in Faro's series were infected with *N. gonorrhoeae* and/or *C. trachomatis.* However, endometrial cultures yielded *M. hominis* from 63.4% of women, *G. vaginalis* from 36.6%, *U. urealyticum* from 31.7%, and *P. bivia* from 21.9% of studied women. All these microorganisms are characteristic of bacterial vaginosis. Authorities now recommend routine empirical therapy for bacterial vaginosis–associated anaerobes during the treatment of pelvic inflammatory disease.[119]

Abnormal Bleeding and Endometritis

Abnormal reproductive tract bleeding (e.g., metrorrhagia or menometrorrhagia) occurs among 40% to 60% of women with clinically recognized pelvic inflammatory disease and is considered indicative of endometrial infection.[120–123] Abnormal reproductive tract bleeding may be the only sign of endometritis.[124] Histologic findings of endometritis have been reported among 3% to 10% of women being evaluated for irregular bleeding.[125] Such abnormal bleeding is thought to result (1) from impaired responsiveness of the infected endometrium to ovarian hormones, or (2) from direct physical disruption of the endometrium due to infection and inflammation.[123]

Both circumstantial and direct evidence link bacterial vaginosis and endometritis. A case series in which *G. vaginalis* was recovered in pure culture from the uterine cavity of three patients who underwent hysterectomy for persistent irregular bleeding initially suggested a link between bacterial vaginosis and abnormal bleeding.[126] Work by Wolner-Hanssen and co-workers[123] identified bacterial vaginosis 3.8 times more often among women not using oral contraceptives who were examined for menorrhagia (hypermenorrhea) compared with women who did not report this complaint. Two studies by Larsson and co-workers[7, 127] demonstrate resolution of metrorrhagia following successful treatment of bacterial vaginosis and *Mobiluncus* spp. infection with oral metronidazole.

Most recently, work from Korn and colleagues[128] supports the association between bacterial vaginosis and upper genital tract infection. Women attending an urban STD clinic for complaints of vaginal discharge were examined for histologic plasma cell endometritis. Among the 60 women with symptomatic vaginal complaints, 36.7% (n = 22) were found to have Gram stain finding of bacterial vaginosis without microbiologic findings of *N. gonorrhoeae,* or *C. trachomatis,* or clinical evidence of upper genital tract tenderness. Pipelle biopsy detected plasma cell endometritis among 45% of bacterial vaginosis–positive women.[128]

Postoperative Infections Following Gynecologic Surgery

Bacterial vaginosis has been shown to significantly increase the risk of postsurgical infection up to four times among women undergoing pregnancy termination and three to six times among women having abdominal hysterectomy.[5, 6, 129] Larsson and co-workers[130] further demonstrated that effective treatment of bacterial vaginosis prior to pregnancy termination significantly reduced the risk of postoperative pelvic inflammatory disease by 70%. Preoperative examination and treatment of bacterial vaginosis could effectively reduce the occurrence of costly postoperative infections following other gynecologic surgical procedures.

Cervical Cancer

Bacterial vaginosis has been suggested as a potential co-factor in the pathogenesis and progression of cervical intraepithelial neoplasia, based largely on epidemiologic associations and theoretical biochemical mechanisms.[131] Early information identified bacterial vaginosis more frequently among women with Papanicolaou (Pap) smears classified as cervical intraepithelial neoplasia (grades I to III).[132] Subsequently, two separate studies evaluated women using colposcopy and endocervical canal cytology as well as Pap smears, or Pap smears and human papillomavirus testing, and found no association between bacterial vaginosis and cervical intraepithelial neoplasia.[133, 134] Further large,

TABLE 19-3 ▶ EXPANDED DISEASE BURDENS AND CLINICAL CONSEQUENCES OF ASYMPTOMATIC AND SYMPTOMATIC BACTERIAL VAGINOSIS (BV)

I. Pregnancy
  A. First-trimester loss
  B. Second-trimester loss
  C. Preterm birth
  D. Intra-amniotic fluid infection (IAI), chorioamnionitis, placentitis
  E. Puerperal infection
  F. Postcesarean wound infection or endometritis
  G. Newborn colonization, genital mycoplasmas
  H. Possible periventricular leukomalacia (PVL), cerebral palsy (CP)
  I. Possible scalp electrode abscess
II. Nonpregnancy
  A. Endometritis
  B. Salpingitis
  C. Presumed infertility, subfertility
  D. Postoperative pelvic infection after termination
  E. Hysterectomy febrile morbidity
  F. Increased susceptibility to sexual HIV transmission
  G. Abnormal cervical cytology (ASCUS, etc.), possible susceptibility to cervical neoplasia

ASCUS = atypical squamous cells of uncertain significance.

well-designed studies are required for the evaluation of the relationship between bacterial vaginosis and cervical intraepithelial neoplasia.

Transmission of HIV Infection

A number of genital tract infections, which presumably alter the integrity of the reproductive tract mucosa, are known to increase the risk of heterosexual HIV transmission.[135] Initially, bacterial vaginosis was also considered a potential risk factor for increased HIV transmission because of the elevated vaginal pH and other biochemical properties thought to impair host defense mechanisms. HIV and lymphocytes are inactivated at low pH levels, such as those found in the healthy vagina.[135] Conversely, as pH increases, survival of HIV increases, and transmission may be favored.[135] The link between bacterial vaginosis and an increased risk of HIV infection is further suggested by Saracco's finding[136] of a 30% (95% CI, 0.3 to 5.8) increased risk of seroconversion among female partners of HIV-infected men with a history of prior "vaginitis" and by a cross-sectional study in Thailand[116] demonstrating an increased likelihood of HIV infection among commercial sex workers with bacterial vaginosis (odds ratio [OR], 2.7; 95% CI, 1.3 to 5.0). Most recently, Sewankambo's findings[137] from a cross-sectional, population-based study of HIV risk factors in rural Uganda demonstrate an increased likelihood of HIV seropositivity among women with increasingly abnormal vaginal flora. The odds ratio of HIV infection increased from 1.5 (95% CI, 1.18 to 1.89) for bacterial vaginosis

Gram stain scores of 7 to 8, to 2.08 (95% CI, 1.48 to 2.94) for bacterial vaginosis scores of 9 to 10.[137]

OBSTETRIC COMPLICATIONS

Many studies from diverse areas of the world link bacterial vaginosis directly to a number of obstetric complications. These include second-trimester pregnancy loss, preterm birth, preterm labor, preterm premature rupture of membranes, amniotic fluid infection, postpartum endometritis, and postcesarean wound infections (Table 19-3).[8-21, 23-26, 46, 138-141] Bacterial vaginosis represents a potentially preventable cause of common and costly adverse obstetric outcomes.

Preterm Birth

Bacterial vaginosis is a well-documented risk factor for preterm birth. Numerous case-control, cross-sectional, prospective cohort studies, and randomized controlled treatment trials, demonstrate an increased risk of preterm labor, preterm premature rupture of membranes, and preterm birth in the presence of bacterial vaginosis (Tables 19-4 and 19-5).[8-21, 23-26, 46, 137a-418] Of great importance, bacterial vaginosis and associated microorganisms appear to increase the risk of preterm birth at the lowest viable gestational ages.[13] This finding is

TABLE 19-4 ▶ PROSPECTIVE STUDIES OF PRETERM BIRTH, PRETERM PREMATURE RUPTURE OF MEMBRANES, AND PRETERM LABOR

Outcome	Study	Weeks of Gestation at Enrollment	Relative Risk (95% CI)
Preterm birth	Minkoff et al[87]		
	Kurki et al[15]	13 (mean)	2.3 (1.0–5.5)
	Hay et al[16]	8–17	7.3 (1.8–29.4)
	Fischbach et al[16a]	<16	5.3 (2.0–13.5)
	Joesoef et al[17]	16–26	5.6 (ND)
	McGregor et al[46]	16–20	2.0 (1.0–3.9)
	McGregor et al[49]	16–26	3.3 (1.2–9.1)
	Hay et al[16]	20–34	3.2 (1.1–9.6)
	McDonald et al[14]	<24	3.3 (1.5–7.4)
	Hauth et al[25]	22–28	1.8 (1.0–3.2)
	Hillier et al[18]	22.9	1.6 (1.3–2.0)
	Meis et al[89]	23–26	1.4 (1.2–1.7)
	Meis et al[89]	24	1.4 (0.9–2.0)
	Meis et al[89]	28	1.8 (1.2–3.0)
	McGregor et al[12]	26–30	NS
	Joesoef et al[17]	28–32	1.5 (0.7–3.0)
Preterm PROM	Kurki et al[15]	8–17	6.9 (2.5–18.8)
	Minkoff et al[87]	13 (mean)	1.5 (0.9–2.6)
	McGregor et al[46]	16–26	5.7 (0.9–36.1)
	Hillier et al[18]	23–26	1.1 (0.8–1.6)
	McDonald et al[14]	22–28	2.7 (1.1–6.5)
	Gravett et al[10]	32 (mean)	
Preterm labor	Minkoff et al[87]	13 (mean)	1.5 (0.8–2.8)
	Gravett et al[9, 10]	32 (mean)	2.2 (1.3–3.8)
	McGregor et al[12]	24 (mean)	2.6 (1.1–6.5)
	Kurki et al[15]	8–17	2.6 (1.3–4.9)
	McGregor et al[46]	16–26	1.5 (0.8–2.6)

CI = confidence interval; ND = not done.

TABLE 19-5 ▶ SUMMARY OF CONTROLLED TREATMENT TRIALS FOR PREVENTING BACTERIAL VAGINOSIS–ASSOCIATED COMPLICATIONS

Patients	Outcome	Treated (%)	Control (%)	Relative Risk (95% CI)	Reference
Oral Antibiotic Treatments					
Unselected antenatal patients	Preterm birth	9.8	18.8	0.52 (0.3–0.9)	McGregor et al[24]
	Preterm labor	1.8	8.8	0.2 (0.1–0.7)	McGregor et al[24]
	Preterm PROM	3.5	6.9	0.5 (0.2–1.4)	McGregor et al[24]
	Preterm birth	4.9	6.1	0.79 (0.4–1.5)	McDonald et al[26]
	Preterm PROM	3.1	3.6	0.87 (0.37–2.02)	McDonald et al[26]
Selected patients					
Prior preterm birth	Preterm birth	18	39	0.4 (0.2–0.8)	Morales et al[23]
	Preterm PROM	5	33	0.14 (0.03–0.6)	Morales et al[23]
Prior preterm birth	Preterm birth	9.1	41.7	0.14 (0.01–0.84)	McDonald et al[26]
Prior preterm birth	Preterm birth	39	57	0.67 (0.5–0.91)	Hauth et al[25]
Maternal weight <50 kg	Preterm birth	14	33	0.42 (0.18–1.0)	Hauth et al[25]
Surgical abortion	Postabortion PID	3.6	12.2	0.3 (0.1–1.0)	Larsson et al[22]
Intravaginal Antibiotic Treatments					
Unselected patients	Preterm birth	15	7.2	2.0 (0.7–5.8)	McGregor et al[46]
	Preterm PROM	5	4.4	1.1 (0.2–5.4)	McGregor et al[46]
	Preterm labor	21.7	14.5	1.5 (0.7–3.2)	McGregor et al[46]
	Preterm birth	15	13.5	1.1 (0.7–1.7)	Joesoef et al[140]

PID = pelvic inflammatory disease; PROM = premature rupture of membranes.

further supported by recent information that documents associations between second-trimester, previable pregnancy loss and bacterial vaginosis.[16, 141]

Eschenbach, Gravett and colleagues[8–11] were the first to implicate bacterial vaginosis as a risk factor for preterm labor and low birthweight. The presence of bacterial vaginosis was identified with the use of gas-liquid chromatography among 19% of women in mid-third trimester (mean 32.6 weeks) and was associated with an increased risk for preterm labor (OR, 2.0; 95% CI, 1.1 to 3.5) and preterm premature rupture of membranes (OR, 2.0; 95% CI, 1.1 to 3.7).[9] McDonald and colleagues[14] examined bacterial vaginosis (culture for high-grade colonization with *G. vaginalis*) earlier in gestation (22 to 28 weeks) and demonstrated similar risks for preterm birth following labor (OR, 1.8) and preterm premature rupture of membranes (OR, 2.7). Work by McGregor and colleagues[24] demonstrated that 22% of preterm births in their inner-city population were attributable to bacterial vaginosis. The largest, prospective U.S. study examined 10,397 parturients and detected bacterial vaginosis among 16% of studied women between 23 and 26 weeks of gestation. The presence of bacterial vaginosis was associated with a 40% increase in risk (95% CI, 1.1 to 1.8) of delivering a preterm–low-birth-weight infant (born before 37 weeks of gestation and weighing less than 2,500 g).[18]

The strongest association between bacterial vaginosis and preterm birth is found in studies that examine for bacterial vaginosis at the earliest points of gestation and carefully control for intervening antimicrobial treatment. Among a large cohort of Finnish women examined for bacterial vaginosis between 8 and 17 weeks of gestation and followed prospectively without treatment, the risks of preterm birth (OR = 6.9),

preterm premature rupture of membranes (OR = 7.3), and preterm labor (OR = 2.6) were significantly increased.[15] Similar high risks of preterm birth are reported by Hay[16] for British women with Gram stain findings of bacterial vaginosis prior to 16 weeks of gestation (calculated from data provided, RR 5.2; 95% CI, 2.0 to 13.5).

The presence of bacterial vaginosis early in pregnancy may determine risks of subsequent adverse effects. In an innovative analysis, Joesoef and colleagues[17] noted that women with findings of bacterial vaginosis at 16 to 20 weeks of gestation were at increased risk for preterm birth, even if their conditions spontaneously resolved and they no longer had findings of bacterial vaginosis at the later follow-up visit (20.5% preterm birth among women with bacterial vaginosis at both visits, and 20.5% preterm birth among women with bacterial vaginosis only at the first visit vs. 11.8% preterm birth among women without bacterial vaginosis). Conversely, the 7% of women who developed bacterial vaginosis between the screening intervals (i.e., those negative at 16 to 20 weeks of gestation and positive at 28 to 32 weeks of gestation) were not at increased risk for preterm birth (10.7% preterm birth among women developing bacterial vaginosis vs. 11.8% among women never positive for bacterial vaginosis; calculated OR, 0.9). These authors concluded that "only bacterial vaginosis in early pregnancy plays a major role as a risk factor for preterm delivery."[17] Most recently, Gratacos and co-workers[142] noted similarly that Swedish women who resolve bacterial vaginosis spontaneously continue to have high rates of preterm birth. These findings suggest that physiologic processes present or initiated at, or prior to, 16 to 20 weeks of gestation are important for the subsequent development of preterm birth.

Conversely, Meis and colleagues[89] reported the greatest bacterial vaginosis–associated increase in risk for preterm birth (defined as birth <35 weeks of gestation) among women who developed bacterial vaginosis between screenings at 22 to 24 weeks of gestation and 26 to 29 weeks of gestation (OR, 2.53; 95% CI, 1.3 to 4.8). Although these authors discussed the information that women who received "antibiotics" between the first and second screening visits tended to have a lower risk of preterm birth (OR, 0.44; 95% CI, 0.11 to 1.9), the risk of preterm birth among untreated women with bacterial vaginosis is not presented separately.[89] Effective intervening antimicrobial treatment and/or population differences may account for these conflicting results.

Antimicrobial Treatment Trials for the Prevention of Preterm Birth

Most importantly, several recent, well-controlled treatment trials for preventing preterm birth demonstrate reductions in the rate of preterm birth among women with asymptomatic bacterial vaginosis during pregnancy (see Table 19–4).[23–26] McGregor and colleagues[24] identified bacterial vaginosis using standard clinical criteria among 32% of inner-city pregnant women. The risk of preterm birth was reduced by 50% among women with bacterial vaginosis who received oral clindamycin treatment (300 mg twice daily for 1 week) compared with untreated observational control subjects.[24] McDonald and colleagues[26] similarly examined all women attending prenatal care for bacterial vaginosis and randomized consenting women with positive findings to receive oral metronidazole (400 mg twice daily for 2 days) or oral placebo. Subset analysis, which excluded women with preterm birth due to obstetric or maternal indications and evaluated those who took the medication, indicated a 21% (RR, 0.79; 95% CI, 0.4 to 1.5) reduction in preterm birth among treated women.[26] Similarly, among women with spontaneous preterm birth who had had a prior preterm birth, metronidazole treatment reduced the risk of preterm birth by 86% (RR, 0.14; 95% CI, 0.01 to 0.84).[26] These findings confirm prior work by Morales and coworkers[23] demonstrating a nearly 60% reduction in spontaneous preterm birth (RR, 0.41; 95% CI, 0.2 to 0.8) among treated U.S. women with bacterial vaginosis and prior preterm birth compared with those receiving placebo. Strong confirmatory evidence that treatment of bacterial vaginosis reduces the risk of preterm birth comes from a large study designed to evaluate the benefits of prophylactic metronidazole and erythromycin versus dual placebos among women considered at increased risk for preterm birth because of a prior preterm birth or because of low maternal weight.[25] In the total study group, antimicrobial treatment was associated with a 28% reduction in the risk of preterm birth (RR, 0.71; 95% CI, 0.56 to 0.9). Subgroup analysis revealed that the benefit from antimicrobial treatment occurred only among women with bacterial vaginosis. Women with bacterial vaginosis achieved a 40% reduction (RR, 0.6; 95% CI, 0.5 to 0.9) in the rate of preterm birth from antimicrobial treatment compared to women given placebos.[25]

The route and timing of treatment are important factors in preventing bacterial vaginosis–associated preterm birth. In contrast to studies that used oral antimicrobial agents, preterm birth was not reduced among women with bacterial vaginosis who received 2% clindamycin vaginal cream between 16 and 26 weeks of gestation in two randomized, placebo-controlled trials despite apparently adequate treatment of bacterial vaginosis.[46, 140] Indeed, data suggest that the outcomes of women treated with active intravaginal drug tended to have higher rates of preterm births (15%) than those of women receiving placebo (7.2% to 13.5%).[46, 140] Several reasons are suggested to explain why relatively late-gestation intravaginal treatment might not be effective in preventing preterm birth: (1) bacterial vaginosis–associated, susceptible microorganisms may already be present within the decidual tissues, and systemic treatment is required for effective eradication and reduction in the risk of preterm birth; (2) women receiving placebo may be more likely to continue to have bacterial vaginosis and have this condition detected by their careproviders and, thus, receive oral antimicrobial therapy; and (3) a transient increase in the recovery of *Escherichia coli* and *Enterococcus* spp. following intravaginal clindamycin treatment may increase risk of preterm birth.[46, 140, 143]

Taken together, these findings support the idea that screening for and standard oral treatments of bacterial vaginosis can prevent significant numbers of preterm births mediated by bacterial vaginosis. Conversely, midgestational antenatal intravaginal treatment does not appear to prevent bacterial vaginosis–associated preterm birth.

There remain important questions whose answers will refine recommendations regarding screening and therapy for bacterial vaginosis as a means of preventing preterm birth. These issues include (1) the timing and type of treatment in women diagnosed with bacterial vaginosis in early pregnancy or in women preparing for pregnancy, (2) the most appropriate intervals for follow-up, (3) mechanisms of beneficial effect, and (4) cost accounting of preventing preterm birth and short- and long-term related morbidity and costs. Despite these unanswered questions, considerable knowledge demonstrates that important benefits for women, babies, and families can be obtained by routine screening for and (oral) treatment of bacterial vaginosis during pregnancy.

Intrapartum and Postpartum Infections

Other bacterial vaginosis–associated complications may be avoided by treating bacterial vaginosis during or prior to pregnancy. Bacterial vaginosis has been linked with clinical amniotic fluid infection as well as postpartum endometritis.[19, 20, 144, 145] The microorganisms recovered from women with these complications often include the common constituents of bacterial vaginosis; that is, *Prevotella bivia, G. vaginalis, M. hominis,* and *Peptostreptococcus* spp.[144, 145] Clinical studies have examined bacterial vaginosis, identified by either Gram stain or gas-liquid chromatography, and have shown that women with clinical amniotic fluid infection more commonly have findings of bacterial vaginosis compared with women who do not have clinical infection.[10, 20, 21] Among the 286 (2.4%) women from the Vaginal Infections and Prematurity Study who developed amniotic fluid infection, antenatal carriage (23 to 26 weeks of gestation) of bacterial vaginosis (RR = 1.5; 95% CI, 1.2 to 2.2) and bacterial vaginosis–associated microorganisms were significantly associated with amniotic fluid infection.[144] This increase in the risk of amniotic fluid infection associated with bacterial vaginosis was independent of other commonly associated factors.[144]

Postpartum endometritis occurs following 2% to 5% of vaginal births and 10% to 20% of cesarean deliveries. More than 80% of cases are polymicrobial in nature.[145] In a series of 161 women with postpartum endometritis described by Watts and colleagues,[145] the common constituents of bacterial vaginosis (i.e., *G. vaginalis, P. bivia, Peptostreptococcus* spp., and *Bacteroides* spp.) were recovered from endometrial cultures in as many as 60% of women. Wound infections developed among 18% (16 of 79) of women with endometrial bacterial vaginosis–associated flora and among 8% (4 of 53) of women with other bacteria recovered from the endometrium.[145] Watts demonstrated a 5.8-fold increased risk of postcesarean section endometritis among women with bacterial vaginosis.[145] Treatment of bacterial vaginosis prior to birth may reduce the risks of postdelivery febrile morbidity and wound infections.

Diagnosis

The diagnosis of bacterial vaginosis is complicated by the polymicrobial nature of the condition. Culture for single microorganisms such as *G. vaginalis* does not provide an accurate diagnosis of the clinical condition.[3, 34] Currently, the clinical "gold standard" for the diagnosis of bacterial vaginosis is based on the observation of three of the four following clinical criteria:

1. Homogeneous, thin, adherent gray-white discharge
2. Vaginal fluid pH > 4.5
3. Release of amine odor, with alkalinization of vaginal fluid, the "whiff test"
4. Presence of vaginal epithelial cells with borders obscured with adherent, small bacteria called "clue" cells

Increased pH (>4.5) is the most sensitive but least specific of these clinical criteria. Normal vaginal pH ranges between 3.8 and 4.2 during the years from menarche through menopause.[34] Some clinicians recommend routine screening for bacterial vaginosis with the use of pH paper (easy to use, inexpensive) and then the performance of further tests of choice if the pH is greater than 4.5. Identification of pH over 4.5 is generally considered the best discriminator for distinguishing between bacterial vaginosis and the normal vaginal ecosystem.[34] Elevated pH is highly sensitive (92%) for the diagnosis of bacterial vaginosis, but it is not specific (62%).[3, 34, 146] Other factors commonly present in the vagina, such as semen, cervical mucus, menses, other infectious agents, and, possibly, recent douching fluids, also may increase pH. Samples for examination of vaginal fluid pH should be obtained from the lateral vaginal side wall or posterior fornices. Only pH indicator paper that allows distinction between the normal vaginal pH (3.8 to 4.2) and pH over 4.5 should be used. Do not use Nitrazine paper, which detects pH around 7.0.

The presence of "clue" cells on saline wet-mount examination is the most specific and sensitive indicator of bacterial vaginosis. Microscopic examination of a saline wet-mount preparation of vaginal fluid is essential for the accurate clinical assessment of bacterial vaginosis. The identification of clue cells accurately predicts 85% to 90% of women with clinical bacterial vaginosis (positive predictive value).[146]

Clue cells, with their characteristic stippled and ragged appearance (Fig. 19–2), may be distinguished from normal vaginal epithelial cells, whose cell borders are distinct and clearly seen (Fig. 19–3). Observation of the background bacterial flora aids in the identification of bacterial vaginosis.[146, 147] When bacterial vaginosis is present, background bacterial flora appears greatly increased in number, and short rods and coccobacillary forms predominate. In addition, the characteristic long rods, or normal *Lactobacillus* morphotypes, are absent or rare. *Mobiluncus* spp. may be identified by their characteristic spiral or serpent-like motility.[147]

The characteristic unpleasant, "fishy" or sharp, odor distinctive of bacterial vaginosis results from release of volatile amines (e.g., putrescine, cadaverine, and trimethylamine) by alkalinization of vaginal fluid.[43] This odor also may be released by agents that raise the vaginal pH, such as semen and menstrual fluid. Addition of a drop of potassium hydroxide to vaginal fluid volitalizes amines and yields a sharp or fishy amine odor. The presence of an amine odor is highly

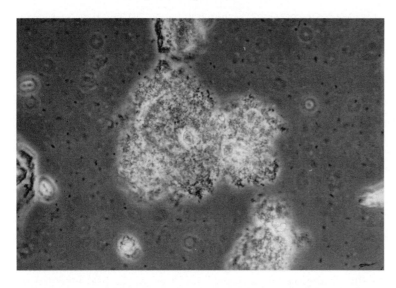

FIGURE 19-2 ▶ Clue cells.

predictive of bacterial vaginosis (positive predictive value 94%).[146, 148] However, putrescine is also present in semen, and other anaerobic infections may result in positive amine tests.[43] In addition, release of odor is the least sensitive (84%) of the criteria; therefore, the absence of odor does not negate the presence of bacterial vaginosis.[3]

The characterization of vaginal fluid as increased, thin, "milky," homogeneous, and adherent is the most subjective indicator of bacterial vaginosis. The quantity of vaginal fluid often differs and may range from scant, to moderate, to profuse. In addition, vaginal fluid may appear "frothy" in as many as 27% of women with bacterial vaginosis.[29] Owing to low sensitivity (52%) and specificity (71%), characterization of vaginal fluid should be used only in conjunction with other clinical diagnostic criteria, and not as the sole indicator of bacterial vaginosis.[146] This stipulation is especially true in pregnancy, when the normal leukorrhea of pregnancy may interfere with the recognition of bacterial vaginosis–associated vaginal fluid.

Laboratory-Based Diagnostic Tests

Several diagnostic strategies and tests have been developed to provide the clinician with more objective means of detecting bacterial vaginosis. When microscopy is unavailable, the combination of an elevated pH and the release of an amine odor may be used to support a presumptive diagnosis of bacterial vaginosis. A commercially available icon-based test card indicates the presence of pH greater than 4.5 and the presence of trimethylamine (FemExam Testcard [Litmus Concepts, Santa Clara, CA]). A similarly well-evaluated test confirms the diagnosis of bacterial vaginosis, *T. vaginalis* infection, and candidiasis with the use of nucleic acid probes (The Affirm VP III Microbial Identification Test [Becton Dickinson and Company, Sparks, MD]). Bacterial vaginosis is presumptively diagnosed, based on the detection of high concentrations of *G. vaginalis*.[149] This test accurately detected 95% to 97% of women with clinical criteria for bacterial vaginosis (sensitivity) and 71% to 98% of women without bacterial vaginosis.[149, 150]

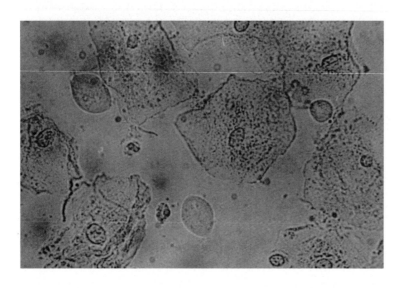

FIGURE 19-3 ▶ Normal vaginal epithelial cells.

Papanicolaou Smear Diagnosis. The sensitivity, specificity, and positive predictive value of Pap smear findings suggestive of bacterial vaginosis can be similar to those of the standard clinical criteria. A possible diagnosis of bacterial vaginosis and trichomoniasis may "add value" to these frequently performed tests.[151]

Platz-Christensen and colleagues[117] reported excellent agreement between Pap smear detection of clue cells and the standard clinical diagnosis of bacterial vaginosis. The sensitivity, specificity, and positive predictive value were 90%, 97%, and 94%, respectively, in this study by Platz-Christensen.[117] However, a vaginal sample from the posterior vaginal fornix is part of routine cytologic screening in this setting, and the vaginal sample was reviewed for clue cells.[117, 152] Davis and co-workers[153] examined Pap smear samples using standard ectocervical and endocervical scrappings and demonstrated low sensitivity (55%), indicating that the diagnosis in large numbers of women with bacterial vaginosis would be missed if Pap smears findings were used for screening. Conversely, standard Pap smear samples that had high specificity (98%) and high positive predictive value (96%) suggested that Pap smears findings of bacterial vaginosis reliably indicate the presence of bacterial vaginosis but do not rule out the condition.[153]

Gram Stain Diagnosis. Bacterial vaginosis is characterized by a shift from predominance of *Lactobacillus* morphotypes to predominance of coccobacillary morphotypes and gram-negative rods. Dunkelberg[154] first examined vaginal fluid Gram stains for the presence of clue cells and adjacent dense bacteria. Spiegel and colleagues[155] reintroduced the idea of Gram stain detection of bacterial vaginosis. Normal fluid is described by a predominance of large gram-positive rods considered *Lactobacillus* morphotypes, with or without smaller gram-variable bacilli considered *Gardnerella* morphotypes (Fig. 19–4).[155] A pattern of mixed vaginal flora that includes *Gardnerella* morphotypes, gram-negative rods, fusiforms curved rods, and gram-positive cocci and absent or reduced numbers of *Lactobacillus* morphotypes (less than 5 per high power field [HPF]) is consistent with bacterial vaginosis (Fig. 19–5).[155] Subsequent work by Nugent, Krohn, and Hillier[156] provides a method of further standardizing Gram stain interpretation for bacterial vaginosis. This technique specifically examines four bacterial morphotypes and assigns a summary score to the vaginal specimen based on the semiquantitative assessment for *Lactobacillus*, *G. vaginalis*, and *Prevotella* spp. morphotypes and *Mobiluncus* spp. morphotypes. A score of 7 to 10 is considered diagnostic of bacterial vaginosis.[156] Compared with other diagnostic methods, this standardized scheme has demonstrated superior reproducibility in comparing examinations by separate individuals and duplicate examinations by the same individual.[157, 158] In addition, comparison of this technique with Amsel's clinical criteria demonstrates a sensitivity of 89% but a specificity of 83%.[159] This finding suggests that standard clinical diagnosis of bacterial vaginosis may miss an important proportion of women with abnormal vaginal flora.[159]

Bacterial Metabolic Byproducts. Measurements of prolineaminopeptidase activity, diamine concentration, and organic acid metabolites have been utilized to diagnose bacterial vaginosis, but these tests are not commercially available.[31, 43, 160]

Microbial Culture. Culture for *G. vaginalis* is an inappropriate means of diagnosing bacterial vaginosis. Comparisons of sensitive culture for *G. vaginalis* with clinical criteria or Gram stain for bacterial vaginosis demonstrate the presence of this microorganism in as many as 60% of women without bacterial vaginosis.[3, 65] Therefore, culture for *G. vaginalis* falsely overestimates up to 60% of healthy women as having bacterial vaginosis.[3, 34, 65] Quantitative aerobic and anaerobic vaginal

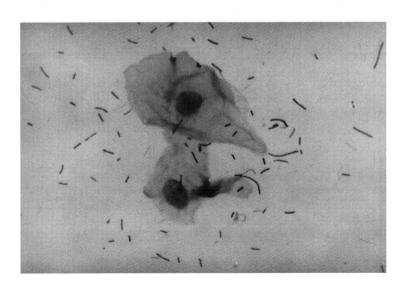

FIGURE 19–4 ▶ Normal vaginal fluid Gram stain.

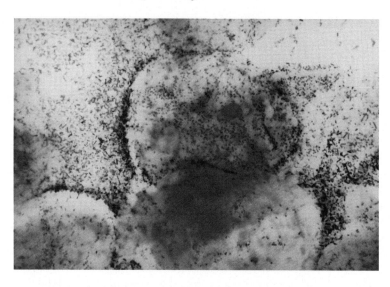

FIGURE 19-5 ▶ Gram stain of bacterial vaginosis.

cultures have been used in clinical research studies to evaluate bacterial vaginosis, but these techniques are expensive and impractical for clinical use.[14, 15]

TREATMENTS

Clinicians and women can choose from many oral or topical treatment regimens that use metronidazole or clindamycin. Efficacy rates reported for the various treatments often differ between studies and reflect primarily population differences or methodologic differences, such as differing diagnostic criteria for bacterial vaginosis, inclusion criteria, and criteria for "cure." Duration of follow-up is probably the most important variable in determining effectiveness. Examinations 1 to 2 weeks following the 1-week treatment courses generally show resolution of bacterial vaginosis among 85% to 100% of women.[161–166] Follow-ups that extend for 4 to 5 weeks after treatment generally show resolution rates that are 25% to 35% lower, or resolution of bacterial vaginosis among 60% and 95% of women (Table 19–6).[161–166] Few studies have followed women for longer intervals of time.

The efficacy of oral metronidazole for the treatment of bacterial vaginosis was demonstrated in 1978 by Pheifer and colleagues;[161] since then a number of different regimens of oral metronidazole have been examined.[161] Oral metronidazole, 500 mg twice daily for 7 days, continues to be the standard therapy recommended by the Centers for Disease Control and Prevention in the United States for the treatment of bacterial vaginosis.[119] Early follow-up "cure" rates with this regimen average above 95%; follow-up that extends longer shows resolution of bacterial vaginosis among approximately 80% of women.[161–168] The use of a single 2-g oral dose of metronidazole is a popular treatment of bacterial vaginosis. Open (nonblinded) treatment trials report 4-week cure rates of approximately 80% (range 68% to 90%).[107, 165–171] Conversely, in three ran-

domized, blinded studies, cure rates at 4 weeks post dosing with a single 2-g dose of metronidazole were 45%, 47%, and 69%.[163, 164, 172] A few authors have examined the efficacy of a 2-g dose of oral metronidazole given on days 1 and 3. Cure rates for this regimen and for single-dose regimens are similar (range 73% to 94%).[107, 161–174] In general, when the single-dose regimens are compared with the standard 7-day regimen in the same populations, cure rates with single 2-g dose of metronidazole are lower.[41, 107]

Clindamycin also is active against anaerobic bacteria, *M. hominis* and *G. vaginalis*. Greaves and co-workers[167] examined 49 women, 7 to 10 days following completion of a 7-day course of oral clindamycin, 300 mg twice daily, and demonstrated a 94% cure rate. McGregor and colleagues[24] examined 194 pregnant women and found a 92% cure rate 2 to 4 weeks post treatment.

Local therapy with either 2% clindamycin vaginal cream or 0.75% metronidazole gel provides high medication levels at the site of the infection and low systemic levels. Clindamycin vaginal cream (2%), used once daily for 7 days, provides a cure for bacterial vaginosis among 72% to 94% of women at 4 to 10 days following treatment and 50% to 75% of women examined at 1 month post treatment.[143, 176–179] Microorganisms associated with bacterial vaginosis (i.e., *G. vaginalis*, *M. hominis*, *Prevotella* spp., and *Peptostreptococcus* spp.) are greatly reduced in numbers, and *Lactobacillus* spp. colonization is greatly increased following treatment with clindamycin vaginal cream, even though clindamycin is also effective against lactobacilli.[143] As previously mentioned, recovery of *Escherichia coli* increased from 13% to 66% of women and that of *Enterococcus* spp. from 0% to 62% of women at 1 week after completing vaginal clindamycin cream treatment. Although *E. coli* colonization did not persist to the 1-month follow-up visit, recovery of *Enterococcus* spp. continued in as many as 50% of women at 1 month following treatment.[143]

TABLE 19-6 ▶ EFFECTIVENESS OF TREATMENT FOR BACTERIAL VAGINOSIS

Antimicrobial	Dose	Follow-Up		
		7 Days (%)	14–21 Days (%)	3–6 Weeks (%)
Metronidazole—oral	2 g × 1 dose			
Blackwell et al[32]		80	—	62
Eschenbach[2]		—	100	58
Swedberg et al[164]		87	47	—
Metronidazole—oral				
Blackwell et al[32]	400 mg bid × 7 days	100	—	60
Nayagam[177a]	400 mg bid × 7 days	56	55	—
McDonald et al[139]	400 mg bid × 2 days	—	—	76
Eschenbach[2]	500 mg bid × 1 day	—	21	—
	500 mg bid × 3 days	—	100	56
	500 mg bid × 5 days	—	92	56
Metronidazole—oral				
Eschenbach[2]	500 mg bid × 7 days	—	100	94
Pheifer et al[161]		99	—	85
Greaves et al[167]		96	—	—
Swedberg et al[164]		—	97	87
Fischbach et al[178]		—	87	81
Anders et al[179]		—	74	71
Schmitt et al[177]		—	87	61
Nayagam[177a]		56	—	55
Covino et al[188]		—	85	—
Morales et al[23]		—	—	89
Ferris et al[187]		—	84	—
Hanson et al[186]		—	85	71
Larsson et al[7]	500 mg tid × 10 days	—	—	76
	750 mg qd × 7 days	—	—	61
Clindamycin—oral				
Greaves et al[167]	300 mg bid × 7 days	94	—	—
McGregor et al[24]	300 mg bid × 7 days	—	—	94
0.75% MetroGel-Vaginal	0.75% bid × 7 days			
Hillier et al[59]		—	87	85
Livengood et al[185]		—	78	68
Ferris et al[187]		—	75	—
Hanson et al[186]		—	84	71
2% Clindamycin vaginal cream	2% qd × 7 days	—	85	84
Fischbach et al[178]		—	91	79
Anders et al[179]		—	94	92
Livengood et al[176]		—	94	94
Hillier[184]		—	72	61
Schmitt et al[177]		77	—	79
Stein[178a]		—	86	85
Joesoef et al[140]		95	—	90
McGregor et al[46]		—	86	—
Ferris et al[187]		—	—	59
Other Antimicrobials				
Pheifer et al[161]	Sulfa cream	14	0	—
Pheifer et al[161]	Ampicillin, 500 mg qid × 7 days	28	—	—
Duff et al[86]	Amoxicillin, 500 mg tid × 14 days	—	59	28
Nayagam[177a]	Ofloxacin, 200 mg bid × 7 days	23	—	—
	Ofloxacin, 300 mg bid × 7 days	—	43	—
Placebo—cream/gel				
Livengood et al[176]	Cream, qd × 7 days	—	25	18
Hillier & Holmes[41]	Cream	—	25	—
Hillier et al[59]	Gel	—	17	9
Livengood et al[185]	Gel	—	27	—
Placebo—oral				
McDonald et al[139]	Oral	—	—	28
Larsson et al[7]	Oral	—	—	5
Morales et al[23]	Oral	—	—	14

Intravaginal metronidazole treatment has been achieved with vaginal tablets (400- or 500-mg tablets) and metronidazole-containing vaginal sponges.[180-183] These preparations currently are not available in the United States. Intravaginal metronidazole gel (0.75%), formulated at a pH of 4.0, is approved within the United States for bacterial vaginosis treatment. Several randomized, double-blind, controlled trials demonstrate equivalent efficacy rates for metronidazole vaginal gel and oral metronidazole or clindamycin vaginal cream. The efficacy of this medication was first documented among symptomatic women, with 78% to 87% cured at 1 to 2 weeks post treatment.[184–187] Four to five weeks post treatment, 69% to 73% of studied women were free from bacterial vaginosis.[184, 185] Hanson and co-workers[186] compared metronidazole vaginal gel with oral metronidazole and again demonstrated equivalent efficacies for the two treatments. Bacterial vaginosis was eliminated by 1 week post treatment among 83.7% (36 of 43) of women randomized to metronidazole vaginal gel and 85.1% (40 of 47) of women randomized to oral metronidazole.[186] Similarly, bacterial vaginosis was absent at 4 weeks post treatment among 70.7% and 71% of women who received intravaginal and oral metronidazole, respectively.[186]

Other treatments of bacterial vaginosis include ampicillin, amoxicillin-clavulanic acid, ofloxacin, and erythromycin, triple sulfa cream, and vaginal acidification.[86, 161, 188, 189] These treatments are less effective than either oral or vaginal preparations of metronidazole or clindamycin and are not recommended.

Despite evidence that suggests that bacterial vaginosis is linked to sexual activity, a number of randomized controlled trials that examined co-treatment of male partners failed to demonstrate reduced recurrence rates of bacterial vaginosis in women.[173, 174]

Treatment During Pregnancy

Cure rates for bacterial vaginosis during pregnancy are similar to those obtained among nonpregnant women. McDonald and colleagues[168] reported that 76% of women were cured of bacterial vaginosis findings 4 weeks following treatment with oral metronidazole. This rate is similar to the 70% resolution of bacterial vaginosis approximately 4 weeks post treatment reported by Hauth and colleagues[25] for women who received metronidazole and erythromycin. Oral treatment with clindamycin may be used throughout pregnancy, including the first trimester, and provides resolution of bacterial vaginosis equivalent to that of oral metronidazole. Two studies, which examined 2% clindamycin vaginal cream, demonstrated cure rates of 85% to 95% at examinations 1 to 2 weeks after treatment.[46, 140] The efficacy of metronidazole vaginal gel has not been examined among pregnant women.

Traditionally, metronidazole has been avoided during early pregnancy, owing to laboratory evidence that the drug is mutagenic in bacteria and oncogenic and teratogenic in selected animal models given high doses. After 30 years of clinical use, carcinogenic effects of metronidazole in humans have not been detected. Similarly, several retrospective studies and a recent meta-analysis have examined the pregnancy outcomes for women who received metronidazole during different stages of pregnancy. No evidence of increased birth defects has been detected.[190, 191]

Adverse Effects from Treatment

An unpleasant metallic taste is the most common complaint after metronidazole treatment, occurring in 35% to 50% of patients.[177] Nausea, vomiting, abdominal pain, headache, and dizziness have also been noted. The incidence of yeast vaginitis following oral metronidazole treatment varies from 5% to 22%.[119, 177, 178]

Among studied women receiving oral treatment with clindamycin, nausea (12%) and yeast vaginitis (8.5% to 24%) were the most common complaints.[24, 167] Complaints of loose stools or diarrhea occurred in similar numbers of women who were receiving oral clindamycin (6.3%) and among women given a single 2-g dose of oral metronidazole (8.8%). Systemic side effects from intravaginal treatments occur less often than among orally treated women, with the exception of yeast vaginitis.[184–187]

Probiotic Treatments

Interest in vaginal infection treatment and vaginal recolonization with *Lactobacillus* preparations has continued throughout this century. Attempts to reestablish normal vaginal "Döderlein's bacillus" with bacterial therapy have been described in the medical literature since 1917.[192–194] Metchnikoff's work promoting ingestion of *Lactobacillus*-containing foods for relief of gastrointestinal problems is credited as the first use of probiotic *Lactobacillus* to restore or maintain health.[192] In a recent randomized, controlled clinical trial, Hallen and co-workers[195] examined twice-daily treatment with H_2O_2-producing *L. acidophilus* intravaginal suppositories versus placebo among 57 Danish women with bacterial vaginosis. Initially, 57% (16 of 28) of treated women appeared successfully treated, but bacterial vaginosis recurred in most subjects after the next menses.[195]

Commercial preparations of *L. acidophilus* are available as powders and capsules as well as live culture in yogurt and acidophilus milk. These preparations have either not been systematically examined for their effectiveness or have been shown not to provide long-term relief from bacterial vaginosis. Studies show that only isolates derived from human sources demonstrated adherence to vaginal epithelial cells, whereas isolates from yogurt demonstrate low adherence.[196] Many non-dairy *Lactobacillus*-containing products are contaminated with potentially harmful bacteria, including *Clostridium sporogenes* and *Enterococcus* spp.[196]

Work continues to develop strains of *Lactobacillus* that can readily adhere to vaginal epithelial cells and establish mucosal colonization. This may lead to reestablishing a persistently "healthy" vaginal microecology. The use of probiotics following or in conjunction with proven antimicrobial agents in the treatment of bacterial vaginosis may increase the chances of long-term cure and reduce recurrences in women with bacterial vaginosis.

CONCLUSION

Bacterial vaginosis is the most common cause of vaginal discharge. Bacterial vaginosis is best understood as a massive expansion of an abnormal "bacterial-vaginosis" set of microorganisms featuring *G. vaginalis*, anaerobes, and genital mycoplasmas. This abnormal "bloom" ("red tide") of microorganisms is associated with vaginal discharge and odor. The clinical consequences of bacterial vaginosis in pregnant women include preterm birth, intra-amniotic infection, and postpartum infections. Bacterial vaginosis is similarly associated with endometritis and salpingitis, as well as post-termination and posthysterectomy infections among nonpregnant women. The presence of bacterial vaginosis also appears to amplify the risk of HIV transmission among exposed women. Authorities now suggest screening and treating bacterial vaginosis routinely prior to and during pregnancy and in reproductive-age women receiving gynecologic care. Care providers now have new evidence-based opportunities, as well as imperatives and obligations, to screen and treat women at risk for serious obstetric and gynecologic sequelae because of bacterial vaginosis.

REFERENCES

1. Thomason JL, Gelbart SM: Bacterial Vaginosis: Current Concepts. Kalamazoo, MI, The Upjohn Company, 1990.
2. Eschenbach DA: Vaginal infection. Clin Obstet Gynecol 1983; 26:186.
3. Eschenbach DA, Hillier SL, Critchlow C, et al: Diagnosis and clinical manifestations of bacterial vaginosis. Am J Obstet Gynecol 1988; 158:819.
4. Paavonen J, Teisala K, Heinonen PK, et al: Microbiological and histopathological findings in acute pelvic inflammatory disease. Br J Obstet Gynaecol 1987; 94:454.
5. Soper DE, Bump RC, Hurt WG: Bacterial vaginosis and trichomoniasis vaginitis are risk factors for cuff cellulitis after abdominal hysterectomy. Am J Obstet Gynecol 1990; 163:1016.
6. Larsson P-G, Bergman B, Försum U, et al: Mobiluncus and clue cells as predictors of pelvic inflammatory disease after first trimester abortion. Acta Obstet Gynecol Scand 1989; 68:217.
7. Larsson P-G, Bergman B, Försum U, Påhlson C: Treatment of bacterial vaginosis in women with vaginal bleeding complications of discharge and harboring *Mobiluncus*. Gynecol Obstet Invest 1990; 29:296.
8. Eschenbach DA, Gravett MG, Chen KCS, et al: Bacterial vaginosis during pregnancy: An association with prematurity and post partum complications. In: Mårdh PA, Taylor-Robinson D (eds): Bacterial Vaginosis Stockholm, Almqvist and Wiksill, 1984, pp. 213–222.
9. Gravett MG, Nelson HP, DeRouen T, et al: Independent associations of bacterial vaginosis and *Chlamydia trachomatis* infection with adverse pregnancy outcome. JAMA 1986; 256:1899.
10. Gravett MG, Hummel D, Eschenbach DA, Holmes KK: Preterm labor associated with subclinical amniotic fluid infection and with bacterial vaginosis. Obstet Gynecol 1986; 67:229.
11. Martius J, Krohn MA, Hillier SL, et al: Relationships of vaginal *Lactobacillus* species, cervical *Chlamydia trachomatis*, and bacterial vaginosis to preterm birth. Obstet Gynecol 1988; 71:89.
12. McGregor JA, French JI, Richter R, et al: Antenatal microbiologic and maternal risk factors associated with prematurity. Am J Obstet Gynecol 1990; 163:1465.
13. Hillier SL, Martius J, Krohn MA, et al: A case-control study of chorioamnionic infection and histologic chorioamnionitis in prematurity N Engl J Med 1988; 319:972.
14. McDonald HM, O'Loughlin JA, Jolley P, et al: Prenatal microbiological risk factors associated with preterm birth. Br J Obstet Gynaecol 1992; 99:190.
15. Kurki T, Sivonen A, Renkonen O-V, et al: Bacterial vaginosis in early pregnancy and pregnancy outcome. Obstet Gynecol 1992; 80:173.
16. Hay PE, Lamont RF, Taylor-Robinson D, et al: Abnormal bacterial colonization of the genital tract and subsequent preterm delivery and late miscarriage. Br Med J 1994; 308:295.
16a. Fischbach F, Kolben M, Thurnay R: Genital infection in the course of pregnancy: A prospective study. Geburtshilfe Favenheilkd 1988; 48:409.
17. Joesoef MR, Hillier SL, Utomon B, et al: Bacterial vaginosis and prematurity in Indonesia: Association in early and late pregnancy. Am J Obstet Gynecol 1993; 169:175.
18. Hillier SL, Nugent RP, Eschenbach DA, et al, for the Vaginal Infections and Prematurity Study Group: Association between bacterial vaginosis and preterm delivery of a low-birth-weight infant. N Engl J Med 1995; 333:1737.
19. Watts DH, Krohn MA, Hillier SL, Eschenbach DA: Bacterial vaginosis as a risk factor for postcesarean endometritis. Obstet Gynecol 1990; 75:52.
20. Silver HM, Sperling RS, St Clair P, Gibbs RS: Evidence relating bacterial vaginosis to intraamniotic infection. Am J Obstet Gynecol 1989; 161:808.
21. Hillier SL, Krohn MA, Cassen E, et al: The role of bacterial vaginosis and vaginal bacteria in amniotic fluid infection in women in preterm labor with intact fetal membranes. Clin Infect Dis 1995; 20(suppl 2):S276.
22. Larsson P-G, Platz-Christensen J-J, Thejls H, et al: Incidence of pelvic inflammatory disease after first-trimester legal abortion in women with bacterial vaginosis after treatment with metronidazole: A double-blind, randomized study. Am J Obstet Gynecol 1992; 166:100.
23. Morales WJ, Schorr S, Albritton J: Effects of metronidazole in patients with preterm birth in preceding pregnancy and bacterial vaginosis: A placebo-controlled, double-blind study. Am J Obstet Gynecol 1994; 171:345.
24. McGregor JA, French JI, Parker R, et al: Prevention of premature birth by screening and treatment for common genital tract infections: Results of a prospective controlled evaluation. Am J Obstet Gynecol 1995; 173:157.
25. Hauth JC, Goldenberg RL, Andrews WW, et al: Reduced incidence of preterm delivery with metronidazole and erythromycin in women with bacterial vaginosis. N Engl J Med 1995; 333:1732.
26. McDonald HM, O'Loughlin JA, Vigneswaran R, et al: Impact of metronidazole therapy on preterm birth in women with bacterial vaginosis flora (*Gardnerella vaginalis*): A randomized, placebo-controlled trial. Br J Obstet Gynaecol 1997; 104:1391.
27. Doderlein A: Das Scheidensekret und seine bedeutung fur das puerperalfieber. Leipzig, O. Durr, 1892.
28. Thomason JL, Gelbart SM, Broekhuizen FF: Advances in the understanding of bacterial vaginosis. J Reprod Med 1989; 34:581.
29. Gardner HL, Dukes CD: *Haemophilus vaginalis* vaginitis. Am J Obstet Gynecol 1955; 69:962.
30. Greenwood JR, Pickett MJ: Transfer of *Haemophilus vaginalis* Gardner and Dukes to a new genus *Gardnerella: G. vaginalis* (Gardner and Dukes) comb. nov. Int J Syst Bacteriol 1980; 30:170.
31. Spiegel CA, Amsel R, Eschenbach D, et al: Anaerobic bacteria in nonspecific vaginitis. N Engl J Med 1980; 303:601.
32. Blackwell AL, Phillips I, Fox AR, Barlow D: Anaerobic vaginosis (non-specific vaginitis): Clinical, microbiological, and therapeutic findings. Lancet 1983; 2:1379.

33. Weström L, Evaldson G, Holmes KK, et al: Taxonomy of vaginosis: Bacterial vaginosis—a definition. In: Mårdh P-A, Taylor-Robinson D (eds): Bacterial Vaginosis. Uppsala, Sweden; Almqvist & Wiksell, 1984, pp 259–260.

34. Amsel R, Totten PA, Spiegel CA, et al: Nonspecific vaginitis: Diagnostic criteria and microbial and epidemiologic associations. Am J Med 1983; 74:14.

35. Sobel JD: Bacterial vaginosis—an ecologic mystery. Ann Intern Med 1989; 111:551.

36. Mårdh P-A: The vaginal ecosystem. Am J Obstet Gynecol 1991; 165:1163.

37. Spiegel CA: Bacterial vaginosis. Clin Microbiol Rev 1991; 4:485.

38. Giorgi A, Torriani S, Dellaglio F, et al: Identification of vaginal lactobacilli from asymptomatic women. Microbiologica 1987; 10:377.

39. Eschenbach DA: Bacterial vaginosis: Emphasis on upper genital tract complications. Obstet Gynecol Clin North Am 1989; 16:593.

40. Paavonen J, Miettinen A, Stevens CE, et al: *Mycoplasma hominis* in nonspecific vaginitis. Sex Transm Dis 1983; 10(suppl):271.

41. Hillier SL, Holmes KK: Bacterial vaginosis. In: Holmes KK, Mårdh P-A, Sparling PF, et al (eds): *Sexually Transmitted Diseases*, 2nd ed. New York, McGraw-Hill Information Services Co. 1990, pp 547–559.

42. Piot P, VanDyke E, Godts P, Vanderheyden J: The vaginal microbial flora in non-specific vaginitis. Eur J Clin Microbiol 1982; 1:301.

43. Chen KCS, Amsel R, Eschenbach DA, Holmes KK: Amine content of vaginal fluid from untreated patients with nonspecific vaginitis. J Clin Invest 1979; 63:828.

44. Pybus V, Onderdonk AB: Evidence for a commensal, symbiotic relationship between *Gardnerella vaginalis* and *Prevotella bivia* involving ammonia: Potential significance for bacterial vaginosis. J Infect Dis 1997; 175:406.

45. Briselden AM, Moncla BJ, Stevens CE, Hillier SL: Sialidases (neuraminidases) in bacterial vaginosis and bacterial-vaginosis—associated microflora. J Clin Microbiol 1992: 30:663.

46. McGregor JA, French JI, Jones W, et al: Bacterial vaginosis is associated with prematurity and vaginal fluid sialidase: Results of a controlled trial of topical clindamycin cream. Am J Obstet Gynecol 1994; 170:1048.

47. Glasson JH, Woods WH: Immunoglobulin proteases in bacteria associated with bacterial vaginosis. Austr J Med Lab Sci 1988; 9:63.

48. McGregor JA, French JI, Jones W, et al: Association of cervico/vaginal infections with increased vaginal fluid phospholipase A_2 activity. Am J Obstet Gynecol 1992; 167:1588.

49. McGregor JA, Lawellin D, Franco-Buff A, Todd JK: Phospholipase C activity in microorganisms associated with reproductive tract infection. Am J Obstet Gynecol 1991; 164:682.

50. McGregor JA, Lawellin D, Franco-Buff A, et al: Protease production by microorganisms associated with reproductive tract infection. Am J Obstet Gynecol 1986; 154:109.

51. Platz-Christensen JJ, Mattsby-Baltzer I, Thomsen P, Wiqvist N: Endotoxin and interleukin-1-α in the cervical mucus and vaginal fluid of pregnant women with bacterial vaginosis. Am J Obstet Gynecol 1993; 169:1161.

52. Platz-Christensen JJ, Brandberg A, Wiqvist N: Increased prostaglandin concentrations in the cervical mucus of pregnant women with bacterial vaginosis. Prostaglandins 1992; 43:133.

53. Redondo-Lopez V, Cook RL, Sobel JD: Emerging role of lactobacilli in the control and maintenance of vaginal bacterial microflora. Rev Infect Dis 1990; 12:856.

54. Eschenbach DA, Davick PR, Williams BL, et al: Prevalence of hydrogen peroxide–producing *Lactobacillus* species in normal women and women with bacterial vaginosis. J Clin Microbiol 1989; 27:251.

55. Paavonen J: Physiology and ecology of the vagina. Scand J Infect Dis 1983; 40:31.

56. Peeters M, Piot P: Adhesion of *Gardnerella vaginalis* to vaginal

epithelial cells: Variables affecting adhesion and inhibition by metronidazole. Genitourin Med 1985; 61:391.

57. Mårdh P-A, Soltesz LV: In vitro interactions between lactobacilli and other microorganisms occurring in the vaginal flora. Scand J Infect Dis 1983; 40(suppl):47.

58. Klebanoff SJ, Hillier SL, Eschenbach DA, Waltersdorph AM: Control of the microbial flora of the vagina by H_2O_2-generating lactobacilli. J Infect Dis 1991; 164:94.

59. Hillier SL, Krohn MA, Rabe LK, et al: The normal vaginal flora, H_2O_2-producing lactobacilli, and bacterial vaginosis in pregnant women. Clin Infect Dis 1993; 16(suppl 4):S273.

60. Hillier SL, Krohn MA, Klebanoff SJ, Eschenbach DA: The relationship of hydrogen peroxide–producing lactobacilli to bacterial vaginosis and genital microflora in pregnant women. Obstet Gynecol 1992; 79:369.

61. Hawes SE, Hillier SL, Benedetti J, et al: Hydrogen peroxide–producing lactobacilli and acquistion of vaginal infections. J Infect Dis 1996; 174:1058.

62. Rosenstein IJ, Fontaine EA, Morgan DJ, et al: Relationship between hydrogen peroxide–producing strains of lactobacilli and vaginosis-associated bacterial species in pregnant women. Eur J Clin Microbiol Infect Dis 1997; 16:517.

63. Boris J, Pahlson C, Larsson P-G: Six years observation after successful treatment of bacterial vaginosis. In Dis Obstet Gynecol 1997; 5(4):297.

64. Hill LH, Ruparelia H, Embil JA: Nonspecific vaginitis and other genital infections in three clinic populations. Sex Transm Dis 1983; 10:114.

65. Krohn MA, Hillier SL, Eschenbach DA: Comparison of methods for diagnosing bacterial vaginosis among pregnant women. J Clin Microbiol 1989; 27:1266.

66. Centers for Disease Control: Nonreported sexually transmissible diseases—United States. MMWR 1979; 28:61.

67. Embree J, Caliando JJ, McCormack WM: Nonspecific vaginitis among women attending a sexually transmitted diseases clinic. Sex Transm Dis 1984; 11:81.

68. Lossick JG: The descriptive epidemiology of vaginal trichomoniasis and bacterial vaginosis. In: Horowitz BJ, Mårdh P-A (eds): Vaginitis and Vaginosis. New York, Wiley-Liss, 1991, pp 77–84.

69. Rosenberg MJ, Davidson AJ, Chen J-H, et al: Barrier contraceptives and sexually transmitted diseases: A comparison of female dependent methods and condoms. Am J Public Health 1992; 82:669.

70. Hart G: Factors associated with trichomoniasis, candidasis, and bacterial vaginosis. Int J STD AIDS 1993; 4:21.

71. Moi H: Epidemiologic aspects of vaginitis and vaginosis in Scandinavia. In: Horowitz BJ, Mårdh P-A (eds): Vaginitis and Vaginosis. New York, Wiley-Liss, 1991, pp 85–91.

72. Hallén A, Påhlsson C, Försum U: Bacterial vaginosis in women attending STD clinic: Diagnostic criteria and prevalence of *Mobiluncus* spp. Genitourin Med 1987; 63:386.

73. Moi H: Prevalence of bacterial vaginosis and its association with genital infections, inflammation, and contraceptive methods in women attending sexually transmitted disease and primary health clinics. J STD AIDS 1990; 1:86.

74. Bell TA, Farrow JA, Stamm WE, et al: Sexually transmitted diseases in females in a juvenile detention center. Sex Transm Dis 1985; 12:140.

75. Hill LVH, Luther ER, Young D, et al: Prevalence of lower genital tract infections in pregnancy. Sex Transm Dis 1988; 15:5.

76. Lefevre JC, Averous S, Bauriaud R, et al: Lower genital tract infections in women: Comparison of clinical and epidemiologic findings with microbiology. Sex Transm Dis 1988; 15:110.

77. Hay PE, Taylor-Robinson D, Lamont RF: Diagnosis of bacterial vaginosis in a gynaecology clinic. Br J Obstet Gynecol 1992; 99:63.

78. Riordan T, Macaulay ME, James JM, et al: A prospective study of genital infections in a family planning clinic. Epidemiol Infect 1990; 104:47.

79. Larsson P-G, Platz-Christensen JJ: Enumeration of clue cells in rehydrated air-dried vaginal wet smears for the diagnosis of bacterial vaginosis. Obstet Gynecol 1990; 76:727.

80. Stevens-Simon C, Jamison J, McGregor JA, Douglas JM: Racial

variations in vaginal pH among healthy sexually active adolescents. Sex Transm Dis 1994; 21:168.

81. Bump RC, Zuspan FP, Buesching WJ, et al: The prevalence, six-month persistence and predictive values of laboratory indicators of bacterial vaginosis (nonspecific vaginitis) in asymptomatic women. Am J Obstet Gynecol 1984; 150:917.

82. Gardner HL, Damper TK, Dukes CD: The prevalence of vaginitis: A study in incidence. Am J Obstet Gynecol 1957; 73:1080.

83. Schmidt H, Hansen JG: A wet smear criterion for bacterial vaginosis. Scand J Prim Health Care 1994; 12:233.

84. Singh V, Gupta MM, Satyanarayana L, et al: Association between reproductive tract infections and cervical inflammatory epithelial changes. Sex Transm Dis 1995; 22:25.

85. Paavonen J, Hienonen PK, Aine R, et al: Prevalence of nonspecific vaginitis and other cervicovaginal infections during the third trimester of pregnancy. Sex Transm Dis 1986; 13:5.

86. Duff P, Lee ML, Hillier SL, et al: Amoxicillin treatment of bacterial vaginosis during pregnancy. Obstet Gynecol 1991; 77:431.

87. Minkoff H, Grunebaum AN, Schwarz RH, et al: Risk factors for prematurity and premature rupture of membranes: A prospective study of the vaginal flora in pregnancy. Am J Obstet Gynecol 1984; 150:965.

88. McGregor JA, French JI, Richter R, et al: Cervicovaginal microflora and pregnancy outcome: Results of a double-blind, placebo-controlled trial of erythromycin treatment. Am J Obstet Gynecol 1990; 163:1580.

89. Meis PJ, Goldenberg RL, Mercer B, et al, and the National Institute of Child Health and Human Development Maternal-Fetal Medicine Units Network: The preterm prediction study: Significance of vaginal infections. Am J Obstet Gynecol 1995; 173:1231.

90. Platz-Chritensen JJ, Pernevi P, Hagmar B, et al: A longitudinal follow-up of bacterial vaginosis during pregnancy. Acta Obstet Gynecol Scand 1993; 72:99.

91. Thorsen P, Jensen IP, Jeune B, et al: An epidemiologic study of bacterial vaginosis in a population of 3600 pregnant women: Am J Obstet Gynecol 1998; 178:580.

92. Hillier SL, Krohn MA, Nugent RP, Gibbs RS, for the Vaginal Infections and Prematurity Study Group: Characteristics of three vaginal flora patterns assessed by Gram stain among pregnant women. Am J Obstet Gynecol 1992; 166:938.

93. Bump RC, Buesching WJ III: Bacterial vaginosis in virginal and sexually active adolescent females: Evidence against exclusive sexual transmission. Am J Obstet Gynecol 1988; 158:935.

94. Goldenberg RL, Iams JD, Mercer BM, et al, and the NICHD MFMU Network: The preterm prediction study: The value of new vs standard risk factors in predicting early and all spontaneous preterm births. Am J Public Health 1998; 88:233.

95. Thomason JL, Gelbart SM, Wilcoski LM, et al: Proline aminopeptidase activity as a rapid diagnostic test to confirm bacterial vaginosis. Obstet Gynecol 1988; 71:607.

96. Holst E, Wathne B, Hovelius B, Mårdh P-A: Bacterial vaginosis: Microbiological and clinical findings. Eur J Clin Microbiol 1987; 6:536.

97. Barbone F, Austin H, Louv WC, Alexander WJ: A follow-up study of methods of contraception, sexual activity, and rates of trichomoniasis, candidiasis and bacterial vaginosis. Am J Obstet Gynecol 1990; 163:510.

98. Hammerschlag MR, Cummings M, Doraiswamy B, et al: Nonspecific vaginitis following sexual abuse in children. Pediatrics 1985; 75:1028.

99. Berger BJ, Kolton S, Zenilman JM, et al: Bacterial vaginosis in lesbians: A sexually transmitted disease. Clin Infect Dis 1995; 21:1402.

100. Keane FE, Thomas BJ, Whitaker L, et al: An association between non-gonococcal urethritis and bacterial vaginosis and the implications for patients and their sexual partners. Genitourin Med 1997; 73:373.

101. Holst E: Reservoir of four organisms associated with bacterial vaginosis suggests lack of sexual transmission. J Clin Microbiol 1990; 28:2035.

102. Piot P, Van Dyck E, Peeters M, et al: Biotypes of *Gardnerella vaginalis*. J Clin Microbiol 1984; 22:677.

103. Vejtorp M, Bollerup AC, Vejtorp L, et al: Bacterial vaginosis: A double-blind randomized trial of the effect of treatment of the sexual partner. Br J Obstet Gynaecol 1988; 95:920.

104. Vutyavanich T, Pongsuthirak P, Vannareumol P, et al: A randomized double-blind trial of tinidazole treatment of the sexual partners of females with bacterial vaginosis. Obstet Gynecol 1993; 82:550.

105. Cook RL, Redondo-Lopez V, Schmitt C, et al: Clinical, microbiological, and biochemical factors in recurrent bacterial vaginosis. J Clin Microbiol 1992; 30:870.

106. Hay PE, Morgan DJ, Ison CA, et al: A longitudinal study of bacterial vaginosis during pregnancy. Br J Obstet Gynecol 1994; 101:1048.

107. Larsson P-G: Treatment of bacterial vaginosis. Int J STD AIDS 1992; 3:239.

108. Sobel JD, Schmitt C, Meriwether C: Long-term follow-up of patients with bacterial vaginosis treated with oral metronidazole and topical clindamycin. J Infect Dis 1993; 167:783.

109. Mou SM, Pavlova SI, Kilic AO, Tao L: Phage infection in vaginal Lactobacilli: An in vitro model. Presented at Infection Disease Society for Obstetricians and Gynecologists annual meeting. Beaver Creek, CO, 1996.

110. Tao L, Pavlova SI, Mou SM, et al: Analysis of *Lactobacillus* products for phages and bacteriocins that inhibit vaginal lactobacilli. Infect Dis Obstet Gynecol 1997; 5(3):244.

111. Tao L, Pavlova SI, Mou SM: Factors affecting phage induction in vaginal lactobacilli. Presented at the 2nd Annual Infectious Disease Society of OB/GYN-USA Meeting. Las Vegas, Nevada, April 25–27, 1997.

112. Mårdh P-A: An overview of infectious agents in salpingitis, their biology, and recent advances in methods of detection. Am J Obstet Gynecol 1980; 138:933.

113. Eschenbach DA, et al: Polymicrobial etiology of acute pelvic inflammatory disease. N Engl J Med 1975; 293:166.

114. Soper DE, Brockwell NJ, Dalton HP, Johnson D: Observations concerning the microbial etiology of acute salpingitis. Am J Obstet Gynecol 1994; 170:1008.

115. Sweet RL: Role of bacterial vaginosis in pelvic inflammatory disease. Clin Infect Dis 1995; 20(suppl 2):S271.

116. Cohen CR, Duerr A, Pruithithada N, et al: Bacterial vaginosis and HIV seroprevalence among female commercial sex workers in Chiang Mai, Thailand. AIDS 1995; 9:1093.

117. Platz-Christensen J-J, Sundström E, Larsson P-G: Bacterial vaginosis and cervical intraepithelial neoplasia. Acta Obstet Gynecol Scand 1994; 73:586.

118. Faro S, Martens M, Maccato M, et al: Vaginal flora and pelvic inflammatory disease. Am J Obstet Gynecol 1993; 169:470.

119. Centers for Disease Control and Prevention: 1998 Guidelines for treatment of sexually transmitted diseases. MMWR 1998; 47(No. RR-1):70.

120. Wolner-Hanssen P, Mårdh P-A, Moller B, Weström L: Endometrial infection in women with chlamydial salpingitis. Sex Transm Dis 1982; 9:84.

121. Wolner-Hassen P, Mårdh P-A, Svensson L, Westrom L: Laparoscopy in women with chlamydial infection and pelvic pain: A comparison of patients with and without salpingitis. Obstet Gynecol 1983; 61:299.

122. Mårdh P-A, Moller BR, Ingerselv HJ, et al: Endometritis caused by *Chlamydia trachomatis*. Br J Vener Dis 1981; 57:191.

123. Wolner-Hanssen P, Kiviat NB, Holmes KK: Atypical pelvic inflammatory disease: Subacute, chronic, or subclinical upper genital tract infection in women. In: Holmes KK, Mårdh P-A, Sparling PF, et al (eds): Sexually Transmitted Diseases, 2nd ed. San Francisco, CA, McGraw-Hill, 1990, pp 615–620.

124. Greenwood SM, Moran JJ: Chronic endometritis: Morphologic and clinical observations. Obstet Gynecol 1981; 58:176.

125. Greenwood SM, Rotterdam H: Chronic endometritis: A clinical pathologic study. Pathol Annu 1978; 13:209.

126. Kristiansen FV, Oster S, Frost L, et al: Isolation of *Gardnerella vaginalis* in pure culture from the uterine cavity of patients with irregular bleeding. Br J Obstet Gynaecol 1987; 94:979.

127. Larsson P-GB, Bergman BB: Is there a causal connection

between motile curved rods, *Mobiluncus* species, and bleeding complications? Am J Obstet Gynecol 1986; 154:107.

128. Korn AP, Bolan G, Padian N, et al: Plasma cell endometritis in women with symptomatic bacterial vaginosis. Obstet Gynecol 1995; 85:387.

129. Larsson P-G, Platz-Christensen J-J, Försum U, Påhlson C: Clue cells in predicting infections after abdominal hysterectomy. Obstet Gynecol 1991; 77:450.

129a. Persson E, Bergstrom M, Larsson PG, et al: Infections after hysterectomy: A prospective nation-wide Swedish study. Acta Obstet Gynecol Scand (Denmark) 1996; 75:757.

130. Larsson P-G, Platz-Christensen J-J, Thejls H, et al: Incidence of pelvic inflammatory disease after first-trimester legal abortion in women with bacterial vaginosis after treatment with metronidazole: A double-blind, randomized study. Am J Obstet Gynecol 1992; 166:100.

131. Pavic N: Is there a local production of nitrosamines by vaginal microflora in anaerobic vaginosis/trichomoniasis. Med Hypotheses 1984; 15:433.

132. Guijon F, Paraskevas M, Rand F, et al: Vaginal microbial flora as a cofactor in the pathogenesis of uterine cervical intraepithelial neoplasia. Int J Gynecol Obstet 1992; 37:185.

133. Peters N, van Leeuwen AM, Pieters WJLM, et al: Bacterial vaginosis is not important in the etiology of cervical neoplasia: A survey on women with dyskaryotic smears. Sex Transm Dis 1995; 22:296.

134. Frega A, Stentella P, Spera G, et al: Cervical intraepithelial neoplasia and bacterialvaginosis: Correlation or risk factor? Eur J Gynaecol Oncol 1997; 18:76.

135. Voeller B: Heterosexual transmission of HIV. JAMA 1992; 267:1917.

136. Saracco A, Musicco M, Nicolosi A, et al: Man-to-woman sexual transmission of HIV: Longitudinal study of 343 steady partners of infected men. J Acquir Immune Defic Syndr 1993; 6:497.

137. Sewankambo N, Gray RH, Wawer MJ, et al: HIV-1 infection associated with abnormal vaginal flora morphology and bacterial vaginosis. Lancet 1997; 350:546.

138. McDonald HM, O'Loughlin JA, Jolley P, et al: Vaginal infection and preterm labour. Br J Obstet Gynaecol 1991; 98:427.

139. McDonald HM, O'Loughlin JA, Jolley PT, et al: Changes in vaginal flora during pregnancy and association with preterm birth. J Infect Dis 1994; 170:724.

140. Joesoef MR, Hillier SL, Wiknjosastro G, et al: Intravaginal clindamycin treatment for bacterial vaginosis: Effects on preterm delivery and low birth weight. Am J Obstet Gynecol 1995; 173:1527.

141. Llahi-Camp JM, Rai R, Ison C, et al: Association of bacterial vaginosis with a history of second trimester miscarriage. Hum Reprod 1996; 11:1575.

142. Gratacos E, Figuera F, Barranco M, et al: Spontaneous recovery of bacterial vaginosis during pregnancy is not associated with an improved perinatal outcome. Acta Obstet Gynecol Scand 1998; 77:37.

143. Hillier S, Krohn MA, Watts DH, et al: Microbiologic efficacy of intravaginal clindamycin cream for the treatment of bacterial vaginosis. Obstet Gynecol 1990; 76:407.

144. Krohn MA, Hillier SL, Nugent RP, et al, for the Vaginal Infections and Prematurity Study Group: The genital flora of women with intraamniotic infection. J Infect Dis 1995; 171:1475.

145. Watts DH, Eschenbach DA, Kenny GE: Early postpartum endometritis: The role of bacteria, genital mycoplasmas, and *Chlamydia trachomatis*. Obstet Gynecol 1989; 73:52.

146. Thomason JL, Gelbart SM, Anderson RJ, et al: Statistical evaluation of diagnostic criteria for bacterial vaginosis. Am J Obstet Gynecol 1990; 162:155.

147. Thomason JL, Schreckenberger PA, Spellacy WN, et al: Clinical and microbiological characterization of patients with non-specific vaginosis having motile, curved anaerobic rods. J Infect Dis 1984; 149:801.

148. Erkkola R, Järvinen H, Terho, P, Meurman I: Microbial flora in women showing symptoms of nonspecific vaginosis: applicability of KOH test for diagnosis. Scand J Infect Dis Suppl 1983; 40:59.

149. Sheiness D, Dix K, Watanabe S, Hillier SL: High levels of *Gardnerella vaginalis* detected with an oligonucleotide probe combined with elevated pH as a diagnostic indicator of bacterial vaginosis. J Clin Microbiol 1992; 30:642.

150. Briselden AM, Hillier SL: Evaluation of Affirm VP microbial identification test for *Gardnerella vaginalis* and *Trichomonas vaginalis*. J Clin Microbiol 1994; 32:148.

151. Schnadig VJ, Davie KD, Shafer SK, et al: The cytologist and bacterioses of the vaginal-ectocervical area: Clues, commas and confusion. Acta Cytol 1988; 33:287.

152. Platz-Christensen JJ, Larsson P-G, Sundstrom E, Bondeson L: Detection of bacterial vaginosis in Papanicolaou smears. Am J Obstet Gynecol 1989; 160:132.

153. Davis JD, Connor EE, Clark P, et al: Correlation between cervical cytologic results and Gram stain as diagnostic tests for bacterial vaginosis. Am J Obstet Gynecol 1997; 177:532.

154. Dunkelberg WE Jr: Diagnosis of *Hemophilus vaginalis* vaginitis by gram-stained smears. Am J Obstet Gynecol 1965; 91:998.

155. Spiegel CA, Amsel R, Holmes KK: Diagnosis of bacterial vaginosis by direct gram stain of vaginal fluid. J Clin Microbiol 1983; 18:170.

156. Nugent RP, Krohn MA, Hillier SL: Reliability of diagnosing bacterial vaginosis is improved by a standardized method of gram stain interpretation. J Clin Microbiol 1991; 29:297.

157. Joesoef MR, Hillier SL, Josodiwondo S, Linnan M: Reproducibility of a scoring system for gram stain diagnosis of bacterial vaginosis. J Clin Microbiol 1991; 29:1730.

158. Mazzulli T, Simor AE, Low DE: Reproducibility of interpretation of gram-stained vaginal smears for the diagnosis of bacterial vaginosis. J Clin Microbiol 1990; 28:1506.

159. Schwebke JR, Hillier SL, Sobel JD, et al: Validity of the vaginal gram stain for the diagnosis of bacterial vaginosis. Obstet Gynecol 1996; 88:573.

160. Thomason JL, Gelbart SM, Wilcoski LM, et al: Proline aminopeptidase activity as a rapid diagnostic test to confirm bacterial vaginosis. Obstet Gynecol 1988; 71:607.

161. Pheifer TA, Forsyth PS, Durfee MA, et al: Nonspecific vaginitis: Role of *Haemophilus vaginalis* and treatment with metronidazole. N Engl J Med 1978; 298:1429.

162. Blackwell AL, Phillips I, Fox AR, Barlow D: Anaerobic vaginosis (non-specific vaginitis): Clinical microbiological and therapeutic findings. Lancet 1983; 2:1379.

163. Eschenbach DA, Critchlow CW, Watkins H, et al: A dose-duration study of metronidazole for the treatment of nonspecific vaginosis. Scand J Infect Dis Suppl 1983; 40:73.

164. Swedberg J, Steiner JF, Deiss F, et al: Comparison of single-dose vs one-week course of metronidazole for symptomatic bacterial vaginosis. JAMA 1985; 254:1046.

165. Jerve F, Berdal TB, Bohman P, et al: Metronidazole in the treatment of non-specific vaginitis (NSV). Br J Vener Dis 1984; 60:171.

166. Jones BM, Geary I, Alawattegama AB, et al: In-vitro and in-vivo activity of metronidazole against *Gardnerella vaginalis*, *Bacteroides* spp. and *Mobiluncus* spp. in bacterial vaginosis. J Antimicrob Chemother 1985; 16:189.

167. Greaves WL, Chungafung J, Morris B, et al: Clindamycin versus metronidazole in the treatment of bacterial vaginosis. Obstet Gynecol 1988; 72:799.

168. McDonald HM, O'Loughlin JA, Vigneswaran R, et al: Bacterial vaginosis in pregnancy and efficacy of short-course oral metronidazole treatment: A randomized controlled trial. Obstet Gynecol 1994; 84:343.

169. Balsdon MJ: Treatment of *Gardnerella vaginalis* syndrome with a single 2-gram dosage of metronidazole. Scand J Infect Dis Suppl 1983; 40:101.

170. Mohanty KC, Deighton R: Comparison of two different metronidazole regimens in the treatment of *Gardnerella vaginalis* infection with or without trichomoniasis. J Antimicrob Chemother 1985; 16:799.

171. Blackwell A, Fox A, Phillips I, Barlow D: Metronidazole in treatment of non-specific vaginitis: Clinical and microbiological findings in ten patients given 2 grams of metronidazole. Scand J Infect Dis 1983; 40:103.

172. Ison CA, Taylor RFH, Link C, et al: Local treatment for bacterial vaginosis. BMJ 1987; 295:886.

173. Moi H, Erkkola R, Jerve F, et al: Should male consorts of women with bacterial vaginosis be treated? Genitourin Med 1989; 65:263.

174. Vejtorp M, Bollerup AC, Vejtorp L, et al: Bacterial vaginosis: A double-blind randomized trial of the effect of treatment of the sexual partner. Br J Obstet Gynaecol 1988; 95:920.

175. Flagyl®-ER (metronidazole extended-release tablets) 750 mg Prescribing Information. Skokie, IL, G.D. Searle, 1998.

176. Livengood CH III, Thomason JL, Hill GB: Bacterial vaginosis: Treatment with topical intravaginal clindamycin phosphate. Obstet Gynecol 1990; 76:118.

177. Schmitt C, Sobel JD, Meriwither C: Bacterial vaginosis: Treatment with clindamycin cream versus oral metronidazole. Obstet Gynecol 1992; 79:1020.

177a. Nayagam AT, Smith MD, Ridgeway GL, et al: Comparison of ofloxacin and metronidazole for the treatment of bacterial vaginosis. Int J STD AIDS 1992; 32:204.

178. Fischbach F, Petersen EE, Weissenbacher ER, et al: Efficacy of clindamycin vaginal cream versus oral metronidazole in the treatment of bacterial vaginosis. Obstet Gynecol 1993; 82:405.

178a. Stein GE, Christensen SL, Mummaw NL, Soper DE: Placebo-controlled trial of intravaginal 2% cream for the treatment of bacterial vaginosis. Ann Pharmacol 1993; 27:1343.

179. Anders FJ, Parker R, Hosein I, Benrubi GI: Clindamycin vaginal cream versus oral metronidazole in the treatment of bacterial vaginosis: A prospective double-blind clinical trial. S Med J 1995; 85:1077.

180. Bistoletti P, Fredricsson B, Hagström B, Nord C-E: Comparison of oral and vaginal metronidazole therapy for nonspecific bacterial vaginosis. Gynecol Obstet Invest 1986; 21:144.

181. Bro F: Metronidazole pessaries compared with placebo in the treatment of bacterial vaginosis. Scand J Prim Health Care 1990; 8:219.

182. Brenner WE, Dingfelder JR: Metronidazole-containing vaginal sponges for the treatment of bacterial vaginosis. Adv Contracept 1986; 2:363.

183. Edelman DA, North BB: Treatment of bacterial vaginosis with intravaginal sponges containing metronidazole. J Reprod Med 1989; 34:341.

184. Hillier SL, Lipinski C, Briselden AM, Eschenbach DA: Efficacy of intravaginal 0.75% metronidazole gel for the treatment of bacterial vaginosis. Obstet Gynecol 1993; 81:963.

185. Livengood CH III, McGregor JA, Soper DE, et al: Bacterial vaginosis: Efficacy and safety on intravaginal metronidazole treatment. Am J Obstet Gynecol 1994; 170:759.

186. Hanson JM, McGregor JA, Hillier SL, et al: Metronidazole vaginal gel versus oral metronidazole for the treatment of bacterial vaginosis: Results of a multi-center trial (in press).

187. Ferris DG, Litaker MS, Woodward L, et al: Treatment of bacterial vaginosis: A comparison of oral metronidazole, metronidazole vaginal gel, and clindamycin vaginal cream. J Fam Pract 1995; 41:443.

188. Covino JM, Black JR, Cummings M, et al: Comparative evaluation of ofloxacin and metronidazole in the treatment of bacterial vaginosis. Sex Transm Dis 1993; 20:262.

189. Durfee MA, Forsyth PS, Hale JA, Holmes KK: Ineffectiveness of erythromycin for treatment of Haemophilus vaginalis–associated vaginitis: Possible relationship to acidity of vaginal secretions. Antimicrob Agent Chemother 1979; 16:635.

190. Piper JM, Mitchel EF, Ray WA: Prenatal use of metronidazole and birth defects: No association. Obstet Gynecol 1993; 82:348.

191. Burtin P, Taddio A, Ariburnu O, et al: Safety of metronidazole in pregnancy: A meta-analysis. Am J Obstet Gynecol 1995; 172:525.

192. Bibel DJ: Elie Metchnikoff's bacillus of long life. Am Soc Microbiol News 1988; 54:661.

193. Block FB, Llewelyn TH: The treatment of leukorrhea with lactic acid bacilli. JAMA 1917; 6:2025.

194. Mohler RW, Brown CP: Döderlein's bacillus in the treatment of vaginitis. Am J Obstet Gynecol 1933; 25:718.

195. Hallen A, Jarstrand C, Påhlson C: Treatment of bacterial vaginosis with lactobacilli. Sex Transm Dis 1992; 19:146.

196. Hughes VL, Hillier SL: Microbiologic characteristics of Lactobacillus products used for colonization of the vagina. Obstet Gynecol 1990; 75:244.

20 Trichomonas Vaginalis

SUSAN M. MOU ▶ SEBASTIAN FARO

Trichomonas vaginitis is one of the more common sexually transmitted diseases (STDs) and accounts for approximately one fourth of vaginitis cases. It is estimated that there are 3 million cases of *Trichomonas* vaginitis in the United States annually.[1]

Donne first described the protozoan *Trichomonas vaginalis* in 1836. In 1936, Hohne established a relationship between the presence of the protozoan and vaginal symptoms and described the association between an increase in vaginal discharge and the presence of *T. vaginalis* in the vagina. Trussell and Plass[2] established *T. vaginalis* as the etiologic agent by fulfilling Koch's postulates. This was accomplished by inoculating the vaginas of healthy, uninfected volunteers with pure cultures of *T. vaginalis*. In 1947, Trussell[3] published a monograph describing the infection of the lower genital tract caused by *T. vaginalis*.

Although this infection is not regarded as serious, significant effort has been expended in studying this organism because of the related complications associated with *T. vaginalis* vaginitis. *T. vaginalis* vaginitis has been associated with premature labor, low-birth-weight infants, other STDs, and increased transmission and acquisition of human immunodeficiency virus. Approximately one half of women with *T. vaginalis* have a symptomatic infection.

Although metronidazole is effective in treating most cases of vaginal trichomoniasis, urogenital infection continues to be a significant worldwide problem, and is one of the world's most preventable STDs. A significant contributing factor to the continuing dilemma is that men often do not obtain treatment because they have an asymptomatic infection. In addition to some women having a symptomatic infection, other factors include the following: many people become chronically infected, strains that are resistant to metronidazole develop, and the patient is or becomes allergic to metronidazole. The emergence of resistant strains, although somewhat uncommon, can contribute to the organism's survival.

Trichomonads that parasitize humans have evolved to occupy a specific body site. Each species has evolved a specific structure and function, and relationship to the host. *T. vaginalis* has evolved to a level where it is

rather hardy and can withstand fairly extreme changes in the vaginal environment. The vaginas of pregnant women appear to favor colonization and growth of *T. vaginalis*, as well as being readily infected sites. However, the reasons why *T. vaginalis* appears to favor the vaginal conditions associated with pregnancy are not well understood. Although *T. vaginalis* has been recognized for many decades, it continues to be surrounded by many perplexing problems. A significant problem is the lack of information regarding the organism's life cycle. Another poorly understood area is the relationship between *T. vaginalis* and endogenous vaginal bacteria, and the possible synergistic role played by endogenous flora in causing serious pelvic infections (e.g., pelvic inflammatory disease), infertility, premature labor, premature rupture of amniotic membranes, and postoperative infections.

Resistance to metronidazole, the only agent approved for the treatment of trichomoniasis in the United States, continues to be low. The agent is well tolerated by most patients, and significant allergic reactions are uncommon. Although it remains one of the most common causes of vaginitis, the incidence of vaginal trichomoniasis in the United States and Scandinavia has decreased since 1976.[4]

MICROBIOLOGY

There are five known species belonging to the genus *Trichomonas*: *T. tenax, T. vaginalis, T. fecalis, Pentatrichomonas,* and *Dientamoeba fragilis.* They are all members of the order Trichomonadida and the family Trichomonadida. *Pentatrichomonas* and *Dientamoeba* belong to the subfamily Dientamoeba of the family Monocercomonadida.[5] *T. vaginalis* infects the vagina, urethra, and paraurethral glands. This is important because it dictates the use of systemic treatment in place of intravaginal medication when one treats vaginal trichomoniasis.

The morphology of *T. vaginalis* depends on the pH, temperature, and oxygen concentration of the specific environment it is infecting (e.g., urethra, Skene's glands, Bartholin's gland, and vagina). All these factors play a significant role in determining the structural configuration of the organism at a given moment in

240

the environment. Therefore, it is important to understand the role the vaginal ecosystem plays in maintaining the status of the vaginal microflora. The microsystem of the vagina exists in a delicate balance that is influenced by a variety of factors: host factors, including hormones, immunoglobulins, and metabolic products; microbial metabolic products; and factors introduced by the environment. Exogenous factors that also exert an influence on the vaginal ecosystem include chemicals such as douching agents and antimicrobials; and sexual activity, which can introduce additional microorganisms as well as influence the pH because of the alkalinity of semen.

Trichomonas vaginalis has four anteriorly placed flagella that are easily seen during microscopic examination of the organism from vaginal discharge or culture (Fig. 20–1). The organism measures 10 to 20 μm in length, is fusiform in shape, and is slightly larger than a white blood cell (WBC).[6] The nucleus is located in the anterior portion of the cell. Movement is carried out by an undulating membrane that extends from the anterior pole of the protozoan and is attached for a distance of one half to two thirds of its body. It grows best under anaerobic conditions at a pH of 5 or more (e.g., a shift in the vaginal microflora giving rise to a pH ≥ 5, the presence of semen or menstrual blood).[7] Infection is usually seen in reproductive-age women and in women on estrogen therapy. Vertical transmission has been reported in neonates who received estrogen stimulation from their mothers.[8]

There are eight serotypes of *T. vaginalis* that possess shared and unshared antigens not associated with pathogenicity.[9, 10] *T. vaginalis* colonizes and infects mucosal surfaces and, therefore, it would be expected that immunoglobulin A (IgA) would be invoked and be of considerable importance. However, IgA does not function to initiate complement-mediated cytotoxicity and therefore does not have a lethal effect on *T. vagi-*

nalis. Additional studies are needed to understand the response to and effect of IgA on trichomonads. Direct killing of *T. vaginalis* appears to reside with polymorphonuclear leukocytes.[11] The process depends on the oxygen concentration and activation of the C3b pathway. The C3b fragment binds to *T. vaginalis*, which in turns allows binding of the fragment to the polymorphonuclear leukocyte.[12, 13] *T. vaginalis* vaginitis stimulates antibody production but does not confer transient or lasting immunity in the patient. This is readily borne out in clinical practice because recurrent infection is common.

Although *T. vaginalis* infects the vagina, it must coexist with the vaginal microflora and develop a new ecosystem to ensure its survival. Approximately 20% to 50% of vaginal trichomoniasis cases are asymptomatic. Therefore, the protozoan establishes a synergistic relationship in the ecosystem that enables it to thrive but not assume a dominant role. Once the trichomonads assume dominance, they deplete their source of nourishment and eventually create an environment hostile to their survival.

The relationship between invading organisms and the endogenous microflora is one of delicate balance. In a healthy vaginal ecosystem, the microflora is dominated by *Lactobacillus* species that produce hydrogen peroxide and bacteriocin. One species, *Lactobacillus acidophilus*, when dominant produces lactic acid to maintain the pH at less than 4.5. This inhibits the growth of *Gardnerella* and obligate anaerobes. *Gardnerella* is sensitive to hydrogen peroxide and bacteriocin. Thus, all three factors, pH, hydrogen peroxide, and bacteriocin, function to inhibit the growth of *Gardnerella*, *Escherichia coli*, and *Streptococcus agalactiae*, as well as other bacteria. This effect is particularly pronounced on the bacteria that cause the condition known as bacterial vaginosis (BV). The absence of voluminous bacterial growth also works against the survival of *T. vaginalis*. The complexity of the vaginal bacteriology remains intact, although the numbers of pathogenic bacteria are kept low ($<10^3$ bacteria/mL of vaginal fluid) by the action of *Lactobacillus*. Once the balance is tipped in favor of *Gardnerella*, *Lactobacillus* loses its dominance and the ecosystem changes. This not only allows for conditions that favor emergence of an altered endogenous bacteriology, but facilitates the establishment of infection by organisms from the external environment (e.g., *T. vaginalis*, *Neisseria gonorrhoeae*, and *Chlamydia trachomatis*).

Several investigators have studied the relationship between *T. vaginalis* and the endogenous vaginal microflora. In a study comparing 104 women with trichomoniasis with 232 women known not to have the infection, no differences were found in isolation of *Mycoplasma*, *Ureaplasma*, *Lactobacillus*, *Candida*, *S. agalactiae*, or *Enterococcus faecalis*.[14] Levenson and colleagues,[15] in a similar study, found that altering the number of

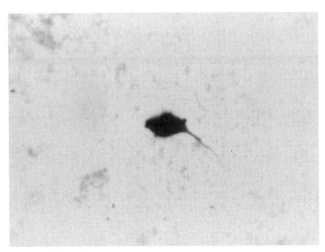

FIGURE 20–1 ▶ Gram-stained preparation of *Trichomonas vaginalis* showing flagella.

lactobacilli resulted in changes in the isolation rates of *T. vaginalis*. These investigators found that when the concentration of lactobacilli was decreased and *T. vaginalis* was present, there was an increase in the number of obligate anaerobic bacteria. Hawes and co-workers[16] followed 182 women over a 2-year period and found that when there was a decrease in hydrogen peroxide-producing lactobacilli, there was an associated increase in vaginitis. However, vaginal trichomoniasis was associated with a new sexual partner, not with the concentration of hydrogen peroxide-producing lactobacilli. The role of lactobacilli is further clouded by the results of Stefanovic,[17] who examined 1,562 premenarchal children and found vaginal trichomoniasis in 3% to 8%. The presence or absence of lactobacilli did not correlate with *T. vaginalis* infection or appear to place the child at risk for acquisition of trichomoniasis.

Microorganisms such as *E. coli* and *Mycoplasma hominis* can attach to *T. vaginalis* and be carried to distant places such as the fallopian tube and the peritoneal cavity. *M. hominis* and *Ureaplasma urealyticum* have been found inside vesicles in the protozoan.[18, 19] *T. vaginalis* has been isolated from the peritoneal cavity at the time of laparoscopy in women with pelvic inflammatory disease.[20] These studies, if proven accurate, will have a significant impact on our understanding of the potential role of *T. vaginalis* in causing damage to the fallopian tubes, thus placing the patient at risk for infertility or ectopic pregnancy. *T. vaginalis* may contribute to the development of asymptomatic pelvic inflammatory disease.

Another contributing factor is the concentration of estrogen in the vagina and vaginal tissue. The presence of estrogen provides an environment that permits *T. vaginalis* to exist in a motile state, which is the apparent vegetative and reproductive state. In the absence of estrogen, *T. vaginalis* assumes a nonflagellated spheroid state that is seen in premenarchal and postmenopausal women.[21] Sharma and colleagues[7] reported on the cure of a postmenopausal woman with vaginal trichomoniasis who was allergic to metronidazole after the discontinuation of estrogen replacement therapy.

EPIDEMIOLOGY

Trichomonas vaginalis is a fastidious organism and, in some respects, has the characteristics of a true parasite completely dependent on its host for survival. There is no known cyst stage, although there is strong suspicion that such a stage exists. The absence of a cyst stage is difficult to understand because the organism seems to exist in the host in an asymptomatic state. Therefore, it appears able to withstand periods of dryness, high temperature, and increasing hydrogen ion concentrations. However, the protozoan has been found to survive outside the human host if the humidity is high. *T. vaginalis* has been isolated from baths

and poorly chlorinated water such as that found in whirlpools, hot tubs, and swimming pools.[22, 23] Studies have documented recovery of *T. vaginalis* from vaginal fluid outside the body at 10°C for up to 48 hours.[23] Viable *T. vaginalis* has also been isolated from urine for up to 3 hours and from ejaculated semen for up to 6 hours.[24] The organism has also survived in water on washcloths at a temperature of 35°C.[25, 26] One third of washcloths contaminated with *T. vaginalis* contained viable trichomonads after 2 to 3 hours, and 10% had viable organisms up to 24 hours after being contaminated.[19] Kessel and associates[27] found that 37% of women with vaginal trichomoniasis left urine and vaginal discharge on toilet seats after use, and 36% of the samples contained viable trichomonads. Toilet seats seeded with exudates containing trichomonads were found to have viable organisms up to 45 minutes after the exudates were deposited.[28]

Experimental data strongly suggest that *T. vaginalis* can exist outside the human host. It has not been documented that the organism can be acquired through a route other than sexual contact, however. The current consensus is that *T. vaginalis* infection is an STD and is almost exclusively acquired through sexual intercourse.[29–32] However, one report documents transmission of *T. vaginalis* between a lesbian couple through mutual masturbation.[33] This couple stated that they were in a monogamous relationship, did not have sex with men, and did not use penetrating sexual instruments.[33] The critical factor in acquiring *T. vaginalis* infection, or any infection, is the inoculum size—that is, there must be a critical number of organisms deposited at a suitable site for infection to occur. Therefore, the mere presence of a few organisms is not likely to be sufficient to induce infection.

Neonatal acquisition of trichomoniasis can occur during delivery as the infant passes through the birth canal and is contaminated with maternal vaginal discharge. Three cases of *T. vaginalis* pneumonia have been documented.[34, 35] No other pathogen was recovered from the respiratory tract.

The risk of contracting trichomoniasis depends on the number of sexual partners in the pool of contacts infected with *T. vaginalis*. People between 20 and 30 years of age are at greatest risk because this is the age group that engages in the most frequent heterosexual activity and is most likely to acquire an STD. One difference between the acquisition of *T. vaginalis* and *N. gonorrhoeae* infection is that the latter tends to decrease in the older population, whereas the former tends to increase among sexually active women between the ages of 30 to 40 years.[25, 31]

Transmission of *T. vaginalis* is greater from men to women. In one study, 14% to 60% of exposed men acquired infection, whereas the disease developed in 67% to 100% of exposed women.[29] Men also clear *T. vaginalis* spontaneously at a rate greater than women.

Krieger[29] reported spontaneous clearance rates of 17% to 70%. This raises the concern that men can serve as an asymptomatic reservoir and vector for transmitting the disease to their sexual partners. Another theory is that the man may actually present with nongonococcal, nonchlamydial urethritis or prostatitis.[36–38] Meares[39] isolated *T. vaginalis* from 50 of 447 men (11.2%), of whom 9 of 50 (18%) were known contacts of women with trichomoniasis and 27 of 50 (54%) had symptoms of urethritis. Men tend to become asymptomatic within 24 hours after contact with an infected partner and acquisition of the disease. A pure trichomonal infection in the man produces a clear to slightly purulent discharge.

CLINICAL PRESENTATION AND PATIENT EVALUATION

Vaginal trichomoniasis is asymptomatic in up to 50% of infected patients. Approximately one third of asymptomatic patients become symptomatic within 6 months. The symptomatic patient typically presents with a malodorous discharge; occasional vaginal itching or soreness, or dyspareunia is also present. The discharge is dirty gray to green or yellow, may be frothy, and is usually liquid.[40] Petechial hemorrhages (strawberry cervix or colpitis macularis) can be detected with macroscopic examination on the cervix and vagina in 25% of cases. Approximately 90% of patients have petechial hemorrhages of the cervix on colposcopic examination.[41]

Trichomonas vaginalis vaginitis can be diagnosed in approximately 75% of cases by careful microscopic examination of the vaginal discharge. A patient with a dirty gray to green or yellow discharge and a pH of 5 or more should be suspected of having trichomoniasis. Microscopic examination of a diluted aliquot of vaginal discharge under 40× magnification should reveal the presence of trichomonads, if they are present. Trichomonads can easily be identified by noting the characteristic whipping of the flagella on the ovoid or elliptical cells. Carefully focusing the fine adjustment reveals the presence of the four anterior flagella. The trichomonads are larger than WBCs but smaller than estrogenized squamous epithelial cells. The investigator should note any other abnormality present in the vaginal discharge, such as clue cells suggesting the presence of BV. The patients should also be evaluated for the presence of other STDs.

Women presenting with a vaginal discharge characterized by the presence of many WBCs, the absence or presence of clue cells, and the absence of yeast should be evaluated for trichomoniasis. In those instances where the vaginal pH is 5 or more and microscopic examination of the vaginal discharge does not reveal the presence of a specific pathogen, a specimen of the vaginal discharge should be used to inoculate Diamond's medium for the growth of *T. vaginalis*. In addition, cervical specimens should be obtained for the detection of *N. gonorrhoeae* and *C. trachomatis*. Diamond's medium can detect approximately 88% of positive *Trichomonas* infections.[41] Another available culture system is the Pouch *T. vaginalis* (InPouch TV) culture system (BioMed Diagnostics, Santa Clara, CA), which consists of culture medium in a clear plastic envelope. The pouch is inoculated with vaginal secretions and examined daily for the presence of trichomonads. It has a sensitivity comparable with that of Diamond's medium, approximately 81%.[42] The InPouch TV system is less labor intensive than other culture methods and, in one study, detected *T. vaginalis* in 97.6% of cases within 24 hours, which is earlier than with Diamond's or Trichosel media.[43]

Although the most widely used test for diagnosing vaginal trichomoniasis is microscopic examination of the vaginal discharge, the specificity and sensitivity are low. In a study of 600 women at risk for trichomoniasis, only 60% of culture-proven *T. vaginalis* infections were detected by microscopic examination of the vaginal discharge.[41] Papanicolaou (Pap) smears have only 56% to 78% sensitivity for the detection of *T. vaginalis* vaginitis and, therefore, may provide a significant number of false-positive results.[40, 41] Mason and colleagues[44] diagnosed trichomoniasis in 126 patients by Pap smear, but could not confirm the diagnosis in all cases by other methods. Perl[45] studied 1,199 patients and diagnosed 666 positives on Pap smear, but could not confirm the diagnosis in 37%. Thus, Pap smear is not a reliable technique for establishing a diagnosis of trichomoniasis.

There is significant concern among investigators that many cases of *T. vaginalis* vaginitis go undiagnosed, leaving the patient open to more serious upper genital tract infections. This may expose the patient undergoing gynecologic surgery to a greater risk of postoperative infection and the obstetric patient to complications early in the pregnancy. This concern is based on the following: (1) many physicians do not have the time to examine vaginal discharge thoroughly because of the pressures placed on them under the current insurance system; (2) not all physicians are able to obtain reimbursement for performing office evaluations; (3) the physician may be inexperienced in evaluating vaginal discharge; and (4) the wet preparation (wet prep) method lacks significant sensitivity and specificity. One group of investigators found that microscopic examination of the vaginal discharge (wet prep) when the Pap smear is obtained may be beneficial in the management of the patient and thus reduce the need for repeat Pap smears. They found that a Pap smear with inflammatory characteristics was associated with BV ($P < .0001$), excess WBCs ($P < .0001$), positive cervical cultures for *N. gonorrhoeae* and *C. trachomatis*

TABLE 20-1 ▶ DIAGNOSTIC TESTS FOR TRICHOMONIASIS		
Test	Sensitivity (%)	Comments
Microscopy	36–80	Low cost, immediate office Dx, 100% sensitivity with motile trichomonads
Diamond's medium	88	Can use isolated organisms for susceptibility studies, delay in establishing the Dx
InPouch *Trichomonas vaginalis*	81–97.6	1 to 7 days for Dx
Papanicolaou smear	56–78	Needs confirmation
Monoclonal antibody	80	Delay in Dx, false-positive results
Monoclonal enzyme-linked immunosorbent assay	89	Delay in Dx
Probes (Affirm VP)	83	Can be performed in the office, requires 30 minutes, patient must wait, delay in Dx
Polymerase chain reaction		Research

Dx = diagnosis.

(P < .001), trichomoniasis (P < .0001), and abnormal wet preps in general (P < .0001).[46]

The monoclonal antibody test used in direct immunofluorescence is 86% sensitive and the monoclonal enzyme-linked immunosorbent assay is 89% sensitive in detecting *T. vaginalis* compared with culture.[41] Synthetic oligonucleotide probes (Affirm VP) are 83% sensitive compared with wet-mount examination and culture.[47] A polymerase chain reaction assay has also been developed to establish a diagnosis of trichomoniasis. This technology can be used on vaginal swabs, such as tampons, that are self-inserted and sent to a laboratory.[48] The polymerase chain reaction test is costly and there is, as with other so-called rapid tests, a delay in making the diagnosis. What is needed is a rapid, highly sensitive and specific test that can be performed quickly in the physician's office. This will ensure that treatment is instituted and not delayed. A comparison of the available tests is provided in Table 20–1.

TREATMENT

Metronidazole is the only antiprotozoal agent approved in the United States for the treatment of *T. vaginalis* vaginitis. Metronidazole, when taken orally, is 95% absorbed, achieving peak serum levels in 1 to 3 hours. If taken with a meal or shortly after eating, absorption is delayed and peak serum levels are not attained for 3 hours.[49, 50] The drug is metabolized in the liver into at least five different metabolites.[51] Approximately 20% to 30% of the daily dose is excreted in the urine and feces. When administered vaginally, as a cream or suppository, systemic absorption occurs. The peak level achieved after a 500-mg dose within 12 to 24 hours is 0.2 μg/L.[52] Patients taking metronidazole should refrain from consuming alcohol-containing liquids because they may experience abdominal pain (a disulfiram-like reaction).[53] Metronidazole should be administered with care to patients taking anticonvulsant medication and warfarin because it can enhance the action of these medications.[54] Common side effects of metronidazole are listed in Table 20–2.

There are a variety of regimens for the treatment of *T. vaginalis* vaginitis, all involving metronidazole (Table 20–3). The key to successful treatment is ensuring that the patient is compliant and that her sexual partner is treated. The latter becomes problematic if the patient has more than one sexual partner. Therefore, the patient should be advised to have either her partner or herself wear a condom during sexual intercourse. This recommendation should apply to all sexual encounters, but especially until it can be established that the trichomonads have been eradicated and the vaginal ecosystem has returned to a healthy state.

Metronidazole does enter breast milk, and therefore a breast-feeding infant can acquire metronidazole from its mother. Erickson and colleagues[55] demonstrated that a single 2-g dose administered to a nursing

TABLE 20-2 ▶ ADVERSE REACTIONS TO METRONIDAZOLE
1. Nausea   6. Dizziness
2. Vomiting   7. Peripheral neuropathy
3. Gastric distress   8. Seizures
4. Metallic taste   9. Ataxia
5. Headache   10. Disulfiram-like reaction

TABLE 20-3 ▶ METRONIDAZOLE TREATMENT REGIMENS FOR *TRICHOMONAS VAGINALIS* VAGINITIS
1. Oral regimens:
a. 2 g as a single dose
b. 750 mg qd for 7 days
c. 500 mg bid for 7 days
d. 250 mg tid for 7 days

mother would result in a concentration of 25 mg/L of metronidazole in her breast milk.

Metronidazole is well tolerated by most patients; however, some people are truly allergic to this antibiotic. The allergic reaction is characterized by urticaria, pruritus, rash, vasodilation, flushing, and bronchospasm.[56] Typically, hypersensitivity reactions occur within 60 minutes of exposure to the allergen, but the allergic reaction to metronidazole can occur as long as 24 hours after exposure to the drug. The severity of the reaction can vary from mild to a true anaphylactoid reaction with hypotension, cardiac arrhythmias, syncope, seizures, loss of consciousness, shock, and death.

Patients who are truly allergic to metronidazole and have trichomoniasis, but do not respond to lesser treatments, should be sensitized to the antibiotic. Desensitization should be carried out in a setting where the patient's vital signs can be continuously monitored and immediate resuscitation can be carried out (Table 20–4). An anesthesiologist should be consulted and available for immediate assistance. The anesthesiologist should be prepared to assist in the resuscitation effort during the desensitization process and up to 24 hours after the procedure.

Pearlman and co-workers[56] reported on two women with a documented allergy to metronidazole. Each patient was tested to determine if a true allergy to metronidazole existed. A 0.2-mm layer of 0.75% metronidazole gel was applied to the vaginal epithelium along the lateral vaginal wall. The presence of an erythematous wheal at the site of metronidazole application was taken to mean that the patient was indeed allergic to metronidazole. The patient then proceeded to desensitization (Table 20–5).

PREGNANCY

Vaginal trichomoniasis has been epidemiologically linked to premature rupture of membranes, preterm

TABLE 20-4 ▶ EQUIPMENT NECESSARY FOR DESENSITIZING A PATIENT TO METRONIDAZOLE

1. Automated blood pressure cuff
2. Continuous monitoring of oxygen saturation
3. Continuous cardiac monitoring
4. Intravenous fluids
5. Epinephrine
6. Oxygen
7. Metaproterenol
8. Hydrocortisone
9. Diphenhydramine
10. Aminophylline
11. Cimetidine
12. Resuscitation equipment

TABLE 20-5 ▶ PROTOCOL FOR DESENSITIZATION TO METRONIDAZOLE

Dose	Fluid Infused
1. 5 μg	1 mL
2. 15 μg	1 mL
3. 50 μg	1 mL
4. 150 μg	3 mL
5. 500 μg	1 mL
6. 1.5 mg	3 mL
7. 5 mg	1 mL
8. 15 mg	3 mL
9. 30 mg	6 mL
10. 60 mg	12 mL
11. 125 mg	25 mL
Oral dose administered at 1-h intervals.	
12. 250 mg	1 tablet
13. 500 mg	1 tablet
14. 2 g	4 tablets

Data from Pearlman MD, Yashar C, Ernst S, Solomon W: An incremental dosing protocol for women with severe vaginal trichomoniasis and adverse reaction to metronidazole. Am J Obstet Gynecol 1996; 174:934.

delivery, and low birth weight.[57] Cotch and associates[58] found, in a multicenter, prospective study of 13,816 pregnant women, that those with *T. vaginalis* vaginitis were 30% more likely to have a low-birth-weight infant, and 40% were more likely to have a preterm and low-birth-weight infant than women without trichomoniasis. A prospective study of pregnant women with *T. vaginalis* vaginitis treated with metronidazole has not been performed. However, the risk of metronidazole in pregnancy is low, and withholding this antibiotic may not be in the patient's best interest.[57, 59–61] *T. vaginalis* has also been linked to an increased risk of febrile morbidity in the puerperium and perioperative period. Therefore, screening the patient for trichomoniasis and treating with metronidazole may reduce postoperative infections after high-risk procedures such as cervical cerclage, cesarean section, and transcervical chorionic villus sampling.

GYNECOLOGY

Trichomoniasis has been associated with postoperative vaginal cuff cellulitis after hysterectomy. A preoperative or perioperative antibiotic that includes coverage against trichomoniasis has not been studied. A reasonable approach might be to screen patients before surgery for the presence of trichomoniasis and BV, and to treat them before performing the operative procedure.

Trichomonas vaginalis is also associated with other STDs. Therefore, patients with a diagnosis of trichomoniasis should be screened for *N. gonorrhoeae* and *C. trachomatis*. If the patient is in a high-risk behavior group, screening for other STDs should also be carried out, including hepatitis B, hepatitis C, and human immunodeficiency virus infection.

References

1. Lossick JG, Kent HL: Trichomoniasis: Trends in diagnosis and management. Am J Obstet Gynecol 1991; 165:1217.
2. Trussell RE, Plass ED: The pathogenicity and physiology of a pure culture of *Trichomonas vaginalis*. Am J Obstet Gynecol 1940; 40:833.
3. Trussell RE. *Trichomonas vaginalis* and Trichomoniasis. Springfield, IL, Charles C Thomas, 1947.
4. Kent HL: Epidemiology of vaginitis. Am J Obstet Gynecol 1991; 165:1168.
5. Honigberg BM: Taxonomy and nomenclature. In: Honigberg BM (ed): Trichomonads Parasitic in Humans. New York, Springer-Verlag, 1990, pp 3–35.
6. Krieger JN, Alderete JF: *Trichomonas vaginalis* and trichomoniasis. In: Holmes KK, et al (eds): Sexually Transmitted Diseases, 3rd ed. New York, McGraw-Hill Health Professions Div 1999, pp 587–604.
7. Sharma R, Pickering J, McCormack WM: Trichomoniasis in a postmenopausal woman cured after discontinuation of estrogen replacement therapy. Sex Transm Dis 1997; 24:543.
8. Danesh IS, Stephen JM, Gorbach J: Neonatal *Trichomonas vaginalis* infection. J Emerg Med 1995; 13:51.
9. Kott H, Adler S: A serological study of *Trichomonas* sp. parasitic in man. Trans R Soc Trop Med Hyg 1961; 55:333.
10. Su-Lin E-K, Honigberg BM: Antigenic analysis of *Trichomonas vaginalis* strains by quantitative fluorescent antibody methods. Z Parasitenkd 1983; 69:161.
11. Rein MF, Sullivan JA, Mandell GL: Trichomonacidal activities of human polymorphonuclear neutrophils: Killing by disruption and fragmentation. J Infect Dis 1980; 142:575.
12. Gillin FD, Sher A: Activation of the alternative complement pathway by *Trichomonas vaginalis*. Infect Immun 1981; 34:268.
13. Holbrook TW, Boackle RJ, Vesely J, Parker BW: *Trichomonas vaginalis*: Alternative pathway activation of complement. Trans R Soc Trop Med Hyg 1982; 76:473.
14. Mason PR, MacCallum MJ, Poynter B: Association of *Trichomonas vaginalis* with other microorganisms. Lancet 1982; 1:1067.
15. Levison ME, Trestman I, Quach R, et al: Quantitative bacteriology of the vaginal flora in vaginitis. Am J Obstet Gynecol 1979; 133:139.
16. Hawes S, Hillier SL, Benedetti J, et al: Hydrogen peroxide-producing lactobacilli and acquisition of vaginal infections. J Infect Dis 1996; 174:1058.
17. Stefanovic J: *Trichomonas* in girls during the period of hormonal inactivity. Bratisl Lek Listy 1990; 91:780.
18. Soszka S, Kazanowska W, Kuczynska K, et al: *Trichomonas* vaginitis at different life stages of women. Wiad Parazytol 1990; 36:211.
19. Rein MF, Muller M: *Trichomonas vaginalis*. In: Holmes KK, Mardh PA, Sparling PF, Weisner PJ (eds): Sexually Transmitted Diseases. New York, McGraw-Hill, 1984, pp 525–535.
20. Santler R, Thurner J, Poitscher C: Trichomoniasis. Z Hautkr 1976; 51:757.
21. Keith LG, Berger GS, Edelman DA, et al: On the causation of pelvic inflammatory disease. Am J Obstet Gynecol 1984; 149:215.
22. Kozlowska D, Wichrowska B: The effect of chlorine and its compounds used for disinfection of water on *Trichomonas vaginalis*. Wiad Parazytol 1976; 22:433.
23. Whittington MJ: The survival of *Trichomonas vaginalis* at temperatures below 37°C. J Hyg 1951; 22:400.
24. Gallai Z, Sylvestre L: The present status of urogenital trichomoniasis: A general review of the literature. Appl Ther 1966; 8:773.
25. Jirovec O, Petru M: *Trichomonas vaginalis* and trichomoniasis. Adv Parasitol 1968; 6:117.
26. Soszka S, Kuczynska K: Effect of *T. vaginalis* on the physiological vaginal flora. Wiad Parazytol 1977; 23:519.
27. Kessel JF, Thompson CF: Survival of *Trichomonas vaginalis* in vaginal discharge. Proc Soc Exp Biol Med 1950; 74:755.
28. Whittington JM: Epidemiology of infections with *Trichomonas vaginalis* in the light of improved diagnostic methods. Br J Vener Dis 1957; 33:80.
29. Krieger JN: Trichomoniasis in men: Old issues and new data. Sex Transm Dis 1995; 22:83.
30. Krieger JN: Urologic aspects of trichomoniasis. Invest Urol 1981; 18:411.
31. Catterall RD, Nicol CS: Is trichomonal infection a venereal disease? BMJ 1960; 1:1177.
32. Catterall RD: Trichomonal infections of the genital tract. Med Clin North Am 1972; 56:1203.
33. Kellock D, O'Mahony CP: Sexually acquired metronidazole-resistant trichomoniasis in a lesbian couple. Genitourin Med 1996; 72:60.
34. Hiemstra I, Van Bel F, Berger HM: Can *Trichomonas vaginalis* cause pneumonia in newborn babies? BMJ 1984; 289:355.
35. McLaren LC, Davis LE, Healy GR, James CG: Isolation of *Trichomonas vaginalis* from the respiratory tract of infants with respiratory disease. Pediatrics 1983; 71:888.
36. Gardner WA Jr, Culberson DE, Bennett BD: *Trichomonas vaginalis* in the prostate gland. Arch Pathol Lab Med 1986; 110:430.
37. Kuberski T: *Trichomonas vaginalis* associated with nongonococcal urethritis and prostatitis. Sex Transm Dis 1980; 7:135.
38. Mardh PA, Colleen S: Search for uro-genital tract infections in patients with symptoms of prostatitis. Scand J Urol Nephrol 1975; 9:8.
39. Meares EM Jr: Prostatitis syndromes: New perspectives about old woes. J Urol 1980; 123:141.
40. Wolner-Hanssen P, Krieger JN, Stevens CE, et al: Clinical manifestations of vaginal trichomoniasis. JAMA 1989; 261:571.
41. Krieger JN, Tam MR, Stevens CE, et al: Diagnosis of trichomoniasis: Comparison of conventional wet-mount examination with cytologic studies, cultures, and monoclonal antibody staining of direct specimens. JAMA 1988; 259:1223.
42. Ohlemeyer CL, Hornberger LL, Lynch DA, Swierkosz EM: Diagnosis of *Trichomonas vaginalis* in adolescent females: InPouch TV culture versus wet-mount microscopy. J Adolesc Health 1998; 22:205.
43. Borchardt KA, Zhang MZ, Shing H, Flink K: A comparison of the sensitivity of the InPouch TV, Diamond's and Trichosel media for the detection of *Trichomonas vaginalis*. Genitourin Med 1997; 73:297.
44. Mason PR, Super H, Fripp PJ: Comparison of four techniques for the routine diagnosis of *Trichomonas vaginalis* infection. J Clin Pathol 1976; 29:154.
45. Perl G: Errors in the diagnosis of *Trichomonas vaginalis* infections as observed among 1199 patients. Obstet Gynecol 1972; 39:7.
46. Eltabbakh GH, Eltabbakh GD, Broekhuizen FF, Griner BT: Value of wet mount and cervical cultures at the time of cervical cytology in asymptomatic women. Obstet Gynecol 1995; 85:499.
47. Briselden AM, Hillier SL: Evaluation of Affirm VP microbial identification test for *Gardnerella vaginalis* and *Trichomonas vaginalis*. J Clin Microbiol 1994; 32:148.
48. Paterson BA, Tabrizi SN, Garland SM, et al: The tampon test for trichomoniasis: A comparison between conventional methods and a polymerase chain reaction for *Trichomonas vaginalis* in women. Sex Transm Infect 1998; 74:136.
49. Houghton GW, Smith J, Thorne PS, Templeton R: The pharmacokinetics of oral and intravenous metronidazole in man. J Antimicrob Chemother 1979; 5:621.
50. Levison ME: Microbiological agar diffusion assay for metronidazole concentrations in serum. Antimicrob Agents Chemother 1974; 5:466.
51. Stambaugh JE, Feo LG, Manthei RW: The isolation and identification of the urinary oxidative metabolites of metronidazole. J Pharmacol Exp Ther 1968; 161:373.
52. Alper MM, Barwin BN, McLean WM, et al: Systemic absorption of metronidazole by the vaginal route. Obstet Gynecol 1985; 65:781.
53. Winter D, Stanescu C, Sauvard S: The effect of metronidazole on the toxicity of ethanol. Biochem Pharmacol 1969; 18:1246.
54. O'Reilly RA: The stereoselective interaction of warfarin and metronidazole in man. N Engl J Med 1976; 295:354.
55. Erickson SH, Oppenheim GL, Smith GH: Metronidazole in breast milk. Obstet Gynecol 1981; 57:48.
56. Pearlman MD, Yashar C, Ernst S, Solomon W: An incremental

dosing protocol for women with severe vaginal trichomoniasis and adverse reaction to metronidazole. Am J Obstet Gynecol 1996; 174:934.

57. Saurina GR, McCormack WM: Trichomoniasis in pregnancy. Sex Transm Dis 1997; 24:361.

58. Cotch MF, Pastorek JG II, Nugent RP, et al: *Trichomonas vaginalis* associated with low birth weight and preterm delivery. Sex Transm Dis 1997; 24:353.

59. Piper JM, Mitchel EF, Ray WA: Prenatal use of metronidazole and birth defects: No association. Obstet Gynecol 1993; 82:348.

60. Heinonen OP, Slone D, Shapiro S: Birth Defects and Drugs in Pregnancy. Littleton: Publishing Sciences Group, 1977, pp 326–335.

61. Struthers BJ: Metronidazole appears not to be a human teratogen: Review of the literature. Infect Dis Obstet Gynecol 1997; 5:326.

21 Pediatric Vulvovaginitis

MELISA M. HOLMES

From birth until the onset of puberty, most girls experience some degree of vulvar or vulvovaginal irritation. Although many cases are transient and resolve spontaneously, occasionally the inflammation becomes severe enough to cause significant discomfort, pruritus, or discharge, resulting in the diagnosis of pediatric vulvovaginitis. In pediatric gynecology referral centers, vulvovaginitis is one of the most common reasons for evaluation or consultation.[1] It is frequently related to a combination of predisposing anatomic, physiologic, or behavioral factors that lead to a disturbance in vulvovaginal homeostasis. Although the etiology is usually benign, vaginal discharge or vulvar inflammation in a young girl evokes concern about the possibility of more serious causes such as sexual abuse or a vaginal foreign body. Furthermore, it is a condition that has important psychological implications that should be addressed.

To evaluate and treat vulvovaginitis in a child, it is important to understand normal physiologic genital changes that occur with advancing age and to recognize common prepubertal vulvovaginal conditions that are associated with vulvovaginal inflammation (Table 21–1). A methodical approach to the problem helps prevent misdiagnosis and reduces the potential for iatrogenic physical or emotional trauma.

PATHOPHYSIOLOGY

Most cases of pediatric vulvovaginitis represent a primary vulvitis that may extend to the distal vagina and secondarily cause vaginal inflammation and discharge. Less commonly, a primary vaginitis is the inciting event that secondarily causes vulvar irritation. The microorganisms that cause vulvovaginitis in girls are not typically the same organisms responsible for vaginitis in adults, but are usually normal inhabitants of the anorectal region or the upper respiratory tract.[2–5] However, numerous other pathologic organisms, including parasites, sexually transmitted microbes, and viruses, have also been isolated.[6]

Regardless of the specific causative organisms, the occurrence of pediatric vulvovaginitis is related to multiple factors. Prepubertal genital anatomy and physiol-

ogy play an important role. Compared with adults, the prepubertal genital anatomy offers less protection against contamination and infection of the vulvovaginal area. With flattened labia and no pubic hair, the introitus is more exposed. Also, the distance between the anus and vagina is relatively shorter than in adults, making fecal contamination more likely. Although very little is known about local immune effects in the prepubertal vulva and vagina, individual variations in im-

TABLE 21-1 ▶	PEDIATRIC VULVOVAGINITIS: CAUSES AND DIFFERENTIAL DIAGNOSIS

Bacterial
  Nonspecific mixed infections related to
    Poor perineal hygiene and coliform bacteria
    Respiratory flora
    Vaginal foreign body
    Urinary tract infection
    Dermatologic infections
  Specific pathogens
    Sexually transmitted infections
    Enteric pathogens
    Oropharynx/respiratory pathogens
Viral infections
  Herpes simplex
  Human papilloma virus
  Varicella
Fungal infections
  Candida species
    Vulvar: diaper rash
    Vaginal: immunocompromised/chronic antibiotic use/
      pubertal
Parasite/protozoal infections
  Trichomoniasis
  Amebiasis
  Pinworm
Anatomic abnormalities
  Trauma
  Hymenal variants/tags
  Neoplasia
  Ectopic ureter
  Crohn's disease
Skin disorders
  Allergic contact reactions
  Psoriasis
  Lichen sclerosus
  Lichen planus
  Eczema
  Seborrhea
  Impetigo
  Intertrigo

249

mune responses may also affect the severity of symptoms experienced with vulvovaginitis.

RISK FACTORS

Common childhood behaviors can also increase the risk of vulvovaginitis. The suboptimal toileting habits of children increase the risk for fecal contamination of the vagina. Other hygiene-related behaviors lead to contamination of the area by unclean hands that may carry organisms from the respiratory or gastrointestinal tracts. Playing in sand or dirt can cause irritation of the sensitive vulvar tissues and initiate a local inflammatory reaction sometimes referred to as *sandbox bottom*. Similarly, wearing leotards, tights, or bathing suits that maintain excessive moisture may cause mild maceration and irritation of exposed and sensitive vulvar skin.[6] Local chemical irritants such as bubble baths, detergents, dyes, perfumes, and soaps can also cause significant irritation and inflammation.[7]

In addition to these common predisposing factors, sexual abuse or molestation puts young girls at risk for contracting sexually transmitted diseases (STDs) that affect the prepubertal vagina and vulva rather than the upper genital tract. Vulvar trauma or irritation can also result from abuse and present as a vulvovaginitis.

PHYSIOLOGIC HORMONAL INFLUENCES

An understanding of normal physiologic hormonal influences on the prepubertal genitalia is important in the evaluation and treatment of pediatric vulvovaginitis. The tissues of the vulva and vagina are very sensitive to estrogen and undergo predictable age-related changes that are influenced by varying levels of estrogenization. In the newborn, recent exposure to transplacental maternal estrogens results in the normal findings of breast buds, prominent labia, a thickened hymen, and mature vaginal mucosa. As a result of the estrogen exposure, the vaginal secretions are acidic and the vaginal microflora is similar to that of a normal adult. The estrogen acts on the endocervical glands and vaginal mucosa to cause the white-to-clear mucoid discharge frequently seen in the newborn. As estrogen levels decline, the discharge decreases, and the newborn may have a small amount of estrogen-withdrawal bleeding from the uterus.[8, 9]

As the effects of neonatal estrogenization disappear, the genitalia undergo "atrophic" changes and take on the typical prepubertal appearance. The labia become flattened and sometimes wrinkled; the hymen becomes very thin and translucent; the genital mucosa becomes thin and atrophic.[9, 10] Because the mucosal epithelium has thinned, it takes on a reddened appearance as the capillaries become relatively superficial. Occasionally, this relative "hyperemia" may be misinterpreted as

an inflammatory process. In the absence of estrogen, lactobacilli are also absent, and the vaginal environment and secretions become neutral or alkaline, resulting in an excellent "culture medium" for respiratory, gastrointestinal, and other pyogenic organisms.

In late childhood, at approximately 8 years of age increasing activity of the hypothalamic-pituitary-ovarian axis results in intermittent follicle-stimulating hormone secretion with resultant estrogen release and subtle changes in the female reproductive tract. Gradually, and sometimes intermittently, the mons and labia become more prominent, the genital mucosa and hymen become thicker, and the vagina lengthens and develops rugae.[9, 11] As thelarche begins under the influence of estrogen, genital changes also become more pronounced.[12] Estrogen stimulation of the endocervical glands and vaginal mucosa produces a white-to-yellow discharge made up of desquamated epithelial cells, cervical mucus, and vaginal transudate.[13] *These physiologic vaginal secretions are not malodorous, do not cause vaginal irritation, and usually do not cause clinically evident vulvar irritation.* It is important to recognize this normal physiologic discharge to provide appropriate reassurance and avoid unnecessary treatment of a presumed vulvovaginitis.

As girls enter puberty, cyclic hormonal influences exert estrogenic effects on the genitalia that result in anatomically adult proportions, mature genital mucosa, and an acidic vaginal ecosystem.[10] At this point, vulvovaginal problems in young girls should be evaluated and treated as they would be in adults. With maturity, the reproductive tract becomes more susceptible to bacterial vaginosis, candidiasis, and upper gential tract infections, but the anatomic changes and acidic environment provide protection against many of the problems that cause vulvovaginitis in children.

MICROBIOLOGY

The vaginal environment is a dynamic ecosystem in which alterations in estrogen exposure, glycogen content, and vaginal pH affect the populations of specific microorganisms. In pubertal girls, an estrogenized vaginal environment promotes the growth of organisms such as lactobacilli that offer protective antibiosis through the production of lactic acid and hydrogen peroxide.[14] In *pre*pubertal girls, the neutral to alkaline environment allows the growth of many of the same organisms found in the mature vagina, but does not confer the same protection as the acidic environment of the mature vagina. This also leaves the vagina and vulva more susceptible to overgrowth of local contaminants or infection by pathogens. Because of factors related to the neutral pH and lack of glycogen, the prepubertal vagina does not support the growth of candidal species, and yeast vaginitis is rare before puberty unless the child is immunosuppressed or has been on chronic antibiotics. Thus, one of the more important distinctions in evaluating and treating pediatric vulvovaginitis is whether the girl is prepubertal or pubertal.

The normal flora of the *prepubertal* vagina was explored by Hill and colleagues[15] in a prospective observational study. Vaginal cultures were obtained from 19 healthy prepubertal girls (average age, 2.8 years) who were undergoing an elective surgical procedure and had no history of genitourinary complaints, sexual abuse, antibiotic use, or immunosuppressive therapy. All cultures were positive for at least one organism, and an average of 12 species were isolated from each subject. Table 21–2 lists the normal prepubertal vaginal flora identified. Although specifically sought, there were no cultures positive for *Gardnerella vaginalis*, *Mobiluncus* species, *Mycoplasma hominis*, *Neisseria gonorrhoeae*, *Trichomonas vaginalis*, *Chlamydia trachomatis*, or human papilloma virus (HPV).

There are no studies specifically on the normal flora of *pubertal* girls. However, once a girl enters puberty (as evidenced by the initiation of breast development), the genital mucosa becomes estrogenized, glycogen is available to promote the growth of lactobacilli, and the pH becomes more acidic, as in the adult vagina. As puberty progresses, the vaginal pH and the microflora should be the same as in other normal women of reproductive age. At this developmental stage, susceptibility to candidal vaginitis also increases.

Two other controlled, prospective, microbiologic studies have attempted to identify common "normal flora" and various etiologic pathogens in pediatric vulvovaginitis; however, both studies were limited by the inclusion of both prepubertal and pubertal girls.

Paradise and colleagues[2] performed vaginal cultures on girls 5 months to 12.6 years of age with vulvovaginits diagnosed by history or clinical examination, and on a control group without symptoms. Bacterial or candidal infection was identified in 52% of the patients with a visible discharge and in none of the patients without discharge. *Candida* was identified only in pubertal (although premenarcheal) girls and not in any prepubertal girls. No etiologic diagnosis was made in 22%, but most of these improved with increased attention to perineal hygiene.

In a similar microbiologic study, Gerstner and coworkers[3] used vaginoscopy in girls 3 months to 16 years of age to obtain vaginal cultures and decrease the likelihood of contamination from the vulva. Vaginal cultures from asymptomatic control subjects revealed a wide variety of aerobic and anaerobic bacteria, including colonic bacteria. Subjects with vaginal discharge or vulvovaginitis showed a similar pattern of aerobes and anaerobes, but bacterial counts were higher than for the asymptomatic control subjects. The authors conclude that the quantity of bacteria, and not just the identity, is significant in the development of an infection. Thus, quantitative bacteriologic studies may provide valuable information not elicited by qualitative methods alone.

PRESENTATION

A child with vulvovaginitis may present with a wide variety of symptoms. In an infant or young child, the problem is identified by the caretaker during diaper changes or baths. For preverbal children, irritability may be the only reported symptom, or the child may

TABLE 21–2 ▶ VAGINAL MICROFLORA IN PREPUBERTAL GIRLS

Category of Organism	Prevalence (n = 19)	Mean No. of Species	Mean Count (log$_{10}$)
Anaerobes	100	8.7 ± 3.8	7.4 ± 1.3
Gram-positive rods	95	2.7 ± 1.1	6.9 ± 1.3
Actinomyces species	>32	—	6.8 ± 1.0
Lactobacillus species	>21	—	6.4 ± .58
Gram-negative rods	89	4.7 ± 2.3	6.9 ± 1.1
Black-pigmenters	47	—	5.6 ± .86
Bacteroides ureolyticus	26	—	6.6 ± .85
Fusobacterium species	>26	—	5.7 ± .97
Bacteroides fragilis group	21	—	5.0 ± .88
Gram-positive cocci	89	2.2 ± 1.0	6.9 ± 1.1
Gram-negative cocci	21	—	6.3 ± 1.2
Aerobes	95	3.4 ± 1.6	6.1 ± .94
Gram-positive cocci	84	2.0 ± .97	5.9 ± 1.1
Coagulase-negative *Staphylococcus*	68	—	5.3 ± 1.0
Streptococcus viridans	42	—	6.1 ± 1.4
Enterococcus faecalis	32	—	5.4 ± .67
Gram-negative rods	58	1.6 ± .92	5.2 ± .72
Lactose fermenters	32	—	5.3 ± .84
Gram-positive rods	53	1.2 ± .42	5.3 ± .63
Diphtheroids	42	—	5.2 ± .57

From Hill GB, St Claire KK, Gutman LT: Anaerobes predominate among the vaginal microflora of prepubertal girls. Clin Infect Dis 1995; 20:S269, with permission of the University of Chicago.

be seen rubbing or pulling at the genital area. In an older child, vulvar pruritus, burning, dysuria, or a combination of these symptoms may be reported. It is not uncommon for a child with vulvovaginitis to be inappropriately treated for a urinary tract infection because dysuria is a common presenting complaint, and a voided urine specimen contains leukocytes from the associated vaginal discharge. The dysuria that occurs with pediatric vulvovaginitis is different from the typical dysuria that occurs with urinary tract infections; it is a "contact dysuria" or "splash dysuria" caused by urine flowing over inflamed vulvar tissues. Occasionally, the child with vulvovaginitis has no complaints, but has been noted to have blood or discharge in her underwear.

History

A carefully taken history provides guidance for the subsequent physical examination. For young children, the history must come from the parent or caretaker, but the child should always be included as much as possible. Important historical considerations are listed in Table 21–3.

Because of the potential for vulvovaginitis related to sexual abuse, the child should be interviewed alone with sensitive but direct questions addressing the possibility of inappropriate touching of the genital area. The parent or caretaker should also be asked whether he or she suspects any sexual molestation or abuse.

TABLE 21–3 ▶ IMPORTANT HISTORICAL CONSIDERATIONS FOR ASSESSING PEDIATRIC VULOVAGINITIS

General history (from caretaker and child)
  History of present illness: quality, quantity, duration, pain, associated symptoms
  Associated history
    Soaps, detergents, bubble baths, shampoos
    Toileting habits
    Masturbation
    Enuresis/encopresis
    Anal pruritus
    Behavioral changes
      Nightmares, fears, aches, school performance
      Inappropriate sexual behavior
    Sexual contact
  Recent health: respiratory, gastrointestinal symptoms
  Recent medications: antibiotics, immunosuppressives
Past medical/surgical history
  Delivery and neonatal period
    Abnormalities noted or treated
    Maternal infections—condyloma, herpes simplex, other sexually transmitted diseases
  Immunizations
  Childhood illnesses
Family history
  Recent viral or bacterial infections
  Atopic dermatoses
  Bleeding diathesis
  Alcohol or drug abuse

Simple screening questions are appropriate initially, but if the history or examination supports the possibility of abuse, a more thorough assessment is necessary and is optimally performed by a professional specifically trained in conducting and interpreting this type of interview. The medical evaluation and management of suspected childhood sexual abuse should also be provided by a clinician with experience in performing child sexual abuse examinations.

Examination

The components of the physical examination are similar for all prepubertal girls, but the approach to the examination varies according to the child's age and developmental level. The most important step in the examination is to develop rapport with the child and to gain her trust. Sometimes, if the child is not ready to proceed with the examination, this means delaying it to a second visit later in the day or even to another day. It is important for the child to feel a sense of control both as the examination is initiated and while it is ongoing. This can be accomplished by explaining what the child should expect, by giving the child choices, such as choosing a gown color, or choosing to be examined in her parent's lap or on the table, and by asking permission before touching the child.

Because vulvitis can be the initial manifestation of a systemic disease, a general physical examination should be performed first. Examination of the ears, nose, and throat should rule out infection as well as oral mucocutaneous lesions that could indicate a problem such as lichen planus or Behçet's syndrome (both of which can also involve the vulvar mucosa). The chest should be examined for other evidence of respiratory tract infection. Breast examination should include Tanner staging to assess estrogen exposure. The abdomen should be evaluated for pain or masses that could indicate a problem such as inflammatory bowel disease; vulvar fistulas have been documented in children as the initial presentation of Crohn's disease.[16] Similarly, a müllerian obstruction or abnormality may present with an abdominal or pelvic mass. Costovertebral angle tenderness should be evaluated to assess for signs of an upper urinary tract infection. Finally, a very thorough examination of the skin should be performed to look for vascular lesions, pigmented lesions, traumatic injuries, and any dermatologic condition or eruption that could also affect the vulva.

The prepubertal genital examination includes inspection of the mons, labia majora, labia minora, clitoris, urethra, fourchette, hymen, distal vagina, and anus. In most cases, this can be accomplished in the office. Occasionally, inspection of the entire vagina is necessary and is accomplished through vaginoscopy. Although an older, cooperative child can tolerate office vaginoscopy with topical anesthetics and a small-diame-

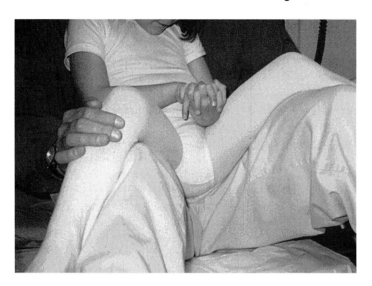

FIGURE 21-1 ▶ Lithotomy position in a caretaker's lap allows the child to feel more secure.

ter scope, examination under anesthesia is required for the young child. A child should never be restrained for a genital examination, and sedation is rarely necessary. In a totally uncooperative child who clearly needs a genital examination, it is best performed under general anesthesia or deep conscious sedation.

Positioning for the examination also depends on the child's age, but several positions are extremely useful and provide good visualization of the external genitalia. For young children, the parent or caretaker can assist by cradling the child either in his or her lap (Fig. 21–1) or on an examination table. Most children can be examined in a frog-legged position or in stirrups. The knee-chest position is also extremely useful for visualizing the distal vagina and posterior hymen (Fig. 21–2). If there is any question about the appearance of the posterior hymen or any difficulty visualizing the distal vagina, the examination should always be repeated in the knee-chest position.[17]

To provide the best visualization of the hymen and distal vagina with the least discomfort, the labia majora should be gently grasped and pulled outward and slightly posterior. Spreading the labia laterally places excessive tension on the fourchette and is painful. A child may be more cooperative if she is allowed to help separate and "hold" the labia open. The appearance of the hymen should always be documented, preferably with a simple illustration or magnified photograph. Improved visualization of the premenarcheal hymen can be achieved using a colposcope, and colposcopic photographs can be very useful for documentation and preventing repeat examinations if necessary for forensic evidence. There are many normal variants of hymenal shape, and the appearance varies depending on the amount of traction, the degree of relaxation, and the position of the child.[18] It is important for the clinician seeing pediatric patients to recognize normal and abnormal variants of the prepubertal hymen.[18, 19] Although a digital vaginal examination is not indicated, a gentle digital rectal examination is well tolerated and can be very helpful in assessing for vaginal discharge and palpating for a solid foreign body. Using

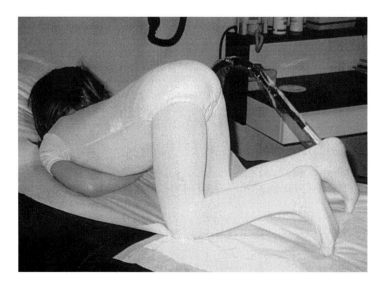

FIGURE 21-2 ▶ The knee-chest position allows excellent visualization of the distal vagina and posterior hymenal rim.

a gentle "milking" motion through the rectovaginal septum, vaginal discharge, if present, can be brought into the distal vagina for visualization and access for cultures.

If cultures are indicated, they should be obtained as the last part of the examination. Cultures should be obtained from the vagina rather than the vulva. Vulvar cultures are less helpful because of heavy contamination from rectal or skin flora. A useful technique for obtaining vaginal washings for multiple swabs was originally described by Pokorny and Stormer.[20] Their catheter-within-a-catheter system has since been patented as the Pedi Vaginal Aspirator (Cook Ob/Gyn, Spencer, IN). This device provides a narrow catheter within a catheter that allows for atraumatic irrigation and retrieval of vaginal secretions that can then be applied to culture swabs for testing. The examiner can stand to the side of the patient, quickly and gently insert the aspirator, inject 1 mL of sterile, nonbacteriostatic saline, and aspirate the vaginal secretions. Culture results from vaginal washings obtained in this manner provide accurate results compared with vaginal swab specimens.[21, 22] If this type of device is not available, only small swabs such as the male urethral swab or nasopharyngeal microswab should be used in the prepubertal vagina.

DIAGNOSIS AND TREATMENT OF PEDIATRIC VULVOVAGINITIS

Nonspecific Vulvovaginitis

Most cases of pediatric vulvovaginitis are related to suboptimal perineal hygiene and are termed *nonspecific vulvovaginitis.* The associated microbiologic findings may reveal an overgrowth of both anaerobic and aerobic bacterial flora rather than a single specific causative organism.[2, 3, 15] The presenting complaint is usually vulvar irritation with a discharge and odor. Occasionally the discharge is noted in the child's underwear without other evidence of local inflammation. More commonly, the inflammation is obvious and involves the labial mucosa, the introitus, the hymen, and the distal vagina. The discharge may be infectious or inflammatory, and it is characteristically yellow to green, but not bloody. It may be scant or copious. The inflammatory process can cause vulvar erythema and edema. Excessive moisture from the discharge may also lead to maceration of the vulvar tissues or allow for overgrowth of candidal species on the vulva. Local irritation may cause vulvovaginal pruritus. Excoriations from scratching are often seen.

The diagnosis is usually based on the clinical examination, but additional laboratory testing may be helpful in ruling out more specific causes. A saline wet mount reveals a predominance of white blood cells and bacteria. The presence of fungal elements, clue cells, or trichomonads is rare in children, but should be specifically ruled out. Clue cells have been noted in virginal adolescents, and have also been associated with child sexual abuse.[23, 24] Therefore, their presence in a prepubertal child has uncertain implications. If the discharge is copious, vaginal cultures can be helpful in identifying the predominant organism or a specific pathogen. However, if the discharge is scant, cultures are of little clinical use.[2, 3]

Initial treatment is conservative and aimed at improving local hygiene, decreasing the bacterial contamination of the area, and providing symptomatic relief of irritation and pruritus. Increased supervision of toileting habits with appropriate instruction in front-to-back wiping should be encouraged. Sitz baths with warm water or colloidal oatmeal can remove bacteria-laden discharge and provide relief of pruritus and irritation. Ointments or creams such as petrolatum, zinc-based diaper rash creams, or even vegetable shortening can provide a protective skin barrier and prevent further irritation of the vulvar tissues.[25] It is also important to break the "itch–scratch" cycle by providing topical or oral antihistamines or mild corticosteroid preparations such as 1% hydrocortisone ointment. Most cases resolve within 2 weeks with the measures listed in Table 21–4.

After conservative treatment for nonspecific pediatric vulvovaginitis, follow-up is indicated in 2 to 3 weeks

TABLE 21–4 ▶ INITIAL TREATMENT FOR NONSPECIFIC PEDIATRIC VULVOVAGINITIS

General hygiene measures
When urinating, sit with legs spread and labia separated
Wipe from front to back after urinating and bowel movements
Wash the vulva with plain water or a mild unscented soap (Basis, unscented Dove)
Avoid bubble baths and shampooing while sitting in the tub
After bathing, pat the area dry then dry completely with a blow dryer on cool setting
Wear cotton underwear, avoid tight clothing, nylon, and spandex
Wear loose-fitting skirts or dresses; avoid tights or tight blue jeans
Do not wear a wet bathing suit longer than necessary
Symptomatic treatment
For irritated vulva
Sitz baths three to four times/day in plain water (no soap)
Pat vulva dry then air dry or dry completely with blow dryer on low setting
Apply bland emollient/skin barrier such as:
Zinc-based diaper rash creams, A&D ointment, Crisco, Maalox liquid (can pour over vulva if child doesn't tolerate contact application), petrolatum
Topical lidocaine 5% ointment before urination or as needed
Witch hazel pads or baby wipes may give soothing relief and may be used in place of toilet paper for wiping.
For oozing lesions, soak soft linen or cotton cloth with Burrow's solution and apply to vulva; remove when dry and reapply as needed.
For vulvar pruritus
Colloidal oatmeal sitz bath
Oral hydroxyzine or diphenhydramine
Topical hydrocortisone ointment (1%–2.5%)

to confirm resolution of the problem. If symptoms persist or recur soon after treatment, the child should be re-examined and cultures obtained to identify specific pathogens, including sexually transmitted infections. General aerobic and anaerobic cultures should be obtained as described previously. Cultures for gonorrhea and chlamydial infection are also indicated for persistent vulvovaginitis and can be taken from the vagina rather than the endocervix.[26, 27] Antibiotic therapy may be warranted for persistent cases, but should not be initiated before appropriate cultures have been obtained because of the possibility of treating an unrecognized STD.[28]

In children, individual cultures for gonorrhea and chlamydial infection should be used rather than enzyme-linked immunoassays or DNA amplification techniques. The nonculture tests, particularly for chlamydiae, carry a slight risk of false positivity.[29, 30] Obviously, the inaccurate diagnosis of an STD in a child could have a devastating outcome. In adult women, the newer DNA amplification techniques, specifically ligase chain reaction, used on first-voided urine have demonstrated higher detection rates than endocervical swabs.[29] This technology may have a role in screening at-risk children and adolescents.[13] However, all positive results require confirmation by the gold standard, culture. Furthermore, these techniques have so far been applied only to detection of gonorrhea and chlamydial infection, and are not helpful with other STDs.

Objective studies on the effectiveness or necessity of antibiotic therapy for the treatment of pediatric vulvovaginitis are not available. However, many expert clinicians advocate the use of antimicrobial treatment for persistent cases that have not responded to conservative measures. When cultures are taken, the laboratory should be requested to identify specific organisms, quantify heavy or light growth, and avoid the term *normal vaginal flora*. In general, growth of aerobes warrants antibiotic therapy only if there is heavy growth. Broad-spectrum oral antibiotics such as amoxicillin or cephalexin usually provide adequate coverage. Cultures with light aerobic growth or no growth often respond to conservative symptomatic treatment and usually do not require antibiotic therapy.[2] If the cultures grow anaerobes, treatment and follow-up should be more aggressive because heavy anaerobic growth can be associated with more refractory vaginitis or a vaginal foreign body. When culture results are not available, the presence of a strong anaerobic odor provides sufficient clinical support for using an antimicrobial agent with better anaerobic coverage, such as amoxicillin plus clavulanic acid. Finally, if initial antibiotic treatment is not successful or if the vaginitis is recurrent, vaginoscopy is indicated to search for a vaginal foreign body or a vaginal abnormality such as an ectopic ureter or other anatomic abnormality.

Because recurrences are common, the importance of prevention by maintaining the recommended changes in hygiene and perineal care should be stressed. Providing the child's caretakers with detailed written instructions that describe the recommended treatment and hygiene measures can enhance compliance and understanding.

Specific Vulvovaginitis

When the primary site of infection is the vagina rather than the vulva, a specific pathologic organism or other specific cause is usually identified. As in nonspecific vulvovaginitis, the route of infection may be due to hygiene or autoinnoculation, but it may also occur through systemic infection, direct contact infection, or a retained foreign body. The vaginal discharge is characteristically profuse and sometimes bloody. Pruritus may not be an intial complaint, but the persistence of a heavy discharge can lead to vulvar inflammation and associated pruritus.

The history in these cases often reveals a recent upper respiratory tract infection, urinary tract infection, skin infection, or diarrhea. Vaginal culture often reveals the organism that was likely responsible for the primary infection. Treatment is aimed at providing appropriate antimicrobial therapy along with local symptomatic treatment and attention to perineal hygiene. Occasionally, however, a second course of antibiotic therapy may be necessary to clear the vulvovaginitis completely. Recommended treatments and dosing for specific causes of vulvovaginitis are listed in Table 21–5. Again, if antimicrobial and symptomatic treatments do not clear the vulvovaginitis, vaginoscopy is indicated.

Candidal Vulvovaginitis

Antifungal creams are commonly prescribed for pediatric vulvovaginitis; however, candidal vulvovaginitis is uncommon in childhood. The most common candidal infection in children occurs in relation to diaper rash, particularly in combination with oral thrush. Children in diapers may acquire a candidal rash with the typical erythema and satellite lesions, but there is no associated vaginal discharge because extension into the vagina is rare. In childhood, the vagina does not support the growth of candidal species; therefore, yeast vaginitis does not usually occur unless the child is immunocompromised or has been on long-term antibiotic therapy. Once a girl enters puberty (pubertal, not necessarily menarcheal) and has estrogenized vaginal mucosa, vulvovaginal candidiasis becomes a common cause of vulvovaginitis.

The primary symptom of vulvovaginal candidiasis is vulvar pruritus; the typical "cottage cheese" vaginal discharge seen in women is unusual in children, and there may not be any report of discharge. The diagno-

TABLE 21-5 ▶ SUGGESTED TREATMENTS FOR SPECIFIC CAUSES OF PEDIATRIC VULVOVAGINITIS

Etiology	Treatment

Bacterial	Antimicrobial per culture results and sensitivities
	Commonly prescribed:
	    Amoxicillin 40 mg/kg/day in three divided doses
	    Augmentin 40 mg (amoxicillin portion)/kg/day in three divided doses
	    Cephalexin 25–50 mg/kg/day in four divided doses
	    Azithromycin 10 mg/kg load, then five mg/kg/day

Foreign body	Removal of foreign body Antibiotics are not necessary.

Candida	Vulvitis
	    Topical nystatin cream applied twice daily for 7–10 days
	    Topical miconazole cream applied twice daily
	With oral thrush
	    Fluconazole 3 mg/kg/day daily for 7–14 days
	Vaginitis
	    Fluconazole 6 mg/kg single dose

Labial agglutination	Estrogen cream applied with cotton-tipped applicator to line of agglutination two to three times daily for 2–3 wk
Urethral prolapse	Sitz bath three to four times daily Estrogen cream to urethra two to three times daily for 2–3 wk Recurrent or recalcitrant cases may require surgical management.
Lichen sclerosus	Initial treatment with potent fluorinated topical steroid (e.g., clobetasol) applied to affected area bid for 2–4 weeks followed by less potent steroid (e.g., cutavate) qHS to bid for 2–4 wk, followed by mild steroid (e.g., hydrocortisone 2.5%) qHS to every other night for 3–4 wk. May require longer-term maintenance therapy or reinititiation of high-dose therapy for flares and recurrences.
Pinworms	Mebendazole 100 mg orally, for one dose Repeat same dose in 1 week. Treat other family members.
Contact allergy	Topical steroids, cold compresses Prednisone 0.5–2 mg/kg/day divided daily to qid
Contact sensitivity	Sitz baths, Burow's compresses, bland ointments
Superinfected dermatoses	Dermatologic treatment for primary condition (e.g., impetigo) Topical mupirocin 2% ointment tid for 5–14 days or penicillin VK 25–50 mg/kg/day in three to four divided doses

sis should be confirmed by preparing a suspension of the vaginal washings or discharge in a drop of potassium hydroxide and identifying the classic fungal elements. Candidal vulvitis related to simple diaper rash can be treated with topical antifungal creams. If oral thrush is also present, systemic treatment is usually necessary. In children with confirmed candidal vulvovaginitis, topical antifungals provide the most rapid symptomatic relief. Intravaginal preparations obviously are not appropriate. Systemic therapy with fluconazole or nystatin is well tolerated and effective. Immunocompromised girls may require more frequent or chronic antifungal therapy.

Pinworms

If pruritus, particularly nighttime or perianal pruritus, is a significant symptom, it is important to evaluate for pinworms by looking for larvae or eggs that may be captured by touching the anus with a piece of cellophane tape and then placing it on a glass slide for microscopy. For the best results, the tape test should be obtained by the child's caretaker in the early morning, before the child awakens. If the evaluation remains negative, but symptoms are significant, some clinicians recommend empiric treatment for pinworms.

Other Specific Infectious Organisms

Bloody discharge is most commonly associated with a vaginal foreign body, but it may also occur with infections caused by hemolytic streptococci, *Shigella*, and *Yersinia*.[31–33] Vaginal cultures are important in making the appropriate diagnosis and guiding treatment. If the vaginitis follows a course of diarrheal illness, vaginal cultures should be sent to the laboratory with a specific request to identify possible enteric pathogens.

Severe vulvovaginitis can also be caused by contact irritants or true allergic reactions. For treatment purposes, it is important to distinguish between the two etiologies. With irritant reactions, burning or stinging usually begins immediately after contact with the inciting agent. Erythema and edema may occur transiently, but itching or blistering do not occur. Common irritants include soaps, topical medications such as lidocaine, and other medication or lotion ingredients such as propylene glycol and alcohol. Treatment is aimed at providing symptomatic relief with sitz baths, Burow's compresses, and bland emollients.[25]

A true contact allergy is less common and implicates a cell-mediated reaction that takes approximately 48 hours to develop and persists for up to 3 to 4 weeks. Blistering, erythema, and pruritus occur wherever the skin was touched by the allergen. Symptomatic treatment with topical steroids and cool compresses can provide immediate relief, but a course of systemic steroid therapy with prednisone is often necessary.[25]

Secondary vulvar infections can also result from scratching or rubbing vulvar lesions related to eczema, psoriasis, or allergic or contact reactions. Systemic illness such as chickenpox, measles, or Crohn's disease can also manifest initially on the vulva and create symptoms consistant with vulvovaginitis, or even mimic vulvar trauma. Similarly, dermatologic conditions, including seborrhea, psoriasis, and eczema, can involve the vulva. Treatment of the vulvovaginitis resulting from these types of systemic or secondary infections should be aimed at treating the primary condition and providing local symptomatic treatment.

Sexually Transmitted Diseases

The diagnosis of an STD in a child should initiate a thorough evaluation for abuse. Nonsexual transmission of an STD is rare in children.[34] However, it is important to keep in mind all possible sources of infection, including vertical transmission, direct sexual contact, nonsexual casual contact, and fomites. All states have mandatory reporting requirements for cases of suspected child sexual abuse. Clinicians who see this age group should be very familiar with their state protocols and local resources for child abuse victims. Accurate documentation and appropriate testing are critical, and follow-up should be arranged with a professional who is experienced in evaluating and treating childhood sexual abuse.

Vulvovaginal signs or symptoms occur with most STDs in prepubertal girls.[35] If left untreated, however, the symptoms of vaginal discharge or vulvar irritation lessen in severity and can eventually disappear.[5] Because the prepubertal genital tract lacks estrogen, the vaginal portio of the cervix does not expose endocervical glands, and therefore the upper genital tract is protected from ascending infections.[36] Pelvic inflammatory disease is extremely rare in prepubertal girls, and has not been reported in the modern literature. If a discharge is present and a primary vaginitis is suspected, cultures for STD are indicated before any antibiotic therapy is initiated.[21] Treatment should follow Centers for Disease Control and Prevention recommendations for the treatment of STD with antimicrobial therapy that is appropriate for the age group[37] (Table 21–6). A complete discussion of sexually transmitted infections in prepubertal girls is beyond the scope of this chapter, and comprehensive reviews are available elsewhere.[38]

Human Papilloma Virus

The presence of genital HPV infection in a child deserves special mention. Because of the latency of symp-

TABLE 21–6 ▶ RECOMMENDED TREATMENT FOR SEXUALLY TRANSMITTED INFECTIONS IN CHILDREN*	
Infection	**Treatment**

Gonorrhea	<45 kg: Ceftriaxone 125 mg IM
	>45 kg and >7 y of age:
	  Ciprofloxacin 500 mg PO, single dose
	  Cefixime 400 mg PO, single dose
	  Doxycycline 100 mg PO bid for 7 days

Chlamydial infection	<45 kg: Erythromycin base 50 mg/kg/day PO in four divided doses/day for 10–14 days >45 kg: <8 y of age: Azithromycin 1 g PO single dose >45 kg: >8 y of age: Azithromycin 1 g PO single dose or doxycycline 100 mg PO bid for 7 days
Trichomoniasis	Metronidazole 40 mg/kg/day (max. 2 g) PO single dose or 15 mg/kg/day (max. 1 g/day) in three divided doses/day for 7 days
Bacterial vaginosis	Metronidazole 15 mg/kg/day (max. 1 g/day) in three divided doses/day for 7 days
Human papilloma virus/genital warts	Laser or electrical ablation Surgical excision Trichloroacetic or bichloroacetic acid; best if used with topical anesthetic Cryotherapy
Genital herpes simplex (primary outbreak)	Acyclovir 400 mg PO tid for 7–10 days Famciclovir 250 mg PO tid for 7–10 days Valacyclovir 1 g PO bid for 7–10 days

*The diagnosis of a sexually transmitted disease in a child should initiate an investigation into the possibility of sexual abuse.

toms of HPV infection, children as old as 18 to 24 months of age can manifest genital HPV infection that was acquired perinatally through an infected birth canal. However, the same clinical picture can also arise from sexual abuse. It is critical, therefore, that a thorough evaluation be performed by someone who can make the appropriate diagnosis when sexual abuse has occurred, but can also forestall false accusations of abuse. Studies by experts in child and adolescent sexual abuse suggest that most children older than 12 to 18 months of age with anogenital warts acquired their infection through direct sexual contact.[39, 40]

Human papilloma virus infection in the prepubertal girl may present with genital bleeding, discharge, or pain. Often, it is noticed incidentally during diapering or routine physical examinations. The clinical appearance of HPV lesions on the prepubertal genital mucosa is different from the typical hyperkeratotic genital wart seen in adolescents or adults. In girls, the lesions are fluffy, soft, and friable. The diagnosis can be made visually. Tissue biopsy is not necessary but may be helpful when the diagnosis is uncertain. Concern about the relationship between specific HPV subtypes and subsequent vulvar and cervical epithelial malignancies have led some clinicians to recommend viral subtyping.[41] However, there are no guidelines to direct how this type of information should be used in the treatment or follow-up of children, and viral subtyping has little clinical use at present. Regardless of viral subtyping, children with genital warts should be followed at least annually for recurrences.

A wide variety of treatments are available for genital warts, but many of these are not approved or are not appropriate for use in young children. Podophyllin- or podofilox-based topical treatments have not been approved for use in children because of the potential for absorption with systemic toxicity and serious complications. Imiquimod has not been approved for use in young children because there have been no clinical trials. Topical trichloroacetic or bichloroacetic acid is probably of limited use in children because of discomfort and the need for repetitive applications. For small warts that would be expected to respond to one or two applications, trichloroacetic or bichloroacetic acid may be appropriate if applied after providing local anesthesia with an effective topical anesthetic such as EMLA (eutectic mixture of local anesthetics). Cryotherapy, similarly, can be painful and most children do not tolerate repetitive treatments. For small warts, however, some clinicians advocate cryotherapy. To minimize discomfort, caution must be taken to freeze only the wart and not the surrounding tissue. Surgical treatment is commonly used to treat young or older children with more than a few scattered warts. Surgical treatments include CO_2 laser ablation, surgical excision, and, in some cases, electrocautery. The CO_2 laser is especially useful for extensive warts and is the treatment of choice for periurethral or intraurethral warts. Performed properly, it also provides the best cosmetic result.

NONINFECTIOUS CAUSES OF PEDIATRIC VULVOVAGINITIS

Vaginal Foreign Body

The most common cause of bloody vaginal discharge in a child is a vaginal foreign body. In the prepubertal vagina, any type of foreign object induces an intense inflammatory reaction with a foul-smelling, bloody or brown vaginal discharge. Often, a vaginal foreign body can be visualized in the distal vagina and removal accomplished in the office setting. The most commonly found foreign object is toilet tissue. Small, rolled-up pieces inadvertently trapped in the vagina look like small, gray clumps of matter; there are usually multiple pieces. These can easily be irrigated from the vagina with warm water briskly flushed through a long, small-diameter tube such as a pediatric feeding tube or intrauterine inseminator catheter. A solid foreign body can occasionally be "milked" out of the vagina through a digital rectal examination (which is well tolerated in most children). If these measures are not successful, vaginoscopic retrieval of the object is necessary. Once the object is removed, the vaginal discharge clears within several days, and antibiotics are not necessary.

Lichen Sclerosus

Lichen sclerosus is a skin condition with an unclear etiology that primarily affects the vulva of prepubertal girls and postmenopausal women. Symptoms may include vulvar itching, irritation, and "contact" dysuria, but without a significant discharge. Ulcerations and subepithelial hemorrhage may also occur. Genital examination reveals hypopigmentation and thin, parchment-like skin in a figure-of-eight distribution that encircles the vulva and anus. During flares, skin blisters and subepithelial hemorrhage can be easily mistaken for trauma or sexual abuse. Biopsy is not necessary when the diagnosis can be made clinically based on the classic findings; however, a biopsy can confirm an uncertain diagnosis. The severity of symptoms tends to fluctuate throughout childhood, but most girls have complete resolution of symptoms by menarche. Chronic or severe cases left untreated can result in labial or clitoral atrophy, fissures of the vulva and anus, and stenosis of the urethra, vagina, or anus.

Initial treatment includes topical therapy with a medium- to high-potency corticosteroid ointment (clobetasol proprinate 0.05%, or betamethasone valerate 0.1%) once or twice daily for 2 to 3 weeks, followed by a gradual taper to a less potent steroid (triamcinolone acetonide 0.1%, alclometasone dipropionate 0.05%, or hydrocortisone 2.5%). Many girls with lichen sclerosus require long-term maintenance with once- or twice-weekly application of topical steroid ointment, and intermittent treatment with more potent ointments for recurrent symptomatic flares.[42] Alternate therapy includes topical progesterone in oil (100 mg in 1 oz. Aquaphor) applied twice daily until symptoms resolve, then tapered to a maintenance treatment once or twice a week.[25] Topical testosterone is no longer recommended for the treatment of licen sclerosus and specifically should not be used in children. Furthermore, there is no evidence to support the use of laser "brushing" or surgical treatment for lichen sclerosus in children.

Labial Adhesions

Agglutination of the labia minora may occur as a result of dry, hypoestrogenic vulvar mucosa or from chronic inflammation from any cause. It is usually asymptomatic and often noted incidentally on routine genital examinations of young children. In the absence of symptoms, no treatment is necessary because most cases resolve spontaneously. Occasionally, the agglutination becomes extensive enough to divert or obstruct urinary outflow or allow urine to become trapped in the distal vagina. This may initiate a distal vaginitis or lead to urinary tract infections. Trapped urine may also dribble onto the perineum, causing irritation and symptoms of vulvovaginitis.

For symptomatic cases, treatment includes application, two to three times daily, of estrogen cream or a bland ointment using a cotton-tipped applicator and applying gentle pressure to the line of agglutination. Over 2 to 3 weeks, the agglutination weakens and the labia either separate spontaneously or can be easily separated with gentle traction (after application of a topical anesthetic). Separating the adhesion by traction is painful and traumatic, and should be avoided. Rarely, the agglutination becomes severe enough to cause acute urinary retention and require immediate separation. This can be accomplished under anesthesia or in the office setting using a topical anesthetic cream (EMLA). If the agglutination must be separated, the area should be treated subsequently for 1 to 2 weeks with topical estrogen cream to aid healing. *Traumatic separation should be avoided* because the scarring can lead to more severe recurrences. The patient or caretaker should be advised that labial adhesions frequently recur until the child approaches puberty. Recurrences can be avoided by having the caretaker or child apply a bland ointment to the area two to three times a week.

Urethral Prolapse

Vulvar bleeding and pain is occasionally the result of urethral prolapse. The cause is often unknown, but it can be associated with chronic irritation, chronic cough, masturbation, or sexual abuse. It involves protrusion of the urethral mucosa through the meatus, creating a hemorrhagic, edematous, friable mass. It is easily mistaken for a vaginal mass, but the distinction is made by visualizing the urethral orifice in the center of the mass that is separate from the vaginal opening or by passing a catheter through the orifice in the center of the mass and obtaining urine. If urination is not impaired, treatment should consist of warm sitz baths and topical estrogen cream two to three times daily until the mass resolves. In rare cases, urine outflow is obstructed or the mass may be large and necrotic. This type of presentation requires placement of an indwelling catheter, ligation, and resection or ablation of the redundant tissue.

SEQUELAE

Most causes of pediatric vulvovaginitis are not associated with long-term physical sequelae, but recurrences may be common. Preventive education for the patient and her caretaker and continued attention to perineal hygeine are both crucial elements in avoiding recurrences.

For some causes, particularly sexually transmitted infections, long-term sequelae are a concern. There are no data indicating any long-term effect of prepubertally acquired STD on reproductive function. There has never been a reported case of pelvic inflammatory disease in a prepubertal girl. For viral diseases, including HPV and the herpes viruses, long-term follow-up is warranted because of the potential neoplastic risks associated with these diseases. The young girl who has experienced sexual abuse or molestation is at great risk for future psychological and behavioral problems as well as recurrent abuse. These girls should always be referred to an appropriate agency or person with expertise in addressing childhood sexual abuse.

For a girl diagnosed with a vulvovaginitis, the most serious sequelae are usually psychological. Becoming hypervigilant to genital symptoms and pain can induce an unhealthy "genital fixation" for the girl or her caretaker. For the child's parent or caretaker, regardless of the presenting complaint, there is usually an underlying (or obvious) concern about the possibility of sexual abuse. This concern should always be addressed, regardless of whether it is voiced by the caretaker. By approaching pediatric vulvovaginits in a matter-of-fact manner and providing reassurance that the problem can be treated and will not likely cause any long-term effects, clinicians can help young girls and their caretakers maintain an appropriate perspective and attitude toward a common problem.

REFERENCES

1. Koumantakis EE, Hassan EA, Deligeoroglou EK, Creatsas GK: Vulvovaginitis during childhood and adolescence. J Pediatr Adolesc Gynecol 1997; 10:39.

2. Paradise JE, Campos JM, Freidman HM, et al: Vulvovaginitis in premenarcheal girls: Clinical features and diagnostic evaluation. Pediatrics 1982; 70:193.

3. Gerstner GJ, Grunberger W, Boschitsch E, Rotter M: Vaginal organisms in prepubertal children with and without vulvovaginitis. Arch Gynecol 1982; 231:247.

4. Cox RA: *Haemophilus influenzae*: An underrated cause of vulvovaginitis in young girls. J Clin Pathol 1997; 50:765.

5. Hammerschlag MR, Alpert S, Rosner I, et al: Microbiology of the vagina in children: Normal and potentially pathogenic organisms. Pediatrics 1978; 62:57.

6. Altcheck A: Vulvovaginitis, vulvar skin disease, and pelvic inflammatory disease. Pediatr Clin North Am 1981; 28:397.

7. Brown JL: Hair shampooing technique and pediatric vulvovaginitis. [Letter.] Pediatrics 1989; 83:146.

8. Heller ME, Savage MO, Dewhurst J: Vaginal bleeding in childhood: A review of 51 patients. Br J Obstet Gynaecol 1978; 85:721.

9. Huffman JW: Premenarcheal growth and development. In: Huffman JW (ed): The Gynecology of Childhood and Adolescence. Philadelphia, WB Saunders, 1968, pp 47–54.

10. Marshall WA: Growth and secondary sexual development and related abnormalities. Clin Obstet Gynecol 1974; 1:593.

11. Styne D: Normal growth and pubertal development. In: Sanfilippo JS (ed): Pediatric and Adolescent Gynecology. Philadelphia, WB Saunders, 1994, pp 26–33.

12. Rohn RD: Papilla (nipple) development during female puberty. J Adolesc Health Care 1982; 2:217.

13. Huggins GR, Preti G: Vaginal odors and secretions. Clin Obstet Gynecol 1981; 24:355.

14. Mardh P: The vaginal ecosystem. Am J Obstet Gynecol 1991; 165:1163.

15. Hill GB, St Claire KK, Gutman LT: Anaerobes predominate among the vaginal microflora of prepubertal girls. Clin Infect Dis 1995; 20:S269.

16. Lally MR, Orenstein SR, Cohen BA: Crohn's disease of the vulva in an 8 year old girl. Pediatr Dermatol 1988; 5:103.

17. Emans SJ, Goldstein DP: The gynecologic examination of the prupubertal child with vulvovaginitis: Use of the knee-chest position. Pediatrics 1980; 65:758.

18. Heger A, Emans SJ (eds). Evaluation of the Sexually Abused Child: A Medical Textbook and Photographic Atlas. New York, Oxford University Press, 1992, pp 79–112.

19. Berenson AB, Heger AH, Hayes JM, et al: Appearance of the hymen in prepubertal girls. Pediatrics 1992; 89:387.

20. Pokorny SF, Stormer J: Atraumatic removal of secretions from the prepubertal vagina. Am J Obstet Gynecol 1987; 156:581.

21. Embree JE, Lindsay D, Williams T, et al: Acceptability and usefulness of vaginal washes in premenarcheal girls as a diagnostic procedure for sexually transmitted diseases. Pediatr Infect Dis J 1996; 15:662.

22. Pokorny SF, Hammill H: Clinical correlates of vaginal cultures in the prepubertal female. [Abstract.] Adolesc Pediatr Gynecol 1995; 8:156.

23. Bump RC, Bueshing WJ: Bacterial vaginosis in virginal and sexually active adolescent females: Evidence against exclusive sexual transmission. Am J Obstet Gynecol 1988; 158:935.

24. Gardner JJ: Comparison of the vaginal flora in sexually abused and nonabused girls. J Pediatr 1992; 120:872.

25. McKay M: Vulvitis and vulvovaginitis: Cutaneous considerations. Am J Obstet Gynecol 1991; 165:1176.

26. Bump RC: *Chlamydia trachomatis* as a cause of prepubertal vaginitis. Obstet Gynecol 1985; 65:384.

27. Fuster DC, Neinstein LS: Vaginal *Chlamydia trachomatis* prevalence in sexually abused prepubertal girls. Pediatrics 1987; 79:235.

28. Shapiro RA, Schubert CJ, Myers PA: Vaginal discharge as an indicator of gonorrhea and *Chlamydia* infection in girls under 12 years old. Pediatr Emerg Care 1993; 9:341.

29. Hammerschlag MR, Rettig PH, Shields ME: False positive result with the use of *Chlamydia* antigen detection tests in the evaluation of suspected sexual abuse in children. Pediatr Infect Dis 1988; 7:11.

30. Lee HH, Chernesky MA, Schachter J, et al: Diagnosis of *Chlamydia trachomatis* genitourinary infection in women by ligase chain reaction assay of urine. Lancet 1995; 345:213.

31. Ginsburg CM: Group A streptococcal vaginitis in children. Pediatr Infect Dis 1982; 1:36.

32. Murphy TV, Nelson JD: *Shigella* vaginitis: Report of 38 patients and review of the literature. Pediatrics 1979; 63:511.

33. Watkins S, Quan L: Vulvovaginitis caused by *Yersinia enterocolitica*. Pediatr Infect Dis 1984; 3:444.

34. Neinstein LS, Goldenring J, Carpenter S: Nonsexual transmission of sexually transmitted disease: An infrequent occurrence. Pediatrics 1984; 74:67.

35. Muram D, Speck PM, Dockter M: Child sexual abuse examination: Is there a need for routine screening for *N. gonorrhoeae*? J Pediatr Adolesc Gynecol 1996; 9:79.

36. Huffman JW: Anatomy. In: Huffman JW (ed): The Gynecology of Childhood and Adolescence. Philadelphia, WB Saunders, 1968, pp 26–46.

37. Centers for Disease Control and Prevention: 1998 Guidelines for treatment of sexually transmitted diseases. MMWR Morb Mortal Wkly Rep 1997; 47(RR-1):7.

38. Mulchahey KM: Sexually transmitted diseases in childhood. In: Sanfilippo JS (ed): Pediatric and Adolescent Gynecology. Philadelphia, WB Saunders, 1994, pp 336–355.

39. Boyd AS: Condyloma acuminata in the pediatric population. Am J Dis Child 1990; 144:817.

40. Herman-Giddens ME, Gutman LT, Berson NL: Association of coexisting vaginal infections and multiple abusers in female children with genital warts. Sex Transm Dis 1988; 15:63.

41. Bender ME: New concepts of condyloma acuminata in children. Arch Dermatol 1986; 122:1121.

42. Dalziel KL, Wojnarowska F: Long-term control of vulvar lichen sclerosus after treatment with a potent topical steroid cream. J Reprod Med 1993; 38:25.

22

Cervicitis

JORMA PAAVONEN

Cervicitis can be infectious or noninfectious. Infectious cervicitis is caused by *Chlamydia trachomatis, Neisseria gonorrhoeae,* herpes simplex virus (HSV), or combinations of these sexually transmitted pathogens. Infectious cervicitis represents a reservoir for sexual and perinatal transmission of pathogenic microorganisms. Cervicitis may lead to at least three types of complications: ascending intraluminal spread of pathogenic organisms from the cervix, producing pelvic inflammatory disease (PID); ascending infection during pregnancy, resulting in premature rupture of the membranes, chorioamnionitis, premature delivery, and puerperal and neonatal infections; and the development of cervical neoplasia.

Noninfectious cervicitis has not been well defined, but usually there is inflammation of the ectopic endocervical columnar epithelium.

The clinical diagnosis of cervicitis has been impeded by the lack of wide acceptance of objective criteria for cervicitis or cervical inflammation. This is best illustrated by the confusing nomenclature for cervicitis. Such terms as acute cervicitis, chronic cervicitis, cervical erosion, cervical ectropion, cervical discontinuity, follicular cervicitis, hypertrophic cervicitis, and mucopurulent cervicitis have all been used. This confusion results in part from changes that occur in the cervix over the reproductive years, and in part from difficulties in differentiating normal physiologic cervical ectopy from true cervicitis.

DYNAMIC ANATOMY OF CERVICAL EPITHELIUM

Because the cervix is a hormonally responsive organ, the appearance of the epithelium changes with age, pregnancy, and oral contraceptive use. These major physiologic alterations in the appearance of the epithelium markedly affect the anatomy of the cervix and its susceptibility to pathogenic microorganisms. Two types of epithelium are commonly found on the ectocervix: peripheral stratified squamous epithelium and a centrally located, single-cell layer of columnar epithelium continuous with the endocervical columnar epithelium (Fig. 22–1). In young women, the squamocolumnar junction often lies well out on the ectocervix, forming a bright red central zone of ectopic columnar epithelium termed *ectopy.* With increasing age, sexual activity, and during pregnancy, squamous metaplasia occurs along the squamocolumnar junction, progressively replacing the columnar epithelium with metaplastic and maturing squamous epithelium (Fig. 22–2). The original squamocolumnar junction is apparent even when

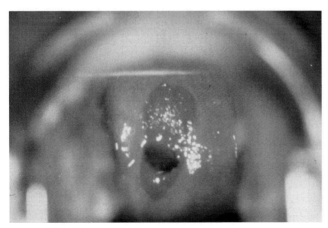

FIGURE 22-1 ▶ Cervical ectopy consisting of normal physiologic columnar epithelium.

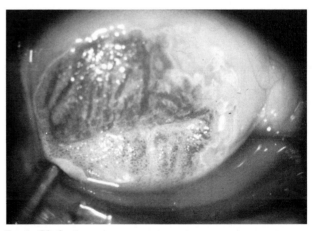

FIGURE 22-2 ▶ Cervical squamous metaplasia progressively replacing central columnar epithelium. Note the original squamocolumnar junction marked by gland openings, and the more centrally located new squamocolumnar junction showing faint acetowhiteness.

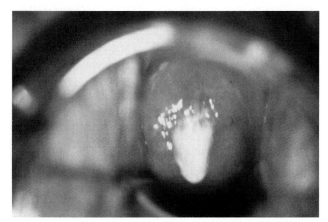

FIGURE 22–3 ▶ Mucopurulent cervicitis caused by *Chlamydia trachomatis.*

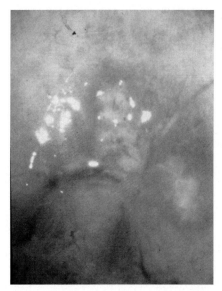

FIGURE 22–4 ▶ Ulcerative ectocervicitis caused by herpes simplex virus type 2.

the new metaplastic squamous epithelium has completely covered the exposed columnar area because small retention cysts and gland openings mark its site. This border is indicated by the "last" gland on the cervix. In older women, the squamocolumnar junction lies high up in the endocervical canal and is usually not visible from the vagina on speculum examination.

ETIOLOGY OF CERVICITIS

The principal recognized infectious causes of cervicitis are the sexually transmitted pathogens *C. trachomatis,* *N. gonorrhoeae,* and HSV.[1] Other common infectious causes of cervicitis are *Trichomonas vaginalis* and *Treponema pallidum.* Rare causes are *Mycobacterium tuberculosis,* *Staphylococcus aureus,* and *Calymmatobacterium granulomatis.*

Two types of cervicitis can be distinguished, endocervicitis and ectocervicitis. *Chlamydia trachomatis* and *N. gonorrhoeae* cause endocervicitis (Fig. 22–3), whereas *T. vaginalis* and HSV primarily cause ectocervicitis (Fig. 22–4). Cervical ulcer is common in primary first-episode genital herpes (Fig. 22–5), but rare in recurrent herpes. The role of genital mycoplasmas in the etiology of cervicitis is controversial, although *Ureaplasma urealyticum* has been linked to mucopurulent cervicitis.[2]

To provide a guide for therapy, patient counseling, and management of sex partners, a specific microbiologic diagnosis should be obtained in patients with suspected cervicitis. Patients with mucopurulent cervicitis should have Gram's stain or wet-mount examination, culture for *N. gonorrhoeae,* and a test for *C. trachomatis.* A test for HSV is indicated if genital ulcer disease is suspected. The development of the nucleic acid amplification based diagnostic tests for *C. trachomatis* has been a major breakthrough. Studies have shown that first-void urine can replace endocervical swab in the diagnosis of *C. trachomatis* infection.

Noninfectious causes of cervicitis include malignant disease, rare autoimmune diseases, mechanical

trauma, chemical injury, and irradiation. Bacterial vaginosis has also been associated with mucopurulent cervicitis and PID,[2-4] suggesting that changes in the cervicovaginal environment might foster the development of cervicitis.

DIAGNOSIS

Clinical Diagnosis

The simple objective criterion for the clinical diagnosis of infectious cervicitis is demonstration of mucopurulent endocervical discharge. The presence of mucopurulent endocervical discharge can be confirmed by visualization of cloudy or yellow endocervical mucopus on a white swab (swab test).[1] However, mucopus is not always present in proven cases of infectious cervicitis, and may represent only the "tip of the iceberg" of all cervicitis.

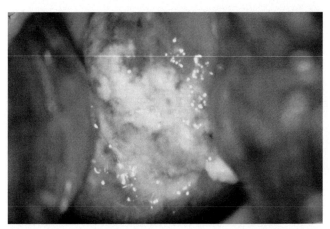

FIGURE 22–5 ▶ Cervical ulcer caused by primary first-episode genital herpes.

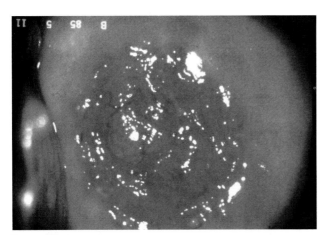

FIGURE 22–6 ▶ Severe (3+) edema of an ectopy consistent with cervicitis.

Cervicitis Severity Score

Deriving a cervicitis severity score based on the presence of cervical erythema and edema and induced mucosal bleeding is useful in clinical studies monitoring the response of cervicitis to antimicrobial therapy.[5] The severity of inflammation of the cervical epithelium can be assessed by scoring the degree of (1) mucosal bleeding induced by swabbing the cervix, (2) erythema, and (3) edema (Fig. 22–6) in the zone of ectopy and the transformation zone as observed with the unaided eye. Each finding is scored as 0 (none or normal), 1+ (mild), 2+ (moderate), or 3+ (severe), and the sum of these scores represents the cervicitis severity score. When chlamydial and nonchlamydial cases with mucopurulent cervicitis were compared, those with chlamydial cervicitis had higher cervicitis severity scores.[5]

Endocervical Gram Stain

For quantitation of polymorphonuclear (PMN) leukocytes in endocervical secretions, the swab should be rolled onto a glass microscopic slide, air dried, and Gram stained. The slide should be scanned at a magnification of 100× to identify cervical mucus containing inflammatory cells. The number of PMNs per 1,000× microscopic field in five nonadjacent fields can then be established using an oil immersion lens. The presence of large numbers of vaginal squamous cells and vaginal flora mixed with inflammatory cells suggests that the specimen includes ectocervical material and that inflammatory cells might originate in the vagina, indicating vaginitis rather than cervicitis. Ectocervical specimens are unsatisfactory for the diagnosis of endocervicitis. In menstruating women, neither the swab test nor the quantitation of PMN leukocytes can be used. There is no evidence of significant variation in PMN counts between women with and those without

mucopus over the menstrual cycle, except during menses.

The aforementioned criteria for the clinical diagnosis of cervicitis have been developed and implemented in a high-risk sexually transmitted disease (STD) clinic population, but have not been properly evaluated in low-risk populations.

Vaginal Wet Mount

Vaginal wet-mount examination is a bedside procedure and easier to perform than cervical Gram's stain. A vaginal wet mount showing more leukocytes than vaginal epithelial cells (per 400× microscopic field) with no apparent vaginal infection (e.g., yeast, T. vaginalis) is suggestive of cervicitis[6] (Fig. 22–7).

Cytology

Although cervical cytologic analysis by Papanicolaou (Pap) smear was introduced for detection of cervical neoplasia, there is growing interest in the use of this method for the diagnosis of specific cervical and vaginal infections. The Pap smear is useful in the diagnosis of several cervicovaginal infections, including bacterial vaginosis, T. vaginalis, yeast, human papilloma virus, HSV, and Actinomyces (intrauterine device users).

Cytologic manifestations of cervical and vaginal infection include both epithelial and inflammatory cellular changes. A study performed in an STD clinic setting[7] showed that increased numbers of lymphocytes, histiocytes, and PMN leukocytes best correlated with C. trachomatis and T. vaginalis cervical infection (Fig. 22–8). PMN leukocytes also correlated with HSV infection. Transformed lymphocytes and plasma cells correlated with C. trachomatis. Of epithelial cellular changes, reactive endocervical cells correlated with C. trachomatis infection. Atypical metaplastic cells correlated with C. trachomatis and N. gonorrhoeae. Thus, specific inflammatory patterns can be used to identify women

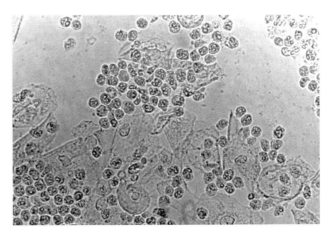

FIGURE 22–7 ▶ Vaginal wet mount showing increased number of white cells suggestive of cervicitis.

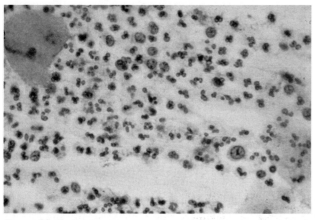

FIGURE 22–8 ▶ Papanicolaou smear showing increased numbers of histiocytes, lymphocytes, and polymorphonuclear leukocytes, consistent with cervicitis.

likely to have chlamydial cervicitis. Knowledge of the association of a specific genital infection with specific cytologic atypias may help to interpret such abnormalities and improve the control of genital infections, particularly *C. trachomatis* infections.

Colposcopy

Colposcopy is usually used to evaluate women from whom directed cervical biopsies will be obtained because of cytologic atypia. Thus, colposcopy has not been extensively used as a screening procedure for cervical infections. However, bright light and magnification greatly improve the diagnosis of cervicovaginal infections as well. Many colposcopic features are associated with specific cervical or vaginal infections.[8] Apparent endocervical mucopus is associated with *C. trachomatis*, *N. gonorrhoeae*, and HSV, "strawberry cervix" (colpitis macularis) is associated with *T. vaginalis*, hypertrophic ("follicular") cervicitis with *C. trachomatis* (Fig. 22–9), immature metaplasia with *C. trachomatis*

and cytomegalovirus, ulcers and necrotic areas with HSV, and increased cervical surface vascularity with *C. trachomatis*, *T. vaginalis*, and HSV. Obviously, the colposcope cannot be a substitute for specific microbiologic tests. However, awareness of the association of colposcopic features with specific infections is important for colposcopists to identify patients who need specific microbiologic studies, just as awareness of cytologic manifestations of cervical infections is important to cytopathologists examining Pap smears obtained from women at high risk for such infections.

Histopathology

Most histologic features of cervical inflammation (i.e., intraepithelial or luminal PMN leukocytes, reactive endocervical cells, dense subepithelial inflammation, edema, necrotic ulceration, granulation tissue, germinal centers, spongiosis) are more frequent in patients with cervicitis and proven cervical infection with *C. trachomatis* (Fig. 22–10), *N. gonorrhoeae*, HSV, or *T. vaginalis* than in patients without. Histopathologic studies[9] of endocervical infection have shown that intraepithelial PMN leukocytes, dense subepithelial endocervical inflammation, a predominance of plasma cells in stromal tissue, and well-formed germinal centers are associated with chlamydial cervicitis (see Fig. 22–10); necrotic ulcers and a predominance of lymphocytes are associated with cervical HSV; and spongiosis is associated with cervical *T. vaginalis* infection.

TREATMENT

The recognition and treatment of infectious mucopurulent cervicitis is important to prevent PID and its sequelae. The current guidelines[10] recommend treatment of mucopurulent cervicitis as recommended for uncomplicated chlamydial infection (doxycycline 100 mg orally twice daily for 7 days, or azithromycin 1 g

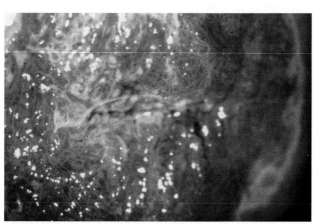

FIGURE 22–9 ▶ Hypertrophic cervicitis caused by *Chlamydia trachomatis*.

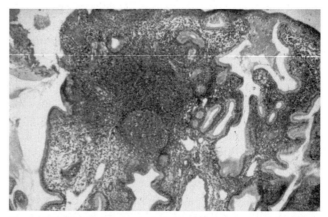

FIGURE 22–10 ▶ Histopathologic findings, consisting of dense inflammation and a well-formed germinal center of the cervical stroma, associated with cervicitis caused by *Chlamydia trachomatis*.

orally in a single dose). Empirical treatment for gonorrhea should be considered, depending on the prevalence of this infection in the population. Sex partners of women with cervicitis should be evaluated for STD and treated with an appropriate regimen.

Many cervicitis treatment studies have left several issues unresolved. First, cure usually has been defined as the eradication of specific organisms such as *C. trachomatis* or *N. gonorrhoeae*. However, only approximately half of the women with mucopurulent cervicitis have *C. trachomatis* or *N. gonorrhoeae* isolated from the cervix. For instance, in men with nongonococcal urethritis, conventional practice has been to demonstrate a reduction in clinical symptoms and urethral PMNs as measures for therapeutic response. In contrast, the effects of antibiotic therapy on mucopus per se or on cervical PMNs usually have not been assessed in women with chlamydial, gonococcal, or nonchlamydial nongonococcal mucopurulent cervicitis. Second, long-term follow-up has not been used to study late recurrences. There is a growing concern that late recurrences may be common and can cause PID, ectopic pregnancy, and tubal factor infertility.

PREVENTION

Pelvic inflammatory disease is a frequent complication of cervicitis. Evidence for upper genital tract infection in patients without clinical findings suggestive of PID has been obtained in several studies.[11] It is likely that symptomatic acute PID represents only a small fraction of all upper genital tract infections. Silent or atypical PID accounts for a significant proportion of cases of tubal factor infertility and tubal pregnancy. Therefore, screening for cervicitis and for cervicitis-causing microorganisms, most notably *C. trachomatis*, is of paramount importance in the prevention of long-term sequelae associated with PID. STD control programs should include development of diagnostic services with proper quality control, guidelines for clinicians in the clinical diagnosis and management of cervicitis, screening to identify asymptomatic carriers of *C. trachomatis*, establishment of surveillance systems, training of health care workers, periodic monitoring and evaluation of control measures, routine evaluation of sex partners, and effective patient education in behavioral aspects and contraception.

Because *C. trachomatis* is the most common sexually transmitted pathogen and a major cause of PID, it is logical to focus prevention efforts on chlamydial infection. The asymptomatic nature of cervicitis makes screening for chlamydial infection the mainstay for prevention of PID.

Disease prevention can be primary, secondary, or tertiary. Tertiary prevention of acute and chronic chlamydial infections of the upper genital tract has largely failed because substantial tubal damage has already occurred by the time symptoms develop. Delay of care is another critical factor predicting permanent tubal damage.[12] Although patients respond to antimicrobial therapy, the risk for development of tubal factor infertility or ectopic pregnancy may still be high.

Primary prevention involves preventing both exposure to and acquisition of chlamydial infection through lifestyle counseling and health education. Clinicians play an important role in primary prevention by asking questions about high-risk sexual behavior, encouraging screening tests for those at risk, ensuring that male sex partners are evaluated and treated, and counseling about safe sex practices. Primary prevention of STDs through health education has not yet proven to be very effective. However, studies of the efficacy of primary prevention are slow and extremely complicated to conduct. Clearly, more emphasis should be directed to primary prevention. Effective health education programs should be implemented among adolescents.

Secondary prevention by universal screening is likely to play a critical role in the prevention of PID and long-term sequelae,[13] although this still needs to be proved in randomized, controlled intervention trials. Secondary prevention means early detection of subclinical disease by screening to prevent lower genital tract infection from becoming upper genital tract infection. Chlamydial infection meets the general prerequisites for disease prevention by screening because chlamydial infections are highly prevalent, associated with significant morbidity, and can be diagnosed and treated.

Emerging evidence suggests that systematic screening of asymptomatic populations decreases the incidence of *C. trachomatis* infection. This has been documented both in nationwide screening programs and in screening programs performed in other defined populations with stable screening activity. One randomized, controlled trial has provided strong evidence that intervention with selective screening for chlamydial infection effectively reduces the incidence of PID.[13] Technological advances should further enhance efforts to prevent chlamydial infection.[14] These include single-dose therapy using azithromycin, amplification tests, and the first-void urine specimens for the diagnosis.[15, 16] However, it remains to be seen whether such intervention will also have a significant effect on the incidence of ectopic pregnancy and tubal factor infertility.

REFERENCES

1. Brunham RC, Paavonen J, Stevens CE, et al: Mucopurulent cervicitis: The ignored counterpart in women of urethritis in men. N Engl J Med 1984; 311:1.
2. Paavonen J, Critchlow C, DeRouen T, et al: Etiology of cervical inflammation. Am J Obstet Gynecol 1986; 154:556.
3. McCormack WM. Pelvic inflammatory disease. N Engl J Med 1994; 330:115.
4. Paavonen J, Teisala K, Heinonen PK, et al: Microbiological and histopathological findings in acute pelvic inflammatory disease. Br J Obstet Gynaecol 1987; 94:454.

5. Paavonen J, Roberts PL, Stevens CE, et al: Randomized treatment of mucopurulent cervicitis with doxycycline or amoxicillin. Am J Obstet Gynecol 1989; 161:128.

6. Weström L: Clinical manifestation and diagnosis of pelvic inflammatory disease. J Reprod Med 1984; 23(suppl):703s.

7. Kiviat N, Paavonen J, Brockway J, et al: Cytologic manifestation of cervical and vaginal infections. 1: Epithelial and inflammatory cellular changes. JAMA 1985; 253:989.

8. Paavonen J, Kiviat N, Wölner-Hanssen P, et al: Colposcopic manifestation of cervical and vaginal infections. Obstet Gynecol Surv 1988; 43:373.

9. Kiviat N, Wölner-Hanssen P, Echenbach DA, et al: Endometrial histopathology in patients with culture-proved upper genital tract infection and laparoscopically diagnosed acute salpingitis. Am J Surg Pathol 1990; 14:67.

10. STD treatment guidelines. MMWR Morb Mortal Wkly Rep 1998; 47:RR-1.

11. Paavonen J, Lehtinen M: Chlamydial pelvic inflammatory disease. Hum Reprod 1996; 2:519.

12. Hillis SD, Joesoef R, Marchbanks PA, et al: Delayed care of pelvic inflammatory disease as a risk factor for impaired fertility. Am J Obstet Gynecol 1993; 168:1503.

13. Scholes D, Stergachis A, Heidrich FE, et al: Prevention of pelvic inflammatory disease by screening for cervical chlamydial infection. N Engl J Med 1996; 334:1362.

14. Black CM: Current methods of laboratory diagnosis of *Chlamydia trachomatis* infection. Clin Microbiol Rev 1997; 10:160.

15. Davies PO, Ridgway GL: The role of polymerase chain reaction and ligase chain reaction for the detection of *Chlamydia trachomatis*. Int J STD AIDS 1997; 8:731.

16. Martin DH, Mroczkowski TF, Dalu ZA, et al: A controlled trial of a single dose of azithromycin for the treatment of chlamydial urethritis and cervicitis. N Engl J Med 1992; 327:921.

23 Pelvic Inflammatory Disease

DAVID E. SOPER

EPIDEMIOLOGY

In 1988, more than 10% of American women of reproductive age reported that they had received treatment for pelvic inflammatory disease (PID).[1] This is probably an underestimate of the true magnitude of this disease because of the poor reliability of the diagnosis and the realization that many women with it show only atypical symptoms or no symptoms at all.[2] These high rates of PID are alarming and underscore its importance as the most common and serious complication of cervicovaginal sexually transmitted diseases (STDs). Direct costs for PID and its associated sequelae of ectopic pregnancy and infertility approach 3 billion dollars a year. These costs are projected to approach 10 billion dollars annually by the year 2000, with an increasing proportion of that sum being covered by public payment sources.[3] Although there has been a decreased incidence of hospitalization for acute PID since 1983, the average annual number of women visiting private physicians' offices for this disorder has increased, suggesting a higher proportion of women with clinically mild disease associated with *Chlamydia trachomatis*.[4] *Chlamydia trachomatis* infection remains the most common bacterial STD in America, whereas rates of *Neisseria gonorrhoeae* infection have been decreasing since the 1970s.[5]

The settings in which patients are seen are likely to have a significant effect on the clinical manifestations and microbiology of PID. Women evaluated in an urban emergency room usually exhibit classic signs and symptoms of this disease, including fever and the "chandelier sign" associated with gonococcal PID, whereas women selected from an STD clinic or college population may have more benign clinical presentations associated with chlamydial PID.[6–8] However, universal risk assessment for the development of PID and its sequelae depends primarily on the identification of variables associated with the acquisition of an STD (gonorrhea, chlamydial infection, bacterial vaginosis [BV]). These clinical variables relate both to the ability of a patient to become infected with pathogenic microorganisms (i.e., host susceptibility) as well as to environmental factors that may promote the ascending spread of these pathogens. Risk markers include

younger age, lower socioeconomic status, substance abuse, and certain contraceptive practices. Risk factors associated with ascending infection include failure to seek adequate health care (allowing more prolonged STD infection), intrauterine device (IUD) use, and douching.[9]

Younger age predicts PID risk by being correlated with sexual behavior and potential acquisition of STD. It may also reflect biologic characteristics conducive to the development of PID, such as lower prevalence of protective chlamydial antibodies, larger zone of cervical ectopy, and greater permeability of cervical mucus.[10] Low socioeconomic status and substance abuse appear to be conducive to an increased prevalence of STDs in the population as well as failure to seek adequate health care and risky sexual behavior.

When properly used, mechanical and chemical contraceptive barriers are associated with decreased risk of STD, PID, and infertility.[9] These methods of contraception appear to exert their protective effect by decreasing the risk of acquisition of STD. In addition, the use of condoms may decrease the risk for development of PID after acquisition of an STD by eliminating a vehicle, the sperm, for ascending spread. Oral contraceptives (OCs) have a variable effect on the risk of PID. They appear to increase the risk of endocervical infection with *C. trachomatis*, probably by increasing the zone of cervical ectopy and thereby offering a larger area of endocervical cells for attachment. However, OCs are associated with a decreased risk of symptomatic PID. It is postulated that the progestin component of combination OCs induces changes in cervical mucus, making it thicker and less penetrable by bacteria. Also, decreased menstrual blood loss may lead to less retrograde menstruation and a less-than-optimal environment for bacterial proliferation. Last, OCs may modify the immune responses to chlamydial infections. The observation that OCs exert no significant effect on the risk of tubal infertility despite a decreased risk of symptomatic PID suggests that women using OCs may still acquire PID but in a milder, possibly asymptomatic form ("silent salpingitis"). This explanation has been confirmed by Ness and colleagues,[11] who noted that women with unrecognized endometritis were 4.3 times more likely than women with clinically recognized PID to use OCs.

Most studies have found an increased risk of PID and its sequelae, ranging from twofold to ninefold, among IUD users.[9] This risk of PID in IUD users appears to be highest in the first 4 months of use and not significantly elevated above baseline at 5 months.[12] This temporal sequence supports the hypothesis that introduction of vaginal and cervical microorganisms into the endometrial cavity during IUD insertion accounts for most cases of IUD-related PID. Preliminary data have suggested that prophylactic use of doxycycline at the time of insertion may reduce the risk for development of PID.[13] However, a more recent randomized, clinical trial in 1,833 women at low risk for sexually transmitted infection has shown no benefit from azithromycin prophylaxis compared with placebo.[14] In fact, there was only one case of PID in each study group, making the risk for PID in this population negligible.

Vaginal douching may be associated with acute PID and ectopic pregnancy. Several studies have noted that women with PID are more likely to have a history of douching than women without PID. One case-control study included a multivariate analysis to adjust for confounding variables and found that douching within the previous 2 months was associated with an adjusted relative risk of 1.7 (95% confidence interval = 1.02, 2.82).[15] The risk of PID was positively correlated with frequency of douching. Two hypotheses explain these associations: (1) douching could alter the vaginal environment and make it less protective against pathogenic organisms, and (2) douching might flush vaginal and cervical microorganisms into the uterine cavity and increase the risk of upper genital tract infection. Further study is needed to define more clearly the precise relationship between douching and PID. The first hypothesis was confirmed when douching was linked with an increased risk for the development of BV.[16]

MICROBIOLOGY AND PATHOGENESIS

The microbial etiology of PID can be divided into three categories: sexually transmitted microorganisms, vaginal ("BV") microorganisms, and respiratory microorganisms (Table 23–1). In North America, the microbial etiology of PID has been defined by the use of endocervical cultures for the STD microorganisms: gonococcal PID, chlamydial PID, and nongonococcal nonchlamydial PID. Studies that use culdocentesis specimens in hospitalized patients with the clinical diagnosis of PID suggest that as many as 80% of cases are associated with mixed infections of both aerobic and anaerobic microorganisms.[17–20] However, it has become apparent that culdocentesis is an unreliable method for defining the microbiology of the upper genital tract and in fact may even contaminate the cul-

TABLE 23–1 ▶ MICROBIAL PATHOGENESIS OF PELVIC INFLAMMATORY DISEASE
Sexually transmitted microorganisms
Neisseria gonorrhoeae
Chlamydia trachomatis
Vaginal microorganisms
"Bacterial vaginosis microorganisms"
Prevotella spp.
Peptostreptococcus spp.
Mycoplasma hominis
Escherichia coli
Respiratory pathogens
Haemophilus influenzae
Streptococcus pyogenes
Streptococcus pneumoniae

de-sac and yield false-positive cultures.[21, 22] Subsequent reports in which only laparoscopically obtained isolates were used and the use of culdocentesis was restricted have confirmed a polymicrobial etiology in only 30% to 40% of cases.[6, 7, 23, 24] *N. gonorrhoeae* remains the single most frequent pathogen recovered. *C. trachomatis* can be detected in up to 40% of women with PID in some populations. Studies done in Scandinavia reflect a different bacterial pathogenesis in that *C. trachomatis* is the most frequently recovered pathogen and anaerobic bacteria are conspicuously absent.[25]

Respiratory pathogens are isolated from the fallopian tube in approximately 5% of cases of acute salpingitis.[24] *Haemophilus influenzae* is the most commonly isolated microorganism in this category and is commonly associated with pyosalpinx formation.[26] In addition, *Streptococcus pyogenes*, *Neisseria meningitidis*, and *Streptococcus pneumoniae* have all been isolated from the upper genital tract of women with PID. That respiratory pathogens can be initiators of PID should come as no surprise because there is substantial similarity between the histology of the respiratory and upper genital tracts.[27]

Bacteria isolated from the upper genital tract of women with PID have usually been BV microorganisms. These are predominantly anaerobic bacteria such as *Prevotella* and *Peptostreptococcus* species commonly found in high concentrations in the vagina of women with BV. An increased concentration of *Mycoplasma hominis*, a genital mycoplasma, is also found in women with BV. BV has been associated with adnexal tenderness and, therefore, presumptive PID.[28] Moreover, the recovery of BV microorganisms has been shown to be associated with histologic endometritis in women with clinical signs of PID.[29] Uncommonly, microorganisms found in the gut may translocate across the bowel wall in cases involving significant bowel inflammation in patients with tubo-ovarian abscess (TOA). Cases of PID may be secondary to direct extension of an inflammatory process due to appendicitis or Crohn's disease. Only rarely do women using an intrauterine contraceptive device contract PID due to *Actinomyces israelii*.

Although it is clear that the pathogenesis of PID involves an ascending infection, the precise mechanisms determining the spread of microorganisms from the lower to the upper genital tract are poorly understood. The female genital tract is an open system. Particulate matter and dyes have been observed to ascend to the fallopian tubes after being placed in the vagina or endometrium.[30] Investigators using real-time sonography have demonstrated the ascending spread, enhanced by uterine contractions, of albumin placed in the vagina.[31] These observations suggest that a vehicle is unnecessary for the transportation of potential pathogenic microorganisms into the upper genital tract. This may be particularly true when the functional barrier afforded by the cervical mucus is attenuated by the changing of its rheologic properties during ovulation or its absence during menstruation. Evidence suggests, however, that spermatozoa may play a role in enhancing ascending spread. Sexual activity is a prerequisite for PID, and high coital frequency has been associated with an increased risk of acquiring the disease.[9] Bacteriospermia in men and adherence of bacteria to spermatozoa have been documented, suggesting that sperm may allow bacteria to piggyback their way to the fallopian tube.[30] Another mechanism by which bacteria may be propelled into the fallopian tube relates to the common occurrence of retrograde menstruation. Microorganisms may spread with this blood, contributing to the development of PID. Direct inoculation of the upper genital tract by gynecologic procedures such as IUD insertion, hysterosalpingography, and uterine curettage can also occur.

Once the gonococcus ascends to the fallopian tube, it selectively adheres to nonciliated mucus-secreting cells. After traversing these cells, the bacteria are released from the basal surface by exocytosis and invade the subepithelial space. Despite invasion of the gonococcus into the nonciliated epithelial cells, the major damage occurs in uninfected ciliated epithelial cells. It has been suggested that two structural components of the gonococcal surface, lipo-oligosaccharides and peptidoglycan, may exert a toxic effect, either directly or indirectly by the release of cytokines, on the ciliated epithelial cells. In addition, an acute, complement-mediated inflammatory response occurs involving the migration of polymorphonuclear leukocytes, vasodilation, and transudation of plasma into the tissues. This inflammatory reaction causes extensive cell death and tissue damage. The process of tissue repair, with the removal of dead cells and ingrowth of fibroblasts, goes on simultaneously with the inflammatory process, resulting in scarring and tubal adhesions.[32]

Cell-mediated immune mechanisms appear to be important in the tissue destruction associated with chlamydial tubal infection. Primary chlamydial tubal infection appears to be a self-limited disease associated with a mild to moderate tubal inflammatory response and little permanent damage.[33] Although cell-mediated immune responses often protect the host, chlamydial reinfection in some women is followed by more severe disease. Repeated genital challenges with *C. trachomatis* in experimental animals can induce a chronic hypersensitivity response to chlamydial antigens (particularly to a genus-specific 57-kD stress response protein) that can cause irreversible damage to tissues through immunopathologically mediated phenomena. These observations suggest that tubal inflammation with resulting tissue destruction in genital chlamydial infections might be the result of a delayed (hyper)immune reaction to repeated exposures to chlamydial antigens in a proportion of immunologically "primed" women.[32] The chronic exposure to *C. trachomatis* that occurs in asymptomatic women with silent chlamydial tubal infection might be especially conducive to the development of this immune response. Moreover, the presence of homologous regions in the chlamydial 57-kD protein and the human 60-kD heat shock protein suggests that sensitization of the immune system to chlamydial protein might lead to the development of an autoimmune response to the homologous human protein. Once this autoimmune circuit becomes established, host tissue damage may continue even if *C. trachomatis* is no longer present.[34]

Fitz-Hugh–Curtis Syndrome

The Fitz-Hugh–Curtis syndrome (FHCS) is an extrapelvic manifestation of PID.[35] FHCS is composed of two phases, acute and chronic. In the acute phase, a perihepatitis and a focal peritonitis result from the transport of inflammatory peritoneal fluid either directly or by lymphatics to the subphrenic and subdiaphragmatic space. Laparoscopically, these patients have a purulent exudate visible on the liver capsule but no adhesions. Both *N. gonorrhoeae* and *C. trachomatis* have been isolated from the liver surface of women with FHCS. Microscopic examination of the liver parenchyma reveals acute inflammation of the capsule without parenchymal involvement. The chronic phase is characterized by "violin-string" adhesions between the anterior surface of the liver and the anterior abdominal wall (Fig. 23–1).

Fitz-Hugh–Curtis syndrome tends to be an incidental finding in patients with a clinical diagnosis of PID because their pelvic symptoms and signs are usually more dramatic than those related to perihepatitis. Patients with pleuritic upper abdominal pain and PID are presumed to have FHCS. Uncommonly, patients with FHCS may primarily complain of a sudden onset of upper quadrant pain. This pain is usually on the right side and is exacerbated by breathing or coughing. There may be some radiation of this pain to the shoulder or back. When the right upper quadrant pain is severe, clinicians may overlook the possibil-

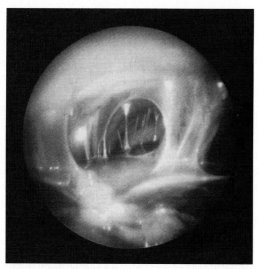

FIGURE 23-1 ▶ "Violin-string" adhesions in a patient with Fitz-Hugh–Curtis syndrome.

ity of PID-associated FHCS as an etiology for these complaints. Physical signs of PID are present as previously described. In addition, patients with FHCS demonstrate upper abdominal tenderness and guarding. Liver enzymes and bilirubin determinations are usually normal or slightly elevated, excluding the possibility of a viral hepatitis as an etiology of the patient's symptoms.

Atypical Pelvic Inflammatory Disease ("Silent Salpingitis")

More than half of women with tubal factor infertility (TFI) give no history of PID.[36, 37] In addition, antibodies to *C. trachomatis* or *N. gonorrhoeae* are noted in most of these patients, suggesting that prior infection has occurred. Moreover, both gross and microscopic examination of the fallopian tubes of women with TFI fail to differentiate between those patients with or without a history of PID.[38] These data indirectly suggest that women may contract salpingitis and subsequent tubal damage without manifesting the typical clinical symptoms, primarily lower abdominal pain and fever, associated with the traditional diagnosis of PID.

Women with atypical PID may display abdominal or pelvic discomfort such as dysmenorrhea or dyspareunia, which clinicians commonly associate with an alternative gynecologic diagnosis such as endometriosis. Others may have symptoms previously associated with PID (metrorrhagia and vaginal discharge), but in the absence of a concurrent complaint of abdominal pain, clinicians may not relate these symptoms to a sexually transmitted genital infection.[39] The absence of significant abdominal pain in these patients most likely relates to the lack of an associated peritonitis.[40]

Women with mucopurulent endocervicitis (MPC) often have histologic evidence of endometritis.[41] This

is direct evidence that upper genital tract inflammation may be present in the absence of signs and symptoms suggesting PID. In addition, almost half of women with chlamydial endocervical infections may have concurrent endometrial infections without evidence of pelvic organ tenderness on physical examination.[42] Many women with infertility and positive chlamydial serology also have silent but active chlamydial infections of the endometrium.[43]

DIAGNOSIS

The goal of the clinical diagnosis of PID is to establish diagnostic guidelines that are sufficiently sensitive to avoid missing mild cases, but sufficiently specific to avoid antibiotic therapy in women with no infection. Because symptoms are what bring the patient to the physician, the first step in treating the patient is to define symptoms that are potential indicators of upper genital tract infection. As has already been mentioned, any number of genital tract symptoms may be indicators of PID, but none has sufficient specificity to warrant a diagnosis of PID on historical grounds alone. However, all patients with any genitourinary symptoms should have the diagnosis of PID considered. These symptoms include, but are not limited to, lower abdominal pain, menorrhagia, metrorrhagia, fever/chills, and urinary symptoms. Also, if the physical findings described as follows are noted, a diagnosis of PID may be made even in the asymptomatic woman.

The next crucial step is an evaluation of the lower genital tract secretions, both vaginal and endocervical. The vaginal secretions should be evaluated for the presence of increased numbers of polymorphonuclear leukocytes (leukorrhea). Leukorrhea is present when more than one polymorphonuclear leukocyte per epithelial cell is seen during microscopy of a wet mount of the vaginal secretions (the inflammatory cells are the predominant cell observed on the slide; Fig. 23–2).

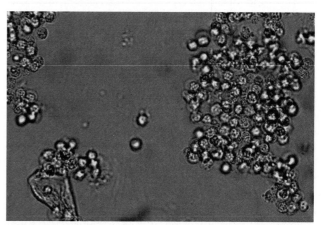

FIGURE 23-2 ▶ Microscopic examination of a saline mount of the vaginal secretions shows an increased number of leukocytes (leukorrhea). (Magnification 400×.)

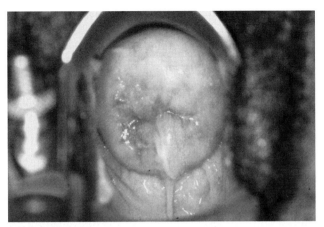

FIGURE 23-3 ▶ Evidence of mucopus documents lower genital tract inflammation.

The endocervix should be evaluated for the presence of MPC. Endocervicitis is characterized by a mucopurulent (green or yellow) endocervical discharge and an endocervix that is erythematous, edematous, and friable (Fig. 23–3). Tests from the endocervix for the detection of *N. gonorrhoeae* and *C. trachomatis* should be performed. A bimanual pelvic examination should then be performed and any pelvic organ tenderness or uterine, adnexal, or cervical motion tenderness should be noted. Management of the patient can then be based on findings of this evaluation.

The clinical criteria for the diagnosis of PID have never been validated in large prospective studies[44] (Table 23–2). Two similar sets of guidelines for the diagnosis have been suggested. Jacobson and Westrom[45] were the first to evaluate the accuracy of conventional signs and symptoms of PID as assessed by the visual confirmation of acute salpingitis. Diagnostic accuracy was improved by increasing the number of positive param-

eters. Westrom and Mardh[46] suggested that the basis for the diagnosis of PID should include at least three criteria, with supportive signs, laboratory tests, or both improving the specificity of the diagnosis. Of particular importance is Westrom's[47] uniform finding of a marked increase in the number of inflammatory cells (leukorrhea) in the wet smear of the vaginal secretions of women with PID. It appears that this simple test can be used to exclude the possibility of PID in women with abdominal pain. In other words, women with PID almost always have leukorrhea, but women with leukorrhea do not necessarily have PID.

In a separate analysis of Westrom's data, purulent vaginal discharge, an elevated erythrocyte sedimentation rate, positive culture for *N. gonorrhoeae*, adnexal swelling on bimanual examination, and a temperature greater than 38°C were good predictors of laparoscopically confirmed salpingitis.[48] Hager and colleagues[49] published similar guidelines suggesting that clinicians rely on three major clinical signs and at least one of five supportive parameters. Their guidelines eliminate the necessity for a chief complaint of abdominal pain, an important improvement if we accept the possibility that many patients with atypical PID may not have abdominal pain. Unfortunately, they diminish the importance of assessing the patient's vaginal secretions, although a Gram's stain of the endocervix revealing gram-negative diplococci is an adjunctive criterion. A comprehensive analysis of symptoms, physical signs, laboratory data, and combinations of these indicators failed to reveal an algorithm that would reliably predict PID.[50] In light of these findings, adnexal tenderness or cervical motion tenderness was thought to be sufficient to allow a diagnosis of mild PID in the absence of strong evidence for a competing diagnosis. For women with a more serious degree of clinical illness, addi-

TABLE 23-2 ▶ CLINICAL CRITERIA FOR THE DIAGNOSIS OF PELVIC INFLAMMATORY DISEASE

Westrom and Mardh[46]	Hager and Colleagues[49]	Suggested
Major criteria (all must be present)		
Symptoms		
Abdominal pain	None required	None required
Signs		
Adnexal tenderness	Abdominal tenderness	Pelvic organ tenderness
Signs of a lower genitourinary tract infection	Cervical motion tenderness Adnexal tenderness	Leukorrhea or mucopurulent endocervicitis
Minor criteria (additional criteria increase the specificity of the diagnosis)		
Palpable adnexal mass	Gram's stain of endocervix =	Endometrial biopsy = endometritis
ESR ≥15 mm/h	positive for gram-negative	Elevated C-reactive protein or ESR
Temperature >38°C	diplococci	Temperature >38°C
	Temperature >38°C	Leukocytosis
	Leukocytosis (>10,000/mm³)	Positive test for chlamydial
	Purulent material by culdocentesis	infection or gonorrhea
	Pelvic complex by examination or sonography	

ESR = erythrocyte sedimentation rate.
Modified from Soper DE: Diagnosis and laparoscopic grading of acute salpingitis. Am J Obstet Gynecol 1991; 164:1370.

tional evaluation, including invasive tests such as endometrial biopsy and laparoscopy, was recommended.

Women without pelvic organ tenderness and with no evidence of MPC need not be treated with antibiotics unless a history suggests the need for epidemiologic therapy (exposure to a known carrier of gonorrhea or chlamydial infection). Women with pelvic organ tenderness and no evidence of MPC should have other diagnoses considered, such as a ruptured ovarian cyst, mittelschmerz, or other lower abdominal disorders. These women should not require antibiotic treatment. Women with pelvic organ tenderness and evidence of MPC should be started on antibiotic therapy for a presumed diagnosis of PID. A complete blood count and C-reactive protein should be drawn, but the results need only be used retrospectively to support the presumptive diagnosis. Follow-up reveals which of these women have positive tests for gonorrhea or chlamydial infection. This procedure allows the women who have no evidence of lower genital tract inflammation and who were not started on antimicrobial therapy for gonorrhea or chlamydial infection to be treated for these endocervical infections.

These recommendations are an attempt to provide a rationale for the institution of antimicrobial therapy in women with or at risk for PID. These guidelines should provide a "low threshold for diagnosis" of PID but not allow indiscriminate use of antibiotic treatment for any woman presenting with lower abdominal pain or pelvic organ tenderness. Note that women without evidence of lower genital tract inflammation (leukorrhea or MPC) are not considered to have PID. These guidelines will still result in substantial overtreatment for the diagnosis of PID because at least a third of these women would not have acute salpingitis if examined laparoscopically. Indeed, because many of these patients do not have a chief complaint of pelvic pain, their chance of having laparoscopically verified salpingitis is even lower. However, a substantial number of these women have lower genital tract infections, as manifested by the increase in inflammatory cells in their vaginal secretions, requiring antimicrobial treatment even if they do not have salpingitis. Moreover, those patients without lower genital tract inflammation have still been tested for gonorrhea and chlamydial infection. If these tests are positive, call-back and treatment are appropriate.

Endometrial Biopsy

Endometritis is uniformly associated with salpingitis.[51-53] Endometrial biopsy and subsequent histologic confirmation of acute or chronic endometritis confirm the diagnosis of PID. The procedure is technically uncomplicated and can be performed by both gynecologists and primary care physicians. Although not imperative in the evaluation of the woman with suspected

PID, the procedure allows the clinician to evaluate objectively the upper genital tract for inflammation, but stops short of requiring general anesthesia and laparoscopy. When performed with the Pipelle endometrial suction curet, only minor discomfort is experienced by the patient.

Ultrasound

Endovaginal sonography has been shown to correlate well with laparoscopic findings of patients with severe PID; however, sonographic findings are only minimal in women with mild salpingitis.[54] The lack of diagnostic endovaginal sonographic findings in patients with mild disease limits its usefulness in evaluating women with atypical or mild clinical presentations. For the most part, sonographic findings in women with PID are not specific enough to add to the overall diagnosis of the patient with suspected PID.

Laparoscopy

Laparoscopy remains the gold standard for the diagnosis and grading of acute salpingitis. The minimum criteria for the visual confirmation of acute salpingitis include (1) pronounced hyperemia of the tubal surface, (2) edema of the tubal wall, and (3) a sticky exudate on the tubal surface and from the fimbriated ends when patent[44, 45] (Fig. 23–4). In some cases erythema and edema can be overinterpreted because of observer bias.[55] For this reason, visual confirmation of salpingitis without the presence of exudate may be erroneous (false-positive). Evaluation of the peritoneal exudate is suggested to document the presence of inflammatory cells. Peritoneal fluid in normal patients and in those with endometriosis contains predominantly macrophages. Peritoneal fluid cytologic exami-

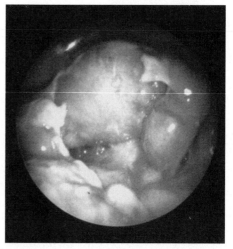

FIGURE 23–4 ▶ Laparoscopy visually confirms the presence of edematous, erythematous fallopian tubes and a sticky, purulent exudate documenting upper genital tract inflammation.

nations in patients with acute salpingitis inevitably reveals a predominance of neutrophils. It is also imperative that an endometrial biopsy be performed during the diagnostic laparoscopy to add objective evidence of endometrial inflammation.

The severity of clinical disease is unrelated to laparoscopic findings.[7, 56] Women with more indolent symptoms who delay in seeking health care tend to have more severe tubal abnormalities noted at laparoscopy than their benign clinical presentation would suggest.[8] Alternatively, patients admitted with four-quadrant rebound and significant temperature elevation are more likely to have a laparoscopically mild salpingitis rather than a ruptured TOA.

Treatment issues are discussed in the context of the severity of clinical disease in the next section.

Tubo-ovarian Abscess

The diagnosis of TOA is made when the bimanual pelvic examination reveals a palpable adnexal mass in the patient with a clinical diagnosis of PID. Further characterization of this mass can be undertaken with endovaginal sonography. In addition, some patients are too tender to allow adequate evaluation of the adnexa when admitted to the hospital. Sonography can help determine the presence of inflammatory complexes in these patients.

TREATMENT

Treatment of the patient with PID encompasses more than just prescribing the appropriate antimicrobial regimen. Determining the need for hospitalization, patient education, management of sexual partners, and careful follow-up are key treatment issues.

Although most women with PID are treated as outpatients, data on the treatment of PID in an outpatient setting is limited.[57] Moreover, the microbial etiology of PID seen in this setting is not well established. It is assumed that it mirrors the bacterial pathogenesis observed in patients undergoing laparoscopy and hospital admission. The recommended regimen of a beta-lactam antibiotic and doxycycline (Table 23–3) has been used extensively in the treatment of outpatient PID since 1984.[58] One study revealed rather poor coverage by doxycycline of facultative bacteria and anaerobic microorganisms isolated from women with PID.[59] In addition, a single dose of a beta-lactam antibiotic should not be sufficient to treat a significant anaerobic soft tissue infection. Despite this, clinical efficacy varies from 81% to 94%.[60–63] Ofloxacin is effective against both *N. gonorrhoeae* and *C. trachomatis*. Limited study of this quinolone suggests that it is useful in treating women with PID in an outpatient setting.[64] Despite the results of this trial, there is concern related to ofloxacin's lack of anaerobic coverage; the addition of clinda-

TABLE 23–3 ▶	1998 CENTERS FOR DISEASE CONTROL AND PREVENTION GUIDELINES FOR TREATMENT OF PELVIC INFLAMMATORY DISEASE

Outpatient treatment
  Regimen A
Ofloxacin 400 mg PO bid for 14 days
PLUS
Metronidazole 500 mg PO bid for 14 days
  Regimen B
Ceftriaxone* 250 mg IM once, or cefoxitin 2 g IM plus
    probenecid, 1 g PO concurrently or equivalent cephalosporin
PLUS
Doxycycline 100 mg PO bid for 14 days
Inpatient treatment
  Regimen A
Cefotetan 2 g IV q12h or cefoxitin IV 2 g q6h
PLUS
Doxycycline 100 mg q12h PO or IV
  Regimen B
Clindamycin IV 900 mg q8h
PLUS
Gentamicin loading dose IV or IM (2 mg/kg) followed by a
    maintenance dose (1.5 mg/kg) q8h. Single daily dosing may be
    substituted.

One of the preceding regimens is given for at least 24 h after the patient clinically improves.

After discharge from hospital, continue doxycycline 100 mg bid to a total of 14 days or clindamycin 450 mg orally qid to a total of 14 days

---

IM = intramuscular; IV = intravenous; PO = oral.
*Other cephalosporins such as ceftizoxime, cefotaxime, and ceftriaxone, which provide adequate gonococcal, other facultative gram-negative aerobic, and anaerobic coverage may be used in appropriate doses.
  Data from Centers for Disease Control and Prevention: 1998 Guidelines for treatment of sexually transmitted diseases. MMWR Morb Mortal Wkly Rep 1993; 47:79.

mycin or metronidazole provides this coverage (see Table 23–3). Amoxicillin-clavulanate with or without doxycycline has been evaluated in the treatment of 63 women with suspected PID who were treated as outpatients.[65] All women completing therapy were either cured or improved, although 20% experienced gastrointestinal side effects necessitating the discontinuation of therapy. Azithromycin, the first available antibiotic from a new class of azalide antimicrobials, has been shown to be an effective single-dose (1 g orally) treatment for chlamydial MPC, but it has not been studied in the treatment of PID.[66]

The patient's need for hospitalization can be based on the severity of the clinical illness, likelihood of compliance with an outpatient regimen, suspicion of anaerobic infection, and certainty of the diagnosis (Table 23–4). It is not known whether parenteral regimens are superior to oral regimens for the treatment of PID. However, the high cost of in-hospital treatment prevents routine hospitalization of all patients who are diagnosed with PID.

Patients with severe clinical disease require hospitalization to monitor their early response to therapy and to rule out the possibility of a rupturing TOA. These

TABLE 23-4 ▶ INDICATIONS FOR HOSPITALIZATION

Noncompliance with outpatient regimen
   Addicts
   Adolescents
   Nausea/vomiting precludes oral therapy
Severe clinical disease
   Temperature >101°F
   White blood cell count >15,000/mm³
   Upper peritoneal signs
   Septic shock
Suspected anaerobic infection
   History of intrauterine instrumentation
   Intrauterine device use
   Suspected pelvic or tuboovarian abscess
Uncertain diagnosis
   Failure to respond to outpatient treatment
   Pregnancy and pelvic inflammatory disease (rule out ectopic)
   Rule out appendicitis

patients usually have high white blood cell counts (>15,000/mm³), significant fever (>101°F), or upper peritoneal signs. Patients with significant nausea and vomiting that precludes oral therapy also require admission for parenteral antimicrobial therapy. Other concerns about compliance with oral antibiotic regimens may make the hospitalization of adolescents and addicts appropriate.[67] Patients with a history of intrauterine instrumentation, IUD use, or a pelvic mass noted during bimanual pelvic examination should be considered for parenteral therapy with inpatient antimicrobial regimens that more effectively cover anaerobic bacteria. Those women with PID and an IUD in situ should also have the IUD removed soon after the initiation of antimicrobial therapy.[68]

Patients with an uncertain diagnosis also warrant admission for observation and possible diagnostic laparoscopy. Laparoscopy is especially recommended for women with a history of recurrent, outpatient-treated PID. These women may have an alternative etiology such as endometriosis that accounts for their recurrent symptoms. This is also the case in most women failing to respond to outpatient antibiotic treatment. Patients with a positive pregnancy test and a diagnosis of PID should have the possibility of ectopic pregnancy ruled out.

Treatment is based on a consensus that PID is polymicrobial in cause, and currently recommended antimicrobial regimens are broad-spectrum in coverage[60, 68] (see Table 23-3). Treatment usually must be initiated before the microbial cause is established and is usually empiric. The two recommended inpatient regimens have been studied extensively (over 1,000 patients studied), and those studies strongly suggest that both regimens are clinically effective. In one regimen (a combination of cefoxitin and doxycycline), cefoxitin was selected for coverage of N. gonorrhoeae, the Enterobacteriaceae, and anaerobes. Doxycycline was chosen primarily to cover C. trachomatis. In the other regimen (a

combination of clindamycin and gentamicin), clindamycin was selected to cover anaerobes and gram-positive aerobes. The aminoglycosides were chosen to cover gram-negative aerobes, including N. gonorrhoeae. The second regimen is thought to be potentially more useful than the first for patients with pelvic abscesses, but it provides less coverage for C. trachomatis. However, one study suggests that the effectiveness of extended-spectrum antibiotic coverage, including single-agent broad-spectrum antibiotics such as cefoxitin used in conjunction with doxycycline, is equivalent to that of clindamycin-containing regimens for the treatment of TOA.[69] More than 75% of patients with TOAs respond to antibiotic treatment alone and do not require surgical intervention.

A number of alternative regimens appear to have promise for the treatment of PID. Penicillins with beta-lactamase inhibitors (ampicillin-sulbactam, ticarcillin-clavulanate, amoxicillin-clavulanate) appear to be effective in the treatment of PID, but use of these agents in treating those infections attributable to C. trachomatis remains in question. Quinolones such as ofloxacin have in vitro activity against some facultative gram-positive cocci, gram-negative organisms including N. gonorrhoeae, and C. trachomatis; however, they have limited activity against anaerobes. Quinolones appear to be effective in the treatment of salpingitis not complicated by TOA.[7, 64]

There has been considerable interest in the use of anti-inflammatory agents as adjunctive therapy for PID. The prominent role of the immune system in the pathogenesis of tubal inflammation and scarring has prompted interest in this area. However, data supporting the efficacy of either steroids or nonsteroidal anti-inflammatory agents in decreasing the morbidity of PID are lacking. Falk[70] studied the effect of prednisone on the clinical course and end results of PID. Although prednisone accelerated the normalization of body temperature, erythrocyte sedimentation rate, and resolution of adnexal swelling, it had no effect on hysterosalpingographic findings, fertility, or tubal disease found in a subsequent laparotomy. Likewise, in a murine chlamydial salpingitis model, no apparent benefit resulted from the addition of anti-inflammatory agents.[71]

Antibiotic therapy should be continued to complete a 10- to 14-day course. Patients should be followed for criteria indicative of a therapeutic response, including lysis of fever, normalization of the white blood cell count, total disappearance of rebound tenderness, and marked amelioration of pelvic organ tenderness. Although prompt response is common in women with even severe clinical manifestations of PID, patients with laparoscopically severe disease or TOA tend to require a longer hospitalization. Patients failing to show a response to antimicrobial treatment within 96 hours should be re-evaluated to determine the accuracy of diagnosis and the possibility of the presence of a TOA that may require surgical intervention. In some cases, percutaneous drainage of the abscess can be effected under computed tomographic or sonographic guidance, obviating the need for surgical intervention.[72]

Surgical Treatment

The initial surgical approach usually involves laparoscopy to confirm the diagnosis and establish the severity of the disease. Laparoscopy is especially helpful in ruling out the possibility of acute appendicitis. Patients with severe disease may benefit from operative endoscopy to lyse adhesions, aspirate pyosalpinges, dissect and drain loculations of pus, and irrigate the pelvic and abdominal cavities.[73] Laparotomy is recommended in cases of generalized peritonitis associated with signs of sepsis due to a suspected ruptured TOA or when severe PID is refractory to medical therapy. A great deal of judgment must be used to determine the extent of extirpative surgery necessary to cure the patient. In patients who want to preserve fertility, unilateral adnexectomy may be elected if the disease is predominantly one-sided. In some cases, bilateral salpingectomy or bilateral salpingo-oophorectomy may be necessary. Patients without adnexa may still be able to conceive with the help of in vitro fertilization and ovum donation as long as the uterus is intact. Total abdominal hysterectomy with bilateral salpingo-oophorectomy remains the procedure of choice for severe PID refractory to medical therapy in women finished with their childbearing.

Adjunctive Therapy

Bed rest and avoidance of sexual intercourse during therapy are an integral part of the treatment of PID. Bed rest in the semi-Fowler position allows purulent material to pool in the cul-de-sac and promotes patient comfort. Sexual abstinence should continue until all signs and symptoms of PID have disappeared and until male sexual partners have completed treatment.

The sexual partners of women with PID should be tested for *N. gonorrhoeae* and *C. trachomatis* and treated empirically with ceftriaxone, 250 mg intramuscularly, and doxycycline 100 mg orally every 12 hours for 7 days or azithromycin 1 g PO in a single dose. Over half of male sexual partners of women with gonococcal PID have cultures positive for *N. gonorrhoeae*, even though many are asymptomatic.[74, 75] Chlamydial infection has also been found in approximately one third of male sexual partners of women with PID.[76] In women with PID in whom neither *N. gonorrhoeae* nor *C. trachomatis* is cultured, testing the male sexual partner may disclose a sexually transmitted cause for the episode of acute salpingitis.

LONG-TERM SEQUELAE

It is well known that the reproductive sequelae of TFI and ectopic pregnancy are common consequences of PID. In a longitudinal study of over 1,800 women, TFI was shown to be related to the severity of salpingitis and to the number of episodes of PID.[77] For patients with only one episode of PID, incidence of proven TFI increased significantly with the severity of the infection as visually judged at the time of the index laparoscopy. The rate of TFI was 0.6% after a case of mild salpingitis, 6.2% after a case of moderate salpingitis, and 21.4% after severe salpingitis. Each repeated episode of PID roughly doubled the rate of TFI. Overall, after one, two, and three or more episodes, the rates were 8.0%, 19.5%, and 40.0%, respectively.

Damage to the fallopian tubes after PID is a well-documented etiologic risk for tubal pregnancy. Westrom and co-workers[77] confirmed Westrom's earlier population study, noting that the rate of ectopic pregnancy was increased by almost a factor of four in women with a visually documented case of salpingitis compared with control subjects. Such an increased risk is extended beyond an eventual intrauterine pregnancy.[78]

In a retrospective study, Safrin and colleagues[79] noted that 24% of women with PID had pelvic pain for 6 months or more after hospitalization. This confirms earlier work by Westrom,[80] in which he reported an 18% incidence of chronic pelvic pain after an episode of PID. Patients may also complain of longer and more painful menstruation and pain during sexual intercourse.[81]

PREVENTION

All available evidence suggests that by the time a patient is diagnosed with PID, those events that will lead to tubal scarring and other sequelae have probably already occurred. For this reason, prevention of PID becomes of utmost importance. Prevention options focus primarily on avoiding either exposure to STDs or acquisition of infection after exposure. This requires people to practice healthy sexual behavior, such as postponing one's sexual debut, choosing uninfected sex partners, and limiting the number of sex partners. Women need to recognize that they are the ones who pay the price of PID, chronic pelvic pain, and infertility for their partner's promiscuity. Women, empowered by the knowledge of what behaviors put them at risk, can then play a major role in preventing infection by modifying their own high-risk sexual behaviors, refusing to have coitus with a high-risk partner, or insisting on the use of mechanical or chemical barriers that can be used for personal prophylaxis against acquiring an STD. In addition, if a woman participates in risky coitus, the knowledge of this risk, coupled with access to medical care, can lead to prompt recognition and treatment of STDs.[82]

Most chlamydial and gonococcal lower genital tract infections and many upper genital tract infections are asymptomatic. Therefore, increasing symptom awareness in women will have only a minor impact on the morbidity associated with ascending infections. Patient education, with a focus on risk and screening rather than on symptoms associated with disease, is an important tool in the overall fight against STDs and PID. In a randomized, controlled trial, Scholes and colleagues[83] showed that a strategy of identifying, testing, and treating women at increased risk for cervical chlamydial infection was associated with a reduced incidence (relative risk = 0.44) of PID.

The male sex partner also must be brought into this equation. It is not uncommon to see a monogamous woman with PID infected by her promiscuous male sex partner. It is important not only to contact, trace, and treat infected male sexual partners, but to educate these men with respect to the morbidity they cause by their reckless sexual behavior. Education concerning these issues should be incorporated into the public sex education curriculum.

Health care providers play an obvious role in prevention strategies. Increasing the amount of clinical training in STDs will lead to appropriate screening of high-risk people as well as improve recognition and treatment of clinically recognizable infections. Aggressive identification and treatment of uncomplicated lower genital tract infections in women should reduce the risk for development of PID. Counseling to reduce further STD risk is an important adjunct to treatment of any STD.

REFERENCES

1. Aral SO, Mosher WD, Cates W: Self-reported pelvic inflammatory disease in the United States, 1988. JAMA 1991; 266:2570.
2. Wolner-Hanssen PW, Kiviat NB, Holmes KK: Atypical pelvic inflammatory disease: Subacute, chronic, or subclinical upper genital tract infection in women. In: Holmes KK, Mardh P-A, Sparling PF, et al. (eds): Sexually Transmitted Diseases, 2nd ed. New York: McGraw-Hill, 1990, pp 615–620.
3. Washington AE, Katz P: Cost of and payment source for pelvic inflammatory disease: Trends and projections, 1983 through 2000. JAMA 1991; 266:2565.
4. Rolfs RT, Galaid EI, Zaidi AA: Pelvic inflammatory disease: Trends in hospitalizations and office visits, 1979 through 1988. Am J Obstet Gynecol 1992; 166:983.
5. Centers for Disease Control and Prevention: Summary of notifiable diseases, United States 1997. MMWR Morb Mortal Wkly Rep 1997; 46:34.
6. Wasserheit JN, Bell TA, Kiviat NB, et al: Microbial causes of proven pelvic inflammatory disease and efficacy of clindamycin and tobramycin. Ann Intern Med 1986; 104:187.
7. Soper DE, Brockwell NJ, Dalton HP: Microbial etiology of urban emergency department acute salpingitis: Treatment with ofloxacin. Am J Obstet Gynecol 1992; 167:653.
8. Svennson L, Westrom L, Ripa KT, Mardh P-A: Differences in some clinical and laboratory parameters in acute salpingitis related to culture and serologic findings. Am J Obstet Gynecol 1980; 138:1017.
9. Washington AE, Aral SO, Wolner-Hanssen P, et al: Assessing risk for pelvic inflammatory disease and its sequelae. JAMA 1991; 266:2581.
10. Cates W, Rolfs RT, Aral SO: Sexually transmitted diseases, pelvic inflammatory disease, and infertility: An epidemiologic update. Epidemiol Rev 1990; 12:199.
11. Ness RB, Keder LM, Soper DE, et al: Oral contraception and the recognition of endometritis. Am J Obstet Gynecol 1997; 176:580.
12. Grimes DA: Intrauterine devices and pelvic inflammatory disease: Recent developments. Contraception 1987; 36:97.
13. Sinei SKA, Schulz KF, Lamptey PR, et al: Preventing IUCD-related pelvic infection: The efficacy of prophylactic doxycycline at insertion. Br J Obstet Gynaecol 1990; 97:412.
14. Walsh T, Grimes D, Frezieres R, et al: Randomised controlled trial of prophylactic antibiotics before insertion of intrauterine devices: IUD Study Group. Lancet 1998; 351:1962.
15. Wolner-Hanssen P, Eschenbach DA, Paavonen J, et al: Association between vaginal douching and acute pelvic inflammatory disease. JAMA 1990; 263:1936.
16. Hawes SE, Hillier SL, Benedetti J, et al: Hydrogen peroxide-producing lactobacilli and acquisition of vaginal infections. J Infect Dis 1996; 174:1058.
17. Eschenbach DA, Buchanan TM, Pollock HM, et al: Polymicrobial etiology of acute pelvic inflammatory disease. N Engl J Med 1975; 293:166.
18. Cunningham FG, Hauth JC, Gilstrap LC, et al: The bacterial pathogenesis of acute pelvic inflammatory disease. Obstet Gynecol 1978; 52:161.
19. Chow WC, Malkasian KL, Marshall JR, Guze LB: The bacteriology of acute pelvic inflammatory disease: Value of cul-de-sac cultures and relative importance of gonococci and other aerobic and anaerobic bacteria. Am J Obstet Gynecol 1975; 122:876.
20. Monif GRG, Welkos SL, Baer H, Thompson RJ: Cul-de-sac isolates from patients with endometritis-salpingitis-peritonitis and gonococcal endocervicitis. Am J Obstet Gynecol 1976; 126:158.
21. Sweet RL, Draper DL, Schachter J, et al: Microbiology and pathogenesis of acute salpingitis as determined by laparoscopy: What is the appropriate site to sample? Am J Obstet Gynecol 1980; 138:985.
22. Soper DE, Brockwell NJ, Dalton HP: False-positive cultures of the cul-de-sac associated with culdocentesis in patients undergoing elective laparoscopy. Obstet Gynecol 1991; 77:134.
23. Sweet RL, Draper DL, Hadley WK: Etiology of acute salpingitis: Influence of episode number and duration of symptoms. Obstet Gynecol 1981; 58:62.
24. Brunham RC, Binns B, Guijon F, et al: Etiology and outcome of acute pelvic inflammatory disease. J Infect Dis 1988; 158:510.
25. Mardh P-A, Moller BR, Paavonen J: Chlamydial infection of the female genital tract with emphasis on pelvic inflammatory disease: A review of Scandinavian studies. Sex Transm Dis 1981; 8:140.
26. Teisala K, Heinonen PK, Punnonen R: Laparoscopic diagnosis and treatment of acute pyosalpinx. J Reprod Med 1990; 35:19.
27. McGee ZA, Pavia AT: Is the concept, "agents of sexually transmitted disease" still valid? [Editorial.] Sex Transm Dis 1991; 18:69.
28. Eschenbach DA, Hillier S, Critchlow C, et al: Diagnosis and clinical manifestations of bacterial vaginosis. Am J Obstet Gynecol 1988; 158:819.
29. Hillier SL, Kiviat NB, Hawes SE, et al: Role of bacterial vaginosis-associated bacteria in endometritis. Am J Obstet Gynecol 1996; 175:435.
30. Keith LG, Berger GC, Edelman DA, et al: On the causation of pelvic inflammatory disease. Am J Obstet Gynecol 1984; 149:215.
31. Lund KJ, Williamson C, Parsons A, McGregor JA: Active uterine transport of ultrasound contrast medium during the ovarian cycle: A key to upper reproductive tract infection? [Abstract.] Annual Meeting of the Infectious Disease Society for Obstetrics and Gynecology, Jackson Hole, Wyoming, August 5–8, 1998. Infect Dis Obstet Gynecol 1998; 6:100.

32. Rice PA, Schachter J: Pathogenesis of pelvic inflammatory disease: What are the questions? JAMA 1991; 266:2587.

33. Patton DL, Halbert SA, Kuo CC, et al: Host response to primary *Chlamydia trachomatis* infection of the fallopian tube in pig-tailed monkeys. Fertil Steril 1983; 40:829.

34. Witkin SS, Ledger WJ: New directions in the diagnosis and treatment of pelvic inflammatory disease. J Antimicrob Chemother 1993; 31:197.

35. Lopez-Zeno JA, Keith LG, Berger GS: The Fitz-Hugh-Curtis syndrome revisited: Changing perspectives after half a century. J Reprod Med 1985; 30:567.

36. Sellors JW, Mahony JB, Chernesky MA, Rath DJ: Tubal factor infertility: An association with prior chlamydial infection and asymptomatic salpingitis. Fertil Steril 1988; 49:451.

37. Tjiam KH, Zeilmaker GH, Alberda AT, et al: Prevalence of antibodies to *Chlamydia trachomatis, Neisseria gonorrhoeae,* and *Mycoplasma hominis* in infertile women. Genitourin Med 1985; 61:175.

38. Patton DL, Moore DE, Spadoni LR, et al: A comparison of the fallopian tube's response to overt and silent salpingitis. Obstet Gynecol 1989; 73:622.

39. Curran JW, Rendtorff RC, Chandler RW, et al: Female gonorrhea: Its relation to abnormal uterine bleeding, urinary tract symptoms, and cervicitis. Obstet Gynecol 1975; 45:195.

40. Wolner-Hanssen P, Kiviat NB, Holmes KK: Atypical pelvic inflammatory disease: Subacute, chronic, or subclinical upper genital tract infection in women. In: In: Holmes KK, Mardh P-A, Sparling PF, et al. (eds): Sexually Transmitted Diseases, 2nd ed. New York: McGraw-Hill, 1990, pp 760–778.

41. Paavonen J, Kiviat NG, Brunham RC, et al: Prevalence and manifestations of endometritis among women with cervicitis. Am J Obstet Gynecol 1985; 152:280.

42. Jones RB, Mammel JB, Shepard MK, Fisher RR: Recovery of *Chlamydia trachomatis* from the endometrium of women at risk for chlamydial infection. Am J Obstet Gynecol 1986; 155:35.

43. Cleary RE, Jones RB: Recovery of *Chlamydia trachomatis* from the endometrium in infertile women with serum antichlamydial antibodies. Fertil Steril 1985; 44:233.

44. Soper DE: Diagnosis and laparoscopic grading of acute salpingitis. Am J Obstet Gynecol 1991; 164:1370.

45. Jacobson L, Westrom L: Objectivized diagnosis of acute pelvic inflammatory disease: Diagnostic and prognostic value of routine laparoscopy. Am J Obstet Gynecol 1969; 105:1088.

46. Westrom L, Mardh P-A: Salpingitis. In: Holmes KK, Mardh P-A, Sparling PF, et al. (eds): Sexually Transmitted Diseases. New York: McGraw-Hill, 1984, pp 615–632.

47. Westrom L: Diagnosis and treatment of salpingitis. J Reprod Med 1983; 28:703.

48. Hadgu AH, Westrom L, Brooks CA, et al: Predicting acute pelvic inflammatory disease: A multivariate analysis. Am J Obstet Gynecol 1986; 155:954.

49. Hager WD, Eschenbach DA, Spence MR, Sweet RL: Criteria for the diagnosis and grading of salpingitis. Obstet Gynecol 1983; 72:7.

50. Kahn JG, Walker CG, Washington AE, et al: Diagnosing pelvic inflammatory disease: A comprehensive analysis and considerations for developing a model. JAMA 1991; 266:2594.

51. Paavonen J, Aine R, Teisala K, et al: Comparison of endometrial biopsy and peritoneal fluid cytologic testing with laparoscopy in the diagnosis of acute pelvic inflammatory disease. Am J Obstet Gynecol 1985; 151:645.

52. Kiviat NB, Wolner-Hanssen P, Eschenbach DA, et al: Endometrial histopathology in patients with culture-proved upper genital tract infection and laparoscopically diagnosed acute salpingitis. Am J Surg Pathol 1990; 14:167.

53. Sellors J, Mahony J, Goldsmith C, et al: Accuracy of clinical findings and laparoscopy for pelvic inflammatory disease. Am J Obstet Gynecol 1991; 164:113.

54. Patten RM, Vincent LM, Wolner-Hanssen P, Thorpe E: Pelvic inflammatory disease: Endovaginal sonography with laparoscopic correlation. J Ultrasound Med 1990; 9:681.

55. Sellors J, Mahony J, Goldsmith C, et al: The accuracy of clinical findings and laparoscopy for pelvic inflammatory disease. Am J Obstet Gynecol 1991; 164:113.

56. Livengood CH, Hill GB, Addison WA: Pelvic inflammatory disease: Findings during inpatient treatment of clinically severe, laparoscopy-documented disease. Am J Obstet Gynecol 1992; 166:519.

57. Rolfs RT, Galaid EI, Zaidi AA: Pelvic inflammatory disease: Trends in hospitalizations and office visits, 1979 through 1988. Am J Obstet Gynecol 1992; 166:983.

58. Wolner-Hanssen P, Eschenbach D, Paavonen J, Holmes KK: Treatment of pelvic inflammatory disease: Use of doxycycline with an appropriate B-lactam while we wait for better data. [Editorial.] JAMA 1986; 256:3262.

59. Hasselquist MB, Hillier S: Susceptibility of upper genital tract isolates from women with pelvic inflammatory disease to ampicillin, cefodoxime, metronidazole, and doxycycline. Sex Transm Dis 1991; 18:146.

60. Peterson HB, Walker CK, Kahn JG, et al: Pelvic inflammatory disease: Key treatment issues and options. JAMA 1991; 266:2605.

61. Brunham RC: Therapy for acute pelvic inflammatory disease: A critique of recent treatment trials. Am J Obstet Gynecol 1984; 148:235.

62. Soper DE. Treatment. In: Berger GS, Westrom L (eds): Pelvic Inflammatory Disease. New York, Raven Press, 1992, pp 150–165.

63. Wolner-Hanssen P, Paavonen J, Kiviat N, et al: Outpatient treatment of pelvic inflammatory disease with cefoxitin and doxycycline. Obstet Gynecol 1988; 71:595.

64. Wolner-Hanssen P, Paavonen J, Kiviat N, et al: Ambulatory treatment of suspected pelvic inflammatory disease with Augmentin, with or without doxycycline. Am J Obstet Gynecol 1988; 158:577.

65. Wendel GC, Cox SM, Bawdon RE, et al: A randomized trial of ofloxacin versus cefoxitin and doxycycline in the outpatient treatment of acute salpingitis. Am J Obstet Gynecol 1991; 164:1390.

66. Martin DH, Mroczkowski TF, Dalu ZA, et al: A controlled trial of a single dose of azithromycin for the treatment of chlamydial urethritis and cervicitis. N Engl J Med 1992; 327:921.

67. Katz BP, Zwickl BW, Caine VA, Jones RB: Compliance with antibiotic therapy for *Chlamydia trachomatis* and *Neisseria gonorrhoeae.* Sex Transm Dis 1992; 19:351.

68. Centers for Disease Control and Prevention: Pelvic inflammatory disease: Guidelines for prevention and management. MMWR Morb Mortal Wkly Rep 1991; 40:1.

69. Reed SD, Landers DV, Sweet RL: Antibiotic treatment of tuboovarian abscess: Comparison of broad-spectrum β-lactam agents versus clindamycin-containing regimens. Am J Obstet Gynecol 1991; 164:1556.

70. Falk V: Treatment of acute non-tuberculous salpingitis with antibiotics alone and in combination with glucocorticoids. Acta Obstet Gynecol Scand 1965; 44:1.

71. Landers DV, Sung ML, Bottles K, Schachter J: Does addition of anti-inflammatory agents to antimicrobial therapy reduce infertility after murine chlamydial salpingitis? Sex Transm Dis 1993; 20:121.

72. Casola G, vanSonnenberg E, D'Agostino HB, et al: Percutaneous drainage of tubo-ovarian abscesses. Radiol 1992; 182:399.

73. Reich H: Laparoscopic treatment of tuboovarian and pelvic abscess. J Reprod Med 1987;32:747.

74. Gilstrap LC, Herbert WNP, Cunningham FG, et al: Gonorrhea screening in the male consorts of women with pelvic infection. JAMA 1977; 238:965.

75. Potterat JJ, Phillips L, Rothenberg RB, et al: Gonococcal pelvic inflammatory disease: Case-finding observations. Am J Obstet Gynecol 1980; 138:1101.

76. Moss TR, Hawkswell J: Evidence of infection with *Chlamydia trachomatis* in patients with pelvic inflammatory disease: Value of partner investigation. Fertil Steril 1986; 45:429.

77. Westrom L, Joesoef R, Reynolds B, et al: Pelvic inflammatory disease and fertility: A cohort study of 1,844 women with laparoscopically verified disease and 657 control women with normal laparoscopic results. Sex Transm Dis 1992; 19:185.

78. Joesoef R, Reynolds G, Westrom L, et al: Recurrence of ectopic

pregnancy: The role of salpingitis. Am J Obstet Gynecol 1991; 165:46.

79. Safrin S, Schachter J, Dahrouge D, Sweet RL: Long-term sequelae of acute pelvic inflammatory disease: A retrospective cohort study. Am J Obstet Gynecol 1992; 166:1300.

80. Westrom L: Pelvic inflammatory disease: Bacteriology and sequelae. Contraception 1987; 36:111.

81. Adlet MW, Belsey EH, O'Connor BH: Morbidity associated with pelvic inflammatory disease. Br J Vener Dis 1982; 58:151.

82. Washington AE, Cates W, Wasserheit JN: Preventing pelvic inflammatory disease. JAMA 1991; 266:2574.

83. Scholes D, Stergachis A, Heidrich, et al: Prevention of pelvic inflammatory disease by screening for cervical chlamydial infection. N Engl J Med 1996; 334:1362.

24 Infection and Infertility

In 1900, Albert Neisser gave a graphic description of a link between upper genital tract infection, sexually transmitted diseases, and subsequent infertility. He wrote that "should the infection reach the tubes, an acute febrile condition with severe attacks of pain, combined with tumor-like swelling of the tubes, occurs, which even in the most favorable cases keeps the patient in bed for weeks and requires the most careful treatment. Even after this, the condition usually is not entirely cured but leads to chronic persistent ill health with frequent acute exacerbations. These recurrent attacks may become a danger to life, so that operative interference and removal of the collections of pus by laparotomy becomes inevitable. When both tubes are infected, there is every prospect of lasting sterility."[1] Neisser would lend his name to one of the infectious agents that cause upper genital tract disease, *Neisseria gonorrhoeae*. Two of Neisser's assistants, Halberstaedter and von Prowazek, were involved in the discovery of *Chlamydia trachomatis*.[2] Contemporary research has established *Chlamydia* as a cause of genital tract infection and infertility.

Neisser made the above comments at the turn of the twentieth century. The last few decades of this century have seen epidemic levels of *Chlamydia* and gonorrhea. In 1996, *Chlamydia* and gonorrhea were the two most commonly reported infections in the United States. Tubal factor infertility (TFI) is a common gynecologic condition and the purpose of this chapter is to review the link between this type of infertility and sexually transmitted diseases. Although tuberculosis can also cause damage to fallopian tubes, this infection will not be discussed here.

EPIDEMIOLOGY

It is difficult to determine the true prevalence of infertility. The women who eventually seek care for infertility are likely a small, self-selected part of the whole. One British study asked people by mail survey about infertility. Twenty to 35% of couples failed to conceive after one year at some point in their reproductive lives.[3] Based on data like these, it is estimated that 5 million couples in the United States have infertility.

Approximately 1.5 million physician visits are made each year for infertility, and this number may rise over the next two decades.[5] Infertility due to prior infection with damaged fallopian tubes is usually referred to as TFI or postinfectious infertility. This type of infertility is among the most common. One review gave the following reasons for female infertility: tubal factor, 36%; ovulatory disorders, 33%; endometriosis, 6%; and no demonstrable problem in the female partner, 40%.[6]

Much of what we understand about the epidemiology of upper genital tract infection and subsequent infertility is derived from the large prospective study of pelvic inflammatory disease (PID) in Lund, Sweden[7] (Table 24-1). From 1960 to 1984, all women presenting with signs and symptoms of PID underwent laparoscopic examination. Approximately 3,000 women underwent laparoscopy and in 1,800 the diagnosis of PID was confirmed. Women were then followed prospectively. These authors noted that the number of episodes of PID and the severity of those cases influenced the rate of TFI after PID. After one episode of PID the risk of TFI was 11.4%. One episode of severe PID entailed a 30% risk. An increasing number of episodes approximately doubled the risk of infertility. This group has also reported that a diagnosis of PID at an older age was associated with a worse fertility prognosis.[8] A similar but smaller study from Winnipeg, Canada, found a worse prognosis when PID was caused by chlamydial infection when compared with gonorrhea.[9]

Three additional risk factors should be considered for the development of TFI. Smoking increases the risk of TFI in a dose-dependent fashion.[5] Smoking may also be a risk factor for PID. Contraceptive choices also affect the rate of TFI. Barrier contraceptives, such as condoms, prevent the initial infection with *C. trachomatis* and *N. gonorrhoeae* and thus are protective against PID and subsequent infertility. Oral contraceptives are likely to have a mixed effect. Women who are sexually active and rely on hormonal contraception may be more likely to be exposed to sexually transmitted infections. However, symptomatic PID is less common in women taking oral contraceptives.[7] One recent study

279

TABLE 24-1 ▶   RISK FACTORS FOR TUBAL FACTOR INFECTION

Pelvic inflammatory disease—risk increases with increasing number of episodes and increasing severity of episodes
Age
Contraception choices
Smoking

---

has associated the use of oral contraceptives with a risk of "unrecognized" endometritis.[10] Animal models of genital tract infection and exposure to oral contraceptives have likewise given mixed results. The overall effect on the development of tubal factor infertility is unknown. The intrauterine device (IUD) has long been cited as a risk factor for the development of PID and TFI. However, many of these studies are riddled with biases and inappropriate control groups. For example, if women in the control group are using condoms and are subsequently protected from PID, women using the intrauterine device will have a spurious elevation in PID rates. Most cases of PID associated with intrauterine device usage are related to contamination during insertion. Grimes[11] has eloquently reviewed this literature and concluded that exposure to sexually transmitted diseases is the threat to fertility, not the intrauterine device.

Not all cases of tubal factor infertility are preceded by a case of symptomatic PID. One multicenter trial found that 84% of women with TFI did not report a history of PID.[12] These authors attempted to find epidemiologic markers that might identify women at risk for TFI without a history of PID. They concluded that these women resemble their fertile control patients and that clinical predictors are lacking (Table 24–2).

PATHOGENESIS

The pathogenesis of tubal factor infertility is incompletely understood. In *in vitro* models of infection, *C. trachomatis* is relatively benign and does not cause tissue damage per se. The host immunologic response to chlamydial infection apparently initiates a cascade of

events leading to fallopian tube damage. Recent research has concentrated on the 60-kD chlamydial heat shock protein (hsp 60) as the target antigen for these pathogenic responses.[13, 14] These "stress" or "heat shock" proteins act as chaperonins at times of increased intracellular stress. These proteins are highly conserved across species, both eukaryotes and prokaryotes. There is 50% homology between the *Escherichia coli* and human 60-kD heat shock protein. More recently, a second 10-kD chlamydial heat shock protein has been described.[15] Antibodies to hsp 60 have been associated with PID and ectopic pregnancy; this literature has been reviewed by Brunham and Peeling.[14] Three studies have used this protein as an antigen in an enzyme-linked immunoassay to test the sera of women with TFI.[16–18] The results of these three studies are remarkably consistent with antibodies in 76%–81% of women with TFI. In one study, antibodies to hsp 60 were the only risk factor present in a majority of women with TFI.

There is considerable debate about the exact mechanisms of how host responses to chlamydial heat shock proteins lead to fallopian tube damage. At least three theories have been put forward. One theory is that there is a highly polarized lymphocyte response to hsp 60.[19] In this model, helper T-cell type 1 (T_H1) responses are protective against genital tract infections with *C. trachomatis*. T_H2 responses would lead to an inability to clear the microorganism and persistent infection of the fallopian tube. T_H1 responses are known to be critical in resolving genital tract infection in murine models of chlamydial infection.[20] Data from women with TFI are lacking, although in one study with trachoma, an ocular disease caused by repetitive infections with *C. trachomatis*, this mechanism appeared to be at work. These authors found that patients with scarring trachoma had T_H2 responses as determined by interleukin-4–producing lymphocytes.[21] Another theory is that the hsp 60 antigen causes a delayed hypersensitivity response. Data from animal models of ocular and genital tract infection support this idea.[22] The histologic changes in these studies are similar to the mononuclear infiltrates seen in women with TFI. Witkin and colleagues[23] have presented data that these

---

TABLE 24-2 ▶   DEMOGRAPHIC VARIABLES IN WOMEN WITH TUBAL FACTOR INFERTILITY WITH AND WITHOUT A HISTORY OF PELVIC INFLAMMATORY DISEASE

	Fertile Control Subjects (%)	TFI Without a History of PID (%)	TFI with a History of PID (%)
Unmarried	4.7	4.2	24.4
Education ≤12 y	24.0	29.8	40.0
Current cigarette smoker	14.8	31.1	55.6
Number of lifetime sexual partners >10	13.3	17.2	28.9
History of gonorrhea	1.9	2.5	24.4

PID = pelvic inflammatory disease; TFI = tubal factor infertility

antibodies recognize both hsp 60 and their analogues, both the human heat shock protein and the *E. coli* heat shock protein. In this theory, antibodies that recognized conserved epitopes of heat shock proteins cause the destruction of the fallopian tube through an autoimmune mechanism.

Gonorrhea has a different pathogenic effect on the fallopian tubes. There are no-well accepted animal models of gonococcal upper genital tract infection, and much of what we know is based on the human fallopian tube organ culture.[24] In this model, gonococci adhere to non-ciliated epithelial cells of the epithelium and induce phagocytosis. In this intracellular environment, gonococci are sequestered from attack from host complement, antibodies and neutrophils. Damage is also done to adjacent ciliated cells although they are not directly infected. Decreased beating of the cilia and eventual sloughing can be observed. Purified gonococcal lipo-oligosaccharide (LOS) has the same effect in this model.[25] Peptidoglycan may also have direct toxic effects on infected tissues. Under the electron microscope, small blebs of cell wall containing lipo-oligosaccharide and peptidoglycan can be visualized breaking off from the gonococci.

Bacterial vaginosis appears to be involved in the pathogenesis of upper genital tract infection.[26] However, whether these interactions play a role in the development of TFI as a sequela of PID is unknown.

CLINICAL MANIFESTATIONS AND DIAGNOSIS

As stated above and shown in Table 24–2, there are really no clinical predictors of TFI. It would seem prudent to inquire about a history of sexually transmitted diseases and PID in the initial evaluation of an infertile woman, but the information gained will probably not influence further infertility testing. Glatstein and coworkers[27] have surveyed reproductive endocrinologists to determine a standardized approach to the infertility evaluation. They found that these specialists rely heavily on five traditional infertility tests: the semen analysis, an assessment of ovulation, a postcoital test, hysterosalpingogram (HSG) and laparoscopy. The latter two tests are assessments of tubal patency. In HSG, radiopaque dye is introduced through the cervix into the lower uterine segment. A normal study shows uniform filling of the uterine cavity and spill from the distal fallopian tubes into the abdominal cavity. Unfortunately, HSG will not show more subtle changes associated with TFI, such as tubo-ovarian adhesions. Laparoscopy can more fully assess the pelvic anatomy; however, this test is more expensive and entails the risk of anesthesia.

Laparoscopy is considered the gold standard for visualization of the pelvis in the infertile woman, and HSG is performed as a preliminary test prior to laparoscopy.[28] This approach makes it difficult to give a true estimate of the accuracy of HSG. Women who become pregnant after an HSG but before a planned laparoscopy will bias a study toward decreased specificity of HSG. Hysterosalpingogram has prognostic value with a 70% reduction in fecundity with bilateral obstruction of the fallopian tubes. Similar data for the prognostic value of laparoscopy do not exist. Swart and colleagues[29] have done a meta-analysis of the diagnostic accuracy of HSG. Twenty studies were included in this review and the gold standard was laparoscopy. They estimate the sensitivity at 65% and specificity at 83%, and conclude that the high specificity makes HSG a good choice for ruling in tubal disease.

Because of the close association of chlamydial infection and TFI, serologic evidence of prior infection with *C. trachomatis* may also be a diagnostic test for TFI. A serologic test would be less invasive than the other procedures for testing tubal patency outlined earlier. Meikle and associates[30] have reported on a series of 208 women, all of whom had HSG, laparoscopy, and antibody titers against *C. trachomatis* using a commercially available kit. In this report, the sensitivity was 78% for detecting tubal disease for both the *C. trachomatis* antibody test and HSG. The specificity of the tests was 64% for *C. trachomatis* antibodies and 84% for HSG. Mol and colleagues[31] have performed a meta-analysis of 23 similar studies and reported that these sensitivity and specificity values are typical. However, a single point estimate of specificity and sensitivity could not be calculated due to the wide disparities in study design and technique for determining antibody status.

TREATMENT OF TUBAL FACTOR INFERTILITY

In vitro fertilization is the treatment of choice for TFI. Simply put, this procedure amounts to "tubal bypass." Multiple follicles are produced by ovulation induction; these oocytes are fertilized in the laboratory and transferred into the uterus. This approach will achieve a live birth within four cycles in greater than 70% of women with TFI.[32] The delivery per transfer rate was 48.4% in women younger than 30 years of age and this rate declined with advancing age. This approach to the treatment of TFI is the most cost-effective as well.[33] However, in vitro fertilization is technology-intensive, expensive, and not always covered by insurance, and involves extensive monitoring of ovarian stimulation. In addition, TFI is a risk factor for an ectopic pregnancy after in vitro fertilization. The series cited previously reported an ectopic pregnancy rate of 2.4%.

Surgical repair of distal tubal obstruction has been a therapy for women with TFI. Penzias and DeCherney[34] have reviewed the major reported series in this area, reporting a pregnancy rate of 18%–33% after surgical repair of distal tubal obstruction. The subsequent rate can be as high as 14%. These surgeries will relieve the mechanical obstruction of the fallopian tube and release adhesions from the ovaries and tubes. However, nothing can be done to repair or treat the underlying damage to the fallopian tube epithelium. This is the weakness of a surgical approach to TFI. These authors and others have convincingly argued that tubal surgery is "obsolete," especially when the alternative of in vitro fertilization is considered.

PREVENTION OF TUBAL FACTOR INFERTILITY

There are no clinical trials that would indicate that any certain antibiotic or combination of antibiotics will protect women from TFI after PID. The Lund study used multiple different antibiotics and found no differences in outcomes.[7] There are no prospective, randomized studies of PID treatments and fertility outcomes. Some animal studies have indicated that antibiotics have little effect on eventual tubal damage. Patton and coworkers[35] have reported a study using a macaque monkey model of chlamydial PID. There were four treatment groups studied—doxycycline alone, doxycycline plus the steroid triamcinolone, doxycycline plus the nonsteroidal anti-inflammatory ibuprofen, and placebo. The intention was to discover if these anti-inflammatory combinations had any effect on the outcome of PID. One endpoint of their study was adhesion scores at hysterectomy 12 to 16 weeks post treatment. No significant differences were found among any of the four groups. In other words, the administration of antibiotics had no effect on the development of adhesions in well-established upper genital tract infections, even when compared with untreated control subjects.

The Lund data were reanalyzed by Hillis and colleagues,[36] who reported on the effect of the delay of care on the development of infertility. Basically, delaying care for three days or longer led to a threefold increase in infertility. This effect is more pronounced in upper genital tract infections involving *C. trachomatis*. This study has led many experts to recommend empiric therapy for PID in any clinical setting where PID is in the differential diagnosis.

The best strategy for preventing TFI would be preventing the initial acquisition of chlamydial infection and gonorrhea. A national screening program for chlamydial infection has started in the United States, and some initial success has been reported at lowering the prevalence of this sexually transmitted disease.[37] Screening is also effective in preventing PID. A randomized, controlled trial of 2,607 women enrolled in a health maintenance organization was reported in 1996.[38] Enrollment was based on a set of risk factors for chlamydial infection in women 18 to 34 years of age. The PID rate was reduced by 56% in the intensively screened group.

Tubal factor infertility is a common gynecologic problem. Prospective studies have yielded a set of risk factors for this type of infertility; however, many women have silent infection and tubal damage. Much research is needed to understand the pathogenesis of TFI. Several recent studies have indicated that screening for chlamydial infection may decrease the prevalence of this disease and, it is hoped, prevent TFI.

REFERENCES

1. Neisser A: Gonorrhoea: Its dangers to society. Med News NY 1900; 2:41.
2. Oriel J: Eminent venereologists: Albert Neisser. Genitourin Med 1989; 65:229.
3. Page H: Estimation of the prevalence and incidence of infertility in a population: A pilot study. Fertil Steril 1989; 51:571.
4. Stephen E, Chandra A: Updated projections of infertility in the United States: 1995–2025. Fertil Steril 1998; 70:30.
5. Cates W, Wasserheit J: Genital chlamydial infections: Epidemiology and reproductive sequelae. Am J Obstet Gynecol 1991; 164:1771.
6. Healy D, Trounson A, Andersen A: Female infertility: Causes and treatment. Lancet 1994; 343:1539.
7. Westrom L, Joesoef R, Reynolds G, et al: Pelvic inflammatory disease and fertility. Sex Transm Dis 1992; 19:185.
8. Westrom L: Sexually transmitted diseases and infertility. Sex Transm Dis 1994; 21(suppl 2):s32.
9. Brunham R, Binns B, Guijon F, et al: Etiology and outcome of acute pelvic inflammatory disease. J Infect Dis 1988; 158:510.
10. Ness R, Keder L, Soper D, et al: Oral contraceptives and the recognition of endometritis. Am J Obstet Gynecol 1997; 176:580.
11. Grimes D: The intrauterine device, pelvic inflammatory disease and infertility: The confusion between hypothesis and knowledge. Fertil Steril 1992; 58:670.
12. Cates W, Joesoef R, Goldman M: Atypical pelvic inflammatory disease: Can we identify clinical predictors? Am J Obstet Gynecol 1993; 169:341.
13. Peeling R, Brunham R: Chlamydiae as pathogens: New species and new issues. Emerg Infect Dis 1996; 2:307.
14. Bruham R, Peeling R: *Chlamydia trachomatis* antigens: Role in immunity and pathogenesis. Infect Agents Dis 1994; 3:218.
15. LaVerda D, Byrne G: Use of monoclonal antibodies to facilitate identification, cloning and purification of *Chlamydia trachomatis* hsp 10. J Clin Microbiol 1997; 35:1209.
16. Toye B, Laferriere C, Claman C, et al: Association between antibody to the chlamydial heat shock protein and tubal infertility. J Infect Dis 1993; 168:1236.
17. Arno J, Yuan Y, Cleary R, et al: Serological responses of infertile women to the 60 kDa chlamydial heat shock protein. Fertil Steril 1995; 48:787.
18. Ault K, Statland B, Smith King MM, et al: Antibodies to the chlamydial 60 kilodalton heat shock protein in women with tubal factor infertility. Infect Dis Obstet Gynecol 1998; 6:163.
19. Peeling R, Kimani J, Plummer F, et al: Antibody to chlamydial hsp 60 predicts an increased risk for chlamydial pelvic inflammatory disease. J Infect Dis 1997; 175:1153.
20. Cotter T, Byrne G: Immunity to *Chlamydia*: Comparison of human infections and murine models. Res Immunol 1996; 147:587.
21. Holland M, Bailey R, Conway D, et al: T helper type-1 (Th1)/Th2 profiles of peripheral blood mononuclear cells: Responses to antigens of *Chlamydia trachomatis* in subjects with severe trachomatous scarring. Clin Exp Immunol 105:429, 1996.
22. Beatty W, Byrne G, Morrison R: Repeated and persistent infection with *Chlamydia* and the development of chronic inflammation and disease. Trends Microbiol 1994; 2:94.
23. Witkin S, Askienazy-Elbhar M, Henry-Suchet J, et al: Circulating antibodies to a conserved epitope of the *Chlamydia trachomatis* 60 kDa heat shock protein (hsp 60) in infertile couples

and its relationship to antibodies to *C. trachomatis* surface antigens and the *Escherichia coli* and human hsp 60. Hum Reprod 1998; 13:1175.

24. McGee Z, Johnson A, Taylor-Robinson D: Pathogenic mechanism of *Neisseria gonorrhoeae*. J Infect Dis 1981; 143:413.
25. Gregg C, Melly M, Hellerqvist CG, et al: Toxic activity of the purified lipopolysaccharide of *Neisseria gonorrhoeae* for the human fallopian tube mucosa. J Infect Dis 1981; 143:432.
26. Sweet R: Role of bacterial vaginosis in pelvic inflammatory disease. Clin Infect Dis 1995; 20(suppl 2):s271.
27. Glatstein I, Harlow B, Hornstein M: Practice patterns among reproductive endocrinologists: The infertility evaluation. Fertil Steril 1997; 67:443.
28. Mol B, Swart P, Bossuyt P, et al: Is hysterosalpingogram an important tool in predicting fertility outcome? Fertil Steril 1997; 67:663.
29. Swart P, Mol B, van der Veen F, et al: The accuracy of hysterosalpingography in the diagnosis of tubal pathology: A meta-analysis. Fertil Steril 1995; 64:486.
30. Meikle S, Zhang O, Marine W, et al: *Chlamydia trachomatis* antibody titers and hysterosalpingography predicting tubal disease in infertility patients. Fertil Steril 1994; 62:305.
31. Mol B, Dijkman B, Wertheim P, et al: The accuracy of serum chlamydial antibodies in the diagnosis of tubal pathology: A meta-analysis. Fertil Steril 1997; 67:1031.
32. Bendiva C, Kligman I, Davis O, et al: In vitro fertilization versus tubal surgery: Is pelvic reconstructive surgery obsolete? Fertil Steril 1995; 64:1051.
33. Van Voorhis B, Sparks A, Allen B, et al: Cost effectiveness of infertility treatments: A cohort study. Fertil Steril 1997; 67:830.
34. Penzias AS, DeCherney A: Is there ever a role for tubal surgery? Am J Obstet Gynecol 1996; 174:1218.
35. Patton D, Sweeney Y, Bohannon N, et al: Effects of doxycycline and anti-inflammatory agents on experimentally induced chlamydial upper genital tract infection in female macaques. J Infect Dis 1997; 175:648.
36. Hillis S, Joesoef R, Marchbanks P, et al: Delayed care of pelvic inflammatory disease as a risk factor for impaired fertility. Am J Obstet Gynecol 1993; 168:1503.
37. Addis D, Vaughn M, Ludka D, et al: Decreased prevalence of *Chlamydia trachomatis* infection associated with a selective screening program in family planning clinics in Wisconsin. Sex Transm Dis 1992; 20:24.
38. Scholes D, Stergachis A, Heidrich F, et al: Prevention of pelvic inflammatory disease by screening for cervical chlamydial infection. N Engl J Med 1996; 334:1362.

25 Posthysterectomy Infections

Hysterectomy is the second most frequently performed major surgical procedure among reproductive-aged women in the United States according to surveillance data covering the years 1980 to 1993.[1] Approximately 600,000 procedures were performed annually. Women between the ages of 40 and 44 years were the most likely to undergo hysterectomy, and the most frequent preoperative diagnosis was uterine leiomyoma. Hysterectomy rates and patient ages did differ by geographic region of the United States, being lowest and for older women in the Northeast, and highest and among younger women in the South. Table 25–1 presents indications for hysterectomy by patient age group.

Sampling design changes precluded comparison between the two different periods comprising the survey; the first was 1980 to 1987, and the second from 1988 to 1993. The rate of hysterectomy declined from 7.1/1,000 female civilians 15 years of age or older in 1980 to 5.3/1,000 in 1993. As less invasive measures for treating abnormal bleeding and other gynecologic diagnoses resulting in hysterectomy are developed, this rate will undoubtedly continue to decrease.

Most (51%) women undergoing hysterectomy had removal of their ovaries at the time of their hysterectomy. If the surgical approach was abdominal, bilateral oophorectomy was more than three times more common (63% vs. 18%). Oophorectomy was age related, occurring in only 18% of women 15 to 24 years of age, and increasing to 62% among women older than 55 years (Fig. 25–1). During the last half of the surveillance period, however, there was a significant increase in the performance of bilateral oophorectomy; it almost tripled between 1988 and 1993. During the surveillance period, only approximately one fourth of hysterectomies were performed vaginally. The percentage of vaginal hysterectomies associated with laparoscopy was significantly increased from less than 1% during the 1980s to 14.2%; in 1993, it was 15.3%. Infection is the most common morbidity observed after hysterectomy.

Soon after the introduction of antibiotics into clinical medicine, physicians performing surgery began to administer them to prevent infection, regardless of procedure variables and without defined risk factors.

Antibiotic administration began when the patient was admitted to the hospital, usually the day before the surgical procedure, and was continued until the patient was discharged, whether 5 or 10 days after the procedure. It became apparent that objectivity was required in selecting surgical procedures that required antibiotic administration to decrease postoperative infection, because all procedures certainly did not. In 1964, a committee investigating ultraviolet irradiation in the operating room and other variables classified surgical procedures depending primarily on predictive risk factors for infection after observation of infection rates in thousands of patients.[2] Four separate categories were defined: (1) clean, (2) clean-contaminated, (3) contaminated, and (4) dirty.

If the surgical incision was nontraumatic, and there was neither inflammation encountered in the operative site nor a break in surgical technique, the wound was classified as *clean*. The infection rate observed in this group of patients without prophylaxis was only approximately 5%; urinary tract operations meeting the aforementioned criteria, appendectomies, and hysterectomies were included. No antibiotic prophylaxis was required for the cases in this category. If an established gynecologist's patient infection rate after hysterectomy was no more than 5% to 8%, prophylaxis was not indicated. Most such practitioners have retired.

A wound was classified *clean-contaminated* if there was a minor break in surgical technique or entry into the respiratory, genitourinary, or gastrointestinal tract without significant spillage. These wounds also had to be nontraumatic. The infection rate observed in this category was 10.1%. Hysterectomy has been reclassified as a clean-contaminated procedure because of the inoculation of vaginal flora into the operative site during surgery. At vaginal hysterectomy, the contamination begins with the vaginal incision and continues throughout the procedure. Crossing of vaginal planes does not occur until the end of an abdominal hysterectomy, theoretically decreasing the infection rate. Perioperative antibiotic administration for this class of procedures would be considered prophylactic.

The vaginal flora has been eloquently summarized in Chapter 1, and is the source of contaminating po-

TABLE 25-1 ▶	MOST FREQUENT DIAGNOSIS BY AGE GROUP FOR WOMEN UNDERGOING HYSTERECTOMY
Age Ranges (y)	**Principal Diagnoses**
<30	Abnormal bleeding
	Cervical dysplasia
30–34	Endometriosis
35–54	Uterine leiomyoma
>55	Uterine prolapse
	Cancer

tential pathogens inoculated into the surgical site during the procedure. Alterations in this flora may alter the postoperative infection rate. According to work presented by Soper and colleagues[3] and Larsson and associates,[4] preoperative bacterial vaginosis and *Trichomonas vaginalis* infection were associated with an increased infection rate after abdominal hysterectomy. This risk factor could be eradicated by preoperative evaluation and treatment.

If the surgical procedure was one in which there was a gross break in surgical technique, a large spillage from the gastrointestinal tract, or entry into the biliary or genitourinary tract in the presence of infected bile or urine, the procedure was considered to be *contaminated*. Surgery performed in an inflamed area was also believed best classified as contaminated. The infection rate in this subset of patients was approximately 20%. Hysterectomy performed in the presence of pelvic cellulitis would fall into this category of procedures. Anti-

biotic administration in these cases would be therapeutic and ongoing, and not prophylactic.

Dirty procedures were ones in which trauma was present, there was a perforated viscus, or it was necessary to operate in a field contaminated by purulent material. Women having hysterectomy for ruptured tubo-ovarian abscess would certainly qualify for this category. The infection rate for this patient population was 25% or above. Antibiotic administration in these cases was therapeutic.

The Centers for Disease Control and Prevention (CDC) proposed definitions of surgical wound infection[5] that were modified in 1992 by Horan and colleagues.[6] This system is used by most hospital infection-control survey teams. It divides infections into two major categories: (1) *an organ/space surgical site infection (SSI)*, and (2) *superficial and deep incision infection*. The former is any anatomy that is opened or manipulated during a surgical procedure other than the incision. This category encompasses most of the infections that develop after hysterectomy and are described individually later. Although there were 23 specific organ or space SSI described in the 1992 revision, only "vaginal cuff," "other male or female reproductive tract," or "intra-abdominal nonspecified elsewhere" categories would apply to infection after hysterectomy.

The organ/space SSI must develop within 30 days of the hysterectomy and must be accompanied by one of the following: (1) diagnosis by a surgeon or attending physician; (2) an abscess or other evidence of infection identified during reoperation or by radio-

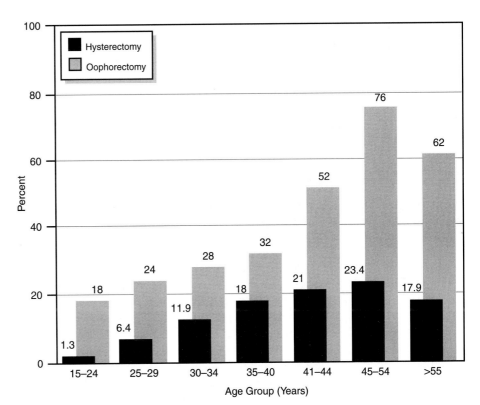

FIGURE 25-1 ▶ Hysterectomy and oophorectomy by age group.

logic or histopathologic examination; (3) aseptically obtained organ/space fluid or tissue, the culture of which resulted in bacterial isolates; or (4) purulent drainage from a drain placed through a stab wound into the organ/space.

It is difficult to obtain tissue or fluid from a pelvic infection site transvaginally with confidence in an aseptic technique. Percutaneous samples obtained by an interventional radiologist are acceptable, but such is rarely called for in most women who have infection after hysterectomy. An uncontaminated specimen from an infected site should be submitted for aerobic and anaerobic culture. It cannot guide the empiric antibiotic regimen selected for initial therapy, but it will be useful if the original regimen is unsuccessful in curing the infection. Sonography is helpful in differentiating infected hematoma or abscess from cellulitis.

Infection diagnosis is usually made based on patient symptomatology, vital signs, including a temperature elevation, and physical examination of the abdomen and pelvis. Before the administration of antibiotic for a pelvic infection after hysterectomy, a complete history and physical examination, including the abdomen and pelvis, must be conducted, and a diagnosis made. Administering antibiotic for "presumed pelvic infection" without history and physical examination evidence to confirm the diagnosis is not appropriate. Administering antibiotic for temperature elevation only in an asymptomatic patient without positive physical findings is difficult to justify, with few exceptions. Other infections, such as upper respiratory tract infections, pneumonia, phlebitis, atelectasis, pyelonephritis, and so forth, may cause fever.

In addition to infection of the vaginal surgical margin, or "cuff cellulitis," pelvic cellulitis, pelvic phlegmon, cellulitis or abscess in a retained adnexa, and an infected hematoma or abscess in the pelvis qualify as organ/space SSI diagnoses. Parenteral antimicrobial therapy is indicated for all but perhaps mild cuff cellulitis. *Cuff cellulitis* is the mildest of postoperative infections. In fact, cellulitis at that incision site after hysterectomy is uniform, but it usually is not associated with symptoms. If the vagina is examined during the first several days after a hysterectomy, an indurated, erythematous, edematous cuff is a "normal" finding. There are purulent secretions in the vagina; this is the normal host response to the vaginal surgical incision. This area is usually somewhat tender at bimanual examination, as would be an incision anywhere during this interval after a surgical procedure. These findings obtain regardless of whether there is temperature elevation or symptomatology, and they diminish with time in the absence of clinical infection.

Patients with these findings, in the absence of temperature elevation and symptoms, require no antibiotic treatment. Patients with temperature elevation and symptoms of increasing lower abdominal or back pain,

pelvic pain, or pelvic pressure have enhanced tenderness at the area of the vaginal cuff and perhaps have suprapubic tenderness at gentle abdominal wall depression. Such a patient requires antimicrobial therapy, the type being determined by the degree of infection. Women with this infection have no parametrial or adnexal tenderness and there is no evidence of mass formation. Many times, patients with this infection are treated successfully as outpatients.

This is the infection most frequently observed in women after they are discharged from the hospital after hysterectomy in our indigent patient population. Commonly, this infection develops within 7 to 10 days after discharge from the hospital. This infection also may be responsible for the asymptomatic temperature elevation that develops soon after hysterectomy and disappears without treatment. This temperature elevation is frequently ascribed to atelectasis, which is most frequently observed during the first 48 hours after surgery. If the temperature elevation does not prolong hospitalization, it is not significant.

Surgical site infections are arbitrarily divided into *early* or *late* depending on whether the infection develops during the initial hospitalization or after discharge from the hospital. It is extremely important to include all infections, especially those that develop after discharge from the hospital, to determine an accurate infection rate. Determining the infection rate is less problematic in hospital-based practices, where patients return to the emergency department for treatment as an outpatient or are admitted to the hospital. It is more difficult in a private practice setting, where postoperative care is directed from the physician's office, and that information may not find its way to the patient's inpatient record. In 1995, Gravel-Trooper and co-workers[7] reported that 67% of infections that developed after pelvic surgery did so after the patient went home. Of these, 38% were detected at readmission for inpatient antimicrobial therapy, but most women did not require admission. These infections were detected only by physician survey.

Pelvic cellulitis is the organ/space SSI resulting from inadequate host defense mechanisms, enhanced bacterial virulence factors, increased bacterial inoculum, or insufficient prophylactic antibiotic. The inflammatory response is not contained at the cuff, and infection spreads into the parametrial pelvic soft tissues. Women with this infection have recurring temperature elevations and increasing pain as detailed earlier, except that it is usually predominant on one side. Again, gentle, deep abdominal palpation reveals tenderness over the infected area that was not there at previous examination. Bimanual examination discloses tenderness lateral to the vaginal apex and usually accentuated on one side. No masses are present.

This infection usually develops on the second or third day after surgery. Because patients are now discharged from the hospital on their first to third post-operative day, it is extremely important that they understand the symptomatology of these infections so that the physician may be notified as quickly as possible to allow prompt initiation of parenteral antimicrobial therapy, which results in decreased morbidity.

Phlegmon is a potentially more serious infection consisting of areas of intense cellulitis with edema, induration, and microabscesses. It usually develops in the soft tissues of the parametria. Patients with this uncommon infection have recurring temperature elevations and symptomatology as described previously. At examination, not only are the aforementioned findings present, but now there is a firm, tender nonfluctuant mass. Sonography does not reveal evidence of an infected hematoma or abscess.

The infection that develops in a retained adnexa may be cellulitis involving the tube or ovary, or it may be an abscess. The features of recurring temperature elevation and increasing symptoms as described previously, as well as physical findings at abdominal and pelvic examination, are similar to those seen with pelvic cellulitis, except that the maximum tenderness is not in the parametrial areas, but is usually anterior and cephalad. Infections are not mutually exclusive, so it is possible that a patient may have infection in an adnexa as well as other pelvic soft tissues.

With current prophylactic antibiotic regimens, an adnexal abscess rarely develops after hysterectomy. Historically, a potentially life-threatening event was the development of an ovarian abscess after discharge from the hospital after hysterectomy, and particularly vaginal hysterectomy. The patient had relatively few symptoms until abscess rupture at home, at which time the patient would become dramatically ill in a short time. Immediate surgical therapy was necessary in addition to antimicrobial therapy for these patients. This phenomenon was first described by Ledger and colleagues[8] in 1969 and revisited by Livengood and Addison[9] in 1982.

Potentially the most morbid organ/space SSI after hysterectomy is a *pelvic abscess*. The most frequent location for an abscess is in the space between the peritoneum and the closed vaginal surgical margin. This infection usually develops around day 4 or 5 after hysterectomy, now a time when most patients are at home. Patients with this infection have increasing lower abdominal and pelvic pain and recurring temperature elevation (perhaps including fever and chills), and usually complain of increase in vaginal discharge. On examination, there are more purulent secretions in the vagina than are seen with the other posthysterectomy pelvic infections, and they may be seen issuing between vaginal margins at the cuff. Intra-abdominal rupture does not occur.

At examination, abdominal and pelvic tenderness is present and a fluctuant mass can be palpated cephalad

to the vaginal cuff. Although it is usually central, the abscess can be lateral. There have been instances in which antibiotic therapy alone was administered to women with this infection, with infection resolution; therapy duration is shortened by mechanically draining the abscess space. Draining can be effected by cutting the sutures centrally and using the resultant aperture of 2 to 3 cm. It may be necessary to spread the vaginal margins with a uterine dressing forceps or ring forceps, which usually results in prompt drainage of the space; insertion of a drain is not necessary. Fluid collected from such a space should be cultured because it can be obtained without contamination. A passive drain should not be inserted into that area and left in the vagina. These infections are rare.

All women in whom a hematoma develops after hysterectomy will not become infected. *Infected hematoma* often is a diagnosis of exclusion, and the presence of a hematoma is confirmed by pelvic ultrasonography. Most women with a hematoma located in the same space as a pelvic abscess have no symptoms initially. The hematoma is nonpalpable, and the only way to predict its presence is by a significant drop in serum hemoglobin in the absence of an operative estimated blood loss that could explain the hemoglobin decrease. Initial evidence of the presence of an infected hematoma is asymptomatic temperature elevation.

The examination of such a patient reveals neither abdominal nor pelvic tenderness, nor masses. These women are upset because they feel well and want to be discharged from the hospital—if they are still in the hospital. In 24 to 48 hours, however, lower abdominal and pelvic/back pain develops. As time passes, pain increases and a tender mass becomes palpable as the clot undergoes further organization. Opening this space for clot evacuation does not seem to be as beneficial as does drainage of a pelvic abscess. Antibiotic administration should begin if a temperature elevation develops in a woman with a pelvic hematoma before she becomes symptomatic.

Appropriate surgical technique with small tissue pedicles, as little suture as possible, as little cautery as possible, hemostasis, and gentle handling of tissues contributes to reducing the incidence of postoperative infection, especially when combined with administration of prophylactic antibiotic. Before the routine administration of prophylactic antibiotics, whether the vaginal surgical margin was closed or left open played a role in, and was a risk factor for, the development of operative site infection after hysterectomy. With the advent of antibiotic prophylaxis, this is no longer true.[10] Swartz and Tanaree[11] reported that serum collected in the space between the vaginal surgical margin and the peritoneum in all women after hysterectomy was contaminated with bacteria, and that mechanical drainage of this space using a closed technique was as effective as antibiotic in reducing the postoperative infection rate.[11, 12] This finding has not been reproduced by several other investigators.

Abdominal incision infection, which was divided by the CDC into the categories of *superficial* and *deep SSI,* is much less common than pelvic infection after abdominal hysterectomy. Both must occur within 30 days of the hysterectomy. Superficial infections are those that develop above the rectus fascia. A surgeon's or attending physician's diagnosis confirms these infections. Other variables that confirm the diagnosis of superficial incisional infection are purulent drainage from the incision or from a drain placed above the fascia, bacteria recovered from fluid obtained from a wound that was primarily closed, or a wound that a surgeon deliberately opens (unless it is culture negative).

Deep incisional infections involve the fascia and tissues deep to the fascia. Subfascial or deep infections are rare. The various types of fasciitis also are classified in this category of wound infection. Confirmation variables include purulent drainage from a subfascial drain, and spontaneous dehiscence or deliberate wound opening by a surgeon in a patient who has localized pain or tenderness and a temperature over 38°C, unless the wound culture does not grow pathogens. A third variable is the presence of an abscess or other evidence of infection observed directly or by histopathologic examination.

An incisional infection does not usually develop until the fourth or fifth postoperative day, and may present with pain, fever, and an erythematous surgical margin with or without purulent drainage. Patients with this infection may also present with incisional drainage only. Uncontaminated culture of the wound fluid is possible when wound edges are separated; this should be performed regardless of whether or not the material appears to be purulent. What appears to be a seroma may be an early abscess. Unless there is significant cellulitis in the incision margins, mechanical therapy only with wet-to-dry dressings using fine-mesh gauze three to four times a day is usually sufficient to treat the infection. When the infection is eradicated and there is abundant, healthy granulation tissue, these incisions can be closed secondarily or allowed to heal by secondary intention. Gallup and colleagues[13] demonstrated that closed drainage of the subcutaneous space and antibiotic prophylaxis decreased wound breakdown in obese women undergoing abdominal hysterectomy.

In 1944, Richards[14] reported that locally applied sulfonamide at the time of hysterectomy did not significantly reduce postoperative infection. Six years later, Turner[15] reported that an endocervical penicillin suppository was superior to parenteral penicillin for infection prevention in women undergoing vaginal hysterectomy. It was not until 25 years later that Ledger and co-workers[16] proposed guidelines to decrease postoperative infection after hysterectomy. These guidelines were modified in 1983 by Johnson and associates,[17] and both are presented in Table 25–2.

It has been established that the infection rates after both vaginal and abdominal hysterectomy without antibiotics are high enough to warrant antibiotic prophylaxis; however, it took meta-analyses in 1993[18] and 1994[19] to confirm that women undergoing abdominal hysterectomy also should routinely be given antimicrobial prophylaxis. Early studies evaluating this indication for prophylactic antibiotic administration established that vaginal hysterectomy was more frequently associated with infection than abdominal hysterectomy, and that prophylaxis was more beneficial for that procedure. Initial studies involved administration of antibiotic from before surgery to 7 days after surgery, or when the patient went home. With experience, the administration period decreased to the generally accepted current regimen of a single preoperative dose. Table 25–3 presents in alphabetic order many of the U.S. Food and Drug Administration (FDA)–approved regimens for hysterectomy prophylaxis. Newer agents are approved for both vaginal and abdominal procedures, and usually at a single dose.

Initial studies evaluated intramuscular antibiotics on the nursing ward before the patient left for the operating room. Currently, the preoperative dose is given intravenously in the operating room, when it is certain that the patient's surgery will occur. It may be necessary to administer a second prophylactic dose of any antibiotic if the procedure lasts more than 3 hours.[20] Excessive blood loss (>1,500 mL) may be an equally important reason to administer a second dose because of loss of antibiotic.

Many studies have attempted to identify risk factors for infection after either vaginal or abdominal hysterectomy to identify a subgroup of patients for whom antibiotic prophylaxis was necessary. Evaluated risk factors included menopausal status, prolonged duration

---

TABLE 25–2 ▶ GUIDELINES FOR PREVENTING OPERATIVE SITE INFECTION

1. The operation should have a significant risk for operative site infection after surgery.
2. The operation should be accompanied by endogenous bacterial contamination.
3. The prophylactic antibiotic should have laboratory and clinical evidence of effectiveness against some of the contaminating organisms.
4. The prophylactic antibiotic should be present in the wound, preferably before incision, and should reach a therapeutic concentration in operative site tissues.
5. A short course of prophylactic antibiotics should be used.
6. Therapeutic agents should be reserved for therapy unless proven superior to other agents.
7. Benefits of antibiotic prophylaxis should outweigh the risks.
8. Hospitals should have a functioning infection surveillance program.

TABLE 25-3 ▶ FOOD AND DRUG ADMINISTRATION–APPROVED* HYSTERECTOMY PROPHYLAXIS REGIMENS

| Antimicrobial Name | | | | |
Generic	Trade	Dose (g)	Regimen	Procedure
Cefamandole	Mandol	1 or 2	IV/IM 30–60 min preop then q6h for 24–48 h	TVH
Cefazolin	Ancef/Kefzol	1	IV/IM 30–60 min preop then 0.5–1 g IV/IM intraop q6–8h for 24 h	TVH
Cefotaxime	Claforan	1	IV/IM 30–90 min preop	TVH/TAH
Cefotetan	Cefotan	1 or 2	IV 30–60 min preop	TVH/TAH
Cefoxitin	Mefoxin	2	IV 30–60 min preop then q6h up to 24 h	TVH/TAH
Ceftriaxone	Rocephin	1	IV 30–120 min preop	TVH/TAH
Cefuroxime	Zinacef	1.5	IV 30–60 min preop	TVH
Mezlocillin	Mezlin	4	IV 30–90 min preop then 6 and 12 h later	TVH
Piperacillin	Pipracil	2	IV 30–60 min preop then 6 and 12 h later	TVH/TAH

*Physicians' Desk Reference, 54th ed. Montvale, NJ, Medical Economics Co., 2000.

IM = intramuscular; IV = intravenous; preop = preoperatively; TAH = transabdominal hysterectomy; TVH = transvaginal hysterectomy.

of procedure, surgeon experience, additional surgical procedures, preceding surgery (conization of the cervix), excessive blood loss, menstrual cycle phase, urinary catheter placement, obesity, diabetes, anemia, socioeconomic status, and patient age. Results were varied enough that prophylaxis administration has essentially become uniform. Even with prophylaxis, infection rates are higher in patients who are debilitated, immunocompromised, or of a lower socioeconomic status, the only identified uniform risk factors. Administration of multiple doses of antibiotic does not seem to alter this increased risk.

As outlined in Chapter 1, the potential pathogens for these polymicrobial pelvic infections include a variety of gram-positive and gram-negative aerobic and anaerobic bacteria. For that reason, an agent with an expanded antibacterial spectrum should be more effective for prophylaxis than one with a narrower spectrum. The cephalosporin family of antibiotics has been very successful in decreasing the morbidity due to infection after hysterectomy. Cefazolin, a first-generation agent, fulfills many of the criteria for an ideal agent for prophylaxis with hysterectomy (see Table 25-2). Its antianaerobic activity is limited compared with newer cephalosporins, but its ability to prevent operative site infection after hysterectomy was comparable with that of the newer cephalosporins in small studies. Small sample size may have contributed to lack of power to detect a clinically significant protective effect, however. Spectrum of activity was proven to be important in at least one large, randomized, blind clinical trial in women undergoing abdominal hysterectomy.[21] The rate of infection and the number of

women with postoperative abscess were significantly greater in patients given cefazolin before abdominal hysterectomy than in women given cefotetan.

Pharmacokinetic variables do not seem to play an important role in infection prevention. In theory, administration of an agent with a longer half-life should provide enhanced protection and prevent the necessity of a second dose. It has been shown that multiple dosing does significantly alter the lower reproductive tract flora, as does the family of antibiotic selected for prophylaxis.[22] As indicated in Ledger's guidelines, the benefits of antibiotic administration to prevent infection should outweigh the risks. The risks of single-dose antibiotic administration are low, but at least in theory are life-threatening. Anaphylaxis is always a potential risk any time an antibiotic is administered, and has been reported after single-dose prophylaxis.[23]

As mentioned earlier, altering the vaginal flora is a potential risk. In prospective studies in which the vaginal flora was identified before hysterectomy and again when the patient went home, even when the flora was altered by surgery and prophylaxis, there was no increase in the infection rate. Delayed infection was once believed to be a risk with antibiotic prophylaxis at hysterectomy. The theory was that the lower tract bacterial inoculum would be decreased but not eradicated by antibiotics given at surgery, and it would then increase after the patient was discharged home, where it would cause clinical infection. This was shown not to be true during prospective, blinded clinical trials, and at a time when patients stayed in the hospital long enough that the phenomenon could be detected.[24] Flora alteration and overgrowth of *Clostridium difficile* with resultant colitis is a known risk of prolonged antibiotic administration; it also has been reported after single-dose cephalosporin administration.[25]

Table 25–3 lists many of the antibiotics approved by the FDA for prophylactic administration to women undergoing hysterectomy. Many of these FDA-approved indications are old and have not been revised because a pharmaceutical company has not conducted the expensive clinical trials required to revise their indications or doses. Many agents in this list also have been evaluated in clinical trials as therapeutic agents for women with acute postoperative pelvic infection. Given the safety associated with single-dose prophylaxis, guideline 6 in Table 25–2 becomes less important. The concern was that with prophylactic administration over a period of years, bacteria would acquire resistance to the antibiotics, which then would render the antibiotics ineffective as therapeutic agents. Prospective clinical trials in our hospital indicated that after short-course administration, cefoxitin was as successful as other single-agent and combination regimens in treating women with a posthysterectomy infection.[26, 27]

Hysterectomy as a surgical procedure was given an A-1 rating for prophylaxis justification in a quality standards paper by the Infectious Diseases Society of America (IDSA).[28] The rating reflected the fact that there was good evidence from properly randomized, controlled clinical trials to support the recommendation. The goal was "to make available to infectious disease specialists and other physicians clear, logical, discrete standards that could be applied without controversy in most hospital settings to the care of patients with certain infectious disease problems." Members of the Subcommittee represented the IDSA, the Surgical Infection Society, the Pediatric Infectious Diseases Society, the CDC, the Obstetrics and Gynecology Infectious Diseases Society, and the Association of Practitioners of Infection Control. The standard was endorsed by IDSA.

Operative site infection rates after hysterectomy ranged from 5% to 70% without prophylaxis. In most prospective clinical trials evaluating prophylaxis since then, infection rates have been less than 10%, with few exceptions. A single dose of preoperative prophylactic antibiotic has significantly reduced the postoperative infection rate, hospital stay, and cost of and need for antibiotic therapy. With less exposure to potentially critically ill women, there appears to be an increased tendency to treat a temperature elevation only with therapeutic antibiotics. In evaluating a patient with temperature elevation, history and physical examination are the most important criteria.

Because the white blood cell count commonly is elevated after hysterectomy, that test is not helpful. Women have purulent vaginal discharge contaminated with blood from the vaginal cuff, so a voided urine sample gives the appearance of infection that is not present. The fact that the patient was catheterized may also give false indications of the presence of urinary tract infection. Women may have cystitis after hysterectomy, but it is not associated with temperature elevation. The catheter frequently causes mechanical irritation with resultant trigone and urethral symptoms. Therefore, a standard urinalysis and culture with sensitivity testing is not indicated in the absence of a clinical diagnosis of pyelonephritis.

Clinical evaluation of the lung is usually adequate to suggest normality or the presence of atelectasis or pneumonia. Atelectasis usually disappears within 24 to 36 hours after surgery and is observed more frequently after abdominal hysterectomy. Pneumonia is not clinically evident before 48 hours after hysterectomy, with the exception of aspiration pneumonia, which is diagnosed in the recovery room in most instances. In general, therefore, laboratory testing is not helpful.

Once the clinical diagnosis of a space/organ infection is made, antimicrobial therapy is appropriate. Table 25–4 presents the single-agent regimens that have been evaluated in clinical trials and proven effective in the treatment of women with posthysterectomy operative site infection. Parenteral therapy should be continued until the patient has been afebrile for 24 to 36 hours. Oral antibiotic therapy after successful parenteral antimicrobial therapy is unnecessary.[29]

Table 25–5 lists the combination regimens administered to patients who are clinically more ill than those treated with single-agent regimens. Administration of single-dose gentamicin, 5 to 7 mg/kg once daily, is replacing the schedule of a loading and maintenance dose every 8 hours presented in Table 25–5. Once-daily dosing appears to be as or more effective, less expensive, less time consuming, and also perhaps safer than the multiple-dosing regimens. Peak and trough determinations are not required, but dosing should be reduced if there is decreased glomerular filtration, as

TABLE 25-4 ▶ SINGLE-AGENT PARENTERAL TREATMENT FOR OPERATIVE SITE INFECTIONS AFTER HYSTERECTOMY

Antimicrobial Name		
Generic	Trade	Dose/Interval
Ampicillin/sulbactam	Unasyn	3 g q6h
Cefoperazone	Cefobid	2 g q12h
Cefotaxime	Claforan	1 g q8h
Cefotetan	Cefotan	2 g q12h
Cefoxitin	Mefoxin	2 g q6h
Imipenem/cilastatin	Primaxin	500 mg q8h
Meropenem	Merem	500 mg q8h
Piperacillin	Pipracil	4 g q6h
Piperacillin/tazobactam	Zosyn	3.375 g q6h
Ticarcillin/clavulanate potassium	Timentin	3.1 g q4–6h

IV = intravenous.

TABLE 25-5 ▶ COMBINATION PARENTERAL TREATMENTS FOR OPERATIVE SITE INFECTIONS AFTER HYSTERECTOMY

Antimicrobial Name		Dose/Interval
Generic	*Trade*	
Clindamycin	Cleocin	900 mg q8h
Gentamicin	Garamycin	2 mg/kg loading dose
		1.5 mg/kg q8h as maintenance or 5–7 mg/kg qd
Metronidazole	Flagyl	15 mg/kg loading dose
		7.5 mg/kg maintenance q6h
Gentamicin	Garamycin	As above
Ampicillin	Polycillin-N	2 g q6h

is true for many antibiotics. A nomogram for such dosing was developed by Nicolau.[30]

In patients admitting a questionable allergy to penicillin, cephalosporins have been given safely. If a patient admits a type I anaphylactic-type reaction to a penicillin, a cephalosporin, or a penem and requires coverage for gram-positive aerobic bacteria, she should be treated with vancomycin 500 mg every 6 hours or 1 g every 12 hours. Clindamycin does have gram-positive aerobic as well as anaerobic antibacterial activity. *Enterococcus faecalis*, a species of the normal lower reproductive tract flora, is acquiring resistance to vancomycin, leaving no successful antimicrobial therapy. Caution should be used to prevent the emergence of resistant strains.

For women with cuff cellulitis and who appear to have mild infection, an oral regimen such as amoxicillin with sodium clavulanate (Augmentin), 250 to 500 mg every 8 hours or 875 mg two times daily, is successful for non–penicillin-allergic patients. If patients have a penicillin allergy, clindamycin 450 mg orally every 6 hours should provide adequate coverage.

Because hysterectomy is primarily an elective procedure, the surgeon has time to optimize risk reduction. One of the most frequently observed complications after hysterectomy is operative site infection. Advances in anesthesia technology have significantly reduced posthysterectomy morbidity, but not infectious morbidity. The development of newer sutures, however, has accomplished this. Although the importance of excellent surgical technique cannot be overemphasized, antibiotic administration has been the most significant factor in reducing operative site infection after hysterectomy.

REFERENCES

1. Centers for Disease Control and Prevention: Hysterectomy surveillance: United States, 1980–1993. MMWR Morb Mortal Wkly Rep 1997; 46(SS-4):1.
2. Ad Hoc Committee of the Committee on Trauma, Division of Medical Sciences, National Academy of Sciences, National Research Council: Postoperative wound infections: The influence of ultraviolet irradiation of the operating room and various other factors. Ann Surg 1964; 1(suppl):1.
3. Soper DE, Bump RC, Hurt WG: Bacterial vaginosis and trichomoniasis vaginitis are risk factors for cuff cellulitis after abdominal hysterectomy. Am J Obstet Gynecol 1990; 163:1016.
4. Larsson PG, Platz-Christensen J-J, Forsum U, et al: Clue cells in predicting infections after abdominal hysterectomy. Obstet Gynecol 1991; 77:450.
5. Garner JS, Jarvis WR, Emori TG, et al: CDC definitions for nosocomial infections, 1988. Am J Infect Control 1988; 16:128.
6. Horan TC, Gaynes WP, Martone WJ, et al: CDC definitions of nosocomial surgical site infections. 1992: A modification of CDC definitions of surgical wound infections. Infect Control Hosp Epidemiol 1992; 13:606.
7. Gravel-Trooper D, Oxley C, Memish Z, et al: Underestimation of surgical site infection rates in obstetrics and gynecology. Am J Infect Control 1995; 23:22.
8. Ledger WJ, Campbell C, Taylor D, et al: Adnexal abscess as a late complication of pelvic operations. Surg Gynecol Obstet 1969; 129:973.
9. Livengood CH III, Addison WA: Adnexal abscess as a delayed complication of vaginal hysterectomy. Am J Obstet Gynecol 1982; 143:596.
10. Colombo M, Maggioni A, Zanini A, et al: A randomized trial of open versus closed vaginal vault in the prevention of postoperative morbidity after abdominal hysterectomy. Am J Obstet Gynecol 1995; 173:1807.
11. Swartz WH, Tanaree P: Suction drainage as an alternative to prophylactic antibiotics for hysterectomy. Obstet Gynecol 1975; 45:305.
12. Swartz WH, Tanaree P: T-tube suction drainage and/or prophylactic antibiotics: A randomized study of 451 hysterectomies. Obstet Gynecol 1976; 47:665.
13. Gallup DC, Gallup DG, Nolan TE, et al: Use of a subcutaneous closed drainage system and antibiotics in obese gynecologic patients. Am J Obstet Gynecol 1996; 175:358.
14. Richards WR: An evaluation of the local use of sulfonamide drugs in certain gynecologic operations. Am J Obstet Gynecol 1944; 46:541.
15. Turner SJ: The effect of penicillin vaginal suppositories on morbidity in vaginal hysterectomy and on the vaginal flora. Am J Obstet Gynecol 1950; 60:806.
16. Ledger WJ, Gee C, Lewis WP: Guidelines for antibiotic prophylaxis in gynecology. Am J Obstet Gynecol 1975; 121:1038.
17. Johnson FR, Ohm-Smith M, Galask RP: Prophylactic antibiotics in obstetrics and gynecology. In: Zuspan FP, Christian CD (eds): Controversies in Obstetrics and Gynecology, Vol. 3. Philadelphia, WB Saunders, 1983, pp 450–465.
18. Tanos V, Rojansky N: Prophylactic antibiotics in abdominal hysterectomy. J Am Coll Surg 1994; 179:593.
19. Mittendorf R, Aronson MP, Berry RE, et al: Avoiding serious infections associated with abdominal hysterectomy: A meta-analysis of antibiotic prophylaxis. Am J Obstet Gynecol 1993; 169:1119.
20. Shapiro M, Munoz A, Tager IB, et al: Risk factors for infection in the operative site after abdominal or vaginal hysterectomy. N Engl J Med 1982; 307:1661.
21. Hemsell DL, Johnson ER, Hemsell PG, et al: Cefazolin inferior to cefotetan for single-dose prophylaxis in women undergoing hysterectomy. Clin Infect Dis 1995; 20:677.
22. Hemsell DL, Heard MC, Hemsell PG, et al: Alterations in lower reproductive tract flora after single-dose piperacillin and triple-dose cefoxitin at vaginal and abdominal hysterectomy. Obstet Gynecol 1988; 72:875.
23. Bloomberg RJ: Cefotetan-induced anaphylaxis. Am J Obstet Gynecol 1988; 159:125.
24. Ohm MJ, Galask RP: The effect of antibiotic prophylaxis on patients undergoing vaginal operations. I: The effect on morbidity. Am J Obstet Gynecol 1975; 123:590.
25. McNeeley SG Jr, Anderson GD, Sibai BM: *Clostridium difficile* colitis associated with single-dose cefazolin prophylaxis. Obstet Gynecol 1985; 66:737.
26. Hemsell DL, Cunningham FG, Kappus S, et al: Cefoxitin for prophylaxis in premenopausal women undergoing vaginal hysterectomy. Obstet Gynecol 1980; 56:629.
27. Hemsell DL, Hemsell PG, Heard M, et al: Preoperative cefoxi-

tin prophylaxis for elective abdominal hysterectomy. Am J Obstet Gynecol 1985; 153:225.

28. Dellinger EP, Gross PA, Barrett TL, et al: Quality standard for antimicrobial prophylaxis in surgical procedures. Clin Infect Dis 1994; 18:422.

29. Hager WD, Pascuzzi M, Vernon M: Efficacy of oral antibiotics following parenteral antibiotics for serious infections in obstetrics and gynecology. Obstet Gynecol 1989; 73:326.

30. Nicolau D: Once daily aminoglycosides. Conn Med 1992; 56:561.

26

Wound Infection

MAHMOUD A. ISMAIL ▸ CATHLEEN M. HARRIS ▸ TAMMIE T. ISMAIL

Surgical wound infection remains a frequent complication after gynecologic and obstetric procedures in spite of modern surgical practices.[1, 2] Indeed, wound infections are the most common causes of serious postoperative morbidity, leading to increases in length of hospital stay and cost. Wound infections consume a considerable proportion of health care resources.[3] The frequency of such infection depends on multiple host factors, as well as factors related to the operator and procedure itself. In this chapter, we discuss the epidemiology, clinical diagnosis, and management of wound infections in obstetrics and gynecology.

EPIDEMIOLOGY

Classification of Surgical Wounds

Study of the epidemiology of wound infection[4, 5] resulted in a classification of operative wounds in relation to contamination and increasing risk of infection, as shown in Table 26–1.[5] Cruse and Foord,[4] who studied 62,930 wounds over a 10-year period, reported infection rates of 1.5%, 7.7%, 15.2%, and 40% for clean, clean-contaminated, contaminated, and dirty cases, respectively.

Using the National Nosocomial Infection Surveillance system, Culver and colleagues[6] reported the percentage of operations in the United States by wound class and surgical wound infection rate per 100 operations. They found the infection rates to be 2.1% for clean cases, 3.3% for clean contaminated cases, 6.4% for contaminated cases, and 7.1% for dirty or infected cases.[6]

In 1992, the Centers for Disease Control and Prevention modified the previous definition of surgical wound infection and changed the name to *surgical site infection* (SSI).[1, 2] SSIs are not limited to the incision but may occur anywhere in the operative field.[1, 2]

For surveillance purposes, SSIs are divided into incisional SSIs and organ/space SSIs. Incisional SSIs are further classified as involving only the skin and subcutaneous tissue (superficial incisional SSIs) or involving deep soft tissues of the incision. Organ/space SSIs involve any part of the anatomy (organs or spaces) other than the incision opened or manipulated during the operative procedure (Fig. 26–1).

Superficial incisional SSIs must meet the following criteria: infection occurs within 30 days after the operative procedure and involves only skin or subcutaneous tissue of the incision, and at least one of the following is present:

1. Purulent drainage from the superficial incision
2. Organisms isolated from an aseptically obtained culture of fluid or tissue from the superficial incision
3. At least one of the following signs or symptoms of infection: pain or tenderness, localized swelling, redness, or heat—and superficial incision is deliberately opened by surgeon, unless culture of incision is negative
4. Diagnosis of superficial incisional SSI by the surgeon or attending physician

TABLE 26–1 ▸ CLASSIFICATION OF WOUND INFECTIONS

Clean
Uninfected operative wounds in which no inflammation is encountered and the respiratory, alimentary, genital, or uninfected urinary tracts are not entered.
Clean wounds are primarily closed and, if necessary, drained with closed drainage. Operative incisional wounds that follow nonpenetrating (blunt) trauma should be included in this category if they meet the criteria.

Clean-Contaminated
Operative wounds in which the respiratory, alimentary, genital, or urinary tract is entered under controlled conditions and without unusual contamination. Operations involving the biliary tract, appendix, vagina, and oropharynx are included in this category, provided no evidence of infection or a major break in technique is encountered.

Contaminated
Open, fresh, accidental wounds, operations with major breaks in sterile technique or gross spillage from the gastrointestinal tract, and incisions in which acute, nonpurulent inflammation is encountered.

Dirty-Infected
Old traumatic wounds with retained devitalized tissue and wounds that involve existing clinical infection or perforated viscera.
This definition suggests that the organisms causing the postoperative infection were present before the operation.

From Garner JS: CDC guidelines for prevention of surgical wound infections, 1985. Infect Control 1986; 7:193, with permission.

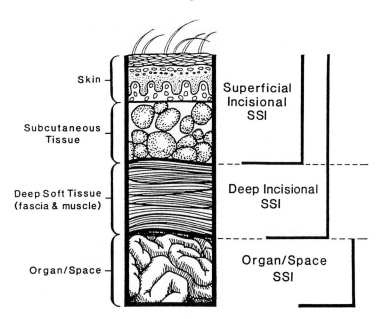

FIGURE 26–1 ▶ Schematic of the anatomy of surgical site infections (SSI) and their appropriate classifications.

Deep incisional SSIs must meet the following criteria: infection occurs within 30 days after the operative procedure if no implant is left in place or within 1 year if an implant is in place, the infection appears to be related to the operative procedure and infection involves deep soft tissues (e.g., fascial and muscle layers) of the incision, and at least one of the following is present:

1. Purulent drainage from the deep incision but not from the organ/space component of the surgical site
2. A deep incision spontaneously dehisces or is deliberately opened by a surgeon when the patient has at least one of the following signs or symptoms: fever (>38°C), localized pain, or tenderness, unless culture of the incision is negative
3. An abscess or other evidence of infection involving the deep incision found on direct examination, during reoperation, or by histopathologic or radiologic examination
4. Diagnosis of a deep incisional SSI by a surgeon or attending physician

An organ/space SSI involves any part of the anatomy (e.g., organs or spaces), other than the incision, opened or manipulated during the operative procedure. Specific sites are assigned to organ/space SSIs to identify the location of the infection. Figure 26–1 shows the specific sites that must be used to differentiate organ/space SSIs. For example, appendectomy with subsequent subdiaphragmatic abscess would be reported as an organ/space SSI at the intra-abdominal site.

Organ/space SSIs must meet the following criteria: infection occurs within 30 days after the operative procedure if no implant is left in place or within 1 year if an implant is in place, the infection appears to

be related to the operative procedure and infection involves any part of the anatomy (e.g., organs or spaces) other than the incision opened or manipulated during the operative procedure, and at least one of the following is present:

1. Purulent drainage from a drain that is placed through a stab wound into the organ/space
2. Organisms isolated from an aseptically obtained culture of fluid or tissue in the organ/space
3. An abscess or other evidence of infection involving the organ/space found on direct examination, during reoperation, or by histopathologic or radiologic examination
4. Diagnosis of an organ/space SSI by a surgeon or attending physician

Surgical site infections may involve more than one site. In these cases, infection that involves both superficial and deep incision sites is classified as deep incisional SSI. Occasionally, an organ/space infection drains through the incision. Such infection usually does not involve reoperation and is considered a complication of the incision. It is therefore classified as a deep incisional SSI.

Risk Factors

Microbiology

Endogenous bacteria are a more important cause of SSI than exogenous bacteria. Bacterial characteristics and size of inoculum also are important in the establishment of wound infections. For example, bacteria with antibiotic resistance can be associated with significant increases in SSI.[7, 8]

Pathogens isolated from surgical wound infections vary with the type of procedure. In clean surgical procedures that do not involve entry of the gastrointestinal, gynecologic, or respiratory tract, *Staphylococcus aureus* from the patient's exogenous skin flora is the usual cause of infection.[9] In other categories of surgical procedures (clean-contaminated, contaminated, and dirty), constituents of the polymicrobial aerobic–anaerobic flora—closely resembling the normal endogenous microflora of the surgically resected organ—are the most frequently isolated pathogens.[10]

Knowledge of the specific bacteria that constitute the exogenous (environmental) flora, together with knowledge of bacteria constituting the endogenous flora at various body sites is the basis on which an empiric choice of antibiotics for prophylaxis or treatment can be made.

EXOGENOUS FLORA

The environmental flora is composed mainly of aerobic organisms because most anaerobes are unable to survive and multiply in the oxygen concentrations of room air. The most pathogenic members of the environmental flora are *S. aureus*, the coliforms (especially *Escherichia coli*), *Staphylococcus epidermidis*, *Pseudomonas* sp., *Citrobacter* sp., *Enterobacter* sp., and *Clostridium* sp. Other microorganisms present in the environment usually do not act as pathogens in humans.

ENDOGENOUS FLORA

The endogenous microflora of the operative site most often is responsible for postoperative infection. Primary pathogens are those species of bacteria normally present in relatively small numbers at a body site that have the capacity of tissue invasion. These bacteria typically elaborate toxins, enzymes, and other products that promote their capacity to invade.[10, 11] Secondary pathogens are also normally present in various body flora in relatively small numbers. These pathogens have relatively low virulence and usually do not elaborate products that might promote an ability to invade tissue. Rather, they possess intrinsic resistance to antibiotics or rapidly acquire resistance through a variety of extrachromosomal mechanisms. Thus, when primary pathogens have been killed, these antibiotic-resistant secondary pathogens may persist. If host defenses are impaired, or if the concentration of these bacteria becomes high enough, the secondary pathogen crosses defensive barriers and becomes invasive.[11]

The organisms that contaminate and invade surgical incisions typically are those that normally colonize the cervix, vagina, and perineum.

The vagina is colonized by large numbers of a variety of bacteria that normally exist in a symbiotic relationship. Several factors influence the vaginal flora, including age, sexual activity, stage of menstrual cycle, and use of antibiotics or immunosuppressive agents.[12–14] The mean bacterial counts in vaginal secretions are 10^8 to 10^9 bacteria/mL, with three to six different species present.[12–14]

The bacteria of the vaginal ecosystem are a mixture of aerobic and anaerobic organisms.[13, 14] Aerobes includes *S. aureus*, *S. epidermidis*, group B streptococci, *Streptococcus* sp., *Enterococcus faecalis*, *E. coli*, *Klebsiella* sp., *Gardnerella vaginalis*, and other organisms considered nonpathogenic, including lactobacilli, *Corynebacterium* sp., and diphtheroids. Anaerobic organisms include *Peptostreptococcus* sp., *Peptococcus* sp., *Bacteroides* sp., *Fusobacterium* sp., *Prevotella bivia*, *Prevotella distens*, and the *Bacteroides fragilis* group.[13, 14]

Surgery itself alters both the number and type of bacteria in the vagina and cervix. After vaginal and abdominal hysterectomy, the number of lactobacilli decreases, and the number of facultative gram-negative rods, *Bacteroides* sp., and enterococci increases.[15, 16] The bacterial colonization rate also has been found to change with the stage of the menstrual cycle, but no concrete data exist to support the concept that timing gynecologic surgery relative to menses alters infection rates. In fact, preoperative hospitalization on the gynecology ward alters vaginal flora in the direction of more virulent bacteria. Antibiotic prophylaxis also alters the vaginal flora, selecting for more pathogenic organisms (e.g., *Enterococcus faecalis*, *E. coli*, and *Enterobacter cloacae*) when infection does occur.[15–18]

Local Environmental Factors

The surgical skills involved in achieving hemostasis, making a sharp, anatomic dissection, placing fine sutures, and handling tissues gently are important to ensure a better healing process and lower rate of infection.[7] The presence of necrotic tissue, hematomas, seromas, large sutures, and foreign material serves to increase the size of the inoculum of bacteria. It also provides a medium for the growth of bacteria, leading to higher rates of SSIs.[7]

▶ Drains: proper indication for use are necessary because drains can function as an access route for pathogens to the patient.[6] The operative site should not be drained through the wound, and the use of closed-suction drains further reduces the potential for contamination and infection.
▶ Electrocautery devices have been clearly associated with increases in superficial SSI. When the electrocautery is properly used to provide pinpoint coagulation or divide tissue under tension, there is minimal tissue destruction, no charring, and no change in the wound infection rate.[6]

Host Defense Mechanisms

The systemic response is designed to control and eradicate infection. Factors that inhibit systemic host mechanisms may be related to the surgical disease or the patient's underlying disease and events surrounding the operation.[8]

Minimal blood loss, avoidance of shock, and maintenance of blood volume, tissue perfusion, and tissue oxygenation minimize trauma and reduce the secondary immunologic effects of major operative procedures.[8] The timing of the operation is crucial if the surgical disease is the cause of the patient's abnormal host defenses.

Older patients with primary pathologic conditions tend to undergo lengthy major abdominal surgery with contamination. This puts them at risk for wound infection. Maintenance of blood volume, hemostasis, and oxygen-carrying capacity has significant implications for all patients. Shock has both an immediate and late effect on the risk of infection because systemic responses are blunted as local factors return to normal.[7, 8, 19]

Advanced age, transfusion, the use of shunts, and the administration of immunosuppressive drugs, including chemotherapeutic agents, are associated with an increased risk of SSI.[19, 20] The air in the operating room and other operating room sources is occasionally implicated in clean cases.[7, 8]

Surgeons also influence the SSI rate. Careful attention to asepsis in the preparation and conduct of the operation is important.[21] The measurement and publication of data about individuals or hospitals with high SSI rates have been associated with a diminution of these rates.[6] Such surveillance provides objective data that contribute to improved patient care.

WOUND INFECTION AFTER CESAREAN DELIVERY

The incidence of abdominal incisional infections after cesarean section has been reported to range from 3% to 15%, with an average of 7%.[22] When prophylactic antibiotics are given, the incidence is decreased to 2% or less. Wound infection is the most common cause of antibiotic therapy failure in patients with metritis after cesarean delivery, as reported by Soper and co-workers.[23]

Risk factors for wound infection after cesarean include obesity, diabetes, corticosteroid therapy, immunosuppression, anemia, and poor hemostasis. In addition, wound thickness, surgical expertise, and proper tissue handling can influence wound infection rates.[22, 23]

Multiple species of bacteria, both aerobes and anaerobes, are commonly responsible for wound infection (Table 26–2). Although these bacteria are normally of low virulence, changes in the wound (e.g., hematomas/devitalized tissue) enhance the virulence of these organisms, rendering them capable of causing SSIs. Indeed, invasion of the amniotic cavity and uterine cavity with a combination of aerobic and anaerobic

---

TABLE 26–2 ▶ BACTERIA COMMONLY RESPONSIBLE FOR FEMALE GENITAL INFECTIONS

Aerobes
  Group A, B, and D streptococci
  Enterococcus
  Gram-negative rods—*Escherichia coli, Klebsiella,* and *Proteus* spp.
  aureus
Anaerobes
  Peptococcus species
  Peptostreptococcus species
  Bacteroides bivius, B. fragilis, B. disiens
  Clostridium species
  Fusobacterium species
Other
  Mycoplasma hominis
  Chlamydia trachomatis

From American College of Obstetricians and Gynecologists: Antimicrobial therapy for obstetric patients. Tech Bull No. 117, June, 1988.

---

bacteria from the cervix and lower genital tract is well recognized as a cause of infection in laboring patients with prolonged ruptured membranes.[24, 25] The polymicrobial nature of genital tract infection associated with cesarean section has been amply described.[24–26]

Clinical Manifestations

Fever beginning on the fourth postoperative day is an indication of incisional abscess. Erythema and drainage may be present. Organisms causing the infection are usually the same as those isolated from amniotic fluid at the time of cesarean section, but hospital-acquired pathogens should also be suspected.[24, 27]

The diagnosis of wound infection is usually a clinical one. Often, patients were given prophylactic antibiotics or antimicrobial therapy for metritis with persistent fever. Ultrasound can be a useful adjunct in making the diagnosis of SSI.

Treatment

Most women with wound infections have already been treated for other pelvic-related infections. Persistent fever and obvious failure of adequate antimicrobial therapy are indications of either infected hematoma or abscess formation—both of which require adequate drainage. Treatment of an abscess includes surgical drainage of all purulent material. In most cases, the entire wound must be explored, with disruption of all layers to the fascia. Careful inspection for fascial integrity is paramount when the wound is first explored. If the fascia is intact, wound débridement and local wound care is appropriate. In some cases, general anesthesia may be required for extensive débridement and exploration of the fascial layer.

After vigorous débridement of all necrotic tissue and drainage of all purulent material, the wound cavity is packed with moistened sterile gauze. Some prefer to use sterile gauze soaked in povidone–iodine solution. The dressing should be changed once or twice daily, and further débridement done as needed during dressing change. Whirlpool hydrotherapy may also be useful in achieving effective débridement and hastening time to reclosure. Hydrotherapy is carried out once or twice weekly.

The ideal dressing does not exist; there is no panacea for all wounds of different causes at different stages of the healing process.[28] A moist environment, however, encourages granulation tissue formation and re-epithelization and allows wound fluid containing bactericidal and growth factors to promote "auto-débridement." Katz and colleagues[29] compared six commercially available semiocclusive dressings for their effect on the growth of bacteria and pre-epithelization of experimentally induced wounds in human volunteers. None of the dressings prevented clinical infection, and all provided microenvironments conducive to the growth of bacteria.

An open wound may be allowed to heal by second intention or can be reclosed at the surgeon's discretion. However, healing by secondary intention takes several weeks to months, depending on the size and depth of the wound. Several studies[30–36] have described early reclosure of laparotomy incisions after wound infection. Howe[33] reported that severe, deep-seated septic wounds could be managed with wide excision of all infected and necrotic tissue followed by immediate reclosure. Such an approach shortened hospital stay as well as eradicated infections and the hazards of cross-contamination. Herman and associates[34] reclosed wounds under general anesthesia 2 days after opening, using en bloc closure after curettage of the wound base and excision of the wound edges. The median time to complete healing was 15 days in the reclosure group, compared with 50 days in the patients allowed to heal by second intention. Robson and colleagues[37] used culture of the subcutaneous tissue as guidance to the time of wound reclosure. When subcutaneous tissue revealed 10^5 or fewer bacteria per gram of tissue, the wounds were reclosed at an average of 4.6 days after wound drainage.

Walters and co-workers[35] prospectively evaluated a technique of delayed closure of disrupted abdominal incisions. Forty-one consecutive postoperative obstetric and gynecologic patients with abdominal incisions that had opened because of infection, hematoma, or seroma and had intact fascia participated in the study. All wounds were first managed identically with surgical drainage and débridement for a minimum of 4 days. The patients were then randomized to either wound reclosure by a standardized en bloc technique (35 patients; Fig. 26–2) or healing by secondary intentions (6 patients). Reclosure was successful in 30 of 35 patients (85.7%). The mean time to complete healing was 15.8 days in successful cases, 67.2 days in failed

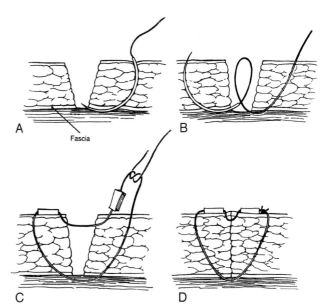

FIGURE 26-2 ▶ Technique of en bloc wound reclosure. *A*, The needle is passed from a point on the skin 3 to 4 cm from the wound edge through the superior part of the fascia at the wound base. *B*, The needle is withdrawn from the wound base, reintroduced into the fascia at the point from which it emerged with the first pass, and brought out through the skin at a point 3 to 4 cm from the opposite wound edge. *C*, Rubber suture guards are loaded onto the suture, the suture is brought across the incision, incorporating the dermis and epidermis of the wound margins, and a second suture guard is loaded. *D*, The suture is tied, closing the wound. (Modified from Walters MD, Dembroski RA, Davidson SA, et al: Reclosure of disrupted abdominal incisions. Obstet Gynecol 1990; 76:597, with permission.)

cases, and 23.2 days for all patients who were reclosed. Failure to heal after reclosure was due to subcutaneous infection in two patients and seroma in three. These women were significantly heavier than those in whom closure was successful. Patients randomized to healing by second intention required a mean of 71.8 days of wound care. The time to complete healing in the wound reclosure group was significantly shorter compared with the group that healed by secondary intention. The authors conclude that en bloc reclosure of disrupted surgical incisions compared with nonsurgical treatment significantly decreases the time required for wound healing and has minimal morbidity. All patients in the study received perioperative antibiotic prophylaxis for reclosure with intravenous cefazolin 1 g before surgery, and again at 6 and 12 hours after surgery. This technique is a modification of the en bloc technique described by Moesgaard and colleagues[31] and Lykkegaard-Nielsen and associates.[32]

POSTHYSTERECTOMY WOUND INFECTION

Abdominal hysterectomy is considered a clean-contaminated operative wound. Patients undergoing such procedure experience a 7.7% wound infection rate according to Cruse and Foord's data.[4]

Clinical Manifestations

Wound infections may be early or late.[38] Early-onset infections are characterized by temperature elevation and cellulitis that develop within the first 48 hours of surgery. Wound breakdown and dehiscence occurs if treatment is not initiated rapidly. The causative organisms are usually group A beta-hemolytic streptococci, but occasional group B beta-hemolytic streptococci are present. Parenteral therapy with penicillin-based antibiotics and aggressive wound care are the essentials of management.

Late-onset infections usually occur on or after the fourth postoperative day. Patients usually have persistent low-grade fever and occasionally purulent drainage from the incision. If an abscess has formed, the patient's temperature will have daily high spikes and be characteristic of abscess fever gram. The causative organisms are S. aureus in 25% of cases and polymicrobial vaginal contaminants in 75%.

Diagnosis

Careful history taking is essential to find clues to the cause of postoperative infection. Time of onset of the complicating infection is important. Early postoperative fevers are usually noninfectious in origin.[39] Possible noninfectious causes include pulmonary atelectasis, hypersensitivity, reactions to antibiotics or anesthetics, pyrogenic reactions to tissue trauma, or hematoma formation. Other important factors in the history include the surgical procedure performed, presence of risk factors, use of prophylactic antibiotics, symptoms, and other ancillary illness.

Erythema and tenderness of skin edges with a purulent discharge indicate simple cellulitis. Fever does not usually appear until the fourth postoperative day; it is often recurrent and associated with increased incision-related symptoms.

Laboratory evaluation includes a complete blood count with a differential, a catheterized urine analysis, and cultures of urine, blood, and the surgical site. In some cases, a chemistry panel is helpful in evaluating hepatic and renal function. The best material for culture is obtained by wound tissue biopsy or aspiration of pus. Transportation to the laboratory should be immediate. Nutritive media should be avoided and anaerobic transport media should be used.

Treatment

Active management of both cellulitis and wound abscess is the same as that discussed earlier for cesarean section wound infections.

NECROTIZING FASCIITIS

This rare and potentially fatal infection is characterized by rapid and progressive necrosis of subcutaneous tissue and fascia. The first clinical description of necrotizing fasciitis was made by Jones, a Confederate army surgeon during the Civil War.[40] Meleney,[41] in a series of 20 cases, was the first to describe a role for beta-hemolytic streptococci in hemolytic streptococcal gangrene. Necrotizing fasciitis of a variety of sites has been described in the literature.[42, 43] In the gynecologic literature, necrotizing fasciitis has been reported in association with both operative and nonoperative conditions, mostly involving the vulva and perineum.[44–54] Cases of necrotizing fasciitis also have been described after cesarean delivery.[54–58] Although this complication is infrequent (1.8 per 1,000 wounds),[58] it does result in appreciable morbidity and mortality. The mortality rate for necrotizing fasciitis is approximately 50% in surgically treated cases, and is much higher in cases with delayed surgery or medical treatment only.

Risk Factors

Risk factors for necrotizing fasciitis include[59, 60] diabetes mellitus, obesity, age older than 50 years, alcoholism, malnutrition, immunocompromised state, operative trauma, peripheral vascular disease, previous radiation therapy, hypertension, and drug abuse. However, as many as 10% of patients diagnosed with necrotizing fasciitis have no predisposing conditions.[61, 62] Necrotizing fasciitis has been reported after minor skin trauma, such as insect bites, and after minor procedures such as episiotomy repair.

Bacteriology

Guiliano and colleagues[63] divided necrotizing fasciitis into two distinct groups. Type I is caused by non–group A streptococci, anaerobes, or facultative anaerobes, often in mixed cultures that include Enterobacteriaceae. Type II is caused by group A beta-hemolytic streptococci or staphylococci. Group A streptococcal necrotizing fasciitis is a highly aggressive, rapidly spreading infection with a mortality rate of 30% to 60%.[64] McHenry and co-workers[46, 65] reported on a variant of monomicrobial necrotizing fasciitis in cases without a wound. Streptococcus pyogenes is the major causative organism in these cases. The more virulent nature of monomicrobial necrotizing fasciitis is related to the production of potent bacterial exotoxins. Pyrogenic exotoxins A and B are thought to be mediators of the rapid tissue destruction, shock, and multisystem organ failure seen in soft tissue infections caused by S. pyogenes. The M proteins of S. pyogenes, type I and III, confer bacterial resistance to phagocytosis, allow bacteria to multiply rapidly, and are responsible for local tissue invasion and bacteremia. Stevens[65] and others postulated that patients who lack antibodies to these exotoxins and M proteins are particularly susceptible to local tissue destruction.

Diagnosis

Early diagnosis and aggressive surgical treatment are critical in the management of necrotizing fasciitis. High mortality rates have been associated with delayed diagnosis. In most cases, definitive diagnosis is made most rapidly by surgical exploration and identification of necrotic subcutaneous tissue and fascia.[66] In 1979, Fisher and associates[67] provided the following diagnostic criteria for necrotizing fasciitis: (1) extensive necrosis of the superficial fascia with peripheral undermining of normal skin; (2) moderate to severe systemic toxic reactions; (3) absence of muscle involvement (clostridial myonecrosis); (4) absence of clostridia in wound and blood culture; (5) absence of major vascular occlusion; and (6) intensive leukocyte infiltration, necrosis of subcutaneous tissue, and microvascular thrombosis on pathologic examination of débrided tissues. Various diagnostic techniques have been advocated to make an earlier diagnosis of this condition, including abdominal roentgenography,[67] computed tomography (CT),[68] magnetic resonance imaging (MRI),[69] and aspiration cytology.[70] Radiographs, although not particularly sensitive, may reveal gas in the soft tissues, which suggests clostridial infection, type I necrotizing fasciitis, or nonclostridial anaerobic fasciitis. CT and MRI may show involvement of the fascia before obvious symptoms or signs. MRI is more sensitive than CT and does not require administration of intravenous agents.[71] Frozen-section biopsy for the rapid diagnosis of necrotizing fasciitis in its early stages was found to provide a definitive and life-saving diagnosis.[72]

Use of nonsteroidal anti-inflammatory agents may delay diagnosis by attenuating the cardinal manifestation of inflammation.[54, 73] Because such agents impair phagocytic function and alter the host's humoral immune responses, a minor infection may develop into a fulminant one.[64, 73]

Clinical Features

The clinical presentation of necrotizing soft tissue infections depends on the infectious etiology, location of the infection, and predisposing factors. The clinical spectrum of necrotizing fasciitis has been described as subacute, acute, and fulminant.[74] Others have divided necrotizing fasciitis into type I, caused by mixed organisms, and type II, mainly caused by group A streptococci.[76]

The clinical signs of *subacute* necrotizing fasciitis are initially indistinguishable from those of cellulitis.[74, 75] A localized area of skin is involved. The skin is tender, red, hot, and swollen. Within a few days, the skin color changes to dusky blue and black. At the same time, bullae may form over the area. Initially the fluid is clear, but it then becomes hemorrhagic. A foul odor may be present, and the skin becomes gangrenous and anesthetic. If left untreated, eventually a black eschar forms over the site and recovery is prolonged, if the patient survives.

Wound pain and discharge may be the only early features of infection. Skin discoloration or blistering may occur later, but these manifestations are only the minor part because the infection spreads extensively along fascial planes.[59] In the case of abdominal surgery, this complication has been reported to occur 3 to 14 days after surgery.[76] Within a few days, the local process spreads to adjacent fat and muscle tissue. At this stage, despite nonspecific, minimal local presenting signs, the patient may appear severely ill with fever, confusion, coma, swelling of the affected area, and rapid fluid and electrolyte changes.[65] Usually on the fourth to fifth day, cutaneous gangrene and desquamation appears as a result of thrombosis of nutrient vessels. Later, burn-like vesicles are noted, and the whole area, which initially was very tender, becomes painless because of subcutaneous nerve terminal injury. The subcutaneous fat and fascia become swollen and necrotic, accompanied by serosanguineous exudate. The skin separates from the underlying tissue as if in an anatomic dissection. In the severe form of the disease, necrotizing fasciitis can also involve the extremities, lower abdomen, chest wall, and perineum.

The *acute* disease has a more rapid course. The symptoms occur over one or several days. The presenting symptoms are similar to those of the subacute disease, but larger areas of the skin are involved and the progress is more rapid. The *fulminant* form presents with symptoms over hours. The patient is toxic, and extensive involvement of the skin is observed. Evidence of early multiple organ failure may be present, including coagulopathy, renal impairment, liver failure, and respiratory distress. This form usually has a high mortality rate despite extensive surgical and medical treatment.

An uncommon cause of necrotizing fasciitis is toxic shock syndrome. Necrotizing fasciitis with or without myonecrosis is present in approximately 50% of patients with streptococcal toxic shock syndrome.[77] A portal of entry from the skin or vaginal mucosa is observed in nearly 60% of patients. In others, the seeding of infection to deeper tissues is caused by a transient bacteremia originating in the pharynx.[64] Early symptoms of streptococcal toxic shock syndrome include myalgia, malaise, fever, chills, nausea, vomiting, and diarrhea. In those with necrotizing fasciitis, pain at the site of minor trauma may be the initial symptom.[64] This is followed by tachycardia, fever, tachypnea, and, in patients who subsequently have necrotizing fasciitis, increasing pain at the site of infection.[75] As the condition progresses, it is characterized by fever, excruciating pain at the infection site, and evidence of shock and multiple organ failure. Hypotension may be present in 50% of patients on admission, and renal impairment usually precedes hypotension. However, cutaneous evidence of necrotizing fasciitis may be absent even in patients who are hypotensive. Laboratory results that may indicate streptococcal toxic shock syndrome include a leftward shift in the granulocytic series (i.e., 40% to 50% immature granulocytes, including myelocytes and metamyelocytes), azotemia, hypocalcemia, hypoalbuminemia, thrombocytopenia, hematuria, and elevated levels of creatine kinase.

Differential Diagnosis

As shown in Table 26–3, the different types of necrotizing infections of the soft tissue can be caused by group A streptococci, S. aureus, Clostridium perfringens, mixed aerobes and anaerobes, and other clostridial species. Predisposing causes include surgery, trauma, diabetes mellitus, crush injuries, epinephrine injection sites, or spontaneous cases related to cancer and cancer chemotherapies, peripheral vascular disease, and minor cuts, burns, and varicella infection. The clinical manifestations (see Table 26–3) include superficial ulceration, gas in skin, fascia, and tissues, myonecrosis and gas formation, destruction of fat and fascia, involvement of the perineum, systemic toxicity, and multiorgan failure.

Treatment

The cornerstone of treatment of necrotizing fasciitis is aggressive surgical management with radical débridement. Delay in diagnosis and improper treatment is associated with higher mortality.[67] Thus, high clinical suspicion and early, aggressive surgical débridement

in patients with postpartum necrotizing fasciitis may decrease mortality.[77, 78]

Operative site wounds should be examined frequently. Marking the skin to document the extent of erythema and induration may be helpful in following the progression of infection. Once the possibility of necrotizing fasciitis is considered, the wound should be explored with the patient under anesthesia. If necrotic subcutaneous tissue and fascia are identified, the diagnosis is confirmed, and radical surgical débridement should be performed. Cultures for both aerobes and anaerobes should be obtained and débridement of all necrotic tissue must be performed regardless of the extent of the resulting defect. Adequate débridement is accomplished by blunt dissection along the fascial planes until the resistance of viable tissue is met, or with sharp dissection to bleeding tissue.[42, 43, 58] Mortality rates increase when multiple operative wound débridements are needed, so aggressive surgical excision of all necrotic tissue at the initial exploration is essential.[76]

Although necrotizing fasciitis usually spares the underlying muscle, deeper involvement of the pelvic organs, especially the uterus and uterine incision, has been reported in infection after cesarean delivery.[68] In such cases, exploration of the abdominal cavity is recommended.

Treatment with broad-spectrum antibiotics is a necessary adjunct to surgical treatment of this disease. A combination of penicillin, gentamicin, and clindamycin or metronidazole is recommended.[43] The postoperative fluid and electrolyte balance should be followed closely, and nutritional support should be initiated. Wound dressings should be changed frequently, with further débridement as necessary.[64] There are few objective reports of the efficacy of hyper-

TABLE 26–3 ❱ NECROTIZING INFECTIONS OF THE SOFT TISSUES

Type	Usual Etiologic Agents	Predisposing Causes	Clinical Manifestations
Meleney's synergistic gangrene	Staphylococcus aureus, microaerophilic Streptococci	Surgery	Slowly expanding ulceration confined to superficial fascia
Clostridial cellulitis	Clostridium perfringens	Local trauma or surgery	Gas in skin; fascia spared; little systemic toxicity
Nonclostridial anaerobic cellulitis	Mixed aerobes and anaerobes	Diabetes mellitus	Gas in tissues
Gas gangrene	Clostridial species (C. perfringens, C. histolyticum, or C. septicum)	Trauma, crush injuries, epinephrine injections, spontaneous cases related to cancer, neutropenia, cancer chemotherapy	Myonecrosis, gas formation, evident systemic toxicity, shock
Necrotizing fasciitis type I	Mixed anaerobes, gram-negative aerobic bacilli, enterococci	Surgery, diabetes mellitus, peripheral vascular disease	Destruction of fat and fascia; skin may be spared; involvement of perineal area in Fournier's gangrene
Necrotizing fasciitis type II	Group A streptococci	Penetrating injuries, surgical procedures, varicella, burns, minor cuts, trauma	Systemic toxicity, severe local pain, rapidly extending necrosis of subcutaneous tissues and skin, gangrene, shock, multiorgan failure

baric oxygen treatment in streptococcal necrotizing fasciitis. One report suggested that in all types of necrotizing fasciitis, hyperbaric oxygen therapy reduced mortality and the need for additional débridement.[79] Depending on the extent of the resulting defect, consultation with reconstructive surgeons may be required for skin grafting. Aggressive surgical management of necrotizing fasciitis with wide excision and débridement, along with antibiotic coverage and support of systemic effects of the disease, serve to decrease morbidity and mortality.[80]

PREVENTION OF WOUND INFECTIONS

Meticulous surgical technique is an essential element in reducing the rates of deep and superficial wound infections. In addition, surveillance for nosocomial infection must be carried out by the hospital infection control team so that every surgeon is aware of his or her individual rate of postoperative infection. Several studies have shown that surgeon-specific wound infection rates can be effectively reduced by such supporting mechanisms.[81, 82] Same-day admission surgery is the routine for all elective gynecologic procedures and is good policy from an infection control perspective.

The old shaving practice should be abandoned and patients must be instructed not to shave themselves the night before. Hair clipping or depilatory is a sound alternative if hair removal is necessary because they do not cause skin cuts and infections. Bowel preparation for major procedures is encouraged because bowel entry is a major cause of contamination and subsequent wound or SSI.

The use of povidine–iodine douches or insertion of gel has been recommended for the night before admission or the day of surgery.

Treating patients with bacterial vaginosis[38] with metronidazole is beneficial in decreasing postoperative infections after hysterectomy. Screening all hysterectomy patients before surgery for bacterial vaginosis and treating those who are infected may be of benefit because these anaerobes play a significant role in postoperative gynecologic infections.

Careful hand-washing techniques[39] should be used by all members of the surgical team. Hand-washing policy should be implemented. Proper gowning, gloving, and eye covering should be observed. Double gloving is recommended to decrease the chances of intraoperative needle sticks and percutaneous injury.

Careful tissue handling, hemostasis, asepsis, and approximation of tissue layers remain the basic elements of sound surgical practice. In an observational study of 635 consecutive cases spanning a 20-year period, using a strict surgical technique and meticulous pinpoint cautery, Lyons and colleagues[83] reported a very low infectious morbidity rate. Iffy and co-workers[84] reported on their institution's success in decreasing wound infections and postcesarean section endometritis morbidity using a strict surveillance protocol.

Fascial Closure and Drains

Reapproximation of the fascia with either continuous or interrupted sutures is appropriate for most cesarean section wounds and is associated with an extremely low incidence of evisceration or late hernia formation.[85] Newer synthetic, absorbable materials such as polyglactin 910 (Vicryl; Ethicon, Somerville, NJ) and polydioxanone are currently used for fascial closures because most of their tensile strength is maintained for 3 weeks.[86] In high-risk and morbidly obese patients, an aggressive closure method is warranted.[87] Compared with interrupted Smead-Jones closure, a continuous running en bloc closure has the advantage of requiring fewer sutures and can be accomplished rapidly.[88] It also has the theoretic advantage of spreading tension more evenly across the wound and reducing the time needed for wound closure, thereby reducing the chance of wound infection. Injudicious cinching of the suture before closure is one potential complication in continuous fascial closure, leading to strangulation of the enclosed tissue and predisposing to dehiscence.

Intraoperative placement of either subfascial or subcutaneous drains is another possible strategy to decrease wound morbidity.[89] Saunders and associates,[90] in a randomized, controlled study of wound suction drainage after transverse suprapubic incision for lower segment cesarean section, found no significant advantage for routine drainage in terms of wound infection, hematoma formation, duration of hospital stay, or analgesic requirements. Loong and colleagues[91] found that the incidence of clinical wound infection was significantly reduced if a Redivac suction drain was placed beneath the rectus sheath, but reported no advantage with use of subcutaneous corrugated drains.

Closure of the subcutaneous tissues (Camper's fascia) at cesarean section has been addressed in a few prospective studies.[92–94] One study[93] used a medical chart review to determine the incidence of wound complications. The authors concluded that a running closure with absorbable suture (usually 3–0 plain gut) was associated with a lower incidence of superficial wound disruption (2.7% compared with 7.4%; $P = .03$). However, the authors did not separately report the incidence of wound infections compared with other causes of dehiscence. Another trial[94] was conducted in gravidas with 2 cm or more of subcutaneous adipose tissue to test whether closing Camper's fascia with a single horizontal running stitch of 3–0 polyglycolic acid would decrease the rate of superficial wound disruption, and to determine whether subcutaneous closure increased the risk for wound infection. Two hundred and forty-five patients were randomized to either subcutaneous closure or no closure. The overall incidence of wound disruption in their study of high-risk patients was 21% (51 of 245). The overall incidence of wound disruption was lower in the closure group (14.5% compared with 26.6%; $P = .02$). The incidence of seromas also was lower in the closure group (6% compared with 19%; $P = .003$).

The use of antibiotic prophylaxis for surgical procedures has increased tremendously and constitutes up to 30% of antibiotic use in general hospitals.[95] However, postoperative wound sepsis continues to be relatively common, comprising 14% of adverse events in hospitalized patients[96] and resulting in significant morbidity and expense.[97] One dose of a first-generation cephalosporin after clamping the umbilical cord is the standard prophylaxis for women undergoing cesarean section with risk factors for postoperative infection.

Short courses of antibiotic prophylaxis are cost-effective.[98] There are concerns, however, over dangerous changes in the microbial qualities of the host and hospital with use of prophylactic antibiotics.[99] Pseudomembranous colitis has been reported in association with a short course of prophylactic antibiotics.[100] Despite these reports, short courses of antibiotic prophylaxis, used appropriately, have no significant adverse effects on the microbial etiology of the host or hospital and do not result in a substantial incidence of adverse effects.

Controversy remains regarding the types of cases in which prophylactic antibiotics are indicated. Their use in contaminated and dirty-infected cases is considered therapeutic.[101] Extensive medical literature documents that appropriate perioperative use of antimicrobial agents can reduce the incidence of postoperative wound infections[101-104]; hundreds of articles on trials of antimicrobial prophylaxis in surgical procedures have been published in the 1990s. The agent chosen should be effective against the pathogens most often recovered from infections occurring after that specific procedure and against the endogenous flora of the region of the body being operated on. Cefazolin has been recommended for obstetric and gynecologic procedures. Any operations that involve the distal ileum, appendix, or colon require agents that cover both aerobic and facultative enteric bacteria and are effective against the obligate anaerobes of the colon, including *B. fragilis*, such as cefoxitin or cefotetan. Newer-generation cephalosporins are not more effective than cefazolin, cefoxitin, or cefotetan.[105] Preoperative prophylaxis should be given to the patient as close to incision time as possible,[15-17] except in cesarean section, where it may be given after clamping the umbilical cord.

Although infections after gynecologic operations, especially hysterectomy, often involve anaerobic bacteria, combinations that include drugs specific for anaerobic bacteria have not been shown to be superior to cefazolin alone.[15-17]

In 1994, Mittendorf and colleagues[105] conducted a meta-analysis of antibiotic prophylaxis and concluded that it should be used routinely with total abdominal hysterectomies. Others[106] consider antibiotic prophylaxis for total abdominal hysterectomies to be a standard of care on the basis of cost–benefit analysis. Quality standards for antimicrobial prophylaxis in surgical procedures were developed by the Quality Standards Subcommittee of the Clinical Affairs Committee of the Infectious Diseases Society of America. The recommendation was that all patients for whom prophylactic antimicrobial agents are recommended should receive them. The agents given should be appropriate in light of published guidelines. A short duration of prophylaxis (usually <24 hours) is recommended.[107, 108]

REFERENCES

1. Society for Hospital Epidemiology of America; Association for Practitioners in Infection Control; Centers for Disease Control and Prevention; Surgical Infection Society: Consensus paper on the surveillance of surgical wound infections. Infect Control Hosp Epidemiol 1992; 13:599.
2. Horan TC, Gaynes PR, Martone WJ, et al: CDC definitions of nosocomial surgical site infections, 1992: A modification of CDC definitions of surgical wound infections. Infect Control Hosp Epidemiol 1992; 13:606.
3. Byrne DJ, Lynch W: Wound infection rates: The importance of definition and post discharge follow up. J Hosp Infect 1994; 26:37.
4. Cruse PJE, Foord R: The epidemiology of wound infection. Surg Clin North Am 1980;60:27.
5. Garner JS: CDC Guidelines for prevention of surgical wound infections, 1985. Infect Control 1986; 7:193.
6. Culver DH, Horan TC, Gaynes RF: Surgical wound infection rates by wound class, operative procedure and patient risk index. Am J Med 1991; 91:152.
7. Nichols RL, Smith JW, Klein DB, et al: Risk of infection after penetrating abdominal trauma. N Engl J Med 1984; 311:1065.
8. Menkins JL: Surgeons, surgery and immunomodulation. Arch Surg 1991; 126:494.
9. Nichols RL, Smith JW: Anaerobes from a surgical perspective. Clin Infect Dis 1994; 18(suppl):S280.
10. Nichols RL: Surgical wound infection. Am J Med 1991; 9(suppl 3B):545.
11. Ulualp K, Condon R: Antibiotic prophylaxis for scheduled operative procedures. Infect Dis Clin North Am 1992; 6:613.
12. Bartlett J, Moon N, Goldstein P, et al: Cervical and vaginal bacterial flora: Ecologic niches in the female lower genital tract. Am J Obstet Gynecol 1978; 130:658.
13. Gorbach WL, Menda K, Thadepalli H, et al: Anaerobic microflora of the cervix in healthy women. Am J Obstet Gynecol 1973; 117:1053.
14. Ohm M, Galask R: Bacterial flora of the cervix from 100 prehysterectomy patients. Am J Obstet Gynecol 1975; 122:683.
15. Faro S, Pastorek JG, Aldridge KE, et al: Randomized double-blind comparison of mezlocillin versus cefoxitin prophylaxis for vaginal hysterectomy. Surg Gynecol Obstet 1988; 166:431.
16. Benigno BB, Evrard J, Faro S, et al: A comparison of piperacillin cephalothin and cefoxitin in the prevention of postoperative infections in patients undergoing vaginal hysterectomy. Surg Gynecol Obstet 1986; 163:421.
17. Hemsell DL: Prophylactic antibiotics in gynecologic and obstetric surgery. Rev Infect Dis 1991; 13(suppl 10):S821.
18. Hemsell DL, Johnson ER, Hemsell PG, et al: Cefazolin is inferior to cefotetan as single-dose prophylaxis for women undergoing elective total abdominal hysterectomy. Clin Infect Dis 1995; 203:677.
19. Olson MM, Lee JT Jr: Continuous 10 year wound infection surveillance results, advantages, and unanswered questions. Arch Surg 1990; 125:794.

20. Ad Hoc Committee of the Committee of Trauma, Division of Medical Sciences, National Academy of Sciences National Research Council: Postoperative wound infection: The influence of ultraviolet irradiation of the operating room and of various other factors. Ann Surg 1964; 160(suppl):1.

21. Hemsell D: Infection after gynecologic surgery. Obstet Gynecol Clin North Am 1989; 16:381.

22. Faro S: Soft tissue infections. In Gilstrap LC, Faro S (eds): Infections in Pregnancy. New York, Wiley-Liss, 1990, p 75.

23. Soper DE, Brockwell WJ, Dalton HP: The importance of wound infection in antibiotic failures in the therapy of postpartum endometritis. Surg Gynecol Obstet 1992; 174:265.

24. Gilstrap LC III, Cunningham FG: The bacterial pathogenesis of infection following cesarean section. Obstet Gynecol 1979; 53:545.

25. Gibbs RS: Microbiology of the female genital tract. Am J Obstet Gynecol 1987; 156:491.

26. Walmer D, Walmer KR, Gibbs RS: Enterococci in post-cesarean endometritis. Obstet Gynecol 1988; 71:159.

27. Emmons SL, Krohn M, Jackson M, et al: Development of wound infections among women undergoing cesarean section. Obstet Gynecol 1988; 72:559.

28. Leaper DJ: Surgical management of wounds. In: Proceedings of the 1st European Conference on Antibiotics in Wound Management. London, Macmillan Magazines, 1992, pp 131–134.

29. Katz S, McGinley K, Leyden J: Semipermeable occlusive dressings: Effect on growth of pathogenic bacteria and re-epithelization in superficial wounds. Arch Dermatol 1986; 122:58.

30. Dineen P: Prevention and treatment of deep wound infections. In: Dineen P, Hidkick-Smith G (eds): The Surgical Wound. Philadelphia, Lea & Febiger, 1981, pp 146–149.

31. Moesgaard F, Larsen PN, Lykkegaard-Nielsen ML, et al: New approaches to treatment of severe incisional abscesses following laparotomy. Dis Colon Rectum 1983; 26:701.

32. Lykkegaard-Nielsen M, Moesgaard F, Larsen PN, et al: Early reclosure versus conventional secondary suture of severe wound abscesses following laparotomy. Scand J Infect Dis Suppl 1984; 43:67.

33. Howe CW: Technique of conversion and closure of postoperative septic wounds. Surg Gynecol Obstet 1967; 125:123.

34. Hermann GG, Bagi P, Christoffersen I: Early secondary suture versus healing by second intention of incisional abscesses. Surg Gynecol Obstet 1988; 167:16.

35. Walters MD, Dembroski RA, Davidson SA, et al: Reclosure of disrupted abdominal incisions. Obstet Gynecol 1990; 76:597.

36. Dodson MK. Magann EF, Mecks CR: A randomized comparison of secondary closure and secondary intention in patients with superficial wound dehiscence. Obstet Gynecol 1992; 80:321.

37. Robson MC, Shaw RC, Hegger JP: The reclosure of postoperative incisional abscesses based on bacterial quantification of the wound. Ann Surg 1970; 171:297.

38. Hager WD: Postoperative infections: prevention and management. In: Rock JA, Thompson JD (eds): Te Linde's Operative Gynecology, 8th ed. Philadelphia, Lippincott-Raven, 1997, pp 233–243.

39. Garibaldi RA, Brodine S, Matsumiya S, et al: Evidence for the non-infectious etiology of early postoperative fever. Infect Control 1985; 6:273.

40. Jones J: Investigation upon the nature, cause and treatment of hospital gangrene as it prevailed in confederate armies mission. Surgical memoirs of the War of Rebellion 1871. Quoted by Meleney FL: Treatise on Surgical Infection. New York, Oxford University Press, 1948, p 15.

41. Meleney FL: Hemolytic streptococcus gangrene. Arch Surg 1924;9:317–364.

42. Wilson B: Necrotizing fasciitis. Am Surg 1952; 18:416.

43. Janevocois RV, Hann S, Batt MD: Necrotizing fasciitis. Surg Gynecol Obstet 1982; 154:97.

44. Cederma JP, Davies BW, Farkas SA, et al: Necrotizing fasciitis of the total abdominal wall after sterilization by partial salpingectomy: Case report and review of the literature. Am J Obstet Gynecol 1990; 163:138.

45. Thompson CD, Brekken AL, Kutteh WH: Necrotizing fasciitis: A review of management guidelines in a large obstetrics and gynecology teaching hospital. Infect Dis Obstet Gynecol 1993; 1:16.

46. McHenry CR, Azar T, Ramahi AJ, et al: Monomicrobial necrotizing fasciitis complicating pregnancy and puerperium. Obstet Gynecol 1996; 87:823.

47. Stephenson H, Dotters DJ, Katz V, et al: Necrotizing fasciitis of the vulva. Am J Obstet Gynecol 1992; 166:1324.

48. Loscar M, Shelling G, Haller M, et al: Group A streptococcal toxic shock syndrome with severe necrotizing fasciitis following hysterectomy: A case report. Intensive Care Med 1998; 24:190.

49. Hewitt PM, Kwong KH, Lau WY, et al: Necrotizing fasciitis after laparosopic surgery. Surg Endosc 1997; 11:1032.

50. Roberts DB, Hester LL: Progressive synergistic bacterial gangrene arising from abscess of the vulva and Bartholin's gland duct. Am J Obstet Gynecol 1972; 114:285.

51. Henderson WH: Synergistic bacterial gangrene following abdominal hysterectomy. Obstet Gynecol 1977; 49:24.

52. Sotrel G, Hirsch E, Edelin KC: Necrotizing fasciitis following diagnostic laparoscopy. Obstet Gynecol 1983; 62:675.

53. Sutton GP, Smirz LR, Clark DH, et al: Group B streptococcal necrotizing fasciitis arising from an episiotomy. Obstet Gynecol 1985; 66:733.

54. Shy KK, Eschenbach DA: Fatal perineal cellulitis from an episiotomy site. Obstet Gynecol 1979; 54:292.

55. Pauzner D, Wolman I, Abramov L, et al: Post-cesarean necrotizing fasciitis: Report of a case and review of the literature. Gynecol Obstet Invest 1994; 37:59.

56. Golde S, Ledger WJ: Necrotizing fasciitis in postpartum patients: A report of four cases. Obstet Gynecol 1977; 50:670.

57. Lowthian JT, Gillard LJ: Postpartum necrotizing fasciitis. Obstet Gynecol 1980; 56:661.

58. Goepfert AR, Guinn DA, Andrews WW, et al: Necrotizing fasciitis after cesarean delivery. Obstet Gynecol 1997; 89:409.

59. Pessa ME, Howard RJ: Necrotizing fasciitis. Surg Gynecol Obstet 1983; 161:357.

60. Francis KR, Lamante HR, Davis JM, et al: Implications of risk factors in necrotizing fasciitis. Am Surg 1993; 59:304.

61. Golshani S, Simons AJ, Der R, et al: Necrotizing fasciitis following laparoscopic surgery: A case report and review of the literature. Surg Endosc 1996; 10:751.

62. Sudarsky LA, Laschinger JC, Coppa GF, et al: Improved results from a standardized approach in treating patients with necrotizing fasciitis. Ann Surg 1987; 206:661.

63. Guiliano A, Lewis F, Hadley K, et al: Bacteriology of necrotizing fasciitis. Am J Surg 1977; 134:32.

64. Stevens DS: Invasive group A streptococcus infection. Clin Infect Dis 1992;14:2.

65. McHenry CR, Brandt CP, Piotrowski JJ, et al: Idiopathic necrotizing fasciitis: Recognition, incidence and outcome of therapy. Am Surg 1997; 60:490.

66. Majeski JA, Alexander JW: Early diagnosis, nutritional support, and immediate extensive debridement improve survival in necrotizing fasciitis. Am J Surg 1983; 145:784.

67. Fisher JR, Conway MJ, Takeshita RT, et al: Necrotizing fasciitis: Importance of roentgenographic studies for soft tissue gas. JAMA 1979; 241:803.

68. Rogers JM, Gibson JW, Farrar WE, et al: Usefulness of computerized tomography in evaluating necrotizing fasciitis. South Med J 1984; 77:782.

69. Sharif HS, Clark DC, Aabed MY, et al: MR imaging of thoracic and abdominal wall infections: Comparison with other imaging procedures. AJR Am J Roentgenol 1990; 154:989.

70. Hirokawa M, Manabe T, Takasu N: Necrotizing fasciitis rapidly diagnosed by aspiration cytology. Acta Pathol Jpn 1991; 41:467.

71. Lille ST, Sato TT, Engrav LH, et al: Necrotizing soft tissue infections: Obstacles in diagnosis. J Am Coll Surg 1996; 182:7.

72. Stamenkovic I, Lew PD: Early recognition of potentially fatal necrotizing fasciitis: The use of frozen-section biopsy. N Engl J Med 1984; 310:1689.

73. Stevens DL: Invasive group A streptococcal infections: The past, present and future. Pediatr Infect Dis J 1994; 321:1.

74. Jarrett P, Rademaker M, Duffill M: The clinical spectrum of necrotizing fasciitis: A review of 15 cases. Aust N Z J Med 1997; 27:29.

75. Bisno AL, Stevens DL: Streptococcal infection soft skin and soft tissues. N Engl J Med 1996; 334:240.

76. Rouse TM, Melangoni M, Schulte WJ: Necrotizing fasciitis: A preventable disaster. Surgery 1982; 92:765.

77. The Working Group on Severe Streptococcal Infections: Defining the group A streptococcal toxic shock syndrome: Rationale and consensus definition. JAMA 1993; 269:390.

78. Shorge JO, Granter R, Lerner LH, et al: Postpartum and vulvar necrotizing fasciitis: Early clinical diagnosis and histopathological correlation. J Reprod Med 1994; 43:586.

79. Riseman JA, Zamboni WA, Curtis A, et al: Hyperbaric oxygen therapy for necrotizing fasciitis reduces mortality and the need for debridements. Surgery 1990; 108:847.

80. Bilton BD, Zibari GB, McMillan RW, et al: Aggressive surgical management of necrotizing fasciitis serves to decrease mortality: A retrospective study. Am Surg 1998; 64:397.

81. Haley RW, Culver H, White JW, et al: The efficiency of infection surveillance and control programs in preventing nosocomial infections in US hospitals. Am J Epidemiol 1985; 121:182.

82. Mead PB, Pories SE, Hall P, et al: Decreasing the incidence of surgical wound infections: Validation of a surveillance-notification program. Arch Surg 1986; 121:458.

83. Lyon JB, Richardson AC: Careful surgical technique can reduce infectious morbidity after cesarean section. Am J Obstet Gynecol 1987; 157:557.

84. Iffy L, Kaminetzky HA, Maidman JG, et al: Control of perinatal infection by traditional preventive measures. Obstet Gynecol 1979; 54:403.

85. Owen J, Andrews W: Wound complication after cesarean sections. Clin Obstet Gynecol 1994; 37:842.

86. Bennett RG: Selection of wound closure materials. Am J Acad Dermatol 1988; 18:619.

87. Hoffman MS, Vila A, Roberts WS, et al: Mass closure of the abdominal wound with delayed absorbable suture in surgery for gynecologic cancer. J Reprod Med 1991; 36:356.

88. Sutton G, Morgan S: Abdominal wound closure using a running looped and polybutester suture: Comparison to Smead-Jones closure in historic controls. Obstet Gynecol 1992; 80:650.

89. Gallup DG, Talled BE, King LA: Primary mass closure of midline incision with a continuous running monofilament suture in gynecologic patients. Obstet Gynecol 1989; 73:675.

90. Saunders NJSTG, Barclay C: Closed suction drainage and lower segment cesarean section. Br J Obstet Gynaecol 1988; 95:1060.

91. Loong RLC, Rogers MS, Cheng AMZ: A controlled trial on wound drainage in cesarean section. Aust N Z J Obstet Gynaecol 1988; 29:266.

92. Hussain SA: Closure of subcutaneous fat: A prospective randomized trial. Br J Surg 1990; 77:107.

93. Del Valle GO, Combs P, Qualls C, et al: Does closure of Camper's fascia reduce the incidence of post cesarean superficial wound disruption? Obstet Gynecol 1992; 80:1013.

94. Naumann RW, Harth JC, Owen J, et al: Does approximation of the subcutaneous tissue lower the incidence of wound complications after cesarean section? [Abstract.] Am J Obstet Gynecol 1994;170:341.

95. Shapiro M, Townsend TR, Rosner B, et al: Use of antimicrobial drugs in general hospitals. Patterns of prophylaxis. N Engl J Med 1979; 301:351.

96. Leaper DJ: Prophylactic and therapeutic role of antibiotics in wound case. Am J Surg 1994; 167:155.

97. Wenzell PR: Preoperative antibiotic prophylaxis. N Engl J Med 1992; 326:337.

98. Iams JD, Chawla A: Patient costs in the prevention and treatment of post cesarean section infection. Am J Obstet Gynecol 1984; 149:363.

99. Kunin CM: Antibiotic accountability. N Engl J Med 1979; 301:380.

100. Block BS, Mercer LJ, Ismail MA, et al: *Clostridium difficile* associated diarrhea follows perioperative prophylaxis with cefoxitin. Am J Obstet Gynecol 1985; 153:835.

101. Anonymous: Antimicrobial prophylaxis in surgery. Med Lett Drugs Ther 1992; 34:5.

102. Kaiser AB: Antimicrobial prophylaxis in surgery. N Engl J Med 1986; 315:1129.

103. Page CP, Bohnen JM, Fletcher JR, et al: Antimicrobial prophylaxis for surgical wounds: Guidelines for clinical care. Arch Surg 1993; 128:79.

104. ASHP Commission on Therapeutics: ASHP therapeutic guidelines on antimicrobial prophylaxis in surgery. Clin Pharm 1992; 11:483.

105. Mittendorf R, Aronson M, Berry R, et al: Avoiding serious infections associated with abdominal hysterectomy: A meta-analysis of antibiotic prophylaxis. Am J Obstet Gynecol 1994; 171:281.

106. Droegemueller W: Preoperative management. In: Herbst AL, Mishell DR Jr (eds): Comprehensive gynecology, 2nd ed. St. Louis, Mosby–Yearbook, 1992, pp 729–732.

107. Dellinger EP, Gross PA, Barrett JL, et al: Quality standard for antimicrobial prophylaxis in surgical procedures. Clin Infect Dis 1994; 18:422.

108. Classen DC, Evans RS, Pestotnik SL, et al: The timing of prophylactic administration of antibiotics and the risk of surgical wound infection. N Engl J Med 1992; 326:281.

27 Hidradenitis Suppurativa

SEBASTIAN FARO

Hidradenitis suppurativa is a complex condition that is considered a chronic infection of the apocrine glands. More recently, it has been considered noninfectious and acneiform. It is usually found in the axillae, buttocks, and groin. Obstetricians/gynecologists commonly observe this condition in the groin and vulva, and it is usually bilateral. Clinically, it initially appears as a red papule on an erythematous base. It is often painful and develops in a localized abscess that can rupture spontaneously, draining foul, purulent, thick exudates.

CLINICAL PRESENTATION

The disease is commonly seen in people 20 to 40 years of age. It occurs more frequently in women than in men, with African Americans having a higher incidence than women of other races. Hidradenitis suppurativa is suppressed by estrogen and stimulated by androgens. Mortimer and colleagues[1] demonstrated that women with hidradenitis tend to have an increase in serum testosterone compared with unaffected women. These investigators hypothesized that the increased testosterone results in overactivity of the apocrine gland and renders it incapable of extricating its product, thereby resulting in occlusion of the gland. Bacteria that normally reside in the area are trapped in the gland and an inflammatory reaction ensues.

Multiple sites of involvement characterize the disease, with red papular lesions progressing to painful nodules or cysts. The lesion is often mistaken for a furuncle or boil. Early indication of impending hidradenitis suppurativa is the presence of twin comedones originating in a single follicle, causing it to divide at the surface into a "Y"-like split[2] (Fig. 27–1). The presence of twin comedones is considered pathognomic for hidradenitis suppurativa.[2]

It is not uncommon to find evolution of the disease in a patient. Careful inspection of the vulva of a patient with hidradenitis suppurativa often reveals the presence of red nodules, a local pyodermitis-type or furuncle-like lesion, a draining sinus, and a healed lesion (Fig. 27–2). Healed lesions are scarred with a pitted center (Fig. 27–3). Therefore, this is a chronic, recurring disease, often causing emotional distress as well as physical discomfort.

PATHOGENESIS

Initially, one follicle is involved in the disease process. However, the inflammation often involves nearby follicles, causing the disease to spread. The nodule develops into an abscess that can assume a chronic state or rupture spontaneously, releasing a foul-smelling, purulent fluid. Inguinal lymphadenopathy can develop and, if the disease is extensive, a systemic response can occur. The patient can become febrile and manifest a flu-like syndrome.[2] Some patients with hidradenitis suppurativa have also had Crohn's disease; however, no direct association has been demonstrated between these two chronic conditions.[3]

Shortly after the duct of the apocrine gland becomes occluded, polymorphonuclear leukocytes migrate into the area, initiating a noticeable inflammatory reaction. The polymorphonuclear leukocytes infiltrate the gland and surrounding tissue, leading to the development of an erythematous papule and subsequently a nodule or cyst. Bacteria from the follicle become trapped in this plug of apocrine secretion (sweat, keratinous material,

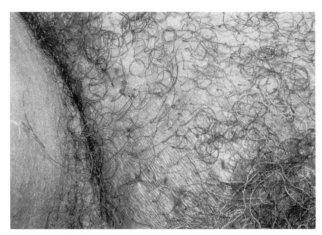

FIGURE 27–1 ▶ Striking comedones, some with a double outlet that represents the initial lesion of the disease. Keratin, sebum, and bacteria trapped below the comedones expand the follicular epithelium into a cyst wall. (From Lynch PJ, Edwards L (eds): Genital Dermatology. New York, Churchill Livingstone, 1994, p 109.)

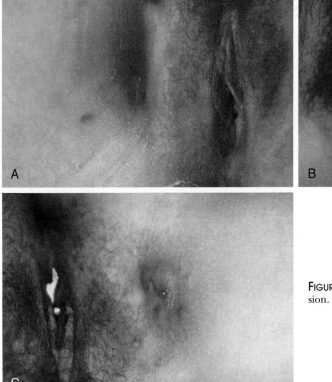

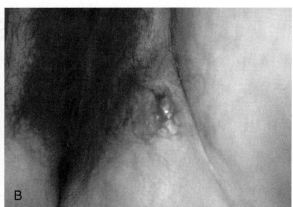

FIGURE 27-2 ▶ *A*, Pyderma-like lesion. *B*, Furuncle-like lesion. *C*, Draining sinus.

and bacteria) and polymorphonuclear leukocytes. After the migration of polymorphonuclear leukocytes, lymphocytes, plasma cells, and giant cells become dominant (Fig. 27–4).

Apocrine glands are found in several locations in the human body, including the axillae, areolae, periumbilical and perianal regions, mons pubis, and vulva. The apocrine gland consists of two components, a coiled secretory segment found in the lower dermis or subcutaneous tissue, and a straight excretory portion that empties into the infundibulum of the hair follicle just above the entrance of the sebaceous duct (Fig. 27–5). Inflammation of the follicle just distal to the junction of the apocrine gland and the follicular infundibulum results in occlusion of the follicle and apocrine gland.[4] This apocrine plug blocks the egress of the gland, causing it to become distended and, eventually, an abscess. The apocrine gland draws bacteria from the adjacent communicating hair follicle; these bacteria are normally found as part of the hair follicle ecosystem. The bacterial Flora of the vulvar skin and its appendages consists of a large variety of gram-posi-

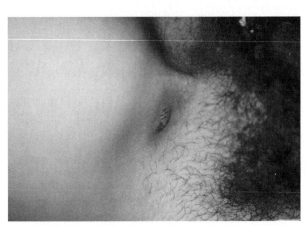

FIGURE 27-3 ▶ Healed lesion with pitted center.

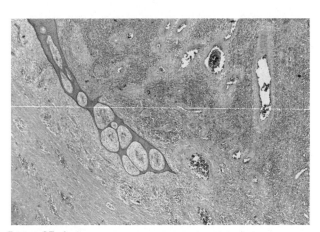

FIGURE 27-4 ▶ Numerous acute and chronic inflammatory cells infiltrate the papillary and reticular dermis. Several ectatic blood vessels are adjacent to reactive squamous epithelium. (Magnification ×200; courtesy of Dr. Pincas Bitterman, Departments of Pathology and Obstetrics and Gynecology, Chicago, IL, Rush Medical College.)

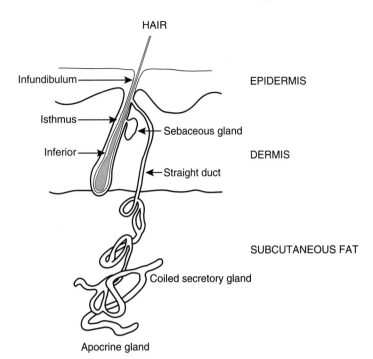

FIGURE 27-5 ▶ Relationship of the apocrine gland to hair follicle. The apocrine gland empties into the infundibular part of the hair follicle. The bacteria colonizing the hair follicle can become trapped below the epidermis. Inflammation in this area can result in the shaft of the follicle becoming blocked. This allows bacteria residing below the area of occlusion to enter the apocrine gland, causing infection. (Adapted from Moschella SL, Hurley HJ [eds]: Dermatology, Vol 1. Philadelphia: WB Saunders 1985, p 60.)

tive and gram-negative facultative and obligate anaerobic bacteria, such as *Staphylococcus aureus, Streptococcus pyogenes, Pseudomonas aeruginosa,* microaerophilic streptococci, *Staphylococcus epidermidis,* enterococci, members of the Enterobacteriaceae *(Escherichia coli), Bacteroides, Prevotella, Fusobacterium, Staphylococcus hominis, Corynebacterium, Acinetobacter,* and *Lactobacillus.*[5]

There is some debate as to whether hidradenitis suppurativa is a true infection. However, it does appear that infection is involved in the process and may be a secondary consequence. The fact that antibiotic therapy rarely results in a cure supports the hypothesis that this is not a condition that results from a primary infection. Nevertheless, there is no doubt that infection plays a role in the condition. Bacteria can be recovered from aspirates of follicular-apocrine abscesses. This infection is typically polymicrobial and can induce a toxic reaction in the patient. The presence of a bacterial abscess and occurrence of a toxic reaction supports the role of infections in hidradenitis suppurativa.

There may be a genetic factor that predisposes some people toward development of hidradenitis suppurativa. The primary abnormality appears to be an abnormally developed follicle, called *twin comedones.*[2, 6] The fact that there are racial differences also lends support to a genetic predisposition for African Americans because, as a rule, they have numerous apocrine gland–associated hair follicles.[2]

Other factors associated with an increase in the occurrence of hidradenitis are obesity, smoking, and endogenous hormones. Obese patients tend to have an increased risk for development of hidradenitis suppurativa because it is common for these people to have

parts of their anatomy in close contact; for example, the thigh and vulva essentially hide the groin, allowing the area to accumulate significant moisture and presenting a hygienic problem. Konig and co-workers[7] reported that cigarette smoking was significantly associated with development of hidradenitis suppurativa compared with nonsmokers, with an odds ratio of 9.4 and a calculated 95% confidence interval of 3.7 to 23.7 ($P<.001$). Panniculus of the abdominal wall also can create an environment suitable for the development of hidradenitis suppurativa. A large panniculus creates an overhanging abdominal wall, forming a large crease just above the mons pubis. This crease or fold of tissue remains warm and moist, and the tissue covered in these areas can easily become macerated, resulting in obstruction of the follicular–apocrine unit.

Elevated testosterone has been considered to be a contributing factor in the development of hidradenitis suppurativa. However, a study by Barth and associates[8] found no supporting evidence for hyperandrogenism in women with hidradenitis suppurativa compared with matched control subjects. These investigators found no difference in testosterone and dehydroepiandrosterone sulfate serum levels between patients with hidradenitis suppurativa and control subjects.

TREATMENT

The treatment of hidradenitis suppurativa has been approached from various vantage points. Antibiotics administered early in the development, before the onset of multiple lesions, can be of benefit. Because the infection is polymicrobial, the use of broad-spectrum agents is indicated, such as metronidazole 500 mg plus ofloxacin 300 mg orally administered twice daily for 7 to 10 days, or L-ofloxacin 500 mg administered orally, daily for 7 to 10 days. Antibiotics can also be used in the same manner as for the treatment of acne, primarily as anti-inflammatory agents, such as tetracycline or erythromycin, 500 mg twice daily administered for several months.[2] Another approach is to culture the lesions, isolate the bacteria, and determine the microbes' antibiotic sensitivity.[9] Triamcinolone acetonide injected intralesionally, 5 mg/0.5 mL weekly, has proved useful.[2] Oral prednisone can be administered, 20 to 40 mg/day for up to 14 days, although long-term use of prednisone is associated with significant side effects. Topical application of steroids is of no value.

Hormonal therapy with oral contraceptive pills that have a low androgenic profile can be useful. Antiandrogen therapy such as cyproterone acetate, 50 μg, ethinyl estradiol 50 μg, and norgestrel, 500 μg daily has also been shown to be effective.[1, 10] Spironolactone, 50 mg twice a day, can be administered until the condition resolves, but, as with all therapy, recurrence is common.

The retinoid isotretinoin, which is used for the treatment of acne, has also been used in the treatment of hidradenitis suppurativa, but with limited success. Treatment is usually prolonged and the patient must be placed on oral contraceptive pills, which should be used because of their estrogenic and antiandrogenic effects. The disadvantages of the retinoids are that only 50% of the patients respond and relapses are frequent.[11, 12] Boer and van Gemert[13] treated 68 patients with isotretinoin for 4 to 6 months and reported that 23.5% of patients had resolution of their disease. Patients must be warned to avoid pregnancy while taking this medication because it is teratogenic.

When all medically attempted therapy fails or if the disease appears to be progressing, surgical intervention should be instituted. There are several possible approaches to operative intervention, but the choice of procedure depends on the stage of disease, whether there are multiple lesions, the depth of suspected involvement, and whether lesions are communicating by fistulas between follicular–apocrine complexes.

In the presence of one to three relatively small lesions and a process that has not been ongoing for a long time (e.g., <6 months), incision, drainage, and curettage or electrocauterization of the base of the lesion can be done. Carbon dioxide laser ablation of the lesion and sinus tracts has also been reported in 11 patients. The results were good, but the patients experienced considerable pain.[14] Finley and Ratz[15] performed 12 carbon dioxide laser excisions of hidradenitis suppurativa on 7 patients. They allowed the areas to heal by secondary intention and followed the pa-

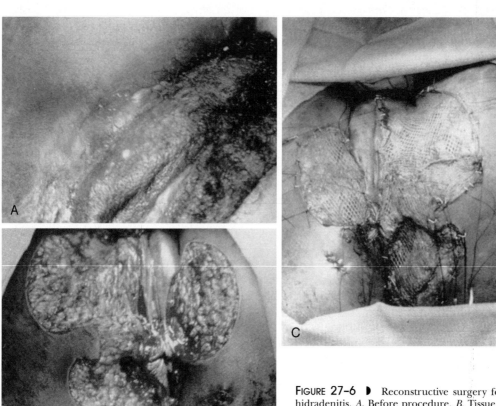

FIGURE 27–6 ▶ Reconstructive surgery for hidradenitis. A, Before procedure. B, Tissue removed. C, Skin graft in place. (From Kaufman RH, Faro S: Benign Diseases of the Vulva and Vagina, 4th ed. 1994, p 253.)

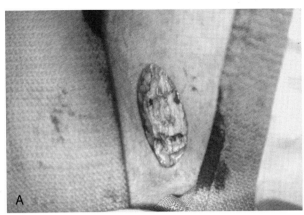 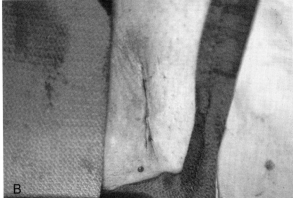

FIGURE 27-7 ▶ *A*, Excision of involved area. *B*, Primary closure.

tients for 10 to 27 months. Healing of all lesions, axillary and inguinoperineal, required 4 to 8 weeks. One patient experienced a recurrence of the disease.[15]

In the presence of chronic disease and multiple lesions, a more extensive approach is necessary. When a surgical approach is taken, the area of involvement must be delineated in all cases. This can be determined by inserting a probe (e.g., a lacrimal duct probe) into the opening of a draining nodule or cyst and gently locating the fistulas. When lesions are close together, they will be connected by fistulas. The skin encompassing the involved areas should be clearly outlined, and the entire area should be excised, leaving a disease-free margin of approximately 1 cm. This margin of normal tissue is necessary to prevent recurrences, although recurrences are frequent.[16–18] The excision should be taken down to the subcutaneous tissue and, in some instances, may require removal of the subcutaneous tissue. A skin graft can be used to repair the surgical defect[19] (Fig. 27–6). If the defect is not too large, primary closure can be performed with typically good results (Fig. 27–7).

SUMMARY

Hidradenitis suppurativa is a chronic disease whose etiology has not been completely determined. It is a complex condition with a hormonal basis that may be responsible for an overproduction of apocrine substances, resulting in occlusion of a hair follicle. Subsequent to this mechanical blockage of both the hair follicle and apocrine gland, infection results. Early recognition of the disease with aggressive management offers the patient the best results.

REFERENCES

1. Mortimer PS, Dawber RP, Gales MA, Moore RA: A double-blind controlled cross-over trial of cyproterone acetate in females with hidradenitis suppurativa. Br J Dermatol 1986; 115:263.
2. Lynch PJ, Edwards L: Red papules and nodules. In: Edwards L (ed): Genital Dermatology. New York, Churchill Livingstone, 1994, pp 107–111.
3. Burrows NP, Jones RR: Crohn's disease in association with hidradenitis suppurativa. Br J Dermatol 1992; 126:523.
4. Yu CC, Cook MG: Hidradenitis suppurativa: A disease of follicular epithelium, rather than apocrine glands. Br J Dermatol 1990; 122:763.
5. Jemec GB, Faber DR, Gutschik E, Wendelboe P: The bacteriology of hidradenitis suppurative. Dermatology 1996; 193:203.
6. Fitzsimmons JS, Guilbert PR, Fitzsimmons EM: Evidence of genetic factors in hidradenitis suppurativa. Br J Dermatol 1985; 113:1.
7. Konig A, Lehmann C, Romple R, Happle R: Cigarette smoking as a triggering factor of hidradenitis suppurative. Dermatology 1999; 198:261.
8. Barth JH, Layton AM, Cunliffe WJ: Endocrine factors in pre- and postmenopausal women with hidradenitis suppurativa. Br J Dermatol 1996; 134:1057.
9. Highet AS, Warren RE, Weekes AJ: Bacteriology and antibiotic treatment of perineal suppurative hidradenitis. Arch Dermatol 1988; 124:1047.
10. Mortimer PS, Dawber RP, Gales MA, Moore RA: Mediation of hidradenitis suppurativa by androgens. BMJ 1986; 292:245.
11. Hogan DJ, Light MJ: Successful treatment of hidradenitis suppurativa with acitretin. J Am Acad Dermatol 1988; 19:355.
12. Norris JF, Cunliffe WJ: Failure of treatment of familial widespread hidradenitis suppurativa with isotretinoin. Clin Exp Dermatol 1986; 11:579.
13. Boer J, van Gemert MJ: Long-term results of isotretinoin of 68 patients with hidradenitis suppurative. J Am Acad Dermatol 1999; 40:73.
14. Sherman AI, Reid R: CO_2 laser for suppurative hidradenitis of the vulva. J Reprod Med 1991; 36:113.
15. Finley EM, Ratz JL: Treatment of hidradenitis suppurativa with carbon dioxide laser excision and second intention healing. J Am Acad Dermatol 1996; 34:465.
16. Harrison BJ, Mudge M, Hughes LE: Recurrence after surgical treatment of hidradenitis suppurativa. BMJ 1987; 294:487.
17. Jemec GB: Effect of localized surgical excisions in hidradenitis suppurativa. J Am Acad Dermatol 1988; 18:1103.
18. Endo Y, Tamura A, Ishikawa OM, Yachi Y: Perianal hidradenitis suppurativa: Early surgical treatment gives good results in chronic or recurrent cases. Br J Dermatol 1998; 139:906.
19. Bhatia NN, Bergman A, Broen EM: Advanced hidradenitis suppurativa of the vulva: A report of three cases. J Reprod Med 1984; 29:436.

28

Septic Shock

MICHAEL R. LEONARDI ▶ BERNARD GONIK

Sepsis is the clinical syndrome that encompasses the spectrum of host responses to systemic infection. *Shock* is a morbid condition in which the functional intravascular volume is inadequate to fill the vascular bed, leading to hypotension and inadequate tissue perfusion. If the course of this process is left unaltered, cellular hypoxia, organ dysfunction, and death ensue.[1] *Septic shock* describes a constellation of infection-mediated clinical findings marked by altered ability to maintain vascular integrity and homeostasis, resulting in inadequate tissue oxygenation and circulatory failure. The spectrum of host response is related to the degree of systemic activation of the inflammatory response and ranges from simple sepsis to septic shock with multiple organ system dysfunction and death.

Septic shock accounts for approximately 10% of admissions to noncoronary intensive care units (ICUs) and is the 13th leading cause of death in the United States. Its incidence appears to be increasing.[2] Even after correcting for the increased age of the population, the rate of septic shock reported by the Centers for Disease Control between 1979 and 1987 more than doubled. This increased rate of septic shock was observed regardless of age group or geographic area.[3] Despite optimal ICU care, the mortality rate from septic shock remains 40% to 50% in most series.[4] Those patients who survive septic shock face increased morbidity and mortality for up to 5 years after the episode, even after accounting for other comorbidities.[5] Although septic shock remains an uncommon event in the obstetric and benign gynecologic population, factors that contribute to the increased rate of sepsis in the general population are becoming more common in women of reproductive age. In addition, because maternal mortality is so uncommon, sepsis will remain an important overall cause of maternal mortality.[6] In the gynecologic population, the incidence and clinical course of septic shock mirror those of a comparable general surgical population. As the population ages and the prevalence of women who were previously thought to be poor candidates for elective surgical procedures because of age or coexisting medical illness increases, septic shock will be a more common occurrence in the gynecologic service. Advanced age along with preexisting medical conditions remain the most important factors in prognosticating operative and postoperative deaths.[7, 8] Newer diseases and therapeutic modalities, such as human immunodeficiency virus infection and organ transplantation, as well as survival of childhood malignancy, have increased the prevalence of patients with immune dysfunction who are potentially at an increased risk for sepsis.[9] Oncology patients in particular are at high risk because of the increased prevalence of advanced age, comorbidities, and immune suppression due to surgery, chemotherapy, radiation, or malignancy.

The etiology of infection in hospitalized patients is commonly the patient's endogenous flora.[10] The reason for hospitalization, medical or surgical procedures performed, and many preexisting diseases combine to limit the host's ability to control her endogenous microflora.[9] The normal vaginal flora, for example, consists predominantly of lactobacilli. Surgery, antibiotics, antifungals, topical bactericidal agents, steroids, hormonal changes, and diabetes all alter the vaginal ecosystem and allow overgrowth of more pathogenic organisms.[11] Similar changes can occur in the gut associated with changes in nutrition status or the selective pressure exerted by broad-spectrum antibiotics.[12] Prolonged hospitalization and use of broad-spectrum antibiotics increase the risk of infection with resistant gram-negative organisms and pseudomonads.[13] Anaerobes are part of the normal genitourinary and gastrointestinal flora but may become pathogens when the normal mechanisms limiting their growth are altered. Antibiotics, decreased local vascular supply, foreign body material, and tissue trauma all favor anaerobic infection.[14] The stomach and small bowel normally have minimal microbiologic contaminants,[13] but the use of nasogastric tubes, suppression of the normally acidic stomach pH, and patient sedation allow overgrowth of the stomach with coliforms and increase the likelihood of their subsequent aspiration.[15, 16]

SYSTEMIC INFLAMMATORY RESPONSE SYNDROME

A consensus conference adopted the term *systemic inflammatory response syndrome* (SIRS) to describe the general inflammatory response to a variety of insults. Its etiology is not limited to infection because burns, trauma, and pancreatitis can elicit a similar clinical picture. SIRS is characterized by two or more of the following: (1) body temperature less than 36°C or more than 38°C; (2) pulse greater than 90 beats per minute; (3) tachypnea manifested as respiratory rate exceeding 20 per minute or a $PaCO_2$ less than 32 mm Hg; and (4) a leukocyte count less than 4,000/mm³, greater than 12,000/mm³, or showing more than 10% immature forms in the differential count. When SIRS is the result of documented infection, it is termed *sepsis*.

Severe sepsis is diagnosed when SIRS is associated with organ dysfunction, hypoperfusion, or hypotension. Useful indicators of hypoperfusion include lactic acidosis, oliguria, or acute alterations in mental status. If abnormalities of blood pressure and perfusion persist despite adequate fluid resuscitation, *septic shock* is present. Hypotension is not necessary for the diagnosis if the patient requires vasopressor support. *Multiple organ system dysfunction syndrome* is the terminal phase of this spectrum represented by the progressive physiologic deterioration of interdependent organ systems such that homeostasis cannot be maintained without active intervention. Commonly affected organ systems include pulmonary and renal dysfunction with adult respiratory distress syndrome (ARDS) and acute renal failure, respectively.[1]

CLINICAL PRESENTATION

The observed clinical spectrum of sepsis represents increasing severity of the host response to infection rather than increasing severity of infection.[17] Although various risk factors have been identified and scoring systems developed, no effective way to predict which patients will progress from bacteremia to septic shock and multiple organ system dysfunction syndrome has yet been identified.[18] More severe inflammatory responses are accompanied by progressively greater mortality rates.[19] Because experimental infusions of endogenous inflammatory mediators such as interleukin (IL)-1, IL-2, and tumor necrosis factor-alpha (TNF-α) reproduce this syndrome, an exaggerated host inflammatory response is thought to be central to its pathophysiology.[20–22]

In the early phase of septic shock (Table 28–1), bacteremia is heralded typically by shaking chills, sudden rise in temperature, tachycardia, and warm extremities. Although the patient may appear ill, the diagnosis of septic shock may be elusive until mild hypotension is documented. In addition, patients may present initially with nonspecific complaints such as malaise, nausea, vomiting, and, at times, profuse diarrhea. Abrupt alterations in mental status also may herald the onset of septic shock; these behavioral alter-

TABLE 28–1 ▶ CLINICAL FEATURES OF SEPTIC SHOCK
Early shock
Altered mental status
Peripheral vasodilation
Tachypnea
Tachycardia
Temperature instability
Hypotension
Increased cardiac output and decreased peripheral resistance
Late shock
Peripheral vasoconstriction (cool, clammy skin)
Oliguria
Cyanosis
Adult respiratory distress syndrome
Decreased cardiac output and increased peripheral resistance
Secondary shock
Obtundation
Anuria
Hypoglycemia
Disseminated intravascular coagulation
Myocardial failure

ations have been attributed to reductions in cerebral blood flow. Tachypnea or dyspnea may be present with minimal findings on physical examination. These findings may represent the endotoxin's direct effect on the respiratory center and may immediately precede the clinical development of ARDS.

Laboratory findings are quite variable during the early stages of septic shock. The white blood cell count may be depressed at first; soon afterward, a marked leukocytosis is usually evident. Although there is a transient increase in the blood glucose level secondary to catecholamine release and tissue underutilization, hypoglycemia may prevail later when a reduction in gluconeogenesis occurs secondary to hepatic dysfunction. Early evidence of disseminated intravascular coagulation (DIC) may be represented by a decreased platelet count, decreased fibrinogen, elevated fibrin split products, and elevated thrombin time. Initial arterial blood gases may show a transient respiratory alkalosis secondary to tachypnea. These parameters later reflect an increasing metabolic acidosis because tissue hypoxia and lactic acid levels increase.

Later clinical manifestations of untreated shock include cold extremities, oliguria, and peripheral cyanosis. Myocardial depression becomes a prominent feature of prolonged septic shock, with marked reductions in cardiac output and systemic vascular resistance (SVR).[23] Overt evidence of prolonged cellular hypoxia and dysfunction includes profound metabolic acidosis, electrolyte imbalances, and DIC. If these symptoms are left untreated, rapid progression to irreversible shock is the rule.

As suggested, progressive cardiac dysfunction features prominently in the clinical presentation of septic shock. Cardiac output and cardiac index are increased because of increased heart rate and the profound decreases in SVR. However, the increased cardiac output is inadequate to meet the patient's metabolic needs. Both the left and right ventricles dilate, and the ejection fractions decrease.[24] The limitation in cardiac performance and ejection fraction is greater than that seen in equally ill, nonseptic patients.[25] Ventricular compliance is also affected as evidenced by a decrease in the ability to increase contractility in response to increases in preload.[26]

In the acute phase of septic shock, the ability to dilate the left ventricle to maintain cardiac output in the face of declining ejection fraction appears to represent an adaptive response that confers a survival advantage.[25] Two subsets of patients have been identified based on response to volume loading: those who respond with ventricular dilation, and those with increased pulmonary capillary wedge pressure (PCWP) rather than increased cardiac output.[27] Cardiac depression of similar magnitude and frequency has been reported in septic obstetric patients managed with pulmonary artery catheters.[28] Extensive study in humans and animal models points to a circulating myocardial depressant factor rather than alterations in coronary flow or myocardial oxygenation as the etiology for myocardial dysfunction.[29] Endotoxin infusion has similar effects on myocardial function and is thought to play a role in the elaboration of a myocardial depressant factor.[24]

PATHOPHYSIOLOGY OF SEPTIC SHOCK

The clinical manifestations of septic shock include both systemic responses such as tachycardia, tachypnea, and hypotension as well as end-organ dysfunction such as ARDS and acute renal failure.[30] The severity of the clinical presentation is determined by the vigor of the host inflammatory response rather than the virulence of the inciting infection.[31] Once septic shock is established, the physiologic derangements induced by systemic activation of inflammatory mediators are more important than the microbial milieu in prognosticating outcome. In those patients who succumb, death is predominantly a function of the host response to the initiating insult.[4]

Endotoxin, a complex lipopolysaccharide present in the cell wall of aerobic gram-negative bacteria, appears to be the critical factor in producing the pathophysiologic derangements associated with septic shock.[6] Endotoxin is released from the bacterium at the time of the organism's death. In patients with gram-positive sepsis, shock can also develop and appears to be closely related to the release of an exotoxin.[32, 33] From a clinical perspective, the overt physiologic alterations induced by either lipopolysaccharide or exotoxins are the same. The ability of both gram-positive and gram-negative organisms to activate the systemic inflammatory cascade has particular relevance in obstetric and gynecologic patients, where mixed polymicrobial infec-

tions are commonly identified.[34] Although gram-negative coliforms make up a significant portion of the organisms recovered in bacteremic obstetric patients, other organisms, including aerobic and anaerobic streptococci, *Bacteroides fragilis*, and *Gardnerella vaginalis*, are found frequently.

Local activation of the immune system and its effector cells is important at the site of infection. The inflammatory process is normally tightly regulated and functions to confine locally the spread of infection. If the ability to regulate this response is lost, systemic activation of effector cells results in the elaboration of proinflammatory cytokines with widespread systemic effects.[35] The syndrome of septic shock represents the culmination of overzealous activation of normal body defense mechanisms in an attempt to eradicate the invading pathogen.[36]

Preliminary evidence suggests that an initial insult may cause simultaneous subclinical injury to multiple organ systems. It is theorized that this initial insult primes the immune system for a disproportionate response to any subsequent insult.[37–40] The immune system, as one of the injury-primed organ systems, responds to a second insult with an outpouring of inflammatory mediators.[41] Activation of the complement cascade also plays a central role in activation of the immune system[42] and can produce the hemodynamic changes characteristic of sepsis in animal models.[43]

A wide variety of proinflammatory mediators has been implicated in the pathogenesis of septic shock. Several lines of experimental evidence in both humans and animal models support the central role of lipopolysaccharide-induced secretion of the cytokine TNF-α in the pathophysiology of the sepsis syndrome.[44] Large amounts of TNF-α are produced in response to endotoxin administration in healthy human subjects,[45, 46] and the administration of either endotoxin or TNF-α provokes similar physiologic derangements.[47] The infusion of TNF-α into experimental animals is associated with shock and lethality and produces the pulmonary, renal, and gastrointestinal histopathologic findings observed at autopsy in septic patients.[48–51] In similar models, antibodies directed against TNF-α provide protection and decrease mortality if given early enough to provide adequate tissue levels.[20, 52] At the cellular level, lipopolysaccharide bound to a carrier protein interacts with the CD14 receptor on cells of the monocyte line. The resulting monocyte activation leads to production of TNF-α and IL-1, either simultaneously or in parallel. Lipopolysaccharide also binds to soluble CD14 to facilitate interaction with tissues lacking the CD14 receptor, such as vascular endothelium.[53] The production of TNF-α stimulates the secretion of interleukins, prostaglandins, leukotrienes, and other inflammatory mediators. These inflammatory products cause the clinical symptoms associated with sepsis as well as capillary leak, hypotension, and activation of the coagulation system.[54]

Vascular endothelium is metabolically active and exerts a pivotal role in the regulation of underlying vascular smooth muscle tone and maintenance of vessel integrity, fluidity of blood, and leukocyte adhesion. Maintenance of vascular homeostasis is regulated in large part by production of nitric oxide (endothelium-derived relaxing factor).[55] TNF-α stimulation of macrophages causes a sustained increase in nitric oxide production, resulting in profound effects on vascular tone and permeability. Cyclooxygenase is also activated, and the elaboration of prostaglandins contributes to the maldistribution of blood flow.[56]

Tumor necrosis factor-alpha and activated complement fragments attract neutrophils, whose products exacerbate endothelial injury.[57] This results in altered ability of the host to maintain tissue perfusion by regulating blood pressure, cardiac output, and SVR.[30] The production of IL-1β by macrophages has the added effect of producing procoagulant activity, which results in fibrin deposition in the microvasculature and leads to further perturbations of organ perfusion.[58–60] Activation of the microvasculature endothelium by TNF-α and IL-1β produces capillary leak and increased leukocyte receptor expression. Leukocyte migration and activation result in the release of vasoactive substances such as histamine, serotonin, and bradykinin. These substances, in turn, increase capillary permeability, induce endothelial damage, and promote vasodilation.[36] A respiratory burst is stimulated by neutrophil activation with increased production and release of lysosomal enzymes and toxic oxygen species such as superoxide, hydroxyl, and peroxide radicals. This has deleterious effects on the vasculature as well as other organs and is especially detrimental in the lung, where it is thought to play a key role in the pathogenesis of ARDS.[55] Stimulation of neutrophils by activated complement fragments also leads to leukotriene secretion, further affecting capillary permeability and blood flow distribution.[58] At the same time, the damage to the vascular endothelium stimulates platelet aggregation. Complement activation ensues with microthrombus formation and fibrin deposition, leading to further derangements of perfusion.[61]

Intact reflex responses to what are initially local events, through sympathetic activation, may produce profound vasoconstriction in some organ systems; this vasoconstriction results in reductions in tissue perfusion.[36] The local loss of control of vascular tone can also result in failure of arterioles and metarterioles to dilate in response to physiologic vasodilating substances such as histamine and bradykinin.[62] Further capillary leak continues and leads to increased intravascular fluid loss. In addition, cellular hypoxia and acidosis disrupt the ability of individual cells to use available oxygen.[63] Marked reductions in peripheral vascular resistance now appear with extensive capillary pooling of blood. Direct effects of bacterial immunologic complexes play an important role in tissue injury.[64] Immune complex precipitants have been identified in the lung vasculature, and they are thought to contribute to the development of ARDS. Likewise, focal areas of acute tubular necrosis seen in the kidney have been associated with the deposition of inflammatory infiltrates.

Disseminated intravascular coagulation frequently complicates septic shock and involves activation of the coagulation cascade as well as fibrinolysis and depletion of circulating coagulation factors. Tissue factor is released by TNF-α stimulation of monocytes and by exposure of subendothelially located tissue factor after injury to the vascular endothelium with activation of the extrinsic pathway. Microvasculature fibrin deposition compromises end-organ perfusion. At the same time, TNF-α also inhibits the production and action of regulatory proteins such as protein C, thereby amplifying the procoagulant state. Although its role in DIC is not significant, activation of the intrinsic pathway provides a powerful stimulus to the production of kinins, such as bradykinin, contributing to the hypotension and disruption of vascular homeostasis. Derangements in the coagulation system are magnified by rapid activation of endotoxin and then suppression of fibrinolysis, which again appears to be mediated by TNF-α.[65]

PREGNANCY AND SEPTIC SHOCK

Although little objective evidence exists comparing the ability of pregnant and nonpregnant women to process bacterial antigens and elicit an appropriate immune response, pregnancy is traditionally considered an immunocompromised state. Pregnant women remain at risk for common medical and surgical illness such as pneumonia and appendicitis, as well as conditions unique to pregnancy, all of which may result in sepsis. Although genital tract infections are common in an obstetric service,[66–68] septic shock in this same population tends to be an uncommon event (Table 28–2). When an obstetric patient has clinical evidence of local infection, the incidence of bacteremia is approximately

---

TABLE 28–2 ▶ POOR PROGNOSTIC INDICATORS IN SEPTIC SHOCK

Delay in initial diagnosis
Underlying debilitating disease process
Poor response to intravenous fluid resuscitation
Depressed cardiac output
Reduced oxygen extraction
Presence of adult respiratory distress syndrome or renal failure
High serum lactate (>4 mmol/L)
Reduced colloid osmotic pressure (<15 mm Hg)

TABLE 28-3 ▶ BACTERIAL INFECTIONS ASSOCIATED WITH SEPTIC SHOCK IN THE PREGNANT PATIENT

Infection	Incidence (%)
Chorioamnionitis	0.5–1
Postpartum endometritis	
Cesarean section	0.5–85
Vaginal delivery	<10
Urinary tract infections	1–4
Pyelonephritis	1–4
Septic abortion	1–2
Postoperative necrotizing fasciitis	<1

8% to 10%.[34, 69–72] Overall, rates of bacteremia of 7.5 per 1,000 admissions to the obstetric/gynecologic services at two large teaching hospitals have been reported.[69, 70] More striking is the fact that obstetric patients with bacteremia rarely progress to development of more significant complications such as septic shock. Ledger and colleagues[70] identified only a 4% rate of shock in pregnant patients with bacteremia. These findings are in agreement with those of other investigators, who have reported a 0% to 12% incidence of septic shock in bacteremic obstetric and gynecologic patients.[69–73]

The physiologic changes that accompany pregnancy may place the gravida at greater risk for morbidity than her nonpregnant counterpart. Elevation of the diaphragm by the gravid uterus, delayed gastric emptying, and the emergent nature of many intubations in obstetrics dramatically increase the risk of aspiration pneumonitis, for example. Pregnancy decreases the gradient between colloid oncotic pressure and PCWP (COP-PCWP), increasing the propensity for pulmonary edema if pulmonary capillary permeability is altered or the PCWP increases.[74] In the critically ill, nonpregnant patient, decreases in the COP-PCWP gradient predict an increased propensity for pulmonary edema,[75–77] and that gradient is already decreased by

normal pregnancy. The intrapulmonary shunt fraction is also increased,[78] which may increase the risk of pulmonary morbidity.

Fortunately, mortality, which is extremely high in the face of septic shock in other medical and surgical specialties, tends to be an infrequent event in obstetrics and gynecology. The incidence of death from sepsis is estimated at 0% to 3% in obstetric patients, compared with 10% to 81% in nonobstetric patients.[69, 70, 79, 80] Suggested reasons for these more favorable outcomes in the parturient include (1) younger age group, (2) transient nature of the bacteremia, (3) type of organisms involved, (4) primary site of infection (pelvis) more amenable to both surgical and medical intervention, and (5) lack of associated medical diseases that could adversely affect the prognosis for recovery.

The peripartum host may be different from the traditional septic shock host in ways other than the presence of different microbiologic pathogens. Physiologic adaptations to pregnancy designed to promote favorable maternal and fetal outcome occur in almost every organ system.[74, 78, 81–83] Certain of these changes—the dramatic increase in pelvic vascularity, for example—promote maternal survival after infection. They can also influence the presentation and course of septic shock in the gravida, although such potential differences have received little attention in the literature. Some physiologic adaptations to pregnancy (e.g., ureteral dilatation) may predispose the gravid woman to more significant infectious morbidity than her nonpregnant counterpart (Table 28–3).

As would be expected in an uncommon condition, the available human data regarding septic shock in pregnancy are limited. The data describing contemporary ICU management, including invasive hemodynamic monitoring in the septic obstetric patient, are even more limited (Table 28–4). The patient populations studied tend to be small and heterogeneous and

TABLE 28-4 ▶ HEMODYNAMIC AND VENTILATORY PARAMETERS IN PREGNANCY

	Nonpregnant	Pregnant	Relative Change (%)
Cardiac output (L/min)	4.3	6.2	43
Heart rate (beats/min)	71	83	17
Systemic vascular resistance (dyne/sec/cm^{-5})	1530	1210	21
Pulmonary vascular resistance (dyne/sec/cm^{-5})	119	78	34
COP (mm Hg)	20.8	18.0	14
COP-PCWP gradient (mm Hg)	14.5	10.5	18
Mean arterial pressure (mm Hg)	86.4	90.3	No change
Central venous pressure (mm Hg)	3.7	3.6	No change
PCWP (mm Hg)	6.3	7.5	No change
Left ventricular stroke work index (g/m/m^{-2})	41	48	No change

COP = colloid oncotic pressure; PCWP = pulmonary capillary wedge pressure.
From Clark SL, Cotton DB, Lee W, et al: Central hemodynamic assessment of normal term pregnancy. Am J Obstet Gynecol 1989; 161:1439.

have a variety of preexisting medical conditions, as well as some degree of ascertainment bias. A multi-institution review of women with sepsis in pregnancy whose management was guided by a pulmonary artery catheter characterized the hemodynamic alterations seen in this patient population. The maternal mortality rate was 20%. As in the nonpregnant patient, septic shock was accompanied by an overall decrease in peripheral SVR. The range of values for this hemodynamic variable was quite wide and depended on the stage of shock at which the pulmonary artery catheter was initially inserted. At presentation, normal to increased cardiac output and decreased SVR were observed. Those patients who ultimately survived had increases in mean arterial pressure, SVR, and left ventricular stroke work index during therapy. Left ventricular stroke work index appeared to be the best measure of cardiac function and predictor of outcome. Longitudinal measurements of SVR also proved to be useful in monitoring the progress of therapy. Response to intervention was reflected in normalization of the SVR to intermediate values.[84] These findings are consistent with physiologic patterns observed in nonpregnant patients in septic shock.[85]

TREATMENT OF SEPTIC SHOCK

Resuscitation goals for the patient in septic shock have been directed toward the aggressive use of volume replacement and inotropes to treat hypotension. Contemporary management has modified these therapeutic goals and emphasizes oxygen delivery and organ perfusion as end points for hemodynamic intervention. Similar manipulations will probably be included in future management algorithms, with the addition of efforts to mediate or neutralize the effects of inflammatory mediators.[86]

Initial intervention should be directed at the following general goals: (1) improvement in functional circulating intravascular volume, (2) establishment and maintenance of an adequate airway to facilitate management of respiratory failure, (3) assurance of adequate tissue perfusion and oxygenation, (4) initiation of diagnostic evaluations to determine the septic focus, and (5) institution of empirical antimicrobial therapy to eradicate the most likely pathogens.

If the patient is pregnant, priorities should be directed toward maternal well-being, even in the face of the potential deleterious effects of septic shock on the fetus. Because fetal compromise results primarily from maternal cardiovascular decompensation, improvements in the maternal status should have positive effects on the fetal condition. Furthermore, attempts to deliver the fetus in a hemodynamically compromised mother may lead to increased risks of fetal distress and the need for more aggressive obstetric intervention. In a mother who is not adequately resuscitated or is unsta-

ble, further decreases in intravascular volume associated with blood loss at abdominal delivery may result in irrecoverable decompensation in maternal hemodynamic status. Maternal interests should take precedence, especially early in the course of resuscitation. This, of course, presumes that the fetal compartment is not the source of sepsis. Under such circumstances, therapy includes initiating delivery while stabilizing the mother.

Volume Expansion

The mainstay of the acute management of septic shock involves volume expansion and correction of absolute or relative hypovolemia.[64, 87–91] Such therapy is always needed and correlates closely with improvement in cardiac output, oxygen delivery, and survival.[92] At times, considerable quantities of fluid are needed because of profound vasodilation, increased capillary permeability, and extravasation of fluid into the extravascular space. Blood pressure, heart rate, urine output, and hematocrit are conventionally used to assess the adequacy of intravascular volume. They do not measure intravascular volume directly, but permit it to be inferred based on secondary changes. Although these criteria are adequate for the initiation of volume resuscitation, they are unreliable in guiding optimal fluid and inotrope management in the patient with septic shock or multiple organ system dysfunction.[93] The best means of monitoring this critical therapy is with the use of a flow-directed pulmonary artery catheter.[94, 95] Although central venous pressure (CVP) monitoring has been suggested as an alternative, reports suggesting erroneous information obtained with CVP monitoring during pregnancy support the use of a flow-directed pulmonary artery catheter.[96] In addition, pulmonary artery catheterization allows determination of cardiac output and the calculation of variables related to oxygen delivery and utilization. These determinations cannot be made with standard CVP systems. Use of a pulmonary artery catheter to optimize oxygen delivery and allow earlier intervention in the event of decompensation has been shown to decrease morbidity and mortality in high-risk surgical ICU patients.[86, 95] In addition, the most significant risks with the use of a CVP line or a pulmonary artery catheter are complications that are associated with placement, and those risks are the same regardless of which line is placed.

Titration of therapy to optimize cardiopulmonary performance is preferable to the use of a specific PCWP value as an end point.[24, 97, 98] Fluid resuscitation is a dynamic process, not an end point, and the value for PCWP that optimizes preload varies by patient. Therapy is optimized for the individual patient by sequentially expanding intravascular volume until a plateau is reached where further volume challenge produces no incremental increase in cardiac output.[24]

Vasoactive Drug Therapy

At times, fluid resuscitation proves inadequate in restoring optimal cardiovascular performance. After restoration of adequate intravascular volume guided by a pulmonary artery catheter, the use of vasoactive agents is indicated. Traditionally, the most commonly used agent in this regard is dopamine, although increasing attention is being focused on the early use of norepinephrine in septic shock. Dopamine is a drug with dose-dependent effects on dopaminergic and alpha- and beta-adrenergic receptors.[99] In very low doses (<5 μg/kg/min), a selective dopaminergic increase in mesenteric and renal blood flow occurs. As the dosage is increased, the predominant effect is to increase myocardial contractility and cardiac output without increasing myocardial oxygen consumption. With doses exceeding 20 μg/kg/min, alpha effects predominate, with marked vasoconstriction and a further reduction in tissue perfusion. Dopamine is administered as a continuous infusion, starting at 2 to 5 μg/kg/min and titrated according to clinical and hemodynamic responses.[100]

Dobutamine is an inotropic agent with fewer chronotropic effects than dopamine. It increases cardiac index and oxygen delivery and decreases SVR, improving perfusion.[101] It is commonly combined with low-dose dopamine to improve myocardial performance and maintain renal perfusion in the ICU setting. Other vasoactive drugs, including norepinephrine[102, 103] and epinephrine,[86, 101, 104, 105] have been suggested as alternatives in dopamine-resistant shock. Epinephrine increases cardiac index, oxygen delivery, blood pressure, and contractility. Oxygen debt is increased, possibly reflecting decreased tissue oxygenation, but hypotension is reversed by a balanced effect on both SVR and cardiac output.[101] These hemodynamic improvements come at the expense of increased myocardial work and oxygen requirement,[86] which has limited epinephrine's use in the past. Significant vasoconstriction and end-organ hypoperfusion is also a concern.

Early experience using norepinephrine as a primary agent for inotropic support in septic shock was disappointing. Fears of excessive vasoconstriction and reversal of hypotension at the expense of organ perfusion limited its use. As newer catecholamines, such as dopamine, became available with more "favorable" side effect profiles, they were used as first-line agents.[106] Some now argue that norepinephrine's poor initial response was related to inadequate monitoring and suboptimal volume replacement, resulting in a need for excessively large vasopressor doses and the development of hypoperfusion.[107] As a second-line drug reserved for cases of dopamine-resistant or refractory

shock, additional adverse outcomes were reported for norepinephrine.[102, 103]

Until recently, little attempt was made to compare the effects of dopamine and norepinephrine on hemodynamic parameters and oxygen delivery in septic shock in a randomized, controlled fashion. In one such study, Martin and colleagues[106] demonstrated that norepinephrine more reliably reversed hypotension and oliguria than did dopamine. Likewise, oxygen delivery and consumption were more favorably improved with norepinephrine. In addition, norepinephrine effectively reversed shock in those patients who failed dopamine therapy.[106] Dopamine has also been demonstrated adversely to affect the balance between splanchnic oxygen delivery and utilization compared with norepinephrine. Both agents comparably increased mean arterial pressure, but dopamine decreased gastric intramucosal pH, suggesting detrimental effects on splanchnic perfusion.[108] Unfortunately, microvascular shunting and hypoperfusion associated with any vasoactive agent is at times difficult to recognize, and only becomes apparent with deterioration of the patient's overall condition or with increased serum lactic acid concentrations.[24] Despite well-described limitations to this biochemical test, serially following lactic acid levels may be useful as an indicator of end-organ perfusion. Changes in calculated oxygen delivery and extraction are also helpful in assessing adequacy of tissue perfusion and response to therapy.

The ability spontaneously to generate a hyperdynamic state in response to sepsis is associated with a lower mortality rate.[37, 85, 93, 109] It is unclear whether the beneficial effect on mortality reflects the impact of therapeutic intervention or better underlying cardiovascular function in a host who is more responsive to intervention. Survivors are clearly more responsive to inotropic therapy,[109] but this may just reflect underlying hemodynamic differences in survivors versus nonsurvivors. The observation that better cardiovascular performance was associated with survival has led many intensivists to conclude that titration of inotropic support to supranormal values should improve outcome.[110–115]

This approach to management is controversial and has been questioned in two large, prospective series. The controversy surrounding end points for inotropic support is in part attributable to differences in the populations studied and indications for ICU admission. Initially, this approach was evaluated as prophylaxis in high-risk surgical patients. More recent work that questions this management scheme randomized patients after shock and organ failure were established. These prospective, randomized series found no benefit to normalization of the mixed venous oxygen saturation ($S\bar{v}O_2$) or supraphysiologic goals for hemodynamic manipulation. Hayes and co-workers[116] were unable to demonstrate a decrease in mortality as long as volume replacement was adequate and perfusion pressure was maintained. A large, multicenter European trial found that the targeted parameters were difficult to achieve, and the propensity to achieve them was a function of the patient's age. No decrease in mortality was found in patients who achieved supraphysiologic levels of cardiovascular performance, regardless of group or reason for ICU admission.[117]

These series should not be interpreted as advocating a conservative approach to hemodynamic therapy in septic shock, however. The apparently contradictory findings may be viewed as complementary. In susceptible patients, oxygen delivery, intravascular volume, and perfusion should be optimized to prevent progression to organ failure. In patients in whom shock develops, inotropic therapy should be directed toward maintenance of adequate cardiac output and blood pressure to maintain perfusion and oxygenation.[118] Responsiveness to inotropic support and the ability spontaneously to generate a hyperdynamic state may allow some prognostication regarding outcome.

Oxygenation

Septic patients have increased metabolic needs for oxygen and a simultaneously decreased ability to extract the oxygen that is delivered.[119] Peripheral tissue utilization of oxygen is frequently reduced, resulting in tissue hypoxia.[120] Although oxygenation at the lungs can be assessed easily by arterial blood gas determinations, oxygen consumption or utilization is a more difficult parameter to evaluate. The use of a pulmonary artery catheter allows direct measurement and calculation of parameters relevant to oxygen delivery and consumption. Early in the course of shock, blood pressure may actually be normal owing to peripheral vasoconstriction, because perfusion is disproportionately diverted from the renal and splanchnic circulations to maintain central blood pressure. Impairment of splanchnic perfusion permits translocation of bacteria and toxins across the gastrointestinal mucosa, worsening septic shock.[41, 121] Oxygen delivery and tissue extraction are decreased in all forms of shock. Untreated, anaerobic metabolism and progressive oxygen debt develop, with the development of lactic acidemia, organ dysfunction, and death.[115]

Decreased tissue extraction can be indirectly measured by elevations in $S\bar{v}O_2$ or by the determination of a reduced arteriovenous oxygen content difference.[119] Actual peripheral oxygen consumption can be calculated using the Fick equation; the normal range is 120 to 140 mL/min/m².[122] Oxygen consumption is normally independent of oxygen delivery because delivery far exceeds consumption. In the septic patient, oxygen delivery should be increased until lactic acid concentrations return to normal.[86, 109] Even in the absence of lactic acidosis, it is prudent to maintain excess

oxygen delivery to avoid local reduction in tissue perfusion and subsequent organ dysfunction.[41] The gut, for example, demonstrated anaerobic metabolism (implying inadequate perfusion) in an animal model of sepsis with supranormal cardiac output and oxygen delivery adequate for the rest of the body.[35]

Adult Respiratory Distress Syndrome

The diagnosis of ARDS is made on the basis of progressive hypoxemia, a normal PCWP, diffuse infiltrates on chest radiography, and decreased pulmonary compliance.[36] Pathophysiologically, increased capillary permeability leads to extravasation of fluid into interstitial spaces with the development of progressive oxygen debt that contributes to multiple organ system dysfunction and death. The cornerstone of the treatment of ARDS involves intubation and ventilatory support to maintain adequate gas exchange at nontoxic levels of inspired oxygen. Positive end-expiratory pressure (PEEP) is often necessary to accomplish this goal. Even in the face of overt pulmonary capillary leakage, intravenous hydration should be continued and adequate intravascular volume maintained to promote systemic perfusion. PEEP generates increased intrathoracic pressure and may impede venous return and consequently cardiac output, depending on volume status and amount of PEEP. The effect of PEEP of artificially increasing PCWP measurements should be borne in mind when interpreting hemodynamic readings and assessing intravascular volume status.

Antimicrobial Therapy

In concert with attempts at restoring normal cardiovascular function and tissue oxygenation, a careful investigation into the underlying etiology of sepsis should be initiated. Because the course of septic shock can be short and fulminant, such a work-up must be carried out without delay, and empirical antimicrobial therapy started. The diagnostic work-up should include the microbiologic evaluation of specimens from blood, urine, sputum, and wound. Even though mixed flora is usually identified in transvaginal cultures, a careful sampling of the endometrial cavity may be helpful if this is the suspected source of infection.[123] In patients thought to have chorioamnionitis, transabdominal amniocentesis or cultures taken from a free-flowing internal pressure transducer catheter may be useful.[124] Selected radiographic studies are helpful in arriving at a diagnosis. Both ultrasound and computed tomography are helpful, for example, in the search for an intra-abdominal abscess. Ultrasound can be performed at the bedside, and in experienced hands is reliable. Resolution may be limited by obesity, air-filled loops of bowel, as well as abdominal wounds, dressings, and drains. Computed tomography scanning does not share the same limitations, but it cannot be performed as a bedside study in the critically ill patient.

The likelihood of survival is increased when patients are treated with antibiotics that demonstrate activity against the pathogens ultimately cultured from the patient.[7] Empirical therapy in the septic patient should therefore include coverage for a wide variety of both aerobic and anaerobic gram-negative and gram-positive bacteria. Institution-specific sensitivities of common nosocomial pathogens and specific patient factors should be considered in the choice of empirical therapy until culture results are available. Broad-spectrum parenteral therapy active against the expected pathogens should be instituted. In patients who previously received cephalosporin therapy, additional coverage specifically directed against enterococci may be warranted. When available, culture results and organism sensitivities should be used to guide more selectively subsequent antimicrobial therapy. Appropriate monitoring for efficacy and toxicity of a given antimicrobial agent should be instituted as a matter of routine. Aminoglycosides, for example, have well-known nephrotoxic effects, especially in the patient with potentially compromised renal function. An iatrogenic complication that may limit the clinical effectiveness of aminoglycosides is their consistent underdosing attributable to the significant increase in their volume of distribution in trauma and septic patients.[10] Each clinician must be familiar with the administration and potential toxic effects of these drugs.

The critically ill patient is at high risk for sources of infection not commonly encountered by the obstetrician-gynecologist, and careful physical examination and selected imaging studies are important in excluding uncommon sources. Sinusitis may develop secondary to prolonged intubation or nasogastric suction, for example. Nosocomial pneumonia commonly develops in patients admitted to the ICU and is independently associated with increased risk of mortality.[125] When broad-spectrum antibiotics are used, routine surveillance for resistant organisms and fungal infection is imperative.

Surgical Therapy

Extirpation of infected tissues is vital and enhances survival. In patients with suspected septic abortion, evacuation of the uterus should begin promptly after initiating antibiotics and stabilizing the patient. Septic shock in association with chorioamnionitis in a viable fetus is treated by delivery; this can be accomplished vaginally if maternal hemodynamic parameters are stable and delivery is imminent. Under certain circumstances, after initial maternal resuscitation, cesarean section may be appropriate, given the increased chance of survival of the fetus and the uncertain risks to the mother if the nidus for infection is not removed

rapidly. In the postpartum patient, hysterectomy may be indicated if microabscess formation is identified within myometrial tissues or if there is clinical evidence of deterioration in the patient's condition despite appropriate antibiotic therapy. When the diagnosis of septic pelvic thrombophlebitis is entertained, treatment with heparin in combination with broad-spectrum antibiotics is appropriate. If this proves unsuccessful, surgical evaluation may be necessary.[126]

Abscess formation is common when sepsis follows extensive pelvic surgery. In fact, fluid and fibrin are secreted in response to peritoneal inflammation to localize the insult and entrap bacteria. Local blood flow and capillary permeability increase, promoting the extravasation of large amounts of fluid, which may contribute to the patient's intravascular volume depletion and hypotension.[13, 127] The conditions found in an abscess favor anaerobes and limit antibiotic function, making drainage mandatory. Such factors include low pH, low redox potential, debris, increased bacterial concentration, and secretion of bacterial enzymes that degrade antibiotics. Abscess should be suspected in the presence of failure to improve clinically or repeatedly positive blood cultures despite appropriate antibiotic therapy.[13, 128] Simple abscesses with a percutaneously accessible route for drainage can be managed with radiographically directed catheter placement. If unsuccessful, the clinician can then proceed to laparotomy. Multiloculated abscesses and those containing debris or hematomas are less amenable to catheter drainage.[13, 127]

Gastrointestinal Tract and Nutrition

Although commonly underemphasized, the gastrointestinal tract can be a reservoir of infection and a source of considerable morbidity to the ICU patient. Provision for adequate nutrition, preventing or minimizing the effect of translocation of bacteria from the gut to the systemic circulation, and stress ulcer prophylaxis are directly related to efforts to maintain adequate splanchnic circulation and the integrity of the gastrointestinal mucosa.

Sepsis provokes a catabolic state, but the metabolic alterations provoked by sepsis differ from those of starvation in that the compensatory mechanisms invoked to preserve lean body mass in starvation are absent.[129] Provision for adequate nutrition early in the patient's ICU course is vital. In addition to providing adequate calories, carbohydrates, lipids, protein, vitamins, and trace elements to prevent catabolism, restoration of adequate nutritional support has other beneficial effects. Inadequate nutrition is associated with significant immune impairment with suppression of both cellular and humoral immunity. Animal and preliminary human data suggest that specific nutrients such as glutamine, arginine, and omega-3 fatty acids may have significant immunomodulatory functions.[130]

Malnutrition has additional deleterious effects. It alters gut mucosal integrity and promotes increases in endogenous gut flora. By itself, malnutrition does not promote translocation of bacteria and bacterial toxins into the circulation.[131] Sepsis increases the permeability of gastrointestinal mucosa, and permeability increases with increasing severity of infection, an effect probably mediated by endotoxin.[131, 132] Because of its high metabolic rate, gastrointestinal mucosa is highly susceptible to injury from hypotension. It is affected early when perfusion is redirected away from the gut to maintain central nervous system and cardiac perfusion. Ischemia interferes with the barrier function of the mucosa, which prevents bacterial translocation into the systemic circulation.[35, 133]

When providing nutritional supplementation, the adage "if the gut works, use it" should be borne in mind. Even in the face of nutritionally adequate replenishment, total parenteral nutrition (TPN) is associated with impairment of host defenses and intrinsic gut immunity. Excluding complications associated with central access and line sepsis, infectious complications are increased with TPN.[130] The enteral route slows atrophy and maintains integrity of the mucosal barrier, especially if glutamine is provided. If adequate caloric replacement cannot be provided enterally, even small-volume feedings with the remaining nutrition provided by TPN are better than TPN alone in promoting mucosal integrity and preventing atrophy.[129] Enteral nutrition can be provided to the intubated patient either through a needle catheter jejunostomy or through a small nasogastric tube advanced well into the duodenum.

Alterations in splanchnic perfusion, the patient response to stress, and medications commonly administered to ICU patients all promote ulceration and upper gastrointestinal bleeding. Prophylaxis is commonly provided in the form of either regular administration of antacids, histamine-2 (H_2) receptor antagonists, or cytoprotective agents such as sucralfate. More than 50 trials have been performed with various end points, and have found a comparable protective effect regardless of which type of prophylaxis is used. A relative disadvantage of antacids and H_2 receptor antagonists is that they increase gastric pH, promoting overgrowth of the normally sterile stomach with gram-negative enteric pathogens. The risk of aspiration and nosocomial pneumonia is increased significantly by their use and has led some to recommend sucralfate over antacids or H_2 blockers.[15, 16, 134–138] Although sucralfate is associated with a reduction in nosocomial pneumonias in intubated patients, adequate trials have not been conducted to demonstrate conclusively a reduction in mortality.

CONTROVERSIAL TREATMENT MODALITIES

Historically, the most controversial modality in the treatment of septic shock was the use of high-dose steroids. Their use is theoretically appealing, with potential benefits including stabilization of lysosomal membranes, inhibition of complement-induced inflammatory changes, and attenuation of the effects of cytokines and other inflammatory mediators. Two large, randomized, placebo-controlled, prospective studies subsequently demonstrated neither benefit of early administration of corticosteroids in the treatment of severe sepsis and septic shock nor prophylactic value of steroids in preventing clinical evolution to septic shock.[139, 140] Currently, there is no compelling reason to use corticosteroids in the therapy of septic shock; their use should be reserved for those patients with documented adrenal insufficiency. Other potential roles for steroids in the management of the septic patient may include their use in the late fibroproliferative phase of ARDS to prevent lung injury from evolving to fibrosis. Several small series have suggested that although progression from lung injury to ARDS is not prevented, steroids may be of some benefit in the prevention of pulmonary fibrosis and may accelerate recovery in this subgroup of patients.[141–144]

Lachman and colleagues[145] administered anti-lipopolysaccharide immunoglobulin to obstetric and gynecologic patients in septic shock. In treated patients, a reduction in both morbidity and mortality rates was observed. Despite these initial favorable results, anti-endotoxin and anti-cytokine therapies are of questionable benefit in the treatment of septic shock. Preliminary studies showed that antibodies specifically directed against endotoxin or inflammatory mediators such as TNF-α reduced mortality in animal models and human patients with septic shock.[52] Clinical trials have unfortunately produced inconsistent results. Although initially promising, the clinical experience has not been as good as expected.[146–150] Circulating natural inhibitors of proinflammatory cytokines have been described. In animal models, these circulating inhibitors decrease mortality in endotoxic shock. The interactions between these circulating antagonists and the proinflammatory cytokines on the molecular level and their impact on the clinical course of sepsis are only beginning to be investigated. Their presence may explain the inconsistent results observed in clinical trials of exogenously administered inflammatory mediators.[151]

Beta-endorphins are a group of polypeptides present in the central nervous system. They are derived from the precursor molecule pro-opiomelanocortin, which is produced in response to stress. Studies have suggested that there is a release of this opiate-like substance in the presence of septic shock. After release, this peptide is thought to produce a profound blood pressure reduction, which can be reversed by narcotic antagonists such as naloxone.[152] Several anecdotal reports in the literature support these preliminary observations. It is interesting to note that beta-endorphin levels have been shown to increase progressively throughout gestation.[153] This specific pregnancy-related effect on septic shock remains to be elucidated.

CONCLUSION

Septic shock is a morbid event with high lethality. In survivors, the increased risk for death extends from 1 to 5 years after the episode of sepsis. Its incidence can be expected to increase as the population ages and the prevalence of patients with compromised immune function who undergo gynecologic procedures increases. The optimal therapy of septic shock involves a high index of suspicion, prompt recognition, early and aggressive treatment in an ICU, and the prevention of subsequent insult or injury. Meticulous attention by the clinician directed toward the maintenance of perfusion and tissue oxygenation, the eradication of focuses of infection, management of electrolyte imbalances, correction of metabolic acidosis, stabilization of coagulation defects, prophylaxis for deep venous thrombosis, and monitoring of renal function will optimize the chances for good outcome. The episode of sepsis may be limited or prevented with infection control procedures and meticulous attention toward preserving and optimizing the patient's host defenses, including skin, glottis and upper esophageal sphincter, and gastrointestinal mucosa, and by the avoidance of actions that alter the endogenous flora.

REFERENCES

1. Bone RC, Balk RA, Cerra FB, et al: Definitions for sepsis and organ failure and guidelines for the use of innovative therapies in sepsis. Chest 1992; 101:1644.
2. Centers for Disease Control and Prevention, National Center for Health Statistics: Mortality patterns—United States, 1990. Mon Vital Stat Rep 1993; 41:5.
3. Progress in Chronic Disease Prevention, Chronic Disease Reports: Deaths from nine chronic diseases—United States, 1986. MMWR Morb Mortal Wkly Rep 1990; 39:30.
4. Brun-Buisson C, Doyon F, Carlet J, et al: Incidence, risk factors, and outcome of severe sepsis and septic shock in adults: A multicenter prospective study in intensive care units. JAMA 1995; 274:968.
5. Quartin AA, Schein RMH, Kett DH, Peduzzi PN: Magnitude and duration of the effect of sepsis on survival. JAMA 1997; 277:1058.
6. Gibbs CE, Locke WE: Maternal deaths in Texas, 1969 to 1973. Am J Obstet Gynecol 1976; 126:687.
7. Freid MA, Vosti KL: The importance of underlying disease in patients with gram-negative bacteremia. Arch Intern Med 1965; 121:418–423.
8. Ledger WJ, Child MA: The hospital care of patients undergoing hysterectomy: An analysis of 12,026 patients from the Professional Activity Study. Am J Obstet Gynecol 1973; 117:423.
9. Ledger WJ, Reite AM, Headington JT: Ideas and actions: A system for infectious disease surveillance on an obstetric service. Obstet Gynecol 1971; 37:769.
10. Reed RL: Antibiotic choices in surgical intensive care unit patients. Surg Clin North Am 1991; 71:765.
11. Mardh PA: The vaginal ecosystem. Am J Obstet Gynecol 1991; 165:1163.
12. Ledger WJ, Campbell C, Taylor D, Willson JR: Adnexal abscess as a late complication of pelvic operations. Surg Gynecol Obstet 1969; 129:973.
13. McClean KL, Sheehan GJ, Harding GKM: Intraabdominal infection: A review. Clin Infect Dis 1994; 19:100.
14. Sweet RL: Anaerobic infections of the female genital tract. Am J Obstet Gynecol 1975; 122:891.
15. Craven DE, Kunches LM, Kilinshy V, et al: Risk factors for pneumonia and fatality in patients receiving continuous mechanical ventilation. Am Rev Respir Dis 1986; 133:792.
16. Cook DJ, Reeve BK, Guyatt GH, et al: Stress ulcer prophylaxis in critically ill patients: Resolving discordant meta-analyses. JAMA 1996; 275:308.
17. Bone RC: Sepsis syndrome: New insights into its pathogenesis and treatment. Infect Dis Clin North Am 1991; 5:793.
18. Bone RC, Sibbald WJ, Sprung CL: The ACCP-SCCM consensus conference on sepsis and organ failure. Chest 1992; 101:1481.
19. Rangel-Frausto MS, Pittet D, Costigan M, et al: The natural history of the systemic inflammatory response syndrome (SIRS). JAMA 1995; 273:117.
20. Tracey KJ, Fong Y, Hesse DG, et al: Anti-cachectin/TNF monoclonal antibodies prevent septic shock during lethal bacteraemia. Nature 1987; 330:662.
21. Okusawa S, Gelfand JA, Ikejima T, et al: Interleukin 1 induces a shock-like state in rabbits: Synergism with tumor necrosis factor and the effect of cyclooxygenase inhibition. J Clin Invest 1988; 81:1162.
22. Sculier JP, Bron D, Verboven N, et al: Multiple organ failure during interluekin-2 and LAK cell infusion. Intensive Care Med 1988; 14:666.
23. Parker MM, Parillo JE: Septic shock: Hemodynamics and pathogenesis. JAMA 1983; 250:3324.
24. Porembka DT: Cardiovascular abnormalities in sepsis. New Horiz 1993; 2:324.
25. Parker MM, Shelhamer JH, Bacharach SL, et al: Profound but reversible myocardial depression in patients with septic shock. Ann Intern Med 1984; 100:483.
26. Ognibene FP, Parker MM, Natanson C, et al: Depressed left ventricular performance: Response to volume infusion in patients with sepsis and septic shock. Chest 1988; 93:903.
27. Parrillo JE: Cardiovascular dysfunction in septic shock: New insights into a deadly disease. Int J Cardiol 1985; 7:314.
28. Lee W, Clark SL, Cotton DB, et al: Septic shock during pregnancy. Am J Obstet Gynecol 1988; 159:410.
29. Marksad AK, Ona CJ, Stuart RC, et al: Myocardial depression in septic shock: Physiologic and metabolic effect of a plasma factor on an isolated heart. Circ Shock 1979; 1(suppl):35.
30. Parrillo JE: Mechanisms of disease: Pathogenetic mechanisms of septic shock. N Engl J Med 1993; 328:1471.
31. Lynn WA, Cohen J: Science and clinical practice: Management of septic shock. J Infect 1995; 30:207.
32. Kwaan HM, Weil MH: Differences in the mechanism of shock caused by infections. Surg Gynecol Obstet 1969; 128:37.
33. Cleary PP, Kaplan EL, Handley JP, et al: Clonal basis for resurgence of serious Streptococcus pyogenes disease in the 1980s. Lancet 1992; 339:518.
34. Monif GRG, Baer H: Polymicrobial bacteremia in obstetric patients. Obstet Gynecol 1976; 48:167.
35. Pinsky MR, Matuschak GM: Multiple systems organ failure: Failure of host defense homeostasis. Crit Care Clin 1989; 5:199.
36. Sugerman HJ, Peyton JWR, Greenfield LJ: Gram-negative sepsis. Curr Probl Surg 1981; 18:405.
37. Moore FA, Haenel JB, Moore EE, et al: Incommensurate oxygen consumption in response to maximal oxygen availability predicts postinjury multiple organ failure. J Trauma 1992; 33:58.
38. Van Bebber PT, Boekholz WKF, Goris RJA, et al: Neutrophil function and lipid peroxidation in a rat model of multiple organ failure. J Surg Res 1989; 47:471.
39. Daryani R, Lalonde C, Zhu D, et al: Effect of endotoxin and

a burn injury on lung and liver lipid peroxidation and cata-lase activity. J Trauma 1990; 30:1330.

40. Poggetti RS, Moore FA, Moore EE, et al: Liver injury is a re-versible neutrophil-mediated event following gut ischemia. Arch Surg 1992; 127:175.

41. Demling RH, Lalonde C, Ikegami K: Physiologic support of the septic patient. Surg Clin North Am 1994; 74:637.

42. Fearon DT, Ruddy S, Schur PH, et al: Activation of the pro-perdin pathway of complement in patients with gram-negative bacteremia. N Engl J Med 1975; 292:937.

43. Schirmer WJ, Schirmer JM, Naff GB, et al: Systemic comple-ment activation produces hemodynamic changes characteris-tic of sepsis. Arch Surg 1988; 123:316.

44. Tracey KJ, Lowry SF, Cerami A: The pathophysiologic role of cachectin/TNF in septic shock and cachexia. Ann Inst Pasteur 1988; 139:311.

45. Hesse DG, Tracey KJ, Fong Y, et al: Cytokine appearance in human endotoxemia and primate bacteremia. Surg Gynecol Obstet 1988; 166:147.

46. Michie HR, Manogue KR, Spriggs DR, et al: Detection of cir-culating tumor necrosis factor after endotoxin administra-tions. N Engl J Med 1988; 318:1481.

47. Michie HR, Spriggs DR, Manogue KR, et al: Tumor necrosis factor and endotoxin induce similar metabolic responses in human beings. Surgery 1988; 104:280.

48. Tracey KJ, Lowry SF, Fahey TJ III, et al: Cachectin/tumor ne-crosis factor induces lethal shock and stress hormone re-sponses in the dog. Surg Gynecol Obstet 1987; 164:415.

49. Mayoral JL, Schweich CJ, Dunn DL: Decreased tumor necrosis factor production during the initial stages of infection corre-lates with survival during murine gram-negative sepsis. Arch Surg 1990; 125:24.

50. Tracey KJ, Beutler B, Lowry SF, et al: Shock and tissue injury induced by recombinant human cachectin. Science 1986; 234:470.

51. Remick DG, Kunkel RG, Larrick JW, et al: Acute in vivo ef-fects of human recombinant tumor necrosis factor. Lab Invest 1987; 56:583.

52. Beutler B, Milsark IW, Cerami AC: Passive immunization against cachectin/tumor necrosis factor protects mice from le-thal effect of endotoxin. Science 1985; 229:869.

53. Lynn WA, Golenbock DT: Lipopolysaccharide antagonists. Im-munol Today 1992; 13:271.

54. Hageman JR, Caplan MS: An introduction to the structure and function of inflammatory mediators for clinicians. Clin Perinatol 1995; 22:251.

55. Hollenberg SM, Cunnion RE: Endothelial and vascular smooth muscle function in sepsis. J Crit Care 1994; 9:262.

56. Dinerman JL, Lowenstein CJ, Snyder SH: Molecular mecha-nisms of nitric oxide regulation: Potential relevance to cardio-vascular disease. Circ Res 1993; 73:217.

57. Sriskandan S, Cohen J: Science and clinical practice: The pathogenesis of septic shock. J Infect 1995; 30:201.

58. Jacobs RF, Tabor DR: Immune cellular interactions during sepsis and septic injury. Crit Care Clin 1989; 5:9.

59. Bonney RJ, Humes JL: Physiological and pharmacological reg-ulation of prostaglandin and leukotriene production by mac-rophages. J Leukoc Biol 1984; 35:1.

60. Goetzl EJ, Payan DG, Goldman DW: Immunopathogenic roles of leukotrienes in human diseases. J Clin Immunol 1984; 4:79.

61. Lee W, Cotton DB, Hankins GDV, et al: Management of sep-tic shock complicating pregnancy. Obstet Gynecol Surv 1989; 16:431.

62. Altura BM, Gebrewold A, Burton RW: Failure of microscopic metarterioles to elicit vasodilator responses to acetylcholine, bradykinin, histamine and substance P after ischemic shock, endothelial cells. Microcirc Endoth Lymph 1985; 2:121.

63. Duff JH, Groves AC, McLean LPH, et al: Defective oxygen consumption in septic shock. Surg Gynecol Obstet 1969; 128:1051.

64. Knuppel RA, Papineni SR, Cavanagh D: Septic shock in ob-stetrics. Clin Obstet Gynecol 1984; 27:3.

65. Levi M, ten Cate H, van der Poll T, et al: Pathogenesis of dis-seminated intravascular coagulation in sepsis. JAMA 1993; 270:975.

66. Balk RA, Bone RC: The septic syndrome: Definition and clini-cal implications. Crit Care Clin 1989; 5:1.

67. Duff P: Pathophysiology and management of postcesarean en-domyometritis. Obstet Gynecol 1986; 67:269.

68. Gibbs RS, Jones PM, Wilder CJ: Antibiotic therapy of endome-tritis following cesarean section: Treatment successes and fail-ures. Obstet Gynecol 1978; 52:31.

69. Blanco JD, Gibbs RS, Castaneda YS: Bacteremia in obstetrics: Clinical course. Obstet Gynecol 1981; 58:621.

70. Ledger WJ, Norman M, Gee C, et al: Bacteremia on an obstet-ric-gynecologic service. Am J Obstet Gynecol 1975; 121:205.

71. Reimer LG, Reller LB: *Gardnerella vaginalis* bacteremia: A re-view of thirty cases. Obstet Gynecol 1984; 64:170.

72. Bryan CS, Reynolds KL, Moore EE: Bacteremia in obstetrics and gynecology. Obstet Gynecol 1984; 64:155.

73. Chow AW, Guze LB: Bacteroidaceae bacteremia: Clinical expe-rience with 112 patients. Medicine (Baltimore) 1974; 53:93.

74. Clark SL, Cotton DB, Lee W, et al: Central hemodynamic as-sessment of normal term pregnancy. Am J Obstet Gynecol 1989; 161:1439.

75. Rackow EC, Fein IA, Leppo J: Colloid osmotic pressure as a prognostic indicator of pulmonary edema and mortality in the critically ill. Chest 1977; 72:709.

76. Weil MH, Henning RJ, Morissette M, et al: Relationship be-tween colloid osmotic pressure and pulmonary artery wedge pressure in patients with acute cardiorespiratory failure. Am J Med 1978; 64:643.

77. Rackow EC, Fein IA, Siegel J: The relationship of the colloid osmotic-pulmonary artery wedge pressure gradient to pulmo-nary edema and mortality in critically ill patients. Chest 1982; 82:433.

78. Hankins G, Clark S, Uckan E: Intrapulmonary shunt (QS/QT) and position in healthy third-trimester pregnancy. Am J Obstet Gynecol 1996; 174:322A.

79. Cavanagh D, Knuppel RA, Shepherd JH, et al: Septic shock and the obstetrician/gynecologist. South Med J 1982; 75:809.

80. Wernstein MP, Murphy JR, Retter LB, et al: The clinical sig-nificance of positive blood cultures: A comparative analysis of 500 episodes of bacteremia and fungemia in adults. Rev In-fect Dis 1983; 5:54.

81. Metcalfe J, Ueland K: Maternal cardiovascular adjustments to pregnancy. Prog Cardiovasc Dis 1974; 16:363.

82. Maternal adaption to pregnancy. In: Pritchard JA, MacDonald PC, Gant NF (eds): Williams Obstetrics, 17th ed. Norwalk, CT, Appleton-Century-Crofts, 1985, p 181.

83. Fletcher AP, Alkjaersig NK, Burstein R: The influence of preg-nancy upon blood coagulation and plasma fibrinolytic enzyme function. Am J Obstet Gynecol 1979; 134:743.

84. Lee W, Clark SL, Cotton DB, et al: Septic shock during preg-nancy. Obstet Gynecol 1984; 159:410.

85. Shoemaker WC, Montgomery ES, Kaplan E, et al: Physiologic patterns in surviving and nonsurviving shock patients. Arch Surg 1973; 106:630.

86. Lindeborg DM, Pearl RG: Recent advances in critical care medicine: Inotropic therapy in the critically ill patient. Int An-esthesiol Clin 1993; 31:49.

87. Rackow EC, Weil MK: Recent trends in diagnosis and manage-ment of septic shock. Curr Surg 1983; 40:181.

88. Packman MI, Rackow EC: Optimum left heart filling pressure during fluid resuscitation of patients with hypovolemic and septic shock. Crit Care Med 1983; 11:165.

89. Kaufman BS, Rackow EC, Falk JL: The relationship between oxygen delivery and consumption during fluid resuscitation of hypovolemic and septic shock. Chest 1984; 85:33.

90. Hawkins DF: Management and treatment of obstetric bacter-emia shock. J Clin Pathol 1980; 33:895.

91. Roberts JM, Laros RK: Hemorrhagic and endotoxic shock: A pathophysiologic approach to diagnosis and management. Am J Obstet Gynecol 1971; 110:1041.

92. Weil MN, Nishijima H: Cardiac output in bacterial shock. Am J Med 1978; 64:920.

93. Shippy CR, Appel PL, Shoemaker WC: Reliability of clinical monitoring to assess blood volume in critically ill patients. Crit Care Med 1984; 12:107.

94. Swan HJ, Ganz W, Forrester J, et al: Catheterization of the

heart in man with use of a flow-directed balloon-tipped catheter. N Engl J Med 1970; 283:447.

95. Shoemaker WC, Kram HB, Appel PL, et al: The efficacy of central venous and pulmonary artery catheters and therapy based upon them in reducing mortality and morbidity. Arch Surg 1990; 125:1332.

96. Cotton DB, Gonik B, Dorman K, et al: Cardiovascular alterations in severe pregnancy-induced hypertension: Relationship of central venous pressure to pulmonary capillary wedge pressure. Am J Obstet Gynecol 1985; 151:762.

97. Packman MI, Rackow EC: Optimum left heart filling pressure during fluid resuscitation of patients with hypovolemic and septic shock. Crit Care Med 1983; 11:165.

98. Rackow EC, Kaufman BS, Falk JL, et al: Hemodynamic response to fluid repletion in patients with septic shock: Evidence for early depression of cardiac performance. Circ Shock 1987; 22:11.

99. Rao PS, Cavanagh D: Endotoxic shock in the primate: Some effects of dopamine administration. Am J Obstet Gynecol 1982; 144:61.

100. Goldberg LI: Dopamine: Clinical uses of an endogenous catecholamine. N Engl J Med 1974; 291:707.

101. Bollaert PE, Bauer P, Audibert G, et al: Effects of epinephrine on hemodynamics and oxygen metabolism in dopamine-resistant septic shock. Chest 1990; 98:949.

102. Desjars P, Pinaud M, Poptel G, et al: A reappraisal of norepinephrine therapy in human septic shock. Crit Care Med 1987; 15:134.

103. Meadows D, Edwards JD, Wilkins RG, et al: Reversal of intractable septic shock with norepinephrine therapy. Crit Care Med 1988; 16:663.

104. MacKenzie SJ, Kapadia F, Nimmo GR, et al: Adrenaline in treatment of septic shock: Effects on hemodynamics and oxygen transport. Intensive Care Med 1991; 17:36.

105. Moran JL, O'Fathartaign MS, Peisach AR, et al: Epinephrine as an inotropic agent in septic shock: A dose-profile analysis. Crit Care Med 1993; 21:70.

106. Martin C, Papazian L, Perrin G, et al: Norepinephrine or dopamine for the treatment of hyperdynamic septic shock? Chest 1993; 103:1826.

107. Lucas CE: A new look at dopamine and norepinephrine for hyperdynamic septic shock. Chest 1994; 105:7.

108. Marik PE, Mohedin M: The contrasting effects of dopamine and norepinephrine on systemic and splanchnic oxygen utilization in hyperdynamic sepsis. JAMA 1994; 272:1354.

109. Shoemaker WC, Appel PL, Kram HB: Oxygen transport measurements to evaluate tissue perfusion and titrate therapy: Dobutamine and dopamine effects. Crit Care Med 1991; 19:672.

110. Shoemaker WC, Appel PL, Kram HB, et al: Prospective trial of supranormal values of survivors as therapeutic goals in high-risk surgical patients. Chest 1988; 94:1176.

111. Tuchschmidt J, Fried J, Astiz M, et al: Elevation of cardiac output and oxygen delivery improves outcome in septic shock. Chest 1992; 102:216.

112. Boyd O, Grounds RM, Bennett ED: A randomized clinical trial of the effect of deliberate perioperative increase of oxygen delivery on mortality in high-risk surgical patients. JAMA 1993; 270:2699.

113. Bishop MH, Shoemaker WC, Appel PL, et al: Prospective, randomized trial of survivor values of cardiac index, oxygen delivery, and oxygen consumption as resuscitation endpoints in severe trauma. J Trauma 1995; 38:780.

114. Yu M, Levy MM, Smith P, et al: Effect of maximizing oxygen delivery on morbidity and mortality rates in critically ill patients: A prospective, randomized, controlled study. Crit Care Med 1993; 21:830.

115. Shoemaker WC, Appel PL, Kram HB: Role of oxygen debt in the development of organ failure sepsis, and death in high-risk surgical patients. Chest 1992; 102:208.

116. Hayes MA, Timmins AC, Yau EHS, et al: Elevation of systemic oxygen delivery in the treatment of critically ill patients. N Engl J Med 1994; 330:1717.

117. Gattinoni L, Brazzi L, Pelosi P, et al: A trial of goal-oriented hemodynamic therapy in critically ill patients. N Engl J Med 1995; 333:1025.

118. Hinds C, Watson D: Manipulating hemodynamic and oxygen transport in critically ill patients. N Engl J Med 1995; 333:1074.

119. Tuchschmidt J, Oblitas D, Fried JC: Oxygen consumption in sepsis and septic shock. Crit Care Med 1991; 19:664.

120. Duff JH, Groves AC, McLean APH, et al: Defective oxygen consumption in septic shock. Surg Gynecol Obstet 1969; 127:1051.

121. Fiddian-Green RG, Haglund U, Gutierrez G, et al: Goals for the resuscitation of shock. Crit Care Med 1993; 21:S25.

122. Shoemaker WC, Appel PL, Bland R, et al: Clinical trial of an algorithm for outcome prediction in acute circulatory failure. Crit Care Med 1983; 11:165.

123. Duff P, Gibbs RS, Blanco JD, et al: Endometrial culture techniques in puerperal patients. Obstet Gynecol 1983; 61:217.

124. Gibbs RS, Blanco JD, Hrilica VS: Quantitative bacteriology of amniotic fluid. J Infect Dis 1982; 145:1.

125. Fagon JY, Chastre J, Vuagnat A, et al: Nosocomial pneumonia and mortality among patients in intensive care units. JAMA 1996; 275:866.

126. Collins CG: Suppurative pelvic thrombophlebitis. Am J Obstet Gynecol 1970; 108:681.

127. Malangoni MA, Shumate CR, Thomas HA, Richardson JD: Factors influencing the treatment of intra-abdominal abscesses. Am J Surg 1990; 159:167.

128. Landers DV, Sweet FL: Tubo-ovarian abscess: Contemporary approach to management. Rev Infect Dis 1983; 5:876.

129. Wojnar MM, Hawkins WG, Lang CH: Nutritional support of the septic patient. Crit Care Clin 1995; 11:717.

130. Mainous MR, Deitch EA: Nutrition and infection. Surg Clin North Am 1994; 74:659.

131. Deitch EA, Winterton J, Li M, et al: The gut as a portal of entry for bacteremia: Role of protein malnutrition. Ann Surg 1987;681–92.

132. Ziegler TR, Smith RJ, O'Dwyer ST, et al: Increased intestinal permeability associated with infection in burn patients. Arch Surg 1988; 123:1313.

133. Riddington DW, Venkatesh B, Boivin CM, et al: Intestinal permeability, gastric intramucosal pH, and systemic endotoxemia in patients undergoing cardiopulmonary bypass. JAMA 1996; 275:1007.

134. Sauve JS, Cook DJ: Gastrointestinal hemorrhage and ischemia: Prevention and treatment. Int Anesthesiol Clin 1993; 31:169.

135. Cannon LA, Heiselman D, Gardner W, et al: Prophylaxis of upper gastrointestinal tract bleeding in mechanically ventilated patients. Arch Intern Med 1987; 147:2101.

136. Driks MR, Craven DE, Celli BR, et al: Nosocomial pneumonia in intubated patients given sucralfate as compared with antacids or histamine type 2 blockers. N Engl J Med 1987; 317:1376.

137. Bresalier RS, Grendell JH, Cello JP, et al: Sucralfate suspension versus titrated antacid for the prevention of acute stress-related gastrointestinal hemorrhage in critically ill patients. Am J Med 1987; 83:110.

138. Tryba M: Risk of acute stress bleeding and nosocomial pneumonia in ventilated intensive care unit patients: Sucralfate versus antacids. Am J Med 1987; 83:117.

139. Bone RC, Fisher CJ Jr, Clemmer TP, et al: A controlled clinical trial of high-dose methylprednisolone in the treatment of severe sepsis and septic shock. N Engl J Med 1987; 317:653.

140. The Veterans Administration Systemic Sepsis Cooperative Study Group: Effect of high-dose glucocorticoid therapy on mortality in patients with clinical signs of systemic sepsis. N Engl J Med 1987; 317:659.

141. Hooper RG, Kearl RA: Established ARDS treated with a sustained course of adrenocortical steroids. Chest 1990; 97:138.

142. Weigelt JA, Norcross JF, Borman KR, et al: Early steroid therapy for respiratory failure. Arch Surg 1985; 120:536.

143. Meduri GU, Belenchia JM, Estes RJ, et al: Fibroproliferative phase of ARDS: Clinical findings and effects of corticosteroids. Chest 1991; 100:943.

144. Ashbaugh DG, Maier RV: Idiopathic pulmonary fibrosis in adult respiratory distress syndrome: Diagnosis and treatment. Arch Surg 1985; 120:530.

145. Lachman E, Pitsoe SB, Gaffin SL: Antilipopolysaccharide immunotherapy in management of septic shock of obstetric and gynaecologic origin. Lancet 1984; 1:981.

146. Natanson C, Hoffman WD, Suffredini AF, et al: Selected treatment strategies for shock based on proposed mechanisms of pathogenesis. Ann Intern Med 1994; 120:771.

147. Greenman RL, Schein RMH, Martin MA, et al: A controlled clinical trial of E5 murine monoclonal IgM antibody to endotoxin in the treatment of gram-negative sepsis. JAMA 1991; 266:1097.

148. Ziegler EJ, Fisher CJ Jr, Sprung CL, et al: Treatment of gram-negative bacteremia and septic shock with HA-1A human monoclonal antibody against endotoxin. N Engl J Med 1991; 324:429.

149. Warren HS, Danner RL, Munford RS: Anti-endotoxin monoclonal antibodies. N Engl J Med 1992; 326:1153.

150. Wenzel RP: Monoclonal antibodies and the treatment of gram-negative bacteremia and shock. N Engl J Med 1991; 324:486.

151. Goldie AS, Fearon KCH, Ross JA, et al: Natural cytokine antagonists and endogenous antiendotoxin core antibodies in sepsis syndrome. JAMA 1995; 274:172.

152. Holaday JW, Faden AI: Naloxone reversal of endotoxin hypotension suggests role of endorphins in shock. Nature 1978; 275:450.

153. Genazzani AR, Facchinetti F, Parrini D: β-lipotropin and β-endorphin plasma levels during pregnancy. Clin Endocrinol 1981; 14:409.

29 Necrotizing Fasciitis

DAVID E. SOPER

Necrotizing fasciitis is an uncommon but life-threatening infection primarily involving the superficial fascia of the extremities, abdominal wall, or vulva. The cutaneous manifestations of this disorder were originally described by a Confederate Army surgeon, Joseph Jones, in 1871, while he was caring for soldiers with wounds in their extremities.[1] Meleney[2] subsequently reported twenty cases of streptococcal gangrene that we now recognize as being cases of streptococcal necrotizing fasciitis. The sine qua non for the diagnosis of this disease is extensive necrosis of superficial fascia and fat, with widespread undermining of the skin. The obstetrician and gynecologist encounter this disease most commonly in the perineum or the anterior abdominal wall. Early diagnosis, allowing aggressive surgical débridement combined with broad-spectrum antibiotic therapy, offers the patient the best chance of survival.

NOMENCLATURE

A rather confusing nomenclature has evolved over the years with respect to categorizing necrotizing fasciitis and related entities. In reporting on the importance of roentgenographic studies for the demonstration of soft tissue gas in diagnosing necrotizing fasciitis, Fisher and colleagues[3] established six criteria for identifying the disease: (1) extensive necrosis of the superficial fascia with widespread undermining of the surrounding tissue; (2) a moderate to severe systemic toxic reaction including altered mental status; (3) absence of muscle involvement (vs. the prominent myonecrosis seen in certain clostridial infections and in synergistic necrotizing cellulitis); (4) failure to demonstrate clostridia in wound and blood cultures; (5) absence of major vascular occlusion; and (6) débrided tissue showing intense leukocytic infiltration, focal necrosis of fascia and surrounding tissues, and microvascular thrombosis on pathologic examination.

Synergistic necrotizing cellulitis (or gangrene) is identical to necrotizing fasciitis except that there is prominent involvement of the muscle and skin as well as the subcutaneous tissue and fascia. Clostridial cellulitis is the same disease as necrotizing fasciitis except that its microbiology involves clostridia as the primary pathogen. Anaerobic cellulitis is an anaerobic infection of the subcutaneous tissues that has not progressed to necrosis; it is similar to what Shy and Eschenbach[4] have called superficial fascial infection. Myonecrosis, or gas gangrene, is associated with significant necrosis of the pelvic or rectus musculature and is most commonly due to clostridial infection. Practically speaking, anaerobic cellulitis is the only entity that can be treated initially with antibiotic therapy alone. Once necrosis has occurred, surgical excision of necrotic (dead) tissue is crucial for clinical improvement to occur.

PATHOPHYSIOLOGY

Although there are reports of patients with necrotizing fasciitis in the absence of underlying disease, the disease most commonly affects those with diabetes or atherosclerosis.[5–7] Indeed, over 70% of cases reported in the gynecologic literature have been diabetic women. Patients with underlying chronic diseases that require long-term treatment with steroids or nonsteroidal anti-inflammatory agents[8–10] (i.e., autoimmune diseases) are also at risk. The exception to this rule involves the postpartum patient. The puerperium should be considered another risk factor for the development of this disease. Necrotizing fasciitis after cesarean delivery is not associated with the aforementioned purported risk factors.[11] Less commonly, postpartum patients acquire necrotizing fasciitis of an episiotomy. None of the seven patients reported in the literature with necrotizing fasciitis associated with episiotomy infections was diabetic. Initially, simple infection occurs when bacteria enter the subcutaneous tissue through a surgical wound, by way of a trivial injury such as an abrasion or after what appears to be an insignificant infection (e.g., furuncle).[9] Rarely, necrotizing fasciitis may follow the development of a Bartholin duct abscess.[12] The patient may complain of pain, and the affected area is initially erythematous, swollen, without sharp margins, hot, and extremely tender. The course of this infection may be fulminant, with rapid extension into surrounding tissues. Conversely, it may remain quiescent for weeks only to be followed by an explosive spread along tissue planes. Rarely, the infection may progress slowly over a period of several weeks. Lymphangitis and lymphadenitis are infrequent. The process progresses with sequential changes in skin color from red-purple to patches of blue-gray. In most cases, skin breakdown with bullae (containing thick pink or purple fluid) and frank cutaneous gangrene (resembling a thermal burn) occurs within 3 to 5 days. By the time these symptoms occur, the involved area is no longer tender but has become anesthetic because of thrombosis in small blood vessels and destruction of superficial nerves located in the necrotic, undermined subcutaneous tissues.[13] The development of anesthesia may precede the appearance of skin necrosis and may provide a clue to the presence of necrotizing fasciitis rather than simple cellulitis.[9]

Despite variations in the rate of development of necrotizing fasciitis, most patients are acutely ill when they see a physician. Systemic signs of sepsis are present; a temperature in excess of 102°F is not uncommon. Significant leukocytosis with a significant left shift (>20% bands) is the rule; however, in severe cases neutropenia can occur. A severe deficiency in intravascular fluid volume may occur as a result of significant third spacing of fluid in the infected compartment. Anemia may also be present as a result of the action of bacterial hemolysins. In addition, blood may be lost in extensive subcutaneous venous thromboses and cutaneous ecchymoses. Disseminated intravascular coagulation may also occur. Ionic calcium deficits occur as the result of calcium sequestration in the areas of fat necrosis; as a result of the fat being degraded by bacterial lipases, calcium combines with fatty acids to form insoluble soap.[9]

The microbiology of necrotizing fasciitis may be divided into two distinct microbial groups.[14] The first includes a polymicrobial flora involving both anaerobic and facultative aerobic bacteria (Table 29–1). These organisms are responsible for most of the cases of necrotizing fasciitis seen in obstetric and gynecologic patients. The second floral group consists of *Streptococcus pyogenes* (group A streptococcus), with or without *Staphylococcus aureus*.[15] Clinically, the microbiologic groups responsible for necrotizing fasciitis are indistinguishable. However, certain clinical findings correlated with some bacteria: edema with the *Bacteroides fragilis* group, *Clostridium* spp., *S. aureus*, *Prevotella spp.*, and group A streptococci; gas and crepitation in tissues with members of the family Enterobacteriaceae and *Clostridium* spp.; and foul odor with *Bacteroides* spp.[16] Virulence factors elaborated by both groups of organisms enhance the spread of infection along fascial planes. The prototype organism for this disease is *S. pyogenes*.

The group A streptococcus produces more than 20 extracellular products. The most important of these is hyaluronidase, an enzyme that splits hyaluronic acid,

TABLE 29–1 ▶ MICROORGANISMS CULTURED FROM OBSTETRIC-GYNECOLOGIC PATIENTS WITH NECROTIZING FASCIITIS*

Microorganisms	No. of Isolates
Aerobic	
Streptococcus sp.	22
Group A (3)†	
Group B (2)	
Enterococci (8)	
Staphylococcus sp.	12
S. aureus (5)	
Diphtheroids	3
Escherichia coli	13
Proteus sp.	7
Klebsiella sp.	5
Pseudomonas aeruginosa	1
Citrobacter sp.	2
Enterobacter cloacae	3
Anaerobic	
Peptococcus	8
Peptostreptococcus	4
Bacteroides sp.	11
Bifidobacterium sp.	1
Fusobacterium symbiosum	1
Gaffkya anaerobium	1
Propionibacterium avidum	1

* N = 41.
† Number of specific microorganisms in parentheses.

an important component of connective tissue. This enzyme is also known as *spreading factor*.[17] In addition, the aerobic and anaerobic flora, which are found in the genital tract and are responsible for the polymicrobial type of necrotizing fasciitis, can manufacture proteases that break down collagen and elastin and therefore allow spread of the infection along tissue planes.[18]

Although myonecrosis may occur in association with a severe necrotizing fasciitis (progressive synergistic necrotizing cellulitis) caused by a polymicrobial flora, it is not commonly associated with clostridial infection. *Clostridium perfringens* is the most common and most easily cultured and recognized of the clostridia causing such infection. This organism produces more than 17 virulence factors, including phospholipases, hyaluronidase, hemolysins, and toxins that increase capillary permeability.[19] Despite a high frequency of clostridial contamination of major traumatic, open wounds, the incidence of gas gangrene is only 1% to 2%. This underscores the important role of devitalized tissue, as well as the presence of a foreign body, in the pathogenesis of clostridial myonecrosis. *Clostridium perfringens* is present in large numbers in the normal flora of human feces, but is uncommon in the female genital tract.

Clostridium sordellii is the microorganism most commonly identified with serious episiotomy infections. Infection caused by this bacterium is associated with massive, malignant edema, probably due to the elaboration of a lethal edema-producing toxin.[20] There are several case reports of maternal deaths associated with vulvar edema.[21, 22] These cases more than likely represent cases of necrotizing fasciitis.[23] Patients with vulvar edema due to *C. sordellii* die from cardiovascular collapse after marked third spacing of fluids.[24]

ANATOMIC SITE

Vulva

Obstetrician-gynecologists most frequently encounter necrotizing fasciitis involving the vulva. This is probably due to several causes. Because this is an area in which it is difficult for women to examine themselves, they may not recognize the early symptoms of infection and therefore do not seek medical help. Also, physicians may overlook early signs of cellulitis involving the vulva. If cellulitis is diagnosed, the severity of the disease may not be recognized and patients may be treated with antibiotics alone, without surgical intervention. Episiotomy pain is common and highly variable; the beginning of infection may be overlooked until systemic signs of infection, such as fever, occur. The vulvar area is bathed with microorganisms normally found in the vagina, and is also close to the anal region. It is amazing that more women do not have significant infection from episiotomies. Moreover, it is not difficult to imagine how a small abrasion or surgical wound may become infected with the polymicrobial flora present in the area of the vulva. If the right mix of virulent organisms is present, especially in a susceptible host (e.g., a patient with diabetes), necrotizing fasciitis may occur.

The superficial fascia of the vulva is continuous with that of the anterior abdominal wall. The shallow layer (Camper's fascia) of the superficial fascia is loose, areolar tissue containing much adipose tissue in its meshes. This comprises most of the labia majora and is contiguous with the subcutaneous fat of the anterior abdominal wall and with the same fascia on the inner side of the thighs. The deeper layer of superficial fascia of the vulva (Colles' fascia) is a thin, aponeurotic structure contiguous with Scarpa's fascia in the abdominal wall.[25] This deep layer of superficial fascia usually acts as a plane on which the spreading infection advances from the vulva to the abdominal wall, or vice versa, and to the inner thighs. The fascia overlying the pelvic musculature is usually spared in this infectious process. However, deep fascial infection, even with involvement of the underlying muscles, may occur in severe cases.

Abdominal Wall

Necrotizing fasciitis has been reported as a complication of abdominal incision after cesarean section,[11, 26] hysterectomy,[27] suprapubic catheter insertion,[28] and diag-

nostic laparoscopy.[29] The spread of infection in all of these instances followed the planes of the superficial fascia in the anterior abdominal wall, but in three cases it also involved the deep fascia. In addition, necrotizing fasciitis after cesarean section may be associated with significant necrosis of the uterus requiring either hysterectomy or at least resection of a necrotic uterine incision.[24] The incidence of necrotizing fasciitis after cesarean delivery in one series of nine patients diagnosed in an 8-year period was 1.8 per 1,000.[11] Two (22.2%) of these nine patients died from their disease.

Subgluteal and Retropsoal Spaces

Rarely, infection may occur in the subgluteal and retropsoal spaces. This is invariably associated with the administration of paracervical or transvaginal pudendal anesthesia. The hallmark of this infection is severe hip pain associated with limitation of motion. In addition, when a retropsoas abscess is present, there is unmistakable psoal spasm, causing the patient to hold her ipsilateral thigh flexed.[30, 31] Pain can be elicited when the thigh is fully extended as the patient lies on her contralateral side. Bacteria are apparently introduced into the paracervical and paravaginal tissues at the time of anesthetic administration. The subsequent infection spreads along the paths of least resistance posteriorly toward the hollow of the sacrum. Cellulitis surrounding the hip capsule or formation of a subgluteal abscess may occur.

DIAGNOSIS

The clinical diagnosis of necrotizing fasciitis is based on a constellation of symptoms and signs in association with a high index of suspicion (Table 29–2). Unfortunately, most of these telltale signs are indicative of

TABLE 29–2 ▶	CLINICAL DIAGNOSIS OF NECROTIZING FASCIITIS

Predisposing factors
  Diabetes
  Atherosclerosis
  Steroid therapy
  Postpartum
Symptoms
  Superficial skin lesion
  Swelling of the affected area
  Pain followed by anesthesia
  Fever
Signs
  Skin changes (bullae and dark discoloration)
  Subcutaneous gas
  Temperature = 102°–105°F
Laboratory abnormalities
  Anemia
  Leukocytosis
  Hypocalcemia
  Radiography showing soft tissue gas

advanced disease. The diagnosis should be considered in those patients with progressive edema and erythema involving any abdominal incision, vulvar abrasion or furuncle, or episiotomy site. The hallmark of necrotizing fasciitis affecting the vulva is a woody induration extending into the inner thighs. Fisher and co-workers'[3] diagnostic criteria for the condition can be used only retrospectively, after surgery has been performed and the histologic type and microbiology involved are known. Roentgenograms, exposed for maximum soft tissue visualization, commonly show gas in the affected tissues.[3] Obstacles to the diagnosis of necrotizing fasciitis include negative findings (no pus or bacteria by Gram's stain) after fine-needle aspiration of the affected area, nondiagnostic radiographs, and admission to a nonsurgical service.[32] In those patients not exhibiting clear-cut signs of necrotizing fasciitis, an incisional biopsy performed under local anesthesia at the bedside may be helpful. The volume of the tissue sample should be at least 1 mL. Frozen-section analysis of this biopsy should be able to differentiate between necrotizing fasciitis and nonspecific ulcers, abscesses, or ischemic necrosis. The patient should be transferred to the operating room immediately for surgical débridement if microscopy demonstrates necrosis of the superficial fascia, infiltration of the deep dermis and fascia by polymorphonuclear leukocytes, fibrinoid thrombi and angiitis of the arteries and veins passing through the fascia, and the presence of microorganisms in the destroyed fascia and dermis.[33, 34] If severe systemic manifestations are present or resolution of the infection does not occur after 24 to 48 hours of treatment with broad-spectrum parenteral antibiotics, the patient should be taken to the operating room.[4] This should occur despite negative findings as noted previously.

Both ultrasound and computed tomography have been used in the evaluation of patients with necrotizing fasciitis. The ultrasonographic findings of necrotizing fasciitis include (1) irregularity of the fascia, (2) abnormal fluid collections along the fascia plane, and (3) diffuse thickening of the fascia compared with the control site.[35] Computed tomography demonstrates subcutaneous and fascial edema early and delineates its degree and extent, which are often underestimated clinically.[36]

The single most impressive finding at surgery for necrotizing fasciitis is a bloodless operative site until normal tissue is reached. Obvious abscess formation is not present. Necrotic superficial fascia appears dull and gray compared with the bright yellow, bloody appearance of normal subcutaneous tissue. A "dishwater" exudate is present. The subcutaneous tissue is easily separated from the underlying deep fascia as well as from the overlying skin.

Clinically, it is difficult to differentiate between necrotizing fasciitis and myonecrosis. A definitive diagnosis depends on findings in the operating room. Although the involved muscles may initially exhibit only pallor, edema, and loss of elasticity, they undergo rapid disintegration. They fail to contract on stimulation and do not bleed from a cut surface. Later they become discolored and friable. Histologically, the muscle fibers show coagulation necrosis and the supporting connective tissue is destroyed; numerous gram-positive bacilli may be present.[37]

MANAGEMENT

Surgical débridement is the mainstay of therapy for the patient with necrotizing fasciitis. In fact, a delay in surgical intervention, usually due to a delay in diagnosis, increases the mortality rate (from 4% to 38%) associated with this disease.[38] Once the diagnosis is made, the patient should be prepared for surgery. Correction of fluid imbalance, anemia, electrolyte abnormalities, and hypocalcemia should be rapidly accomplished. Broad-spectrum antibiotic therapy to cover both anaerobic and aerobic bacteria should be started.

Because these patients are critically ill, it is important to maintain a broad spectrum of antimicrobial coverage of their infections until culture results are available. This coverage should include activity against the organisms most commonly isolated in necrotizing fasciitis (e.g., streptococci, enterococci, gram-negative aerobic organisms, and beta-lactamase–producing anaerobes) as well as uncommon but particularly virulent organisms (e.g., *C. perfringens* and *C. sordellii*). This can be accomplished by using combination antibiotic therapy (Table 29–3). A single agent that affords broad enough coverage for this polymicrobial disease process is imipenem/cilastatin. Other broad-spectrum single

TABLE 29–3 ▶ ANTIBIOTICS USEFUL IN THE TREATMENT OF NECROTIZING FASCIITIS		
Antibiotic		**Dosage**
Combination therapy		
Clindamycin		900 mg q8h
	OR	
Metronidazole		1,000 mg q6h
	PLUS	
Ampicillin		1,000 mg q6h
	OR	
Penicillin G		2.5 million units q6h
	PLUS	
Gentamicin		1 mg/kg q8h
	OR	
Other aminoglycosides dosed by weight		
	OR	
Aztreonam		2,000 mg q8h
Single-agent therapy		
Imipenem/cilastatin		500 mg q6h
	OR	
Other carbapenems		

TABLE 29-4 ▶ **ANTIMICROBIAL SUSCEPTIBILITIES OF SELECTED MICROORGANISMS ASSOCIATED WITH NECROTIZING FASCIITIS AND MYONECROSIS**

| Organism | Strains Susceptible to Various Antibiotics (%) | | | | | | |
	Penicillin	Ampicillin	Gentamicin	Other Aminoglycosides	Clindamycin	Metronidazole	Imipenem/ Cilastatin
Streptococcus sp.	100	100	86	64	100	NT	100
Enterococcus sp.	26	96	NT	NT	NT	NT	100
Escherichia coli	NT	55	95	100	NT	NT	99
Klebsiella sp.	NT	2	99	100	NT	NT	81
Peptostreptococcus	100	NT	NT	NT	100	76	100
Prevotella bivia	58	NT	NT	NT	96	99	100
Clostridium perfringens	100	NT	NT	NT	98	100	100

NT = not tested.

agents have important deficits in their coverage (e.g., enterococci are resistant to cephalosporins, and some gram-negative aerobes remain resistant to antibiotics combined with beta-lactamase inhibitors). Table 29–4 shows the antimicrobial susceptibilities of selected isolates associated with necrotizing fasciitis and myonecrosis.[39]

Surgical débridement should consist of incision over the areas involved. In so doing, the surgeon should keep in mind which incision or incisions will allow the best exposure of the involved area, as well as allow for thorough wound inspection and dressing changes once the patient is stabilized and on the postoperative ward. Tunneling incisions should not be attempted to salvage overlying skin because they are difficult to pack and inspect. All necrotic subcutaneous tissue should be removed. The deep fascia should be inspected, and if it is involved, resected. All nonviable muscle should be excised, as well as all necrotic skin. In general, normal tissue is easily identified. Tissue should be resected to bleeding edges; however, if the extent of fascial necrosis is in question, a frozen-section biopsy may aid in establishing appropriate surgical margins. Specimens of the resected tissue should be submitted for Gram staining and aerobic and anaerobic cultures.

Once adequate débridement has been accomplished, the wound should be packed with povidone-iodine-impregnated gauze and the patient should be transferred to the intensive care unit. For more severe cases, reoperation should be routinely scheduled in 24 hours to permit reassessment of the extent of necrosis and to simplify changing the dressing on the wound. After it has been established that the progressive nature of the disease in under control, the dressing may be changed in the intensive care unit or on the ward, depending on the patient's status.

Antibiotics should be continued until wound induration and systemic signs of sepsis have resolved. The wound should appear beefy red, with granulation tissue. Continued dressing changes allow many wounds to heal by secondary intention. However, in some cases, secondary closure or skin grafting is necessary.

Consultation with a plastic surgeon may be appropriate to obtain the best cosmetic result in patients with extensive vulvar or abdominal incisions.

REFERENCES

1. Jones J: Investigation upon the nature, causes and treatment of hospital gangrene as it prevailed in the Confederate armies 1861–1865. New York: U.S. Sanitary Commission, Surgical Memoirs of the War of Rebellion, 1871.
2. Meleney FL: A differential diagnosis between certain types of infectious gangrene of the skin. Surg Gynecol Obstet 1933; 56:847.
3. Fisher JR, Conway MJ, Takeshita RT, Sandoval MR: Necrotizing fasciitis: Importance of roentgenographic studies for soft-tissue gas. JAMA 1979; 241:803.
4. Shy KK, Eschenbach DA: Fatal perineal cellulitis from an episiotomy site. Obstet Gynecol 1979; 54:292.
5. Rea WJ, Wyrick WJ: Necrotizing fasciitis. Ann Surg 1970; 172:957.
6. Addison WA, Livengood CH, Gill GB, et al: Necrotizing fasciitis of vulvar origin in diabetic patients. Obstet Gynecol 1984; 63:473.
7. Roberts DB: Necrotizing fasciitis of the vulva. Am J Obstet Gynecol 1987; 157:568.
8. Rimailho A, Riou B, Richard C, Auzepy P: Fulminant necrotizing fasciitis and nonsteroidal anti-inflammatory drugs. J Infect Dis 1987; 155:143.
9. Wilson B: Necrotizing fasciitis. Am Surg 1952; 18:416.
10. Kahn LH, Styrt BA: Necrotizing soft tissue infections reported with nonsteroidal antiinflammatory drugs. Ann Pharmacother 1997; 31:1034.
11. Goepfert AR, Guinn DA, Andrews WW, Hauth JC: Necrotizing fasciitis after cesarean delivery. Obstet Gynecol 1997; 89:409.
12. Roberts DB, Hester LL: Progressive synergistic bacterial gangrene arising from abscesses of the vulva and Bartholin's gland duct. Am J Obstet Gynecol 1972; 114:285.
13. Swartz MN: Subcutaneous tissue infection and abscesses. In: Mandell GL, Douglas RG Jr, Bennett JE (eds): Principles and Practice of Infectious Diseases, 2nd ed. New York, John Wiley & Sons, 1985, pp 609–613.
14. Giuliano A, Lewis F, Hadley K, Blaisdell FW: Bacteriology of necrotizing fasciitis. Am J Surg 1977; 134:52.
15. McHenry CR, Azar T, Ramahi AJ, Collins PL: Monomicrobial necrotizing fasciitis complicating pregnancy and the puerperium. Obstet Gynecol 1996; 87:823.
16. Brook I, Frazier EH: Clinical and microbiological features of necrotizing fasciitis. J Clin Microbiol 1995; 33:2382.
17. The streptococci. In: Jawetz E, Melnick JL, Adelberg EA (eds): Review of Medical Microbiology, 17th ed. Norwalk, CT, Appleton & Lange, 1987, pp 224–225.
18. McGregor JA, Lawellin D, Franco-Buff A, et al: Protease production by microorganisms associated with reproductive tract infection. Am J Obstet Gynecol 1986; 154:109.

19. Smith LDS: Virulence factors of *Clostridium perfringens.* Rev Infect Dis 1979; 1:254.
20. Arseculeratne SN, Panabokke RG, Wizesundera S: The toxins responsible for the lesions of Clostridium sordellii gas gangrene. J Med Microbiol 1969; 2:37.
21. Ewing TL, Smale LE, Elliott FA: Maternal deaths associated with postpartum vulvar edema. Am J Obstet Gynecol 1979; 134:173.
22. Finkler NJ, Salon LE, Ryan KJ: Bilateral postpartum vulvar edema associated with maternal death. Am J Obstet Gynecol 1987; 156:1188.
23. Sutton G: Necrotizing fasciitis. [Letter.] Am J Obstet Gynecol 1988; 159:267.
24. Soper DE: Clostridial myonecrosis arising from an episiotomy. Obstet Gynecol 1986; 68:26S.
25. Gray H: Anatomy, Descriptive and Surgical, 6th ed. New York, Crown, 1977, p 370.
26. Golde S, Ledger WJ: Necrotizing fasciitis in postpartum patients: A report of four cases. Obstet Gynecol 1977; 50:670.
27. Loscar M, Schelling G, Haller M, et al: Group A streptococcal toxic shock syndrome with severe necrotizing fasciitis following hysterectomy: A case report. Intensive Care Med 1998; 24:190.
28. Bearman DM, Livengood CH, Addison WA: Necrotizing fasciitis arising from a suprapubic catheter site: A case report. J Reprod Med 1988; 33:411.
29. Storel G, Hirsch E, Edelin KC: Necrotizing fasciitis following diagnostic laparoscopy. Obstet Gynecol 1983; 62:67S.
30. Hibbard LT, Snyder EN, McVann RM: Subgluteal and retropsoas infection in obstetric practice. Obstet Gynecol 1972; 39:137.
31. Svancarek W, Chirino O, Schaefer G, Blythe JG: Retropsoas and subgluteal abscesses following paracervical and pudendal anesthesia. JAMA 1977; 237:892.
32. Lille ST, Sato TT, Engrav LH, et al: Necrotizing soft tissue infections: Obstacles in diagnosis. J Am Coll Surg 1996; 182:7.
33. Stamenkovic I, Lew PD: Early recognition of potentially fatal necrotizing fasciitis. N Engl J Med 1984; 310:1689.
34. Majeski J, Majeski E: Necrotizing fasciitis: Improved survival with early recognition by tissue biopsy and aggressive surgical treatment. South Med J 1997; 90:1065.
35. Tsai CC, Lai CS, Yu ML, et al: Early diagnosis of necrotizing fasciitis by utilization of ultrasonography. Kao Hsiung I Hsueh Ko Hsueh Tsa Chih 1996; 12:235.
36. Walshaw CF, Deans H: CT findings in necrotizing fasciitis: A report of four cases. Clin Radiol 1996; 51:429.
37. Swartz MN: Myositis. In: Mandell GL, Douglas RG Jr, Bennett JE (eds): Principles and Practice of Infectious Diseases, 2nd ed. New York, John Wiley & Sons, 1985, pp 613–616.
38. Bilton BD, Zibari GB, McMillan RW, et al: Aggressive surgical management of necrotizing fasciitis serves to decrease mortality: A retrospective study. Am Surg 1998; 64:397.
39. Musial CE, Rosenblatt JE: Antimicrobial susceptibilities of anaerobic bacteria isolated at Mayo Clinic during 1982 through 1987: Comparison with results from 1977 through 1981. Mayo Clin Proc 1989; 64:392.

Other Infections

30 Respiratory Infections

Maurizio L. Maccato ▶ Sebastian Faro

UPPER RESPIRATORY INFECTIONS

This section deals with infections of the upper respiratory tract that are common to the adult—the common cold, pharyngitis, and sinusitis. These infections are quite common, often not serious, but do account for considerable economic loss because of absences from work, resulting in a decrease in productivity. Although these infections are frequently vital in origin, bacteria play a significant role and can cause serious morbidity.

Common Cold

The "common cold" is a misnomer. Although the term is used frequently by both the lay population and medical professionals, the clinical entity is caused by a group of five viruses (Table 30–1). It is typically mild in severity and self-limited, and causes significant inflammation of the upper respiratory mucosa. The common cold was reported, in 1976, as a major reason for school and work absenteeism in the United States.[1] It most likely continues to be a major cause for absenteeism in the United States today.

The first cold virus to be isolated was the parainfluenza virus in 1955.[2] In 1956, rhinoviruses were isolated from adults with syndromes resembling the common cold.[3] In 1958, coxsackievirus A21 was isolated from military recruits.[4] The coronaviruses were the last group of viruses to be isolated from people with symptoms of the common cold, in the 1960s.[5] Other viruses, such as the adenovirus and influenza virus, can also cause symptoms resembling the common cold. However, these viruses frequently cause lower respiratory infections that tend to be more severe.

Thus, the common cold is caused by a variety of viruses that cause a similar complex of clinical symptoms. Patients presenting with this complex of symptoms often cannot be distinguished from those with a virus that is likely to cause a lower respiratory infection until the symptom complex is more severe.

Etiology

Five major groups of viruses account for most common colds: the myxoviruses, paramyxoviruses, adenoviruses,

picornaviruses, and coronaviruses.[6–8] Viruses such as the enteroviruses (listed as "Other" in Table 30–1) commonly produce inflammation of the upper respiratory tract, coryza, as do viruses such as rubeola, rubella, and varicella. However, the latter viruses are also associated with an exanthem. Makela and colleagues[9] found that among 200 patients diagnosed with a cold, 138 were found to have a viral etiology. The most common virus isolated was the rhinovirus (105 patients). This was followed by the coronaviruses (17 patients), influenza A or B (12 patients), and single isolates of the parainfluenza virus, respiratory syncytial virus, adenovirus, and enterovirus.[9] Thus, the rhinovirus causes approximately 50% of cases of the common cold. Seven patients were found to have a bacterial infection; *Chlamydia pneumoniae* antibodies were detected in four patients, antibodies to *Haemophilus influenzae* were found in one patient, one patient had antibodies against *Streptococcus pneumoniae*, and one had antibodies to *Mycoplasma pneumoniae*.[9]

Common colds are frequent illnesses, worldwide in distribution, because of the many varieties of viral agents that can cause a similar clinical illness. In addition, recurrent infection with the same virus type is

TABLE 30–1 ▶ VIRUSES ASSOCIATED WITH THE COMMON COLD

Virus	Antigenic Types	Percentage of Cases*
Rhinovirus	100 types and 1 subtype	30–35
Coronavirus	≥3 types	≥10
Parainfluenza	4 types	10–15
Respiratory syncytial	1 type	10–15
Influenza	3 types	10–15
Adenovirus	33 types	10–15
Other		5
Unknown		30–35
Group A beta-hemolytic streptococci†		5–10

* Estimated percentage of colds annually.
† Included because differentiation of streptococcal and viral pharyngitis is not possible by clinical means.
Adapted from Gwaltney JM Jr: The common cold. In: Mandell GL, Douglas RG Jr, Bennett JE (eds): Principles and Practice of Infectious Diseases, 3rd ed. New York, Churchill Livingstone, 1990, p 489.

333

not uncommon. Reinfection with the same viral type appears to be quite common; for example, approximately 80% of people infected with coronavirus OC43 have had a prior infection with this virus and have a neutralizing antibody to the virus.[10]

Upper respiratory infections can occur at any time during the year but tend to be seasonal. In the United States, the season begins in late August to mid-September, rises sharply as colder weather sets in, and peaks in the winter months. The incidence levels off as spring approaches and reaches low levels in the summer months. It appears that specific viruses have their own seasonal predilection. Rhinoviruses tend to have their highest attack rates in early fall and mid-spring, whereas coronaviruses favor the winter months.[10, 11]

The attack rate for upper respiratory tract infection during peak season is 6 to 8 colds per 1,000 people per day.[11] During the nadir season, the attack rate is 2 to 3 per 1,000 people per day.[11, 12] The average number of colds per adult is two to four per year.[11, 12] The main factors contributing to the acquisition of colds are crowded conditions and exposure to children. Children tend to acquire more colds in a year than adults, but adults living with children tend to have more frequent colds than those without constant exposure to children.[12, 13]

Children are the reservoir for respiratory viruses. Transmission most likely occurs in the home and in school. Transmission can occur through direct contact with secretions from a child with a cold, transportation of infected respiratory droplets through the air, and, possibly, contact with an object with which a child has had close contact. High titers of virus are present in nasal secretions and, typically, occur on the second to fourth day of a symptomatic cold.[14] It has been demonstrated that wiping nasal secretions with an unprotected hand can result in the virus being present on the skin. If such a person shakes hands with someone, the virus can be transmitted to the recipient's hand. Thus, if the uninfected person brings the virus-colonized hand in contact with nasal and conjunctival mucosa, infection can occur.[15]

Pathogenesis

Once the virus gains entrance to the epithelium of the upper respiratory tract, sloughing of this epithelium, which includes ciliated epithelial cells, begins. Virus is also found along with this epithelium; for example, shedding of rhinovirus lasts for 3 weeks, whereas shedding of coronaviruses lasts for approximately 1 to 4 days.[10, 16, 17] Asymptomatic carriage of viruses causing the common cold does not occur. However, people can have a subclinical infection and still shed virus.[18, 19]

Although infection causes sloughing of the nasal epithelium with progressive pyknotic changes in the nuclei and inclusion bodies in the cytoplasm, there do not appear to be destructive changes in the retained nasal epithelium. Biopsy specimens of nasal epithelium obtained from people with common colds have not demonstrated any significant cellular changes,[20, 21] and electron microscopic studies of nasal biopsy specimens obtained from people with common colds have not revealed any destructive changes.[22, 23] A polymorphonuclear leukocytic infiltrate is seen, but there is no increase in mast cells.[22] This histologic picture is in contrast to that seen in association with influenza.

The establishment of the common cold alters the local environment of the upper respiratory tree, leading to a change in the resident bacterial flora. This often results in the development of a secondary bacterial infection of areas that are normally sterile (e.g., sinuses, pharynx, middle ear, and tracheobronchial tree). In association with this potentially natural change in the microbial ecology of the upper respiratory system is the addition of antibiotics for the treatment of the common cold. This condition is the second most common reason that antibiotics are prescribed.[24, 25] A study by Kaiser and associates[26] demonstrated that 20% of patients evaluated for the common cold were found to be culture positive for *H. influenzae*, *Mortierella catarrhalis*, or *S. pneumoniae*.

Diagnosis and Management

The incubation period is 48 to 72 hours and the patient usually presents with nasal discharge, nasal obstruction, sneezing, sore or scratchy throat, and cough. Typically, the adult patient does not have a significant elevation in body temperature. The duration of the common cold is 1 to 2 weeks, with an average of 5 to 7 days.

The patient usually makes the diagnosis. Difficulty arises when the symptoms last more than a week, or other areas of the respiratory tree become involved (e.g., sinuses, middle ear, or throat). People whose symptoms extend beyond 1 week and have a significant elevation in temperature should be evaluated for a secondary bacterial infection. Those complaining of a sore throat with a fever should be examined for the presence of streptococcal infection ("strep throat"). However, simply examining the throat and identifying a marked erythema, lymphadenopathy, and even the presence of an exudate does not establish the diagnosis of a streptococcal infection. The differential diagnosis for this presentation should include streptococcal infection, adenovirus infection, Vincent's angina, and mononucleosis. A specimen should be obtained for culture and appropriate antibiotics should be administered. The presence of fever ($\geq$101°F), should alert the physician that the patient may have a condition warranting evaluation to determine whether (1) there is a bacterial infection present, (2) the condition is

---

TABLE 30–2 ▶ TREATMENT FOR THE COMMON COLD

I. Rhinorrhea and nasal congestion
  A. Oral decongestants
    1. Pseudoephedrine (Sudafed) 60 mg q4h
    2. Phenylpropanolamine 25 mg q4h
  B. Topical decongestants
    1. Oxymetazoline (Afrin, Dristan) 0.025% or 0.05%, two to three drops or sprays bid
    2. Phenylephrine (Neo-Synephrine) 0.125% or 0.5%, one to two drops or sprays q4h
II. Cough
  A. Antitussives
    1. Codeine, 10–20 mg q4h
    2. Dextromethorphan (Delsym) 10–30 mg q4h
    3. Benzonatate (Tessalon Perles) one to two capsules tid
  B. Expectorants
    1. Guaifenesin (Robitussin, Humibid LA) 100–400 mg q3–6h

---

limited to the upper respiratory tree, or (3) the lower respiratory tract is involved.

Treatment for the common cold is supportive and antibiotics should not be prescribed without examining and evaluating the patient. Treatment directed against specific complaints may be beneficial (Table 30–2).

Pharyngitis

Acute pharyngitis is a common condition heralded by the onset of a scratchy sensation at the back of the throat. It is an acute inflammatory process that can be precipitated by a variety of microorganisms. Viruses cause most cases of acute pharyngitis. However, it is important to distinguish between a viral etiology and streptococcal infection. The latter can lead to rheumatic fever and acute glomerulonephritis. Streptococcal pharyngitis also responds well to antibiotic therapy.

Pharyngitis tends to occur in colder months and coincides with the common cold and lower respiratory infection seasons. Rhinoviruses are most common in fall and spring, whereas coronaviruses tend to be seen more in the winter months, and influenza tends to occur in the winter and early spring. Streptococcal pharyngitis mainly occurs during the winter and early spring. The variety of microorganisms that can cause pharyngitis are listed in Table 30–3.

Pathogenesis

Biopsies obtained from people with rhinovirus pharyngitis have shown little cytopathic effect.[6, 27] Bradykinin and lysyl-bradykinin are released in the nasal passages

---

TABLE 30–3 ▶ MICROBIAL ETIOLOGIC AGENTS THAT CAN CAUSE PHARYNGITIS

Microbe	Infection	Approximate Percentage
Viral		
1. Rhinovirus (89 types and 1 subtype)	Common cold	20
2. Coronavirus (≥4 types)	Common cold	≥5
3. Adenovirus (types 3, 4, 7, 14, 21)	Pharyngoconjunctival fever, ARD	5
4. Herpes simplex (types 1 and 2)	Gingivitis, stomatitis, pharyngitis	4
5. Parainfluenza (types 1–4)	Common cold, croup	2
6. Influenza (types A and B)	Influenza	2
7. Coxsackie (types 2, 4–6, 8, 10)	Herpangina	<1
8. Epstein-Barr	Infectious mononucleosis	<1
9. Cytomegalovirus	Infectious mononucleosis	<1
10. HIV	Primary HIV infection	<1
Bacterial		
1. *Streptococcus pyogenes**	Pharyngitis, tonsillitis, scarlet fever, rheumatic fever, glomerulonephritis	15–30
2. Mixed anaerobic infection	Gingivitis, pharyngitis (Vincent's angina) peritonsillitis, peritonsillar abscess	<1
3. *Neisseria gonorrhoeae*	Pharyngitis	<1
4. *Corynebacterium diphtheriae*	Diphtheria	<1
5. *Corynebacterium ulcerans*	Pharyngitis, diphtheria	<1
6. *Corynebacterium hemolyticum* (*Arcanobacterium hemolyticum*)	Pharyngitis, scarlatiniform rash	<1
7. *Yersinia enterocolitica*	Pharyngitis, enterocolitis	<1
8. *Treponema pallidum*	Secondary syphilis	<1
9. *Chlamydia psittaci*	ARD, pneumonia	?
10. *Mycoplasma pneumoniae*	Pneumonia, bronchitis, pharyngitis	<1
11. *Mycoplasma hominis* (type 1)	Pharyngitis in volunteers	?
12. Unknown		40

ARD = adult respiratory disease; HIV = human immunodeficiency virus.
*Group A beta-hemolytic streptococci.
Adapted from Gwaltney JM Jr: Pharyngitis. In: Mandell GL, Douglas RG Jr, Bennett JE (eds): Principles and Practice of Infectious Diseases, 3rd ed. New York, Churchill Livingstone, 1990, p 494.

of people with rhinovirus infection.[7] These agents are inflammatory mediators and stimulate pain nerve endings. Support for the role of these agents comes from experiments demonstrating that when volunteers are administered intranasal bradykinin, they experience symptoms of sore throat.[28] Infection with coxsackievirus and adenovirus leads to direct invasion of the pharyngeal mucosa.[29] Edema and hyperemia characterize viral infection of the pharyngeal mucosa and tonsils. Infection with the Epstein-Barr virus and adenovirus may be accompanied by exudates. Infection with herpes virus and coxsackievirus may be accompanied by the development of vesicles and mucosal ulcerations.

Streptococcus pyogenes (a group A beta-hemolytic *Streptococcus*) is a common inhabitant of the posterior pharynx, and conditions that activate the virus to become pathogenic are not understood. There is undoubtedly a relationship between *S. pyogenes* and other bacteria comprising the pharyngeal microbial ecosystem that allows them to coexist in an asymptomatic state. Host immunity must also play a role in maintaining *S. pyogenes* in an asymptomatic state. Activation of the bacterium results in symptomatic infection characterized by a marked inflammatory response in the pharyngeal tissue. The surface tissue of the pharynx and tonsils may be covered with an exudate or hemorrhage, and there may be noticeable lymphedema.

Diagnosis and Management

It is impossible to differentiate viral and bacterial pharyngitis, and it is possible for two infections to coexist. However, patients with a sore throat and fever cannot be distinguished as having a viral or bacterial etiology for their condition. The patient typically presents with fever, which may be low grade and insidious in onset, or it may be high grade and acute in onset. Physical findings are listed in Table 30–4 and laboratory tests in Table 30–5.

Patients documented to have, or strongly suspected of having, streptococcal pharyngitis should receive a 10-day course of penicillin V, 250 mg every 6 hours, or benzathine penicillin, 1.2 million units intramuscularly one time. Patients allergic to penicillin can be treated with azithromycin, 500 mg as the initial dose, followed by 250 mg daily on days 2, 3, 4, and 5, or erythromycin 500 mg four times daily for 10 days. The availability of rapid tests for streptococcal infection virtually eliminates the use of empiric antibiotic therapy. This reduces the risk of the patient having an adverse reaction to the antibiotic.

Patients who have pharyngitis secondary to infection with *Chlamydia* or *Mycoplasma* can be adequately treated with tetracycline, 500 mg four times daily for 10 days. Doxycycline, 100 mg twice daily for 10 days is also suitable. Erythromycin, 500 mg four times a day

TABLE 30–4 ▶ CLINICAL FINDINGS ASSOCIATED WITH PHARYNGITIS

I. Physical examination
   A. Edema of the posterior pharynx may be present.
   B. Tonsils can be enlarged, appear edematous.
   C. Uvula is not positioned in the center of the palate.
   D. An exudate may be present.
   E. A pseudomembrane may be present.
   F. An enanthema (eruption on the mucosal surface) may be present.
   G. Postnasal drip may be seen.
   H. Mucosal ulcerations can be seen with herpes simplex virus and coxsackievirus infection.
II. Palpable physical findings
   A. The presence of anterior tender cervical lymph nodes is suggestive of bacterial infection.
   B. The presence of posterior enlarged, tender cervical lymph nodes is suggestive of viral infection.

for 10 days, or azithromycin, 500 mg on day 1, followed by 250 mg on days 2, 3, 4, and 5, can be substituted for tetracycline or doxycycline (e.g., in the pregnant patient).

Sinusitis

Acute sinusitis is usually caused by a bacterium or virus in patients who had a common cold or other upper respiratory infection. Acute sinusitis may occur secondary to a dental infection, allergic rhinitis, or intracranial infection, or in a patient whose normal mucociliary function is hampered.

TABLE 30–5 ▶ LABORATORY TESTS TO ESTABLISH THE ETIOLOGY OF PHARYNGITIS

Organism	Test
Group A beta-hemolytic streptococci	Throat culture, rapid tests performed on a 2- to 4-h culture can be performed, direct immunofluorescence, latex agglutination
Neisseria gonorrhoeae	Thayer-Martin culture; nucleic acid probes; polymerase chain reaction
Corynebacterium diphtheriae	Culture on Loeffler's medium
Epstein-Barr virus	Heterophile IgM antibodies in 90% of patients by the third week of illness
Vincent's angina	A specimen from the pharyngeal or tonsillar exudate stained with crystal violet showing numerous fusiform bacteria and spirochetes
Chlamydia psittaci	Isolation of the organism. Serologic tests; fourfold rise in complement-fixing antibody in acute and convalescent serum specimens
Mycoplasma pneumoniae	Cold agglutinins, IgM antibodies that exhibit specificity for I antigen of red blood cells. These are detected at 4°C[30, 31]

IgM = immunoglobulin M.

TABLE 30-6 ▶ MICROBIAL ETIOLOGY OF ACUTE SINUSITIS

Organism	Percentage of Cases*
Community-acquired bacteria	
Streptococcus pneumoniae	33 (20–35)
Haemophilus influenzae (unencapsulated)	21 (6–26)
S. pneumoniae and *H. influenzae*	5 (1–9)
Anaerobic bacteria	6 (0–10)
Staphylococcus aureus	4 (0–8)
Streptococcus pyogenes	2 (1–3)
Branhamella catarrhalis	2
Gram-negative bacteria	9 (0–24)
Nosocomially acquired bacteria	
Pseudomonas aeruginosa	
Klebsiella pneumoniae	
Enterobacter sp.	
Proteus mirabilis	
Viruses	
Rhinovirus	15
Influenza virus	5
Parainfluenza virus	3
Adenovirus	

* Mean (range).
Adapted from Gwaltney JM Jr: Sinusitis, In: Mandell GL, Douglas RG Jr, Bennett JE (eds); Principles and Practice of Infectious Diseases, 3rd ed. New York, Churchill Livingstone, 1990, p 510.

Etiology

A variety of bacterial and viral agents are responsible for acute sinusitis (Table 30-6). The most common organisms are *S. pneumoniae* and *H. influenzae*. However, mixed anaerobic infections account for approximately 6% of the cases of acute sinusitis. Viruses, such as rhinoviruses, influenza virus, and parainfluenza virus, were involved in acute sinusitis either alone or in combination with bacteria in approximately 20% of cases.[32] The fungi have also been isolated from patients with acute sinusitis, including *Aspergillus, Mucor,* and *Exserohilum.*[33–39]

Acute sinusitis makes its appearance during the months that upper respiratory infections are prevalent. Approximately 0.5% of upper respiratory tract infections are complicated by the development of sinusitis.[32] During the summer months, occurrence of sinusitis is associated with swimming.

Pathology

It has been postulated that most cases of sinusitis follow from viral respiratory infections.[40, 41] Because the sinuses are normally sterile and maintained in this state by the mucociliary action of the cells lining the sinus cavity, it is hypothesized that viruses are able to avoid this defense mechanism and cause infection. The inflammatory response initiated by the viral infection results in disruption of mucociliary function, thus allowing bacteria to gain entrance to the sinus cavity and cause infection.

Once infection develops, the mucosa becomes in-

flamed and edematous. The sinus cavity begins to accumulate a polymorphonuclear leukocytic infiltrate, with leukocyte counts in excess of $5,000/mm^3$.[42] Bacterial counts range from 10^5 to 10^8 colony-forming units/mL of exudate.[32] Failure to properly treat acute episodes is likely to lead to chronic sinusitis. The ciliated epithelium becomes replaced with stratified squamous epithelium, which eventually obstructs the lumen of the sinus. The sinus cavity is no longer sterile, but contains a variety of gram-positive and gram-negative bacteria.[43]

Infection is important in acute sinusitis and is the initiating event; however, repeated episodes or exacerbation of acute sinusitis can lead to structural damage. It is the latter event that leads to the development of chronic sinusitis. The bacteria involved in chronic sinusitis are secondary factors resulting from the structural changes in the sinus cavity.

Diagnosis and Management

The preceding clinical symptoms and signs in sinusitis are those of the common cold or other upper or lower respiratory infections. The most common clinical features are facial pain and rhinitis. In addition, the patient may complain of headache, nasal obstruction, disorders of smell, and a nasal quality to her voice.[32] The patient typically has a purulent nasal and postnasal discharge. Examination of the nares frequently reveals the presence of pus in the middle meatus when the maxillary sinus is involved.[32]

Involvement of the ethmoid sinus is usually indicated by edema of the eyelids and excessive tearing. Chemosis, proptosis, and restricted extraocular movement are indicative of orbital involvement extending from the ethmoid sinus.[32] Maxillary sinusitis is usually independent of the other sinusitises and, therefore, occurs alone. However, involvement of the other sinuses usually indicates that they are also infected. Frontal or ethmoid sinus infection may progress to osteomyelitis. The patient can acquire a collection of pus underneath the periosteum of the frontal bone. This results in swelling and edema over the forehead, a condition known as Pott puffy tumor.[44]

The diagnosis is established by taking a detailed history and examination. Transillumination of the frontal maxillary sinuses should be conducted in a darkened room. Complete opacity is evidence that the patient has sinusitis.[32] The patient should have radiographs of the sinus cavities. The presence of air–fluid levels in the sinus cavities, radiologic opacity, and mucosal thickening is indicative of sinusitis.[32, 33, 45, 46]

Specimens for culture can be obtained by aspirating the sinus cavity. This should not be performed on a routine basis, but only for those unusual cases or in patients who have not responded to appropriate antimicrobial therapy. The goal of treatment is to drain the sinus cavity and eliminate the offending organism.

TABLE 30-7 ▶	ANTIMICROBIAL THERAPY FOR THE TREATMENT OF ACUTE SINUSITIS

Trimethoprim-sulfamethoxazole (Bactrim, Septra) 1 tablet bid
Amoxicillin 500 mg tid
Amoxicillin/clavulanate 500 mg tid
Cefaclor (Ceclor) 250 mg tid
Cefuroxime axetil (Ceftin) 250 mg bid
Azithromycin (Zithromax) 500 mg day 1, 250 mg a day days 2 to 5

An antibiotic should be administered for 7 to 10 days (Table 30–7). The patient may benefit from the use of decongestants, mucolytics, and cilia activators (e.g., guaifenesin).

LOWER RESPIRATORY INFECTIONS

Infections of the lower respiratory tract (i.e., alveoli and respiratory bronchioles) are serious conditions that require rapid diagnosis and prompt and appropriate therapy to ensure the best possible outcome for the patient. In the female patient, of particular concern is the development of pneumonia during pregnancy. A variety of etiologic agents have been associated with infections of the lower respiratory tract. New patterns of antimicrobial resistance in respiratory tract pathogens have compelled a re-evaluation of therapeutic options for this set of infections. During pregnancy, the prevalence of pneumonia is between 0.04% and 1%. A mortality rate of 20% was reported before the availability of broad-spectrum antibiotics. With the development of effective antimicrobial agents and the improvement of supportive therapy, mortality is now rare. During pregnancy, a significant incidence of preterm labor has been associated with the development of pneumonia.[47–49]

Pathogenesis

Infection of the lower respiratory tract occurs when pathogenic organisms succeed in overcoming the numerous host defenses. The alveoli and respiratory bronchioles are essentially sterile in the normal patient. The host defenses protecting the lower airways include (1) trapping of a particle larger than 10 μm in the upper airways and clearing of those particles by the motion of the ciliated epithelium; (2) protection from aspiration by the epiglottic and cough reflex; (3) the presence of a mucociliary escalator, which helps to move secretions from the tracheal/bronchial tree by the motion of the ciliated epithelium; and (4) both cell-mediated and humoral immunity, which come into play if pathogenic organisms succeed in invading the lung parenchyma.

Polymorphonuclear leukocyte infiltration develops in association with increased permeability of the involved capillaries. IgA antibodies in the secretions and IgG antibodies in the alveoli and lung parenchyma are responsible for opsonization of the pathogens, leading to more efficient phagocytosis by the lung macrophages.

A variety of factors that predispose to pneumonia have been identified in adults. Smoking is perhaps the most common. Smoking reduces the effectiveness of the mucociliary escalator and depresses immune function. Any condition that leads to a diminution of the ability of the upper airway to shield the lung parenchyma from bacterial inoculation results in an increased likelihood of pneumonia, therefore, endotracheal tubes, depressed epiglottic or cough reflexes, a variety of neurologic disorders, and altered mental status have all been linked to increased risk. Alcoholism also reduces the effectiveness of alveolar macrophages, in combination with altering mental status. Of course, any depression of immune function secondary to associated medical conditions, immunosuppressive agents, or anemia or chronic disease increases the likelihood of infection.

Microbiology

A large number of bacteria, viruses, fungi, and parasites have been associated with infection of the lower respiratory tract. It is therefore critical that a careful diagnostic evaluation with a detailed history, careful physical examination, and supportive radiologic and microbiologic studies be carried out to ensure that an appropriate therapeutic regimen is rapidly instituted. Antibiotic therapy can be optimized once microbiologic results are obtained. However, as a rule, empiric broad-spectrum antibiotic therapy is necessary while awaiting final identification and sensitivities of the cultured pathogens. The most common bacterial pathogens in pneumonia are *S. pneumoniae*, *H. influenzae*, *Staphylococcus aureus*, *Klebsiella pneumoniae*, and *Legionella pneumophila*. In aspiration pneumonia, anaerobic bacteria must be considered. *Mycoplasma pneumoniae* is the most common organism causing atypical pneumonia.[50, 51]

Streptococcus pneumoniae has been associated with 30% to 50% of cases. This same percentage appears to hold among the pregnant population as well. This gram-positive, encapsulated diplococcus requires opsonization for phagocytosis. As a rule, the pneumococcus does cause destruction of lung parenchyma. Pneumococcal pneumonia has a sudden onset with fever, chills, pleuritic chest pain, and a productive cough with rusty sputum. In patients who have undergone splenectomy, severe pneumococcal pneumonia is common. Pneumococcal vaccination therefore plays a role in the prevention of this condition.

Haemophilus influenzae causes approximately 10% of acute community-acquired pneumonias. During pregnancy, it is the second most common bacterium identified. Opsonization is necessary for phagocytosis because of the polysaccharide capsule of this small, gram-negative coccobacillus. As with the pneumococcus, tissue destruction and abscess formation are rare.

Staphylococcus aureus is a gram-positive coccus frequently recovered after a pulmonary infection with influenza. The organism causes fever and chills, purulent sputum, pleuritic chest pain, cavitations, and pleural effusions. The exotoxins produced by *S. aureus* lead to extensive tissue necrosis and destruction. *S. aureus* has been implicated in the development of hematogenously spread infection, frequently from a focus of infective endocarditis or related to the presence of an intravenous catheter.

Klebsiella pneumoniae has been associated with pneumonia in alcoholic patients. Infection with this gram-negative encapsulated rod frequently leads to tissue destruction and abscess formation. An upper lobe pneumonia with pleural effusion and cavitations is the hallmark of the organism.

Legionella pneumophila is a bacterium that does not take up the Gram stain reagents. Because of its ability to necrose the intraveolar septa, infection with *L. pneumophila* leads to fibrosis after resolution of the disease. Fever, chills, and nonproductive cough with gradual onset over 2 to 3 days in association with headache and sore throat is the typical presentation of *L. pneumophila* pneumonia.

Mycoplasma pneumoniae is the most common agent of atypical pneumonia. Mycoplasmas are bacteria that lack a rigid cell wall. Atypical pneumonia develops over time with a low-grade fever, mildly elevated white blood cell count, and nonproductive cough. Symptoms usually remain mild to moderate, but the chest radiograph may show significant infiltrates. *Mycoplasma* pneumonia is associated with bullous myringitis, cervical lymphadenopathy, and, occasionally, a skin rash. Recovery from *Mycoplasma* pneumonia occurs in 10 to 14 days after onset of symptoms, and mortality is uncommon.

Pathogens that are seldom associated with lower respiratory infections include opportunistic bacteria, such as *Acinetobacter* or *Pseudomonas*. These organisms require very large inoculums to establish the infection, and therefore are associated with pneumonia in patients with inadequate upper airway protective mechanisms (i.e., hospitalized patients who are intubated or have altered mental status). A rare, gram-negative aerobic pneumonia is associated with hematogenous spread to the lungs from intra-abdominal or pelvic abscesses or septic pelvic thrombophlebitis. Multiple infiltrates in the lung fields are seen in the chest radiograph.

Francisella tularensis causes a rapid onset of disease with fever, chills, and nonproductive cough after exposure to infected animals or after a tick bite. The organism is difficult to identify on Gram stain. Tissue destruction is frequent and lymphadenopathy is the norm. The chest radiograph may reveal a characteristic oval infiltrate near the hilus of the lung.

Yersinia pestis may cause a pneumonia as well. Together with *M. pneumoniae*, several different species of chlamydiae have been associated with pneumonia. *Chlamydia psittaci* causes psittacosis. The organism is an obligate intracellular parasite acquired by inhalation of contaminated fecal particles from host birds, usually parakeets. The disease may be severe, with nonproductive cough and influenza-like symptoms. Human-to-human transmission is rare, but has been reported. *Chlamydia trachomatis* and *Chlamydia pneumoniae* can cause an atypical pneumonia as well. Another organism that has been linked to atypical pneumonia is *Coxiella burnetii*. Like the chlamydiae, it is an obligate intracellular parasite; infection results from inhalation of the spores, which are very resistant to drying. The infection is found among personnel involved in the care of livestock.

Viruses likely to cause pneumonia in adults include influenza virus and adenovirus. Several others, including Epstein-Barr virus, cytomegalovirus, herpes virus, and varicella have been associated with a pneumonia. Influenza type A is the most common type of viral pneumonia. It develops 24 to 36 hours after the development of the upper respiratory tract symptoms of influenza. It is a pneumonia of particular importance in pregnancy because an increased risk of mortality appears to be associated with development of influenza pneumonia in the third trimester of pregnancy. Pneumonia is a rare complication of varicella infection. It is associated with significant risks of serious morbidity and even mortality when it develops in adults. Measles is caused by an RNA virus that also may cause a nodular infiltrate pneumonia. A pharyngitis associated with pneumonia frequently confined only to the lower lung fields is characteristic of adenovirus infection. Adenovirus is a DNA virus; types 4 and 7 have been linked to pneumonia in military recruits.[52]

Fungal infections with *Aspergillus*, *Candida*, *Histoplasma*, and other fungi are most common in immunocompromised hosts. A handful of parasites, specifically *Pneumocystis carinii* and *Toxoplasma gondii*, are frequent causes of pneumonia in immunocompromised patients. The helminths *Ascaris lumbricoides* and *Strongyloides stercoralis* have been linked to a lower respiratory infection as well.

Evaluation and Treatment

Because the causative agents of pneumonia cause different clinical syndromes and are more likely to be found in specific populations, to initiate properly a satisfactory antimicrobial therapy, a careful review of the patient history and a thorough physical examination are indispensable. It is important to obtain a history of underlying medical conditions, such as alcoholism, and possible antecedent infection, usually an upper respiratory tract disease. Any history of altered mental status, loss of consciousness, or intubation is of critical importance for suspicion of anaerobic and opportunistic infections. Therapy of pneumonia in the setting of influenza must consider the possibility of superinfection with *S. pneumoniae* or *S. aureus*. Immunosuppressed patients must be screened for pneumonia caused by uncommon pathogens like *P. carinii* as well as the more common ones. Travel history, occupational history, and history of exposure to potential sources of infection must be obtained. The physical examination must not be confined to auscultation of the lungs. Bullous myringitis has been associated with *M. pneumoniae*. Pneumococcal pneumonia is frequently associated with herpes labialis. Poor dentition has been associated with anaerobic pneumonia.

Because optimal microbiologic evaluation of patients leads to the most satisfactory antibiotic therapy, it is important to obtain appropriate culture specimens before initiation of empiric broad-spectrum antimicrobial therapy. The initial steps are the collection of an appropriate sputum sample for culture and Gram stain. The sample of sputum collected has to be evaluated to determine whether it represents lower respiratory tract secretions. If few epithelial cells are noted and many polymorphonuclear leukocytes are present, the sample is probably adequate. It is possible to obtain a sample of the lower respiratory tract if the patient is unable to produce an adequate sputum sample, but invasive methods, including transtracheal aspiration, bronchoscopy, or open lung biopsy are associated with significant potential morbidity, and therefore their use has to be individualized. Culture of some of the responsible organisms may, at times, be difficult from a sputum specimen. *Streptococcus pneumoniae* and *H. influenzae* are notoriously difficult to culture.

Blood cultures should be obtained as well because, although seldom positive, they are very specific.[53–56]

Because of the difficulties in culturing some of the organisms associated with atypical pneumonia, serology is frequently of help. Cold agglutinins are positive in approximately 70% of pneumonias caused by *M. pneumoniae*; however, they have been associated with pneumonias caused by legionellae or pneumococci as well. *Legionella pneumophila* acute and convalescent antibody titers confirm the diagnosis.

Radiologic Evaluation

One of the most helpful adjuncts to the history and physical examination is the chest radiograph. Because of the increased permeability of the capillaries of the lung parenchyma, an increase in alveolar and interstitial fluid develops and, depending on the specific locations of the fluid, three specific patterns of chest radiographs in the patient with pneumonia have been described:

1. *Air space pneumonia.* In this pattern, the lung parenchyma appears consolidated because of inflammatory exudates that fill the alveoli. The bronchi are relatively spared and patent, leading to the development of air bronchograms.
2. *Interstitial pneumonia.* In this case, the inflammation is predominantly confined to the alveolar septa with prominent interstitial markings and development of a reticular appearance to the chest radiograph.
3. *Bronchopneumonia.* In bronchopneumonia, the bronchi themselves are involved in the consolidation of lung parenchyma. Atelectasis is prominent and no air bronchograms can be clearly seen. As stated earlier, lobar consolidation is frequently associated with a bacterial pathogen. In staphylococcal pneumonia, the formation of abscesses, empyema, and cavitations is common. *Mycoplasma pneumoniae* usually causes an interstitial pneumonia.

Therapy

In conjunction with antimicrobic therapy, the general management of patients with pneumonia involves adequate supportive care with hydration, oxygen supplementation if necessary, and close monitoring.[57] In the pregnant patient, admission is warranted. In the nonpregnant patient, outpatient management is appropriate in selected cases. The resolution of bronchospasm with bronchodilators maximizes oxygen transport. Of course, if respiratory insufficiency or respiratory failure occurs, oxygen supplementation and intubation may become necessary. In the pregnant patient, oxygen saturation should be maintained at greater than 95% by pulse oximeter to minimize hypoxia to both mother and fetus.

The cornerstone of pneumonia therapy remains antibiotic therapy. The type of therapy is based on the most likely pathogens involved once the initial evaluation has been performed. Patients who are not immunocompromised, and present with the classic syndrome of pneumonia with a sudden onset of fever, chills, a productive, purulent sputum, and a chest radiograph with lobar consolidation must have antibiotic coverage that includes *S. pneumoniae*, *H. influenzae*, *K. pneumoniae*, and *S. aureus* if the illness has occurred after a bout of influenza. On the other hand, if the patient presents with an atypical pneumonia with slower onset of symptoms, with myalgia, headaches, nonproductive cough, and a low-grade fever over several days, and the chest radiograph reveals a reticular or nonhomogeneous infiltrate, coverage for *M. pneumoniae*, *L. pneumophila*, and *Chlamydia* must be pres-

TABLE 30–8 ▸ EMPIRICAL THERAPY OF PNEUMONIA

1. **Community-acquired pneumonia**
   Macrolides, PO or IV (erythromycin, 500 mg PO q6h; azithromycin, 500 mg PO then 250 mg PO qd for 4 d; clarithromycin, 500 mg PO q12h)
   Alternatives (do not use in pregnancy): doxycycline, fluoroquinolones (levofloxacin, trovafloxacin, sparfloxacin)
   If patient is hospitalized (or pregnant), consider adding second- or third-generation cephalosporin to preceding regimen
2. **Influenza**
   Amantadine or ramantadine 100 mg PO bid ± ribavarin inhalation therapy (all agents contraindicated in pregnancy, but may be used if patient's condition requires it)
3. **After influenza**
   Nafcillin 1–2 g IV q4h or vancomycin 1 g IV q12h if resistant *Streptococcus pneumoniae* is suspected
4. **Nosocomial**
   Aminoglycoside plus third-generation cephalosporin or penicillin with beta-lactamase inhibitor
5. **Aspiration**
   Clindamycin 900 mg IV q8h. If gram-negative organism suspected, add aminoglycoside or third-generation cephalosporin.
6. **Varicella pneumonia**
   Acyclovir 10 mg/kg IV q8h

ent.[58, 59] The specific antibiotic therapy depends on the pattern of antibiotic resistance in the community where the patient lives. Unfortunately, an increase in antimicrobial resistance is making the therapy of lower respiratory tract infection more challenging. In addition, in pregnant patients, consideration of the effect of the antimicrobial on the developing fetus further limits the therapeutic options available. One of the issues of greatest concern in the management of pneumonia is the increased resistance of *S. pneumoniae* to penicillin. High levels of resistance in up to 10% of strains must be kept in mind when choosing appropriate antibiotic coverage.[60–62]

Table 30–8 summarizes options in the empirical therapy of community-acquired pneumonia. In the pregnant patient, the use of the new fluoroquinolones is not appropriate because of the potential for fetal toxicity.

In nosocomial pneumonia, because of the broad spectrum of organisms that may be encountered, both gram-positive and gram-negative and aerobic and anaerobic, therapy with a third-generation cephalosporin and an aminoglycoside, or a penicillin with a penicillinase inhibitor and an aminoglycoside, may be appropriate.[57, 63, 64] Imipenem and fluoroquinolones may also play a role in therapy. If the pneumonia is caused by influenza, amantadine or rimantadine can be used.[65] In varicella pneumonia, acyclovir is of help.[66–69]

If aspiration pneumonia is suspected, therapy must include adequate coverage for anaerobic organisms. The recommended therapy is clindamycin intravenously. Metronidazole does not appear to be as effective as clindamycin. Alternatives include penicillin with a penicillinase inhibitor or a second-generation cepha-

losporin. If an immunocompromised state is present, therapy is individualized and coverage of unusual pathogens such as fungi, *P. carinii*, and others must be considered. Appropriate antibiotic coverage can then be initiated.

Aspiration Pneumonia

The pregnant patient is at especially high risk for aspiration pneumonia because of delayed gastric emptying and weak gastroesophageal sphincter tone associated with pregnancy. The risk of aspiration pneumonia is particularly serious with the induction of general anesthesia.[70, 71] More than 100 maternal deaths per year have been associated with aspiration pneumonia at the time of anesthetic administration.[71, 72] In patients with aspiration pneumonitis, respiratory insufficiency may develop because of mechanical interference with gas exchange, but of greater importance is the chemical pneumonitis secondary to acidic damage to the capillaries from the gastric contents. Rapid damage is noted. The superior segments of both lower lobes are the most commonly involved sites in aspiration pneumonia. Prompt assistance by mechanical ventilation and positive expiratory pressure, if necessary, helps maximize oxygen transport. Although the use of prophylactic antibiotics is controversial, antibiotic therapy should be immediately initiated if a bacterial superinfection is suspected. This superinfection usually develops 2 to 3 days after the original aspiration episode. The therapy therefore involves the use of antibiotics effective against gram-negative aerobes and anaerobic organisms. A third-generation cephalosporin and an aminoglycoside have been recommended. The most important issue in aspiration pneumonia is prevention. Neutralization of gastric acid before induction of general anesthesia, continuous cricoid pressure during intubation, and extubation with patient awake decrease the risk of this complication.[73, 74]

REFERENCES

1. Rice DP, Feldman JJ, White KL: The current burden of illness in the United States. In: Occasional Papers of the Institute of Medicine. Washington, DC, National Academy of Sciences, 1976, p 1.
2. Chanock RM: Association of a new type of cytopathic myxovirus with infantile croup. J Exp Med 1956; 104:55.
3. Pelon W, Mogabgab WJ, Phillips IA, et al: A cytopathic agent isolated from naval recruits with mild respiratory illness. Proc Soc Exp Biol Med 1957; 94:262.
4. Price WH: The isolation of a new virus associated with respiratory clinical disease in humans. Proc Natl Acad Sci U S A 1956; 43:892.
5. Lennete EH, Fox VL, Schmidt NJ, et al: The COE virus: An apparently new virus recovered from patients with mild respiratory disease. Am J Hyg 1958; 68:272.
6. Stuart-Harris CH, Andrews C, Andrews BE, et al: A collaborative study of the etiology of acute respiratory infection in Britain 1961–4: A report of the Medical Research Council working party on acute respiratory virus infections. BM J 1965; 2:319.
7. Hamre D, Connelly AP Jr, Procknow JJ: Virologic studies of

acute respiratory disease in young adults: IV. Virus isolation during four years of surveillance. Am J Epidemiol 1966; 83:238.

8. Monto AS, Ullman BM: Acute respiratory illness in an American community: The Tecumseh study. JAMA 1974; 227:164.

9. Makela MJ, Puhakka T, Ruuskanen O, et al: Viruses and bacteria in the etiology of the common cold. J Clin Microbiol 1998; 36:539.

10. Monto AS: Coronaviruses. In: Evans AS (ed): Viral Infections in Humans: Epidemiology and Control. New York, Plenum, 1982, p 151.

11. Gwaltney JM Jr, Hendley JO, Simon G, Jordan WS Jr: Rhinovirus infections in an industrial population: I. The occurrence of illness. N Engl J Med 1966; 275:1261.

12. Dingle JH, Badger GF, Jordan WS Jr: Illness in the Home: Study of 25,000 Illnesses in a Group of Cleveland Families. Cleveland, The Press of Western Reserve University, 1964.

13. Gwaltney JM Jr, Hendley JO, Simon G, Jordan WS Jr: Rhinovirus infections in an industrial population: II. Characteristics of illness and antibody response. JAMA 1967; 202:494.

14. Gwaltney JM Jr: Epidemiology of the common cold. Ann NY Acad Sci 1980; 353:54.

15. Gwaltney JM Jr, Moskalski PB, Hendley JO: Hand-to-hand transmission of rhinovirus colds. Ann Intern Med 1978; 88:463.

16. Cate TR, Couch JM Jr, Johnson KM: Studies with rhinoviruses in volunteers: Production of illness, effect of naturally acquired antibody, and demonstration of a protective effect not associated with serum antibody. J Clin Invest 1964; 43:56.

17. Winther H, Gwaltney JM Jr, Mygind N, et al: Sites of rhinoviruses recovery after point inoculation of the upper airway. JAMA 1986; 256:1763.

18. Hamre D: Rhinoviruses. In: Melnick JL (ed): Monographs in Virology 1. Basel, Karger, 1968, p 1.

19. Frank AL, Taber LH, Wells CR, et al: Patterns of shedding of myxoviruses and paramyxoviruses in children. J Infect Dis 1981; 144:433.

20. Tuner RB, Hendley JO, Gwaltney JM Jr: Shedding of infected ciliated epithelial cells in rhinovirus colds. J Infect Dis 1982; 145:849.

21. Douglas RG Jr, Alford BR, Couch RB: Atraumatic nasal biopsy for studies of respiratory virus infection in volunteers. Antimicrob Agents Chemother 1968; 8:340.

22. Hamory BH, Hendley JO, Gwaltney JM Jr: Rhinovirus growth in nasal polyp organ culture. Proc Soc Exp Biol Med 1977; 155:577.

23. Winther B, Brofeldt S, Christensen B, Mygind N: Light and scanning electron microscopy of nasal biopsy from patients with naturally acquired common colds. Acta Octolaryngol 1984; 97:309.

24. Gonzales R, Sande M: What will it take to stop physicians from prescribing antibiotics in acute bronchitis? Lancet 1995; 345:665.

25. McCaig LF, Hughes JM: Trends in antimicrobial drug prescribing among office-based physicians in the United States. JAMA 1995; 273;214.

26. Kaiser L, Lew D, Hirschel B, et al: Effects of antibiotic treatment in the subset of common-cold patients who have bacteria in nasopharyngeal secretions. Lancet 1996; 374:1507.

27. Gwaltney JM Jr: Virology of middle ear. Ann Otol Rhinol Laryngol 1971; 80:365.

28. Proud D, Reynolds CJ, Lacapra S, et al: Nasal provocation with bradykinin induces symptoms of rhinitis and a sore throat. Am Rev Respir Dis 1988; 137:613.

29. Gwaltney JM Jr: Pharyngitis. In: Mandell GL, Douglas RG Jr, Bennett JE (eds): Principles and Practice of Infectious Diseases, 3rd ed. New York, Churchill Livingstone, 1990, pp 493–498.

30. Loomes LM, Uemura K, Feizi T: Interaction of Mycoplasma pneumoniae with erythrocyte glycolipids of I and i antigen types. Infect Immun 1985; 47:15.

31. Janney FA, Lee LT, Howe C: Cold hemagglutinin cross-reactivity with Mycoplasma pneumoniae. Infect Immun 1978; 22:29.

32. Gwaltney JM Jr: Sinusitis. In: Mandell GL, Douglas RG Jr,

Bennett JE (eds): Principles and Practice of Infectious Diseases, 3rd ed. New York, Churchill Livingstone, 1990, pp 510–514.

33. McGuirt WF, Harrill JA: Paranasal sinus aspergillosis. Laryngoscope 1979; 898:1563.

34. Rinaldi MG: Invasive aspergillosis. Rev Infect Dis 1983; 5:1061.

35. Padhye AA, Ajello L, Wieden MA, Steinbronn KK: Phaeohyphomycosis of the nasal sinuses caused by a new species of Exserohilum. J Clin Microbiol 1986; 24:245.

36. MacMillin RH III, Cooper PH, Body BA, Mills AS: Allergic fungal sinusitis due to Curvularia lunata. Hum Pathol 1987; 18:960.

37. Parfrey NA: Improved diagnosis and prognosis of mucormycosis: A clinicopathologic study of 33 cases. Medicine (Baltimore) 1986; 65;113.

38. Kern ME, Uecker FA: Maxillary sinus infection caused by the homobasidiomycetous fungus Schizophyllum commune. J Clin Microbiol 1986; 23:1001.

39. Washburn RG, Kennedy DW, Begley MG, et al: Chronic fungal sinusitis in apparently normal hosts. Medicine (Baltimore) 1988; 67:231.

40. Evans FO Jr, Sydnor JB, Moore WE, et al: Sinusitis of the maxillary antrum. N Engl J Med 1975; 293:735.

41. Hamory BH, Sande MA, Syndor A Jr, et al: Etiology and antimicrobial therapy of acute maxillary sinusitis. J Infect Dis 1979; 139:197.

42. Caplan ES, Hoyt NJ:Nosocomial sinusitis. JAMA 1982; 247:639.

43. Frederick J, Braude AI: Anaerobic infection of the paranasal sinuses. N Engl J Med 1974; 290:135.

44. Wells RG, Sty JR, Landers AD: Radiological evaluation of Pott puffy tumor. JAMA 1986; 255:1331.

45. Lusted LB, Keats TE: Atlas of Roentgenographic Measurement, 4th ed. Chicago, Year Book, 1978.

46. Kovatch AL, Wald ER, Ledesma-Medina J, et al: Maxillary sinus radiographs in children with nonrespiratory complaints. Pediatrics 1984; 73:306.

47. Benedetti TJ, Valle R, Ledger WJ: Antepartum pneumonia in pregnancy. Am J Obstet Gynecol 1982; 144:413.

48. Hopwood HG: Pneumonia in pregnancy. Obstet Gynecol 1965; 25:875.

49. Oxorn H: The changing aspects of pneumonia complicating pregnancy. Am J Obstet Gynecol 1955; 70:1057.

50. Bartlett JG, Mundy LM: Community-acquired pneumonia. N Engl J Med 1995; 333:1618.

51. File TM Jr: Etiology and incidence of community-acquired pneumonia. Infect Dis Clin Pract 1996; 5(suppl 4):S127.

52. Luby JP: Southwestern Internal Medicine Conference: Pneumonia in adults due to Mycoplasma, chlamydia and viruses. Am J Med Sci 1987; 294:45.

53. Barrett-Connor E: The non-value of sputum culture in the diagnosis of pneumococcal pneumonia. Am Rev Respir Dis 1971; 103:845.

54. Kalin M: Accuracy of sputum examination for the diagnosis of pneumococcal pneumonia. [Letter.] J Infect Dis 1985; 152:1097.

55. Musher DM: Gram-stain and culture of sputum to diagnose bacterial pneumonia. [Letter.] J Infect Dis 1985; 152:1096.

56. Perlino CH: Laboratory diagnosis of pneumonia due to Streptococcus pneumoniae. J Infect Dis 1984; 150:139.

57. Macfarlane JT: Treatment of lower respiratory infections. Lancet 1987; 2:1446.

58. Lode H: Initial therapy in pneumonia: Clinical, radiographic, and laboratory data important for the choice. Am J Med 1986; 80:70.

59. Woodhead MA, MacFarlane JT: Comparative clinical and laboratory features of Legionella with pneumococcal and mycoplasma pneumonias. Br J Dis Chest 1987; 81:133.

60. Butler JC, Hofmann J, Cetron MS, et al: The continued emergence of drug-resistant Streptococcus pneumoniae in the United States: An update from the Centers for Disease Control and Prevention pneumococcal sentinel surveillance system. J Infect Dis 1986; 174:986.

61. Doem GV, Brueggemann A, Holley HP Jr, Rauch AM: Antimicrobial resistance of Streptococcus pneumoniae recovered from outpatients in the United States during the winter months of 1994 to 1995: Results of a 30-center national

surveillance study. Antimicrob Agents Chemother 1996; 40:1208.

62. Jernigan DB, Cetron MS, Breiman RF, the Drug-Resistant *Streptococcus pneumoniae* Working Group: Defing the public health impact of drug-resistant *Streptococcus pneumoniae*: Report of a working group. MMWR Morb Mortal Wkly Rep 1996; 45 (suppl RR-1): 1.

63. Bartlett JG, Gorbach SL: Treatment of aspiration pneumonia and primary lung abscess: Penicillin G vs. clindamycin. JAMA 1975; 234:935.

64. Grassi GG: Respiratory infections: Established therapy and its limitations. Clin Ther 1985; 7 (suppl A):19.

65. Chow AW, Jewesson PS: Pharmacokinetics and safety of antimicrobial agents during pregnancy. Rev Infect Dis 1985; 7:287.

66. Eder SE, Apussio JJ, Weiss G: *Varicella pneumoniae* during pregnancy: Treatment of two cases with acyclovir. Am J Perinatol 1988; 5:16.

67. Hankins GD, Gilstrap LC, Patterson AR: Acyclovir treatment of varicella pneumonia in pregnancy. [Letter.] Crit Care Med 1987; 15:336.

68. Landsberger EJ, Hager WD, Grossman JH: Successful management of varicella pneumonia complicating pregnancy: A report of three cases. J Reprod Med 1986; 31:311.

69. Straus SE: The management of varicella and zoster infections. Infect Dis Clin North Am 1987; 1:367.

70. Bynum LJ, Pierce AK: Pulmonary aspiration of gastric contents. Am Rev Respir Dis 1976; 114:1129.

71. Kallos T, Lampe KF, Orkin FK: Pulmonary aspiration of gastric contents. In: Orkin FK, Cooperman LH (eds): Complications in Anesthesiology. Philadelphia, JB Lippincott, 1983, pp 152–164.

72. Morgan M: Anesthetic contribution to maternal mortality. Br J Anaesth 1987; 59:842.

73. Malinow AM, Ostheimer GW: Anesthesia for the high-risk parturient. Obstet Gynecol 1987; 69:951.

74. Power KJ: The prevention of the acid aspiration (Mendelson's) syndrome: A contribution to reduced maternal mortality. Midwifery 1987; 3:143.

31

Infectious Diarrhea

JAVIER A. ADACHI ▶ HERBERT L. DUPONT

Worldwide, diarrheal diseases were reported to have caused nearly 1 billion episodes of illness in 1996, ranking this group of disorders second to acute upper respiratory diseases as the most common diseases in men or women.[5] Although in industrialized regions diarrhea causes significant economic loss and is a major cause of absenteeism, it is of greater importance in developing countries, where the illness is not only a leading cause of morbidity in children, but, more important, it is the major cause of infant mortality.[5–7] Also, diarrhea is a cause of serious morbidity in travelers to these areas from areas of lower endemicity.

Diarrhea is usually defined as the passing of a greater number of stools of decreased form than is customary. It is often secondary to a gastrointestinal infection. A more rigid definition is not practical. Diarrhea is considered acute when it lasts less than 14 days, and persistent when lasting more than 2 weeks. Acute diarrhea is the primary focus of this chapter because, with current laboratory techniques, we have evidence that most cases of infectious diarrhea present in this way.[6, 7]

In this chapter, we discuss the pathogenic mechanisms, etiologic agents, specific epidemiologic modes of transmission, and the evaluation, treatment, and prevention of patients with diarrhea.

EPIDEMIOLOGY

The route of transmission of infectious diarrhea is usually fecal-oral, through ingestion of contaminated water or food.[6] Other routes of transmission are through aerosols (viruses), contaminated hands or surfaces, and sexual activity (e.g., proctitis from receptive anal intercourse).[5, 9]

Important epidemiologic factors are detailed in the following sections.

Travel

Travelers' diarrhea is the most common travel-related illness. There is a background rate of diarrhea of 2% to 4% for people who have short trips to low endemic areas (e.g., United States, Canada, and northwestern Europe), possibly related to increased consumption of food in public establishments, to alcohol taken in greater amounts than usual, and to more stress compared with nontravelers. The rate of diarrhea increases to approximately 10% when the destination is northern Mediterranean areas, China, Russia, or certain Caribbean islands, and it occurs at rates as high as 40% to 50% when people travel from industrialized regions to developing tropical and subtropical areas of Latin America, Asia and Africa.[6, 7, 9]

Bacterial pathogens are the most common etiologic agents in travelers' diarrhea among people in high-risk regions: enterotoxigenic *Escherichia coli* (ETEC) is the most common, found in up to 40% of travelers with diarrhea, followed by *Shigella* spp. and *Aeromonas/Plesiomonas* spp. (10% for each), *Salmonella* spp. (4% to 5%), and *Campylobacter jejuni* (3%).[2, 7] Viruses (Norwalk-like or rotavirus; 10% to 12%) and parasites (*Entamoeba histolytica*, *Giardia lamblia*, *Cryptosporidium*, and *Cyclospora*; 2% to 4%) occur less commonly.[6, 7] *Vibrio cholerae* is a concern to travelers to some areas of Latin America and Asia, where it is epidemic, although cholera occurs in only 1 in 500,000 travelers to these areas. Thirty percent of people with travelers' diarrhea do not have a detected etiologic agent in stool samples, but in most of these cases the illness improves with antimicrobial therapy, suggesting that most cases are caused by undetected bacterial pathogens.[6, 7]

In general, female travelers have a reduced risk of contracting travelers' diarrhea compared with men because of their tendency to eat safer food and beverage items.

Location

Rotavirus, *G. lamblia*, *Shigella* spp., *C. jejuni*, and *Cryptosporidium* have been reported to cause outbreaks of infectious diarrhea in day care centers among non–toilet-trained toddlers.[2, 5, 9] Hospitals (especially intensive care units and pediatric wards) and nursing homes are sites of high attack rates of gastrointestinal infections. *Clostridium difficile*–associated diarrhea[11] and diarrhea caused by *Salmonella* spp., rotavirus, and enteropathogenic *E. coli* (EPEC) are the most commonly reported forms of diarrhea in these settings. Diarrhea is common in nursing homes for the elderly and in institutions for the mentally handicapped.[2, 5]

Antimicrobial Therapy

Clostridium difficile–associated diarrhea is frequently related to recent use of an antimicrobial agent by the patient (usually during or within 2 to 4 weeks of use), and it is one of the predominant causes of nosocomial diarrhea.[9, 11]

Age

Children in developing countries younger than 5 years of age have higher diarrhea morbidity rates and, because of more common dehydration and malnutrition, they more often experience mortality from infectious diarrhea. Rotavirus, ETEC and EPEC, *C. jejuni*, and *G. lamblia* are found more often in enteric infections during childhood.[1, 4]

In industrialized regions of the world, including the United States, diarrhea occurs with a frequency of one to two bouts per person per year in all age groups.[5] In these areas, the consequences of diarrhea, including death, are greater in elderly populations.

Incubation Period in Outbreaks of Diarrhea

A short time of incubation (≤7 hours) and reports of multiple cases with a possible common source suggest the possibility of bacterial food intoxication due to *Staphylococcus aureus* or *Bacillus cereus*. An outbreak with an incubation period of 8 hours or more usually is secondary to an enteric infection due to *Clostridium perfringens*, *V. cholerae*, ETEC, *Salmonella* spp., *Shigella* spp., or others.[1, 5, 9]

Immunocompromised Status

Patients with acquired immunodeficiency syndrome (AIDS) or other deficits in their immune defenses have a greater risk of development of diarrhea and infection by a wide variety of enteric pathogens.[2, 5] In advanced human immunodeficiency virus (HIV) infection, a reduction in intestinal immunity occurs. Reduction in intestinal CD4 cells leads to histopathologic changes resulting in malabsorption and diarrhea. With reduced immune function, the gut is also more susceptible to enteric infection. The agents responsible for illness include usual bacterial agents, *Mycobacterium avium-intracellulare* complex, *Cryptosporidium parvum*, *Giardia lamblia*, *Isospora*, *Cyclospora*, *Microsporidium*, cytomegalovirus, herpes simplex virus, or HIV itself. Treatment of enteric infection in AIDS may be associated with improvement in symptomatology. Relapse of infection or reinfection with a new pathogen often occurs in these patients.[5]

PATHOPHYSIOLOGY

There are three general mechanisms that lead to diarrhea. The first is the alteration of fluid and electrolyte movement from the serosal to the mucosal surface. Movement of electrolytes (often chloride ion) may occur as a result of stimulation of cyclic nucleotides by bacterial enterotoxins or by inflammatory pathogens causing a release of cytokines. The second mechanism is malabsorption or presence in the lumen of the gut of nonabsorbed materials. The third is intestinal motility alterations resulting in more rapid transit of intestinal content.[2, 9] In acute infectious diarrhea, the first mechanism is the most important. The second and third mechanisms are important in chronic forms of diarrhea. Tropical and nontropical sprue, Whipple's disease, small bowel scleroderma, advanced AIDS, and other disorders that alter the gut anatomy result in malabsorption. Irritable bowel disease, due to autonomic dysfunction, and inflammatory bowel disease appear to produce diarrhea primarily through alterations in intestinal motility.

ETIOLOGIC AGENTS

The formidable list of microorganisms that cause acute infectious diarrhea is not reviewed completely in this chapter. Instead, the focus is on the most important agents. These microorganisms include bacteria, viruses, and protozoal parasites. Fungal agents are found only occasionally and are not reviewed in this chapter.

Bacterial Agents

Bacterial pathogens are responsible for approximately 30% of cases of infectious diarrhea in developed countries and more than 50% of cases in developing tropical and subtropical nations.[5, 7] Table 31–1 lists the more important bacterial causes of acute diarrhea, with their virulence properties and world distribution. The most common bacteria that cause watery diarrhea through enterotoxin production are ETEC, *V. cholerae*, *C. perfringens*, *C. difficile*, *B. cereus*, *S. aureus*, *Aeromonas hydrophila*, and possibly *Plesiomonas shigelloides*. Invasive agents that cause dysentery or inflammatory diarrhea, responsible for 15% of cases, include *Shigella* spp., *Salmonella* spp., *Campylobacter jejuni*, enterohemorrhagic *E. coli* (EHEC), enteroinvasive *E. coli* (EIEC), and *Yersinia enterocolitica*.[4, 5, 8]

Vibrio cholerae

Cholera results when enterotoxin is released by *V. cholerae* O1. Historically, cholera has been a severe form

TABLE 31-1 ▶ IMPORTANT BACTERIAL ENTEROPATHOGENS, VIRULENCE PROPERTIES, AND WORLD DISTRIBUTION

Pathogen	Virulence Properties	Distribution
Vibrio cholerae	Heat-labile enterotoxin	Endemic areas in Asia, Africa, and Latin America
Enterotoxigenic *E. coli*	Heat-stable and heat-labile enterotoxin, colonization factor antigens	Developing countries, tropical areas, infants, travelers
Enteropathogenic *E. coli*	Enteroadherence	Infants, worldwide
Enteroaggregative *E. coli*	Enteroadherence	Infants, worldwide
Enteroinvasive *E. coli*	Shigella-like invasiveness	Worldwide, endemic in South America and Eastern Europe
Enterohemorrhagic *E. coli*	Shiga-like toxin	Beef, endemic areas
Shigella	Shiga-like toxin, invasiveness	Worldwide
Salmonella	Cholera-like toxin, invasiveness	Worldwide
Campylobacter jejuni	Cholera-like toxin, invasiveness	Worldwide
Aeromonas spp.	Hemolysin, cytotoxin, enterotoxin	Worldwide, especially Thailand, Australia, and Canada
Yersinia enterocolitica	Heat-stable enterotoxin, invasiveness	Worldwide, especially Canada, Scandinavia, and South Africa
Clostridium difficile	Cytotoxin A and B	Worldwide
Clostridium perfringens	Preformed toxin	Worldwide
Bacillus cereus	Preformed toxin	Worldwide
Staphylococcus aureus	Preformed toxins	Worldwide

of watery diarrhea with dehydration that occurred in endemic areas of Asia, Africa, and the Middle East. Since the outbreak of cholera in Peru, in 1991, the disease has become endemic in most countries of Latin America.[2, 5] Since the early 1980s, *V. cholera* O1 biotype El Tor, serotype Inaba has been documented in a small number of cases in the Gulf Coast of the United States. *V. cholerae* non-O1 infection may also occur in patients with diarrhea.[4, 8] The agents may also produce diarrhea and septicemia in immunocompromised patients.

Escherichia coli

Diarrheagenic *E. coli* is a still-growing group of microorganisms that taxonomically belong to one species, but with different virulence properties, epidemiologic characteristics, and clinical manifestations.

ENTEROPATHOGENIC *E. COLI* (EPEC)

Enteropathogenic *E. coli* was the first of the diarrheagenic *E. coli* described in the 1920s to 1940s as causes of outbreaks in hospital newborn nurseries.[5, 9] Initially, the strains were identified by serotypes, but since the early 1980s, they have been shown to exhibit a localized adherence pattern to HEp-2 cells. EPEC have a worldwide distribution, and the most widely accepted pathophysiologic mechanism is that they cause damage to the epithelial surface without intestinal invasion.[5, 8]

ENTEROTOXIGENIC *E. COLI* (ETEC)

These strains were first identified in the 1970s. ETEC produce one or two toxins, heat-labile cholera-like toxin (LT) and heat-stable toxin (ST), that cause transudation of fluid and electrolytes in the intestinal lumen.[5, 8] It is the most important cause of diarrhea in developing countries and among travelers to these regions from industrialized countries.[6, 7]

ENTEROINVASIVE *E. COLI* (EIEC)

Enteroinvasive *E. coli* possess the property of *Shigella*-like invasiveness, with a characteristic clinical presentation of febrile dysentery. EIEC are found worldwide, but they appear to be particularly endemic in areas of South America and Eastern Europe.[5, 8] The strains possess the same invasion plasmid as *Shigella*, and most of them also have other defined *Shigella* antigens.

ENTEROHEMORRHAGIC *E. COLI* (EHEC)

Enterohemorrhagic *E. coli* have been identified in outbreaks associated with consumption of contaminated beef or unpasteurized apple juice and contact with contaminated swimming pools, leading to the occurrence of hemorrhagic colitis (bloody diarrhea from intense colitis).[2, 5] The most common etiologic agent is *E. coli* O157:H7. EHEC produce shiga-like toxin, and the infection may lead to the hemolytic-uremic syndrome.

DIFFUSELY ADHERENT *E. COLI* (ENTEROADHERENT *E. COLI*)

Non-EPEC strains with a diffuse adherent pattern to HEp-2 cells have been identified in some cases of diarrhea, but the importance of these pathogens is uncertain.

ENTEROAGGREGATIVE *E. COLI* (EAEC or EAggEC)

This group of organisms is the most recent addition to the list of diarrheagenic *E. coli*. They are non-EPEC strains that do not produce ETEC LT or ST. These strains adhere to HEp-2 cell in a characteristic aggregative pattern (they adhere generally to cells and the glass cover slip, giving a stacked-brick appearance).[5, 7] They are being recognized as causes of pediatric diarrhea in developing countries, often associated with persistent illness and malnutrition. The pathogenesis of EAEC diarrhea is not completely understood.

Shigella Species

The different strains of *Shigella* characteristically produce an inflammatory, dysenteric form of diarrhea, with blood and leukocytes in stools secondary to extensive mucosal invasion of the colon. These strains have a worldwide distribution and cause infection after exposure to a small inoculum.[2, 8]

Salmonella Species

In salmonellosis or *Salmonella* gastroenteritis, there is local invasion of the mucosa of the colon, followed by development of an intense inflammatory (polymorphonuclear leukocyte) reaction.[2, 8] In typhoid or enteric fever, the intestinal mononuclear leukocyte reaction may facilitate the systemic dissemination of the microorganism.

Campylobacter jejuni

Campylobacter jejuni shows worldwide distribution, with transmission through poultry and unpasteurized milk.[5] The strains produce inflammatory diarrhea like that caused by *Shigella* spp.

Yersinia enterocolitica

This microorganism is distributed worldwide, with a preference for colder regions (e.g., Scandinavia and Canada).[8] It typically produces an inflammatory diarrhea.

Aeromonas and *Plesiomonas* Species

Aeromonas spp. show a worldwide distribution. Most strains produce enterotoxins and cytotoxins. The organisms are excreted by asymptomatic carriers.[5] *Plesiomonas shigelloides* is an occasional cause of diarrhea, and two important epidemiologic factors in *Plesiomonas* diarrhea are recent travel and ingestion of seafood.[7]

Viral Agents

Rotavirus, Norwalk virus, and other small, round-structured, Norwalk-like viruses, adenoviruses, and caliciviruses are responsible for most of the acute, infectious watery diarrhea in young infants.[1, 2]

Rotavirus

This virus is distributed worldwide. In developing regions, it is an important cause of infantile mortality. The organism usually affects children younger than 3 years of age, producing watery diarrhea associated with nausea and vomiting.[1, 5] The infection commonly leads to dehydration because both vomiting and diarrhea occur in a young infant of small body size.

Small Round Structured Viruses

Norwalk virus and the other small, round-structured viruses represent major causes of waterborne and foodborne disease worldwide.[1] In the United States and other industrialized areas, Norwalk virus infects all age groups, whereas in developing countries, this organism infects primarily children up to 3 years of age.[4]

Parasitic Agents

Numerous parasites produce diarrhea and have an ubiquitous distribution. The four most important protozoal parasitic causes of diarrhea are *G. lamblia*, *Cryptosporidium*, *E. histolytica*, and *Cyclospora*.

Giardia lamblia

This organism is found commonly in developing countries. It typically causes acute, watery diarrhea after the first infection, with subsequent development of immunity to symptomatic reinfection.[2, 8] Reinfection without development of clinical symptoms commonly occurs in endemic areas. A small subgroup of highly susceptible people (particularly those with immunoglobulin A deficiency) may acquire a chronic or intermittent giardiasis.

Cryptosporidium parvum

Cryptosporidium is a worldwide pathogen often related to waterborne outbreaks. The parasite is found in infants in day care centers and in patients with AIDS-associated diarrhea. The frequency of AIDS-associated cryptosporidiosis is decreasing because of improved immunity secondary to effective antiretroviral therapy.[3, 4]

Entamoeba histolytica

This organism causes acute inflammatory diarrhea in tropical developing nations, with the frequency of infection showing an inverse relationship with socioeconomic level. Abscess of the liver develops in approximately 3% of patients with intestinal amebiasis.[5, 8] Women during the reproductive years have a reduced occurrence of this complication. However, dissemination of *E. histolytica* may occur during pregnancy.

Cyclospora

Cyclospora is an important cause of acute and persistent diarrhea. It is endemic in many developing regions, although the highest rates appear to be in Nepal and Peru.[5] The organism is spread through contaminated water, soil or berries.

CLINICAL MANIFESTATIONS

There is no typical clinical picture of patients with acute infectious diarrhea, and patients can present a wide variety of signs and symptoms such as diarrhea, nausea, vomiting, abdominal pain, dehydration, or fever. It is impossible to diagnose the etiology of diarrhea on clinical grounds because illnesses due to different etiologic agents share similar clinical features.

Clinical severity of a diarrhea episode can be categorized as follows[5, 6]:

Mild: One or two unformed stools per day with non-distressing, tolerable enteric symptoms that do not interfere with normal activities.

Moderate: Three to five unformed stools per day with distressing symptoms that impair or force a change in activities but do not prohibit them.

Severe: Six or more unformed stools in 24 hours with incapacitating symptoms that prohibit normal activities and force confinement to bed, or any number of unformed stools with concomitant fever and dysentery.

The following clinical features represent important findings that help narrow the diagnostic possibilities and often allow a preliminary diagnosis.

Dehydration

History of decreased urination, dry mucous membranes and low blood pressure are some of the clinical findings in patients with dehydration. Patients with dehydration need fluid and electrolyte replacement. Dehydration is most common in pediatric and elderly populations.

Fever

Fever is usually a reaction to an inflammatory process, and most of the pathogens that produce fever invade the intestinal mucosa. The classic invasive bacterial enteropathogens are *Shigella* spp., *Salmonella* spp. and *C. jejuni*. However, fever can be also produced by EIEC, *Vibrio parahaemolyticus*, *Aeromonas* spp., *C. difficile*, and viral pathogens such as rotavirus and Norwalk and Norwalk-like viruses.

Vomiting

Food intoxication and viral gastroenteritis are the likely processes when vomiting is the predominant symptom. Food poisoning is secondary to the presence of an enterotoxin produced by *S. aureus* or *B. cereus*, with an incubation period of less than 8 hours.[2] Rotavirus in infants and Norwalk and Norwalk-like viruses in any age group are the other major category of agents commonly implicated in patients with significant vomiting.[1]

Dysentery

Dysentery is defined as the passage of small-volume stools that contain blood and often mucus. It can also occur with tenesmus (straining without passing stools) and fecal urgency (inability voluntarily to delay stool evacuation by 15 minutes). In the United States, the most common causes of dysentery are *Shigella* spp. and *C. jejuni* (30% to 50% of cases of either infection are reported to have bloody stools).[5] Other causes of dysentery are *Salmonella* spp., *Aeromonas* spp., *V. parahaemolyticus*, *Y. enterocolitica*, EIEC, EHEC, *E. histolytica*, and inflammatory bowel disease.

Systemic Involvement

A number of enteric pathogens may produce systemic infections.[2, 4] Patients infected with *Shigella* or EHEC may acquire hemolytic-uremic syndrome, patients with *Yersinia* infection may have Reiter's syndrome or glomerulonephritis, and patients with *Salmonella typhi* and *Salmonella paratyphi* infection may get typhoid or enteric fever.

DIAGNOSIS

Patients with mild acute diarrhea usually need only clinical evaluation. An etiologic assessment is unnecessary and treatment can be given empirically. Laboratory tests are reserved for those with moderate to severe diarrhea and for patients with persistent disease (Table 31–2).

Fecal Leukocyte Test

The most rapid and useful test for all patients with moderate to severe diarrhea is the fecal leukocyte examination.[4, 10] In this test, a recently passed stool (if present, a mucus strand) is stained with dilute methylene blue and examined microscopically. A wet-mount preparation under a cover slip or a heat-dried stained sample can be examined by oil immersion microscopy, and the presence of leukocytes and a rough quantification of their number can be determined. The finding of numerous polymorphonuclear leukocytes indi-

TABLE 31-2 ▶	INDICATIONS FOR LABORATORY TESTS AND POSSIBLE DIAGNOSIS	
Laboratory Test	**Indications**	**Probable Diagnosis**
Fecal leukocytes	Moderate to severe cases	Diffuse colonic inflammation
Stool culture	Moderate to severe diarrhea, fever, fecal leukocytes (+), male homosexuals	*Shigella, Campylobacter, Salmonella, Aeromonas*
Blood culture	Enteric fever, sepsis	*Salmonella*, less likely *Campylobacter, Yersinia*
Parasite examination	>2 wk of diarrhea, travel to specific areas, day care centers, male homosexuals	*Giardia, Cryptosporidium, Entamoeba histolytica, Cyclospora*
Rotavirus antigen	Hospitalized infants <3 y of age	Rotavirus
Clostridium difficile toxin	Antibiotic-associated diarrhea	*C. difficile*

cates diffuse colonic inflammation rather than a specific etiology, and stool cultures in these cases are often negative for specific pathogens. The major causes of diffuse colonic inflammation are *Shigella* spp., *Salmonella* spp. and *C. jejuni*. Other etiologic agents and conditions that may lead to many fecal leukocytes in the stools are *C. difficile*–associated diarrhea, *Aeromonas* spp., *Y. enterocolitica, V. parahaemolyticus*, EIEC, idiopathic ulcerative colitis, and allergic colitis.[4] It is important to understand the limitations of this test because not all patients with invasive bacterial diarrhea have leukocyte-positive stools.

Stool Culture

A routine laboratory culture should be able to recover *Shigella, Salmonella*, and *Campylobacter* from a stool culture, and in selected cases on request, the laboratory should be able to detect *V. cholerae, V. parahaemolyticus, Aeromonas* spp., *Y. enterocolitica*, or *C. difficile*.[5] The indications for performing a stool culture are moderate or severe diarrhea, febrile and dysenteric disease, persistent diarrhea, and fecal leukocyte-positive diarrhea.

Blood Culture

A blood culture should be performed in all patients with enteric fever or in any hospitalized patient with gastrointestinal symptoms. Systemic enteric infections that are diagnosed etiologically through blood culture are infections secondary to *S. typhi* and nontyphoid *Salmonella, Clostridium fetus*, and *Y. enterocolitica*.

Parasite Examination

Direct examination of a stool sample to identify a parasite is less useful as a routine test than stool culture. Immunologic techniques to detect antigens of protozoan parasites (*Giardia, Cryptosporidium, E. histolytica*) are more sensitive and specific than traditional methods.[5, 8] Intestinal parasites may be difficult to detect in stool and sometimes are better diagnosed by duodenal aspiration or intestinal biopsy. The few indications for performing parasite examination are (1)

persistent diarrhea, (2) diarrhea in a male homosexual patient, (3) diarrhea with history of regular contact with a day care center, or (4) diarrhea in a traveler to mountainous areas of North America, to Russia or to developing regions of the world.

Special Tests

Serologic diagnosis of typhoid fever (Widal's reaction) is useful only in endemic areas of the developing world. In areas where typhoid fever is unusual (e.g., the United States), exposure to other cross-reacting, gram-negative rods rather than *S. typhi* can explain false-positive serologic results. Commercial rotavirus antigen testing kits are readily available, easy to perform, and sensitive. An appropriate indication for rotavirus testing is screening of hospitalized children younger than 3 years of age with gastroenteritis.[1] An infant with a rotavirus-positive test should receive fluid therapy without antimicrobial therapy. The laboratory test for diagnosing antibiotic-associated colitis is the *C. difficile* toxin assay by tissue culture or serologic procedure.[11] The commercial serologic kits detect only toxin A and are less sensitive than the tissue culture method, but are easier to perform. Young infants and children may have toxin in stools without evidence of any cytopathologic process. The Entero Test, a gelatin capsule affixed to a nylon string, may be useful to sample small bowel mucus in cases of typhoid fever, giardiasis and strongyloidiasis.

Sigmoidoscopy/Colonoscopy

In general, sigmoidoscopy and sometimes colonoscopy are reserved for cases of clinical colitis (dysentery, positive fecal leukocytes) without improvement within 14 days. Mucosal changes may not be specific except when pseudomembranes are sought, and biopsy may be helpful. Examination of the distal colon in patients with acute diarrhea, especially in homosexual men, may show evidence of proctitis (inflammation of the distal 15 cm of the colon), proctocolitis (inflammation beyond 15 cm), or enteritis (no colitis).[4]

TABLE 31–3 ❯	EMPIRICAL TREATMENT OF ACUTE DIARRHEA IN ADULTS
Clinical Manifestations	**Therapy**
Watery diarrhea with mild symptoms (no alteration of itinerary)	Oral fluids and saline crackers
Watery diarrhea with moderate symptoms (change in itinerary but able to function)	Loperamide or bismuth subsalicylate
Watery diarrhea with severe symptoms (incapacitating)	Perform stool culture and fecal leukocytes and consider antimicrobial drugs*
Dysentery or fever	Antimicrobial drugs,* no loperamide
Persistent diarrhea (>14 days)	Perform parasite examination and consider a course of metronidazole
Vomiting, minimal diarrhea	Bismuth subsalicylate
Diarrhea in pregnant women	Fluids and electrolytes; can consider attapulgite

*Antimicrobial drugs recommended: norfloxacin, ciprofloxacin, levofloxacin, or fleroxacin for adults.

TREATMENT

In all cases of diarrhea, fluid and electrolyte replacement should be encouraged. Selected patients may benefit from symptomatic therapy, and others can have their illness shortened by empirical antimicrobial therapy (Table 31–3). In cases of acute diarrhea in pregnant women, it is necessary to know the possible adverse effects of and contraindications of the different drugs in the mother and fetus.

Fluid Replacement

Although this treatment is not usually critical to well nourished adults with mild to moderate diarrhea, rehydration is an important part of therapy, especially in the very young, pregnant women, and the elderly.[5, 6] All patients should drink commercial solutions (Gatorade, Pedialyte, Lytren) or soft drinks with saltine crackers. In dehydrating illness, oral rehydration salts or intravenous fluids should be given.

Dietary Management

During diarrhea, the intestinal tract is unable to process complex dietary material. For infants and young children, breast feeding should be continued but other milk suspended. As the stool rate decreases and appetite improves, staple foods such as cereals, potatoes, noodles, crackers, toasts, and bananas can gradually be added to the diet. These foods facilitate enterocyte renewal. Patients should resume their usual diet once stools retain their shape. In most cases, full diet can be resumed in 2 to 3 days. Milk, milk products, caffeine, and spicy and fried foods should be excluded in all people while passing unformed stools.[6, 7]

Nonspecific Therapy

Symptomatic agents are useful for the treatment of mild to moderate diarrhea. They ameliorate symptoms and allow patients to return to their normal activities. The drugs may improve the form of the stool, decrease the number of stools passed, and decrease the duration of the illness. Although mild symptoms need not be treated with anything other than fluids, moderate illness may improve with a nonspecific drug such as bismuth subsalicylate or loperamide (Table 31–4).

There are three types of symptomatically acting drugs: adsorbents, antisecretory agents, and antimotility drugs. Attapulgite, a nonabsorbable magnesium aluminum silicate, is more active than the combination of kaolin and pectin, the classic adsorbent drug combination.[6] This drug binds to fluid and perhaps toxins, improving the form of the stools. The preparation is intrinsically safe and, although not approved for use in young infants and pregnant women, should be safe in all people.

Bismuth subsalicylate is an antisecretory drug that

TABLE 31–4 ❯	NONSPECIFIC DRUGS FOR PROPHYLAXIS AND THERAPY IN ADULTS	
Agent	**Prophylactic Dose for Travelers**	**Therapeutic Dose**
Attapulgite	Not used	3 g initially, then 3 g after each loose stool or q2h (not to exceed 9 g/d) (should be safe during pregnancy and childhood)
Loperamide	Not used	4 mg initially, then 2 mg after each loose stool (not to exceed 16 mg/d) (do not use in dysenteric diarrhea)
Bismuth subsalicylate	Two 262-mg tablets before meals and at bedtime (do not use for prophylaxis for >3 wk)	30 mL or two 262-mg tablets q30 min for eight doses (may repeat on day 2)

blocks the effect of enterotoxin on intestinal mucosa, apparently secondary to the salycilate moiety. The bismuth portion, because of its antimicrobial effects, is the important constituent acting as a prophylactic agent in the prevention of travelers' diarrhea. When used for therapy of diarrhea, this drug reduces the number of stools passed and the duration of illness by approximately 50%.[7] Other, novel antisecretory drugs are being evaluated in acute diarrhea, and one of the objectives is to find one without constipating effects or the potential for worsening invasive forms of acute infectious diarrhea.

The most common antimotility drug is loperamide. This drug increases segmental contractions of the bowel, resulting in slowing of the movement of the intestinal column and thereby providing more opportunity for fluid absorption. Its weak antisecretory effect is through inhibition of intestinal calmodulin. Loperamide reduces the frequency of stools and the duration of illness by 80% compared with nontreated patients.[7] Diphenoxylate hydrochloride with atropine, paregoric, tincture of opium, and codeine are also effective as antimotility agents, but they have a greater capacity to produce central opiate toxicity. The antimotility drugs can lead to a worsening of clinical manifestations in patients with infection by an invasive pathogen, and they are not recommended in patients with fever or dysentery.

Antimicrobial Agents

All antimicrobial agents are classified B or C in the U.S. Food and Drug Administration pregnancy risk categories (Table 31–5). Class B includes those antimicrobials with animal studies showing no risk in pregnancy, but with no adequate studies in humans, or with animal studies showing toxicity but human studies showing no risk. Category C comprises drugs that cause toxicity in pregnant animals, without adequate human studies, but also with benefits that may exceed their risks.

Empirical Therapy

Tables 31–3 and 31–6 list the conditions for which antimicrobial drugs may be used, along with the rec-

ommended therapy.[6, 7] There are two main indications for empirical antimicrobial therapy: travelers' diarrhea and patients with febrile, dysenteric illness.

The drug of choice for travelers' diarrhea in adults is an oral fluoroquinolone given for 1 to 3 days.[6, 7] For children, trimethoprim (TMP)-sulfamethoxazole (SMX) plus a macrolide may be given. Alternative drugs for children are nalidixic acid or azithromycin.

In cases of dysenteric diarrhea, the most common enteric pathogens are *Shigella* spp. and *C. jejuni*, with *Salmonella* spp. and *Y. enterocolitica* occurring less commonly. Empirical therapy for febrile dysentery in adults should consist of fluoroquinolones in adults and TMP-SMX plus a macrolide or nalidixic acid in children.

Treatment of Bacterial Diarrhea

Ideally, the laboratory can provide information about the presumptive or definitive diagnosis. Table 31–6 shows the current recommendations for the different specific organisms identified by the laboratory. Shigellosis should always be treated with antimicrobials to prevent secondary spread because it takes only few organisms to transmit the infection.[2, 4] The treatment of salmonellosis is more controversial. There is no doubt that systemic salmonellosis (typhoid or enteric fever, osteomyelitis, or septicemia) should be treated for at least 7 to 10 days after blood cultures are performed, and especially in immunocompromised hosts. We also advise treating severe cases of salmonellosis because of the likelihood of the patient having bacteremia. Cases of nontyphoid salmonellosis should also be treated in the patient with inflammatory bowel disease or uremia, patients undergoing hemodialysis, those taking corticosteroids, patients with sickle cell anemia, renal transplantation or any malignancy, those with aortic aneurysm, prosthetic heart valves, or vascular or orthopedic protheses, and those at the extremes of age (≤3 months and ≥65 years of age). A fluoroquinolone is recommended for all patients other than infants, to whom ceftriaxone is given. Patients with mild symptoms and nontyphoid salmonellosis and those who are asymptomatic are best not treated to prevent antibiotic-associated prolongation of excretion of the infecting organism. TMP-SMX or fluoroquino-

TABLE 31–5 ▶ FDA CATEGORIES OF SELECTED ANTIMICROBIALS USED IN TREATMENT OF INFECTIOUS DIARRHEA IN PARTURIENTS

FDA Pregnancy Risk Category	Antimicrobial Drugs
B: No risk in animal study, but no adequate human study; or toxicity in animal study, but no risk in human study	Erythromycin, azithromycin, metronidazole
C: Toxicity in animal study and no adequate human study, but benefit may exceed risk	Quinolones, trimethoprim-sulfamethoxazole, vancomycin, albendazole

FDA = U.S. Food and Drug Administration.

TABLE 31-6 ▶ ANTIBACTERIAL THERAPY FOR INFECTIOUS DIARRHEA IN ADULTS

Diagnosis	Recommended Therapy
Empirical Therapy in Bacteriologically Unconfirmed Disease	
Travelers' diarrhea	Norfloxacin 400 mg bid, ciprofloxacin 500 mg bid, levofloxacin 500 mg qd, or fleroxacin 400 mg qd for 1 to 3 days
Febrile dysenteric disease	Norfloxacin 400 mg bid, ciprofloxacin 500 mg bid, levofloxacin 500 mg qd, or fleroxacin 400 mg qd for 3 days
Persistent diarrhea	Metronidazole 250 mg qid for 7 days
Organism-Specific Diarrhea (Laboratory Confirmed)	
Cholera	Ciprofloxacin 1,000 mg single dose or 500 mg bid for 3 days, norfloxacin 400 mg bid, levofloxacin 500 mg qd, or fleroxacin 400 mg qd for 3 days, or doxycycline 300 mg single dose
Shigellosis	Norfloxacin 400 mg bid, ciprofloxacin 500 mg bid, levofloxacin 500 mg qd, or fleroxacin 400 mg qd for 3 days
Campylobacteriosis	Erythromycin 500 mg qid for 5 days, azithromycin 500 mg qd, norfloxacin 400 mg bid, ciprofloxacin 500 mg bid, levofloxacin 500 mg qd, or fleroxacin 400 mg qd for 3 days
Salmonellosis (typhoid fever and nontyphoid disease)	Norfloxacin 400 mg bid, ciprofloxacin 500 mg bid, levofloxacin 500 mg qd, or fleroxacin 400 mg qd for 7–10 days (controversy [see text] over whether intestinal nontyphoid salmonellosis without systemic infection needs antimicrobial therapy)
Aeromonas spp. or *Plesiomonas* spp.	Norfloxacin 400 mg bid, ciprofloxacin 500 mg bid, levofloxacin 500 mg qd, fleroxacin 400 mg qd, or TMP-SMX 160 mg/800 mg bid for 3 days
Yersiniosis	Norfloxacin 400 mg bid, ciprofloxacin 500 mg bid, levofloxacin 500 mg qd, fleroxacin 400 mg qd, or TMP-SMX 160 mg/800 mg bid for 3 days
Enteropathogenic *Escherichia coli* diarrhea	Susceptibility test necessary
Clostridium difficile colitis	Metronidazole 500 mg tid for 7–14 days

TMP-SMX = trimethoprim-sulfamethoxazole.

lones can also be used for treatment of *V. cholerae, Y. enterocolitica, Aeromonas,* and *Plesiomonas.*

In cases of diarrhea secondary to *C. jejuni,* the treatment of choice is one of the macrolides (especially in children) or fluoroquinolones.[4] *Clostridium difficile*–associated diarrhea should be treated with metronidazole,[11] which is less expensive and has near-equivalent efficacy compared with oral vancomycin.

Outbreaks of EPEC infection in nursery centers should be treated once specific in vitro susceptibility results are available. Antimicrobial therapy of EHEC infection is not advised because of the possibility of precipitating the occurrence of hemolytic-uremic syndrome.

Treatment of Parasitic Infections

Table 31–7 shows the current recommendations for treatment of parasitic diarrhea. In general, treatment of these diseases requires laboratory identification of the parasite, with the exception of anti-*Giardia* empiric treatment.[4, 8] Asymptomatic patients with *E. histolytica*

TABLE 31-7 ▶ ANTIPARASITIC THERAPY FOR INFECTIOUS DIARRHEA IN ADULTS

Diagnosis	Recommended Therapy
Entamoeba histolytica excretion (asymptomatic)	Iodoquinol 650 mg tid for 20 days or paramomycin 500 mg tid for 7 days
E. histolytica diarrhea	Metronidazole 750 mg tid for 5–10 days or tinidazole 1,000 mg bid for 3 days, followed by iodoquinol 650 mg tid for 20 days or paramomycin 500 mg tid for 7 days
Giardiasis	Metronidazole 250 mg tid, albendazole 400 mg qd, or quinacrine 100 mg tid for 7 days, or tinidazole 2,000-mg single dose
Cryptosporidiosis	None. In severe cases or patients with AIDS, consider paramomycin 500–750 mg tid or qid for approximately 2 wk or azithromycin 1,200 mg qd for 4 wk
Cyclospora diarrhea	TMP-SMX 160 mg/800 mg bid for 7 days, followed by 160 mg/800 mg 3×/week in patients with AIDS
Isosporiosis	TMP-SMX 160 mg/800 mg qid for 10 days, followed by 160 mg/800 mg bid for 3 weeks or pyrimethamine 75 mg qd with folinic acid 10 mg qd for 14 days
Microsporidiosis	Albendazole 400 mg bid or atovaquone 750 mg bid, followed by chronic suppression for patients with AIDS

AIDS = acquired immunodeficiency syndrome; TMP-SMX = trimethoprim-sulfamethoxazole.

should be treated to prevent relapsing disease and possible progression to liver abscess, whereas patients with intestinal disease should receive treatment against the trophozoite form (metronidazole) and the cyst form (iodoquinol). Metronidazole is the drug of choice for empiric therapy of giardiasis because it also has activity against other parasites and is effective in the treatment of small bowel bacterial overgrowth. In cryptosporidiosis, the available data are controversial.[3] The current recommendation is no therapy, except in severe cases or in symptomatic patients with HIV infection, for whom paramomycin can be used. Preliminary data suggest the efficacy of high-dose azithromycin in cryptosporidiosis. Finally, in *Isospora belli* or *Cyclospora* infections, the drug of choice is TMP-SMX, whereas in microsporidiosis the recommended drug is albendazole.[5, 6]

PREVENTION

Although diarrheal diseases in developing countries are secondary to many different factors, improvements in personal and food hygiene, and in sanitation could make a significant reduction in their high prevalence.

In the specific case of travelers to high-risk areas, education may reduce the risk of acquiring diarrhea.[6, 7] Safe foods and beverages are those served steaming hot, dry foods like bread, freshly cooked food, fruits that can be peeled, syrups and jelly, and bottled liquids. We believe drug prophylaxis has a role in certain travelers. It may be useful for a small number of people making critical trips, for people with underlying medical problems who will be put at risk for development of a more serious illness or complication, and for short-term use, and always after receiving approval from a physician and after the risks and benefits are completely understood. The drugs currently recognized to prevent travelers' diarrhea are the fluoroquinolones and bismuth subsalicylate.[6, 7, 12]

The antimicrobial agents are 80% to 90% effective in a daily dose (norfloxacin 400 mg, ciprofloxacin 500 mg, or levofloxacin 500 mg) beginning the day of travel and continuing for 1 to 2 days after returning. Bismuth subsalicylate prevents 60% to 65% of cases of diarrhea and is given in a dose of two tablets (525 mg) before meals and at bedtime (four times a day). It may cause temporary harmless darkening of the tongue and stools. In general, prophylaxis is most practical for short-term use and should be restricted to trips of 3 weeks or less. Because of the risk of side effects and the possibility of infection with a more resistant pathogen, cautious food selection and early treatment are the optimum ways to prevent or treat this disease.[6, 7]

Research is ongoing toward the development of effective vaccines against the common enteric pathogens. Promising preliminary data have accrued in vaccine development programs for immunoprophylaxis against rotavirus, *Shigella* spp., *S. typhi*, *V. cholerae*, and ETEC.

REFERENCES

1. Blacklow NR, Greenberg HB: Viral gastroenteritis. N Engl J Med 1991; 25:252.
2. Butterton JR, Calderwood SB: Acute infectious diarrheal diseases and bacterial food poisoning. In: Fauci AS, et al (eds): Harrison's Principles of Internal Medicine, 14th ed. New York, McGraw-Hill, 1998, pp 520–529.
3. Clark DP: New insights into human cryptosporidiosis. Clin Micro Rev 1999; 12:554.
4. DuPont HL: Gastrointestinal infections. In: Stein JH, et al (eds): Internal Medicine, 4th ed. St. Louis, Mosby–Year Book, 1994, pp 1915–1925.
5. DuPont HL: Review article: Infectious diarrhoea. Aliment Pharmacol Ther 1994; 8:3.
6. DuPont HL, Ericsson CD: Prevention and treatment of travelers' diarrhea. N Engl J Med 1993; 328:1821.
7. Ericsson CD, DuPont HL: Traveler's diarrhea: Approaches to prevention and treatment. Clin Infect Dis 1993; 16:616.
8. Guerrant RL, Bobak DA: Bacterial and protozoal gastroenteritis. N Engl J Med 1991; 325:327.
9. Guerrant RL: Principles and syndromes of enteric infection. In: Mandell GL, et al (eds): Mandell, Douglas and Bennett's Principles and Practice of Infectious Diseases, 4th ed. New York, Churchill Livingstone, 1995, pp 945–961.
10. Harris JC, DuPont HL, Hornick RB: Fecal leukocytes in diarrheal illness. Ann Intern Med 1972; 76:697.
11. Johnson S, Gerding DN: *Clostridium difficile*-associated diarrhea. Clin Infect Dis 1998; 26:1027.
12. Steffen R, Heusser R, DuPont HL: Prevention of travelers' diarrhea by non-antibiotic drugs. Rev Infect Dis 1986; 8(suppl 2):S151.

32 Urinary Tract Infections

LOUISE-MARIE DEMBRY ▶ VINCENT T. ANDRIOLE

Urinary tract infections are one of the most common types of infectious diseases encountered in the practice of medicine. Increased frequency of micturition accompanied by the sensation of discomfort before, during, or after voiding is a symptom complex experienced by large numbers of women at some time during their lives.[1] Urinary tract symptoms, particularly dysuria, occur in approximately 20% of women each year. Although only half of these women seek medical attention, they account for six to seven million office visits per year.[1-3] Approximately 25% to 35% of women 20 to 40 years of age have a history of a physician-diagnosed episode of urinary tract infection.[4] On average, each episode of a urinary tract infection in a young woman is associated with 6.1 days of symptoms, 2.4 days of restricted activity, 1.2 days away from school or work, and 0.4 bed days.[5] It has been estimated that the management of a single case of cystitis costs $140 and that the overall costs of evaluation and treatment of ambulatory women with dysuria approximates 1 billion dollars annually in the United States.[6]

Any discussion of urinary tract infections in women must take into account whether the patient is pregnant. Although the epidemiologic and microbiologic characteristics of pregnant women with bacteriuria are similar to those in nonpregnant women, the evaluation and treatment are different. Symptomatic urinary tract infections develop in 1% to 2% of pregnant women, and most are in patients who have persistent bacteriuria.[7] In addition, in a significant proportion of women with asymptomatic bacteriuria during pregnancy, pyelonephritis develops by late pregnancy.

DEFINITIONS

Urinary tract infections encompass a spectrum of clinical and pathologic conditions and may involve various parts of the urinary tract system. Such syndromes range from asymptomatic bacteriuria to perinephric abscesses. Urinary tract infections may be subdivided anatomically into lower and upper tract infections. In women, lower tract infection includes cystitis and urethritis and upper tract infection refers to pyelonephritis and renal abscesses. Most urinary tract infec-

tions are caused by bacteria, but they may occasionally be caused by fungi and viruses. Urine is normally a sterile body fluid, and therefore bacteria in urine is referred to as *bacteriuria*. This may reflect infection or contamination from urethral or periurethral organisms at the time of specimen collection. *Significant bacteriuria* differentiates bacteriuria of true infection from that due to contamination. *Asymptomatic bacteriuria* is a term used to refer to significant bacteriuria in a patient without urinary tract symptoms. This occurs most commonly in pregnant or elderly women. Small numbers of bacteria may enter the urinary stream as contaminants during passage through the distal urethra and over the vaginal introitus in women. The concept of significant bacteriuria differentiates between actual colonization of the bladder urine and contaminants collected during voiding. A clean-catch urine specimen contains either no bacteria or a small number of contaminants in the range of 10^2 to 10^3 bacteria/mL of urine. The recovery of small numbers of *Escherichia coli* and other uropathogens from the urine of asymptomatic women reflects colonization of the urethra or vaginal introitus. However, lower bacterial counts with uropathogens may be clinically meaningful and should not necessarily be disregarded. Bacterial counts may also be reduced by brisk diuresis and the use of suppressive antimicrobial agents.

Urinary tract infection refers to microorganisms present anywhere in the urinary tract. Urinary tract infections are also classified as uncomplicated or complicated. An uncomplicated infection of the bladder or kidney is one occurring in a normal host without structural or functional abnormalities of the urinary tract. A urinary tract infection is considered complicated in the presence of urinary calculi, cystic renal disease, obstruction, anatomic abnormalities, neurologic bladder dysfunction, or a foreign body.[8] The infection may also be classified as complicated based on the presence of host factors such as diabetes mellitus, pregnancy, transplanted kidneys, or other metabolic or immunologic conditions, and in nonambulatory elderly patients.

Recurrent urinary tract infections are divided into reinfections and relapses. In women, a relapse is defined as a recurrence of infection within 2 weeks of completion of treatment with the identical organism. Reinfection refers to infection with an organism different from the preceding infecting strain or recurrence with the same pathogen after an interval of 2 weeks or longer after treatment.[8]

PATHOGENESIS OF BACTERIURIA

Successful invasion of the urinary tract by microorganisms is determined by bacterial virulence factors, inoculum size, and host defenses. Important host factors predisposing to urinary tract infections in women include (1) urinary tract obstruction, stasis, and vesicoureteral reflux; (2) pregnancy and increased age; (3) sexual intercourse; (4) Lewis blood group nonsecretor (Le[a + b −]) and recessive (Le[a − b −]) phenotypes; (6) hyperosmolality of the renal medulla inhibiting mobilization of granulocytes into the medulla; (7) increased receptivity of uroepithelial, periurethral, and vaginal cells for uropathic coliforms in some women with recurrent infections; and (8) immunologic responses to persistence of bacterial antigen and to cross-reactivity between Tamm-Horsfall protein and gram-negative bacteria.[9]

Microorganisms can infect the urinary tract through three routes; ascending, hematogenous, and lymphatic pathways. Virtually all uropathogens enter the urinary tract by the ascending pathway. The urethra is commonly colonized with bacteria; however, these bacteria usually do not multiply in urine and are rarely responsible for urinary tract infections.[10] The female urethra is short and is close to the vulvar and perirectal areas, making contamination likely. It has been shown that the organisms that cause urinary tract infection in women also colonize the vaginal introitus and the periurethral area before urinary tract infection results.[11, 12] Once in the bladder, bacteria may multiply and pass up the ureters, particularly in the presence of vesicoureteral reflux, to the renal pelvis and parenchyma.

Pathogenic gram-negative bacilli normally present in the gut are the source of organisms causing urinary tract infections by the ascending route. The sequence leading to infection includes colonization of the introitus or periurethral area by the gut flora, subsequent extension of colonization into the urethra, and passage along the urethra into the bladder, where infection occurs if the organisms become established. The enterobacteraceae in general, and E. coli (80%) in particular, followed by Klebsiella, Proteus, and Enterobacter, are the most common organisms found in uncomplicated infections. Staphylococcus saprophyticus is the second most common cause of urinary tract infections, particularly in young women.[13] Pseudomonas, enterococci, and streptococci are responsible for the remainder of uncomplicated infections. Noncoliform organisms are more often recovered from patients with complicated

infections. In addition, unusual or fastidious bacteria may occasionally be the cause of urinary tract infections. These bacteria may be difficult to detect without a Gram stain of the urine.

Infections due to Proteus, Providencia, Morganella, strains of Pseudomonas and Klebsiella, S. saprophyticus, Corynebacterium group D2, and Ureaplasma urealyticum are of concern because they produce urease. Urease converts urea into ammonia, which has been shown to have a direct toxic effect on the kidney and inactivates the fourth component of complement in the renal medulla.[14] Ammonia tends to alkalinize the urine, which may lead to crystal formation and precipitation of struvite crystals. Struvite is the predominant component of urinary calculi and encrustations on urinary catheters. The calculi can cause obstruction and convert an uncomplicated infection into a complicated infection.

Only a few serotypes of E. coli cause most urinary tract infections. There appear to be uropathogenic clones of E. coli that are selected from the fecal flora by the presence of virulence factors that enhance both colonization and invasion of the urinary tract and the capacity to produce disease. Strains of E. coli isolated from the urine of patients with acute pyelonephritis adhere in larger numbers to freshly collected human urinary tract epithelial cells in vitro than do either fecal strains or strains recovered from asymptomatic patients.[15] The ability of E. coli to attach to urinary tract epithelial cells seems to correlate with their capacity to produce urinary tract symptoms. However, nonadhering bacteria have also been isolated from patients with acute pyelonephritis and cystitis, and adhering bacteria have been isolated from asymptomatic patients.

The expression and specificity of urovirulence determinants, particularly fimbrial adhesins, hemolysin, and aerobactin, among E. coli isolates recovered from women with urinary tract infections have been studied.[15–24] Fimbrial adhesins mediate attachment to uroepithelial cell receptor molecules. Attachment or adherence can involve a single- or multiple-receptor specificities, and attachment sites in bladder epithelial cells appear to be different from attachment sites in the kidney. Adherence of uropathogenic E. coli to the mucous membranes of the genitourinary tract appears to be necessary for virulence. Specifically, type 1 mannose-sensitive pili, which can be produced by all E. coli, bind mannose-containing glycoproteins on uroepithelial surfaces, and also bind to Tamm-Horsfall glycoprotein (uromucoid) found in human urine. Uromucoid may act as a defense mechanism by entrapping type 1 piliated E. coli, thereby preventing bacterial attachment to urinary mucosa.[19, 25] E. coli possessing P-pili (PAP or pyelonephritis-associated pili) are mannose resistant and bind to uroepithelial cells, but only to target cells containing the globoseries of glycolipids with the common disaccharide alpha-Gal-(1-4)-beta-Gal. They also have a predilection for the kidney and thus produce acute pyelonephritis.[26, 27] *E. coli* expressing P(Gal-Gal)-pili appear to be more virulent than those expressing type 1 pili and are probably essential for the production of pyelonephritis in most women with anatomically normal urinary tracts. Type 1 pili may be important in the production of cystitis.[16]

Polymorphonuclear leukocytes, which play a critical role in localizing and controlling the spread of bacterial infection in the renal parenchyma, contain mannose radicals on their membranes that act as receptors for type 1 pili. This process facilitates bacterial-phagocytic recognition and attachment and enhances nonimmune phagocytosis.[28] The glycopeptide globoseries, which act as receptors for P-pili, are not found on human polymorphonuclear leukocytes.[29] Thus, *E. coli* with P-pili are able to enhance their virulence by avoiding phagocytic cells.[30] Some strains of *E. coli* have the ability to make either or both type I or P-pili, which allows these bacteria to shed their type I pili after tissue invasion, thus avoiding phagocytic cells. The presence of adherence determinants is not typical of strains of *E. coli* associated with asymptomatic bacteriuria in patients who are colonized for long periods.[31]

Women with recurrent urinary tract infection may have more adhesin receptors on their genitourinary mucosa and thus have more binding sites for *E. coli*. Uroepithelial cells from infection-prone women bind more *E. coli* per bacterial cell on average than do cells from women not prone to urinary tract infections.[9] This finding correlates with the Lewis blood group secretor status of the patient. The cells of women with the nonsecretor phenotype (Le[a + b −]) are more readily bound by *E. coli* with Gal-Gal pili than the cells of women with the secretor phenotype. Women with recurrent urinary tract infections are more likely to be nonsecretors than women who are not prone to infections.[32]

SEXUAL ACTIVITY

The increased frequency of urinary tract infections coincident with either the onset of or, in a small subgroup of patients, with alterations in the frequency of sexual activity strongly suggests a causal relationship between these two events. Diaphragm and spermicide use has been shown to be a major contributing factor.[1, 33, 34] These studies have shown diaphragm use to be significantly more common in women with urinary tract infection than in dysuric women without urinary tract infection. *E. coli* vaginal colonization and urinary tract infection are both significantly more frequent among women with a high vaginal fluid pH, an absence of vaginal lactobacilli, or an abnormal vaginal fluid gas or liquid chromotographic pattern characteristic of bacterial vaginosis. In these studies, *E. coli* introital colonization was more frequent in women with

bacterial vaginosis. Vaginal colonization with *E. coli,* as well as the prevalence of *E. coli* bacteriuria, was also increased the morning after sexual intercourse in those women who used either diaphragm–spermicidal jelly or condom–spermicidal foam as contraceptive methods. However, these findings were not significantly increased in women who used oral contraceptives.[34] *E. coli* isolates causing cystitis in women who use diaphragms have fewer virulence determinants than those from women who do not use diaphragms. This suggests that diaphragm use may allow for infection with less virulent strains of *E. coli*.[35] Thus, the use of a diaphragm–spermicidal jelly or of condom–spermicidal foam markedly alters normal vaginal flora because spermicide (nonoxynol-9) suppresses the growth of hydrogen peroxide–producing lactobacilli in the vagina.[36] This appears to predispose the user to *E. coli* vaginal colonization and bacteriuria.

CLINICAL PRESENTATIONS

Infection may involve various parts of the urinary tract. Cystitis is an infection of the urinary bladder with symptoms of dysuria, urgency, and frequency. These symptoms are not specific because inflammation of the bladder without infection and vaginitis can present in the same manner. Of those women who seek medical attention for symptoms of frequency and dysuria, one third have the acute urethral syndrome and two thirds have significant bacteriuria by traditional criteria of greater than 10^5 bacteria/mL of urine. Of those two thirds with significant bacteriuria, half have bladder bacteriuria and the other half have renal parenchymal involvement.[37] However, patients with the acute urethral syndrome cannot be differentiated on clinical grounds alone from those with either bladder or renal bacteriuria. Frequency, burning, and suprapubic pain are found approximately equally in all three groups of patients. Costovertebral angle tenderness and elevated temperature may be present as frequently in patients with the acute urethral syndrome as in patients with renal bacteriuria, and rigors occur in approximately equal numbers of patients (15%) with the acute urethral syndrome as in those with bladder bacteriuria, although less frequently than in patients with renal bacteriuria.[38]

Women who seek medical attention for acute dysuria and frequency (after excluding patients with vaginitis) can be divided into four groups, three of which have potentially treatable infections.[39] One group has typical acute cystitis with greater than 10^5 bacteria/mL of urine on culture, usually coliforms, and pyuria (10 or more leukocytes/mm^3 of urine). The second group has bladder bacteriuria with less than 10^5 bacteria/mL of urine, also usually coliforms or *S. saprophyticus,* and pyuria. A third group has sterile bladder urine but has pyuria, which is consistent with *Chlamydia trachomatis* urethritis. A fourth group has sterile bladder urine, no pyuria, no chlamydial infection, and no recognized cause for their symptoms.[39] Women with low-count bladder bacteriuria ($<10^5$ bacteria/mL of urine) and pyuria cannot be differentiated clinically, in terms of symptoms and signs, from women with typical bacterial cystitis ($>10^5$ bacteria/mL of urine) and pyuria. However, women with the urethral syndrome due to chlamydial infection more often have a history of a new sex partner in the month before onset of symptoms, less frequently have a history of symptoms of urinary tract infections in the preceding 2 years, and more often use oral contraceptives than do women with low-count bladder bacteriuria and pyuria.[39]

These findings can be used as aids in the diagnosis and treatment of the nonpregnant woman who presents with dysuria and frequent urination.[9] Vaginitis and gonorrhea should be excluded first; then, a clean-catch, midstream voided urine specimen should be obtained for quantitative culture and for microscopic analysis of uncentrifuged urine for leukocytes and bacteria. Acute bacterial cystitis is likely if bacteria are seen with or without pyuria. If bacteria are not seen but pyuria is present microscopically, the history may help to separate women with the acute urethral syndrome due to low-count bladder bacteriuria from those with the acute urethral syndrome due to chlamydial infection. Women with low-count bladder bacteriuria are more likely to have a sudden onset of symptoms, microscopic hematuria, and suprapubic pain than those with chlamydial infection, and the culture results show low-count bacteriuria versus sterile pyuria, respectively.[39] Finally, some women have sterile urine and no pyuria and have no recognizable cause for their symptoms. Women with acute cystitis, low-count bladder bacteriuria, or chlamydial infection usually respond to antimicrobial therapy. Those women without pyuria, or the few who may have pyuria but without bladder bacteriuria or chlamydial infection, may or may not respond to antimicrobial therapy.[39]

The prevalence of asymptomatic bacteriuria in nonpregnant women rises with age at a rate of approximately 1% for each decade of life.[40] Urinary tract infection develops in up to 20% of postmenopausal women.[41] The prevalence of bacteriuria increases not only with age but with sexual activity, parity, and sickle cell trait. Other contributing factors include socioeconomic status, a history of recurrent urinary tract infections, diabetes, and anatomic or functional urinary tract abnormalities.[42, 43]

A young, sexually active woman presenting with acute dysuria usually has one of three types of infection: acute cystitis; acute urethritis caused by *C. trachomatis*, *Neisseria gonorrhoeae*, or herpes simplex virus; or vaginitis caused by *Candida* or *Trichomonas vaginalis*. A distinction between these three entities can usually be made from the history and physical examination and

simple laboratory tests. Urinary tract infection is more likely if the patient complains of urgency, suprapubic pain, flank pain, hematuria, or fever ($>38°C$); is a diaphragm–spermicide user; has symptoms that mimic those of a previously confirmed urinary tract infection; has recently undergone urethral instrumentation; has a known functional or anatomic abnormality of the urinary tract; or has suprapubic tenderness, costovertebral tenderness, or hematuria. Approximately 15% to 50% of patients with symptoms of cystitis also have evidence of occult infection of the upper urinary tract.[6] This may explain why single-dose therapy fails in some patients.

Acute pyelonephritis results from infection of the renal parenchyma and collecting system. Symptoms suggestive of pyelonephritis include flank pain, nausea, vomiting, fever ($>38°C$), and costovertebral angle tenderness. Symptoms of cystitis may not be present. The presentation varies from mild to moderate illness to a life-threatening condition with multiple organ system dysfunction and renal failure. The development of an intrarenal or perinephric abscess is uncommon but may occur as a complication of pyelonephritis or as a result of bacteremic seeding of the kidney or perinephric space.

It is important to distinguish uncomplicated from complicated urinary tract infections. The type and extent of evaluation as well as the type and duration of antimicrobial therapy are different for each entity. A complicated urinary tract infection is one associated with a condition that increases the risk for acquiring infection or failing therapy. Acute cystitis is usually considered uncomplicated. Acute pyelonephritis may be considered uncomplicated in a healthy host regardless of the causative pathogen. Patients cannot usually be definitively classified as having complicated or uncomplicated infections on presentation. It can usually be assumed that a premenopausal, sexually active, nonpregnant woman with recent onset of dysuria, frequency, or urgency who has not been instrumented or treated with antibiotics and who has no history of a genitourinary tract abnormality has an uncomplicated lower (cystitis) or upper (pyelonephritis) urinary tract infection.

DETECTION OF BACTERIURIA

A urinalysis to look for pyuria and hematuria is indicated if urinary tract infection is suspected. Pyuria is present in almost all women with acutely symptomatic urinary tract infection and in most women with urethritis caused by *N. gonorrhoeae* or *C. trachomatis*. In the absence of pyuria, an alternative diagnosis should be sought. Pyuria without significant bacteriuria in a dysuric sexually active woman suggests the diagnosis of urethritis. The most accurate method to assess pyuria is to examine an unspun, voided midstream urine specimen. Ten or more leukocytes per cubic millimeter is considered abnormal, and most women with urinary tract infection have hundreds of leukocytes per cubic millimeter.

A single catheterization of the urinary bladder, properly performed to obtain urine for quantitative culture, requires less cooperation from the patient than other methods of urine collection. It also has the advantage of avoiding heavy vaginal contamination of the urine in women. However, a single catheterization carries a 4% to 6% risk of introducing infection and is not justified merely to obtain a urine specimen for diagnostic purposes. The clean-catch method has the important advantage of decreasing the risk of introducing infection compared with catheterization. The patient must be properly instructed in how to obtain the specimen to decrease the chance of contamination. The urine should be refrigerated once collected. The specimen can be refrigerated for up to 1 week without a significant impact on the number of bacteria.[44]

A number of methods are used to quantitate the bacterial count in the urine. The pour plate dilution technique is the most precise and continues to serve as the reference standard with which semiquantitative methods are compared. Its use in clinical laboratories, however, is not practical because of the time required to do this test. More practical tests are commonly used and include the standardized calibrated inoculating loop and the streak plate methods. Relatively accurate results are obtained with these methods. The dip-slide technique is the best available semiquantitative method that is also adaptable to use in the office setting.[45] Modifications of this technique have been developed. These methods are all based on the growth of bacteria on media.

Several indirect chemical tests have been developed to screen for the presence of significant bacteriuria. One such test is the LN strip test (Chemstrip LN), which is simple and rapid. The LN strip detects the presence of both leukocyte esterase (as an indicator of pyuria) and nitrite (as an indicator of bacteriuria). The sensitivity of the LN strip is approximately 89% for specimens with more than 10^5 bacteria/mL of urine. One in every nine patients with high-level ($>10^5$ bacteria/mL of urine) bacteriuria was missed by this test. It also missed one in every five patients with more than 10^4 bacteria/mL of urine.[46] These findings limit the usefulness of the LN strip as a means for routine screening of unselected urine specimens for bacteriuria. The leukocyte esterase test alone has a sensitivity of 75% to 96% and a specificity of 94% to 98% for detecting greater than 10 leukocytes per high-power field. Although the chemical tests are simple to use and provide more rapid results, their sensitivity and specificity are not comparable with those of the semiquantitative culture methods.

Examination of a drop of uncentrifuged urine under the microscope using the high-power lens has been used as a rapid screening tool. Significant bacteriuria is present approximately 20% of the time when no bacteria are seen in the unspun drop of urine.[45] In addition, this technique does not allow for bacteriologic identification and antibiotic susceptibility testing.

Quantitative culture of the urine helps to distinguish significant bacteriuria from contamination. Infection is usually present when 10^5 bacteria/mL of urine or more are present in culture. Bacterial colony counts less than 10^4/mL of urine have traditionally been thought to reflect contamination when the urine is obtained by the clean-catch void technique or catheterization. However, studies have since shown that in women with acute uncomplicated urinary tract infection, the criterion of 10^5 bacteria/mL of urine has a high specificity but a low sensitivity.[47] Up to one third of women with symptoms of acute cystitis have only 100 to 10,000 colonies of *E. coli, S. saprophyticus,* or other pathogens per milliliter of midstream urine on culture. Studies have shown that in women with acute dysuria, frequency, urgency, and pyuria on urinalysis, urine cultures with 100 or more colonies of a uropathogen per milliliter of urine have the highest sensitivity and specificity for identifying acute urinary tract infection.[1, 48] The presence of 100 bacteria/mL of urine can be difficult for most clinical laboratories to detect. Thus, it has been suggested that a minimum colony count of 1,000 bacteria/mL of urine be used in determining the presence of urinary tract infection in women. This cut-off provides a higher specificity and only a slightly lower sensitivity than the cut-off of 100 bacteria/mL of urine.[48]

Approximately 80% of women with acute uncomplicated pyelonephritis have 10^5 bacterial colonies per milliliter of urine. A total of 10% to 15% have between 10^4 and 10^5 bacteria per milliliter of urine, and the remainder have smaller numbers of bacteria isolated from a midstream urine specimen.[49]

Asymptomatic bacteriuria requires more rigid criteria. No change in the traditional criterion is used for this group. Two consecutive midstream urine cultures yielding the same organism with colony counts of greater than 10^5 bacteria/mL of urine in an asymptomatic woman with bacteriuria has a sensitivity and specificity of greater than 95%.

MANAGEMENT OF URINARY TRACT INFECTIONS

Empiric therapy without obtaining a urine culture is a cost-effective approach to the care of selected women with dysuria and frequency.[50–52] Many physicians treat patients for presumptive urinary tract infections without pretreatment urine cultures. Urine cultures probably are not essential in selected young women with clear signs and symptoms of acute dysuria and pyuria and in whom the probability of uncomplicated bacterial cystitis is high.[51] These patients usually respond to short-course therapy that can be given empirically, and urine cultures can be reserved for those who fail therapy.

Based on current evidence, reasonable and practical guidelines for diagnostic urine cultures in the care of patients with urinary tract infections have been suggested.[51] The general arguments in favor of urine culture include accurate diagnosis of infection, determination of antimicrobial susceptibility of the infecting bacteria, and identification of patients with covert bacteriuria in whom treatment prevents complications. Evidence suggests that urine cultures are needed to distinguish urinary tract infections from vaginitis and sexually transmitted diseases caused by *C. trachomatis, N. gonorrhoeae,* or herpes simplex virus urethritis; in infants, children, and the elderly, because clinical manifestations of urinary tract infection are often nonspecific in these patients; in patients with pyelonephritis or complicated urinary tract infections; in relapsing infections; in women who fail short-course therapy; in pregnant patients with covert bacteriuria; in patients about to undergo urologic surgery; and in symptomatic patients with catheter- or instrument-associated nosocomial infection.[51] These guidelines may not apply to all patients in each group.

Post-treatment urine cultures should be obtained in those patients previously mentioned, among whom pretreatment urine cultures are used to establish a diagnosis of urinary tract infection, and when symptoms persist or recur among patients treated empirically without pretreatment culture confirmation of infection.[53]

Therapy for Uncomplicated Urinary Tract Infection

The use of single-dose therapy for uncomplicated lower urinary tract infections in women has been advocated during the past by some investigators,[54, 55] but questioned by others.[1, 48, 56–59] Single-dose therapy is effective in treating many women with acute cystitis if the organism is susceptible. This treatment regimen is less expensive and is associated with significantly fewer side effects. However, infection recurs in a significant proportion of patients.[1, 48, 56–59] Single-dose therapy has been found to be less efficacious in controlled trials than 3 or more days of therapy.[1, 48, 56–59] Also, single-dose therapy with oral beta-lactam antibiotics appears to be less effective than similar regimens with trimethoprim or trimethoprim-sulfamethoxazole.[48] Similar failure rates (approximately 20%) have been observed with the newer quinolones used as oral single-dose agents.[56] This failure rate is comparable with that observed for single-dose therapy with other antimicrobial agents.[60] Based on these observations, single-dose regi-

mens may no longer be the preferred therapy for women with acute cystitis. In contrast, studies have shown that 3-day therapy with trimethoprim-sulfamethoxazole or the newer quinolones predictably cures approximately 95% of women clinically and microbiologically if they are infected with a susceptible pathogen.[56, 60, 61] A 3-day course of therapy appears to be sufficient in most women with uncomplicated lower urinary tract infections because longer courses of therapy do not achieve significantly higher cure rates.[56, 62] Although the quinolones are effective, they are expensive and there is concern about the emergence of bacterial resistance to this group of agents. Unfortunately, increasing numbers of uropathogenic organisms are resistant to ampicillin/amoxicillin. Women with the urethral syndrome due to chlamydial infection respond to a tetracycline given for 7 days or to a single 1-g dose of the newer macrolide azithromycin.

Approximately one third of patients who have typical symptoms of uncomplicated acute cystitis also have occult renal infection.[48] Occult renal infection has been argued to be responsible for single-dose failures or relapses by some investigators, but other studies have failed to confirm these findings.[48, 52, 59] In fact, data suggest that trimethoprim or trimethoprim-sulfamethoxazole eradicates occult renal infection more effectively than single-dose therapy with other agents, although a longer course (e.g., 10 days) of therapy might prove to be more effective.[48] Antimicrobial effects on the fecal and vaginal flora may influence outcome of therapy.[63] Antibiotics that eradicate gram-negative aerobes from the bowel and vagina but have little effect on the anaerobic flora may have an advantage in providing long-term cure of uncomplicated urinary tract infections. The property of colonization resistance may be preserved by maintaining the normal vaginal flora. Amoxicillin and first-generation cephalosporins affect the anaerobic flora, which may allow for reinfection, particularly if gram-negative rods are not eradicated from those sites.

Therapy for Acute Uncomplicated Pyelonephritis

Selected patients with acute uncomplicated pyelonephritis may be candidates for outpatient oral therapy.[64–66] Oral therapy with trimethoprim-sulfamethoxazole or a quinolone for 2 weeks is effective for managing mild acute pyelonephritis in outpatients.[64] This approach is considerably less expensive than inpatient therapy.[65] However, it must be restricted to patients who can be managed in the outpatient setting and should not be used in patients with uncomplicated acute pyelonephritis who are sufficiently ill to require hospitalization. Patients should be considered for hospitalization and administration of parenteral therapy if they are unable to maintain adequate oral hydration or take medications, if there are concerns regarding compliance, or if there is an uncertain diagnosis, severe illness with high fever, severe pain, or marked debility. Patients with known or suspected complicated pyelonephritis such as pregnant women or those with a history of recent urinary catheterization or urinary stones, or a known structural or neurologic abnormality of the urinary tract, should also be admitted and treated with intravenous antibiotics.[64] Intravenous antibiotics are continued until the patient shows significant clinical improvement, at which time oral therapy can be initiated to complete a 14-day course of treatment.

Therapy for Recurrent Urinary Tract Infections

Although short-course antibiotic therapy appears to be the optimal approach to the management of acute episodes of lower urinary tract infection in women, many of these patients have recurrent infections. A number of therapeutic options are available and may be useful in decreasing the frequency of recurrent episodes of infection. Some women have frequent recurrent reinfections caused by new bacterial species or new serotypes; these reinfections tend to occur in clusters.[67] Each infection sets the stage for the next episode, and the longer the interval between infections, the less likely there will be a recurrence.[12] The precise therapy for women with recurrent disease of the reinfection type, whether it is relatively infrequent or highly frequent recurrent disease, has not been well established. Prophylactic therapy in the form of one-half tablet of trimethoprim-sulfamethoxazole (containing 40 mg of trimethoprim and 200 mg of sulfamethoxazole) given three times weekly at bedtime for 6 months is effective prophylaxis for recurrent urinary tract infections of the reinfection type in women.[68] Although this regimen did not predispose to colonization or infection with trimethoprim-resistant Enterobacteriaceae, these women did not lose their propensity for reinfection once prophylaxis was discontinued, and fewer than 10% remained free of infection during a 6-month follow-up period.[68]

Although the role of sexual intercourse in the pathogenesis of recurrent urinary tract infections is not fully understood, some women clearly relate their recurrent episodes to recent intercourse, particularly an increase in the frequency of sexual intercourse. A single dose of an oral antimicrobial agent immediately after coitus has been shown to reduce the incidence of recurrent infections that seem to be associated with sexual intercourse.[69] Prophylaxis should begin only after the current episode of bacteriuria has been eradicated. These patients may also benefit from complete emptying of their bladder at regular intervals and after intercourse.[45]

URINARY TRACT INFECTIONS DURING PREGNANCY

Pregnancy leads to important physiologic and anatomic changes that in turn contribute significantly to the persistence of bacteriuria in pregnancy. Bacteriuria in pregnancy increases the possibility of symptomatic upper tract infection in untreated women, particularly in the third trimester of pregnancy. The significant changes in the urinary tract during pregnancy affect the acquisition and natural history of bacteriuria.[70] In pregnancy, bacteriuria is more likely to be persistent and is associated with subsequent development of symptomatic urinary tract infection. The physiologic changes of the collecting system during pregnancy have the greatest impact on bacteriuria.[71] Hydroureter of pregnancy begins with dilation of the renal pelvis and ureters during the seventh week of gestation, gradually progressing until term. After delivery, the dilated ureter rapidly returns to normal. It is approximately one third of normal by 1 week post partum, another one third by 1 month, and almost completely normal by the second month after delivery. In general, the entire urinary tract reverts to normal by the second month of the puerperium.[72, 73]

Dilatation of the upper collecting system occurs in most pregnancies and extends down to the level of the pelvic brim. The dilated ureters may contain over 200 mL of urine and contribute significantly to the persistence of bacteriuria in pregnancy.[73] These changes are more pronounced on the right than the left because of the drop of the right ureter into the pelvic cavity, although other factors, such as placental placement, may also be important.[70, 74] Hormonal changes also lead to decreased ureteral peristalsis after the second month of gestation, with long periods of complete atony present in the seventh and eighth months of pregnancy.[75] Both mechanical and hormonal changes contribute to the development of hydroureter.

In addition, the kidneys increase in length during the course of gestation by approximately 1 cm, and the bladder undergoes a relative change in position, becoming an abdominal rather than a pelvic organ.[76] The bladder may also have an increased capacity resulting from a progressive decrease in tone secondary to hormonal factors.[77] Late in pregnancy, the bladder may contain double its usual volume without discomfort.[70] These physiologic changes of the urinary tract are more likely to occur during first pregnancies or in women who have had their pregnancies in rapid succession.

Hormonal changes may also lead to other factors that result in an increased susceptibility to urinary tract infections. Estrogen may facilitate infection with *E. coli* strains that have a propensity for upper tract infection.[78] The increased frequency of symptomatic urinary tract infections noted in the third trimester of pregnancy may be caused by physiologic and anatomic effects of estrogens in late pregnancy. Similar physiologic urinary tract changes have also been described in women taking oral contraceptives, who also have a notably increased frequency of bacteriuria.[79-81]

Other physiologic changes may contribute to the increased susceptibility to symptomatic urinary tract infections in pregnancy. For example, urine flow rates may initially be increased in pregnancy but, as the ureters dilate, urinary stasis also increases.[74] A decrease in the concentrating ability of the kidney may also cause a decrease in the natural antibacterial activity of urine and, in the presence of bacteriuria, an increase in susceptibility to upper tract infection.[82] Gestational glucosuria also contributes to bacteriuria in pregnancy.[73]

Epidemiology and Microbiology of Bacteriuria in Pregnancy

The epidemiology of bacteriuria in pregnancy is similar to that in nonpregnant women.[83] The overall prevalence of bacteriuria in pregnancy ranges from 4% to 7%, although in certain subpopulations, rates may vary from as low as less than 2% to as high as over 10%.[84, 85] The prevalence of bacteriuria may be as high as 25% when culturing techniques for fastidious organisms are used.[86] It is not clear whether *Ureaplasma urealyticum* and *Gardnerella vaginalis,* found in the bladder urine of some pregnant women, play significant pathogenic roles. Prevalence rates of bacteriuria as high as 11% have been seen in socioeconomically disadvantaged patients, compared with approximately 2% in patients screened in private clinics.[79] Sickle cell trait has been cited as another association with bacteriuria, likely reflecting renal parenchymal damage.[87, 88] In addition, people with anatomic or functional abnormalities, such as neurogenic bladder secondary to spinal cord injury, have an increased rate of urinary tract infections and also have higher rates of bacteriuria in pregnancy.

Most women with bacteriuria at delivery have been shown to be bacteriuric at the first prenatal visit, although approximately 1% to 2% acquire bacteriuria only later in pregnancy.[84] The optimal time of screening for bacteriuria was evaluated in a large study of 3,254 pregnant women.[85] The risk of acquiring bacteriuria during pregnancy increased with the duration of pregnancy, from 0.8% in the 12th gestational week to 1.93% at the end of pregnancy. Furthermore, the risk for onset of bacteriuria was highest between the 9th and 17th weeks of gestation. Screening at the 16th gestational week seemed to be the optimal time to obtain a single screening for bacteriuria because treatment given at that time provides the greatest number of bacteriuria-free gestational weeks.[85]

Because relatively few women become bacteriuric during the course of pregnancy and because there is no evidence to suggest that bacteriuria present early in pregnancy has been acquired at the time of or since conception, it seems likely that the frequency of symptomatic urinary tract infections during pregnancy reflects asymptomatic bacteriuria acquired earlier in life or later, such as with the onset of sexual activity. The changes that take place in the urinary tract during pregnancy may simply permit urinary colonization established before pregnancy to progress to persistent bacteriuria that may lead to symptomatic upper tract infection. However, although past history of urinary tract infection is more common in bacteriuric patients, it is not possible to identify accurately a subpopulation at risk on that basis alone.[40, 89] Bladder catheterization has been associated with an increased risk for bacteriuria in pregnancy and should be avoided if possible. Bacterial colonization after catheterization may lead to the development of symptomatic infection in those women.

The etiologic agents associated with bacteriuria in pregnant and nonpregnant women are similar. Most organisms recovered by routine culture techniques are coliforms, with *E. coli* the most common. Organisms in the *Klebsiella-Enterobacter* group, *Proteus mirabilis,* and others are much less common.[82] Gram-positive organisms have received increased attention as causes of bacteriuria and urinary tract infections. *S. saprophyticus* and other coagulase-negative staphylococci are seen in a small percentage of pregnant women and are important causes of urinary tract infections and complications, including stone formation.[13, 90] *Streptococcus agalactiae* is also uncommon (<1%) in true infection, and is more commonly isolated as a contaminant from the normal vaginal flora. Enterococci have also been isolated, but are infrequently associated with symptomatic upper urinary tract infection. Many of the gram-positive organisms have been associated with symptomatic low-colony-count (<10^5 organisms/mL of urine) infection in nonpregnant women, but the significance of these low colony counts in asymptomatic pregnant women is not well established.[91]

Improved culture techniques have led to the detection of increased numbers of anaerobic and other fastidious microorganisms. These organisms have been found to be present in an even larger percentage of pregnant women than organisms more commonly associated with bacteriuria.[86, 92, 93] These organisms are often isolated in low (<10^5 bacteria/mL of urine) numbers and include *G. vaginalis,* lactobacilli, microaerophilic streptococci, *C. trachomatis,* and *U. urealyticum.*[94] *Ureaplasma urealyticum* and *G. vaginalis* may be isolated in the bladder urine of an additional 10% to 15% of pregnant women. It is unclear whether these organisms play a significant pathogenic role, although improved outcomes after therapy have been reported.[86, 95, 96]

Significance of Bacteriuria in Pregnancy

Although the risk of development of a symptomatic urinary tract infection in pregnant women with asymptomatic bacteriuria is well established, the relationship of bacteriuria and symptomatic urinary tract infection with other maternal and fetal complications remains unclear.[82, 85, 97, 98] Many complications of pregnancy have been attributed to urinary tract infections during gestation, including preterm labor, low birth weight, and growth retardation. Other associations are less well established, such as the role of bacteriuria in hypertension during pregnancy, anemia, and the long-term risk for maternal renal complications.[96, 99]

Early studies demonstrated that 20% to 40% of women with bacteriuria detected early in pregnancy and not treated have acute symptomatic infection later in pregnancy.[90, 100] Only 1% to 2% of women seen early in pregnancy and found not to have bacteriuria at that time acquire symptomatic urinary tract disease.[84] Postpartum urinary tract infections are also more common in women with bacteriuria during pregnancy. In women who have symptomatic urinary tract infections during pregnancy, the role of acute pyelonephritis and premature delivery is established, with rates of prematurity ranging from 20% to 50% in pregnant women with symptomatic urinary tract infections. The association between acute pyelonephritis during pregnancy and premature delivery was well documented in the preantibiotic era.[40, 101] Most other studies have confirmed the association between pyelonephritis and an increased rate of preterm labor, and have shown that successful treatment of bacteriuria prevents the development of pyelonephritis.[40, 102, 103] Successful treatment of bacteriuria in pregnancy reduces the rate of subsequent symptomatic urinary tract infections by 80% to 90%.[84, 104] Prevention of symptomatic infection is directly related to the success in eradicating bacteriuria. Symptomatic infection is much more likely to develop in those patients who do not have clearance of bacteriuria with antimicrobial therapy.[7]

The mechanisms for premature labor in patients with symptomatic infection are not completely clear. Production of phospholipase A2 by bacteria may in turn initiate labor prostaglandin activation.[43] E. coli and other gram-negative bacteria can produce phospholipase A2.[105] Although these effects occur with intra-amniotic infections, the development of amnionitis in association with symptomatic urinary tract infection could lead to premature labor.[96] There is a well established association between symptomatic urinary tract infections and premature delivery. In contrast, the relationship between asymptomatic bacteriuria and prematurity and fetal mortality remains controversial. Kass[100, 106] reported in 1959 and 1960 that women with asymptomatic bacteriuria had higher rates of prematurity. These studies also suggested that eradicating the bacteriuria significantly reduced the rate of premature delivery. Subsequent studies have evaluated the relationship between bacteriuria and prematurity. Although most of the studies have not supported Kass' initial observations, a meta-analysis of published data supported an association of low birth weight or preterm delivery with untreated bacteriuria during pregnancy, and showed that eradication of bacteriuria improved the outcome of pregnancy.[83, 84, 87, 96, 107, 108] Other coexisting factors may also contribute to an unfavorable outcome, such as socioeconomic status, which is inversely correlated with preterm labor and delivery.[43] Others have noted an increased rate of prematurity in women with bacteriuria, but no alteration in the trend due to treatment.[109] Although some studies have shown an increased rate of prematurity in women with bacteriuria, most studies are small and may not distinguish coexisting risk factors.[108]

The efficacy of therapy is greater, and the consequences of symptomatic infection appear to be less, when bacteriuria is of bladder origin. The difficulty in establishing a renal or bladder origin of bacteriuria has resulted in difficulty in evaluating the effect of treatment on eventual symptomatic infection and increased prematurity.[110] No difference in pregnancy outcome between bacteriuric patients and control subjects was found in one study, regardless of whether the bacteriuria was of bladder or renal origin.[102] However, intrapartum pyelonephritis was associated with preterm labor. Another study found that pregnancies complicated by urinary tract infection were associated with a 2.4-fold increased fetal mortality rate compared with the overall fetal mortality rates in the same geographic area.[111] The same study reported increased risks for prematurity, intrauterine growth retardation, and low birth weight in patients with bacteriuria compared with control subjects. Rates were unchanged when adjusted for age, race, and obstetric history, although no conclusion could be drawn about the influence of treatment of urinary tract infections.

The incidence of prematurity seems to be increased in bacteriuric compared with nonbacteriuric women, and it is probably increased specifically in those women with renal involvement. Most studies have not shown a decreased incidence of prematurity with successful treatment of bacteriuria, an association that does not support bacteriuria as a cause of prematurity. Asymptomatic bacteriuria is only one factor in the complex issue of prematurity. The long-term consequences of renal damage are probably not caused by bacteriuria but rather reflect the degree of underlying renal disease.

Detection of Asymptomatic Bacteriuria in Pregnancy

Asymptomatic bacteriuria in pregnancy is clearly associated with the risk of development of symptomatic pyelonephritis later in pregnancy and may also be associated with other maternal and fetal complications of pregnancy. Rates of bacteriuria vary significantly in certain populations, and no clear predictors of bacteriuria in pregnancy have been established.[112] A strategy for screening pregnant women is warranted to effectively detect bacteriuric pregnant women before the development of symptomatic infection and to provide early treatment. However, because of the large expense in screening all pregnant women and the risks to mother and fetus in receiving antimicrobial therapy during gestation, screening must be done in the most cost-effective manner and treatment should be tailored to minimize the risks of therapy.[113, 114]

Symptomatic infections develop in 20% to 40% of the 4% to 7% of pregnant women with bacteriuria, but screening cultures detect only 40% to 70% of women in whom symptomatic infections develop.[97] Estimates are that as many as 1% to 2% of women with negative initial cultures have symptomatic infection during pregnancy.[70] Although not all women at risk for symptomatic infection are detected, screening and treatment of bacteriuria eliminates a small but definite number of symptomatic infections and the complications that follow. The prevalence of infection in the population to be screened as well as the associated costs must be considered in any recommendations for screening.

The costs associated with screening have been used to argue against screening for bacteriuria during pregnancy. Less costly, nonculture methods for establishing significant bacteriuria, such as nitrite dipstick and urinalysis, are in general less successful than culture-based methods. Women with bacteriuria often give a history of urinary tract infections. However, this information, even in a subgroup at higher risk, is too nonspecific to distinguish a group that should be screened.[112] Similarly, signs of inflammation as determined by pyuria, proteinuria, and urine sediment casts do not necessarily correlate with significant bacteriuria.[115]

A large Swedish study evaluated the timing of bacteriuria screening.[94] The risk of bacteriuria during pregnancy increased from 0.8% in the 12th gestational week to 1.93% by the end of pregnancy. The highest rates were detected during the 9th to 17th weeks of gestation. The optimal time of screening to provide the greatest number of bacteriuria-free gestational weeks was found to be 16 weeks.[85] Screening cultures are recommended for all women early in pregnancy, and consideration should be given to obtaining these cultures during the 16th week of gestation.[96] The initial prenatal visit is a still a reasonable time for screening because few women acquire bacteriuria during the course of pregnancy. Urine cultures are the only satisfactory method for establishing the diagnosis of bacteriuria, and the most cost-effective and reliable means of collecting and culturing the urine should be used.

Women with negative initial cultures usually do not require further testing unless they have a history of recurrent urinary tract infections. Positive screening cultures should be confirmed with a quantitative culture. This allows for the identification of the etiologic agent and the performance of antimicrobial susceptibility testing.

The presence of bacteria on examination of an uncentrifuged drop of urine under high power is rapid, inexpensive, and suggestive of significant bacteriuria. The presence of any bacteria detected in this manner correlates with at least 10^5 bacteria/mL of urine, but it is not sensitive enough to allow its use as a screening procedure for asymptomatic bacteriuria.

Management and Therapy of Urinary Tract Infections in Pregnancy

Studies of the natural history of bacteriuria in pregnancy have provided guidelines for the treatment of asymptomatic bacteriuria in pregnancy. In a significant percentage of pregnant women with asymptomatic bacteriuria, a symptomatic infection develops. Which patients will ultimately have a symptomatic infection usually is unpredictable, although persistent bacteriuria despite treatment is associated with the development of a symptomatic infection. Thus, the recommendation is that all pregnant patients with bacteriuria be treated, and follow-up cultures obtained to document response to therapy. Treatment should be as brief and nontoxic as possible because of the concerns of toxicity to mother and fetus.[116] An initial screening culture should be done on all patients at the first prenatal visit, preferably in the first trimester.[70] Initial screening can be done with a dipstick culture, which is relatively accurate and an inexpensive screening tool. Women with a negative screening culture can be followed up with routine antenatal care. However, women with a history of recurrent urinary tract infections may be at higher risk for development of infection later in pregnancy, despite an initial negative culture.[112] For these women, consideration should be given to reculturing their urine at the beginning of the third trimester. Any positive dipstick culture should be confirmed with a quantitative culture, which also allows for identification of the organism and the performance of antimicrobial susceptibility testing. A serum creatinine measurement should also be obtained in patients with positive urine cultures.

The duration of therapy for bacteriuria of pregnancy has received much attention. Early studies used continuous therapy until term because of the concern about treatment failures after short-course therapy.[100, 109] More recent studies have shown shorter courses of therapy to be as effective as continuous therapy, and they may decrease the potential toxicity of long courses of antimicrobial use to the mother and fetus.[117, 118]

Ideally, therapy should be guided by the results of antimicrobial susceptibility testing. Many short-course regimens have been shown to be effective in eliminating bacteriuria of pregnancy. Approximately 70% to 80% of patients initially treated with 7 to 10 days of antibiotics have clearance of bacteriuria, and similar efficacy rates have been reported after 3-day regimens.[91] Other studies have evaluated single-dose therapy for bacteriuria in pregnant women.[119–122] Initial cure rates in pregnant women were lower (50% to 60%) compared with 7 to 10-day courses of therapy.[120] Short-course therapy (either 3 or 7 to 10 days) seems more effective than single-dose therapy in eradicating bacteriuria in pregnant women, as well as in nonpregnant women, because the drugs are rapidly cleared from the urine. Thus, short-course over single-dose therapy is recommended for bacteriuria in pregnancy.[70] Not only is the length of therapy important, but the appropriate follow-up cultures must be obtained to document the elimination of bacteriuria.[91] Most of the organisms isolated are susceptible to ampicillin, which is not only well tolerated in the non–penicillin-allergic patient but provides high urinary tract concentrations. Ampicillin has been extensively used in pregnancy and does not seem to be harmful to the mother or fetus. Amoxicillin is also effective and well tolerated and can be given as 250 mg three times a day for a 3- or 7-day course for initial therapy. Unfortunately, increasing numbers of urinary isolates are showing resistance to ampicillin/amoxicillin, so treatment should be based on antibiotic susceptibility test results. Nitrofurantoin is an equally effective and nontoxic agent for patients who are allergic to penicillin or infected with ampicillin-resistant organisms. Nitrofurantoin has been given as a single 200-mg dose or 100 mg four times a day for 3 days, but there is more experience in pregnancy with a full 7-day course.[77, 97, 123] One gram of sulfisoxazole followed by 500 mg every 6 hours for 7 days is a traditional regimen and may also be effective in a single, one-time dose of 2 g.[123] However, sulfisoxazole should be avoided near term because of its association with hyperbilirubinemia.[124] Nitrofurantoin and sulfisoxazole are occasionally associated with hemolytic anemia caused by glucose-6-phosphate dehydrogenase deficiency. Short-course therapy with other agents, such as amoxicillin-clavulanic acid and trimethoprim-sulfamethoxazole, is also effective.[125, 126] They are not usually recommended as first-line therapy, however, because of the lack of clinical experience in pregnancy or because of potential or unknown toxicity risks during pregnancy. Treatment failures with short-course therapy may be an indication of the presence of an antimicrobial-resistant infecting organism or renal infection.[72, 122]

A follow-up urine culture should be done approximately 1 week after completion of antimicrobial therapy. If the urine is sterile, the patient should have monthly urine cultures until delivery. Short-course therapy may fail to clear the infection in as many as 20% to 30% of patients. These patients should undergo an additional 7- to 10-day course of therapy with a different agent based on the results of susceptibility testing. Approximately half the patients receiving a second course of therapy still fail to clear their bacteriuria or have a recurrence with the same organism. This is an indication of possible upper urinary tract infection or a structural abnormality.[115]

Only a few patients fail to respond to an initial course of therapy (ampicillin, sulfisoxazole, or nitrofurantoin) followed by a second course with a different agent. In vitro susceptibility data can be used as a guide to the further selection of antimicrobial drugs in the small number of patients who have not responded to two courses of therapy. However, further oral therapy is not likely to be successful. After eradication of recurrent or persistent infection, suppressive therapy with an agent to which the organism is susceptible is recommended. Nitrofurantoin, 50 to 100 mg nightly until delivery, can be used as a suppressive agent.[127] Frequent urine cultures should be obtained to detect the possibility of reinfection by a resistant organism. Follow-up cultures should be done after delivery in all women with recurrent or persistent bacteriuria, and a urologic evaluation of the urinary tract should be undertaken 3 to 6 months after delivery.[128]

The clinical presentation of pyelonephritis in pregnant women is similar to that in nonpregnant women.[115, 129] The therapeutic approaches are also similar for upper tract disease in pregnant women.[77] Intravenous antibiotics, such as ampicillin with an aminoglycoside, should be used for initial therapy. More than 95% of patients have a response within 72 hours.[124] After clinical response to intravenous therapy, therapy may be completed with an oral regimen that should be continued to complete a 14-day course, which should then be followed by suppressive therapy until the time of delivery.[130] If the patient does not respond within 72 hours, other diagnoses should be considered, or the patient should undergo ultrasound imaging of the kidneys.[70]

SUMMARY

Urinary tract infections in women are not uncommon. It is important to distinguish between urinary tract infections occurring during pregnancy and those occurring in nonpregnant women. In addition, the clinician must also distinguish uncomplicated from complicated urinary tract infections because the management and therapy differ. This chapter reviews the epidemiology, pathogenesis, clinical presentation, laboratory diagnosis, and therapy and management of urinary tract infections in women, including those occurring during pregnancy.

REFERENCES

1. Stamm WE, Hooton TM, Johnson JR, et al: Urinary tract infections: From pathogenesis to treatment. J Infect Dis 1989; 159:400.
2. Schappert SM: National ambulatory medical care survey: 1992 summary. In: Advanced Data from Vital Health Statistics. DHHS publication no. 253 (PHS). Hyattsville, MD, National Center for Health Statistics, 1994, p 94.
3. Patton JP, Nash DB, Arbutyn E: Urinary tract infection: Economic considerations. Med Clin North Am 1991; 75:495.
4. Kunin CM: The concepts of significant bacteriuria. In: Detection, Prevention and Management of Urinary Tract Infections, 4th ed. Philadelphia, Lea & Febiger, 1987, p 82.
5. Foxman B, Frerichs RR: Epidemiology of urinary tract infection: I. Diaphragm use and sexual intercourse. Am J Public Health 1985; 75:1308.
6. Johnson JR, Stamm WE: Urinary tract infections in women: Diagnosis and treatment. Ann Intern Med 1989; 11:906.
7. Condie AP, Williams JD, Reeves DS, et al: Complications of bacteriuria in pregnancy. In: O'Grady F, Brumfitt W (eds): Urinary Tract Infection. London, Oxford University Press, 1968, pp 148–159.
8. Ronald AR, Pattullo ALS: The natural history of urinary infections in adults. Med Clin North Am 1991; 75:299.
9. Andriole VT: Urinary tract infections. In: Glass RH (ed): Office Gynecology, 4th ed. Baltimore, William & Wilkins, 1992, pp 387–401.
10. Sobel JD: Pathogens of urinary tract infections. Infect Dis Clin North Am 1997; 11:531.
11. Stamey TA, Timothy M, Millar M, et al: Recurrent urinary infections in adult women: The role of introital enterobacteria. Calif Med 1971; 115:1.
12. Kunin CM, Polyak F, Postel E: Periurethral bacterial flora in women: Prolonged intermittent colonization with Escherichia coli. JAMA 1980; 243:134.
13. Hovelius B, Mardh P: Staphylococcus saprophyticus as a common cause of urinary tract infections. Rev Infect Dis 1984; 6:328.
14. Kunin C: Urinary tract infections in females. Clin Infect Dis 1994; 18:1.
15. Svanborg-Eden C, Hanson LA, Jodal U, et al: Variable adherence to normal human urinary tract epithelial cells of Escherichia coli strains associated with various forms of urinary tract infection. Lancet 1976; 1:490.
16. O'Hanely P, Lark D, Falkow S, et al: Molecular basis of Escherichia coli colonization of the urinary tract in BALB/c mice: Gal-Gal pili immunization prevent Escherichia coli pyelonephritis in the BALB/c mouse model of human pyelonephritis. J Clin Invest 1985; 75:347.
17. Svanborg-Eden C, Jodel U: Attachment of Escherichia coli to urinary sediment epithelioid cells from urinary tract infection–prone and healthy children. Infect Immun 1979; 26:837.
18. Schaeffer AJ, Jones JM, Dunn JK: Association of in vitro Escherichia coli adherence to vaginal and buccal epithelial cells with susceptibility of women to recurrent urinary tract infections. N Engl J Med 1981; 304:1062.
19. Andriole VT: Urinary tract infections: Recent developments. J Infect Dis 1987; 156:865.
20. Fowler JE, Stamey TA: Studies of introital colonization in women with recurrent urinary infections: VII. The role of bacterial adherence. J Urol 1977; 177:472.
21. Svanborg-Eden C, Eriksson B, Hanson LA: Adhesion of Escherichia coli to human uroepithelial cells in vitro. Infect Immun 1977; 18:767.
22. Kallenius G, Winberg J: Bacterial adherence to periurethral epithelial cells in girls prone to urinary tract infections. Lancet 1978; 2:540.
23. Chabanon G, Hartley CL, Richmond MH: Adhesion to human cell line by Escherichia coli strains isolated during urinary tract infections. J Clin Microbiol 1979; 10:563.
24. Bruce AW, Chan RCY, Pickerton D, et al: Adherence of gram-negative uropathogens to human uroepithelial cells. J Urol 1983; 130:293.
25. Orskov I, Ferencz A, Orskov F: Tamm-Horsfall protein or

uromucoid is the normal urinary slime that traps type 1 fimbriated Escherichia coli. Lancet 1980; 1:887.
26. Kallenius C, Molby R, Svensson SB, et al: The p^k antigen as receptor for the haemaglutination of pyelonephritic Escherichia coli. FEMS Microbiol Lett 1980; 7:297.
27. Leffler H, Svanborg-Eden C: Chemical identification of a glycosphingolipid receptor for Escherichia coli attaching to human urinary tract epithelial cells and agglutinating human erythrocytes. FEMS Microbiol Lett 1980; 8:127.
28. Perry A, Ofed I, Silverblatt FJ: Enhancement of mannose-mediated stimulation of human granulocytes by type 1 fimbriae aggregated with antibodies on Escherichia coli surfaces. Infect Immun 1983; 39:1334.
29. Svanborg-Eden C, Bjursten LM, Hull R, et al: Influence of adhesins on the interaction of Escherichia coli with human phagocytes. Infect Immun 1984; 66:672.
30. Bjorksten B, Wadstrom R: Influence of adhesions on the interaction of Escherichia coli with different fimbriae and polymorphonuclear leukocytes. Infect Immun 1982; 32:298.
31. Andersson P, Engberg I, Lidin-Janson G, et al: Persistence of Escherichia coli bacterial adherence. Infect Immun 1991; 59:2915.
32. Sheinfeld J, Schaeffer AJ, Cordon-Cardo C, et al: Association of Lewis blood-group phenotype with recurrent urinary tract infections in women. N Engl J Med 1989; 320:773.
33. Hooton TM, Fihn SD, Johnson C, et al: Association between bacterial vaginosis and acute cystitis in women using diaphragms. Arch Intern Med 1989; 149:1932.
34. Hooton TM, Hillier S, Johnson C, et al: Escherichia coli bacteria and contraceptive method. JAMA 1991; 254:64.
35. Stapleton A, Moseley S, Stamm WE: Urovirulence determinants in Escherichia coli isolates causing first-episode and recurrent cystitis in women. J Infect Dis 1991; 163:773.
36. Hooton TM, Roberts PL, Stamm WE: Effects of recent sexual activity and use of a diaphragm on the vaginal microflora. Clin Infect Dis 1994; 19:274.
37. Sanford JP: Urinary tract symptoms and infections. Annu Rev Med 1975; 26:485.
38. Fairly KF, Grounds AD, Carson NG, et al: Site of infection in acute urinary tract infection in general practice. Lancet 1971; 2:615.
39. Stamm WE, Wagner KF, Amsel R, et al: Causes of the acute urethral syndrome in women. N Engl J Med 1980; 303:409.
40. Savage WE, Hajj SN, Kass EH: Demographic and prognostic characteristics of bacteriuria in pregnancy. Medicine (Baltimore) 1967; 46:385.
41. Raz R, Stamm WE: A controlled trial of intravaginal estriol in postmenopausal women with recurrent urinary tract infections. N Engl J Med 1993; 329:753.
42. Kunin CM (ed): Detection, Prevention and Management of Urinary Tract Infections, 3rd ed. Philadelphia, Lea & Febiger, 1979.
43. Lucas MJ, Cunningham FG: Urinary infection in pregnancy. Clin Obstet Gynecol 1993; 36:855.
44. Andriole VT: Diagnosis of urinary tract infections by urine culture. In: Kaye D (ed): Urinary Tract Infection and Its Management. St. Louis, CV Mosby, 1972, pp 28–42.
45. Andriole VT: Current concepts of urinary tract infections. In: Weinstein L, Fields BN (eds): Seminars in Infectious Disease, Vol. 3. New York: Thieme-Stratton, 1980, pp 89–130.
46. Doern GV, Saubolle MA, Sewell DL: Screening for bacteriuria with the LB strip test. Diagn Microbiol Infect Dis 1986; 4:355.
47. Stamm WE, Counts GW, Running KR, et al: Diagnosis of coliform infection in acutely dysuric women. N Engl J Med 1982; 307:463.
48. Johnson JR, Stamm WE: Urinary tract infections in women: Diagnosis and treatment. Ann Intern Med 1989; 111:906.
49. Roberts FJ: Quantitative urine cultures in patients with urinary tract infection and bacteriuria. Am J Clin Pathol 1986; 85:616.
50. Carlson KJ, Mulley AG: Management of acute dysuria: A decision analysis model of alternative strategies. Ann Intern Med 1985; 102:244.
51. Stamm WE: When should we use urine cultures? Infect Control 1986; 7:431.
52. Schultz HJ, McCaffrey LA, Keys TF, et al: Acute cystitis: A

prospective study of laboratory tests and duration therapy. Mayo Clin Proc 1984; 59:391.

53. Andriole VT: Genitourinary infections in the patient at risk: an overview. Am J Med 1984; 76:155.

54. Rubin RH, Fang LST, Jones SR: Single dose amoxicillin therapy for urinary tract infection. JAMA 1980; 244:561.

55. Bailey RR: Single Dose Therapy of Urinary Tract Infection. Sydney, Australia, ADIS Health Science Press, 1983.

56. Andriole VT: Use of quinolones in treatment of prostatitis and lower urinary tract infections. Eur J Clin Microbiol Infect Dis 1991; 10:342.

57. Andriole VT: Changing treatment patterns in urinary infections. Bull NY Acad Med 1987; 63:433.

58. Philbrick JT, Bracikowski JP: Single dose antibiotic treatment for uncomplicated urinary tract infections. Arch Intern Med 1985; 145:1672.

59. Fihn SD, Johnson C, Roberts PL, et al: Trimethoprim-sulfamethoxazole for acute dysuria in women: A single dose or 10-day course. Ann Intern Med 1988; 108:350.

60. Norrby SR: Short term treatment of uncomplicated lower urinary tract infections in women. Rev Infect Dis 1990; 12:458.

61. Hooton TM, Stamm WE: Management of acute uncomplicated urinary tract infection in adults. Med Clin North Am 1991; 75:339.

62. Naber KG: Use of quinolones in urinary tract infections and prostatitis. Rev Infect Dis 1989; 11:S1321.

63. Hooton TM, Stamm WE: The vaginal flora and UTIs. In: Mobley HLT, Warren JW (eds): UTIs: Molecular Pathogenesis and Clinical Management. Washington, DC, ASM Press, 1996, pp 67–94.

64. Stamm WE, McKevit M, Counts GW: Acute renal infection in women: Treatment with trimethoprim-sulfamethoxazole or ampicillin for two or six weeks. Ann Intern Med 1987; 106:341.

65. Safrin S, Siegel D, Black D: Pyelonephritis in adult women: Inpatient versus outpatient therapy. Am J Med 1988; 85:793.

66. Hooton TM, Stamm WE: Diagnosis and treatment of uncomplicated urinary tract infection. Infect Dis Clin North Am 1997; 11:551.

67. Kraft JK, Stamey TA: The natural history of symptomatic recurrent bacteriuria in women. Medicine (Baltimore) 1977; 56:55.

68. Harding GK, Buckwold FJ, Marrie TJ: Prophylaxis of recurrent urinary tract infection in female patients: Efficacy of low-dose, thrice weekly therapy with trimethoprim-sulfamethoxazole. JAMA 1979; 242:1975.

69. Vosti KL: Recurrent urinary tract infections: Prevention by prophylactic-antibiotics after sexual intercourse. JAMA 1975; 23:934.

70. Patterson TF, Andriole VT: Detection, significance, and therapy of bacteriuria in pregnancy. Infect Dis Clin North Am 1997; 11:593.

71. Fainstat T: Urethral dilation in pregnancy: A review. Obstet Gynecol Surv 1963; 18:845.

72. Hundley JM, Siegel IA, Hatchel FW, et al: Some physiological observations on the urinary tract during pregnancy. Surg Gynecol Obstet 1938; 66:360.

73. Lindheimer MD, Katz AI: The kidney in pregnancy. N Engl J Med 1970; 283:1095.

74. Au KL, Woo JSK, Tang LC, et al: Aetiological factors in the genesis of pregnancy hydronephrosis. Aust N Z J Obstet Gynaecol 1985; 25:248.

75. Traut HF, McLane CM: Physiological changes in the urethra associated with pregnancy. Surg Gynecol Obstet 1936; 62:65.

76. Krieger JN: Complications and treatments of urinary tract infections during pregnancy. Urol Clin North Am 1986; 13:685.

77. Ronald AR: Advances in the treatment of urinary tract infections. Mediguide Infect Dis 1985; 5:1.

78. Sandberg T, Stenquist K, Svanborg-Eden C, et al: Host–parasite relationship in urinary tract infections during pregnancy. Prog Allergy 1983; 33:228.

79. Guyer PB, Delany D: Urinary tract dilation and oral contraceptives. BMJ 1970; 4:588.

80. Marshall S, Lyon RP, Minkler D: Ureteral dilation following the use of oral contraceptives. JAMA 1966; 198:782.

81. Takahashi M, Loveland CM: Bacteriuria and oral contraceptives. JAMA 1974; 227:762.

82. MacDonald P, Alexander D, Catz C, et al: Summary of a workshop on maternal genitourinary infections and the outcome of pregnancy. J Infect Dis 1983; 147:596.

83. Neu HC: Urinary tract infections. Am J Med 1992; 92(suppl 4A):63.

84. Perdue BE, Plaisance KI: Treatment of community-acquired urinary tract infections. American Pharmacy 1995; NS35:37.

85. Stenqvist K, Dahlen-Nilsson, Lidin-Janson G, et al: Bacteriuria in pregnancy. Am J Epidemiol 1989; 129:372.

86. Gilbert GL, Garland SM, Fairley KF, et al: Bacteriuria due to ureaplasmas and other fastidious organisms during pregnancy: Prevalence and significance. Pediatr Infect Dis 1986; 5(suppl):239.

87. Pritchard JA, Scott DE, Whalley PH, et al: The effects of maternal sickle cell hemoglobinopathies and sickle cell trait on reproductive performance. Am J Obstet Gynecol 1973; 117:662.

88. Whalley PJ, Martin FG, Pritchard JA: Sickle cell trait and urinary tract infection during pregnancy. JAMA 1964; 193:903.

89. Little PJ: The incidence of urinary infection in 5,000 pregnant women. Lancet 1966; 2:925.

90. Fowler JE, Hooton TM: Management of urinary tract infections in adults. Ann Intern Med 1985; 102:342.

91. Stamm WE, Hooton TM: Management of urinary tract infections in adults. N Engl J Med 1993; 329:1328.

92. Barr JG, Ritchie JW, Henry O: Microaerophilic/anaerobic bacteria as a cause of urinary tract infection during pregnancy. Br J Obstet Gynaecol 1985; 92:506.

93. McDowall DR, Buchanan JD, Fairley KF, et al: Anaerobic and other fastidious microorganisms in asymptomatic bacteriuria in pregnant women. J Infect Dis 1981; 144:114.

94. Legris M, Hainaut F, Crimail P, et al: Results of detection and early treatment of Chlamydia trachomatis infections in pregnancy. J Gynecol Obstet Biol Reprod 1988; 18:581.

95. Cohen I, Veille JC, Calkins BM: Improved pregnancy outcome following successful treatment of chlamydial infection. JAMA 1990; 263:3160.

96. Naeye RL: Causes of the excessive rates of prenatal mortality and prematurity in pregnancies complicated by maternal urinary tract infection. N Engl J Med 1979; 390:819.

97. Marchant DJ: Urinary tract infections in pregnancy. Clin Obstet Gynecol 1978; 21:921.

98. Zinner SH: Management of urinary tract infections in pregnancy. A review with comments on single dose therapy. Infection 1922; 20(suppl 4):280.

99. Schieve LA, Handler A, Hershow R, et al: Urinary tract infection during pregnancy: Its association with maternal morbidity and perinatal outcome. Am J Public Health 1994; 84:405.

100. Kass EH: Bacteriuria and pyelonephritis of pregnancy. Arch Intern Med 1960; 105:194.

101. Crabtree ED, Prather GC: Clinical aspects of pyelonephritis in pregnancy. N Engl J Med 1930; 202:357.

102. Gilstrap LC, Leveno KJ, Cunningham FG: Renal infection and pregnancy outcome. Am J Obstet Gynecol 1981; 141:709.

103. Sever JL, Elienberg JH, Edmonds D: Urinary tract infections during pregnancy: Maternal and pediatric findings. In: Kass EH, Brumfitt W (eds): Infections of the Urinary Tract. Chicago, University of Chicago Press, 1979, pp 19–21.

104. Harris RE: The significance of eradication of bacteriuria during pregnancy. Obstet Gynecol 1979; 53:71.

105. Andriole VT, Patterson TF: Epidemiology, natural history, and management of urinary tract infections in pregnancy. Med Clin North Am 1991; 75:359.

106. Kass EH: The role of asymptomatic bacteriuria in the pathogenesis of pyelonephritis. In: Quinn EL, Kass EH (eds): Biology of Pyelonephritis. Boston, Little, Brown, 1960, pp 399–412.

107. Beard RW, Roberts AP: Asymptomatic bacteriuria during pregnancy. Br Med Bull 1968; 24:44.

108. Whalley PJ: Bacteriuria of pregnancy. Am J Obstet Gynecol 1967; 97:723.

109. Kincaid-Smith P: Bacteriuria and urinary infection in pregnancy. Clin Obstet Gynecol 1968; 11:533.

110. Romero R, Oyzrzun E, Mazor M, et al: Meta-analysis of the relationship between asymptomatic bacteriuria and preterm delivery/low birth weight. Obstet Gynecol 1989; 73:576.

111. McGrady GA, Darling JR, Peterson DR: Maternal urinary tract infection and adverse fetal outcomes. Am J Epidemiol 1985; 121:377.

112. Chng PK, Hall MH: Antenatal prediction of urinary tract infection in pregnancy. Br J Obstet Gynaecol 1982; 89:8.

113. Campbell-Brown M, McFadyen IR, Seal DV, et al: Is screening for bacteriuria in pregnancy worthwhile? BMJ 1987; 294:1579.

114. Morgan MG, McKenzie H: Controversies in the laboratory diagnosis of community-acquired urinary tract infection. Eur J Clin Microbiol Infect Dis 1993; 12:491.

115. Andriole VT: Urinary tract infections in pregnancy. Urol Clin North Am 1975; 2:485.

116. Neu HC: Optimal characteristics of agents to treat uncomplicated urinary tract infections. Infection 1992; 20(suppl 4):266.

117. Bailey RR: Management of lower urinary tract infections. Drugs 1993; 45(suppl 3):139.

118. Vercaigne M, Zhanel GG: Recommended treatment for urinary tract infection in pregnancy. Ann Pharmacother 1994; 28:248.

119. Bailey RR: Single-dose antibacterial treatment for bacteriuria in pregnancy. Drugs 1984; 27:183.

120. Campbell-Brown M, McFadyen IR: Bacteriuria in pregnancy treated with a single dose of cephalexin. Br J Obstet Gynaecol 1983; 90:1054.

121. Harris RE, Gilstrap LC, Pretty A: Single-dose antimicrobial therapy for asymptomatic bacteriuria during pregnancy. Obstet Gynecol 1982; 59:546.

122. Ronald A, Nicolle LE, Harding G: Single dose treatment failure in women with acute cystitis. Infection 1992; 20(suppl 4):276.

123. Gilstrap LC, Cunningham FG, Whalley PJ: Acute pyelonephritis in pregnancy: An anterospective study. Obstet Gynecol 1981; 57:409.

124. Cunningham FG, Morris GB, Mickal A: Acute pyelonephritis of pregnancy: A clinical review. Obstet Gynecol 1973; 42:112.

125. Pedler SJ, Bint AJ: Comparative study of amoxicillin-clavulanic acid and cephalexin in the treatment of bacteriuria during pregnancy. Antimicrob Agents Chemother 1985; 27:508.

126. Bailey RR, Bishop V, Peddie BA: Comparison of single dose with a 5-day course of cotrimazole for asymptomatic (covert) bacteriuria of pregnancy. Aust N Z J Obstet Gynaecol 1983; 23:139.

127. Pfau A, Sacks TG: Effective prophylaxis for recurrent urinary tract infection during pregnancy. Clin Infect Dis 1992; 14:810.

128. Diokno AC, Compton A, Seski J: Urologic evaluation of urinary tract infection in pregnancy. J Reprod Med 1986; 31:23.

129. Abbott J: Medical illness during pregnancy. Emerg Med Clin North Am 1994; 12:115.

130. Faro S, Pastorek JG, Plauche WC: Short-course parenteral antibiotic therapy for pyelonephritis in pregnancy. South Med J 1984; 77:455.

33 Pyelonephritis

DAVID GONZALEZ ▸ JOSEPH APUZZIO

Pyelonephritis is a bacterial infection of the upper urinary tract affecting the renal pelvis and parenchyma. Clinically, acute pyelonephritis is characterized by both focal and systemic findings that include flank pain, fever, and symptoms of lower urinary tract infection such as frequency and dysuria. Although the true incidence of pyelonephritis in the general population in unknown, women with symptomatic and asymptomatic lower urinary tract disease are at risk for development of pyelonephritis. Because 10% to 20% of women will contract a symptomatic infection of the lower urinary tract during their lifetime, the risk of upper tract infection can be significant.[1]

PATHOGENESIS

Urinary tract infections in women occur primarily as a result of ascending infection of organisms from the urethral area.[2, 3] The proximity of the urethra to the rectum and the short urethral length are two factors that are thought to contribute to the increased risk for urinary tract infection in women. Normally, the distal urethra is colonized by several types of bacteria, including diphtheroids, staphylococci, streptococci, and anaerobic organisms. When urinary tract infections develop in women, bacterial pathogens originating from the fecal flora colonize the vagina and periurethral mucosa. These organisms ascend through the urethra into the bladder and eventually invade the upper urinary tract.[4] Although the kidney is remarkably resistant to infection, once bacteria have invaded the renal parenchyma, the chemical environment of the renal medulla inhibits the normal immunologic processes that act to destroy infection, resulting in increased susceptibility to infection.[5, 6]

Although most infections of the kidney originate from the lower urinary tract, infection of the kidney may also occur hematogenously. A hematogenous etiology should be suspected in patients with urine cultures that grow significant numbers of coagulase-positive staphylococci. Staphylococcal bacteremia secondary to endocarditis, cellulitis, or osteomyelitis may lead to hematogenous invasion of the kidney and the formation of intrarenal or perinephric abscesses. Hematogenous infection is also more common in patients who are immunocompromised or who have chronic illness.

There are also medical conditions that predispose women to lower urinary tract infections and subsequent pyelonephritis. These conditions include renal calculi, anatomic abnormalities in the urogenital tract, vesicoureteral reflux, neurogenic bladder dysfunction, hemoglobinopathies (e.g., sickle cell trait), diabetes mellitus, and genetic factors.

CLINICAL PRESENTATION AND LABORATORY EVALUATION

Women with pyelonephritis present with a variety of focal and systemic signs and symptoms that suggest infection of both the lower and upper urinary tract. Lower urinary tract symptoms may include frequency, urgency, dysuria, suprapubic tenderness, or simply the presence of cloudy, malodorous urine. The symptoms of lower urinary tract infection often precede the development of upper tract symptoms by several days. Systemic symptoms include temperature greater than 101°F, shaking chills, and tachycardia. Gastrointestinal symptoms may also be present, including nausea, vomiting, anorexia, and diarrhea. On physical evaluation, the examiner may be able to illicit costovertebral angle tenderness, tenderness in the area of the kidneys on deep abdominal palpation, and, less commonly, signs of peritonitis. Patients with more severe disease may present with signs and symptoms of gram-negative sepsis and possibly septic shock. Hematuria may also be present.

The presentation of pyelonephritis can be quite variable and may include one, all, or none of the aforementioned findings. Some patients present with nonspecific, isolated complaints such as fatigue, backache, or upper or lower abdominal symptoms. Other patients with documented pyelonephritis may be completely asymptomatic. For example, most elderly patients with significant infection have no specific symptoms of urinary tract infection at the time of presentation. Attempts to distinguish upper from lower urinary tract infection may also prove to be difficult.[1] One third of patients without symptoms of upper urinary tract involvement who present with significant bacteriuria and complaints consistent with cystitis have upper urinary tract infection. Therefore, the absence of fever and costovertebral angle tenderness does not rule out renal infection, but probably reflects less severe upper tract disease.

LABORATORY EVALUATION

The diagnosis of a urinary tract infection usually depends on the presence of clinical symptoms in conjunction with positive laboratory findings. The gold standard for diagnosis of a urinary tract infection is the urine culture. Unfortunately, the urine culture may take 24 to 48 hours to yield a result. Therefore, at the time of initial presentation, quicker and less reliable laboratory tests are used to make a preliminary diagnosis in a symptomatic patient. A urinalysis performed on a clean-catch midstream urine can provide valuable evidence for the presence of infection.[7, 8]

There are several important components to the urinalysis: pH, blood, protein, leukocyte esterase, and nitrite tests. An alkaline pH is usually found in the presence of infection caused by urea-splitting organisms like *Proteus* species. However, *Klebsiella* and *Staphylococcus* may also produce urease. Hematuria, either gross or microscopic, is seen in 30% of patients with urinary tract infections. Persistent hematuria should raise the suspicion of nephrolithiasis or a renal or bladder tumor. Protein in the urine is consistent with the presence of pyelonephritis. It may also indicate a large amount of white blood cells in the urine, the presence of intrinsic renal disease, or contamination with vaginal secretions. Leukocyte esterase is an enzyme produced by white blood cells. A positive leukocyte esterase test is consistent with five or greater white blood cells per high-power field and suggests bacterial infection. The nitrite test is positive in the presence of gram-negative bacteria in the urine that can reduce nitrate to nitrite.

Of the components of the urinalysis, the leukocyte esterase test and nitrite tests are the most specific. When the leukocyte esterase test and nitrite test are positive, the predictive value is approximately 75%. If they are both negative the predictive value is greater than 97%. However, the results of a urinalysis should be interpreted cautiously in women because inappropriately collected specimens yield unreliable results. Contamination of the urine specimen with even a small amount of vaginal secretions may yield a false-positive leukocyte esterase and, less commonly, a positive nitrite test. The nitrite test is negative in the presence of infection if the pathogen is gram-positive or if the frequency of voiding is such that the urine does not remain in the bladder for an adequate time.

In a patient with signs and symptoms consistent with pyelonephritis and a positive urinalysis, microscopic examination of the urine should be performed. The presence of bacteria, white blood cells, and red blood cells suggest infection of the lower urinary tract. The presence of white blood cell casts in the urine is highly specific and suggests infection of the upper urinary tract. However, the absence of white blood cell casts does not rule out pyelonephritis. Microscopic evaluation may also include a Gram stain of the urine, which may provide valuable diagnostic information about the causative organism and also helps in the selection of the initial antibiotic therapy.

Finally, the evaluation of a patient with suspected pyelonephritis must include a urine culture. Traditionally, growth of more than 10^5 colony-forming units of bacteria per milliliter from a properly collected, midstream clean-catch urine has been considered to be diagnostic of a urinary tract infection. However, the interpretation of the results is different depending on the organism identified, the colony count, and the clinical findings. The presence of 10^3 to 10^4 gram-negative bacteria per milliliter in a properly obtained specimen from a patient who is symptomatic is consistent with clinical infection.[9] Similarly, the presence of less than 10^5 gram-positive bacteria or fungi should be regarded as significant because these organisms may not demonstrate the rapid rate of growth of the more common gram-negative organisms grown under the same conditions. Growth of 10^2 to 10^4 bacteria in a specimen obtained through a straight catheter or suprapubic aspiration also suggests infection. Overall, most patients with pyelonephritis have a significant number of bacteria present on urine culture.

In some cases, the quantity of bacteria is not as significant as the organism isolated. Contamination of the urine with vaginal discharge or flora from the distal urethra is common and may yield false-positive culture results. The growth of diphtheroids or *Staphylococcus aureus* in a urine culture, especially when colony counts are less than 10^4/mL, should be interpreted cautiously. Similarly, a urine culture positive for *Lactobacillus* or mixed flora, even in the presence of significant growth, is highly suggestive of contamination with vaginal secretions and should be repeated.

MICROBIOLOGY

Gram-negative bacteria as a group represent the most prevalent organisms responsible for urinary tract infections. *Escherichia coli* is the most common bacterium isolated from patients with symptomatic infection of the lower and upper urinary tract, accounting for 80% to 90% of infections in women. *E. coli* is also the most common cause of nosocomial and recurrent urinary tract infection. Other gram-negative organisms such as *Proteus*, *Klebsiella*, and *Enterobacter* account for only a small portion of community-acquired infections, but are more frequently seen in women with indwelling catheters, urinary obstruction, or recurrent infection.[10] *Proteus* and *Klebsiella* are also more common in patients with nephrolithiasis. *Proteus* infection promotes the formation of renal stones through the production of urease, whereas *Klebsiella* generates extracellular slime and polysaccharides, facilitating the formation of calculi.

Gram-positive bacteria also play a significant role in symptomatic urinary tract disease. *Staphylococcus saprophyticus*, the most common gram-positive urinary pathogen, is responsible for as much as 10% to 20% of urinary tract infections in women of reproductive age in the United States.[11] The infection has a seasonal cycle and is usually more common in the late summer and fall. Infection due to other gram-positive organisms, including *S. aureus*, enterococci, and group B streptococci are less common. Staphylococcal bacteriuria may be seen in patients with renal calculi, urinary tract instrumentation, or hematogenous spread from a distant focus of infection. Enterococci are seen more often in patients with nephrolithiasis or urinary catheters, or as a result of superinfection after antibiotic therapy.

Other, less common organisms responsible for urinary tract infection include anaerobic bacteria, fungi, and viruses. Anaerobes colonize the gut and distal urethra and may cause infection in patients with calculi or tumors. Patients who are immunocompromised, are receiving high doses of corticosteroids, or have diabetes may acquire symptomatic urinary tract infection secondary to *Candida albicans* or, less frequently, *Cryptococcus neoformans*. *C. albicans* may invade the kidney through hematogenous spread, resulting in upper urinary tract disease. Viruses may infect and replicate in the kidney, but have never been shown to be a cause of acute pyelonephritis.

THERAPY

After a complete evaluation, women with clinical and laboratory findings consistent with pyelonephritis should receive antimicrobial therapy. Urine and blood cultures should be obtained before the initiation of antibiotics. Blood cultures are positive in 15% to 20% of patients with pyelonephritis. In patients with evidence of urinary tract obstruction or recurrent infection, consideration should be given to obtaining a sonogram of the kidneys and renal collecting system, or an intravenous pyelogram.

The choice of antibiotics and the need for hospitalization are determined by the clinical symptoms, the suspected organism, and, if performed, the radiologic findings. Inpatient therapy is appropriate for patients with mild to moderate disease who are reliable and able to tolerate oral therapy. Therapy with trimethoprim–sulfamethoxazole or a fluoroquinolone for 10 to 14 days is usually adequate[12] (Table 33–1). Patients with nausea and vomiting and mild to moderate disease may benefit from an initial course of parenteral

TABLE 33–1 ▶	TREATMENT REGIMEN FOR PYELONEPHRITIS (ORAL)

Trimethoprim–sulfamethoxazole 160/800 mg q12h
Ampicillin–clavulanic acid 500 mg q8h
Ciprofloxacin 500 mg q12h
Norfloxacin 400 mg q12h
Ofloxacin 200 mg q12h
Enoxacin 400 mg q12h

Note: Quinolone antibiotics should not be used during pregnancy.

antibiotic therapy and observation. A course of intravenous antibiotics or an intramuscular injection of a third-generation cephalosporin such as ceftriaxone may alleviate some of the symptoms and allow the patient to complete therapy as an outpatient.

Patients with severe disease that includes signs of sepsis require hospitalization and intravenous antibiotic therapy. These patients should be started on broad-spectrum antibiotic coverage pending the results of the urine culture. The choice of antibiotic should be guided by the history and physical findings, including the presence of indwelling catheters, urinary calculi, or suspicion of resistant organisms in patients with recurrent urinary tract infection. Possible antibiotic regimens include cephalosporins, the fluoroquinolones, trimethoprim–sulfamethoxazole, aminoglycosides, aztreonam, a ureido-penicillin, ampicillin–sulbactam, or ticarcillin–clavulanic acid (Table 33–2). Patients with severe disease should be monitored for other possible complications, including respiratory distress syndrome and septic shock.

Most patients respond to the initial course of broad-spectrum antibiotic therapy. Intravenous therapy should be continued until the patient is afebrile for 24 to 48 hours. The patient should then be switched to an oral regimen to complete 14 days of therapy. Patients with positive blood cultures may complete a similar regimen unless other confounding medical problems are present.

If fever, leukocytosis, or flank pain persist after 48 to 72 hours of treatment, the antibiotic regimen should be re-evaluated. A lack of response may indicate a resistant organism, urinary tract obstruction, or the presence of an intrarenal or perinephric abscess. Ra-

TABLE 33–2 ▶	TREATMENT REGIMEN FOR PYELONEPHRITIS (PARENTERAL)

Cefazolin 1–2 g q8h
Ceftriaxone 1–2 g q24h
Ciprofloxacin 400 mg q12h
Ofloxacin 200–400 mg q12h
Ticarcillin–clavulanic acid 3.2 g q6–8h
Gentamicin 1.5 mg/kg q8h
Trimethoprim–sulfamethoxazole 160–800 mg q12h

Note: Quinolone antibiotics should not be used during pregnancy.

diologic studies, including a renal sonogram, should be considered. Computed tomography, magnetic resonance imaging, or intravenous pyelography may also be considered, as clinically appropriate. The results of the urine culture and sensitivity testing should be used to guide a change in antibiotic therapy.

A test of cure should be documented by culture approximately 1 to 2 weeks after the completion of therapy. Obtaining a negative culture is important because patients with acute pyelonephritis may demonstrate resolution of symptoms without the resolution of infection and may require prolonged or alternative antibiotic therapy.

RECURRENT URINARY TRACT INFECTION

Some women, despite appropriate antibiotic therapy, have recurrent urinary tract infection and pyelonephritis.[13] Recurrent infection that presents within 1 to 2 weeks after the completion of antibiotic therapy most probably represents persistent infection and is regarded as a relapse. Recurrence of infection several weeks after therapy or after a negative urine culture should be regarded as reinfection. *E. coli* is the most common bacterium found in patients with recurrence. However, infection is usually secondary to a new serotype of *E. coli* in over 90% of cases. Other, less common bacteria responsible for urinary tract infection become important pathogens in recurrent infection.

In women with recurrent urinary tract infection, the presence of a urinary tract abnormality should be considered. Women at risk include those with a rapid recurrence of infection, recurrent pyelonephritis, renal stones, persistent hematuria, or a history of infection during childhood.[14, 15] Possible anatomic abnormalities include urethral strictures, bladder diverticula, calculi, cystocele, neurogenic bladder, a duplicate collecting system, or vesicoureteral reflux. However, the incidence of urinary tract abnormalities even in these women is extremely low, and therefore most radiologic and urologic studies are negative.

In women with no abnormalities and frequent recurrent infections, defined as four or more episodes per year, the use of antibiotic prophylaxis should be considered. Therapy for these patients should include an extended course of full-dose antibiotics lasting for approximately 2 to 6 weeks.[16] Prolonged therapy may be successful in eradicating bacteria in the upper urinary tract that are responsible for causing persistent infection. After completion of this regimen, trimethoprim, trimethoprim–sulfamethoxazole, nitrofurantoin, or cephalexin may be administered as a single bedtime dose daily or three times per week as prophylaxis.[17] The emergence of resistant strains with these antibiotic regimens is rare. In contrast, the use of penicillins or sulfonamides for prophylaxis has been associated with the rapid emergence of bacterial resistance. Single-dose therapy with the same antibiotics may be used after coitus to decrease the chance of recurrent infection.[18] Voiding after intercourse should also be encouraged. In patients on prolonged therapy, periodic evaluation for signs of antibiotic toxicity should be performed.

PYELONEPHRITIS IN PREGNANCY

Pyelonephritis complicates 1% to 2% of pregnancies. Pregnancy results in physiologic changes of the urinary tract that predispose the patient to the development of urinary tract infection. Hormonal changes lead to decreased bladder and ureteral tone as well as decreased ureteral peristalsis, resulting in the dilatation of the renal collecting system and ureters. Anatomic factors, including compression of the ureters at the pelvic brim by the iliac arteries and the gravid uterus, cause stasis of urine and also promote infection.[19]

The clinical presentation of pyelonephritis in pregnancy is the same as that of the nonpregnant patient, with the exception that the pregnant patient may also present with symptoms of preterm labor. The spectrum of organisms responsible for asymptomatic bacteriuria and pyelonephritis during gestation is also similar to that seen in the nonpregnant state. Coliforms are the most common organisms isolated in women with asymptomatic bacteriuria and pyelonephritis.

Pregnant women with suspected pyelonephritis should be hospitalized for intravenous antibiotic therapy regardless of the severity of the infection. They should also be watched for the development of pneumonitis and adult respiratory distress, which may be a result of pulmonary injury from the infection or overhydration. Cefazolin, a first-generation cephalosporin (or an equivalent cephalosporin), usually provides excellent broad-spectrum coverage and is safe in pregnancy (Table 33–3). Other cephalosporins, such as ceftriaxone, may also be appropriate. Patients with persistent fever and evidence of infection after 48 hours of antibiotic therapy should have an aminoglycoside such as gentamicin added to the regimen. Monitoring of peak and trough levels is suggested to ensure adequate therapy and prevent toxicity. The duration of antibiotic therapy should be 10 to 14 days.

In pregnant women who experience persistent or recurrent urinary tract infection, sonographic evaluation of the urinary tract is recommended. Sonography is the study of choice in pregnancy. Mild hydronephro-

TABLE 33–3 ▶	TREATMENT OF PYELONEPHRITIS DURING PREGNANCY (PARENTERAL)	
Cefazolin 1–2 g q8h	Ceftriaxone 1–2 g q24h	
Cefoxitin 1–2 g q6h	(Or equivalent cephalosporin)	

sis of the collecting system, especially of the right ureter, is a normal finding. As with nonpregnant women, most patients have negative studies. After extended therapy with full-dose antibiotics, prophylactic therapy is recommended for the duration of the pregnancy. A single dose of cephalexin or nitrofurantoin at bedtime has proven to be effective in preventing recurrent infection.[20] In a patient who is taking nitrofurantoin late in the third trimester, consideration should be given to changing the regimen to a cephalosporin, given the theoretic risk of hemolytic anemia in the newborn secondary to the relative lack of glutathione in fetal red blood cells.

PREVENTION

The presence of asymptomatic bacteriuria during gestation is a major contributing factor to the development of upper urinary tract infection. Approximately 2% to 8% of women have asymptomatic bacteriuria during their pregnancy. Risk factors include multiparity, maternal age, frequency of coitus, hemoglobinopathies, diabetes mellitus, and a history of urinary tract infections.[21] Pregnancy itself, however, does not increase the incidence of asymptomatic bacteriuria. Furthermore, it is believed that women with asymptomatic colonization of the urinary tract have infection that is present before pregnancy. Therefore, the physiologic changes that occur in the urinary tract during pregnancy do not cause but rather facilitate the colonization of the upper urinary tract in patients with untreated lower urinary tract infection.

All pregnant women should have urine culture performed at the first prenatal visit.[22] Approximately 90% of upper urinary tract infections in pregnancy can be prevented by screening for and treating asymptomatic bacteriuria. Untreated asymptomatic bacteriuria progresses to pyelonephritis in 20% to 30% of women. In contrast, only 1% of women with a negative urine culture early in pregnancy go on to acquire pyelonephritis in pregnancy.[19]

Antibiotic therapy for the pregnant patient is limited to antibiotics with proven safety in pregnancy.[23] For the treatment of asymptomatic bacteriuria, nitrofurantoin or a cephalosporin like cephalexin are good choices for initial therapy. Although there have not been any adverse effects reported with the use of these antibiotics in early pregnancy, it is probably best to delay treatment of the asymptomatic patient until the second trimester. Ampicillin and amoxicillin should not be used to treat asymptomatic bacteriuria unless sensitivities are available, given the high incidence of resistance among E. coli responsible for urinary tract disease.[24] Sulfonamides are an option but should be avoided in the third trimester because of theoretic concerns with hyperbilirubinemia and kernicterus in the newborn. Fluoroquinolones are associated with ar-

thropathy in immature animals and are therefore contraindicated in pregnancy. Antibiotic therapy should be continued for 7 to 10 days. Three-day therapy in pregnancy may be an option; however, studies evaluating these regimens in pregnancy are lacking. A urine culture should be obtained 1 to 2 weeks after the completion of pregnancy to document a test of cure.

REFERENCES

1. Stamm WE, Hooton TM: Management of urinary tract infections in adults. N Engl J Med 1993; 329:1328.
2. Stamey TA, Timothy M, Millar M, et al: Recurrent urinary infections in adult women: The role of introital bacteria. Calif Med 1971; 115:1.
3. Vivaldi E, Cotran R, Zangwill DP, et al: Ascending infection as a mechanism in pathogenesis of experimental non-obstructive pyelonephritis. Proc Soc Exp Biol Med 1959; 102:242.
4. Bran JL, Levison ME, Kaye D: Entrance of bacteria into the female urinary bladder. N Engl J Med 1972; 286:626.
5. Freedman LR, Beeson PB: Experimental pyelonephritis. IV: Observations on infections resulting from direct inoculation of bacteria in different zones of the kidney. Yale J Biol Med 1958; 30:406.
6. Rocha H, Fekety FR: Acute inflammation in the renal cortex and medulla following thermal injury. J Exp Med 1964; 119:131.
7. Pels RJ, Bor D, Woolhandler S, et al: Dipstick urinalysis screening of asymptomatic adults for urinary tract disorders. JAMA 1989; 262:1221.
8. Pappas PG: Laboratory in the diagnosis and management of urinary tract infections. Med Clin North Am 1991; 75:313.
9. Stamm WE, Counts GW, Running R, et al: Diagnosis of coliform infection in acutely dysuric women. N Engl J Med 1982; 307:463.
10. Turck M, Stamm WE: Nosocomial infection of the urinary tract. Am J Med 1981; 70:651.
11. Hovelius B, Mardh P: Staphylococcus saprophyticus as a common cause of urinary tract infections. Rev Infect Dis 1984; 6:328.
12. Stamm WE, McKevitt M, Counts GW: Acute renal infection in women: Treatment with trimethoprim-sulfamethoxazole or ampicillin for two or six weeks. A randomized trial. Ann Intern Med 1987; 106:341.
13. Foxman B: Recurrent urinary tract infection: Incidence and risk factors. Am J Public Health 1990; 80:331.
14. Piccirello M, Rigsby C, Rosenfield AT: Contemporary imaging of renal inflammatory disease. Infect Dis Clin North Am 1987; 1:927.
15. Fowler JE Jr, Pulaski ET: Excretory urography, cystography, and cystoscopy in the evaluation of women with urinary tract infection: A prospective study. N Engl J Med 1981; 304:462.
16. Nicolle LE, Ronald AR: Recurrent urinary tract infection in adult women: Diagnosis and treatment. Infect Dis Clin North Am 1987; 1:793.
17. Wong ES, McKevitt M, Rnning K, et al: Management of recurrent urinary tract infections with patient administered single dose therapy. Ann Intern Med 1985; 102:302.
18. Vosti K: Recurrent urinary tract infection: Prevention by prophylactic antibiotics after sexual intercourse. JAMA 1975; 231:934.
19. Patterson TF, Andriole VT: Bacteriuria in pregnancy. Infect Dis Clin North Am 1987; 1:807.
20. Pfau A, Sacks TG: Effective prophylaxis for recurrent urinary tract infections during pregnancy. Clin Infect Dis 1992; 14:810.
21. Turck M, Goffe B, Petersdorf RG: Bacteriuria of pregnancy. N Engl J Med 1962; 266:857.
22. Andriole VT, Patterson TF: Epidemiology, natural history, and management of urinary tract infections in pregnancy. Med Clin North Am 1991; 25:359.
23. Krieger JN: Complications and treatment of urinary tract infections during pregnancy. Urol Clin North Am 1986; 13:685.
24. Hooton TM, Stamm WE: Management of acute uncomplicated urinary tract infection in adults. Med Clin North Am 1991; 75:339.

34 Intra-abdominal Infections

JOHN A. WEIGELT ▶ KAREN J. BRASEL

Four common intra-abdominal infections that affect women are appendicitis, cholecystitis, diverticulitis, and secondary peritonitis. The first three involve specific organs, and the fourth can be a complication of the first three or related to other conditions. Each of the infections is discussed and specific concerns related to their presence in women are addressed.

BACTERIOLOGY

The bacteriology of these infections is related to the bacterial population of the gastrointestinal tract. The microorganisms found in the gastrointestinal tract increase in number and types from the stomach to the colon.[1] In healthy people, the stomach and small bowel contain few bacteria. Alterations in the acid environment of the stomach because of an achlorhydric state or acid-reducing medications cause bacterial counts to increase. Once the ileum is entered, bacterial counts of 10^8/mL are present. These increase further as the ileocecal valve is crossed and the colon is entered. The colon can have 10^{12} microorganisms per milliliter of stool. Not only does the concentration increase, but the types of bacteria found change. Organisms that may be present in the stomach and upper small bowel include lactobacilli, enterococci, and a few coliforms. In the ileum, coliforms are common, as are strict anaerobes. The colon is populated primarily by anaerobes, including *Bacteroides*. The anaerobes may outnumber the aerobes by a ratio of 10,000 to 1.[2]

Polymicrobial isolates remain the hallmark of intra-abdominal infections.[3] Both aerobes and anaerobes are commonly present. The average number of isolates ranges from 2.5 to 5. This includes an average of 1.4 to 2 aerobes and 2.4 to 3.8 anaerobes.[4] The most common aerobe isolated is *Escherichia coli*, and the most common anaerobe is *Bacteroides fragilis*.[5] Other *Bacteroides* isolates include *B. distasonis*, *B. ovatus*, *B. thetaiotaomicron*, and *B. vulgatus*.[6] When bacteria are present with cholecystitis, *E. coli*, *Klebsiella*, and enterococci are common.[7, 8] The multiple bacterial isolates indicate that antibiotic therapy must be effective against many different aerobic and anaerobic organisms.

The role enterococci play in intra-abdominal infections is controversial. These bacteria are facultative anaerobes that are indigenous to the gut, oral cavity, vagina, and urethra. *Streptococcus faecalis* is isolated in 90% of cases and *Streptococcus faecium* accounts for the remaining 10%.[9] In a model of intra-abdominal infection, enterococci can only produce abscesses if combined with another organism.[10] This finding supports the contention that specific enterococcal treatment is not necessary if the other bacteria are killed and adequate drainage is performed. Enterococci were isolated from 8% of 330 patients with intra-abdominal infection.[11] They were isolated from 29% of patients with a biliary source of infection, from 28% with a colonic source, and from 9% with an appendiceal source. This study used ciprofloxacin and metronidazole for treatment, and the failure rate was higher among patients with a positive culture for enterococci. Because approximately 70% of patients were successfully treated without specific enterococcal therapy, the routine administration of antibiotics against enterococci was not recommended.

CLINICAL CONDITIONS

Appendicitis

Pathogenesis

Appendicitis is the most common intra-abdominal infection requiring surgical therapy. It occurs most commonly in the second and third decades, although it can occur in patients of all ages. It starts with mechanical obstruction of the base of the appendix from impacted stool (fecalith) or lymphoid hyperplasia of Peyer's patches in the appendiceal submucosa. This leads initially to venous engorgement, edema, and, ultimately, occlusion of the appendiceal artery. This artery is an end artery, and occlusion sets the stage for progressive ischemia, gangrene, and perforation if the disease is left untreated. Increased intraluminal pressure results from continued secretion of the appendiceal mucosa. The bacterial flora multiplies and the ischemic appendiceal mucosa is unable to prevent invasion by these bacteria. Continued unchecked, this process leads to perforation and abscess formation. In many cases, the omentum becomes adherent to the inflammatory mass in an attempt to confine the process to the right lower quadrant. Without containment, generalized peritonitis can occur. This is more likely in patients at the extremes of age, contributing to the higher morbidity and mortality in these age groups.

Clinical Manifestations

The early symptoms of appendicitis are nausea, anorexia, and vague periumbilical pain. These occur as visceral pain fibers are stimulated by the distended appendix. Vomiting can occur, classically after the onset of pain. Bongard and colleagues[12] have suggested that the presence of anorexia, nausea, and vomiting helps distinguish appendicitis from pelvic inflammatory disease. Diarrhea is not usually a prominent complaint. With a retrocecal appendix, the patient may complain of flank pain. As the disease progresses, localized inflammation of the parietal peritoneum results in increased intensity of pain and migration to the right lower quadrant. The point of maximal pain and tenderness was initially described by McBurney[13] as "one and one-half to two inches inside the right anterior spinous process on a line drawn to the umbilicus." Physical examination usually reveals localized rebound and guarding in this location. Pressure on the left lower quadrant may reproduce right lower quadrant pain because of retrograde propagation of colonic air causing distention of the inflamed appendix (Rosving's sign). If the omentum is able to contain the inflammatory process, a palpable right lower quadrant mass may be present. This is often not appreciable until the patient is relaxed under general anesthesia because of involuntary guarding of the abdominal wall muscles. A retrocecal appendix may not produce classic signs of anterior inflammation, but tenderness can be elicited with passive movement of the right leg (psoas and obturator signs) as the appendix is brought against the parietal surfaces with these maneuvers. Rectal and vaginal examinations may elicit tenderness if the appendix lies adjacent to these organs. Fluctuance felt on either of these examinations indicates the presence of a pelvic abscess. A pelvic examination is mandatory in all women with complaints of right lower quadrant pain to exclude the multitude of diagnoses that can mimic appendicitis. Most patients have a low-grade temperature. A high, periodically spiking temperature is characteristic of a pelvic abscess. A rigid abdomen with diffuse involuntary guarding and rebound tenderness indicates generalized peritonitis, suggesting ruptured appendicitis without abscess formation.

Leukocytosis is present in most patients, and an elevated leukocyte count has been shown to have a sensitivity of 81% and specificity of 77% in patients with appendicitis.[14] However, the presence of a leukocyte count greater than 10,000 was unable to distinguish patients with appendicitis in one review.[15] The urine often contains white and red blood cells if the inflamed appendix lies on the ureter. Presence of leukocyte esterase, nitrite, or significant bacteria indicates a urinary tract infection rather than appendicitis.

Diagnosis

Appendicitis is a clinical diagnosis. The presence of nausea, anorexia, vague epigastric pain with migration to the right lower quadrant, a mild leukocytosis, and findings of localized right lower quadrant peritonitis does not need confirmation with further tests, and the patient with these signs and symptoms should be explored for presumed appendicitis. This picture is much more clear-cut in men, where the differential diagnosis is more limited. "Acceptable" rates of negative appendectomies overall range from 13% to 24%, and are higher in women (19% to 32%) than men (9% to 18%).[15, 16] Many conditions that may mimic appendicitis in women have a peak incidence in the same age. Mittelschmerz, ruptured ovarian cyst, ovarian torsion, pelvic inflammatory disease, tubo-ovarian abscess, and ectopic pregnancy can usually be differentiated by a good history, physical examination, and laboratory studies. Pelvic ultrasound can be useful to diagnose right lower quadrant disease when the clinical suspicion is higher for these gynecologic diseases than appendicitis. Right lower quadrant ultrasound has been used in attempts to decrease the negative appendectomy rate with varying success. Its diagnostic accuracy ranges from 72% to 90%,[17–19] and it was found by Jahn and co-workers[17] to offer no improvement over clinical diagnostic accuracy. Computed tomography (CT) is more accurate than ultrasound,[20] with accuracies of 93% to 98%.[21, 22] Rao and associates[22] reported cost savings by using routine appendiceal CT. The actual savings realized in other practices will be affected by the threshold used to send patients for CT and the use of appendiceal, rather than abdominopelvic, CT. Despite high diagnostic accuracies reported by some authors, the advent of ultrasound and CT as diagnostic aids has not changed the incidence of perforated appendicitis or negative appendectomies.[23]

The ultimate diagnostic aid is laparoscopy. In cases of routine appendicitis, laparoscopic appendectomy has no advantage over open appendectomy (see later). However, in young women with abdominal pain of unclear etiology, the use of laparoscopy can have a diagnostic and therapeutic role for both gynecologists and general surgeons.[24, 25]

Appendicitis in Pregnancy

Appendicitis in the pregnant patient deserves special comment. Although it is the most common nonobstetric cause for urgent operation during pregnancy, the common symptoms of nausea and abdominal pain may be due to pregnancy itself. Persistence of symptoms for longer than 24 hours is associated with an increased incidence of perforation.[26, 27] In the pregnant patient, the area of maximal tenderness moves superiorly and laterally as pregnancy progresses. By the third trimester, right upper quadrant pain may be the presenting symptom, making appendicitis difficult to distinguish from cholecystitis. Although maternal mortality is rare and morbidity low, the risk of fetal loss ranges from 3% to 15%.[26–28] Fetal loss can occur with negative laparotomy, but the incidence is much higher in patients with appendicitis and increases further with perforated appendicitis.[27] Laparoscopic appendectomy is possible in pregnant patients.[29]

Treatment

All patients with suspected appendicitis should undergo appendectomy. Preoperative antibiotics should be administered to all patients undergoing appendectomy. The antibiotic used should be active against bacteria normally found in the colon. In uncomplicated acute appendicitis, a single preoperative dose is all that is necessary.[30, 31] In perforated appendicitis with abscess, antibiotics should be administered until the patient is afebrile, has return of gastrointestinal function, and has a normal leukocyte count.[32] A number of antibiotic regimens have been shown to be effective; single-agent therapy is as effective as multidrug therapy.[33–35]

The technique of laparoscopic appendectomy has been credited to Semm and Schreiber.[36, 37] Multiple reports are now available comparing laparoscopic appendectomy with open appendectomy.[38–40] However, the question remains as to which technique should be the preferred treatment.

The technique commonly uses three ports: one infraumbilical, one in the left lower quadrant, and one in the right lower quadrant.[38] Occasionally, a fourth trocar is necessary in the right upper quadrant, especially if the appendix is retrocecal. A number of methods are used to transect the appendix, but most describe either a stapling device or an endoloop. A specimen bag is not routinely used unless the specimen is gangrenous.

A number of issues surrounding laparoscopic appendectomy remain controversial. These include the cost of the procedure, the real benefits for the patient, and the concern that in some cases the infectious complications may be increased.

The cost of laparoscopic appendectomy is greater than that of an open procedure.[38, 39] In one prospective study, open appendectomy was reported as costing more than laparoscopic appendectomy, although the method of cost accounting was not clear.[40] In general,

the operative costs are greater for laparoscopic appendectomy, but the overall costs for the two procedures are not different because patients are presumably discharged sooner after the laparoscopic procedure. The benefit is difficult to identify in patients with simple appendicitis.[41]

The patient benefits include better diagnosis, less pain, shorter hospitalizations, and rapid return to work. Appendicitis remains a clinical diagnosis and a 30% rate of negative appendectomies is not uncommon in a young female population. In 17% of 283 patients, the preoperative diagnosis of appendicitis was corrected by laparoscopic evaluation.[42] Most of these patients were female. Appendectomy was avoided in 23% of the women in this study. A definitive diagnosis is more common in women who are evaluated with laparoscopy.[43] These authors also suggest that early laparoscopy prevents protracted periods of observation and yields very acceptable cosmetic results. However, they caution against its higher cost.

Many reports support claims of less pain, shorter hospitalizations, and rapid return to work.[44–47] One report even discusses outpatient appendectomies for patients with nonperforated appendicitis and normal appendices.[48] However, other reports indicate few differences in these areas between the two procedures.[38–41]

A concern raised in some reports is an increased incidence of infectious complications in patients with complicated appendicitis treated by laparoscopic appendectomy.[49–51] Among 786 patients with perforated appendicitis, intra-abdominal abscesses occurred in 2.6% of patients having an open procedure and 9.0% having a laparoscopic procedure.[49] Other reports found similar results, although the differences do not reach statistical significance.[39, 50, 51]

Laparoscopic appendectomy clearly can decrease the number of negative appendectomies, especially among a female population. It also appears to increase the number of correct diagnoses. It is more costly and unless patient benefits can be documented, it is difficult to recommend as the procedure of choice when the open procedure is very close to minimally invasive surgery. Finally, a concern is raised regarding an increased incidence of infectious complications in patients with perforated appendicitis. These patients are probably best treated by open appendectomy at this time.

Prevention

Prevention of any infectious disease should always be our goal. Some infections lend themselves to a preventive intervention with current technology; others do not. Of the infections covered in this chapter, preventive methods are available for two: appendicitis and diverticulitis. The approaches are different, and some may decide that they are not worthwhile.

Prevention of appendicitis is accomplished by removal of the appendix during other abdominal operations. This is called incidental appendectomy or appendectomy en passant. The purpose of this removal is to prevent appendicitis and possibly colon cancer or other metastatic cancers that could involve the appendix.[52, 53] Two questions are always debated with regard to the validity of incidental appendectomy: does it increase surgical wound infection, and does it really prevent appendicitis?

Some studies suggest that surgical wound infection risk is increased after incidental appendectomy, especially in high-risk patients. A surgical wound infection rate of 1.5% was reported in patients having cholecystectomy alone, compared with 3.7% in patients having a cholecystectomy and appendectomy.[54] This difference was not statistically significant, but patients older than 50 years of age did have a statistically higher surgical wound infection rate compared with patients younger than 50 years of age. A more recent review of elderly Medicare beneficiaries showed an increased risk of wound infection when incidental appendectomy was performed with cholecystectomy.[55] The adjusted odds ratio for wound infection was 83% greater with appendectomy: 1.08 without and 1.93 with appendectomy. In a younger population, surgical wound infection was not different when appendectomy was added to cholecystectomy.[56] Appendectomy also was not reported to increase surgical wound infection or infectious complications in gynecologic procedures, during procedures for ectopic pregnancy, or vaginal surgery.[52, 57–59] The risk of infectious complications is increased slightly with incidental appendectomy, but this may be offset by a decreased rate of appendicitis. The risk of appendicitis decreases with age. It is approximately 20% at birth, decreases to 2% to 3% at 50 years of age, and then to 1% at 70 years of age.[60] The age of 50 years is suggested as the cut-off point after which incidental appendectomy is not beneficial in preventing appendicitis.

Nockerts and associates[61] evaluated the appropriateness of incidental appendectomy in the elderly. They concluded that 100 incidental appendectomies in patients older than 65 years of age are required to avoid 1 case of appendicitis, and that 3,000 cases are necessary to save 1 life from appendicitis. They concluded that incidental appendectomy was not indicated in the elderly. A similar analysis calculated that 4,400 incidental appendectomies were necessary to salvage 1 life from appendicitis.[55]

These data indicate that incidental appendectomy is rarely indicated in patients. This is especially true in patients 50 years of age or older. Because morbidity is low in younger patients and their risk of appendicitis is higher, incidental appendectomy potentially provides more benefit without negative outcomes. This conclusion is only supposition because no specific study addresses this issue directly. When patients are at increased risk for infectious complications based on comorbid factors, incidental appendectomy should not be performed regardless of the patient's age.[53]

Cholecystitis

Pathogenesis

Cholecystitis is an inflammatory process initiated by obstruction of the cystic duct. Obstruction is due to gallstones in most cases, and most gallstones are cholesterol stones. The female-to-male incidence of acute cholecystitis is 3:2, and it most commonly affects people in the fifth decade. As in the pathogenesis of appendicitis, intraluminal pressure rises as the gallbladder mucosa continues to secrete fluid, electrolytes, and proteins. Vascular compromise occurs when the intraluminal pressure becomes greater than the pressure in the capillaries. Normal bile in the absence of obstruction is sterile,[62] attributed in part to high biliary concentrations of immunoglobulins, antibacterial properties of bile salts, and continuous bile flow. With obstruction of the cystic duct, continuous biliary flow is lost and secondary infection can occur. Intraoperative cultures are positive in 42% to 63% of patients undergoing cholecystectomy for acute cholecystitis. The most common pathogens isolated from the bile and gallbladder wall are *E. coli*, *Klebsiella*, and enterococci.[63, 64] Without treatment, progressive ischemia and infarction of the gallbladder wall can lead to frank gangrene and perforation.

Clinical Manifestations

The most common symptom of biliary tract disease is abdominal pain. This typically occurs several hours after a fatty meal. Nausea and vomiting may be present. The pain is constant, not colicky, and severe. It is located in the right upper quadrant and may radiate to the back or scapula. Patients with acute cholecystitis may have a history of previous symptomatic gallstones with attacks that subside after several hours. In contrast, the pain of acute cholecystitis does not remit.

Physical examination may reveal an elevated temperature. There is tenderness in the right upper quadrant, with guarding. A positive Murphy's sign is halting of respiration by the patient with direct pressure over the gallbladder. As the gallbladder distends, it moves laterally and inferiorly, and may be palpable, particularly once the patient is relaxed under general anesthesia. A rigid abdomen is unusual because the process usually remains confined to the right upper quadrant, and the presence of generalized abdominal tenderness should arouse suspicion of a diagnosis other than cholecystitis.

Laboratory testing usually shows a leukocytosis. Liver function tests may be mildly elevated. It is not uncommon to see a bilirubin level of 2 to 3 mg/dL. Bilirubin levels greater than 5 mg/dL or very high liver function test results should raise the suspicion of choledocholithiasis, cholangitis, or hepatitis. Cholangitis is associated with fever, leukocytosis, right upper quadrant pain, and hyperbilirubinemia. It requires urgent resuscitation, antibiotics, and decompression of the biliary tree by some means.[65]

Diagnosis

The gold standard for diagnosis of cholelithiasis is ultrasound. In addition to gallstones, secondary sonographic signs of acute cholecystitis include wall thickening, sonographic Murphy's sign (halting respiration with ultrasound-guided compression directly over the gallbladder), and pericholecystic fluid. The accuracy of ultrasound in the diagnosis of gallstones is 95%. The secondary signs are less accurate when used by themselves; however, in combination with gallstones, a positive sonographic Murphy's sign has a positive predictive value of 92%, and gallbladder wall thickening 95% for acute cholecystitis.[66] A sonographic Murphy's sign may be less helpful in acute gangrenous cholecystitis.[67] Biliary scintigraphy is also used to diagnose biliary tract disease. Nonvisualization of the gallbladder with this test indicates obstruction of the cystic duct and acute cholecystitis. Although most gallbladders fill within 1 hour, the test should be carried out to 4 hours conclusively to demonstrate duct obstruction. Biliary scintigraphy has a positive predictive value of 68% to 97% for acute cholecystitis. Ultrasound is easier, costs less, and takes less time to perform than scintigraphy and should be used as the initial test in acute cholecystitis. Scintigraphy should be reserved for those situations in which ultrasound is technically difficult or equivocal. It should not be used in pregnancy.

Treatment

The treatment of acute cholecystitis is antibiotics and cholecystectomy. The antibiotics should be active against gram-negative bacteria and enterococci. Biliary concentration of antibiotic is not as important as clinical spectrum and achieving bactericidal serum concentrations.[68] A number of antibiotics have been shown to be effective in acute cholecystitis.[69, 70] Most cases of acute cholecystitis resolve with antibiotic therapy alone. However, approximately 10% go on to perforation and gangrene. Cholecystectomy within the first 3 or 4 days is advocated to decrease the incidence and morbidity associated with these complications. Early cholecystectomy is technically easier to perform and decreases the morbidity and length of stay.[71] Simple acute cholecystitis is adequately treated by preoperative antibiotics and cholecystectomy. Patients who have complicated cholecystitis with extensive right upper quadrant inflammation should remain on antibiotics until afebrile with a normal leukocyte count.

Acute cholecystitis is a risk factor for conversion to open cholecystectomy, increasing the likelihood of conversion by 4.6 times (for a conversion rate of 6.1%).[72] However, the safety of laparoscopic cholecystectomy in acute cholecystitis is well documented.[73, 74]

Cholecystitis in Pregnancy

In the pregnant patient, treatment of symptomatic cholelithiasis without cholecystitis should be expectant management, postponing cholecystectomy until after delivery, if possible. Acute cholecystitis may require operative intervention during pregnancy. In the first trimester, the risk of fetal loss is highest with general anesthesia, and acute cholecystitis should be treated medically with antibiotics. If the patient fails to improve as evidenced by normalization of temperature and resolution of abdominal complaints, cholecystectomy is indicated. The same treatment for acute cholecystitis can be used in the second trimester; however, some groups have advocated a more aggressive approach, citing the safety of early laparoscopic cholecystectomy in their hands.[75, 76] Although the technique has been reported, the increase in uterine size in the third trimester makes laparoscopic cholecystectomy technically difficult, and patients who fail to respond to medical management are probably best served with open cholecystectomy. All laparoscopies in pregnancy should use the open technique for placement of the insufflation cannula.

Diverticulitis

Pathogenesis

Diverticula are herniations of colonic mucosa and submucosa through the circular layer of muscle between the taeniae, the longitudinal muscular layers of the colon. These diverticula are classified as pseudodiverticula. The incidence of diverticulosis in the United States increases with age, occurring in approximately one third of people by 50 years and approaching 50% by 80 years of age. There does not seem to be a gender predilection. Increased intraluminal pressure and weakness of the colonic wall that occurs with age contribute to the development of diverticula, which are concentrated in the sigmoid colon. Lack of dietary fiber also plays a significant role, explaining why diverticulosis is much more prevalent in highly industrialized countries such as the United States.[77]

Complications of diverticular disease include bleeding, infection, obstruction, and perforation. These complications occur in an estimated 10% to 20% of patients with diverticulosis.[78, 79] Diverticulitis is a localized inflammation of one or more diverticula that occurs when the base of the diverticulum is obstructed by impacted stool, allowing overgrowth of colonic bacteria. The diverticulum can perforate into the mesentery, between loops of bowel, into the pelvis, or freely into the peritoneal cavity. Erosion of the inflammatory process into adjacent organs can produce coloenteric, colovesical, colocolonic, and colovaginal fistulas.

Clinical Manifestations

Diverticulitis produces crampy lower abdominal pain often localized to the left lower quadrant. The pain is initially crampy, although with progression of disease it becomes more persistent. Altered bowel habits are common, with constipation more usual than diarrhea. Persistent diarrhea may indicate the presence of a coloenteric fistula. Pneumaturia and fecaluria are pathognomonic of a colovesical fistula; dysuria, frequency, and recurrent urinary tract infections are also common.

Findings on physical examination depend on the severity of disease. Patients with mild diverticulitis may have a slightly elevated temperature, whereas those with free rupture and peritonitis can be quite toxic. Abdominal findings range from mild left lower quadrant tenderness, localized rebound and guarding, to the diffuse rigidity of generalized peritonitis. A mass in the left lower quadrant is often palpable. Fluctuance on rectal or pelvic examination indicates a pelvic abscess. Obstruction or ileus secondary to infection can produce abdominal distention.

Diagnosis

In patients with a history of diverticular disease, the presence of fever, left lower quadrant pain and tenderness, and leukocytosis requires no further imaging studies to establish the diagnosis of diverticulitis. In patients without such a history, in whom the diagnosis is uncertain, or in whom a diverticular abscess is suspected, an abdominopelvic CT scan is the preferred initial imaging study.[80] CT can show diverticulosis and signs of inflammation indicating acute diverticulitis. In addition, diverticular abscesses are often amenable to percutaneous drainage once identified by CT scan. Gastrografin or barium enema is not recommended during an acute episode of diverticulitis because of the possibility of ruptured diverticula that could lead to intraperitoneal administration of contrast. Sigmoidoscopy and colonoscopy are often difficult and painful to perform during an acute attack because of the intense spasm of the colon, and are usually unnecessary. However, once an attack has subsided, the entire colon should be evaluated with either colonoscopy or a barium enema to determine the extent of disease and to rule out any other colonic disease. Colovesical fistulas are best diagnosed by cystoscopy, which often shows only an area of inflamed mucosa. Colovaginal fistulas can be diagnosed on pelvic examination or by demonstrating fecal material on a vaginal tampon. Diverticular rupture may not require imaging if the patient has signs of peritonitis mandating emergency operation. However, plain abdominal films show free air, and abdominal CT scan is able to detect smaller amounts of free air.[81, 82]

Treatment

Patients with left lower quadrant pain and no systemic signs of illness (normal temperature and leukocyte count) can often be treated with dietary modification and oral antibiotics. Dietary modification consists of increasing fiber intake. Oral antibiotics should be active against colonic aerobic and anaerobic bacteria. With more intense abdominal pain, fever, or leukocytosis, the patient should be admitted for intravenous antibiotics combined with bowel rest. If the patient shows good clinical response to therapy, diet is slowly advanced and the patient changed to oral antibiotics. Most patients who present with uncomplicated diverticulitis respond to medical therapy. Failure to respond raises suspicion of a diverticular abscess rather than failure of antibiotic therapy, and an abdominal CT scan should be obtained.

Laparoscopic colectomy is an option for surgical treatment of diverticular disease. The methods vary from a total laparoscopic technique to a laparoscopic-assisted technique.[83, 84] The former includes intra-abdominal dissection and anastomosis. The latter usually includes accomplishing the dissection using the laparoscope and creating the anastomosis in an extra-abdominal location. This requires making a small incision to bring the colon onto the anterior abdominal wall.

The technique requires five or six trocar sites.[83, 85] The sites used include an infraumbilical, right and left paramedian at the level of the umbilicus, a left lower quadrant, and a right upper quadrant. When a laparoscopic-assisted procedure is used, the specimen is usually brought out a small incision through the left paramedian trocar site. Other retrieval sites used include a Pfannenstiel incision. The specimen can also be brought out through the rectum if a total laparoscopic procedure is desired.

Advantages for a laparoscopic colon resection mimic those suggested for laparoscopic appendectomy. These include less pain, better cosmesis, fewer complications, shorter hospital stay, and more rapid return to normal activities.[86] The patients do appear to be able to tolerate a regular diet 1 to 2 days earlier, resulting in a 1- to 2-day shorter hospital stay.[84]

The major disadvantage of this procedure is the

increased cost.[87] Once again, the major increase in costs is in the operating room secondary to the increased time spent doing the procedure. The hope that this cost is offset by a decreased length of stay may or may not be realized. This is especially true as conversion rates continue to be approximately 20%.[88, 89] However, in a small group of patients with benign colon disease, the conversion rate was only 2%.[87] The lower rates of conversion are thought to be associated with proper preoperative selection of patients, one-segment colonic resections, and extensive experience. The 20% conversion rate may also represent the limits of current technology.[88]

Patients with diverticulitis requiring surgical therapy can have a laparoscopic colectomy performed safely. These patients may have some benefits related to shorter hospitalization and better cosmesis. However, these procedures do cost more and are hard to justify economically. As technology improves, the cost may fall, and applying this surgical technique more widely would then be possible.

Prevention

Prevention of diverticulitis is based on dietary alterations that it is hoped will decrease the symptoms of diverticular disease, resulting in a decrease in the number of attacks of symptoms consistent with diverticulitis.[90] The recommended dietary alteration is a high-fiber diet based on the observation that diverticular disease is more common in industrialized nations.[77] It has been termed "a disease of Western civilization."[91]

The dietary fiber theory is supported by numerous studies documenting increases in diverticular disease and diverticulitis as fiber was removed and returned to diets.[92, 93] A study of vegetarians and nonvegetarians showed that the incidence of diverticular disease decreased when the fiber was increased.[94] Treatment of patients with a high-fiber diet relieves symptoms in more than 80%.[95, 96] Whether a high-fiber diet actually prevents complications of diverticular disease remains controversial.

When symptomatic patients with diverticulosis were given a high-fiber diet, 91% remained asymptomatic for 5 to 7 years.[97] Among 25 patients who did not adhere to their diet in this study, the recurrence rate of symptoms consistent with diverticulitis was 20%. These authors recommended 40 g of fiber per day. Others suggest as little as 10 to 25 g/day.[90] Symptom relief is usually in the form of decreased pain and possibly decreased number of episodes of diverticulitis.

Unfortunately, whether a high-fiber diet reliably decreases all the complications of diverticulosis is unknown.[98] This is especially true in evaluating the complications other than infection, which include bleeding and obstruction. It seems reasonable to recommend to patients with diverticulosis that a dietary change might be beneficial. The diet should be altered to include as much fiber as possible, which can be obtained from nonabsorbable dietary fiber or hydrophyllic colloid laxatives. Both increase stool bulk, which is the desired result.

As fiber is increased, patients may often complain of abdominal pain, especially in the first 4 to 6 weeks. This subsides as the gastrointestinal tract accommodates to the increased bulk.

Peritonitis

Pathogenesis

Peritonitis is defined as inflammation of the peritoneum. It is classified as primary when there is no source of contamination from the gastrointestinal tract, and secondary when a source is identifiable. Primary peritonitis is not considered here.

Colonic perforation resulting from diverticulitis, cancer, or volvulus accounts for 25% of secondary peritonitis, and perforated appendicitis accounts for an additional 24%. Postoperative peritonitis is responsible for another 20%, with perforated ulcers (11%), pancreatitis and biliary disease (11%), and small bowel disease (7%) occurring less commonly.[99]

The bacteria responsible for peritonitis depend somewhat on the level of perforation. The stomach and duodenum are normally sterile and may produce a chemical peritonitis early in the course of perforated ulcer. However, many patients are treated with antacids or histamine-2 blockers, allowing bacterial overgrowth and polymicrobial peritonitis.[100] Most peritonitis is polymicrobial, with mixed aerobic and anaerobic bacteria.[101, 102]

Clinical Manifestations

The initial symptoms of peritonitis relate to the specific disease responsible. Regardless, pain that may initially have been localized becomes generalized and increases in severity. Any movement, jostling of the bed, or cough aggravates the pain. The patient is febrile and tachycardic, and may become hypotensive as the disease progresses. Mucous membranes are dry and the skin has diminished turgor. Abdominal examination usually reveals hypoactive to absent bowel sounds. Involuntary guarding gives the abdomen a board-like quality, and rebound tenderness is present throughout. Mental status may decline with progressive sepsis and shock.

Laboratory studies in peritonitis reflect the patient's depleted volume status. Leukocytosis with a pronounced left shift is present in most patients with competent immune systems. However, elderly or immunocompromised patients may not be able to mount either fever or leukocytosis, despite the fact that elderly patients are more likely to present with advanced peritonitis.[103] Diagnostic imaging studies are not necessary in the patient with established peritonitis who has a "surgical abdomen," but may reveal free air or other intra-abdominal pathologic processes in patients with less clear-cut clinical signs.

Treatment

The patient must be adequately resuscitated with crystalloid solutions before surgery. In the young, otherwise healthy patient, normal heart rate, urine output of 0.5 to 1 mL/kg, and normal mental status may be used as reliable end points for resuscitation. In elderly patients or those with coexisting chronic medical diseases, invasive monitoring of fluid status may need to begin before surgery.[104] Once adequately resuscitated, patients are taken to the operating room to control the source of the infection.

Antibiotic therapy in intra-abdominal infection is broad-spectrum and empiric, aimed at the mixed aerobic and anaerobic bacteria usually isolated. Routine cultures of the peritoneal cavity are not recommended because results rarely influence clinical decisions.[105] Inappropriate antibiotic choice is associated with increased morbidity and mortality.[105] There are many effective regimens.[106–108] Single-drug therapy has been shown to be equivalent to double- or triple-drug therapy.[102, 105–107] The duration of antibiotic administration should not be fixed, but determined by clinical response. Studies support continuing antibiotics until the patient is afebrile with a normal white blood cell count.[109] Intravenous antibiotics have traditionally been used for the entire course, but the oral route is being investigated as a less costly alternative. Patients are begun on the intravenous form and are switched to oral when appropriate. The intravenous/oral switch approach has been shown to be as effective as the intravenous route alone, although further studies need to be done.[110]

Poor response to antibiotic therapy after adequate source control should raise concern for intra-abdominal abscesses. However, outcome in peritonitis is often related to patient comorbidities and the systemic inflammatory response initiated by intra-abdominal infection.[103, 111]

REFERENCES

1. Yeo CJ, Zinner MJ: Gastrointestinal failure. In: Wilmore DW, Brennan MF, Harlan AH, et al (eds): Surgery, Vol I. New York, Scientific American, 1997, pp 1–16.
2. Donaldson RM, Toskes PP: The relation of enteric bacterial populations to gastrointestinal function and disease. In: Sleisenger MH, Fordtran JS (eds): Gastrointestinal Disease: Pathophysiology, Diagnosis, Management, 4th ed. Philadelphia, WB Saunders, 1989, pp 107–113.
3. Rotstein OD, Pruett TL, Simmons RL: Lethal microbial synergism in intra-abdominal infections. Arch Surg 1985; 120:146.
4. Nichols RL, Holmes JWC: Peritonitis. In: Gorbach SL, Bartlett JG, Blacklow NR (eds): Infectious Diseases. Philadelphia, WB Saunders, 1992, pp 661–668.
5. Dunn DL, Simmons RL: The role of anaerobic bacteria in intraabdominal infections. Rev Infect Dis 1984; 6:S139.
6. Scher KS: Emergence of antibiotic resistant strains. Surg Gynecol Obstet 1988; 167:175.
7. Csendes A, Burdiles P, Maluenda F, et al: Simultaneous bacteriologic assessment of bile from gallbladder and common bile duct in control subjects and patients with gallstones and common duct stones. Arch Surg 1996; 131:389.
8. Muller EL, Pitt HA, Thompson JE, et al: Antibiotics in infections of the biliary tract. Surg Gynecol Obstet 1987; 165:285.
9. deVera ME, Simmons RL: Antibiotic-resistant enterococci and the changing face of surgical infections. Arch Surg 1996; 131:338.
10. Onderdonk AB, Bartlett JG, Louie T, et al: Microbial synergy in experimental intra-abdominal abscess. Infect Immun 1976; 13:22.
11. Burnett RJ, Haverstock DC, Dellinger EP, et al: Defintion of the role of enterococcus in intraabdominal infection: Analysis of a prospective randomized trial. Surgery 1995; 118:716.
12. Bongard F, Landers DV, Lewis F: Differential diagnosis of appendicitis and pelvic inflammatory disease: A prospective analysis. Am J Surg 1985; 150:90.
13. McBurney C: Experience with early operative interference in cases of disease of the vermiform appendix. NY Med J 1989; 50:676.
14. Lau WY, Ho YC, Chu KW: Leucocyte count and neutrophil percentage in appendicectomy for suspected appendicitis. Aust N Z J Surg 1989; 59:395.
15. Hale DA, Molloy M, Pearl RH, et al: Appendectomy: A contemporary appraisal. Ann Surg 1997; 225:252.
16. Korner H, Sondenaa K, Soreide JA, et al: Incidence of acute nonperforated and perforated appendicitis: Age-specific and sex-specific analysis. World J Surg 1997; 21:313.
17. Jahn H, Mathiesen FK, Neckelmann K, et al: Comparison of clinical judgment and diagnostic ultrasonography in the diagnosis of acute appendicitis: Experience with a score aided diagnosis. Eur J Surg 1997; 163:433.
18. Verroken R, Penninckx F, Hoe LV, et al: Diagnostic accuracy of ultrasonography and surgical decision-making in patients referred for suspicion of appendicitis. Acta Chir Belg 1996; 96:158.
19. Puylaert JBCM, Rutgers PH, Lalisang RI, et al: A prospective study of ultrasonography in the diagnosis of appendicitis. N Engl J Med 1987; 317:666.
20. Balthazar EJ, Birnbaum BA, Yee J, et al: Acute appendicitis: CT and US correlation in 100 patients. Radiology 1994; 190:31.
21. Rao PM, Rhea JT, Novelline RA: Sensitivity and specificity of the individual CT signs of appendicitis: Experience with 200 helical appendiceal CT examinations. J Comput Assist Tomogr 1997; 21:686.
22. Rao PM, Rhea JT, Novelline RA, et al: Effect of computed tomography of the appendix on treatment of patients and use of hospital resources. N Engl J Med 1998; 338:131.
23. Sarfati MR, Hunter GC, Witzke DB, et al: Impact of adjunctive testing on the diagnosis and clinical course of patients with acute appendicitis. Am J Surg 1993; 166:660.
24. Taylor EW, Kennedy CA, Dunham RH, et al: Diagnostic laparoscopy in women with acute abdominal pain. Surg Laparosc Endosc 1995; 5:125.
25. Graham A, Henley C, Mobley J: Laparoscopic evaluation of acute abdominal pain. J Laparoendosc Surg 1991; 1:165.
26. Tamir IL, Bongard FS, Klein SR: Acute appendicitis in the pregnant patient. Am J Surg 1990; 160:571.
27. Al-Mulhim AA: Acute appendicitis in pregnancy: A review of 52 cases. Int Surg 1996; 81:295.
28. Masters K, Levine BA, Gaskill HV, et al: Diagnosing appendicitis during pregnancy. Am J Surg 1984; 148:768.
29. Schreiber JH: Laparoscopic appendectomy in pregnancy. Surg Endosc 1990; 4:100.
30. Bauer T, Vennits B, Birger H, et al: Antibiotic prophylaxis in surgery for non-perforated appendicitis: The Danish Multicenter Study—Group III. Ann Surg 1989; 209:307.
31. Yellin AE, Heseltine PNR, Berne TV, et al: The role of Pseu-

domonas species in patients treated with ampicillin and sulbactam for gangrenous and perforated appendicitis. Surg Gynecol Obstet 1985; 161:303.

32. Mosdell DM, Morris DM, Fry D: Peritoneal cultures and antibiotic therapy in pediatric perforated appendicitis. Am J Surg 1994; 167:313.

33. Ceraldi CM, Waxman K: Antibiotic management of surgically treated appendicitis: A review. Infect Surg 1992; p 25.

34. Sirinek KR, Levine BA: Antimicrobial management of surgically treated gangrenous or perforated appendicitis: Comparison of cefoxitin and clindamycin/gentamicin. Clin Ther 1987; 9:420.

35. Heseltine PNR, Yellin AE, Appleman MD, et al: Imipenem therapy for perforated and gangrenous appendicitis. Surg Gynecol Obstet 1986; 162:43.

36. Semm K: Endoscopic appendectomy. Endoscopy 1983; 15:59.

37. Laine S, Rantala A, Gullichsen R, et al: Laparoscopic appendectomy: Is it worthwhile? Surg Endosc 1997; 11:95.

38. Vallina VL, Velasco JM, McCulloch CS: Laparoscopic versus conventional appendectomy. Ann Surg 1993; 218:685.

39. Bonanni F, Reed J, Hartzell G, et al: Laparoscopic versus conventional appendectomy. J Am Coll Surg 1994; 179:273.

40. Martin LC, Puente I, Sosa JL, et al: Open versus laparoscopic appendectomy: A prospective randomized comparison. Ann Surg 1995; 222:256.

41. Hale DA, Molloy M, Pearl RH, et al: Appendectomy a contemporary appraisal. Ann Surg 1997; 225:252.

42. Bouillot JL, Salah S, Fernandez F, et al: Laparoscopic procedure for suspected appendicitis: A prospective study in 283 consecutive patients. Surg Endosc 1995; 9:957.

43. Zaninotto G, Rossi M, Anselmino M, et al: Laparoscopic versus conventional surgery for suspected appendicitis in women. Surg Endosc 1995; 9:337.

44. Attwood SEA, Hill ADK, Murphy PG, et al: A prospective randomized trial of laparoscopic versus open appendectomy. Surgery 1992; 112:497.

45. Kazemier G, de Zeeuw GR, Lange JF, et al: Laparoscopic vs open appendectomy: A randomized clinical trial. Surg Endosc 1997; 11:336.

46. Cox MR, McCall JL, Toouli J, et al: Prospective randomized comparison of open versus laparoscopic appendectomy in men. World J Surg 1996; 20:263.

47. Ortega AE, Hunter JG, Peters JH, et al: A prospective, randomized comparison of laparoscopic appendectomy with open appendectomy. Am J Surg 1995; 169:208.

48. Jain A, Mercado PD, Grafton KP, et al: Outpatient laparoscopic appendectomy. Surg Endosc 1995; 9:424.

49. Paik PS, Towson JA, Anthone GF, et al: Intra-abdominal abscesses following laparoscopic and open appendectomies. J Gastrointest Surg 1997; 1:188.

50. Frazee RC, Bohannon WT: Laparoscopic appendectomy for complicated appendicitis. Arch Surg 1996; 131:509.

51. Kluiber RM, Hartsman B: Laparoscopic appendectomy: A comparison with open appendectomy. Dis Colon Rectum 1996; 39:1008.

52. Westermann C, Mann WJ, Chumas J, et al: Routine appendectomy in extensive gynecologic operations. Surg Gynecol Obstet 1986; 162:307.

53. Fisher KS, Ross DS: Guidelines for therapeutic decision in incidental appendectomy. Surg Gynecol Obstet 1990; 171:95.

54. Andrew MH, Roty AR: Incidental appendectomy with cholecystectomy: Is the increased risk justified? Am Surg 1987; 53:553.

55. Warren JL, Penberthy, Addiss DG, et al: Appendectomy incidental to cholecystectomy among elderly Medicare beneficiaries. Surg Gynecol Obstet 1993; 177:288.

56. El-Sefi TAM, El-Awady HM, Shehata MI: Prophylactic appendicectomy during elective cholecystectomy: Effects on morbidity. A prospective, controlled study. Int Surg 1989; 74:32.

57. Cromartie AD, Kovalcik PJ: Incidental appendectomy at the time of surgery for ectopic pregnancy. Am J Surg 1980; 139:244.

58. Reiner IJ: Incidental appendectomy at the time of vaginal surgery. Tex Med 1980; 76:46.

59. Arnbjörnsson E: Incidental appendectomy: Risks versus benefits. Curr Surg 1983; 40:194.

60. Ludbrook J, Spears GFS: The risk of developing appendicitis. Br J Surg 1965; 52:856.

61. Nockerts SR, Detmer DE, Fryback DG: Incidental appendectomy in the elderly? No. Surgery 1980; 88:301.

62. Csendes A, Fernandez M, Uribe P: Bacteriology of the gallbladder bile in normal subjects. Am J Surg 1975; 129:629.

63. Thompson JE, Bennion RS, Doty JE, et al: Predictive factors for bactibilia in acute cholecystitis: Indications for therapy. Arch Surg 1990; 125:261.

64. Lee W, Chang KJ, Lee CS, et al: Suppurative cholangitis: Bacteriology and choice of antibiotic. Hepatogastroenterology 1992; 39:347.

65. Kadakia SC: Biliary tract emergencies: Acute cholecystitis, acute cholangitis, acute pancreatitis. Med Clin North Am 1993; 77:1015.

66. Ralls PW, Colletti PM, Lapin SA, et al: Real-time sonography in suspected acute cholecystitis: Prospective evaluation of primary and secondary signs. Radiology 1985; 155:767.

67. Simeone JF, Brink JA, Mueller PR, et al: The sonographic diagnosis of acute gangrenous cholecystitis: Importance of the Murphy sign. AJR Am J Roentgenol 1989; 152:289.

68. Keighley MR, Baddeley RM, Burdon DW, et al: A controlled trial of parenteral prophylactic gentamicin therapy in biliary surgery. Br J Surg 1975; 62:275.

69. Muller EL, Pitt HA, Thompson JE, et al: Antibiotics in infections of the biliary tract. Surg Gynecol Obstet 1987; 165:285.

70. Dooley JS, Hamilton-Miller JMT, Brumfitt W, et al: Antibiotics in the treatment of biliary infection. Gut 1984; 25:988.

71. Jarvinen HJ, Hastacka J: Early cholecystectomy for acute cholecystitis. Ann Surg 1980; 191:501.

72. Wiebke EA, Pruitt AL, Howard TJ, et al: Conversion of laparoscopic to open cholecystectomy: An analysis of risk factors. Surg Endosc 1996; 10:742.

73. Miller RE, Kimmelstiel FM: Laparoscopic cholecystectomy for acute cholecystitis. Surg Endosc 1993; 7:296.

74. Bender JS, Zenilman ME: Immediate laparoscopic cholecystectomy as definitive therapy for acute cholecystitis. Surg Endosc 1995; 9:1081.

75. Morrell DG, Mullins JR, Harrison PB: Laparoscopic cholecystectomy during pregnancy in symptomatic patients. Surgery 1992; 112:856.

76. Wishner JD, Zolfaghari D, Wohlgemuth SD, et al: Laparoscopic cholecystectomy in pregnancy: A report of 6 cases and review of the literature. Surg Endosc 1996; 10:314.

77. Morson BC: Pathology of diverticular disease of the colon. Clin Gastroenterol 1975; 4:37.

78. McGowan FJ, Wolff WI: Diverticulosis of the sigmoid colon. Gastroenterology 1952; 21:119.

79. Painter NS, Burkitt DP: Diverticular disease of the colon: A 20th century problem. Clin Gastroenterol 1975; 4:3.

80. Roberts P, Abel M, Rosen L, et al: Practice parameters for sigmoid diverticulitis: Supporting documentation. Dis Colon Rectum 1995; 38:126.

81. Stapakis JC, Thickman D: Diagnosis of pneumoperitoneum: Abdominal CT vs. upright chest film. J Comput Assist Tomogr 1992; 16:713.

82. Earls JP, Dachman AH, Colon E, et al: Prevalence and duration of postoperative pneumoperitoneum: Sensitivity of CT vs left lateral decubitus radiography. AJR Am J Roentgenol 1993; 161:781.

83. Phillips EH, Franklin M, Carroll BJ, et al: Laparoscopic colectomy. Ann Surg 1992; 216:703.

84. Bruce CJ, Coller JA, Murray JJ, et al: Laparoscopic resection for diverticular disease. Dis Colon Rectum 1996; 39:S1.

85. Eijsbouts QAJ, Cuesta MA, de Brauw LM, et al: Elective laparoscopic-assisted sigmoid resection for diverticular disease. Surg Endosc 1997; 11:750.

86. Hoffman GC, Baker JW, Fitchett CW, et al: Laparoscopic-assisted colectomy initial experience. Ann Surg 1994; 219:732.

87. Bergamaschi R, Arnaud JP: Immediately recognizable benefits and drawbacks after laparoscopic colon resection for benign disease. Surg Endosc 1997; 11:802.

88. Wishner JD, Baker JW, Hoffman GC, et al: Laparoscopic-assisted colectomy: The learning curve. Surg Endosc 1995; 9:1179.

89. Agachan F, Joo JS, Weiss EG, et al: Laparoscopic colorectal surgery: Do we get faster? Surg Endosc 1997; 11:331.

90. Naitove A, Almy TP: Diverticular disease of the colon. In: Sleisenger MH, Fordtran JS (eds): Gastrointestinal Disease: Pathophysiology, Diagnosis, Management, 4th ed. Philadelphia, WB Saunders, 1989, pp 1419–1433.

91. Painter NS, Burkitt DP: Diverticular disease of the colon: A disease of Western civilization. BMJ 1971; 2:450.

92. Almy TP, Howell DA: Diverticular disease of the colon. N Engl J Med 1980; 302:324.

93. Manousos O, Day NE, Tzonou A, et al: Diet and other factors in the aetiology of diverticulosis: An epidemiological study in Greece. Gut 1985; 26:544.

94. Gear JS, Fursdon P, Nolan DJ, et al: Symptomless diverticular disease and intake of dietary fibre. Lancet 1979; 1:511.

95. Parks TG: Natural history of diverticular disease of the colon. Clin Gastroenterol 1975; 4:53.

96. Brodribb AJM: Treatment of symptomatic diverticular disease with a high-fibre diet. Lancet 1977; 1:664.

97. Hyland JMP, Taylor I: Does a high fibre diet prevent the complications of diverticular disease? Br J Surg 1980; 67:7.

98. Hackford AW, Veidenheimer MC: Diverticular disease of the colon: Current concepts and management. Surg Clin North Am 1985; 65:347.

99. Solomkin JS, Dellinger EP, Christou NV, et al: Results of a multicenter trial comparing imipenem/cilastatin to tobramycin/clindamycin for intraabdominal infections. Ann Surg 1990; 212:581.

100. Ruddell WSJ, Axon ATR, Findlay JM, et al: Effect of cimetidine on the gastric bacterial flora. Lancet 1980; 1:672.

101. Brook I: A 12 year study of aerobic and anaerobic bacteria in intra-abdominal and postsurgical abdominal wound infections. Surg Gynecol Obstet 1989; 169:387.

102. Hackford AW, Tally FP, Reinhold RB, et al: Prospective study comparing imipenem-cilastatin with clindamycin and gentamicin for the treatment of serious surgical infections. Arch Surg 1988; 123:322.

103. Watters JM, Blakslee JM, March RJ, et al: The influence of age on the severity of peritonitis. J Surg 1996; 39:142.

104. Civetta JM: Clinical decision making. In: Civetta JM, Taylor RW, Kirby RR (eds): Critical Care. Philadelphia, JB Lippincott, 1992, pp 43–52.

105. Mosdell DM, Morris DM, Voltura A, et al: Antibiotic treatment for surgical peritonitis. Ann Surg 1991; 214:543.

106. Chang DC, Wilson SE: Meta-analysis of the clinical outcome of carbapenem monotherapy in the adjunctive treatment of intra-abdominal infections. Am J Surg 1997; 174:284.

107. Wilson SE, Nord CE: Clinical trials of extended spectrum penicillin/beta-lactamase inhibitors in the treatment of intra-abdominal infections: European and North American experience. Am J Surg 1995; 169:21S.

108. Bohnen JMA, Solomkin JS, Dellinger EP, et al: Guidelines for clinical care: Anti-infective agents for intra-abdominal infection. Arch Surg 1992; 127:83.

109. Stone HH, Bourneuf AA, Stinson LD: Reliability of criteria for predicting persistent or recurrent sepsis. Arch Surg 1985; 120:17.

110. Solomkin JS, Reinhart HH, Dellinger EP, et al: Results of a randomized trial comparing sequential intravenous/oral treatment with ciprofloxacin plus metronidazole to imipenem/cilastatin for intra-abdominal infections. Ann Surg 1996; 223:303.

111. Wickel DJ, Cheadle WG, Mercer-Jones MA, et al: Poor outcome from peritonitis is caused by disease acuity and organ failure, not recurrent peritoneal infection. Ann Surg 1997; 225:744.

35

Dermatologic Conditions

Michael J. Hussey ▸ Sebastian Faro

Infectious diseases commonly manifest with dermatologic lesions. These skin lesions often have distinct characteristics that can differentiate a generalized systemic infection from an isolated superficial event. Also, cutaneous signs may guide therapeutic decisions. Furthermore, hormonal changes normally occur in women during puberty, the menstrual cycle, pregnancy, and menopause and such changes can affect dermatologic findings of some infections. For example, there has been increasing information about the effects that estrogen, progesterone, and androgens have on the immune system.[1, 2] Estrogens seem to stimulate the T-cell response and antibody production, whereas progesterone and androgens inhibit T-cell response and decrease antibody production.[3–5] As a result, the net effect of pregnancy is immunosuppression of cell-mediated immunity.[3–5] Therefore, the infectious diseases caused by intracellular organisms, or those controlled by the cell-mediated immune system, can first appear, recur more frequently, or become more severe during pregnancy.[4–7] Pregnancy also poses unique fetal concerns that the clinician treating a pregnant patient with an infectious disease and a rash must keep in mind. This chapter reviews skin manifestations of infectious diseases encountered in the clinical care of women.

GENERAL APPROACH

The approach to the woman with an infectious disease and a rash should include a history, physical examination, and diagnostic tests if necessary. The history should include the initial anatomic site of the rash, the appearance of the initial skin lesions, associated symptoms, the progression or change in the condition, response to therapy, and transmission to family members or sexual partners. The best diagnostic tools for examining the skin are adequate lighting and a magnifying glass. During the initial evaluation, the clinician should determine the pattern of the skin condition by looking for the distribution of the lesions, unique shapes, and the arrangement of the lesions (e.g., linear or annular shape, dermatome, or vascular distribution). Primary skin lesions represent the initial skin change not influenced by superinfection, trauma, or therapy. Secondary lesions represent changes that result from progression of the disease, scratching, infection, or trauma. Often, a careful examination of the skin enables the clinician to make the correct diagnosis.

Sometimes, diagnostic tests are necessary. Magnification that uses a simple magnifying glass can improve viewing of subtle aspects of skin lesions. Transillumination can help detect slight degrees of elevation or depression. Wood's light examination is performed by the operator viewing the skin in a dark room under ultraviolet light filtered through Wood's glass, which is useful in distinguishing color changes. Biopsy is essential for diagnosing any dermatosis of uncertain etiology. Primary lesions should be biopsied. Commonly, a fully developed lesion is chosen for biopsy; however, early lesions provide the best specimens for vesicular, bullous, or pustular lesions. Fungal infections can be demonstrated by microscopic examination of scales taken from the lesion and covered with 10% potassium hydroxide. Gram stain of bacteria and bacterial cultures are extremely important when the primary lesion is a pustule or furuncle. The Tzanck test is rapid and reliable in the diagnosis of vesicular eruptions. Cellular material is scraped from the base of a vesicle and stained with Wright's or Giemsa's stain. Multinucleated giant cells are found in herpes simplex, herpes zoster, and varicella, whereas acantholytic cells are found in pemphigus. Direct and indirect immunofluorescence tests are most useful in diagnosing noninfectious skin diseases.

The patient with an infection and a rash often presents with a fever, a rash, and other nonspecific complaints, such as arthralgias, myalgias, malaise, and headache. Most infectious diseases that involve the skin present with one of the following dermatologic manifestations: pustular lesions, erythematous lesions, purpuric lesions, maculopapular lesions, or vesicular lesions.[8]

PUSTULAR LESIONS

Pustular skin lesions are frequently the result of a staphylococcal skin infection. These gram-positive cocci can produce superficial pustules, erosions with honey-colored crusts, deep abscesses (furuncles, carbuncles), diffuse involvement of the dermis and subcutaneous fat (cellulitis), widespread erythema and desquamation, or purulent purpura. Staphylococci gain access when the superficial epidermis is disrupted either from microscopic breaks in normal skin or as a defect caused by inflammatory dermatoses, vesicular viral infection, or surgical or traumatic wounds.[8]

Extensive staphylococcal infections result in fever, leukocytosis, rigors, and septicemia, whereas systemic manifestations are absent in restricted infections.[8] Septicemia may exist in the absence of an obvious dermatologic focus; however, staphylococcal septicemia is inferred by the presence of skin lesions characteristic of septic emboli. Staphylococcal septic emboli are 1- to 2-mm pustules surrounded by a wide red flare and only rarely form an abscess.[8] If thrombocytopenia is present, the pustules may be surrounded by purpura. Staphylococcal sepsis can initiate disseminated intravascular coagulation (DIC).

ERYTHEMATOUS LESIONS

Erythematous skin lesions can be caused by a wide variety of infectious agents but are often the result of streptococci. Streptococci invade the skin through microscopic breaks in normal skin, inflammatory dermatoses, burns, or surgical or traumatic wounds, or at childbirth.[8] Streptococcal infections may take the form of cellulitis, erysipelas, or scarlet fever.[8]

In cellulitis, the dermis and subcutaneous layer are affected and the skin is red, hot, and edematous. The skin lesion has poorly defined borders.[8] In contrast, in erysipelas, the skin is red and hot but the lesion has more sharply defined edematous borders and the lesion extends more rapidly than in cellulitis.[8] The infection is confined to the dermis. Erysipelas often starts as a solitary lesion and spreads rapidly.

Rarely, streptococci invade the subcutaneous fat and the deep fascial layer, causing thrombosis of deep vessels and gangrene of the overlying tissue (necrotizing fasciitis). Necrotizing fasciitis typically follows surgery or perforating trauma. Within 24 to 48 hours, redness, pain, and edema quickly progress to central patches of dusky blue discoloration, with or without serosanguineous blisters.[8] By the fourth or fifth day, these purple areas become gangrenous.[8] The initial skin condition resembles erysipelas, but within days the skin becomes dusky, evolves into gangrene, and eventually sloughs. Many forms of virulent bacteria have been cultured from necrotizing fasciitis, including streptococci, staphylococci, coliforms, enterococci, Pseudomonas, and Bacteroides. Streptococcal septicemia and metastatic abscesses can be found in association with necrotizing fasciitis.[8] Treatment should include early surgical débridement; intravenous antibiotics, including penicillin, semisynthetic penicillins, and antibiotics with gram-negative coverage; and supportive care. There may be 20% mortality even in the best of circumstances.[8] Poor prognostic indicators include age over 50 years, underlying diabetes, underlying atherosclerosis, or a delay of more than 7 days in diagnosis and surgical intervention.[8]

Streptococci spread through dermal lymphatic vessels in cellulitis and erysipelas. Multiple episodes of cellulitis and erysipelas can impair the lymphatic drainage that predisposes to infections. Recurrent episodes of cellulitis and erysipelas produce dermal fibrosis and lymphedema that can lead to elephantiasis nostras.[8] Affected individuals require daily antibiotic prophylaxis.

The skin lesion of scarlet fever is caused by erythrogenic toxins elaborated by certain strains of beta-hemolytic streptococci.[8] Although the streptococcal infection is usually in the pharynx or tonsils, it can arise in wounds, burns, or the reproductive tract during the puerperium. The rash begins on the upper chest and neck and quickly spreads throughout the trunk and extremities. The rash appears as diffuse erythema with multiple red puncta. The face is flushed with circumoral pallor, and the tongue has a white coating with swollen, red papillae (red strawberry tongue). Petechiae may be present. The skin begins to desquamate any time from 5 days to 2 to 3 weeks after the onset of the rash.[8] The toxins that cause the rash in scarlet fever can also cause fever, changes in the blood-brain barrier, end-organ damage, and enhanced susceptibility to endotoxic shock.[8] Certain strains of staphylococci can produce an erythrogenic toxin, which can cause the same clinical presentation as scarlet fever.[9]

In contrast to staphylococcal sepsis, streptococcal sepsis is not associated with septic emboli. Streptococci can, however, develop suppurative lesions in the joints, pericardium, endocardium, meninges, brain, lungs, and bone.[8] Streptococci can also invade tissues locally. Paranasal sinusitis can lead to meningitis and brain abscess.[8]

PURPURIC LESIONS

Purpura and petechiae are manifestations of infections caused by meningococci, gonococci, and Escherichia coli, and species of Klebsiella, Pseudomonas, and Rickettsia.[8] These lesions can be caused by septic emboli or by DIC.

Acute meningococcemia is characterized by a petechial eruption that coalesces to appear as large areas of purpura.[8] The initial purpuric rash is caused by meningococcal invasion of endothelial cells in dermal and subcutaneous vessels, resulting in endothelial injury, increased capillary permeability, and localized thrombosis and infarction. A serious, usually rapidly fatal variant of meningococcal infection is the Water-house-Friderichsen syndrome, in which gram-negative bacteremia causes a generalized DIC with massive bleeding into the skin, adrenals, and other organs.[8]

Disseminated gonococcemia occurs in 1% to 3% of patients with gonorrhea.[8] This condition is a subacute febrile illness with arthralgias, arthritis, tenosynovitis, and skin lesions. The skin lesions appear as erythematous papules with purpura or as vesicopustules.[8]

Septicemia with gram-negative organisms is usually a life-threatening condition that can be recognized by the characteristic skin lesions. The skin lesion is a wheal or papule with an irregular area of purpura in its center or periphery and is a specific sign of septicemia with gram-negative organisms: *E. coli, Klebsiella, Pseudomonas*, gonococci, or meningococci.[8]

Two rickettsial infections present with purpuric skin eruptions. Rocky Mountain spotted fever is caused by *Rickettsia rickettsii*, is spread by tick bite, and is associated with significant mortality. After an incubation period of 7 days, the patient presents with severe headache, fevers, and myalgias. The cutaneous eruption occurs on approximately the fourth day of illness and is characterized by discrete, rose-colored macules of the wrists, ankles, palms, and soles.[8] The lesions spread to the trunk and head, become petechial, and may slough. Gangrene may occur. Renal insufficiency, meningitis, DIC, and hepatic dysfunction can occur. The treatment of choice is doxycycline. Epidemic typhus is caused by *Rickettsia prowazekii* and is transmitted by the body louse. After a 1- to 2-week incubation period, fever, chills, headache, and weakness develop. A few days later, a truncal macular eruption occurs and then spreads distally. These macular lesions may subsequently become hemorrhagic, often leading to gangrene.[8] The treatment of choice is tetracycline or chloramphenicol.

MACULOPAPULAR LESIONS

Erythematous maculopapular eruptions associated with an infection are usually the result of a viral infection but need to be differentiated from a drug reaction. The two are often differentiated by the evolution of the rash and by associated symptoms. Drug reactions commonly develop simultaneously over the entire body, whereas viral exanthems have characteristic distributions and patterns of spread.[8]

Measles (rubeola) is seen chiefly in children and immunocompromised patients. Fever and malaise usually begin 10 to 11 days following infection. These symptoms are followed by coryza, conjunctivitis, and cough. At the end of this stage, the pathognomonic Koplik spots appear on the lateral buccal mucosa. These are described as small, raised, blue-gray to white lesions surrounded by erythema. The characteristic rash is maculopapular and begins in the head and neck and spreads to the trunk and upper extremities

followed by the lower extremities. The lesions are erythematous macules and papules that coalesce to form erythematous patches and plaques. In severe cases, petechiae or purpura can develop and measles can initiate DIC.[8] If measles occurs during pregnancy, it is unclear whether it carries a worse maternal prognosis. Congenital measles has been associated with a high perinatal mortality; however, the reported cases of mortality occurred before the advent of antibiotics, and secondary bacterial pneumonia was a common cause of death. As a result, the current mortality associated with congenital measles is not known.[10]

Rubella (German measles) has an incubation period of 2 to 3 weeks, followed by a mild prodrome of malaise, anorexia, fever, headache and coryza, and cervical adenopathy. Arthralgias are common in adult women. The rash of rubella consists of pink macules and papules that may become confluent.[8] The eruption begins on the forehead and rapidly spreads to involve the face, trunk, and extremities. The time course of the rubella exanthem is 3 days, which is a differentiating point from the usual 6-day course of the rubeola exanthem. Despite immunization, 10% to 20% of the United States population is susceptible to rubella.[11] A total of 32% of cases of rubella occur in those aged 15 to 29 years.[12] First-trimester rubella infection is believed to cause abortion. Congenital infection may be divided into three categories, based on its manifestations: congenital rubella syndrome (CRS), extended CRS, and delayed CRS. Both CRS and extended CRS are apparent at birth. Delayed manifestations of congenital infection may not be apparent for decades.

Four major defects in CRS are deafness, mental retardation, heart lesions, and ophthalmologic abnormalities. The spectrum of extended CRS includes cerebral palsy, mental retardation, developmental and language delay, seizures, cirrhosis, growth retardation, and immunologic disorders. Delayed manifestations of CRS include endocrinopathies, late-onset deafness and ocular damage, renovascular hypertension, and encephalitis.

Efforts are made to vaccinate susceptible adults as well as young children, but opportunities to do so are missed, including the postpartum period. Almost one half of mothers of infants with CRS have had a previous live birth. All of these cases of CRS could presumably have been prevented by postpartum vaccination after the birth of the first child.[10-12] The goal of immunization should be the eradication of congenital rubella infection. Prevention of in utero infection requires the acquisition of immunity by all persons before the childbearing years.

Parvovirus is known to be the causative agent of erythema infectiosum (fifth disease), a common childhood illness that can also affect adolescents and adults. Fifth disease begins as a warm, red flush on the cheeks that can have raised borders and may have an appearance similar to that of erysipelas.[8] The facial appearance is described as a "slapped cheek." The rash spreads as a maculopapular eruption (often in a reticulated pattern) onto the extremities, buttocks, and trunk. The disease tends to be more severe in adults than in children. Adults commonly develop fatigue, fever, adenopathy, and arthritis.[13] Parvovirus B19 infection may be involved in acute arthralgia and arthritis as well as chronic anemia in immunodeficient patients. This virus is also the primary etiologic agent of transient aplastic crisis in patients with chronic hemolytic anemias. Parvovirus infection during pregnancy may be a cause for concern. In most of the reported parvovirus infections during pregnancy, there has been no adverse outcome. However, in some cases, fetal death, usually involving hydrops fetalis, occurs.[14, 15] Studies suggest that the risk of fetal death in a pregnant woman with documented parvovirus infection is less than 10%.[10] Currently, there is no specific treatment available to patients with parvovirus infection.

Infections caused by enteroviruses (echovirus and coxsackievirus) can sometimes present with maculopapular rashes and fever.[8] Also, the prodromal phase of hepatitis B infection may be associated with a maculopapular or petechial rash.[8] About 5% of cases of infectious mononucleosis (primarily caused by Epstein-Barr virus) are associated with a skin eruption that can resemble rubella. More commonly, essentially all patients with infectious mononucleosis who are treated with ampicillin will develop a pruritic maculopapular eruption 5 to 8 days later.[8, 16]

VESICULAR LESIONS

Infections caused by herpes simplex virus and varicella-zoster virus cause vesicular lesions. Hand-foot-and-mouth disease also presents with vesicular exanthems.

Herpes simplex virus (HSV) infections are caused by herpes simplex virus type 1 or type 2, or both. Traditionally, primary infections of external genitalia have been thought to be symptomatic, but serologic evidence shows that asymptomatic infection is common.[10] Systemic symptoms include fever, malaise, myalgia, and headaches. Local symptoms include pain, discharge, adenopathy, and dysuria. Urinary retention is common. The primary lesions are painful vesicles that appear 2 to 10 days after exposure, then ulcerate and heal without scarring. The diagnosis is made clinically and is confirmed by a Tzanck smear taken from the floor of the vesicle base. Virus identification by the presence of cytopathic effect in tissue culture is the definitive method of making the diagnosis. Recurrent infections are usually milder and of shorter duration than the primary infection. The mean duration of lesions is 11 days in primary infection and 7 days in recurrent infection. Acyclovir and vidarabine are specific antiviral therapies against HSV. When used for primary infection, acyclovir decreases the duration of virus shedding, pain, new lesion formation, and the time to complete healing.[17] Duration of virus shedding may be decreased by 80%. Oral acyclovir is effective in suppressing recurrences with long-term use.[18]

Transplacental infection with HSV is rare.[19] However, infection of the conceptus by transplacental spread has been linked with spontaneous abortion, preterm labor, and congenital malformation.[19] Neonatal transmission occurs intra partum in the vast majority of cases. The virus is encountered in the infected maternal genital tract.[10] Infection acquired intra partum has an average incubation period of 6 to 12 days[20] and may be localized, may be disseminated, or may involve the central nervous system.[10] Neonatal HSV is rarely asymptomatic.[10]

Varicella-zoster virus (VZV) infection causes varicella or herpes zoster, distinct clinical entities dependent on the immune status of the host.[21] Primary infection usually occurs in childhood, clinically presenting as chickenpox, and is generally a self-limited disease characterized by typical skin lesions.[22] It is recognized that when adults contract the disease, both constitutional and pulmonary symptoms may be severe.[10] The varicella exanthem occurs approximately 10 to 21 days following exposure and begins on the head and spreads caudally. The primary lesion is an erythematous papule that evolves into a clear fluid-filled vesicle on an erythematous base. The vesicles evolve into pustules and, eventually, crusts. Lesions in various stages are usually present at the same time. The main complications are staphylococcal or streptococcal impetigo and cellulitis and streptococcal scarlet fever.[8] Chickenpox in adults can be complicated by varicella pneumonitis. Severe cases of chickenpox can initiate DIC.[8] Reactivation of latent zoster infection clinically presents as shingles, which generally occurs in elderly or immunocompromised patients.[10] Zoster presents as painful crops of vesicular lesions occurring along the distribution of segmental dermatomes.[10]

Maternal varicella infection in the first trimester of pregnancy may result in congenital birth defects, including limb hypoplasia, cicatricial skin lesions, atrophic digits, psychomotor retardation, and growth retardation.[23] The risk of the fetus developing these anomalies with first-trimester chickenpox infection is approximately 1% to 2%.[24, 25]

Hand-foot-and-mouth disease is caused by coxsackieviruses and is characterized by the development of vesicles on the buccal mucosa, palate, tongue, hands, feet, palms, and soles. Hand-foot-and-mouth disease is a disease primarily of toddlers.

SPECIFIC DISORDERS

Some systemic infections have distinct morphology and distribution of the cutaneous manifestations, which allows early diagnosis and initiation of appropriate therapy. The following section discusses the dermatologic findings in some of these infections.

Staphylococcal Scalded Skin Syndrome

Staphylococcal scalded skin syndrome (SSSS) is an acute, life-threatening febrile illness caused by exotoxin produced by *Staphylococcus aureus*. SSSS is a disease of children younger than 5 years of age and adults with either renal compromise or immunosuppression.[8, 26, 27]

Patients with SSSS initially present with fever and diffuse, tender blanchable erythema.[26] Frequently, this is preceded by purulent conjunctivitis, rhinorrhea, otitis media, or an erythematous pharynx.[8] The eruption begins around the mouth and rapidly spreads to the remainder of the body. Flaccid blistering occurs within 24 to 48 hours and is followed by exfoliation of large sheets of skin.[26, 27] The palm of the hands, sole of the feet, and mucous membranes are spared.[26] SSSS must be distinguished from toxic epidermal necrolysis (TEN), a disease with a similar presentation but one that occurs most commonly in adults as a reaction to drugs or as a manifestation of graft-versus-host reaction.[8, 27, 28] The clinician can differentiate between the two entities by performing a skin biopsy.[8, 26] Each has a distinct histologic appearance.[26, 28] A toxin causes the lesions; therefore, the organism does not grow from cultures of the bulla fluid.[26, 27] Instead, *S. aureus* may be recovered from the blood, urine, pharynx, nose, conjunctiva, or umbilicus, or other sites, to confirm the diagnosis.[26] Treatment is with penicillinase-resistant penicillin, supportive measures for preventing secondary infection, and attention to fluid balance.[26]

Toxic Shock Syndrome

Toxic shock syndrome was first described in 1978 and is characterized by high fever, erythematous eruption, and profound systemic features (Fig. 35–1).[8, 29, 30] This disorder was first found in children; however, it was soon found in healthy young menstruating women who used highly absorbent tampons made of polyacrylate.[8, 26, 30] Subsequently, cases have been described as associated with infected wounds, contraceptive devices, and nasal packing after rhinoplasty.[26]

This condition is caused by toxin-producing strains of *S. aureus*, and the diagnosis is based on the clinical case definition from the Centers for Disease Control and Prevention (CDC): fever greater than 38.9°C, erythematous macules or erythroderma with acral desquamation, hypotension, and involvement of three or more organ systems.[26] The systemic features include renal, hepatic, and lung dysfunction, encephalopathy, nausea, vomiting, diarrhea, and painful muscles. The eruption varies from diffuse erythroderma, to an erythematous maculopapular patchy eruption of the lower abdomen, perineum, and thighs, or a petechial eruption of the hands, feet, and trunk.[8, 31] In all patients, a full-thickness desquamation of the hand or feet, or both, occurs at 5 to 12 days.[8, 31] Anemia, leukocytosis, and thrombocytopenia also occur.[8] Bacteremia is not associated with staphylococcal toxic shock syndrome.[8] In cases related to tampon use, vaginal cultures are usually positive for *S. aureus*.[26] In 1985, a similar syndrome produced by beta-hemolytic streptococci was described.[32] However, in the syndrome produced by streptococci, a focus of a pyogenic infection was usually identified and bacteremia was present in 60% of cases.[8, 32]

Treatment consists of systemic antistaphylococcal antibiotics, such as penicillinase-resistant penicillin, aggressive fluid and electrolyte therapy, and removal of the tampon or nasal packing or drainage of an infected site.[26]

Bacterial Endocarditis

The dermatologic manifestations of bacterial endocarditis include conjunctival and palatal petechiae, splinter hemorrhages, Roth's spots, Osler's nodes, and Janeway's lesions.[8] Roth's spots are pale areas surrounded by hemorrhage near the optic disc. Osler's nodes are tender, erythematous spots on the fingertips and toes. Janeway's lesions are nontender, red or hemorrhagic macules or nodules in the palms or soles.[8] Osler's nodes and Janeway's lesions are most probably caused by septic emboli in acute bacterial endocarditis caused by *S. aureus*.[8] In contrast, in subacute bacterial endocarditis, Osler's nodes and Janeway's lesions, and probably the petechiae, hemorrhages, and Roth's spots, are immune complex mediated.[8, 33]

Candidiasis

Candidiasis is an infection of the skin, nails, or mucous membranes by one of the yeasts of the genus *Candida*, most commonly *C. albicans*. Patients with acute vulvo-

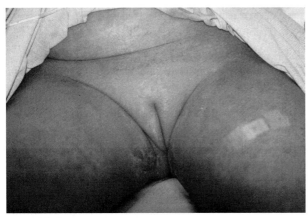

FIGURE 35–1 ▶ Toxic shock syndrome.

vaginal candidiasis present with vulvar and vaginal itching, with or without discharge. If a discharge is present, it is typically yellow-white with a thick, cheesy consistency. Dyspareunia and dysuria are common. On clinical examination, the vulva and vestibule are inflamed, often with fissures and erosion as the result of scratching. The vulva can have erythematous areas with a white discharge, and the infection can spread to the perineum, thighs, and perianal region. The vaginal mucosa can be moist and erythematous. The vaginal pH is less than 4.5. When the vaginal secretions are examined under the microscope (after adding 10% potassium hydroxide), budding yeast cells and hyphae can be seen.

Vulvovaginal candidiasis is 10 to 20 times more frequent during pregnancy than in the nonpregnant state,[34, 35] probably as the result of elevated estrogen levels or progesterone levels, or both. Neonatal candidiasis is acquired during passage through an infected birth canal and presents as diaper dermatitis or oral thrush during the first week of life.[36, 37] Congenital cutaneous candidiasis is the result of an ascending infection of the fetal skin by *Candida* from the birth canal. Infection can occur with intact membranes.[38] The eruption begins within the first 12 hours of life and has macular, papular, vesicular, and pustular phases.[36]

Condyloma Acuminata

Condyloma acuminata (genital warts) are caused by infection with one of the human papillomavirus types. These warts appear as soft, verrucous lesions several millimeters in diameter (Fig. 35–2). They may appear singly or in clusters, and in some patients they multiply and coalesce to form large, exophytic tumors. The warts often have a pebble surface and are soft and round. They are found at the vaginal introitus, in the vagina, at the vaginal vestibule, on the perineum, and in the anus. Infection of the cervix can be recognized at the time of colposcopy. These lesions need to be

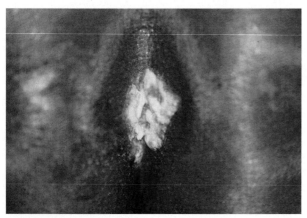

FIGURE 35–2 ▶ Condyloma acuminata.

differentiated from the papular or nodular lesions of secondary syphilis (condyloma lata), which occur at similar sites. This can be accomplished by performing a serologic test for syphilis, or if there is any uncertainty a dark-field examination for spirochetes or a biopsy can be performed.

Lyme Disease

Lyme disease is the result of infection with the spirochete *Borrelia burgdorferi*, which is transmitted by a deer tick. Lyme disease usually begins with a characteristic skin lesion, erythema chronicum migrans, accompanied by a flu-like syndrome and neurologic abnormalities. The rash is an expanding erythematous, annular lesion with central clearing that appears 4 to 21 days after the tick bite. Systemic symptoms may accompany the rash and include arthritis, headache, photophobia, dysesthesias, and a stiff neck. Some patients will later develop cardiac abnormalities, such as atrioventricular heart block or myopericarditis.[10] Because the results of serologic tests for Lyme disease are often negative during the first several weeks of infection, the diagnosis of Lyme disease should be made on the basis of clinical criteria.[10, 39] Lyme disease during pregnancy can cause intrauterine growth restriction, fetal death, prematurity, and malformations.[36, 40]

Coccidioidomycosis

Coccidioidomycosis is a dust-borne disease common in arid regions, including the southwestern United States. It is caused by *Coccidioides immitis*, a dimorphic fungus.[10] Primary infection may be asymptomatic or may resemble a flu-like illness. Disseminated coccidioidomycosis is a progressive, frequently fatal disease.[10] There are three dermatologic manifestations of coccidioidomycosis that, when found with a productive cough, bloody sputum, pleuritic chest pain, or an abnormal chest radiograph result, suggest coccidioidomycosis. The three dermatologic manifestations are toxic erythema, erythema nodosum, and erythema multiforme.[36] Toxic erythema is a diffuse macular rash that occurs during the first few days of infection in approximately 10% of infected individuals.[36] Erythema multiforme and erythema nodosum are more common. Erythema nodosum is characterized by painful erythematous nodules over the extensor surface of the extremities. Erythema multiforme is made up of polymorphous skin lesions (macules, papules, urticaria, and bullae) that range in color from bright red to purple. Iris lesions that consist of a vesicle surrounded by a pale ring, and then a concentric red ring, may develop.

In the nonpregnant state, extrapulmonary dissemination occurs in 0.2% of cases. The rate of dissemination is 23% during the first trimester of pregnancy,

59% during the second trimester, and 68% during the third trimester.[36, 41] Disseminated coccidioidomycosis has a reported maternal mortality rate of 20% to 60% and is a major etiology for maternal mortality in endemic regions.[36, 42] Furthermore, with disseminated disease, the perinatal mortality has been reported to be as high as 50%.[36, 41] Transplacental passage has been reported, although the placenta is thought to limit this method of infection.[43–46]

Syphilis

Syphilis is a chronic systemic infection characterized by exacerbations and caused by the spirochete *Treponema pallidum*. Two major stages are recognized, early and late, and each of these is further divided. The phases of early syphilis are incubating, primary, secondary, and early latent. Late syphilis includes late latent and tertiary. The clinical manifestations are wide-ranging and involve nearly every organ system. The clinical expression depends on the immune status of the host.

The first sign of primary infection is a single, nontender lesion (chancre) at the site of entry. The most common sites of entry in women include the vulva, introitus, or cervix, but lesions may be found at the lips, tongue, tonsils, breasts, or fingers.[47] The chancre is a painless, red macule that becomes a papule, and then ulcerates. The ulcers have a well-defined margin and a rubbery, indurated base. Without treatment, the chancres last 3 to 6 weeks and then heal spontaneously. Painless inguinal adenopathy can develop approximately 1 week after the appearance of the chancre. Both the chancres and the lymph nodes can become tender if they become secondarily infected.[47]

The symptoms of secondary syphilis become apparent approximately 3 to 6 weeks after the disappearance of the chancre. Symptoms include fever, malaise, sore throat, headache, musculoskeletal pain, and weight loss.[47] A macular rash develops over the trunk and flexor surfaces. The lesions are pink, round, and less than 1 cm in diameter.[47] The rash spreads over the whole body, including the palms and soles, and becomes dull red and papular and then squamous. Latent syphilis lacks clinical manifestations. One third of untreated patients develop tertiary syphilis, which is characterized by involvement of the cardiovascular, nervous, or musculoskeletal systems.

Treponema pallidum crosses the placenta and has been associated with preterm delivery, stillbirth, congenital infection, and neonatal death, depending on the timing of infection.[47]

Human Immunodeficiency Virus Infection and Acquired Immunodeficiency Syndrome

Dermatologic manifestations are such significant features of human immunodeficiency virus (HIV) infec-

tion and acquired immunodeficiency syndrome (AIDS) that they can serve as a confirmatory sign of AIDS in an individual who is HIV positive and has an *indicator illness* (severe illnesses that are rare in the absence of compromised cell-mediated immunity, which are described by the Centers for Disease Control and Prevention AIDS surveillance case definition).[48–53] Furthermore, some of these dermatologic findings should alert the clinician to the possibility of HIV infection in the asymptomatic individual.

Oral candidiasis appears as a cheesy-white exudate on the tongue and buccal mucosa. When the exudate is examined under the microscope (after adding 10% potassium hydroxide), budding yeast cells and hyphae can be seen. Oral hairy leukoplakia has a similar appearance and is described as a verrucous plaque on the sides of the tongue.[48, 50, 54] Some patients complain of pain or burning. This represents an Epstein-Barr viral infection of the lingual tissues and responds to zidovudine treatment.[48, 55, 56]

Kaposi's sarcoma in AIDS begins on the trunk, face, and extremities. The initial lesions are flat, indurated patches of a range of colors, including pink, red-brown, blue, and black.[48] The lesions are elongated or slightly irregular. When nodules develop, they may become exuberant and appear as exudative large, pyogenic granulomas.[48]

Bacillary angiomatosis are reddish-purple papules and nodules, measuring a few millimeters to 3 to 4 cm in diameter.[48] They may be pedunculated or sessile and friable. An individual may have one or hundreds of the lesions. The etiologic agent is one of two species of a *Rickettsia*-like organism: *Rochalimaea quintana* and *Rochalimaea henselae*,[48, 57, 58] and antibiotics are highly effective in treating this condition.

A spectrum of papulosquamous disorders occurs in AIDS, including acquired xerosis, acquired ichthyosis, seborrheic dermatitis, and psoriasis.[48] Widespread and recurrent ringworm infections should alert the clinician to the possibility of HIV infection.[48] *Trichophyton rubrum* may produce onychomycosis with severe paronychia and *C. albicans* may produce nail dystrophies. Generalized molluscum contagiosum, extensive condyloma acuminata, and verrucae vulgaris (ordinary warts) should raise the possibility of HIV infection.[48] Herpes zoster occurs seven times more commonly in AIDS patients than in control patients.[59] Herpes simplex infections are common and can manifest as chronic erosions and ulcerations.[48]

Patients with AIDS are vulnerable to cutaneous as well as systemic infections by opportunistic organisms. The cutaneous infections are often chronic and recurrent and usually take the form of impetigo, abscesses, erythematous papules, necrotic nodules, indurated crusted plaques, ulcerations, verrucous papules, molluscum-like papules, cellulitis, and folliculitis.[48] In patients with HIV infection, syphilis may progress rapidly from primary to tertiary within months.[48, 52] Diffuse alopecia, with only fine hairs remaining, may occur either early or late in AIDS.[48]

ACKNOWLEDGMENT

We would like to thank Drs. Michael Tharp and Mireille Chae in the Department of Dermatology at Rush-Presbyterian-St. Luke's Medical Center for providing the photographs used in this chapter.

REFERENCES

1. Lahita RG: The effects of sex hormones on the immune system in pregnancy. Am J Reprod Immunol 1992; 28:136.
2. Berczi I: Prolactin, pregnancy and autoimmune disease. J Rheumatol 1993; 20:1095.
3. Weinberg ED: Pregnancy-associated depression of cell-mediated immunity. Rev Infect Dis 1984; 5:814.
4. Grossman CJ: Regulation of the immune system by sex steroids. Endocr Rev 1984; 5:435.
5. Schuurs AHWM, Verheul HAM: Effects of gender and sex steroids on the immune system. J Steroid Biochem 1990; 35:157.
6. Styrt B, Sugarman B: Estrogens and infection. Rev Infect Dis 1991; 13:1139.
7. Muller HE: Das leistungsfähigere Abwehrsystem der Frau gegen Infektionserreger. Wien Med Wochenschr 1992; 17:389.
8. Braverman IM: Infections. In: Braverman IM (ed): Skin Signs of Systemic Disease, 3rd ed. Philadelphia, WB Saunders, 1998, pp 577–649.
9. Stevens FA: Occurrence of Staphylococcus aureus infection with scarlatiniform rash. JAMA 1927; 88:1957.
10. Gibbs RS: Virus-induced fetal infections. In: Reece EA, Hobbins JC (eds): Medicine of the Fetus and Mother, 2nd ed. Philadelphia, Lippincott-Raven, 1999, pp 369–394.
11. Centers for Disease Control: Rubella and congenital rubella—United States, 1984 to 1986. MMWR 1987; 36:664.
12. Centers for Disease Control: Rubella and congenital rubella syndrome—United States, 1985 to 1988. MMWR 1989; 38:173.
13. Greenwald P, Bashe WJ: An epidemic of erythema infectiosum. Am J Dis Child 1964; 107:30.
14. Anand A, Gray ES, Brown T, et al: Human parvovirus infection in pregnancy and hydrops fetalis. N Engl J Med 1987; 316:183.
15. Torok TJ: Human parvovirus B19 infections in pregnancy. Pediatr Infect Dis 1990; 9:772.
16. Patel BM: Skin rash with infectious mononucleosis and ampicillin. Pediatrics 1967; 40:910.
17. Comy L, Adams HG, Brown ZA, Holmes KK: Genital herpes simplex virus infections: Clinical manifestations, course, and complications. Ann Intern Med 1983; 98:958.
18. Baker DA, Blythe JG, Kaufman R, et al: One-year suppression of frequent recurrences of genital herpes with oral acyclovir. Obstet Gynecol 1989; 73:84.
19. Nahmias AJ, Josey WE, Naib ZM, et al: Perinatal risk associated with maternal genital herpes simplex virus infection. Am J Obstet Gynecol 1971; 110:825.
20. Whitley RJ: Neonatal herpes simplex virus infections: Presentation and management. J Reprod Med 1986; 31:426.
21. Jurecka W: Impact of pregnancy on skin diseases. In: Harahap M, Wallach RC (eds): Skin Changes and Diseases in Pregnancy. New York, Marcel Dekker, 1996, pp 91–127.
22. Young NA, Gershoni AA: Chicken pox, measles, and mumps. In: Remington JS, Klein JO (eds): Infectious Diseases of the Fetus and Newborn. Philadelphia, WB Saunders, 1983, p 375.
23. LaForet E, Lynch CL: Multiple congenital defects following maternal varicella. N Engl J Med 1947; 236:534.
24. Pastuszak AL, Levy M, Schick B, et al: Outcome after maternal varicella infection in the first 20 weeks of pregnancy. N Engl J Med 1994; 330:901.
25. Enders G, Miller E, Cradock-Watson J, et al: Consequences of varicella and herpes zoster in pregnancy: Prospective study of 1739 cases. Lancet 1994; 343:1547.

26. Mercurio MG, Elewski BE: Cutaneous manifestations of systemic viral, bacterial, and fungal infections and protozoan disease. In: Callen JP, Jorizzo JL, Greer KE, et al (eds): Dermatologic Signs of Internal Disease, 2nd ed. Philadelphia, WB Saunders, 1995, pp 253–293.
27. Lyell A: The staphylococcal scalded skin syndrome in historical perspective. J Am Acad Dermatol 1983; 9:285.
28. Ionnides D, Vakali G, Chrysomallis F, et al: Toxic epidermal necrolysis: A study of 22 cases. J Eur Acad Dermatol Venereol 1994; 3:266.
29. Bartter T, Dascal A, Carroll K, et al: Toxic shock syndrome. Arch Intern Med 1988; 148:1421.
30. Todd J, Fishaut M, Kapral F, et al: Toxic-shock syndrome associated with phage-group-1 staphylococci. Lancet 1978; 2:1116.
31. Tofte RW, Williams DN: Toxic shock syndrome: Clinical and laboratory features in 15 patients. Ann Intern Med 1981; 94:149.
32. Bisno AL: Group A streptococcal infections and acute rheumatic fever. N Engl J Med 1991; 325:783.
33. Weinstein L, Schlesinger JJ: Pathanatomic, pathophysiologic and clinical correlations in endocarditis. N Engl J Med 1974; 291:832.
34. Sullivan C, Smith LG: Management of vulvovaginitis in pregnancy. Clin Obstet Gynecol 1993; 36:195.
35. Sobel JD: Candidal vulvovaginitis. Clin Obstet Gynecol 1993; 36:153.
36. Bellman B, Berman B: Skin diseases seriously affecting fetal outcome and maternal health. In: Harahap M, Wallach RC (eds): Skin Changes and Diseases in Pregnancy. New York, Marcel Dekker, 1996, pp 129–182.
37. McCormick WM: Management of sexually transmissible infections during pregnancy. Clin Obstet Gynecol 1975; 18:57.
38. Broberg A, Thiringer K: Congenital cutaneous candidiasis. Int J Dermatol 1989; 18:464.
39. Shrestha M, Grodzichi RL, Steere AC: Diagnosing early Lyme disease. Am J Med 1985; 78:235.
40. Markowitz LE, Steere AC, Benach JL: Lyme disease during pregnancy. JAMA 1986; 255:3394.
41. Walker MPR, Brody CZ: Reactivation of coccidioidomycosis during pregnancy. Obstet Gynecol 1992; 79:815.
42. Peterson CM, Schuppert K, Kelly PC: Coccidioidomycosis and pregnancy. Obstet Gynecol Surv 1993; 48:149.
43. Smale LE, Waechter KG: Dissemination of coccidioidomycosis in pregnancy. Am J Obstet Gynecol 1970; 170:356.
44. Shafai T: Neonatal coccidioidomycosis in premature twins. Am J Dis Child 1978; 132:634.
45. Cohen R: Coccidioidomycosis: Case studies in children. Arch Pediatr 1949; 66:241.
46. Monif GRG: Coccidioides immitis. In: Monif GRG (ed): Infectious Diseases in Obstetrics and Gynecology, 2nd ed. Philadelphia, Harper & Row, 1982, pp 345–348.
47. Sweet RL: Sexually transmitted diseases in pregnancy. In: Reece EA, Hobbins JC (eds): Medicine of the Fetus and Mother, 2nd ed. Philadelphia, Lippincott-Raven, 1999, pp 1307–1327.
48. Braverman IM: Dysproteinemias and immunodeficiency disorders. In: Braverman IM (eds): Skin Signs of Systemic Disease, 3rd ed. Philadelphia, WB Saunders, 1998, pp 161–189.
49. Goodman DS, Teplitz ED, Wishner A, et al: Prevalence of cutaneous diseases in patients with acquired immunodeficiency syndrome (AIDS) or AIDS-related complex. J Am Acad Dermatol 1987; 17:210.
50. Alessi E, Cusini M, Zerboni R: Mucocutaneous manifestations in patients infected with human immunodeficiency virus. J Am Acad Dermatol 1988; 19:290.
51. Cockerell CJ: Cutaneous manifestations of HIV infections other than Kaposi's sarcoma: Clinical and histologic aspects. J Am Acad Dermatol 1990; 22:1260.
52. Friedman-Kien AE: Color Atlas of AIDS. Philadelphia, WB Saunders, 1989.
53. Matis WL, Triana A, Shapiro R, et al: Dermatologic findings associated with human immunodeficiency virus infection. J Am Acad Dermatol 1987; 17:746.

54. Zunt SL, Tomich CE: Oral hairy leukoplakia. J Dermatol Surg Oncol 1990; 16:812.

55. Resnick L, Herbst JS, Raab-Traub N: Oral hairy leukoplakia. J Am Acad Dermatol 1990; 22:1278.

56. Greenspan JS, Greenspan D, Lennette ET, et al: Replication of Epstein-Barr virus with the epithelial cells of oral "hairy" leukoplakia: An AIDS-associated lesion. N Engl J Med 1985; 313:1564.

57. Relman DA, Loutit JS, Schmidt TM, et al: The agent of bacillary angiomatosis: An approach to the identification of uncultured pathogens. N Engl J Med 1990; 323:1573.

58. Koehler JE, Quinn FD, Berger TG, et al: Isolation of *Rochalimaea* species from cutaneous and osseous lesions of bacillary angiomatosis. N Engl J Med 1992; 327:1625.

59. Friedman-Kien AE, LaFleur FL, Gendler E, et al: Herpes zoster: A possible early sign for development of acquired immunodeficiency syndrome in high risk individuals. J Am Acad Dermatol 1986; 14:1023.

Sexually Transmitted Diseases

36 Epidemiology of Sexually Transmitted Infections

GEORGE P. SCHMID

Epidemiology is the study of disease occurrence in populations. Although it is seemingly straightforward to understand the individual physical acts that lead to the occurrence of sexually transmitted infections (STIs) and why infection from one individual to another occurs because of them, this is in fact not the case, and the study of why these acts occur among individuals making up a population is even more complex. Understanding the epidemiology of STIs—why disease occurs in populations—requires an understanding of both individual and group transmission dynamics.

DEFINITION OF SEXUALLY TRANSMITTED INFECTION

Despite what we intuitively know an STI to be, it is difficult to find a definition. Generally, the authors who define the term use definitions such as "the more than 25 infectious organisms that are transmitted through sexual activity, along with the dozens of clinical syndromes that they cause."[1] One problem with this definition is that many more than 25 microorganisms are transmitted via sexual activity (e.g., group B streptococci)[2]; whenever we have sex without a condom, we share organisms with our partner. More important, the definition fails to acknowledge the moral and social implications that accompany an STI in every society. A definition that I prefer is, "An infection that is acquired by the transmission of a microorganism during sexual activity, and in which we would ideally seek to contact the transmitting partner to prevent transmission to others." Prevention might be achieved by medication (for bacterial and parasitic infections) or counseling (for most viral infections). While this definition is also not perfect, it highlights the role of partners in the spread of STIs and eliminates the infections that occur in the reproductive tract that seem to be associated with sexual activity but are not clearly the result of the sexually transmitted organisms we wish to treat in the partner; for example, bacterial vaginosis, or some cases of pelvic inflammatory disease or nongonococcal urethritis.

REPRODUCTIVE TRACT INFECTIONS VERSUS STIs

All infections that occur in the genital tract are reproductive tract infections (RTIs) (Fig. 36–1). Only a por-

tion of these conditions are STIs. That proportion varies by how we define the term *STI* and the frequency of affected infections in individual populations (e.g., monogamous married women have proportionately more nonsexually transmitted RTIs than do commercial sex workers who do not use condoms). Both STIs and non–sexually transmitted RTIs may produce the same clinical syndrome (e.g., vaginal discharge, or pelvic inflammatory disease). Thus, testing of individuals with symptoms or signs compatible with an STI is important for proper treatment, partner notification, counseling, and, therefore, STI control within a population.

THEORETICAL BASIS OF STI TRANSMISSION: THE ANDERSON-MAY EQUATION

More than 10 years ago,[3] Anderson and May proposed a simple formula for explaining the transmission of STIs; this basic formula, subsequently elaborated on in many publications, remains valid:

$$R_0 = \beta cD$$

R_0 = the reproductive rate.
β = the probability of transmission from one person to another for a particular disease.
c = the number of partners over a specific time.
D = the duration of infectiousness.

R_0 refers to the number of new infections that occur, on average, from an individual with an STI. For an infection to spread within a population, R_0 must be greater than 1.0. R_0 is determined by the interaction of three determinants. The probability of transmission from one person to another, β, captures the concept that some infections in populations are more easily transmitted than others, and relates to biologic features such as ID_{50} (the number of organisms that are required for infecting 50% of persons exposed), site of transmission (some modes of sex, e.g., anal, more readily facilitate transmission), and immunity. The number of new partners, c, is a straightforward concept. The duration of infectiousness is how long an individual will remain infectious and is determined by factors such as the biologic nature of the infection (some infections, untreated, remain infectious for longer periods of time than others) and whether people receive treatment (early treatment lessens D).

All material in this chapter is in the public domain, with the exception of any borrowed figures or tables.

395

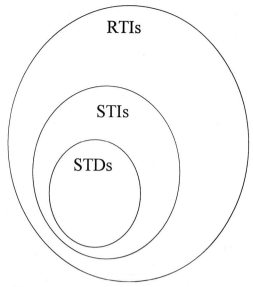

FIGURE 36-1 ▶ The relationships between reproductive tract infections (RTIs), sexually transmitted infections (STIs), and sexually transmitted diseases (STDs), with the area of the circle approximating the relative size of each.

R_0 varies directly as β, c, and D do; the greater these determinants, the greater R_0. The Anderson-May equation captures simply the essence of transmission. Why rates of STIs are so prevalent in one society or population, and not in others, can be simply examined by this equation, as can ways of decreasing these rates. To prevent infection from spreading, we must lower one or all of the determinants of R_0. Successful control and prevention programs will probably attack at least two, and possibly all three. Examples might be programs aimed at decreasing (1) the numbers of partners among sexually active individuals (among the entire population or within segments, e.g., commercial sex workers); (2) the numbers of partners among the sexually uninitiated by delaying the age at which individuals begin having sex (e.g., through school educa-

tion programs); (3) the numbers of infected individuals by screening programs for STIs or the provision of better access to health care, and (4) infectivity (e.g., switching to safer means of sex).

The importance of the rate of sex partner change is evident when one looks at representative parameters, particularly as a control program intervenes (Table 36-1). Indeed, a high rate of sex partner change largely defines a "core group," responsible for the persistence of infection within a population. All populations are a mixture of individuals with varying rates of sex partner change, and these tend to be of a skewed distribution (Fig. 36-2.). The individuals in the tail of the distribution are most responsible for STI transmission because of both numbers of partners and, often, associated high-risk behavior. They thus form the target group for STI control.

HIGH-RISK BEHAVIORS

High-risk behaviors catalyze the epidemiology of STIs, but how these behaviors are defined is imprecise. The Anderson-May model captures some of the essence of this term, by including numbers of partners and duration of illness. The latter factor is affected by things such as condom use, or good or bad health care–seeking behavior. Good health care–seeking behavior is characterized by knowledge of the symptoms of STIs, and the desire to avoid infecting others by, if symptoms appear, immediately ceasing sexual activity and obtaining access to medical care, or through periodic screening for STIs.

While the number ("quantity") of sex partners is one measure of "high-risk," another, less appreciated feature, is the "quality" of the sex partner. Some partners are "riskier" than others, although the features of what makes one partner risky and another less so are inexact. Generally, a risky partner is simply one who has many risk factors for STI acquisition. Certainly, one significant feature that would identify a

TABLE 36-1 ▶	THE DETERMINANTS OF THE ANDERSON-MAY EQUATION—ESTIMATES OF EPIDEMIOLOGIC PARAMETERS NECESSARY TO SUSTAIN TRANSMISSION OF FOUR STIs*		
Agent	**Duration of Infectiousness (D) (in Years)**	**Transmission Efficiency (β)**	**Sex Partner Change Per Year (c)**
Neisseria gonorrhoeae			
No control program†	0.5	0.5	4
Control program	0.15	0.5	13
Chlamydia trachomatis	1.25	0.2	4
Treponema pallidum			
No control program	0.5	0.3	7
Control program	0.25	0.3	13
Haemophilus ducreyi	0.08	0.8	15

*For each row, the numbers when multiplied equal 1; thus, an increase in any will cause infection to expand in a population.

†For *N. gonorrhoeae* and *T. pallidum*, a control program has identified infected individuals and treated them, thus shortening average duration of infectiousness.

Adapted from Brunham RC, Ronald AR: Epidemiology of STDs in developing countries. In: Wasserheit JN, Aral SO, Cates W, Hitchcock P (eds): Reproductive Tract Infections. Washington, DC, American Society of Microbiology, 1991.

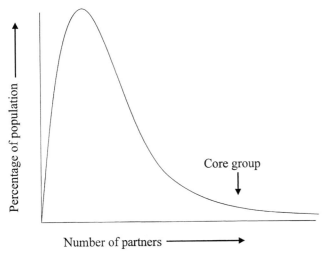

FIGURE 36-2 ▶ Representative distribution of the number of sex partners per individuals in a society. Most individuals have few sex partners, over either a given period of time or a lifetime, but a minority have many partners. Those with many partners are frequently members of the core group.

high-risk partner is the numbers of partners he or she has currently or has had in the past (i.e., quantity). But other features would include whether condoms are used by these partners during sex with others, how well the individuals know one another (people who know one another well are more likely to be concerned about the welfare of one another), or whether the partners are substance abusers.

GLOBAL EPIDEMIOLOGY

In 1995, the World Health Organization estimated the number of four important, curable STIs that occurred in the world: *Treponema pallidum* (12 million), *Neisseria gonorrhoeae* (62 million), *Chlamydia trachomatis* (89 million), and *Trichomonas vaginalis* (170 million).[5] The number of these four infections totaled 333 million and increased from a previous estimate in 1990 of 298 million. The large majority of these infections occurred in the developing world: South and Southeast Asia (116 million; 49%), sub-Saharan Africa (50 million; 21%), and Latin America (23 million; 10%). These numbers of infections ignore population sizes; when these are considered, startling discrepancies in incidence rates remain between the developing and industrialized worlds. It has been estimated that the annual incidence of acquiring a curable STI in the different geographic areas are as follows: Western Europe (1% to 2%), North America (2% to 3%), Latin America (7% to 14%), South and Southeast Asia (9% to 17%), and sub-Saharan Africa (11% to 35%).[6] In addition to these four curable infections, other bacterial and viral infections frequently occur. For example, although genital herpes was once thought to be rare in sub-Saharan Africa, several recent studies show this is not the case. In Uganda, genitally acquired herpes simplex virus (HSV) infection occurred 3 to 4 times as

commonly as chancroid, and about 10 times as commonly as syphilis.[7]

The reasons for the disparity in incidence between industrialized and developing worlds can be found by simply examining the Anderson-May equation. While variation occurs among countries, general features more common to the developing world than to the industrialized world include poorer access to health care facilities, lessened availability of antimicrobials, lessened availability of condoms, and, possibly, increased numbers of sex partners.

The United States, compared to other industrialized countries, has rates of STIs several-fold higher, and rates in some geographic areas of the United States exceed those in some developing countries.[8] In industrialized countries of Europe and Asia, cases of syphilis are rare and those of gonorrhea are focused in segments of the population (e.g., travelers or commercial sex workers). More limited information indicates that the difference is less for viral STIs, HSV having been best studied, where 22% of a cohort of Swedish girls were infected with HSV-2 by age 30 (vs. 25.6% of adult American women[9]) and a 7% infection rate was found in pregnant women in Japan.[10, 11] The reasons for the disparities between the United States and other industrialized countries are varied, but include concerted efforts in some nations to lower their rates. For example, in 1970, Sweden had a rate of gonorrhea of 481 per 100,000, compared to a rate of 297 per 100,000 in the United States. In 1995, the rate in Sweden was about 3 per 100,000, versus 150 per 100,000 in the United States.[1] That other industrialized countries can have rates substantially lower than ours and achieve them through intensive prevention and control programs indicates not only that we have significant progress to make, but also that such programs can be successful.

BIOLOGIC SUSCEPTIBILITY

Youth. Some diseases occur more commonly in young individuals, and lack of immunity and biologic susceptibility are contributory reasons. In general, organisms that cause STIs tend to produce only short-term species-specific immunity,[12] although longer-term, strain- or serotype-specific immunity may occur for some infections (e.g., *C. trachomatis*[13] or *Haemophilus ducreyi*[14]). Even if immunity is not long-term, it may prevent re-infection from occurring during a subsequent high-risk period of several years. Teenagers and young women are also physically more susceptible than are older women to cervical infection with *C. trachomatis*, *N. gonorrhoeae*, and human papillomavirus because of cervical ectopy (i.e., the appearance on the ectocervix of columnar epithelium from the endocervix).[13] This columnar epithelium, to which *C. trachomatis* and *N. gonorrhoeae* preferentially attach,[15, 16] is more exposed on the cervix in adolescent women than in more mature women, as is the squamocolumnar junction, to which human papillomavirus (HPV) preferentially attaches. Cervical ectopy also appears to be a risk factor for acquisition of human immunodeficiency virus (HIV).[17]

Lack of Circumcision. An intact foreskin is associated with STIs characterized by genital ulcers, most likely because of trauma during sex, and HIV.[18, 19] In Africa, rates of HIV generally correlate with the circumcision status of populations, leading to consideration of circumcision in males as a means of HIV control.

BEHAVIOR

Sexual and Reproductive Tract Behaviors. Aral[20] recently identified seven behaviors that place individuals at greater risk for exposure to STIs:

1. *Initiation of sexual intercourse at an early age.* These individuals have longer periods of sexual activity than those of persons who delay intercourse, and tend to have increased numbers of partners and lessened use of barrier contraception
2. *Greater number of sex partners*
3. *Having high-risk partners*
4. *Increased frequency of intercourse and risky types of intercourse.* The more commonly intercourse occurs, the more likely transmission will occur from an infected partner. In addition, the risk of transmission of several STIs (e.g., HIV) is greater with anal intercourse than with vaginal or oral intercourse
5. *Lack of circumcision of the male partner.* An intact foreskin increases the likelihood of STIs characterized by genital ulcers and HIV
6. *Vaginal douching.* Women who douche are at greater risk for developing pelvic inflammatory disease than are women who do not
7. Lack of barrier contraceptive use

Youth. Adolescents are at risk for STIs not only because of biologic reasons but also because of the immaturity of their knowledge and practice of sexual health.[21, 22] Adolescents are often sexually active. The 1997 Youth Risk Behavior Survey found that 48.4% of all youth have had sexual intercourse by grade 12, with black (72.7%) more likely than Hispanic (52.2%) or white (43.6%) teens to have had intercourse.[23] Even by this age, high-risk sex practices are emerging, with 38.5% of black, 15.5% of Hispanic, and 11.6% of white children having four or more partners; 24.7% having used alcohol and only 56.8% a condom at last sexual intercourse. While school and other education programs try to prevent initial infection, additional opportunities to prevent re-infection are not fully utilized. In one clinic, 31% of 562 African-American males with an STI returned with new symptoms.[24] In a teen clinic

serving females aged 14 to 19 years, 112 of 501 teens (23%) returned within 6 months with an additional STI, most commonly *C. trachomatis* (18%); a startling 30% of young women who had only one lifetime sex partner were infected.[25] Each of these settings might have been more fully utilized for partner notification and sexual health counseling, leading to lower re-infection rates. Unfortunately, physicians are not well trained for either effort.

Clinical Status. Individuals with symptoms of an STI are generally socially responsible; that is, they cease having sex and seek care (see later). Almost all diseases (e.g., gonorrhea) are characterized by a large proportion of infected individuals lacking symptoms, although the proportion varies by disease. It is the asymptomatic nature of STIs that largely allows them to be spread widely within a society. In general, the STIs most likely to produce symptoms are found restricted to a smaller portion of the population than those that are characterized by few or no symptoms (Fig. 36–3). For example, infection with *H. ducreyi*, the cause of chancroid, is rarely asymptomatic and, instead, produces with few exceptions painful genital ulcers in men and women alike. As a result, in industrialized societies where health care is relatively available, chancroid is rare—infected individuals cease sex and access care—while chancroid is common in many developing countries. Conversely, infections such as *C. trachomatis*, human papillomavirus, or herpes simplex virus, all of which are frequently asymptomatic (e.g., fewer than 10% of persons seropositive for HSV-2 have a history of genital herpes[9]), are widely spread throughout populations in both the industrialized and the developing worlds.

Women are more likely than men to be asymptomati-

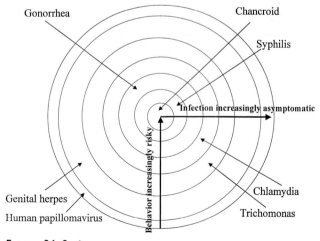

FIGURE 36–3 ▶ Relationship of "educated guesses" of the numbers of cases of individual STIs occurring in a given time period, with the area of the circle approximating the relative size of each. In general, STIs with a higher incidence are characterized by a greater proportion of cases being asymptomatic and less risky sexual practices than those at "the core."

cally infected, owing to the exposed anatomic differences between the two genders. Increasingly appreciated is that men are commonly infected with pathogens that we have thought generally produced symptoms. Prevalences of *C. trachomatis* of 5% to 10% among asymptomatic adolescent males or 2% with *N. gonorrhoeae* in a broader age population, rates not considerably different from those in similar populations of women, occur in sexually active populations in the United States,[26, 27] and a pilot national sample of American adolescents, the 1994 National Survey of Adolescent Males, found 6% to be infected with *C. trachomatis.*[28] In a Ugandan population, if one had relied on symptoms to guide testing, 80% of males and 72% of females with either a gonococcal or a chlamydial infection would not have been detected.[29] Increasingly, efforts to screen men for these infections are occurring in hopes of decreasing rates in women, who suffer the worse consequences of infections with these organisms. A screening program for chlamydial infection in women in Ohio found that although rates in women decreased from 22% to 12% over a 6-year period, rates of nongonococcal urethritis and the proportion of cases of this disorder caused by chlamydia (14% to 15%) remained stable,[30] suggesting that efforts to target men may indeed be necessary for achieving significant further declines in prevalences among women.

Some persons with an STI are not asymptomatic, but they do not recognize their symptoms as indicative of an STI requiring care. Rather, the symptoms are so mild that they are thought to be inconsequential, or to have a different, more unimportant, etiology. Individuals with genital herpes, who frequently shed virus in the absence of characteristic lesions, exemplify this situation. In one study of 27 women with type 2 infection, viral shedding was detected on 28% of 1,410 days, usually without symptoms,[31] while another study found that about half of the women with type 2 antibodies and who did not have a history of genital lesions had clinically recognizable lesions.[32]

Part of our efforts to control STIs must include education about the relative mildness of infection that can occur. If asymptomatic persons do not realize that they have a risk of infection, screening will not occur. If symptoms are present but go unrecognized as possibly being an STI, persons will not cease sexual activity and seek health care.

Health Care Seeking. Not all individuals with an STI who recognize their symptoms as likely to be an STI immediately seek care. A study of individuals attending five U.S. STI clinics found that 35% of men and 37% of women delayed more than a week before seeking care, with the most common reason (half of both genders) being "hoping the symptoms would go away."[33] Delay in seeking care in adolescents may be particularly lengthy among girls.[34] Self-treatment, which was likely to be ineffective, occurred in 21.8%

of attendees at seven STI clinics, was practiced most commonly by women, and delayed health care seeking.[35]

Substance Abuse. Numerous studies have shown that substance abuse, whether socially accepted forms (e.g., alcohol) or not (e.g., cocaine, marijuana, or heroin) are risk factors for the acquisition of STIs.[24, 36] Such behavior is not rare in the U.S. population. The 1996 National Household Survey on Drug Abuse found that 1.7% of the adult population 18 to 59 years of age (1.2 million persons) had substance abuse problems.[37] Even more, 2.8% (3.9 million persons), were deemed at risk for HIV infection because of risky sexual behavior. Individuals with substance abuse problems were more likely to have risky sexual behavior than those without substance abuse, confirming in a population study the numerous individual studies of persons with STIs. Studies of STI prevalence in drug-treatment clinics are generally lacking, even though such individuals practice high-risk behavior.[38]

Incarceration. Individuals who break the law practice high-risk behavior in a variety of ways, including sexual. Only recently has considerable emphasis been placed on identifying and treating infected individuals in correctional settings, who are often core-group members. Although correctional facilities are difficult sites in which to deliver screening and therapeutic sexual health services, they are precisely the sites where high rates are found and services can have a significant public health impact. In 1997, fewer than 5% of women at city and county jail facilities were tested for gonorrhea or chlamydia.[39] Jail screening programs for women have shown high rates of seroreactivity for syphilis: an incidence of 6.5 infections per 100 women-years among women reincarcerated in New York City, a rate greater than 1,000 times that among all women in New York City.[40] Among adolescent and adult women entering jails in three American cities in 1998, rates of chlamydial infection of 6% to 27% and of gonococcal infection of 0 to 17% were found; the rates among women 19 years of age or younger were exceptionally high.[41]

Core Group. The concept of a group of individuals who are high transmitters of infection (the core group) holds for every infection. For infections that are not widely distributed in the population, this group is more easily defined, as they are more "visible." Often, commercial sex workers and substance abusers are characteristic members of the core group.[13] Finding these individuals, and providing accessible and culturally appropriate screening or therapeutic services, can be a challenge, but examples of success are available. Identifying and testing teenagers outside of health care settings identified a prevalence of *C. trachomatis* in young males of 6.1% (with seven of nine female sex partners infected).[27] Rosenberg and colleagues developed a definition of a core group member, finding 14 (16%) of 90 members of a syphilis social network to fit the definition, with 9 of the 14 having current or past syphilis.[42]

INCIDENCE AND PREVALENCE IN THE UNITED STATES

The United States surveillance system for STIs uses numbers of cases provided by state and territory health departments compiled and analyzed at the Centers for Disease Control and Prevention.[43] Six infections are reportable by law in all states and territories: HIV, syphilis, gonorrhea, chancroid, lymphogranuloma venereum, and granuloma inguinale (donovanosis). *Chlamydia* is reportable in 49 states, while surveys conducted by other government agencies or private groups are used to measure the incidence or prevalence of other STIs.

The numbers of cases of bacterial and parasitic STIs have declined markedly in the 1990s. Varying reasons for the decline have been proposed, and there is no consensus on which factors are most important. Putative reasons include the increasing use of barrier contraception, a decrease in the numbers of sex partners, decreased use of drugs, increasing age of sexual debut, and incarceration of high-risk individuals due to tougher incarceration laws (principally for drug possession). Some support for each of these approaches is available, but linking them to a decreasing incidence of STIs is largely conjectural.

Paradoxically, infection with viral STIs remains prevalent, and some evidence indicates that at least one, herpes simplex virus, has increased in the past decade. Why bacterial and parasitic STIs would decline while viral STIs increase is unclear, but the trend might be related to their relatively greater likelihood of asymptomatic infection.

Syphilis. In 1997, the numbers of cases of primary and secondary syphilis (8,550), which are used to measure incidence (because they are the two stages of early syphilis characterized by signs and symptoms), reached the lowest number since 1959, and the rate (3.2 per 100,000) was the lowest since reporting began in 1941. Cases are heavily concentrated geographically (75% of the 3,115 counties reported no cases), with rates in the South (6.6 per 100,000) being considerably higher than elsewhere, and racially (non-Hispanic black Americans having a rate of 22.0 per 100,000, 44-fold higher than that for non-Hispanic whites). As a result of the historically low number of cases, the Center for Disease Control and Prevention (CDC) announced on October 7, 1999, the goal of eliminating syphilis from the United States.

Gonorrhea. In 1997, 324,901 cases of gonorrhea were reported, a decline of 74% since 1975, when a gonorrhea control program was introduced in the mid-1970s. The decline between 1996 and 1997, however, was the third smallest annual decline since 1975, suggesting a leveling off of the decline. Gonorrhea is highly concentrated in non-Hispanic blacks, with a rate of 807.9 per 100,000, 31-fold higher than that among non-Hispanic whites.

Chlamydia. Surveillance for *C. trachomatis* began in 1987. Since then, the number of states reporting has increased from less than 25 to 49. Unsurprisingly, the numbers of cases of chlamydia have increased concomitantly, with 526,653 cases reported in 1997, although 3 million cases are estimated to occur annually.[44] Unlike other STIs (with the exception of trichomoniasis), in which males and females have an approximately equal chance of diagnosis, rates of chlamydia in women (335.8 per 100,000 in 1997) are much greater compared to men (70.4 per 100,000), because that is where screening efforts and testing are concentrated. Unlike syphilis and gonorrhea, chlamydia is widely distributed throughout the population, with rates among women in family planning clinics of 2.0% to 11.2%. The introduction of screening into these clinics has resulted in considerable declines in annual prevalences. The best known of these programs is in the Pacific Northwest, where a program of screening in 160 clinics was accompanied by a 42% decrease in the prevalence of *C. trachomatis*, from 13.2% to 7.6%, over a 5-year period.[45] The expected value of these screening programs is supported by the results of a chlamydia screening program in a health maintenance organization, which showed a 60% decline in pelvic inflammatory disease among women screened compared to those not screened,[46] and a statewide program that showed declines in incidence and prevalence among women, and a decline in hospitalization for pelvic inflammatory disease of 33%.[47]

Chancroid. Following the largest number of cases ever reported, in 1987 (4,986), largely as a result of crack cocaine use, the numbers declined to 243 in 1997, the fewest number since reporting began in 1941. Chancroid is highly localized, with four states (California, New York, South Carolina, and Texas) reporting 85% of reported 1997 cases. Cases are more widespread than these figures indicated, however, because diagnosis is difficult.[48, 49]

Granuloma Inguinale and Lymphogranuloma Venereum. In 1997, 8 cases of granuloma inguinale and 113 cases of lymphogranuloma venereum were reported. It is uncertain how the diagnoses of these diseases are made. It is unlikely that a focus of granuloma inguinale exists in the United States, but clinically compatible, serologically confirmed cases of lymphogranuloma venereum have occurred in New York City.

Trichomoniasis. National surveillance for *T. vaginalis* is not conducted. However, National Disease and Therapeutic Index (NDTI) data (IMS America, Ltd), a result of quarterly sampling of a subset of private physicians, indicate that numbers of infections have declined slowly in recent years. Fewer than 300,000 women were estimated to have had infection diagnosed in private medical care in 1997, although 3 million cases annually among males and females have been estimated.[1]

Genital Herpes. By far, the commonest cause of genital ulcers in the United States is herpes simplex virus, with about 85% of first-episode genital herpes and 95% of recurrent cases caused by type 2 virus. Estimates of the incidence of first-episode genital herpes have been made from the NDTI, with an estimated 175,000 to 200,000 patients seeking private care in 1997 (IMS America, Ltd). The prevalence of infection with HSV type 2 has been estimated from the National Health and Nutrition Survey (NHANES), a periodic sample of the noninstitutionalized American population, using a type-specific serologic test. In NHANES III, conducted from 1988 to 1994, seroprevalence among individuals 12 years of age or older was 21.9%.[9] This is an increase of 30% from NHANES II, conducted from 1976 to 1980,[50] when it was estimated that 31 million Americans 12 years of age or older were infected; this number is now 45 million.[9] The increase occurred principally in the youngest age groups. The NHANES III study showed, as did NHANES II, that women (25.6%) were more likely to be infected than were men (17.8%).

Human Papillomavirus Infection. NDTI data indicate that the numbers of persons seeking initial care for genital warts has declined since 1987, with about 160,000 visits estimated in 1997 (IMS America, Ltd). Papanicolaou (Pap) smear screening to prevent cervical cancer, more than 99.7% of which has been associated with infection by HPV,[51] continues to be widely, although not optimally, practiced. In 1997, 79.7% of American women 18 years of age or older had a Pap smear in the preceding 2 years, and rates of cervical cancer have declined 44.0% between 1973 and 1996.[52] These efforts are important, as an estimated 60% of the American adult population has been infected.[53] The recent development of reliable serologic tests for HPV offers the means of more precisely determining prevalence and incidence of infection.

Hepatitis B Virus. Commonly not recognized as an STI, as many as 60% of cases of hepatitis B virus (HBV) infection are transmitted sexually. Reported numbers of cases of HBV have declined in recent years, in part because of enhanced efforts to vaccinate susceptible adolescents and adults with HBV vaccine. Nevertheless, in 1996, an estimated 65,000 cases of HBV infection

occurred,[54] as did about 3,000 deaths from liver cancer and cirrhosis. The policy of vaccinating newborns with hepatitis B vaccine is widely conducted, with 84% of all children aged 19 to 35 months in the United States receiving vaccine.[55] This program is supplemented by the "catch-up" effort recommended in 1995 to vaccinate all 11- and 12-year-olds, and the recommendation in October 1997 by the Advisory Committee on Immunization Practices to vaccinate all unvaccinated children or adolescents through age 18.[56] Unfortunately, these recommendations are not universally practiced, partly because clinicians do not know them. In addition, parents who believe that their children are not at risk for sexual or intravenous transmission have criticized them. Vaccine is also recommended for adults at high risk for infection, including those who have a current or recent STI or who have had at least two sex partners in the preceding 6 months.[57]

REFERENCES

1. Institute of Medicine (U.S.), Committee on Prevention and Control of Sexually Transmitted Diseases. The Hidden Epidemic: Confronting Sexually Transmitted Diseases. Eng TR, Butler WT (eds). Washington, DC, National Academy Sciences, 1997.
2. Yamamoto T, Nagasawa I, Nojima M, et al: Sexual transmission and reinfection of group B streptococci between spouses. J Obstet Gynaecol Res 1999; 25:215.
3. Anderson RM, May RM: Epidemiologic parameters of HIV transmission. Nature 1988; 333:514.
4. Brunham RC, Ronald AR: Epidemiology of STDs in developing countries. In: Wasserheit JN, Aral SO, Cates W, Hitchcock P (eds): Reproductive Tract Infections. Washington, DC, American Society of Microbiology, 1991.
5. Gerbase AC, Rowley JT, Heymann DH, et al: Global prevalence and incidence estimates of selected curable STDs. Sex Transm Infect 1998; 74S:S12.
6. Dallabetta GA, Laga M, Lamptey PR (eds): Control of STDs. AIDSCAP/Family Health International, 2101 Wilson Blvd., Arlington, VA 22201.
7. Kamali A, Nunn AJ, Malder DW, et al: Seroprevalence and incidence of genital ulcer infection in a rural Ugandan population. Sex Transm Infect 1999; 75:98.
8. Piot P, Islam MQ: Sexually transmitted diseases in the 1990s: Global epidemiology and challenges for control. Sex Transm Dis 1994; 21(2 S):S7.
9. Fleming DT, McQuillan GM, Johnson RE, et al: Herpes simplex virus type 2 in the United States, 1976–1994. N Engl J Med 1997; 337:1105.
10. Christianson B, Bottiger M, Svensson A, Jeansson S: A 15-year surveillance study of antibodies to herpes simplex virus types 1 and 2 in a cohort of young girls. J Infect 1992; 25:147.
11. Hashido M, Lee FK, Nahmias AJ, et al: An epidemiologic study of herpes simplex virus type 1 and 2 infection in Japan based on type-specific serologic assays. Epidemiol Infect 1998; 120:179.
12. Sparling PF, Elkins C, Wyrick PB, Cohen MS: Vaccines for bacterial sexually transmitted infections: A realisic goal? Proc Natl Acad Sci USA 1994; 91:2456.
13. Brunham RC, Kimani J, Bwayo J, et al: The epidemiology of *Chlamydia trachomatis* within a sexually transmitted diseases core group. J Infect Dis 1996; 173:950.
14. Hansen EJ, Lumbley SR, Richardson JA, et al: Induction of protective immunity to *Haemophilus ducreyi* in the temperature-dependent rabbit model of experimental chancroid. J Immunol 1994; 152:184.
15. Draper DL, Donegan EA, James J, et al: Scanning electron microscopy of attachment of *Neisseria gonorrhoeae* colony phenotypes to surfaces of human genital epithelia. Am J Obstet Gynecol 1980; 138:818.

16. Harrison HR, Costin M, Meder JB, et al: Cervical *Chlamydia trachomatis* infection in university women: Relationship to history, contraception, ectopy and cervicitis. Am J Obstet Gynecol 1985; 153:244.

17. Moss GB, Clemetson D, D'Costa L, et al: Association of cervical ectopy with heterosexual transmission of human immunodeficiency virus: Results of a study of couples in Nairobi, Kenya. J Infect Dis 1991; 164:588.

18. Moses S, Bailey RC, Ronald AR: Male circumcision: Assessment of health benefits and risks. Sex Transm Infect 1998; 74:368.

19. Lavereys L, Rakwar JP, Thompson ML, et al: Effect of circumcision on infection of HIV type 1 and other STDs: A prospective cohort study of trucking employees in Kenya. J Infect Dis 1999; 180:330.

20. Aral SO: Sexual behavior in sexually transmitted diseases research: An overview. Sex Transm Dis 1994; 21:S59.

21. D'Souza CM, Shrier LA: Prevention and intervention of sexually transmitted diseases in adolescents. Curr Opin Pediatr 1999; 11:287.

22. Gevelber MA, Biro FM: Adolescents and sexually transmitted diseases. Pediatr Clin North Am 1999; 46:747.

23. CDC: Youth Risk Behavior Survey—United States, 1997. MMWR 1998; 47(No. SS-3).

24. Watstaff DA, Delamater JD, Havens KK: Subsequent infection among adolescent African-American males attending an STD clinic. J Adolesc Health 1999; 25:217.

25. Bunnell RE, Dahlberg L, Rolfs R, et al: High prevalences and incidences of sexually transmitted diseases in urban adolescent females despite moderate risk behavior. J Infect Dis 1999; 80:1624.

26. McNagny SE, Parker RM, Zenilman JM, Lewis JS: Urinary leukocyte esterase test: A screening method for the detection of asymptomatic chlamydial and gonococcal infections in men. J Infect Dis 1992; 165:573.

27. Gunn RA, Podschun GD, Fitzgerald S, et al: Screening high-risk adolescent males for *Chlamydia trachomatis* infection: Obtaining specimens in the field. Sex Transm Dis 1998; 25:49.

28. Ku L, Sonenstein FL, Turner CF, et al: The promise of integrated representative surveys about sexually transmitted diseases and behavior. Sex Transm Dis 1997; 24:299.

29. Paxton LA, Sewankambo N, Gray R, et al: Asymptomatic non-ulcerative genital tract infections in a rural Ugandan population. Sex Transm Infect 1998; 74:421.

30. Schmid G, Mosure D, Berman S, Dorian K: Proceedings of the 3rd European Meeting of Chlamydial Infection. Vienna, 1997.

31. Wald A, Corey L, Cone R, et al: Frequent genital herpes simplex virus 2 shedding in immunocompetent women: Effect of acyclovir treatment. J Clin Invest 1997; 99:1092.

32. Langenberg A, Benedetti J, Jenkins J, et al: Development of clinically recognizable genital lesions among women previously identified as having "asymptomatic" herpes simplex virus type 2 infection. Ann Intern Med 1989; 110:882.

33. Hook EW III, Richey CM, Leone P, et al: Delayed presentation to clinics for sexually transmitted diseases by symptomatic patients: A potential contributor to continuing STD morbidity. Sex Transm Dis 1997; 24:443.

34. Fortenberry JD: Health care–seeking behaviors related to sexually transmitted diseases among adolescents. Am J Public Health 1997; 87:417.

35. Irwin DE, Thomas JC, Spitters CE, et al: Self-treatment patterns among clients attending sexually transmitted disease clinics and the effects of self-treatment on STD symptom duration. Sex Transm Dis 1997; 24:372.

36. Marx R, Aral SO, Rolfs RT, et al: Crack, sex and STDs. Sex Transm Dis 1991; 18:92.

37. Anderson JE, Wilson RW, Barker P, et al: Prevalence of sexual- and drug-related HIV risk behaviors in the U.S. adult population: Results of the National Household Survey on Drug Abuse. J Acquir Immune Defic Syndr 1999; 21:148.

38. Morrison Cl, Ruben SM, Beeching NJ: Female sexual health problems in a drug dependency unit. Int J STD AIDS 1995; 6:201.

39. CDC: Assessment of sexually transmitted disease services in city and county jails—United States, 1997. MMWR 1998; 47:429.

40. Blank S, Sternberg M, Neylans LL, et al: Incident syphilis among women with multiple admissions to jail in New York City. J Infect Dis 1999; 180:1159.

41. CDC: High prevalence of chlamydial and gonococcal infection in women entering jails and juvenile detention centers—Chicago, Birmingham, and San Francisco. MMWR 1999; 48:793.

42. Rosenberg D, Moseley K, Kahn R, et al: Networks of persons with syphilis and at risk for syphilis in Louisiana: Evidence of core transmitters. Sex Transm Dis 1999; 26:108.

43. Division of STD Prevention: Sexually Transmitted Disease Surveillance, 1997. U.S. Department of Health and Human Services, Public Health Service, Atlanta, Centers for Disease Control and Prevention (CDC), September, 1998.

44. Groseclose SL, Zaidi AA, DeLisle SJ, et al: Estimated incidence and prevalence of genital *Chlamydia trachomatis* infections in the United States, 1996. Sex Transm Dis 1999; 26:339.

45. Mosure DJ, Berman S, Fine D, et al: Genital chlamydial infections in sexually active female adolescents: Do we really need to screen everyone? J Adolesc Health 1997; 20:6.

46. Scholes D, Stergachis A, Heidrich FE, et al: Prevention of pelvic inflammatory disease by screening for cervical chlamydial infection. N Engl J Med 1996; 34:1362.

47. Hillis SD, Nakashima A, Amsterdam L, et al: The impact of a comprehensive chlamydia prevention program in Wisconsin. Fam Plann Perspect 1995; 27:108.

48. Schulte JM, Martich FA, Schmid GP: Chancroid in the United States, 1981–1990: Evidence for underreporting of cases. MMWR CDC Surveill Summ 1992; 41:57.

49. Mertz KJ, Trees D, Levine WC, et al: Etiology of genital ulcers and prevalence of human immunodeficiency virus coinfection in 10 U.S. cities: The Genital Ulcer Disease Surveillance Group. J Infect Dis 1998; 178:1795.

50. Johnson RE, Nahmias AJ, Magder LS, et al: A seroepidemiologic survey of the prevalence of herpes simplex virus type 2 infection in the United States. N Engl J Med 1989; 321:7.

51. Walboomers JM, Jacobs MV, Manos MM, et al: Human papillomavirus is a necessary cause of invasive cervical cancer worldwide. J Pathol 1999; 189:12.

52. Blackman DK, Bennett EM, Miller DS: Trends in self-reported use of mammograms (1989–1997) and Papanicolaou tests (1991–1997)—Behavioral Risk Factor Surveillance System. MMWR 1999; 48(SS-6): 1.

53. Koutsky L: Epidemiology of genital human papillomavirus infection. Am J Med 1997; 102:3.

54. Mast EE, Williams IT, Alter MJ, Margolis HS: Hepatitis B vaccination of adolescent and adult high-risk groups in the United States. Vaccine 1998; suppl:S27.

55. CDC: Update: Recommendations to prevent hepatitis B virus transmission—United States. MMWR 1995; 44:574.

56. CDC: Notice to Readers Update: Recommendations to prevent hepatitis B virus transmission—United States. MMWR 1999; 48:33.

57. CDC: 1988 Guidelines for treatment of sexually transmitted diseases. MMWR 1998; 47 (no. RR-1) 1.

37

Syphilis

CHARLES H. LIVENGOOD III

EPIDEMIOLOGY

Transmission of syphilis results from direct contact with one of its moist lesions (e.g., chancre, mucous patch, condyloma latum), which occur during primary and secondary disease. Spirochetes may enter through intact mucosa or skin with epithelial defects. Essentially any exposed body part can be inoculated. Blood is infectious during episodes of spirochetemia, which may manifest as secondary syphilis or may be asymptomatic, and may occur for 4 years or more after primary infection.[1] People with later syphilis are in general held to be noninfectious.

Transmission during sexual activity has been a very consistent theme in the history of syphilis. Approximately 30% (range, 10% to 60%) of casual sexual partners and 90% of steady partners of an infectious person will acquire syphilis.[2, 3] Less intimate contact may also transmit syphilis—primary infection of the fingers is most often seen in medical personnel.[4] Acquisition from blood products has not occurred since screening of donors was implemented, and was uncommon even before because *Treponema pallidum* does not survive in banked blood for more than 48 hours.[5] Needle sharing during illicit drug use seems to be an unusual route of transmission.[6] An important exception to the rarity of transmission in blood is congenital syphilis, in which the fetus is infected by transplacental passage of organisms during an episode of maternal spirochetemia.

The United States experienced an epidemic of syphilis in the years around 1990 that included a profound change in the epidemiology of the disease, best illustrated by events in 1987. Syphilis declined by 15% among homosexual men and rose by over 75% among heterosexual men and women, which in turn fueled a sevenfold increase in congenital syphilis. The epidemic was attributed to routine use of spectinomycin (a drug ineffective against incubating syphilis) to treat gonorrhea because of new resistance patterns in that organism, and diversion of public health resources away from syphilis to deal with the emerging human immunodeficiency virus (HIV) epidemic.[7, 8] Investigation of the epidemic also revealed the extreme importance of the crack cocaine subculture in the epidemiology of

syphilis in the United States. In Miami from 1986 to 1988, 30% of pregnant women with syphilis were crack cocaine users, compared with 4% of control subjects.[9] In New York City, 19% of gravid women using crack cocaine had a positive nontreponemal test, compared with 2% of those with negative urine toxicologic tests for cocaine.[10] Control of syphilis in this population is especially challenging because these people have multiple anonymous partners who are difficult to trace.[11, 12] A practical and apparently successful strategy to resolve this problem has been to take the screening center to the crack house.[13] It is interesting that use of illicit drugs other than crack cocaine carries a much lower increase in risk of acquiring syphilis.[14, 15]

Syphilis in the United States currently is heavily concentrated in the South, and is equally distributed between rural and urban areas.[16, 17] Despite the control of the 1985 to 1990 epidemic, its trend of over-representation of women continues. Among inner-city adolescents attending a comprehensive health center, 84% of cases of syphilis were found in girls, despite a comparable sex representation in the samples.[18] In a case-control study that evaluated syphilis risks relative to sexual behavior, independent risk factors were more than four partners and lack of condom use during the preceding 3 months; however, among all people engaging in these behaviors, women had a significantly higher risk for syphilis than men.[14] Self-reporting of risk factors among inherently high-risk populations is not reliable. Ernst and colleagues[19] evaluated an inner-city emergency department population and found no difference in the prevalence of untreated syphilis among patients at high risk and those at low risk by self-report.

The epidemiology of syphilis in pregnancy is of particular importance because antenatal treatment of infected mothers is necessary to control congenital syphilis. Crack cocaine use retains its importance in this population, and was present in 36% of syphilitic gravidas in a recent large series from Detroit.[20] Ricci and co-workers[9] found that among infants born with congenital syphilis in Miami, 71% were born to crack cocaine users and 67% to women with no prenatal care. Ernst and colleagues[21] found that of inner-city women presenting to an emergency department with no prior prenatal care, 11% had syphilis, compared with 2% of those seen in the obstetrics clinic. In the Detroit series, the greatest risks for congenital syphilis occurred among infants born to women with high nontreponemal titers, those with unknown duration of disease, and those treated for syphilis in the third trimester.[20] In another report from this series, women with syphilis had significantly higher mean parity (4.1) than the general obstetric population there for the year (2.1).[22]

The epidemiology of syphilis represents a complex interplay among human behaviors that serve as surrogate markers for increased risk of sexually transmissible disease, a correlated over-representation among people in relatively disenfranchised segments of society who are less likely to seek medical care, the chronic latent nature of the disease, public health efforts to reach and manage those infected and those at risk, and medical therapies available to treat them. It is now clear that all of those pieces must be considered as we look toward strategies to control syphilis in the future.

MICROBIOLOGY

The family Spirochaetaceae comprises the genera *Treponema*, *Borrelia*, and *Leptospira*. Most species of the genus *Treponema* are nonpathogenic and many are free-living in nature; a number of these species colonize the healthy human gastro-intestinal tract, including the mouth. A number of nonpathogenic species can be grown in culture (e.g., Reiter treponemes), which are valuable for the provision of group antigens used in the treponemal serologic tests to absorb nonspecific antibody. Human pathogens are *T. pallidum* subspecies *pallidum*, *pertenue*, and *endemicum*, and *Treponema carateum*. Curiously, these four organisms are differentiated only by the clinical diseases they cause: syphilis, yaws, bejel or endemic syphilis, and pinta, respectively. No morphologic, biochemical, nutritional, genetic, or immunologic differences among them have been demonstrated.[23, 24] Because of the defined geographic locations in which these diseases occur (syphilis world-wide, yaws in the tropics, pinta in Central and South America, and bejel in the arid Middle East), Hudson[25] and later Hollander[26] and Willcox[27, 28] theorized that climatic differences produce the differences in clinical manifestations. An important practical product of the homology among these organisms is that all uniformly produce positive serologic tests for syphilis.[29]

T. pallidum ranges in length from 10 to 13 μm, tapers at the ends, and is exceptionally thin at a width of 0.05 μm. This narrow width places it below the resolution of light microscopy—hence the need for the indirect light rays it reflects into the microscope lens by dark-field microscopy and the use of silver stains that envelope it in a thick layer to visualize it. The organism exhibits uniform tight spirals with a wavelength of 1.1 μm and amplitude of 0.2 to 0.3 μm, and moves with a rotary corkscrew motion, often flexing and snapping back to linearity with a spring-like motion. *T. pallidum* has an outer membrane consisting of multiple proteins, a middle peptidoglycan layer, and an inner cytoplasmic membrane. All of the known outer membrane proteins are weak antigens[30]; the most antigenic among them is a 47-kD protein.[31] Three fine, spiraling fibrils arise from between the outer two layers at each end; these may be involved in attachment to mammalian cells because it is the organism's ends that are involved in this process. Attachment is prevented by preincubation with specific antibody or trypsin,[32] suggesting that an antigenic protein mediates it. *T. pallidum* lacks the *recA* gene product, crucial to the mechanism for genetic recombination,[33] and therefore lacks the ability to repair damaged DNA.[34] It therefore has a very stable genome. A plasmid in the nucleus has been described,[35] raising the possibility of transmissible penicillin resistance, although none has yet been reported. No toxin production has been reported.

T. pallidum replicates by transverse fission[36] every 30 to 33 hours, although it has been suggested that this interval is considerably prolonged among organisms in lesions of late syphilis.[37–40] Such a phenomenon has implications for therapy because penicillin has killing power only among dividing organisms. Traditional cultivation of treponemes pathogenic in humans has not been possible. The organism is not an obligate anaerobe.[41, 42] A number of animals are susceptible to *T. pallidum* infection, and the rabbit in particular has been a valuable resource in the study of syphilis because infection in this species so closely parallels that in humans.[43] However, no species other than humans manifests the changes of tertiary syphilis. As discussed later, the rabbit infectivity (RIT) test remains the most sensitive assay for viable *T. pallidum*.

T. pallidum is killed by direct contact with soap and water, as in routine hand washing, and by drying. A temperature of 40°C kills *T. pallidum* in 3 hours,[44] lending considerable plausibility to the techniques of fever therapy used in the past.

PATHOGENESIS OF INFECTION

Direct contact with a moist lesion of syphilis during primary and secondary eruptions provides for transfer of the disease to a new host. Organisms traverse intact mucosa or broken skin, but not intact skin, and gain access to superficial vasculature. Within a few hours after infection, vascular and lymphatic dissemination of spirochetes commences, and the disease is systemic. A small number of organisms is capable of seating the infection. Enhanced reproduction of the organism ocurs at the site of entry,[45] and the chancre appears when a critical mass of spirochetes accumulates, 10^7 to

10^8 organisms per gram of tissue.[43] The duration of the incubation period is inversely proportional to the titer of the inoculum, ranging from 3 to 90 days with a median of 21 days. In inmate volunteers inoculated with 10 and 10^4 spirochetes, a chancre developed at the site a mean of 28.7 and 18.6 days later, respectively.[43] The Nichols strain of *T. pallidum*, which is adapted to laboratory growth in rabbits, requires 57 organisms to induce infection in 50% of humans inoculated.[43] It appears that a much higher titer is required to infect by intravenous inoculation; in rabbits, a minimum of 10^7 organisms is necessary.[46] These data are consistent with the predominance of sexual transmission of syphilis, and may be explained in part by the knowledge that normal human serum exerts mild antitreponemal activity in vitro,[47] perhaps because of cross-reactivity of antibody raised against commensal treponemes.

The chancre appears as an erythematous plaque, which is usually singular. It rapidly develops an annular appearance as the borders become raised, and thinning and loss of epithelium within occurs. Ulceration reflects the vascular changes below. Endothelial cell swelling is an early histopathologic change, preceded only by accumulation of polymorphonuclear leukocytes that phagocytose spirochetes but for unknown reasons do not kill them. Vascular and lymphatic proliferation evolves as damage to vessels progresses, evidenced by dense perivascular cuffing by plasma cells and lymphocytes,[48] adventitial proliferation, and eventual obliteration of the lumen. These arteriolar–capillary changes, depicted in Figure 37–1, are the hallmark of the syphilis pathologic process, and are found in every lesion of the disease. With the arrival of activated macrophages, T lymphocytes, and B lymphocytes that elaborate specific antibody,[49] the tide is turned. The population of treponemes declines, and after 1 to 5 weeks the chancre heals.

This scenario is not played out at distant sites to which spirochetes had spread soon after infection, and at some or all of these sites they persist and proliferate.

However, except for rare patients alluded to in the literature with disseminated chancres,[46] these foci of infection are obviously partially controlled. It is well known that colonization of the central nervous system (CNS) occurs early in syphilis. Mills found "abnormal" cerebrospinal fluid (CSF) in 9% of 283 patients with untreated primary syphilis and in 32% of 559 with untreated secondary disease.[50] Viable *T. pallidum* in the CSF of patients with primary syphilis has been demonstrated by rabbit inoculation.[51] In another study,[3] only 1.7% of 2,269 patients with early syphilis had neurologic signs, none of which was documented to be of syphilitic origin, so the presence of spirochetes in the CNS of asymptomatic patients early in syphilis is taken to be benign. Further, despite the high frequency of early CNS colonization, only 5% to 10% of untreated patients with syphilis go on to acquire neurosyphilis.

As implied earlier, the immunology of syphilis is complex and poorly understood. One clinically important fact is that prior treated syphilis, even with persistence of specific antibody, confers no immunity against reinfection. Magnuson and associates[43] first confirmed this by inoculating *T. pallidum* into 11 people with previously treated primary syphilis, all of whom manifested a clinical and serologic response indistinguishable from that in people with no prior exposure. One exception may be variable protection of the person previously treated for long-standing syphilis. These same investigators rechallenged 31 men who had been treated for late latent syphilis or congenital syphilis: 14 showed no clinical or serologic response, 13 responded with primary lesions and nontreponemal titer increases, and 4 had lesions without seroresponse. There may be brief immunity to reinfection during primary syphilis. Other treponematoses, regardless of treatment, provide no protection against syphilis.[52]

However, resistance to reinfection is the rule in *untreated latent* syphilis,[43] which coincides with the development of delayed hypersensitivity to *T. pallidum* antigens.[53, 54] This phenomenon is intuitive, because

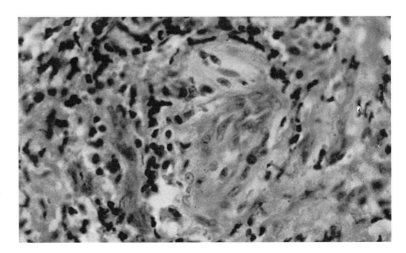

FIGURE 37–1 ▶ Microvascular changes characteristic of the histopathology of syphilitic lesions. (Reprinted from U.S. Public Health Service: Syphilis: A Synopsis. Washington, DC, U.S. Government Printing Office, 1967, p 27.)

latency is defined as seropositivity without evidence of active disease—that is, the infection is controlled (although not cleared) by an immune response that is also adequate to prevent reinfection. This "stand-off" is common with parasitic diseases and is called *premunition*. Unfortunately, protection cannot be transferred by transfusion of T lymphocytes from an immune rabbit (one with established latency) to a susceptible one.[55] There is some evidence that partial treatment may be detrimental by obstructing the assembly of an adequate immune response. For example, syphilitic meningitis and iridocyclitis occur more often among those inadequately treated than those untreated.[3, 56–58] Although antitreponemal antibody inactivates *T. pallidum* in vitro, humoral immunity apparently has little potency in the control or prevention of syphilis. As noted, specific antibody is not protective, and in rabbits administration of specific antibody at the time of inoculation does not prevent infection.[59, 60]

Syphilis may cause alterations in the immune system as a whole—a number of specific defects in cellular and humoral immunity in various stages of the disease have been described.[61–65]

Secondary syphilis occurs in episodes that represent spirochetemia, usually in the first year after infection, but sometimes as long as 4 years later. It is not known whether all episodes of spirochetemia are symptomatic, but based on the delivery of infants with congenital syphilis to women without symptoms during pregnancy,[20] it is probable that they are not. That these episodes occur is evidence that an immune response adequate to contain the infection has not been mustered, but that the lesions are different from chancres implies that some modification of the manifestations of the infection has been achieved by the immune response to that point. Predictably, spirochetes are present in the lesions of secondary syphilis, with one exception, syphilitic nephritis.

Skin manifestations are the most common of the secondary stage, and a good practical rule is that any rash except a vesicular one may represent secondary syphilis (an exception is neonatal congenital syphilis, where vesicular lesions are frequently encountered). The high frequency of skin changes probably represents the preference of *T. pallidum* for cooler temperatures. The histopathologic process of these lesions varies in its epidermal manifestations from complete loss in mucous patches, to normal in some macular lesions, to marked thickening with rete ridge elongation and acanthosis in condylomata lata. The dermal findings, on the other hand, are quite homogeneous, consisting of the vascular abnormalities described previously as the hallmark of the syphilitic pathologic process— endothelial swelling, fibroblastic proliferation, and a dense perivascular infiltrate with chronic inflammatory cells, predominantly plasma cells. A gross description of these lesions is provided later.

Episodes of secondary disease are usually associated with flu-like malaise, myalgia, arthralgia, and often fever. Iritis may also be seen, generalized lymphadenopathy is common, and splenomegaly may be found. In syphilitic hepatitis, histopathologic study reveals granulomatous inflammation with an exudate and infiltrate of lymphocytes and plasma cells in and around portal tracts, and scattered hepatocyte necrosis with frequent acidophilic (Councilman) bodies; the population of spirochetes is sparse.[66] Syphilitic nephritis is exclusively the result of circulating antibody–antigen complex deposition; the antibody is specific anti-treponemal immunoglobulin G (IgG), but the antigen has not been identified.[67–70] Light microscopy may be normal or may show the typical lymphoplasmacytic infiltrate. Electron microscopy reveals subepithelial deposits in the glomerular capillary loops (subepithelial humps) that represent the immune complexes themselves. *T. pallidum* is not found.[66] In fact, animal studies have shown that syphilis can be transmitted in blood, CSF, liver biopsy, and lymph node homogenates from those with secondary disease, but not in renal extracts.[71]

In latent syphilis, there is no manifestation of disease except for seroreactivity. However, most patients are believed to experience ongoing organ damage as spirochetes proliferate and host immune mechanisms act to control them. Latent syphilis persists in this state until the patient's death in approximately one third of cases. Approximately one third experience a tip in the balance that favors the spirochetes, producing tertiary syphilis, which manifests in one or more of three ways: neurosyphilis, cardiovascular syphilis, or late "benign" syphilis (gummas). It is generally believed, although difficult to prove, that approximately one third of patients do eventually clear their infection. The differentiation between early and late latency is frankly confusing. Currently in the United States, it is used mostly to define which cases of latent disease can be expected to respond to the same treatment as primary syphilis (those of less than 1 year's duration). In the past, the same cut-off was used, but the designation's practical use was to identify those cases likely enough to cause transmission that contact investigation was justified. The World Health Organization has used 4 years' duration as the cut-off for contact investigation in the past; more recently, 2 years has been designated as the cut-off. In practice, it often is impossible to determine the duration of latent syphilis because most patients have not had prior serial serologies and do not recall manifestations of early infection.

Neurosyphilis represents the growth of treponemes in the CNS,[45] and is actually a heterogeneous collection of disease states. As discussed, in many cases *T. pallidum* colonizes the CNS during the first year of the infection. Most of these represent asymptomatic neurosyphilis, defined as abnormal CSF in an asymptomatic patient with known syphilis.[72] It has been shown that risk for eventual symptomatic disease in these patients is proportional to the degree of CSF abnormality.[73] Neurosyphilis may develop as late as 44 years after infection,[74] but it usually occurs earlier. Thus, because people usually acquire syphilis early in life, during the peak of sexual activity, it is unusual to find an older patient with neurosyphilis. In the Oslo study, no patients among 169 examined with syphilis of more than 30 years' duration had abnormal CSF.[74] Merritt and colleagues[75] found that only 4.5% of 200 patients with asymptomatic neurosyphilis were older than 61 years of age. These data also imply that people with asymptomatic neurosyphilis are those in whom symptomatic disease later develops. Hook and Marra[76] have provided an excellent overview of the various manifestations of neurosyphilis. The earliest form seen is syphilitic meningitis, which may occur as early as 1 month after infection and most often occurs at 2 to 6 months. The second of the "early" forms of neurosyphilis is meningovascular disease, usually seen 4 to 7 years after acquisition of T. pallidum. It is marked by focal deficits owing to vascular compromise. Histologically, diffuse pia-arachnoid thickening is seen with typical syphilitic changes of the microvasculature. Obstructive hydrocephalus may develop. Both of these early forms of CNS syphilis, like the ocular manifestations cited previously, are associated with inadequate treatment.[3, 73] The more familiar forms of neurosyphilis occur 5 years to decades after infection. Tabes dorsalis results from involvement of the dorsal columns of the lower spinal cord with severe demyelinization, producing a loss of proprioception in the lower extremities and lightning pains. In general paresis, the classic parenchymatous form of CNS syphilis, the brain is shrunken and the lateral ventricles are dilated. There is marked neuronal loss, with an increase in astrocytes and microglia; the latter show a characteristic elongation and orientation perpendicular to the surface, forming the rod cell pathognomonic of the paretic brain. Optic atrophy, a common complication of neurosyphilis, produces blindness and may arise from hydrocephalus, parenchymal gummas, demyelinization, or meningeal disease.

Cardiovascular syphilis has a remarkable affinity for the aortic root, and, like neurosyphilis, represents injury resulting from viable spirochetes. Occlusion of the vasa vasorum is the mechanism, producing necrosis of the tunica media and consequent loss of its integrity. Dilation of the proximal aorta produces the characteristic ascending segment aneurysm and valvular incompetence with left ventricular dilation, and stenosis of the coronary ostea is common. The heart itself is rarely involved. The affected aorta develops a patchy, wrinkled, bark-like internal surface.[77]

Gummas characterize late benign syphilis. These lesions do not contain spirochetes in an appreciable concentration, and are thought to be immunologically mediated.[45] Gummas are the classic granulomatous inflammation and may occur in any organ, and therefore they are by no means always benign. They vary in size from microscopic to over 10 cm in diameter, and consist of caseous necrosis, some giant cells (but fewer than in mycobacterial granulomas), and the typical vascular changes of syphilis. They tend to appear in the skin at sites of trauma (knees, elbows) and in the testis and liver, but not in lymph nodes.

Congenital syphilis is the result of transplacental hematogenous inoculation of the fetus during a maternal episode of spirochetemia that may or may not be symptomatic. Thus, the fetus experiences secondary syphilis as the initial event in the infection, with no primary stage. As a result, essentially every tissue in an affected fetus shows the presence of T. pallidum.[78] Transmission to the fetus may occur as early as the ninth week of pregnancy.[79] A high-titer nontreponemal serology in the mother, which correlates roughly with severity of tissue injury and treponemal burden, is a predictor of increased risk for congenital syphilis and stillbirth in the fetus.[20] The venerable term Kassowitz's law[80] reflects the fact that longer duration of maternal syphilis is associated with progressively less risk of episodes of spirochetemia, and therefore lower risk of fetal infection. Although women with syphilis of less than 4 years' duration have only a 20% chance of a healthy infant, in those with disease of a longer duration the figure is 70%.[81] Fetal infection early in pregnancy is more likely to be associated with stillbirth, that occurring later with liveborn infants who may be grossly normal at birth; presumably, this phenomenon represents evolution of greater fetal immunocompetence during gestation. Because all infants born to syphilitic women are seropositive, identification of those grossly normal at birth (most liveborn syphilitc infants) who are infected and require treatment is problematic. Currently, all of these exposed infants are treated presumptively, but in the past, study of placental pathology was undertaken to attempt to solve this dilemma. Older texts[77] describe affected placentas as enlarged and pale, but more recent evaluations[82, 83] have found no reliable gross change. The "barberpole" umbilical cord of necrotizing funisitis was seen in only 54% of congenital syphilis cases in the Miami series.[9] The constellation of marked proliferative vascular changes, villous immaturity, hypercellularity, and a chronic (histiolymphocytic) villitis with or without microabscess formation correlated well with the presence of spirochetes by silver stain in the Detroit series,[82] but the small number of placentas studied (25) does not provide adequate power to base treatment on these data. As in other entities producing fetal compromise, diminished maternal serum estrone, presumably resulting from fetal adrenal involvement, can be demonstrated in congenital syphilis, whereas pro-

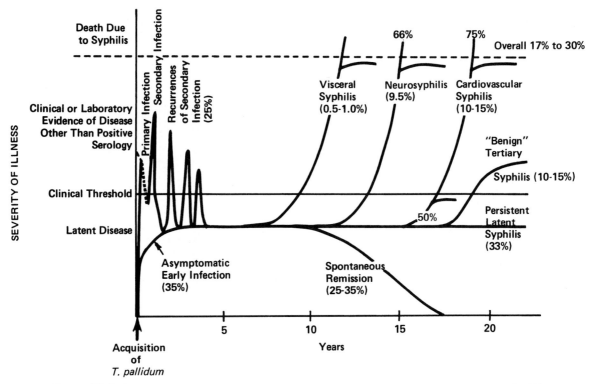

FIGURE 37–2 ▶ Potential outcomes with approximate frequency in the natural history of untreated syphilis. (Reprinted with permission from Livengood CH III: Syphilis. In: Gleicher N [ed]: Principles of Medical Therapy in Pregnancy. New York, Plenum, 1985, p 507.)

gesterone levels remain normal.[84] Fetal liver, bone, and lung are particularly densely affected. The liver is the primary hematopoietic organ of the fetus, and treponemal infection produces anemia (and thrombocytopenia) that causes hydrops, an ominous sign with a historic mortality rate of 100%[85, 86] although more recently, effective treatment has been shown to reverse this process. Among the known causes of nonimmune hydrops, syphilis is rare.[87] In bone, osteochondritis and periostitis of the long bones are common, producing the jagged "sawtooth" appearance of the epiphysis and subperiosteal deposits of osteoid around the shaft. Leukocytic infiltration of the lung parenchyma and airspaces with edema produces the so-called *pneumonia alba* of congenital syphilis.

CLINICAL MANIFESTATIONS

A wide range of clinical manifestations over a long period contributes greatly to the complexity of syphilis, and earned it the reputation as the great imitator of countless other diseases. Figure 37–2 offers an overview of the courses untreated syphilis may follow.

The chancre is the first expression of *T. pallidum* infection, occurring at the site of inoculation (Figs. 37–3 and 37–4). It begins as a dull red macule and rapidly progresses to a papule with a raised, smooth, distinct border. It may be round or oval in shape and is usually 1 to 2 cm in greatest diameter, but may be as

small as 2 to 3 mm. Initially the base is smooth and glistening, but within a few days progresses to ulceration with or without a crusted or shaggy gray exudate. This lesion is usually singular, has a characteristic cartilaginous induration, and is painless unless superin-

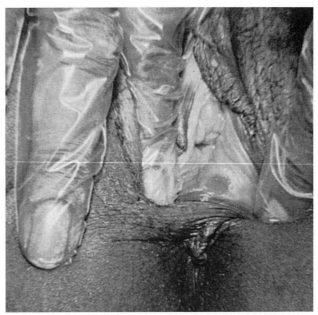

FIGURE 37–3 ▶ Typical chancre of the vaginal vestibule. (Reprinted from U.S. Public Health Service: Syphilis: A Synopsis. Washington, DC, U.S. Government Printing Office, 1967, p 46.)

fected. Regional nodes are enlarged, hard, and pain-less; they do not suppurate, and may be unilateral or bilateral. Unfortunately, almost 50% of chancres are atypical in appearance[88] because of superinfection. These lesions become painful (as do the regional nodes) and acquire a necrotic base with undermined borders. Extragenital chancres are especially prone to superinfection because they are most often found around the mouth or anus. Those of the fingers may resemble paronychia with a nodular, scaling appearance. Unless superinfected, the chancre resolves spontaneously without scarring in 2 to 6 weeks. It is of special importance that chancres in women are often found internally on the mucosa of the vagina or cervix, and therefore may escape detection (Fig. 37–5). The differential diagnosis is extensive, including herpes genitalis, pyoderma, secondary infection of a traumatic lesion, furuncle, chancroid, granuloma inguinale, drug reaction, histoplasmosis, mycobacterial infection, Crohn's disease, ectoparasitic infection, neoplasia, Behçet's syndrome, lichen planus, histiocytosis X, leukemic lesions, cytomegalovirus infections, Paget's disease, lupus syndromes, pellagra, fistula, phycomycosis, psoriasis, and, rarely, lymphogranuloma venereum.

Secondary syphilis occurs in one or more episodes, and is evidence of the systemic involvement of syphilis. The first episode may occur while the chancre is still present, but usually develops several weeks to months after the chancre revolves. It is a variable syndrome with flu-like features of fever, myalgia, arthralgia, malaise, sore throat, headache, and generalized adenopathy. Arthritis, bursitis, periostitis, and osteitis may also be demonstrated. The most characteristic finding is

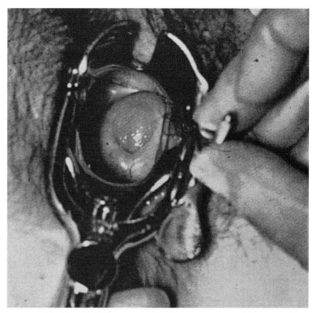

FIGURE 37–5 ▶ Chancre of the cervix. Failure to perform a speculum examination may allow early syphilis to go undiagnosed, resulting in advanced disease and exposure of additional sexual partners. (Reprinted from U.S. Public Health Service: Syphilis: A Synopsis. Washington, DC, U.S. Government Printing Office, 1967, p 50.)

rash—cutaneous or mucosal—and almost any rash type may occur. Evidence of hepatitis is found in 10% of patients,[89] but renal involvement is rare.[70] The earliest form of neurosyphilis, meningitis, is seen during this same time interval, and may occur independent of episodes of secondary syphilis; these patients present with severe headache, stiff neck, nausea, vomiting, and cranial nerve involvement (hearing loss, facial weakness, or visual disturbance). Anterior uveitis representing iritis, retinitis, or optic neuritis may also be seen with syphilitic meningitis.[90]

The rash of secondary syphilis is usually symmetric and dry. Papulosquamous (flaking nodular) lesions are the most common (Fig. 37–6). Macular and maculopapular lesions may have a copper hue in light-skinned people. Palms and soles are not always involved, but when they are the diagnosis of syphilis becomes much more likely (Fig. 37–7). Follicular lesions are the only pruritic variant of the rash. Widespread pustular lesions resembling varicella may occur. Arciform lesions of the scalp, usually of the occiput, produce the patchy or "moth-eaten" alopecia of syphilis, and loss of the distal one third of the eyebrows is common. Annular syphilids bear a resemblance to the chancre without ulceration, and are commonly found on the face. Condylomata lata are moist red to gray placques occurring in intertrigenous areas, most commonly the vulva (Figure 37–8). Mucous patches are rather bland foci of epithelial loss on mucosal surfaces (Fig. 37–9). Although viable *T. pallidum* are present in all of these lesions, the latter two contain the highest concentrations.

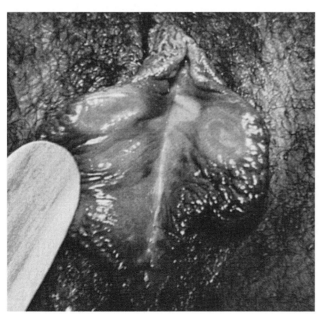

FIGURE 37–4 ▶ Multiple chancres of the vulva. (Reprinted from U.S. Public Health Service: Syphilis: A Synopsis. Washington, DC, U.S. Government Printing Office, 1967, p 47.)

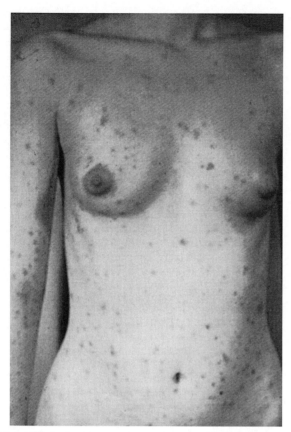

FIGURE 37-6 ▶ The most common rash of secondary syphilis, the papulosquamous. (Reprinted from U.S. Public Health Service: Syphilis: A Synopsis. Washington, DC, U.S. Government Printing Office, 1967, p 58.)

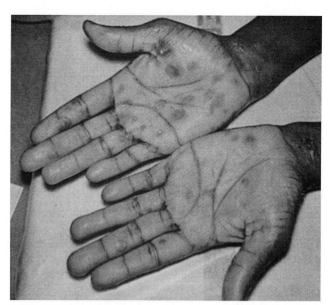

FIGURE 37-7 ▶ A macular rash of secondary syphilis involving the palms. (Reprinted from U.S. Public Health Service: Syphilis: A Synopsis. Washington, DC, U.S. Government Printing Office, 1967, p 39.)

Syphilitic hepatitis presents with hepatomegaly and a disproportionate elevation of alkaline phosphatase, usually without hyperbilirubinemia.[91] The classic triad of nephrotic syndrome (proteinura, hypoalbuminemia, and edema) marks syphilitic renal disease. When the rash is subtle and hepatitis and proteinuria are identified, diagnosis of syphilis is often delayed as evaluation for connective tissue disease, drug reaction, and lymphoma is pursued.[66]

All lesions of secondary syphilis heal without treatment in 2 to 10 weeks. The skin lesions may leave hyperpigmentation or hypopigmentation. Recurrences of clinical secondary syphilis are seen in approximately 25% of patients, usually in the first year of infection, but in some cases for up to 5 years.[92] Lesions that can transmit infection (those of the mouth and anogenital regions) are present in 85% of episodes of secondary syphilis.[92] The differential diagnosis is almost unlimited, including any disease with cutaneous, hepatic, renal, or neurologic manifestations.

Most of what is known about late syphilis is the product of two studies, which complement each other. The Oslo Study consists of a population with primary and secondary syphilis accrued between 1890 and 1910 by Boeck, who withheld the mercurial treatment of the

day because of his sustainable belief that its toxicities exceeded benefits in this setting. A total of 1,978 patients were included, but women were over-represented, so the morbidity for the population is skewed downward because women fared better with the disease. From 1949 to 1951, Gjestland studied this group, obtaining follow-up information on over 80% of the 1,404 original subjects who were permanent Oslo residents, including examining the survivors. Gjestland's

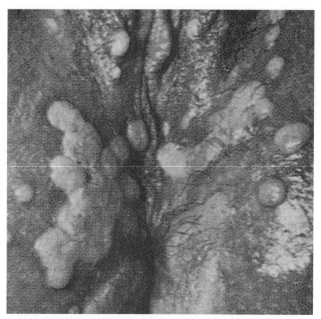

FIGURE 37-8 ▶ Condylomata lata, the lesion of syphilis containing the densest concentration of spirochetes. (Reprinted from U.S. Public Health Service: Syphilis: A Synopsis. Washington, DC, U.S. Government Printing Office, 1967, p 64.)

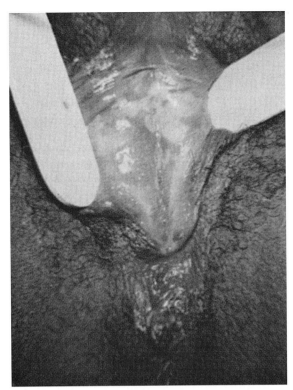

FIGURE 37-9 ▶ Mucous patches of the vaginal vestibule. These relatively subtle, painless lesions are infectious. (Reprinted from U.S. Public Health Service: Syphilis: A Synopsis. Washington, DC, U.S. Government Printing Office, 1967, p 65.)

report[74] is our most valuable source of information on the clinical course of untreated syphilis. The Rosahn Study[93] examined the role of syphilis in almost 4,000 consecutive autopsies at Yale University from 1917 to 1941, providing valuable information about subclinical events in late syphilis. A third study, the Tuskegee Study, enrolled 412 seropositive black men from Macon County, Alabama who were not treated and were compared with 204 matched control subjects. A final report of the study was never written, and little more than frequency of death from any cause can be gleaned from it.[94]

Approximately 70% of people with untreated syphilis live to an apparently healthy old age, 30% acquire symptomatic lesions of late syphilis, and 80% die from a cause other than syphilis. Death from syphilis occurs twice as often in men as women. However, autopsy reveals that 51% of patients with syphilis have anatomic lesions of syphilis at the time of death. Thus, only 40% of lesions of late (tertiary) syphilis cause the death of the patient, and approximately 40% of these lesions are asymptomatic. The three traditional syndromes of tertiary syphilis are late benign, cardiovascular, and neurosyphilis. No manifestation of tertiary syphilis protects against development of another; in fact, 10% to 15% of patients with one of the three syndromes of tertiary syphilis also have another.[77]

Late benign syphilis is defined as the presence of

gummas. The gumma represents a hypersensitivity reaction. It is the most common manifestation of tertiary syphilis, occurring in approximately 15% of untreated syphilitic patients, and the only one that occurs more frequently in women than men. Gjestland[74] found that 70% of gummas involved the skin, 10% bone, and 10% mucosa. Kampmeier's U.S. series[95] from roughly the same time suggests that the skin and skeletal system were involved with an equal frequency of approximately 30%, and the upper respiratory tract and oral mucosa were each involved approximately 10% of the time. Gummas can be found in essentially any body tissue, and are destructive lesions. Thus, particularly when they occur in the brain, heart, liver (where they can be fatal), or eye, the term late "benign" syphilis seems inept.

In the skin, gummas present as uninflamed nodular lesions of 1 to 5 mm diameter that are often multiple and aranged in an arciform pattern (Fig. 37–10). Although they may heal at this stage, more often the overlying skin breaks down and an expanding ulcerative lesion (Fig. 37–11) develops that heals after months or years with an atrophic scar. Skeletal gummas are most often seen in the long bones and skull, and present with bone pain, tenderness, stiffness, and swelling of local soft tissues. Radiographic changes include periostitis, osteitis, and destructive osteomyelitis. In the upper respiratory tract gummas appear as chronic destructive lesions of the nose, palate, pharynx, or larynx, often with perforation.

Cardiovascular syphilis presents with signs and symptoms of aortic regurgitation, and a saccular aneurysm of the ascending aorta is diagnostic of the disease. These aneurysms erode through bone, and have been reported to rupture through the skin. Findings of coronary hypoperfusion are less common. Cardiovascular disease develops in 10% of untreated syphilitic patients overall, in 15% of men and 8% of women. It is diagnosed four times more often at autopsy than in life,

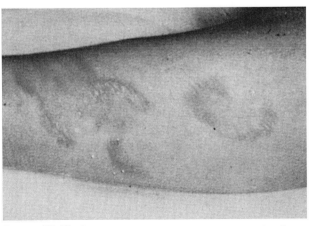

FIGURE 37-10 ▶ Early gummas of the forearm. (Reprinted from U.S. Public Health Service: Syphilis: A Synopsis. Washington, DC, U.S. Government Printing Office, 1967, p 83.)

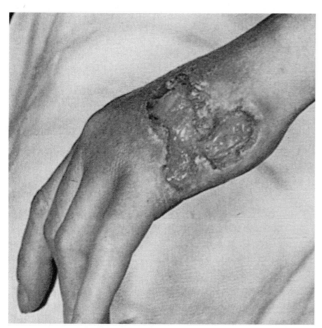

FIGURE 37-11 ▶ An advanced gumma of the hand. (Reprinted from U.S. Public Health Service: Syphilis: A Synopsis. Washington, DC, U.S. Government Printing Office, 1967, p 84.)

suggesting that it is a relatively slow process with a long preclinical course.

Neurosyphilis most commonly exists as asymptomatic disease. Its earliest form of expression, as discussed previously, is meningitis. The second form to appear is meningovascular syphilis, at 1 to 10 years (most often 4 to 7 years) after infection. These patients present with otherwise typical thrombotic cerebrovascular accidents, transient ischemic attacks, or stroke. Meningitis and meningovascular syphilis are reversible diseases. Parenchymatous neurosyphilis (general paresis and tabes dorsalis) is associated with permanent neurologic injury.[73] General paresis appears any time after 5 years of infection with T. pallidum (peak, 10 to 15 years), and presents with myriad symptoms representing diffuse brain deterioration. Progressive dementia from subtle personality change to frank pychosis is the hallmark, and focal neurologic lesions may accompany it. Tabes dorsalis may develop any time after 10 years of syphilis, most often after 20 years, and presents as sensory ataxia (loss of proprioception in the lower extremities, producing the high-stepping, foot-slapping gait), lightning pains, autonomic dysfunction, and optic atrophy. Symptomatic neurosyphilis affects 7% of untreated patients, 10% of men and 5% of women; parenchymatous disease rarely develops in those acquiring syphilis after 40 years of age because of its slow evolution.

Congenital syphilis is largely a function of the management of the gravid woman, and is therefore appropriate for discussion here. Series from Detroit[20, 22] and Miami[9] have modernized the traditional understanding of congenital syphilis. As described earlier, the risk to the fetus is inversely proportional to the duration of maternal syphilis (i.e., directly proportional to the probability of maternal spirochetemia). Unfortunately, as in the distinction between early and late latent syphilis, the practical application of this knowledge is difficult, as was demonstrated in the Detroit series, where 142 of 148 (96%) syphilitic pregnant women presented with asymptomatic disease of unknown duration.[22] Further, all infants born to seropositive mothers are seropositive at birth, and many infants with congenital syphilis have no clinical, laboratory, or radiographic abnormalities. It is therefore not surprising that there is considerable variation in the reported frequency of congenital syphilis in the fetuses of untreated, infected mothers. Older studies suggest that untreated pregnant women with early syphilis infect 70% to 100% of their fetuses, and up to one third of these are stillborn as a result.[57, 96–99] Fetal infection frequency is presented as 30% in a 1986 Centers for Disease Control (CDC) publication,[100] 68% in the 1986 to 1988 Miami epidemic,[9] 12% in a Chicago series from 1976 to 1982,[101] and 22% in the initial report of the Detroit series from 1990.[22] However, in the practical sense these figures are now moot because the CDC now defines probable congenital syphilis in any infant born to a mother with untreated or inadequately treated syphilis at delivery.[102] This strategy ensures treatment of all infants at risk.

Fetal death is the most common outcome of congenital syphilis, and it may occur during any trimester, including the first. Early spontaneous abortion associated with syphilitic endometritis (a lymphoplasmacytic deciduitis with spirochetes identified by silver stain) has been described.[103] The traditional figure for frequency of fetal death as a result of congenital syphilis is 40%.[104] In the Miami series,[9] 34% were stillborn, in the final report of the Detroit series, 14%,[20] and in a series from Mozambique in 1990 to 1991, stillbirth was 5.3 times more common in seropositive pregnancies.[105] It seems clear that high serologic titer in the mother enhances the probability of fetal death.[20, 105]

Among liveborn infants, low birth weight, premature rupture of membranes, preterm labor, and preterm birth (which occurred with a frequency of 28% in the Detroit patients) are more common in syphilitic pregnancies.[9, 20] As indicated earlier, most infected liveborn infants appear normal in all respects except for a positive serology. A few have skin lesions (usually vesicular), hepatosplenomegaly, osteochondritis, and hemopurulent coryza.[78, 106] Nephrotic syndrome also occurs in approximately 15% of infants with congenital syphilis.[107] In some, these lesions of early congenital syphilis develop later, and by definition all occur within the first 2 years. These traditional understandings of findings in congenital syphilis were reconfirmed in the Detroit series. Among 97 liveborn infants with probable congenital syphilis, 3 showed clinical findings of early congenital syphilis, 6 had only radiographic boney changes, and in 11 a reactive CSF Venereal Disease Research Laboratory test (VDRL) was documented.[22] If not treated, approximately 60% of congenital syphilitic children persist with latent disease beyond the age of 2 years, and eventually experience lesions of late congenital syphilis. These include Hutchinson's teeth (notched incisors), mulberry molars, neurosyphilis (most often general paresis), gross bone changes (sabre shins, frontal bossing, palatal perforation), and cutaneous lesions (most often wrinkling at the corners of the mouth, called *rhagades*). Cardiovascular syphilis is rare. The triad of Clutton's joints (painless hydroarthrosis), interstital keratitis, and eighth nerve deafness tends to occur near puberty among children with late congenital syphilis; they probably represent (like gummas) a hypersensitivity reaction because they respond better to cortiocosteroid therapy than to penicillin.[78]

A number of reports involving small numbers of patients during the 1990s suggested that manifestations of syphilis are different (usually enhanced) in human immunodeficiency virus (HIV)-infected patients.[56, 108–119] The issue most frequently raised was that of earlier-onset CNS and eye involvement. However, CNS and eye disease are well known to occur early in HIV-negative syphilitic patients.[58, 120–125] The prevailing opinion is that HIV infection does not significantly affect manifestations of syphilis in most patients.

Finally, it is appropriate briefly to discuss the clinical manifestations of the nonvenereal treponematoses for purposes of differentiation. Pinta *(T. carateum)* begins as an erythematous papule that evolves into a psoriaform plaque, followed by a diffuse rash of multiple similar lesions characterized by marked skin color variations from white to red, blue, brown, or black. Only the skin is involved. Yaws *(T. pallidum* subsp. *pertenue)* begins with a "mother yaw," a papule that evolves into a papillomatous plaque that ulcerates but eventually heals. Months later, a widespread frambesiform (a term specifically reserved for yaws lesions derived from the French *framboise,* "raspberry") rash erupts. Malaise, lymphadenopathy, and bone pain are common cofindings. Over time, destructive lesions of skin and musculoskeletal structures develop. Bejel or endemic syphilis *(T. pallidum* subsp. *endemicum)* is a neonatally acquired disease, usually with an oral primary lesion that goes unnoticed. Over the following years, a syndrome reminiscent of muted congenital syphilis develops with similar lesions of skin, bone, and soft tissue. However, CNS and cardiovascular involvement are rare.

DIAGNOSIS

Sir William Osler's oft-quoted paraphrase, "He who knows syphilis knows medicine," is daunting in its own right.[126] He offered this thought in the late 1890s, before over 200 serologic tests for syphilis had been devised, before HIV disease, and before the complexities of managing syphilis in pregnancy were known. Understanding the diagnosis of syphilis today is more challenging than ever, and efforts to simplify it cause errors. One straightforward principle, however, will serve the practitioner well: in cases of possible syphilis at any stage, the diagnosis requires a *correlation* of physical, serologic, and other findings—no single finding or result is ever enough to rule in or out a diagnosis of syphilis at a given stage.

Inability to grow and isolate *T. pallidum* in artificial media has always been a central obstacle to the diagnosis of syphilis. Fortunately, a number of small animals are susceptible to infection by the organism. The RIT is the oldest technique for identifying *T. pallidum,* having first been described in 1907,[127] and it remains the most sensitive test, with 23 or more organisms producing a positive result in 100% of the tests[43] and 1 or 2 spirochetes in 47%.[38] Unfortunately, it requires both serologic testing and examination of at least two rabbits inoculated serially, so that almost 3 months is required to establish a negative result.[128, 129] Nonetheless, it remains the gold standard.

Dark-field microscopy, which uses reflected light to make this very narrow organism visible, provides for definitive identification of *T. pallidum.* A fresh specimen from a moist lesion (chancre, mucous patch, condyloma latum) is required, and oral and perioral lesions cannot be used because commensal spirochetes in the mouth, most often *T. refringens,* cannot be differentiated from *T. pallidum.* Genital commensal spirochetes can be distinguished by an experienced observer. An aspirate of an affected regional lymph node may also be used. Neither specimen procurement nor dark-field interpretation should be undertaken by the untrained. Details of the procedure may be found in *A Manual of Tests for Syphilis,*[130] an excellent recent review by Larsen and colleagues,[131] and in the original description by Coles in 1909.[132] Briefly, the specimen is obtained by wiping debris from the surface of the lesion and obtaining blood-free fluid from deep in the lesion by squeezing or gentle blunt aspiration against the surface of the lesion. Obtaining a good sample from a superinfected lesion is difficult. A dedicated microscope with single- or double-reflecting dark-field condenser, 40× and 100× objectives, and a funnel stop must be available. The organism is identified by its back-and-forth corkscrew movement and a characteristic spring-like snapping back to linear conformation after bending. It is 10 to 12 μm long, very thin, and has 10 to 12 tight coils. Commensal genital spirochetes are thicker, loosely coiled, and display a shallower wave form.[131] Under optimal conditions (i.e., experienced participants), dark-field examination has a sensitivity of 80%.[133, 134]

Because optimal conditions for dark-field examination are less and less commonly available, this test is being replaced by direct fluorescent antibody—*T. pallidum* staining (DFA-TP). Globulins specific for *T. pallidum* and its subspecies, labeled with fluorescein isothiocyanate (FITC), are applied to the specimen, which is then examined for specific fluorescence. The only disadvantage of this test is the need for a fluorescent microscope, and it has many advantages. Because fresh specimens with live spirochetes are not required, the DFA-TP may be performed at any time after the specimen is obtained, after transport, and at distant locations. Extensive training in interpretation is not required. The stain may be used not only in lesion exudates (which must be obtained using the same technique as for dark-field microscopy),[135-137] but body fluids[138, 139] and tissues.[140, 141] Use of DFA-TP in tissue sections makes the organisms much easier to identify than with silver stains.[136, 140] When an adequate specimen is available (deep tissue fluid from a lesion containing spirochetes), the sensitivity of the DFA-TP is thought to approach 100%.[133, 135] Many experts believe the DFA-TP is currently underused.[142, 143]

Serologic testing for diagnosis of syphilis was introduced by Wasserman and co-workers[144] in 1906. Pangborn[145] in 1941 isolated the active antigen in the reaction, cardiolipin, from beef heart, enhanced its reactivity by addition of cholesterol and lecithin in alcohol, and thus produced the standardized reagent that forms the basis of all nontreponemal tests for syphilis today. Cardiolipin is an acid diphospholipid found on the inner wall of mitochondria in all mammalian cells, and it comprises approximately 10% of the lipid content of *T. pallidum*. People with syphilis, and unfortunately those with a substantial number of other medical conditions, raise a heterogeneous group of antibodies, both IgM and IgG, against cardiolipin, referred to in aggregate as *reagin*. The bulk of reagin in syphilitic patients is thought to arise against autologous cardiolipin liberated by tissue injury, rather than against treponemal cardiolipin. Reagin is the substance tested for in all nontreponemal tests, and all detect both its IgM and IgG moieties. Of the over 200 such tests devised to date, there are 4 currently accepted standard tests: VDRL, USR (unheated serum reagin), RPR (rapid plasma reagin), and TRUST (toluidine red unheated serum test). The accuracy of these four is equivalent, the differences being limited to convenience for individual settings. All four are based on observation of flocculation of immune complex lattices. The reader is referred to Larsen and colleagues[131] for detailed discussion of the mechanisms and details of these tests. Only the VDRL is approved for testing CSF for the presence of reagin. It is of extreme clinical importance to understand not only the nonspecificity of these tests (discussed in detail later), but their insensitivity in most stages of syphilis.

False-negative rates of 25% to 30% in primary syphilis, 30% in untreated latent syphilis, and 30% in late syphilis are well documented, but seem to be subject to passive dismissal in clinical practice.[146]

The treponemal tests, as the name implies, are tests for specific antibody to *T. pallidum*, and are therefore entirely independent of the nontreponemal tests. It is not known how many treponemal antigens these antibodies arise against, but the 47-kD outer membrane protein is thought to be immunodominant. The current standard tests are the fluorescent treponemal antibody—absorbed (FTA-Abs), the FTA-Abs double stain, and the microhemagglutination—*T. pallidum* (MHA-TP). All use *T. pallidum* as the antigen, and all, once positive, remain so indefinitely even after curative therapy in 85% of cases.[147] In the FTA-Abs, the specimen is first diluted 1:5 in sorbent, an extract of the commensal Reiter treponeme, to absorb group-specific antibody raised against nonpathogens; if this step is omitted, over 25% of normal people will have reactive serum.[148] The specimen is then added to a slide to which *T. pallidum* has been fixed, FITC-labeled antihuman globulin is added, and the slide is examined for fluorescing treponemes. Dark-field examination is necessary to confirm the presence of organisms on the slide, a step eliminated by the second stain in the double-stain test. The test is reported as reactive, reactive minimal, nonreactive, or atypical fluorescence. Reactive minimal samples should be retested, serially over time if they are initially unchanged. Atypical fluorescence raises the possibility of connective tissue disease, as discussed later. The MHA-TP begins with an absorption step similar to the FTA-Abs, after which the sample is added to a microwell with sheep erythrocytes coated with sonicated *T. pallidum*. If specific antibody is present, a lattice forms and the erythrocytes are dispersed in a smooth mat on the bottom of the well; if not, a tight button forms. Quantitation by dilution is possible with this test, but provides no data that correlate with clinical behavior of the disease.[149, 150] The MHA-TP is slightly more specific at 99% than the FTA-Abs at 97%. The sensitivity of both is approximately 82% in primary disease and 95% in late syphilis,[151] substantially better than the nontreponemal tests. Nontreponemal tests are used for screening because of the considerably greater resources consumed by the treponemal tests.[76, 152]

All serologic tests for syphilis leave open the possibility for laboratory error. In the nontreponemal tests, the interpreter must determine whether small, medium, large, or no clumps of flocculation are present, and in the FTA-Abs whether fluorescence is minimal, absent, or atypical. This inherent subjectivity forms the basis for the insignificance of a one-tube (twofold) difference in nontreponemal quantitative test results—only a fourfold or greater difference is meaningful. Further, quantitative results are not transferable from one nontreponemal test to another. In the nontreponemal tests, temperature of the specimen and the laboratory is important, with a particular impact on remote field laboratories; a temperature of less than 23°C inhibits reactivity, whereas one more than 29°C enhances it.[131] It has been suggested that one in four false-positive tests result from laboratory error.[153]

The *prozone effect* refers to the immunologic phenomenon wherein a great excess of antibody prevents reactivity. False-negative nontreponemal tests may be seen because of the prozone effect when reagin levels are very high. This circumstance occurs in approximately 2% of patients with secondary syphilis[154] because this stage is associated with the highest reagin levels. Only one prozone-effect specimen was found among 4,328 consecutive screening samples from asymptomatic subjects, confirming its rarity outside of secondary-stage disease.[155] However, Berkowitz and colleagues[156] reported four cases of false-negative nontreponemal tests resulting from the prozone effect in *asymptomatic* pregnant women. All four gave birth to infants with congenital syphilis, raising concern that pregnancy independently carries the risk of a prozone reaction in syphilitic women. All prozone reactions are overridden by testing a 1:16 dilution of the specimen, which is recommended in people with clinical disease suggestive of secondary syphilis or fetal changes suggestive of congenital syphilis when the undiluted specimen is negative.

A biologic false-positive (BFP) result is defined by repeated reactivity in a nontreponemal test with negative treponemal test results in a patient with no evidence of syphilis. The titer is usually 1:8 or less. The various causes of BFP reactions are listed in Table 37–1. The overall prevalence of BFP reactors is 0.3% to 1.0%,[30] although in a 1989 series from Jamaica, 27% of positive nontreponemal test results were BFP reactions, 31% among pregnant women.[157] The duration of a BFP reaction is important, and Moore and Mohr[158] classified them into acute (<6 months) and chronic (>6 months) groups. Acute BFP reactions usually are benign and result from acute infections of bacterial, viral, and protozoal etiologies, vaccination, and pregnancy. They occur in children as well as adults.[159] Chronic reactions are more ominous, suggesting autoimmune disease, diseases associated with atypical antibody production, and malignancy; however, benign/reversible causes of chronic BFP reactions do occur and include aging, intravenous drug use, and possibly leprosy. BFP associated with intravenous drug use is the situation in which higher titers are most commonly found—over 10% are reactive at greater than 1:8 dilution,[160] and in this population 10% to 95% are BFP reactors.[161] Systemic lupus erythematosus (SLE) is particularly associated with BFP reactivity, with 12% or more of patients with SLE exhibiting this finding[157, 162]; up to 80% of positive nontreponemal

test results in patients with SLE represent BFP.[157] Among Finnish patients followed with chronic BFP, development of SLE occurred 1,000-fold more often than in the general population (4 of 59 vs. 7 of 100,000).[163] The presence of lupus anticoagulant in patients with SLE raises the probability of BFP reaction.[164] Autoimmune hemolytic anemia and idiopathic thrombocytopenic purpura may be preceded by many years by BFP reactions.[165] Among women with chronic BFP reactions, an important hazard is penicillin hypersensitivity—up to 20% may have an anaphylactic reaction to penicillin.[30] The significance of the acute BFP reaction in pregnancy is not clear. Although one study[166] found no associated morbidity, another[167] found a higher frequency of obstetric complications among these patients. The management of patients with chronic BFP reactions should include long-term follow-up with testing for SLE, discoid and drug-induced lupus, other rheumatologic disease, hypergammaglobulinemia, Hashimoto's thyroiditis, HIV infection, autoimmune hemolytic anemia, and idiopathic thrombocytopenic purpura. A final consideration in the patient with BFP reaction recalls the complexities of the diagnosis of syphilis. These patients may have syphilis, most likely asymptomatic late syphilis, with false-negative treponemal tests. Therefore, especially in the absence of another explanation, they should undergo evaluation of CSF, chest radiography or echocardiography with attention to the aortic root, and serum referral to a laboratory capable of Western blot testing for antitreponemal antibodies.

False-positive treponemal tests occur in approximately 1% of the population,[168, 169] although one study put the frequency at 0.07%.[170] This result may be due to inadequate absorption of cross-reacting antibodies in patients with Lyme disease or leptospirosis.[171, 172] Repeating the absorption step may resolve some of these cases. The most common cause of false-positive treponemal tests are the lupus syndromes—systemic, discoid, and drug-induced—when serum of these patients is tested in the FTA-Abs assay.[173, 174] Strobel and Kraus[175] have shown that anti-DNA antibodies in these patients (IgG, IgA, and IgM) bind to treponemal DNA at breaks in the outer membrane of the organisms used in the assay. This mechanism explains the beaded-pattern (atypical) fluorescence usually seen in this situation. However, smooth fluorescence may also be seen.[176] With absorption in calf thymus DNA, these specimens become nonreactive if treponemal antibody is absent.[174] The frequency of false-positive treponemal tests in patients with lupus syndromes is unclear; Monson[176] found only 1 case among 54 patients with lupus, whereas Kraus and associates[174] found a high frequency. Alcoholic cirrhosis is associated with false-positive reactivity, with Mackay and colleagues[177] reporting a case, and 6.8% of the population studied by Meyer-Rhon[178] so affected. Studies of patients with leprosy

TABLE 37-1 ▶ POTENTIAL CAUSES OF BIOLOGIC FALSE-POSITIVE RESULTS IN SYPHILIS SEROLOGY

	Acute BFP Reactions	Chronic BFP Reactions
Physiologic	Pregnancy	Advanced age
		Multiple blood transfusions
Infections	Varicella	HIV
	Vaccinia	Tropical spastic paraparesis
	Measles	Leprosy[a]
	Mumps	Tuberculosis[a]
	Infectious mononucleosis	Malaria[a]
	Herpes simplex	Lymphogranuloma venereum[a]
	Viral hepatitis	Trypanosomiasis[a]
	HIV seroconversion illness	Kala-azar[a]
	Cytomegalovirus	
	Pneumococcal pneumonia	
	Mycoplasma pneumonia	
	Chancroid	
	Lymphogranuloma venereum	
	Psittacosis	
	Bacterial endocarditis	
	Scarlet fever	
	Rickettsial infections	
	Toxoplasmosis	
	Lyme disease	
	Leptospirosis	
	Relapsing fever	
	Rat-bite fever	
Vaccinations	Smallpox	
	Typhoid	
	Yellow fever	
Autoimmune disease		Systemic lupus erythematosus
		Discoid lupus
		Drug-induced lupus
		Autoimmune hemolytic anemia
		Polyarteritis nodosa
		Rheumatoid arthritis
		Sjögren's syndrome
		Hashimoto's thyroiditis
		Mixed connective tissue disease
		Primary biliary cirrhosis
		Chronic liver disease
		Idiopathic thrombocytopenic purpura
Other		Intravenous drug use
		Advanced malignancy
		Hypergammaglobulinemia
		Lymphoproliferative disease

[a]BFP reaction resolves with resolution of infection.
BFP = biologic false-positive; HIV = human immunodeficiency virus.
Data from Nandwani R, Evans DTP: Are you sure it's syphilis? A review of false positive serology. Int J STD AIDS 1995; 6:241; and Hook EW III, Marra CM: Acquired syphilis in adults. N Engl J Med 1992; 326:1062.

and positive treponemal tests have come from locales where nonvenereal treponematoses are endemic, and assessing their meaning is therefore infeasible.[179] Case reports of false-positive antitreponemal reactivity in lymphosarcoma, meningioma, rheumatoid arthritis, and autoimmune hemolytic anemia[177] have been published. Two studies have suggested that diabetic patients may display this phenomenon.[178, 180] A study correlating it with herpes genitalis has been refuted.[181] Pregnancy is probably a rare cause of false-positive treponemal tests. Buchanan and Haserick[182] reported a case, Meyer-Rhon[178] found 6.9% so affected in a population, and Manikowska-Lesinska and Zajac[183] found 4 cases among 2,000 pregnant women. The presence of heterophile antibody (as in infectious

mononucleosis) may cause false-positive MHA-TP test results.

Several newer serologic tests for syphilis not yet widely used or in development deserve comment. Western blot techniques for identification of specific antitreponemal antibody that use whole-cell *T. pallidum* as the antigen appear to be impervious to the known factors (group, atypical, and DNA antibodies) that cause false-positive results in the traditional treponemal tests, and have a reported sensitivity of 92% and specificity of 100%.[184] Captia syphilis tests are automated enzyme-linked immunosorbent assay tests designed to detect specific anti-treponemal antibody, with tests for both IgG and IgM under investigation. They use a 1:20 dilution of sample rather than absorption to eliminate group antibody, making them particularly susceptible to false-positive results in patients with Lyme disease and leptospirosis.[185] The IgG test, Captia syphilis G, has been compared with the RPR as a screening test in both obstetric and general populations, revealing a slightly better sensitivity and specificity than the RPR.[186] Its sensitivity in primary syphilis is also comparable with that of the other treponemal tests, at approximately 82%.[187] This may prove to be the first treponemal test whose cost provides for use as a screening test. Polymerase chain reaction (PCR) techniques may provide for actual identification of *T. pallidum*. The exceptional genetic stability of the organism should favor success of this approach. Multiplex PCR testing of genital ulcer samples during the New Orleans chancroid outbreak of 1992 to 1993 showed PCR to have a sensitivity superior to those of dark-field examination and nontreponemal serology.[188] When PCR results were compared with the RIT in neonatal amniotic fluid, serum, and CSF, PCR showed a sensitivity of 78% and specificity of 100%—amniotic fluid samples produced the best sensitivity.[189] Cloned specific *T. pallidum* antigens, which would eliminate test complications resulting from group antibodies, are in development.

Detection of antitreponemal IgM has a special allure. This capability would provide for diagnosis of congenital syphilis in asymptomatic neonates, and differentiation among old, new, and reinfection. The fetus becomes capable of synthesizing IgM at 3 months' gestation. Competitive binding by high-titer IgG and IgA makes a straightforward IgM adaptation of the FTA-Abs insensitive. Using only the 19S (IgM) fraction of serum overcomes this problem. Unfortunately, the 19S-IgM–FTA-Abs remains plagued by inadequate sensitivity (approximately 73%), although its specificity is good,[190] making its most appropriate use a confirmatory test. Use of an IgM-specific conjugate in the Western blot assay has been evaluated in the diagnosis of congenital syphilis, and its specificity and sensitivity appear to be at least 90% and 83%, respectively. The Captia format has also been adapted to an IgM assay. Although the sensitivity of Captia syphilis M seems to be superior to that of the 19S-IgM–FTA-Abs test, it at best equals that of the Western blot IgM, and is inferior to it in cases of late congenital syphilis.[190] A lingering and real concern about the use of tests that identify IgM to make the diagnosis of congenital syphilis is the confirmed finding that the fetus produces homologous IgM in response to exposure to maternal IgG, in the *absence* of exposure to the antigen itself.[131]

Accurate clinical response to primary syphilis has three key elements. The first is that 50% of chancres have an atypical appearance, usually due to superinfection. Therefore, almost any skin lesion, or lesions of apposed surfaces, particularly if open, may represent a chancre. The second is that the nontreponemal sero-logic tests used as the first-line laboratory assessment for syphilis have a false-negative rate of 30% in this setting, and that figure for the FTA-Abs and MHA-TP is 20% and 36%, respectively. Therefore, nonreactive serologies do not rule out primary syphilis. Third, direct examination for spirochetes in a specimen from the lesion is always necessary. Therefore, a lesion raising suspicion of chancre based on its appearance and the epidemiology of the patient should be sampled by obtaining a clean specimen of deep exudate, biopsy, or regional lymph node aspirate, and submitting that for dark-field evaluation, DFA-TP staining, or other appropriate stains to identify the organism. The CDC defines a confirmed diagnosis of primary syphilis as a compatible lesion with *T. pallidum* demonstrated in a clinical specimen (note that serology is not mentioned in this definition).[102] A probable diagnosis is a clinically compatible case with ulcerative skin lesion(s) and a reactive serologic test; in patients with prior positive nontreponemal serology, a fourfold rise in titer is required.

In secondary syphilis, the presence of a skin rash is the usual feature that raises suspicion. However, the rash may be very subtle, and particularly in patients presenting with hepatitis, nephritis, or diffuse lymphadenopathy as the dominant findings, the rash may be overlooked and consideration of syphilis delayed. For practical purposes, the nontreponemal and treponemal tests are always positive in secondary syphilis. A 1:16 dilution of the serum should be ordered in cases clinically suggestive of secondary syphilis where the undiluted serum is nonreactive, to override the prozone effect. The diagnosis of secondary syphilis is effectively ruled out if an undiluted and 1:16 dilution of serum are negative in a nontreponemal test. Biopsy of the skin rash or procurement of exudate from moist lesions or lymph node aspirates for examination for spirochetes should be undertaken in all suspect cases. A skin rash with positive serologies does not make a definitive diagnosis of syphilis because laboratory error, BFP reactions, and prior syphilis may cause false-positive serologies. A confirmed diagnosis of secondary syphilis requires a clinically compatible presentation with demonstration of *T. pallidum* in a lesion sample.[102] A probable diagnosis consists of a clinically compatible case with nontreponemal titer positive at 1:4 or greater dilution; although not included in this CDC definition, a positive treponemal serology to rule out BFP would seem prudent.

In latent syphilis, the only manifestation of disease is reactive serology, and therefore this diagnosis cannot be confirmed. Probable latent syphilis is defined as the presence of reactive nontreponemal and treponemal tests in a person with no prior history of treatment for syphilis, or a fourfold rise in nontreponemal titer when syphilis has been previously treated. Early latent syphilis may be assumed by documentation that the nontreponemal titer rise occurred during the previous 12 months, by a clinical syndrome consistent with early syphilis during that interval, or by documentation of exposure to an infectious person during that interval. Serologic titers run higher in early latent disease than later, but this fact has inadequate consistency to provide for distinction between early and late latency. Late latent syphilis consists of absence of evidence that the disease was acquired during the last 12 months (i.e., failure to satisfy one of the three requirements for diagnosis of early latency). Latent syphilis of unknown duration is defined by absence of criteria for early latent infection in a person 13 to 35 years of age with a nontreponemal titer positive at 1:32 or greater dilution. Those with late and unknown-duration latent syphilis should undergo chest radiography and complete ophthalmologic examination to rule out active tertiary disease. Women in this group should have speculum examination to rule out internal lesions. Some experts advise CSF examination for all of these patients, but it is clearly needed in those with neurologic or ocular findings, other evidence of tertiary syphilis, treatment failure, and HIV infection.[191]

In tertiary (late active) syphilis, the nontreponemal tests are falsely negative in one third of cases, perhaps more often in neurosyphilis.[93] Several authorities suggest that this is the one setting in which a treponemal test should be done when a nontreponemal test is nonreactive because the treponemal tests remain reliably positive in tertiary sphyilis.[76, 131] The diagnosis of cardiovascular syphilis is assumed in a person with a positive treponemal serology, dilatory changes of the proximal aorta on chest radiography or echocardiography, and absence of history of adequate treatment for late syphilis. Confirmation of this diagnosis usually is not possible except at autopsy. Gummatous (late benign) syphilis is diagnosed when characteristic lesions (with classic granulomatous changes on biopsy, if available) are found with a positive nontreponemal serology and absence of adequate treatment for late syphilis. Whenever possible, lesion biopsy should be submitted for specific stains for *T. pallidum*, but, because the organisms are usually scarce, confirmation of the diagnosis often is not possible.

Neurosyphilis is defined as abnormal CSF in a patient with a positive treponemal serology. Specifically, the CSF findings are a mononuclear cell count of more than 5/mL or protein greater than 40 mg/dL. The only serologic test appropriate for use with CSF is the VDRL. A reactive CSF-VDRL is considered confirmatory[102] only if other possible causes are ruled out, but its use requires caution. A certain diagnosis requires demonstration of the organism either in tissue or by rabbit inoculation with CSF. The CSF-VDRL should be done only when the serum treponemal test is positive (the yield is too low to justify the test otherwise). The sensitivity of the CSF-VDRL is low, from 10% to 60%,[72]

and therefore a negative result does not rule out neurosyphilis. However, its high specificity gives a positive result considerable value.[192] False-positive results from blood contamination appear not to be a problem if no grossly visible discoloration of the sample is present.[193] Application of the FTA-Abs to CSF specimens has been examined, and its specificity is poor.[194] However, many experts believe that a negative CSF-FTA-Abs rules out the diagnosis of neurosyphilis,[191] so high is its sensitivity. As noted earlier, asymptomatic neurosyphilis is common, found in 10% to 20% with primary, 30% to 70% with secondary, and 10% to 30% of patients with latent syphilis in classic studies. More recently, Lukehart and colleagues[129] reconfirmed these findings. Further, *T. pallidum* can be identified in CSF by the RIT in up to 30% of syphilitic patients with otherwise normal CSF.[51] It is apparent by the rarity of later symptomatic neurosyphilis in those treated appropriately for early syphilis that special treatment is not necessary for these asymptomatic cases. CSF should be examined in all retreatment candidates, all syphilitic patients with neurologic, ocular, or otic findings, and all children with syphilis.

In pregnancy, the issue of fetal infection compounds the complexity of diagnosis of syphilis. Maternal serology is the mainstay of management in this setting, with neonatal and umbilical cord sera positive in only 63% and 50%, respectively, of pregnancies complicated by syphilis.[195] All pregnant women should have a nontreponemal serology at the initial obstetric visit, and those at high risk should be retested at 28 weeks' gestation and again at delivery, because 3% or more of them will have seroconverted.[196] Nontreponemal titers tend to drift up during pregnancy, sometimes even after treatment. Reinfection, or inadequate treatment if administration of an appropriate regimen cannot be documented, thus becomes a concern. Retreatment is probably not necessary if treatment is known to be adequate, there has been no exposure to a partner with syphilis, the titer rise is less than fourfold, and there are no lesions of early syphilis.[131] Antepartum diagnosis of congenital syphilis has only recently been described. Wendel and associates[197] studied amniotic fluid of five fetuses later confirmed to have congenital syphilis and found dark-field examination to be positive in all five, silver stains in two of five, and DFA-TP in one of three. Hydrops in the fetus of a syphilitic woman is suspect for congenital infection, as are aberrations in amniotic fluid volume.

Necrotizing funisitis (the "barber-pole" umbilical cord) was thought to be accurate in the diagnosis of congenital syphilis by Fojaco and colleagues[198] in their first publication; later, they reported a sensitivity of only 54% for it, and others reported a specificity of approximately 10%. As described previously, placental pathologic processes are not adequately sensitive or specific for making clinical decisions. Similar placental changes may be seen with other bacterial infections, including *Campylobacter* species, *Escherichia coli*, *Proteus* species, and staphylococci, and a normal placenta does not rule out the possibility of congenital syphilis.[82] Further, the interpretation of neonatal serology is fraught with hazards. Not only do almost all infants born to syphilitic women have positive serologies, but the IgG causing BFP reactions crosses the placenta as well and persists for 3 or more months.[30] Passively acquired antibody producing seroreactivity in the neonate persists for 12 to 18 months.[96] After effective antepartum treatment for both mother and fetus, Chang and co-workers[199] found that seronegativity in the nontreponemal test occurred at 6 months for 84% and 12 months for 100% of the neonates; reversion to negative in the treponemal test was also seen in 100% by 12 months. Comparing the titers of the mother and neonate is not useful. A lower neonatal titer does not rule out congenital syphilis, and infected infants have a higher titer than their mothers in 22%.[190] Moreover, infants with congenital syphilis may be seronegative during the first several weeks of life.[151, 200] Late congenital syphilis produces diagnostic difficulties as well, with dramatic fluctuation in nontreponemal test titers,[201] and disappointing accuracy of treponemal tests.[202] Often, changes of bone and teeth are most helpful in diagnosis of late congenital syphilis.

These difficulties in diagnosis of congenital syphilis are apparent in the CDC case definitions of this infection,[102] where emphasis is appropriately placed on ensuring treatment for those neonates at risk. A confirmed case is one in which the organism is demonstrated by dark-field microscopy or appropriate stains in a specimen from a lesion, placenta, umbilical cord, or autopsy material. However, probable cases (for which neonatal treatment is indicated) include those infants born to syphilitic mothers who received no treatment, nonpenicillin treatment, or penicillin treatment 30 days or less before delivery, regardless of signs in the infant. Other criteria for probable congenital syphilis include those with a reactive treponemal test and (1) evidence of congenital syphilis on examination or radiographs of long bones; (2) CSF with elevated cell count or protein, or positive CSF-VDRL; or (3) reactive 19S-IgM–FTA-Abs or Captia syphilis M test.

Human immunodeficiency virus infection has been thought to modify serologic test results for syphilis in some studies, and to have no effect in others.[203-208] Confirmation of an effect of HIV infection on the serologic tests for syphilis remains outstanding. For the present, however, the CDC has concluded that serologic results "can be interpreted in the usual manner" in coinfected patients.[191]

Differentiation of syphilis from the nonvenereal treponematoses is all but impossible in the asymptomatic patient, although in active disease presumptive distinctions can be made on the basis of clinical findings. Only the fact that the nonvenereal treponematoses are mostly childhood diseases of specific geographic regions provides a clue as to which clinical process is present. One scheme suggests that in a locale where one of the nonvenereal treponematoses is endemic, those who have a nontreponemal test titer positive at 1:8 or greater dilution be assigned a diagnosis of syphilis if an adult, and nonvenereal treponematosis if a child.[209] This scheme would have some practical utility assuming the absence of child sexual abuse and that all adults have known childhood serostatus.

All patients with syphilis should be tested for HIV infection, and retreatment candidates should be retested. Testing or presumptive treatment for gonorrhea and genital chlamydial infection is advised at the time of diagnosis. The Papanicolaou smear should be updated in women. Testing for hepatitis B and C should be considered, and vaccination against hepatitis B is strongly encouraged. Sexually transmissible disease counseling should be provided, as well as referral of appropriate personnel for assistance with drug abuse.

At least five major problem areas therefore remain in the diagnosis of syphilis:

1. An accurate method to determine which asymptomatic, seropositive infants born to syphilitic women have congenital syphilis is needed.
2. Current methods of diagnosis of neurosyphilis are inadequate, and the implications of spirochetes and other abnormalities in the CSF of patients with syphilis are poorly understood.
3. There is no rapid, affordable, on-site test to rule in or rule out a diagnosis of primary syphilis in a patient with a genital ulcer.
4. We have no reliable methods for distinguishing between relapsing infection, reinfection, persistent infection, and old infection—dependence on a fourfold titer rise in a test subject to false-positive results is inefficient.
5. We cannot differentiate among treponematoses that have very important differences in their implications.

TREATMENT

The treatment of syphilis has three goals: resolution of current manifestations (except in advanced cardiovascular and neurosyphilis, where permanent injury has already occurred), prevention of transmission (to intimate contacts and to the fetus, if present), and prevention of future progression of syphilis to more severe disease. Eradication of the organism would obviously be a goal if we had the means to determine it, but we do not. Assessing the efficacy of a treatment in the prevention of eventual progression of syphilis takes decades to accomplish, which is the primary reason for the enduring predominance of penicillin in syphilotherapy: it is the only drug with which we have long-term experience. The use of serology as a surrogate for eradication/control of the infection and protection against later severe manifestations of syphilis has limitations that were discussed earlier and that must be respected. Maximal treponemacidal activity of penicillin is reached at 0.1 µg/mL, and sustained serum levels exceeding 0.018 µg/mL for 7 to 10 days without an interruption of greater than 24 hours are adequate for resolution of early syphilis.[210] One intramuscular dose of 2.4 million units (MU) of benzathine penicillin G (BPG) produces penicillin levels above 0.018 µg/mL for almost 3 weeks.[210] Lesion samples reveal the appearance of damaged treponemes within 7 hours after administration of penicillin to the patient.[211] The antimicrobial activity of penicillin depends on active reproduction of the organism, which occurs in *T. pallidum* every 30 to 33 hours. However, some data suggest that its reproductive cycle is prolonged in older syphilitic lesions, so that longer courses of treatment are needed, and animal models have supported this concept.

Rolfs[212] has provided an excellent review of the activity of various agents in the treatment of syphilis. Drugs other than penicillin do have activity in the treatment of syphilis. Amoxicillin has efficacy against *T. pallidum*, although high doses appear to be necessary. Azithromycin showed activity in syphilitic rabbits. Infected humans with early disease given azithromycin 500 mg orally once daily or once every other day for 10 to 11 days seroreverted within 4 months in 90% of cases, with no apparent treatment failures.[213, 214] The related drug clarithromycin showed activity in a hamster model.[215] First-generation cephalosporins and ceftizoxime[216] have antitreponemal action. Ceftriaxone has been most studied among the cephalosporins and appears promising; optimal dosing is not established (although a single dose is known to be inadequate), it has been studied only in early syphilis, and of course its efficacy is preventing late sequelae of syphilis is unknown. Tetracycline and doxycycline are the only agents other than penicillin currently recommended for treatment of syphilis.[191] Their activity in early syphilis is documented, and fully reviewed by Rolfs.[212] However, only one study has compared tetracycline (at 3 g orally daily for 10 days) with penicillin, and the failure rate at 18 months for tetracycline was 13%, twice that of penicillin. Doxycycline has never been systematically studied in comparison with penicillin, but it appears to be on a par with tetracycline. In the past, erythromycin has been used to treat syphilis, but with a failure rate of 30% at 18 months (using a dose of 2 g orally daily for 10 days) in the only study comparing it with penicillin, it is no longer recommended. Further, an erythromycin-resistant strain of *T. pallidum* has been reported, and the drug crosses the placenta poorly. Spectinomycin is not active.

Presumptive treatment of exposed people remains a mainstay of syphilis control measures. Treatment regimens described later for early syphilis, preferably single-dose penicillin because it is believed to be 100% effective in this setting,[217, 218] should be used. Candidates for presumptive treatment after exposure include the following groups,[191] are based on the concept that index case individuals will have been infectious, or will have acquired syphilis from an as-yet untreated sexual partner, for 3 months plus duration of symptoms in primary syphilis, 6 months plus duration of symptoms in secondary syphilis, and for 1 year in early latent syphilis. Those who were exposed less than 90 days before diagnosis of the index case individual should be treated presumptively regardless of serostatus because they may or may not have seroconverted; those whose last exposure was more than 90 days before should all have seroconverted if infected, and need not be treated if seronegative (however, if follow-up is uncertain and negative serologic results are not in hand, these people should be treated presumptively while they are available). People exposed to a person with case-definition latent syphilis of unknown duration (titer positive at 1:32 or greater dilution and age 13 to 35 years) should be treated presumptively. Those chronically exposed to a person with late latent syphilis should be treated on the basis of results of clinical and serologic evaluation.

The preferred treatment for early syphilis (primary, secondary, and early latent) is a single dose of BPG 2.4 MU intramuscularly. Penicillin-allergic, nonpregnant women may instead receive doxycycline 100 mg twice daily orally for 2 weeks or tetracycline hydrochloride 500 mg four times daily orally for 2 weeks, regimens that have lesser efficacy than penicillin. Ceftriaxone 1 g intramuscularly daily for 8 to 10 days may be effective. Erythromycin base or stearate 2 g daily in four divided doses for 2 weeks is the least effective of available treatments. Among penicillin-allergic patients in whom compliance and follow-up cannot be ensured, desensitization and penicillin treatment should be used. Clinicians should also be alert to the possibility that recurrent secondary syphilis may represent disease of more than 1 year's duration. It is prudent to query patients with secondary syphilis regarding previous episodes, and consider additional treatment for those reporting such episodes. After effective treatment, a chancre heals in approximately a week and rash fades to resolution over 4 weeks.[219] These lesions also resolve eventually without treatment or resolution of disease.

Early syphilis is not monolithic in its response to effective treatment. Single-dose BPG therapy resolves primary syphilis in over 99% of cases in the classic studies, and seronegative primary syphilis responds more quickly than seropositive primary syphilis. Secondary syphilis requires retreatment in 5% to 10% (some of these certainly were cases of reinfection, however).[220–222] These figures suggest that apparent failures of BPG therapy in primary syphilis should be intensely investigated for reinfection, evolution of an inducer of BFP reaction, neurosyphilis (meningitis), and possibly for HIV infection. Further, some experts have suggested the use of two doses of BPG 1 week apart in secondary and early latent syphilis, and have noted that such treatment produces more rapid seroreversal.[223] Moreover, efficacy of treatment is judged by a surrogate (serology) in most cases, adding another variable. There are thus no absolute criteria for establishing efficacy of therapy, except that patients having subsequent clinical syndromes of persistent syphilis in the absence of reinfection are treatment failures; otherwise the term *retreatment candidate* is probably more appropriate than *treatment failure.*

A nontreponemal titer should always be obtained on the day of treatment, and the same test should be used for follow-up serologies because RPR titers run slightly higher than those in the VDRL. Patients should be re-examined and retitered at 6 and 12 months after treatment. Traditional criteria have called for a fourfold decline in titer at 6 months in these patients to document efficacy, but a retrospective Canadian study[224] found that 15% to 23% of patients would require retreatment by this criterion, and therefore it is probably too stringent. Hence, patients failing this criterion should at a minimum be followed closely and considered for evaluation of CSF and HIV infection. Those demonstrating a fourfold sustained rise in titer should be retreated, with the considerations listed previously in mind if they were treated for primary syphilis. Retreatment should probably consist of three doses of BPG 2.4 MU given weekly.[191] Most treated for early syphilis are seronegative at 1 year, and the balance should have continued follow-up. Although the treponemal tests are traditionally thought to remain positive for life, Romanowski and colleagues[224] found that 36 months after treatment for early syphilis, the FTA-Abs was negative in 24% and the MHA-TP in 13%.

The Jarisch-Herxheimer reaction (JHR) occurs in approximately 50% of those treated for primary syphilis and in 75% treated for secondary syphilis[225]; it is relatively rare in later syphilis. Given that this reaction results from liberation of endotoxin from dying spirochetes, it is intuitive that those with the greatest burden of organism are at greatest risk for it. The phenomenon was first described by Jarisch[226] in association with mercurial treatment of syphilis in 1895, and has been reported with treatment using several antibiotics in a number of spirochetal diseases, including Lyme disease.[227] It develops 2 to 24 hours after treatment (usually within 4 hours) and occurs only after the first dose of therapy.[219] Flu-like symptoms of fever, chills, headaches, myalgia, and, rarely, nausea and vomiting are seen. Findings include initial vasoconstriction followed by peripheral vasodilation and mild hypotension. The lesions of syphilis appear or worsen during the reaction, and with laryngeal syphilis airway obstruction and death have been reported. Transient elevations in peripheral white blood cell count and liver enzymes may be seen. Klein and associates[228] summarized 12 cases of JHR reported in pregnant women in the 1940s with poor outcomes: 9 patients had preterm labor and 3 experienced intrauterine fetal death. Klein and associates[228] reported more benign results while monitoring 33 gravidas after penicillin treatment for syphilis. Fifteen (45%) had JHR, all of whom had primary or secondary syphilis. Uterine contractions and decreased fetal movement were seen in two thirds, and 3 of 11 (27%) fetuses exhibited late decelerations. No major complications occurred. JHR was more common in women later bearing infants with congenital syphilis, as would be expected. Myles and co-workers[229] also describe a benign outcome among all of 20 pregnant women experiencing JHR. Because no specific treatment or prevention for JHR is clearly efficacious, none is recommended, even in pregnancy. Gravid women should be advised to seek obstetric consultation if contractions or decreased fetal movement occur after treatment, and that fetal death is a rare complication of treatment.[191]

Whereas latent syphilis of unknown duration should be managed like early syphilis with respect to partner notification, it should be managed like late latent syphilis with respect to treatment. These patients should be treated with BPG, 2.4 MU intramuscularly once weekly for a total of three doses.[191] Penicillin-allergic, nonpregnant patients may receive doxycycline, 100 mg orally twice daily, or tetracycline hydrochloride, 500 mg orally four times daily, for 4 weeks, although there are few data to support efficacy of these regimens. Even the penicillin regimen has only successful experience (rather than systematic trials) to recommend it—that is, the development of neurosyphilis or other tertiary manifestations after it is extremely rare. All patients with late/unknown-duration latent syphilis should be closely evaluated for tertiary disease before treatment, including CSF examination if any of the following is identified: (1) neurologic or ocular signs or symptoms, (2) other evidence of tertiary disease, (3) prior "treatment failure," or (4) HIV coinfection. CSF examination in these patients is not discouraged in the absence of these criteria.[191] After treatment, nontreponemal test titers should be repeated at 6, 12, and 24 months. Retreatment candidates are those exhibiting a fourfold titer rise, those with a pretreatment titer of 1:32 or greater dilution that fails to show a fourfold decline within 12 to 24 months, and those in whom the signs or symptoms of persistent/progressive syphilis develop.

Patients with late syphilis may manifest the phenomenon of serofastness in 30% or more of cases,[230] with retention of low-titer (almost always ≤4) seroreactivity in the nontreponemal tests despite otherwise effective treatment. No amount of additional treatment has ever been shown to produce resolution of seroreactivity for these patients. It would seem prudent to retest them annually for several years to document stability of the titer, and to examine them as well for assurance that no evidence of progressive syphilis develops.

Asymptomatic neurosyphilis poses paradoxes. As described previously, early syphilis is commonly associated with abnormalities and treponemes in the CSF, yet these seem to be resolved and progression to symptomatic neurosyphilis reliably avoided by doses of penicillin that fail to achieve treponemacidal levels in the CSF.[231, 232] However, the presence of abnormal CSF in patients with later syphilis clearly carries a risk of progression to symptomatic neurosyphilis when untreated or after inadequate treatment. The series of Smith and colleagues[233] and Hahn and associates[234] respectively studied 47 patients treated with 2.4 to 2.5 MU of BPG and 765 patients treated with various dosages of BPG who showed a significant prevalence of symptomatic neurosyphilis after treatment for abnormal CSF alone in late syphilis. Based on this incomplete information, current therapeutics reflect the belief that asymptomatic neurosyphilis in a patient with late syphilis (disease of more than 1 year's duration) should be treated like symptomatic neurosyphilis, whereas abnormal CSF in an asymptomatic patient requires no special treatment in early syphilis.[191]

Although symptomatic neurosyphilis represents advanced syphilis, it does not necessarily represent late syphilis, and has therefore been declassified as a component of tertiary syphilis.[191] The category of neurosyphilis includes those with ocular and otic disease for treatment purposes. A patient with syphilis at any stage who has neurologic signs or symptoms should have CSF examined using the diagnostic modalities described previously. Those with symptomatic neurosyphilis and late asymptomatic neurosyphilis should be treated with aqueous crystalline penicillin G intravenously 3 to 4 MU every 4 hours for 10 to 14 days. Alternatively, if follow-up can be ensured, procaine penicillin 2.4 MU intramuscularly daily, plus probenecid 500 mg orally four times daily for 10 to 14 days may be used. This course of treatment is short relative to therapy for other categories of late syphilis, so some experts advise a dose of intramuscular BPG 2.4 MU at its completion. The efficacy of these regimens has been established largely by treatment of HIV-positive patients with neuro-ocular disease, as reviewed by Rolfs.[228]

The goal of neurosyphilis therapy is to halt further neurologic destruction because the damage already done usually cannot be reversed. In 1986, the aforementioned regimens replaced three weekly IM doses of BPG 2.4 MU as recommended therapy for neurosyphilis, primarily because of reports of progression of disease after the older regimen.[56, 108] Another reason

cited for this change was failure of the older regimen reliably to produce a treponemacidal level of penicillin in the CSF.[231, 232] In fact, this same problem afflicts the new regimens, but no cases of progression of disease have been reported with them.[235] In the absence of meningeal inflammation, the CSF concentration of penicillin is as little as 1% to 2% of that in serum, whereas CSF levels slightly exceed those in serum with meningeal inflammation. Meningeal inflammation in neurosyphilis is very mild, explaining the difficulty in driving penicillin across the blood–brain barrier in this setting. The finding that *T. pallidum* can persist in the CSF after apparently successful treatment is troubling, but its meaning is unknown.[129, 236]

Cerebrospinal fluid should be re-examined every 6 months until the cell count is normal, which is the earliest and most important indicator of effective therapy.[191] Failure of the cell count to decline after 6 months or to normalize after 2 years is an indication for retreatment. The CSF protein normalizes later, and the CSF-VDRL remains positive for years after successful therapy, although the titer should fall over time. Serologic changes in serum are of little use in evaluating therapy of neurosyphilis.

Tertiary manifestations of syphilis consisting of cardiovascular disease or gummas should be treated with BPG 2.4 MU intramuscularly once weekly for three doses at a minimum.[191] One of the regimens for neurosyphilis is used by some experts for patients with cardiovascular manifestations. All of these patients should have a CSF examination to rule out late asymptomatic neurosyphilis before treatment. Complete management of lesions induced by syphilis in these patients often requires the involvement of a number of consultants, including cardiothoracic and plastic surgeons, hepatologists, otolaryngologists, and others. Follow-up of these patients is important, but is hampered by very little data to direct it and loss of usefulness of even serology in evaluating therapy. Most of these patients have a low or even negative nontreponemal titer at presentation, and among those with reactive serology, up to 50% may be serofast,[230] never achieving seroreversion even after clinically adequate treatment. Careful clinical follow-up is the most appropriate care for these patients.

Like its clinical manifestations and diagnosis, the treatment of syphilis has been re-examined in HIV-infected patients. As stated previously, all patients with syphilis should be tested for HIV. Several reports suggest a decline in efficacy of standard treatment for primary syphilis in HIV-positive patients.[56, 108, 129, 237–239] On the other hand, comparative studies[240–242] have shown no evidence of a significant impact of HIV coinfection on the efficacy of recommended treatments for syphilis. The CDC has concluded that treatment for early syphilis need not be modified for HIV coinfection, except that penicillin only should be used.[191] However, prolongation of the course of treatment and examination of CSF before or after therapy, with modification of treatment in response to positive results, is not discouraged. More frequent follow-up is recommended, with visits at 3, 6, 9, 12, and 24 months. Identification of retreatment candidates is not changed. In HIV-infected patients with late or unknown-duration latent syphilis, a CSF examination is advised before treatment, and if it is negative, no change in treatment is advised, except that again only the penicillin regimen is recommended. Follow-up at 6, 12, 18, and 24 months with clinical and serologic evaluation is indicated. If the titer should rise fourfold or fail to decline fourfold by 24 months after treatment, CSF examination should be performed and, if positive, treatment for neurosyphilis initiated.

Because treatment of the fetus at risk for congenital syphilis is a critical consideration in treatment of syphilis in pregnancy, this issue requires special attention. Penicillin treatment of the gravid woman can prevent and cure fetal syphilis.[96, 97] There are limitations to its efficacy in this application, however, arising from the complex interplay between the inoculum of *T. pallidum* to which the fetus is exposed (a function of the stage of maternal syphilis) and the duration and timing of the infection in the fetus (a host whose immunocompetence is relatively poor overall, but poorer early in gestation than late). To illustrate, the worst-case scenario for the fetus is a mother with active secondary syphilis early in pregnancy who is not treated at all or until late in that pregnancy. In this case, a high-titer inoculum is presented to the fetus at its least immunocompetent age and progresses unchecked over a long period. The best-case scenario for the fetus is a mother with late latent syphilis who is effectively treated early in pregnancy. Here, the fetus is subject to a low-titer or no inoculum, and its infection is prevented or stemmed early by treatment. BPG treatment of the mother early in pregnancy has an efficacy of 98% to 100% in the prevention of congenital syphilis. Later in pregnancy, particularly in the third trimester, efficacy declines dramatically.[9, 20, 22] There are likely two reasons for this decline. First, in this setting, it is more likely that the fetus acquired syphilis at an early, immunoincompetent age and now has extensive organ damage from deeply seated infection with spirochetes that are dividing more slowly and thus are less susceptible to penicillin. Second, the pharmacokinetics of penicillin in the third trimester appear unfavorable. Nathan and colleagues[243] have shown that 7 days after an intramuscular dose of BPG 2.4 MU given to women undergoing cesarean delivery at term, 36% had penicillin levels below 0.018 μg/mL. The half-life of oral phenoxymethyl penicillin is decreased by 50% in the second trimester and 70% in the third.[244] Manifestation of these concepts is seen in the Miami series,[9] in which five patients completed appropriate doses (BPG 7.2 MU) of penicillin in the second and third trimesters, and all delivered infants with congenital syphilis. Mascola and co-workers[245] reported birth of infants with congenital syphilis to four women treated with BPG in the third trimester. In another study,[246] among 64 women delivering infants with congenital syphilis, 72% were treated in the third trimester and 22% in the second. Loss of protection against congenital syphilis by penicillin in later pregnancy was confirmed in the Detroit series,[20] where the authors identified ". . . an alarming rate of failure of current therapy to prevent congenital syphilis." However, in the same population, all of 45 women treated with penicillin in recommended doses more than 30 days before delivery had healthy, apparently uninfected infants.[22]

McFarlin and colleagues[20] concluded that retreatment with BPG during pregnancy was not useful in decreasing the risk of delivering an infant with presumed congenital syphilis, although receipt of the recommended three doses for latent syphilis of unknown duration was superior to one dose. However, five cases in the literature describe hydropic fetuses of syphilitic women treated with high-dose penicillin; the women subsequently delivered infants who survived this otherwise fatal condition.[247–249]

Current recommendations for treatment of syphilis in pregnancy emphasize the use only of penicillin, with skin testing or desensitization for those women reporting allergy. Regimens appropriate to the stage of syphilis described earlier should be used in pregnancy, although an additional dose of BPG 2.4 MU may be given in early syphilis.[191] Sonographic fetal surveillance is appropriate for women at greater risk of fetal treatment failure (those treated after the first trimester, presenting with secondary syphilis or a titer positive at 1:64 or greater dilution, and showing slow serologic response). Management of the risk of JHR was discussed earlier. Particular attention to treatment of sexual partners is needed to diminish risk of reinfection. Serology should be repeated at least once in the third trimester and at delivery, although many practitioners repeat it monthly because of the inherent risk of reinfection in these patients. Many of these patients deliver before a decline in titer is seen.

The safety of oral desensitization of pregnant women with penicillin allergy has been shown in a small series.[250] For detailed discussion of management of infants with congenital syphilis and techniques of penicillin skin testing and desensitization, the reader is referred to the authoritative source,[191] because those topics exceed the scope of this text.

PREVENTION

In 15th-century Scotland, known syphilitic individuals were branded on the cheek to forewarn potential sexual partners of the risk.[251] Catherine the Great passed her potential partners before her own exposure through a series of six women called *les Epreuveuses* ("the testers") over a period of 6 months to observe them for evidence of acquisition of syphilis.[252] Both of these methods of prevention failed.

There is a surprising absence of data on the value of condoms in prevention of syphilis. Because most chancres in men occur on the penis and most in women in the vaginal vault, condoms would be expected to prevent transmission of a considerable proportion of cases if the perineal skin is intact and extragenital contact does not occur. Some topical spermicides have been shown to immobilize *T. pallidum* in vitro, but currently available concentrations of agents are not among them.[253]

It is obvious that syphilis is essentially nonexistent among people in couples where both practice sexual fidelity, and among those sexually abstinant. It is not the nature of all human-kind to be so. Morality is a societal trend that seems to follow a course of its own determination, and efforts to direct it offer a low yield. The control of syphilis therefore has become a matter of identifying infected people, treating them effectively, identifying and treating all people who may have infected or been infected by this index case, and promoting broad public awareness of the existence, dangers, and methods of avoiding syphilis. Individual health care providers can and should be helpful in the initial aspects of this process. Screening for syphilis, and particularly reporting identified index cases, is suboptimal among most practitioners in the United States at present,[254] and this deficiency certainly contributes to the persistence of syphilis.

The balance of the process requires a large-scale organization with adequate numbers of trained personnel who possess the legal authority to trace and treat contacts, and the funding for public awareness. Public health officials have taken on this task, and most progress against syphilis is the result of their efforts. Involvement of other governmental entities, particularly in the control of the crack cocaine subculture that has eluded us to date, is necessary as well.

REFERENCES

1. Fiumara NJ: A legacy of syphilis. Arch Dermatol 1965; 92:676.
2. Hart G: Epidemiologic treatment of syphilis. J Am Vener Dis Assoc 1976; 3:177.
3. Stokes JH, et al: Modern Clinical Syphilogy, 3rd ed. Philadelphia, WB Saunders, 1944, pp 426–522.
4. Tramont EC: *Treponema pallidum* (syphilis). In: Madell GL, Douglas RG, Bennett JE (eds): Principles and Practices of Infectious Diseases. New York, John Wiley & Sons, 1979, pp 1820–1837.
5. Wilcox RR, Guthe T: *Treponema pallidum*: A bibliographical review of the morphology, culture and survival of *T. pallidum* and associated organisma. Bull World Health Organ 1966; 35(suppl): 66.
6. Nelson KE, Vlahov D, Cohn S, et al: Sexually trasmitted diseases in a population of intravenous drug users: Association with seropositivity to the human immunodeficiency virus (HIV). J Infect Dis 1991; 164:457–63.
7. Centers for Disease Control: Continuing increase in infectious syphilis—United States. MMWR Morb Mortal Wkly Rep 1988; 37:35.
8. Felman YM: Repeal of mandated premarital tests for syphilis: A survey of state health officers. Am J Public Health 1981; 71:155.
9. Ricci JM, Fojaco RM, O'Sullivan MJ: Congenital Syphilis: The University of Miami/Jackson Memorial Medical Center experience, 1986–1988. Obstet Gynecol 1989; 74:687.
10. Minkoff HL, McCalla SM, Delke I, et al: The relationship of cocaine use to syphilis and human immunodeficiency virus infections among inner city parturient women. Obstet Gynecol 1990; 163:521
11. Centers for Disease Control and Prevention: Outbreak of primary and secondary syphilis—Baltimore City, Maryland, 1995. MMWR Morb Mortal Wkly Rep 1996; 45:166.
12. Andrus JK, Fleming DW, Harger DR, et al: Partner notification: Can it control epidemic syphilis? Ann Intern Med 1990; 112:539.
13. Centers for Disease Control: Alternative case-finding methods in a crack-related syphilis epidemic—Philadelphia. MMWR Morb Mortal Wkly Rep 1991; 40:77.
14. Finelli L, Budd J, Spitalny KC: Early syphilis: Relationship to sex, drugs, and changes in high-risk behavior from 1987–1990. Sex Transm Dis 1993; 20:89.
15. Ernst AA, Martin DH: High syhilis rates among cocaine abusers identified in an emergency department. Sex Transm Dis 1993; 20:66.
16. Nakashima AK, Rolfs RT, Flock ML, et al: Epidemiology of syphilis in the United States, 1941–1992. Sex Transm Dis 1996; 23:16.
17. Thomas JC: Syphilis in the South: Rural rates surpass urban rates in North Carolina. Am J Public Health 1995; 85:1119.
18. McCabe E, Jaffe LR, Diaz A: Human immunodeficiency virus seropositivity in adolescents with syphilis. Pediatrics 1992; 92:695.
19. Ernst AA, Farley TA, Martin DH: Screening and empiric treatment for syphilis in an inner-city emergency department. Acad Emerg Med 1995; 2:765.
20. McFarlin BL, Bottoms SF, Dock BS, et al: Epidemic syphilis: Maternal factors associated with congenital infection. Am J Obstet Gynecol 1994; 170:535.
21. Ernst AA, Romolo R, Nick T: Emergency department screening for syphilis in pregnant women without prenatal care. Ann Emerg Med 1993; 22:781.
22. Reyes MP, Hunt N, Ostrea EM Jr, et al: Maternal/congenital syphilis in a large tertiary-care urban hospital. Clin Infec Dis 1993; 17:1041.
23. Engelkens HJH, Judanarso J, Oranje AP, et al: Endemic treponematoses. I: Yaws. Int J Dermatol 1991; 30:77.
24. Engelkens HJH, Niemel PLA, van de Stauis JJ, et al: Endemic treponematoses. II: Pinta and endemic syphilis. Int J Dermatol 1991; 30:231.
25. Hudson H: Treponematoses and African slavery. Br J Vener Dis 1964; 40:43.
26. Hollander DH: Treponematosis from pinta to venereal syphilis revisited: Hypothesis for temperature determination of disease patterns. Sex Transm Dis 1981; 8:34.
27. Willcox RR: The treponemal evolution. Trans St Johns Dermatol Soc 1972; 58:21.
28. Willcox RR: Changing patterns of treponemal disease. Br J Ven Dis 1974; 50:169.
29. Benenson AS: Pinta; nonvenereal endemic syphilis; Yaws. In: Benenson AS (ed): Control of Communicable Diseases in Man, 15th ed. Washington, DC, American Public Health Association, 1990, pp 323–324; 425–426; 483–486.
30. Nandwani R, Evans DTP: Are you sure it's syphilis? A review of false positive serology. Int J STD AIDS 1995; 6:241.
31. Norris SJ, and the *Treponema pallidum* Polypeptide Research Group: Polypeptides of *Treponema pallidum*: Progress toward understanding their structural, functional, and immunologic roles. Microbiol Rev 1993; 57:750.
32. Alderete JF, Baseman JB: Surface characterization of virulent *Treponema pallidum*. Infect Immun 1980; 30:814.
33. Stamm LV, Parrish EA, Gherardini FC: Cloning of the recA gene from a free-living leptospire and distribution of RecA-

like protein among spirochetes. Appl Environ Microbiol 1991; 57:183.

34. Steiner BM, Wong GH, Sutrave P, et al: Oxygen toxicity in *Treponema pallidum*: Deoxyribonucleic acid single-stranded breakage induced by low doses of hydrogen peroxide. Can J Microbiol 1984; 30:1467.

35. Norgard MV, Miller JN: Plasmid DNA in *Treponema pallidum* (Nichols): Potential for antibiotic resistance in syphilis bacteria. Science 1981; 213:553.

36. Hovind-Hougen K: *Treponema* and *Borrelia* morphology. In: Johnson RC (ed): The Biology of the Parasitic Spirochetes. New York, Academic Press, 1976, pp 15–25.

37. Eagle H: Speculations as to the therapeutic significance of the penicillin blood level. Ann Intern Med 1948; 28:260.

38. Magnuson HJ, Eagle H, Fleischman R: The minimal infectious inoculum of *Spirochaeta pallida* (Nichols strain), and a consideration of its rate of multiplication in vivo. Am J Syph Gon Vener Dis 1948; 32:1.

39. Yobs AR, Rockwell DH, Clark JW Jr: Treponemal survival in humans after penicillin therapy: A preliminary report. Br J Vener Dis 1964; 40:248.

40. Collart P, Borel L-J, Durel P, et al: Significance of spiral organisms found, after treatment, in late human and experimental syphilis. Br J Vener Dis 1964; 40:81.

41. Fieldsteel AH: Cultivation of virulent *Treponema pallidum* in tissue culture. Infect Immun 1981; 32:908.

42. Jenkin H, Sandok PL: Cultivation of *Treponema pallidum*. In: Schell RF, Musher DM (eds): Pathogenesis and Immunology of Treponemal Infection. New York, Marcel Dekker, 1982, pp 71–98.

43. Magnuson HJ, Thomas EW, Olansky BI, et al: Inoculation of syphilis in human volunteers. Medicine (Baltimore) 1956; 35:33.

44. Boak RA, Carpenter CM, Warren SL: Studies on the physiological effects of fever temperatures. III: The thermal death time of *Treponema pallidum in vitro* with special reference to fever temperature. J Exp Med 1932; 56:741.

45. Fitzgerald TJ: Pathogenesis and immunology of *Treponema pallidum*. Annu Rev Microbiol 1981; 35:29.

46. Musher DM: Biology of *Treponema pallidum*. In: Holmes KK, Mardh PA, Sparling PF, et al (eds): Sexually Transmitted Diseases. New York, McGraw-Hill, 1984, pp 291–298.

47. Bishop NH, Miller JN: Humoral immune mechanisms in acquired syphilis. In: Schell RF, Musher DM (eds): Pathogenesis and Immunology of Treponemal Infections. New York, Marcel Dekker, 1982, pp 241–269.

48. Knox JM, Musher D, Guzick ND: The pathogenesis of syphilis and the related treponematoses. In: Johnson RC (ed): The Biology of Parasitic Spirochetes. New York, Academic Press, 1976, pp 249–259.

49. Soltani K: Detection by direct immunofluorescence of antibodies to *Treponema pallidum* in the cutaneous infiltrates of rabbit syphilomas. J Infect Dis 1978; 138:222.

50. Mills CH: Routine examination of cerebrospinal fluid in syphilis: Its value in regards to more accurate knowledge, prognosis and treatment. BMJ 1927; 2:527.

51. Chesney AM, Kemp JE: Incidence of *Spirocheta pallida* in cerebrospinal fluid during early state of syphilis. JAMA 1924; 83:1725.

52. Yaws or syphilis. [Editorial.] BMJ 1979; 1:912.

53. Marshak LC, Rothman S: Skin testing with a purified suspension of *Treponema pallidum*. Am J Syph Gon Vener Dis 1951; 35:35.

54. Thivolet J: Etude de l'intradermoreaction aux suspensions de treponemes formolees (souche Nichols pathogene) chez les syphilitiques et les sujets normaux. Ann Inst Pasteur Lille 1953; 84:23.

55. Baughn RE: Inability of spleen cells from chancre-immune rabbits to confer immunity to challenge with *Treponema pallidum*. Infect Immun 1977; 17:535.

56. Musher DM, Hamill RJ, Baughn RE: Effects of human immunodeficiency virus (HIV) infection on the course of syphilis and on the response to treatment. Ann Intern Med 1990; 113:872.

57. Stokes JH: Modern Clinical Syphilology, 2nd ed. Philadelphia, WB Saunders, 1934, pp 549–555.

58. Moore JE: Syphilitic iritis. Am J Ophthalmol 1931; 14:110.

59. Turner TB: Effects of passive immunization on experimental syphilis in the rabbit. Johns Hopkins Med J 1973; 133:241.

60. Weiser RS: Immunity to syphilis: Passive transfer in rabbits using serial doses of immune serum. Infect Immun 1976; 13:1402.

61. Pope VS, Larsen SA, Rice RJ, et al: Flow cytometric analysis of peripheral blood lymphocyte immunophenotypes in persons infected with *Treponema pallidum*. Clin Diagn Lab Immunol 1994; 1:121.

62. Baughn RE, Musher DM: Reappraisal of lymphote responsiveness to concanavalin A during experimental syphilis: Evidence that glycosaminoglycans in the sera and tissues interfere with active binding sites on the lectin and not with the lymphocytes. Infect Immun 1982; 35:552.

63. Hayes NS: Parasitism by virulent *Treponema pallidum* of host cell surfaces. Infect Immun 1977; 17:174.

64. Baughn RE: Detection of circulating immune complexes in the sera of rabbits with experimental syphilis: Possible role in immunoregulation. Infect Immun 1980; 29:575.

65. Baughn RE, Musher DM: Altered immune responsiveness associated with experimental syphilis in the rabbit: Elevated IgG and depressed IgA response to sheep erythrocytes. J Immunol 1978; 120:1691.

66. Morrison EB, Norman DA, Wingo CS, et al: Simultaneous hepatic and renal involvement in acute syphilis. Dig Dis Sci 1980; 23:875.

67. Solling J: Circulating immune complexes in syphilis. Acta Derm Venereol 1978; 58:263.

68. Engel S, Diezel W: Persistent serum immune complexes in syphilis. Br J Vener Dis 1980; 56:221.

69. Bhorade MS: Nephropathy of secondary syphilis: A clinical and pathological spectrum. JAMA 1971; 216:1159.

70. Gamble CN, Reardan JB: Immunopathogenesis of syphilitic glomerulonephritis: Elution of antitreponemal antibody from glomerular immune-complex deposits. N Engl J Med 1975; 292:449.

71. Sparling PF: Natural history of syphilis. In: Holmes K, Mardh P-A, Sparling PF, et al (eds): Sexually Transmitted Diseases. New York: McGraw-Hill, 1984, pp 298–305.

72. Jaffe HW, Sherwin AK: Examination of cerebrospinal fluid in patients with syphilis. Rev Infect Dis 1982; 4(suppl):S842.

73. Moore JE, Hopkins HH: Asymptomatic neurosyphilis. VI: The prognosis of early and late asymptomatic neurosyphilis. JAMA 1930; 95:1637.

74. Gjestland T: The Oslo study of untreated syphilis. Acta Derm Venerol Suppl (Stockh) 1955; 34:1.

75. Merritt HH, Adams RD, Solomon HC: Neurosyphilis. New York, Oxford University Press, 1946, pp 72–73.

76. Hook EW III, Marra CM: Acquired syphilis in adults. N Engl J Med 1992; 326:1062.

77. U.S. Public Health Service: Syphilis: A synopsis. Washington, DC, U.S. Government Printing Office, 1967, pp 17–40.

78. U.S. Public Health Service: Syphilis: A Synopsis. Washington, DC, U.S. Government Printing Office, 1967, pp 86–116.

79. Harter CA, Benirschke K: Fetal syphilis in the first trimester. Am J Obstet Gynecol 1976; 124:705.

80. Nabarro D: Congenital Syphilis. London, E. Arnold, 1954, pp 15.

81. Ingall D, Norins L: Syphilis. In: Remington JS, Klein JO (eds): Infectious Diseases of the Fetus and Newborn Infants. Philadelphia, WB Saunders, 1976, pp 414–463.

82. Qureshi F, Jacques SM, Reyes MP: Placental histopathology in syphilis. Hum Pathol 1993; 24:779.

83. Walter P, Blot P, Ivanoff B: The placental lesions in congenital syphilis. Virchows Arch Anat 1982; 397:313.

84. Parker CR Jr, Wendel GD: The effects of syphilis on endocrine function of the fetoplacental unit. Am J Obstet Gynecol 1988; 159:1327.

85. Chawla V, Pandit PB, Nkrumah FK: Congenital syphilis in the newborn. Arch Dis Child 1988; 63:1393.

86. Tan KL: The re-emergence of early congenital syphilis. Acta Paediatr Scand 1973; 62:601.

87. Hallak M, Peipert JF, Ludomirsky A, et al: Nonimmune hydrops fetalis and fetal congenital syphilis. J Reprod Med 1992; 37:173.

88. Chapel TA: The variability of syphilitic chancres. Sex Transm Dis 1978; 5:68.

89. Feher J, Somogyi T, Timmer M, Jozsa L: Early syphilitic hepatitis. Lancet 1975; 2:896.

90. Willcox RR, Goodwin PG: Nerve deafness in early syphilis. Br J Vener Dis 1971; 47:401.

91. Campisi D, Whitcomb C: Liver disease in early syphilis. Arch Intern Med 1979; 139:365.

92. Clark EG, Danbolt N: The Oslo study of the natural course of untreated syphilis: An epidemiologic investigation based on a re-study of the Boeck-Bruusgard material. Med Clin North Am 1964; 48:613.

93. Rosahn PD: Autopsy studies in syphilis. Journal of Venereal Disease Information, supplement no 21, U.S. Public Health Service, Venereal Disease Division, U.S. Government Printing Office, Washington, DC, 1947, pp 1–67.

94. Rockwell DH, Yobs AR, Moore MB Jr: The Tuskegee study of untreated syphilis. Arch Intern Med 1964; 114:792.

95. Kampmeier RH: The late manifestations of syphilis: Skeletal, visceral and cardiovascular. Med Clin North Am 1964; 48:667.

96. Ingraham NR: The value of penicillin alone in the prevention and treatment of congenital syphilis. Acta Derm Venerol Suppl (Stockh) 1951; 24:60.

97. Wammock VS, Carrozzino OM, Ingraham NR, et al: Penicillin therapy of the syphilitic pregnant woman: Its practical application to a large urban obstetrical service. Am J Obstet Gynecol 1950; 59:806.

98. Thomas EW: Syphilis: Its course and management. New York, McMillan, 1949, pp 118–131.

99. Taber LH, Huber TW: Congenital syphilis. Prog Clin Biol Res 1975; 3:183.

100. Centers for Disease Control: Congenital syphilis—United States, 1983–85. JAMA 1986; 256:3206.

101. Srinivasan G, Ramamurthy RS, Bharathi A, et al: Congenital syphilis: A diagnostic and therapeutic dilemma. Pediatr Infect Dis J 1983; 2:436.

102. Centers for Disease Control and Prevention: Case definitions for infectious conditions under public health surveillance. MMWR Morb Mortal Wkly Rep 1997; 46(RR-10):34.

103. Lee WK, Schwartz DA, Rice RJ, et al: Syphilitic endometritis causing first trimester abortion: A potential infectious cause of fetal morbidity in early gestation. South Med J 1994; 87:1259.

104. Centers for Disease Control: Guidelines for the prevention and control of congenital syphilis. MMWR Morb Mortal Wkly Rep 1988; 37(suppl 1):1.

105. Folgosa E, Osman NB, Gonzalez C, et al: Syphilis seroprevalence among pregnant women and its role as a risk factor for stillbirth in Maputo, Mozambique. Genitourin Med 1996; 72:339.

106. Kaufman RE, Jones OG, Blount JH, et al: Questionnaire survey of reported early congenital syphilis: Problems in diagnosis, prevention and treatment. Sex Transm Dis 1977; 4:135.

107. Mehta KP, Gharpure SV: Renal involvement in congenital syphilis: A review and study of 60 cases. Indian Pediatr 1978; 16:611.

108. Johns DR, Tierney M, Felsenstein D: Alteration in the natural history neurosyphilis by concurrent infection with the human immunodeficiency virus. N Engl J Med 1987; 316:1569.

109. Hook EW III: Syphilis and HIV infection. J Infect Dis 1989; 160:530.

110. Radolf JD, Kaplan RP: Unusual manifestations of secondary syphilis and abnormal humoral immune response to Treponema pallidum antigens in a homosexual man with asymptomatic human immunodeficiency virus infection. J Am Acad Dermatol 1988; 18(suppl):423.

111. Katz DA, Berger JR: Neurosyphilis in acquired immunodeficiency syndrome. Arch Neurol 1989; 46:895.

112. McLeish WM, Pulido JS, Holland S, et al: The ocular manifestations of syphilis in the human immunodeficiency virus type 1-infected host. Ophthalmology 1990; 97:196.

113. Veldman E, Bos PJ: Neuroretinitis in secondary syphilis. Doc Ophthalmol 1986; 64:23.

114. Smith JL, Byrne SF, Cambron CR: Syphiloma/gumma of the optic nerve and human immunodeficiency virus seropositivity. J Clin Neuroophthalmol 1990; 10:175.

115. Richards BW, Hessburg TJ, Nussbaum JN: Recurrent syphilitic uveitis. [Letter.] N Engl J Med 1989; 320:62.

116. Zaidman GW: Neurosyphilis and retrobulbar neuritis in a patient with AIDS. Ann Ophthalmol 1986; 118:260.

117. Winward KE, Hamed LM, Glaser JS: The spectrum of optic nerve disease in human immunodeficiency virus infection. Am J Ophthalmol 1989; 107:373.

118. Passo MS, Rosenbaum JT: Ocular syphilis in patients with human immunodeficiency virus infection. Am J Ophthalmol 1988; 106:1.

119. Flood JM, Weinstock HS, Bolan G, et al: Neurosyphilis in San Francisco during the AIDS epidemic of 1985–1989. [Abstract No. 334.] In: Program and Abstracts of the 31st Interscience Conference on Antimicrobial Agents and Chemotherapy (Chicago). Washington, DC, American Society for Microbiology 1991, p 154.

120. Folk JC, Weingeist TA, Corbett JJ, et al: Syphilitic neuroretinitis. Am J Ophthalmol 1983; 95:480.

121. Arruga J, Valentines J, Mauri F, et al: Neuroretinitis in acquired syphilis. Ophthalmology 1985; 92:262.

122. Hira SK, Patel JS, Bhat SG, et al: Clinical manifestations of secondary syphilis. Int J Dermatol 1987; 26:103.

123. Hutchinson CM, Rompalo AM, Reichart CA, et al: Characteristics of patients with syphilis attending Baltimore STD clinics: Multiple, high-risk subgroups and interactions with human immunodeficiency virus infection. Arch Intern Med 1991; 151:511.

124. Centers for Disease Control: Tertiary syphilis deaths—South Florida. MMWR Morb Mortal Wkly Rep 1987; 36:488.

125. Gourevitch MN, Selwyn PA, Davenny K, et al: Effects of HIV infection on the serologic manifestations and response to treatment of syphilis in intravenous drug users. Ann Intern Med 1993; 119:635.

126. Bean RB, Bean WB: Sir William Osler: Aphorisms from His Bedside Teachings and Writings. Springfield, IL, Charles C Thomas, 1961, pp 112.

127. Parodi U: Sulla trasmissione della sifilide al testicole del coniglio. T Accad Torino 1907; 13:288. [Zentralbl Bakteriol 1907; 44:428, German translation.]

128. Turner TB, Hardy PH, Neuman B: Infectivity tests in syphilis. Br J Vener Dis 1969; 45:183.

129. Lukehart SA, Hook EW III, Baker-Zander SA, et al: Invasion of the central nervous system by Treponema pallidum: Implications for diagnosis and treatment. Ann Intern Med 1988; 109:855.

130. Creighton ET: Darkfield microscopy for the detection and identification of Treponema pallidum. In: Larsen SA, Hunter EF, Kraus SJ (eds): A Manual of Tests for Syphilis, 8th ed. Washington, DC, American Public Health Association, 1990, pp 49–62.

131. Larsen SA, Steiner BM, Rudolph AH: Laboratory diagnosis and interpretation of tests for syphilis. Clin Microbiol Rev 1995; 8:1.

132. Coles AC: Spirochaeta pallidia: Methods of examination and detection, especially by means of the dark-ground illumination. BMJ 1909; 1:1117.

133. Daniels KC, Ferneyhough HS: Specific direct fluorescent antibody detection of Treponema pallidum. Health Lab Sci 1977; 14:164.

134. Romanowski BE, Forsey E, Lukehart S, et al: Detection of Treponema pallidum by a fluorescent monoclonal antibody test. Sex Transm Dis 1987; 22:156.

135. Ito FR, George RW, Hunter EF, et al: Specific immunofluorescence staining of pathogenic treponemes with a monoclonal antibody. J Clin Microbiol 1992; 30:832.

136. Ito FE, Hunter RW, George BL, et al: Specific immunofluorescence staining of Treponema pallidum in smears and tissues. J Clin Microbiol 1991; 29:444.

137. Kellogg DS Jr, Mothershed SM: Immunofluorescent detection of Treponema pallidum: A review. JAMA 1969; 107:938.

138. Smith JL, Israel CR: Spirochetes in the aqueous humor in seronegative ocular syphilis: Persistence after penicillin therapy. Arch Ophthalmol 1967; 77:474.

139. Wilkinson AE: Fluorescent treponemal antibody tests on cerebrospinal fluid. Br J Vener Dis 1973; 49:346.

140. Hunter EF, Greer PW, Swisher AR, et al: Immunofluorescent staining of treponema in tissues fixed with formalin. Arch Pathol Lab Med 1984; 108:878.

141. Wilkinson, AE, Cowell LP: Immunofluorescent staining for the detection of T. pallidum in early syphilitic lesions. Br J Vener Dis 1971; 47:452.

142. Yobs AR, Brown L, Hunter EF: Fluorescent antibody technique in early syphilis: As applied to the demonstration of T. pallidum in lesions in the rabbit and in the human. Arch pathol 1964; 77:220.

143. Hook EW III, Roddy RE, Lukehart SA, et al: Detection of Treponema pallidum in lesion exudate with a pathogen-specific monoclonal antibody. J Clin Microbiol 1985; 22:241.

144. Wasserman AA, Neisser A, Bruck C: Eine serodiagnostische Reaktion bei Syphilis. Dtsch Med Wochenschr 1906; 32:745.

145. Pangborn MC: A new serologically active phospholipid from beef heart. Proc Soc Exp Biol Med 1941; 48:484.

146. Felman YM: How useful are the serologic tests for syphilis? Int J Dermatol 1982; 21:79.

147. Schroeter AL, Lucas JB, Price EV, et al: Treatment of early syphilis and reactivity of serologic tests. JAMA 1972; 221:471.

148. Deacon WE, Hunter EF: Treponemal antigens as related to identification and syphilis serology. Proc Soc Exp Biol Med 1962; 110:352.

149. Buist DGP, Pertile R, Morris GJ: Evaluation of the T. pallidum haemagglutination test. Pathology 1993; 5:249.

150. Cox PM, Logan LC, Stout GW: Further studies of a quantitative automated microhemagglutination assay for antibodies to Treponema pallidum. Public Health Lab 1971; 29:43.

151. Felman Y: Syphilis serology today. Arch Dermatol 1980; 116:84.

152. Goodhart GL: Use and interpretation of serologic tests for the diagnosis of syphilis. South Med J 1993; 76:373.

153. U.S. Public Health Service: Syphilis: A Synopsis. Washington, DC, U.S. Government Printing Office, 1967, pp 96–108.

154. Moore MB, Knox JM: Laboratory diagnosis of syphilis. Cutis 1972; 9:172.

155. El-Zaatari M, Martens MG, Anderson GD: Incidence of the prozone phenomenon in syphilis serology. Obstet Gynecol 1994; 84:609.

156. Berkowitz K, Baxi L, Fox HE: False-negative syphilis screening: The prozone phenomenon, nonimmune hydrops, and diagnosis of syphilis during pregnancy. Am J Obstet Gynecol 1990; 163:975.

157. Smikle MF, James OBL, Prabhakar P: Biological false positive serological tests for syphilis in the Jamaican population. Genitourin Med 1990; 66:76.

158. Moore JE, Mohr CF: Biological false-positive serologic test for syphilis: Type, incidence, and cause. JAMA 1952; 150:467.

159. Aaron HCS, Parkhurst GE, Rodriguez J, et al: Further observations on biologic false-positive serologic tests in young children: Possibility of erroneous diagnosis of syphilis. Am J Syphilol 1952; 36:278.

160. Larsen SA: Current status of laboratory tests for syphilis. In: Rippey J, Nakamura R (eds): Diagnostic Immunology: Technology Assessment. Skokie, IL, American College of pathologists, 1983, pp 162–179.

161. Kaufman RE, Weirs S, Moore JD: Biological false positive serological tests for syphilis among drug addicts. Br J Vener Dis 1974; 50:350.

162. Ryuichi Y, Tokugoro T: Application to Japaneese patients of the 1982 American Rheumatism Association revised criteria for the classification of systemic lupus erythematosus. Arthritis Rheum 1985; 28:693.

163. Koskenvuo M, Leikola J, Palasuot VO, et al: False positive seroreactions for syphilis as a harbinger of disease revisited. Clin Exp Rheumatol 1989; 7:75.

164. Shoenfeld Y, Shaulion E, Shaklai M, et al: Circulating anticoagulant and serological tests for syphilis. Acta Derm Venereol 1980; 60:365.

165. Lockyard CC, Savarese DMF: Biologic false positive serologic tests for syphilis and other serologic abnormalities in autoimmune haemolytic anaemia and thrombocytopenic purpura. Medicine (Baltimore) 1989; 68:67.

166. Henriksen R, Sogaard PE, Hansen BU, et al: Autoimmune antibodies and pregnancy outcome in women with false positive syphilis test results. Acta Obstet Gynaecol Scand 1989; 68:537.

167. Thornton JG, Foote GA, Page CE, et al: False positive results for syphilis and the outcome of pregnancy: A retrospective case-control study. BMJ 1987; 295:355.

168. Goldman JN, Lantz MA: FTA-ABS and VDRL slide test reactivity in a population of nuns. JAMA 1971; 217:53.

169. Jaffe HW, Larsen SA, Jones OG, Dans PE: Hemagglutination tests for syphilis antibody. Am J Clin Pathol 1978; 70:230.

170. Lugar AFH: Serological diagnosis of syphilis: Current methods. In: Young H, McMillan A (eds): Immunological Diagnosis of Sexually Transmitted Diseases. New York, Marcel Dekker, 1988, pp 249–274.

171. Hunter EF, Russell H, Farshy CE, et al: Evaluation of sera from patients with Lyme disease in the fluorescent treponemal antibody-absorption tests for syphilis. Sex Transm Dis 1986; 13:232.

172. Magnarelli LA, Miller JN, Anderson JF, et al: Cross-reactivity of nonspecific treponemal antibody in serologic tests for Lyme disease. J Clin Microbiol 1990; 28:1276.

173. Klaus SJ, Haserick JR, Lantz MA: Fluorescent treponemal antibody-absorption test reactions in lupus erythematosus: Atypical beading pattern and probably false-positive reactions. N Engl J Med 1970; 282:1287.

174. Kraus SJ, Haserick JR, Lagan LC, et al: Atypical fluorescence in the fluorescent treponemal antibody-absorption (FTA-ABS) test related to deoxyribonucleic acid (DNA) antibodies. J Immunol 1971; 106:1665.

175. Strobel PL, Kraus SJ: An electron microscopic study of the FTA-ABS "beading" phenomenon with lupus erythematosus sera using ferritin-conjugated anti-human IgG. J Immunol 1972; 108:1152.

176. Monson RAM: Biologic false-positive FTA-ABS test in drug-induced lupus erythematosus: Report of a case. JAMA 1973; 224:1028.

177. Mackay DM, Price EV, Knox IM, et al: Specificity of the FTA-ABS test for syphilis: An evaluation. JAMA 1969; 207:1683.

178. Meyer-Rohn J: Unspezifisch positive Reaktionen im FTA-test. Hautarzt 1974; 25:528.

179. Scotti AT, Mackay DM, Trautman JR: Syphilis and biologic false-positive reactors among leprosy patients. Arch Dermatol 1970; 101:328.

180. Hughes MK, Fusillo MH, Roberson BS: Positive fluorescent treponemal antibody reactions in diabetes. Appl Microbiol 1970; 19:425.

181. Chapel T, Jeffries CD, Brown WJ, et al: Influence of genital herpes on results of fluorescent treponemal antibody absorption test. Br J Vener Dis 1978; 54:299.

182. Buchanan CS, Haserick JR: FTA-ABS test in pregnancy; A probably false-positive reaction. Arch Dermatol 1970; 102:322.

183. Manikowska-Lesinska W, Zajac LB: Specificity of the FTA-ABS and TPHA tests during pregnancy. Br J Vener Dis 1978; 54:295.

184. Bryne RE, Laske S, Bell M, et al: Evaluation of a Treponema pallidum Western immunoblot assay as a confirmatory test for syphilis. J Clin Microbiol 1992; 30:115.

185. Lefevre JC, Bertrand MA, Bauriaud LMB: False positive reactions occurring with the Captia Syphilis G EIA in sera from patients with Lyme disease. Genitourin Med 1992; 68:142.

186. Hooper NE, Malloy DC, Passen S: Evaluation of a Treponema pallidum enzyme immunoassay as a screening test for syphilis. Clin Diagn Lab Immunol 1994; 1:477.

187. Lefevre J, Bertrand M, Baurlaud R: Evaluation of the Captia enzyme immunoassays for detection of immunoglobulins G and M to Treponema pallidum in syphilis. J Clin Microbiol 1990; 28:1704.

188. Orle KA, Martin DH, Gates SR, et al: Multiplex PCR detection of Haemophilus ducreyi, Treponema pallidum, and Herpes simplex virus types -1 and -2 from genital ulcers. [Abstract.] In: Abstracts of the 94th General Meeting of the American Society for Microbiology (Las Vegas). Washington,

DC, American Society for Microbiology, 1994, p 568, abstract No. C437.

189. Grimprel EP, Sanchez GD, Wendel JM, et al: Use of polymerase chain reaction and rabbit infectivity testing to detect *Treponema pallidum* in amniotic fluid. J Clin Microbiol 1991; 29:1711.

190. Stoll BJ, Lee FK, Larsen E, et al: Improved serodiagnosis of congenital syphilis with combined assay approach. J Infect Dis 1993; 167:1093.

191. Centers for Disease Control and Prevention: 1998 Guidelines for treatment of sexually transmitted diseases. MMWR Morb Mortal Wkly Rep 1998; 47 (RR-1):28.

192. Madiedo G, Ho K-C, Walsh P: False-positive VDRL and FTA in cerebrospinal fluid. JAMA 1980; 244:688.

193. Izzat NN, Bartruff JK, Glicksman JM, et al: Validity of the VDRL test on cerebrospinal fluid contaminated by blood. Br J Vener Dis 1971; 47:162.

194. Jaffe HW, Larsen SA, Peters M, et al: Tests for treponemal antibody in CSF. Arch Intern Med 1978; 138:252.

195. Chhabra RS, Brion LP, Castro M, et al: Comparison of maternal sera, cord blood, and neonatal sera for detecting presumptive congenital syphilis: Relationship with maternal treatment. Pediatrics 1993; 91:88.

196. Qolohle DC, Hoosen AA, Moodley J, et al: Serological screening for sexually transmitted infections in pregnancy: Is there any value in re-screening for HIV and syphilis at the time of delivery? Genitourin Med 1995; 71:65.

197. Wendel GD, Maberry MC, Christmas JT, et al: Examination of amniotic fluid in diagnosing congenital syphilis with fetal death. Obstet Gynecol 1989; 74:967.

198. Fojaco RM, Hensley GT, Moskowitz L: Congenital syphilis and necrotizing funisitis. JAMA 1989; 261:1788.

199. Chang SN, Chung KY, Lee JB: Seroreversion of the serological tests for syphilis in the newborns born to treated syphilitic mothers. Genitourin Med 1995; 71:68.

200. Jonna S, Collins M, Abdein M, et al: Postneonatal screening for congenital syphilis. J Fam Pract 1995; 41:286.

201. Olansky S: High serologic titers in late congenital syphilis. JAMA 1976; 236:304.

202. Kaufman RE, Olansky DC, Weisner PJ: The FTA-ABS (IgM) test for neonatal congenital syphilis: A critical review. J Am Vener Dis Assoc 1974; 1:79.

203. Hicks CD, Benson PM, Lupton GP: Seronegative secondary syphilis in a patient infected with the human immunodeficiency virus (HIV) with Kaposi sarcoma. Ann Intern Med 1987; 107:492.

204. Gourevitch MN, Selwyn PA, Davenny D, et al: Effects of HIV infection on the serologic manifestation and response to treatment of syphilis in intravenous drug users. Ann Intern Med 1993; 118:350.

205. Jurado RL, Campbell J, Martin PD: Prozone phenomenon in secondary syphilis: Has its time arrived? Arch Intern Med 1993; 153:2496.

206. Mulhall BP, Naselli G, Whittingham S: Anticardiolipin antibodies in homosexual men: Prevalence and lack of association with human immunodeficiency virus (HIV) infection. J Clin Immunol 1989; 9:208.

207. Haas JG, Bolan S, Larsen M, et al: Sensitivity of treponemal tests for detecting prior treated syphilis during human immunodeficiency virus infection. J Infect Dis 1990; 162:862.

208. Augenbraun MH, DeHovitz JA, Feldman J, et al: Biological false-positive syphilis test results for women infected with human immunodeficiency virus. Clin Infect Dis 1994; 19:1040.

209. Gershman KA, Rolfs RT, Larsen SA, et al: Seroepidemiological characterization of a syphilis epidemic in the Republic of the Marshall Islands, formerly a yaws endemic area. Int J Epidemiol 1992; 21:599.

210. Rein MF: Biopharmacology of syphilotherapy. J Am Vener Dis Assoc 1976; 3:109.

211. Wecke J: *Treponema pallidum* in early syphilitic lesions in humans during high dose penicillin therapy: An electron microscopial study. Arch Dermatol Res 1976; 257:1.

212. Rolfs RT: Treatment of syphilis, 1993. Clin Infect Dis 1995; 20(suppl):S23.

213. Mashkilleyson AL, Gomberg MA, Mashkilleyson N, et al:

Treatment of syphilis with azithromycin. Int J STD AIDS 1996; 7(suppl):13.

214. Verdon MS, Handsfield HH, Johnson RB: Pilot study of azithromycin for treatment of primary and secondary syphilis. Clin Infect Dis 1994; 19:486.

215. Alder J, Jarvis K, Mitten M, et al: Clarithromycin therapy of experimental *Treponema pallidum* infections in hamsters. Antimicrob Agents Chemother 1993; 37:864.

216. Korting HC, Haag R, Walter D, et al: Efficacy of ceftizoxime in the treatment of incubating syphilis in rabbits. Chemotherapy 1993; 39:331.

217. Moore MB: Epidemiologic treatment of contacts to infectious syphilis. In: Proceedings of the World Forum on Syphilis and Other Treponematoses 1962. USDHEW Publication No. 997. Washington, DC, U.S. Department of Health, Education and Welfare, 1964, pp 340–342.

218. Schroeter AL, Turner RH, Lucas JB, et al: Therapy for incubating syphilis: Effectiveness of gonorrhea treatment. JAMA 1971; 218:711.

219. Fiumara NJ: Standards for treatment of primary and secondary syphilis. Am Fam Physician 1983; 27:185.

220. Smith CA, Kamp M, Olansky S, et al: Benzathine penicillin G in the treatment of syphilis. Bull World Health Organ 1956; 15:1087.

221. Nichols L: Treatment of early infectious syphilis with benzathine penicillin G. In: Proceedings of the World Forum on Syphilis and Other Treponematoses 1962. USDHEW Publication No. 997. Washington, DC, U.S. Department of Health, Education, and Welfare, 1964, pp 296–301.

222. Schroeter AL, Lucas JB, Price EV, et al: Treatment for early syphilis and reactivity of serologic tests. JAMA 1972; 221:471.

223. Fiumara NJ: Treatment of primary and secondary syphilis: Serologic response. J Am Acad Dermatol 1986; 14:487.

224. Romanowski B, Sutherland R, Fick G, et al: Serologic response to treatment of infectious syphilis. Ann Intern Med 1991; 114:1005.

225. Aronson IK, Soltani K: The enigma of the pathogenesis of the Jarisch-Herxheimer reaction. Br J Vener Dis 1976; 52:313.

226. Jarisch A: Therapeutic Veruche bei Syphilis. Wien Med Wochenschr 1895; 45:721.

227. Steere AC, Hutchinson GE, Rahn DW, et al: Treatment of the early manifestations of Lyme disease. Ann Intern Med 1983; 99:22.

228. Klein VR, Cox SM, Mitchell MD; et al: The Jarisch-Herxheimer reaction complicating syphilotherapy in pregnancy. Obstet Gynecol 1990; 75:375.

229. Myles TD, Elam G, Park-Huang E, et al: The Jarisch-Herxheimer reaction and fetal monitoring changes in pregnant women treated for syphilis. Obstet Gynecol 1998; 92:859.

230. Fiumara NJ: Serologic responses to treatment of 128 patients with late latent syphilis. Sex Transm Dis 1970; 6:243.

231. Frentz G, Nielsen PB, Espersen F, et al: Penicillin concentrations in blood and spinal fluid after a single intramuscular injection of penicillin G benzathine. Eur J Clin Microbiol 1984; 3:147.

232. Mohr JA, Griffiths W, Jackson R, et al: Neurosyphilis and penicillin levels in cerebrospinal fluid. JAMA 1976; 236:2208.

233. Smith CA, Kamp M, Olansky S, et al: Benzathine penicillin G in the treatment of syphilis. Bull World Health Organ 1956; 15:1087.

234. Hahn RD, Cutler JC, Curtis AC, et al: Penicillin treatment of asymptomatic central nervous system syphilis. I: Probability of progression to symtomatic neurosyphilis. AMA Arch Dermatol 1956; 74:355.

235. Schoth PEM, Wolters ECH: Penicillin concentrations in serum and CSF during high-dose intravenous treatment for neurosyphilis. Neurology 1987; 37:1214.

236. Hay PE, Clarke JR, Strugnell RA, et al: Use of the polymerase chain reaction to detect DNA sequences specific to pathogenic treponemes in cerebrospinal fluid. FEMS Microbiol Lett 1990; 68:233.

237. Rolfs RT: Treatment of syphilis, 1993. Clin Infect Dis 1995; 20(suppl 1):S23.

238. Dowell ME, Ross PG, Musher DM, et al: Response of latent syphilis or neurosyphilis to ceftriaxone therapy in persons

infected with human immunodeficiency virus. Am J Med 1992; 93:481.

239. Malone JL, Wallace MR, Hendrick BB, et al: Syphilis and neurosyphilis in a human immunodeficiency virus type-1 seropositive population: Evidence for frequent serologic relapse after therapy. Am J Med 1995; 99:55.

240. Telzak EE, Greenberg MSZ, Harrison J, et al: Syphilis treatment response in HIV-infected individuals. AIDS 1991; 5:591.

241. Hutchinson CM, Rompalo AM, Reichart CA, et al: Altered clinical presentation of early syphilis in patients with human immunodeficiency virus infection. Ann Intern Med 1994; 121:94.

242. Rolfs RT, Riduan M, Joesoef EF, et al: A randomized trial of enhanced therapy for early syphilis in patients with and without human immunodeficiency virus infection. N Engl J Med 1997; 337:307.

243. Nathan L, Bawdon RE, Sidawi JE, et al: Penicillin levels following the administration of benzathine penicillin G in pregnancy. Obstet Gynecol 1993; 82:338.

244. Heikkila AM, Erkkola RU: The need for adjustment of dosage regimen of penicillin V during pregnancy. Obstet Gynecol 1993; 81:919.

245. Mascola L, Pelosi R, Alexander CE: Inadequate treatment of syphilis in pregnancy. Am J Obstet Gynecol 1984; 150:945.

246. Hallak M, Peipert JF, Ludomirsky A, et al: Nonimmune

247. Galan HL, Yandell PM, Knight AB: Intravenous penicillin for antenatal syphilotherapy. Infect Dis Obstet Gynecol 1993; 1:7.

248. Barton JR, Thorpe EM, Shaver DC, et al: Nonimmune hydrops associated with maternal infection with syphilis. Am J Obstet Gynecol 1992; 167:56.

249. ElTabbakh GH, Elejalde BR, Broekhuizen FF: Primary syphilis and nonimmune fetal hydrops in a penicillin-allergic woman. J Reprod Med 1994; 39:412.

250. Wendel GD Jr, Stark BJ, Jamison RB, et al: Penicillin allergy and desensitization in serious infections during pregnancy. N Engl J Med 1985; 312:1229.

251. Wilcox RR: Venereal disease in the Bible. Br J Vener Dis 1949; 25:28.

252. Rosebury T: Microbes and Morals: The Strange Story of Venereal Disease. New York, Viking, 1971, pp 145–165.

253. Singh B, Cutler JC, Utidjian MD: Studies on the development of a vaginal preparation providing both prophylaxis against venereal disease and other genital infections and contraception. II: Effect in vitro of vaginal contraceptive and non-contraceptive preparations on *Treponema pallidum* and *Neisseria gonorrhoeae*. Br J Vener Dis 1972; 48:57.

254. Fleming, WL, Brown WJ, Donohue JF, et al: National survey of venereal disease treated by physicians in 1968. JAMA 1970; 211:1827.

hydrops fetalis and fetal congenital syphilis. J Reprod Med 1992; 37:173.

38

Herpes

DAVID A. BAKER

Recent advances in the pathophysiology, diagnosis, knowledge of transmission, and treatment of herpes simplex virus (HSV) infections allow the clinician to manage and control them. The significant rise in the number of viral sexually transmitted diseases (STDs) in the United States focuses attention on the need for the health care provider to be able to diagnose, prevent, and appropriately treat these infections. The aim of therapy should be not only to treat the initial infection and medical problems associated with this episode but also to educate the patient and prevent future transmission of HSV (Fig. 38–1).

Forty-five million Americans older than 12 years of age are infected with genital herpes.[1] As with other STDs, HSV type 2 (HSV-2) antibodies usually appear first about the time of sexual activity and show a significant increase during the prime reproductive years. Men and women in their late teens and early twenties show the greatest increase in incidence of genital HSV. One half of 1 million new cases of genital herpes are acquired each year. About 1 in 4 women in the United States is infected with HSV-2, as determined by use of the sensitive HSV type-specific antibodies studies performed on collected and stored sera.[1]

Two different types of HSV have been determined and appear to have different demographic patterns. The majority of genital tract infections in the United States are due to HSV-2. The presentation of the initial infection varies in the female population. Patients may present with clinical disease with severe symptoms, or they may be unaware of their primary infection because it is subclinical.[2] The age of the patient, years of sexual activity, race, one or more episodes of other genital infections, lower annual family income, and multiple sex partners have been associated with genital HSV infection.[3] Recurrent HSV in the genital tract is almost always found after clinically apparent primary genital herpes infection.[4]

Genital herpes in a sexually active and reproductive population translates to an increased risk of exposure of the fetus and newborn to this STD viral infection. Transmission occurs predominantly when there are HSV infectious secretions of the maternal genital tract that a newborn comes into contact with. As is demon-strated by new studies, the majority of mothers who give rise to newborns with neonatal herpes do not know that they are infected and a source of disease to their newborn.[5, 6]

ETIOLOGY

Because of divergent biologic properties, HSV infections have been designated types 1 and 2 (HSV-1 and HSV-2). New serologic testing relies on minor differences in antigenic composition and biochemical characteristics. Because of this, infection with type 1 or 2 viruses results in cross-reacting antibodies capable of extensively neutralizing the heterologous virus type.[7]

Early childhood is the time most commonly associated with exposure to HSV-1. Most infections with HSV-1 are subclinical, and perhaps 10% of primary infections with HSV-1 are clinically overt. In most non–genital herpetic lesions—herpes labialis, gingivostomatitis, and keratoconjunctivitis—HSV-1 is the causative agent.

The genital tract is the most common source of HSV-2 recovered from patients. Transmission of the type 2 strain is primarily contingent on sexual contact.[3] Fleming and co-workers[1] reported the alarming increase in genital HSV infections in the United States, with almost 30% of the female population in the United States infected with HSV-2. A high percentage of susceptible female sexual partners exposed to males with active herpetic lesions of the genitalia (50% to 90%) become infected.

PRESENTATION OF INFECTION

Primary infection with genital lesions occurs with disease on the vulva, vagina, or cervix, or all three between 2 and 14 days following exposure to HSV. Primary infection usually produces many lesions, with a significant surface area involved. Vaginal discharge, discomfort, dysuria, and burning pain occur at this time. Vesicles rupture, producing ulcers that are shallow and painful. Systemic manifestations of disease, such as inguinal lymphadenopathy, malaise, myalgia, and fever as the consequence of virus replication in

430

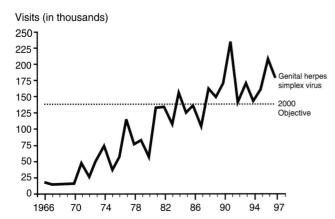

Visits (in thousands)

FIGURE 38-1. ▶ Genital herpes simplex virus infections, initial visits to physicians offices, United States 1966–1999, and the Healthy People year 2000 objective. (Source: Division of STD Prevention. Sexually Transmitted Disease Surveillance 1998. Centers for Disease Control and and Prevention [CDC], 1999.)

the sites of lymphatic drainage and viremia, can be seen.[7] Disease persists for as long as weeks without therapy, but with secondary bacterial or mycotic infections the lesions may persist for up to 6 weeks.

Shedding of virus with a lesion (symptomatic) and without a lesion (subclinical) from the lower genital tract of affected women following healing of primary genital HSV-2 lesions is much more common than previously reported.[4, 8]

Nonprimary First Episode

Prior HSV-1 infection in the oral cavity does not fully protect a patient from initial infection with HSV-2 in the genital tract. With the use of clinical signs and symptoms alone, it is difficult to differentiate primary from nonprimary first-episode disease.[9]

Recurrent Infection

The clinical finding of a few lesions confined to a small anatomic area is more common in recurrent forms of the disease. Lesions and ulcers tend to be limited in size and number. Only local symptoms are reported during a recurrence. All patients experience recurrent disease following a symptomatic primary genital infection.[10]

Subclinical Shedding

Shedding of virus, without a lesion, lasts on average 1½ days, and the quantity of virus shed is low. Sexual partners and the newborn can acquire this virus during times of subclinical shedding. Subclinical shedding makes this viral STD difficult to control and prevent. Shedding of virus during a recurrence can be symptomatic or subclinical. There is significant variation

from patient to patient in the frequency, severity, and duration of symptoms and viral shedding.[8, 11–13]

DIAGNOSIS

Viral isolation in tissue culture and staining techniques are currently being used to diagnose HSV. As HSV replicates, it produces specific cytopathic effects in cells, which allow the diagnosis of herpes to be made. Cells may be large and multinucleated, containing eosinophilic intranuclear inclusion bodies. Cytologic tests have a maximal sensitivity of 60% to 70% when dealing with overt clinical disease. Both the Pap and Zanck smears are poor screening procedures. Biopsy often may lead to a diagnosis, even in the absence of virus isolation studies.[14, 15]

Virus isolation in cell culture remains the standard and the most sensitive test for the detection of infectious herpesvirus from clinical specimens. The percentage of positive culture results varies with the manner in which the culture is obtained and transported, and the time since the onset of the lesion. Studies using more sensitive amplification techniques, such as polymerase chain reaction (PCR) and hybridization methods, have been reported. Slomka and colleagues[16] demonstrated that HSV PCR was significantly more sensitive than viral isolation in culture in both men and women with genital ulceration or symptoms suggestive of genital herpes infection.

Ulcers in the early stages of a recurrence yield virus in 80% of patients. As the lesions heal, the chances of finding culture-positive lesions decrease. Vesicular fluid is obtained by unroofing the lesion, and the fluid is then sampled. Virus isolation can be readily achieved in many primary or continuous human-tissue culture cell lines.[17]

Serologic testing is of relatively limited value because of the frequent presence of cross-reacting antibodies to the heterologous virus. Commercially available serologic tests looking for antibody to genital herpes infection cannot distinguish between HSV-1 and HSV-2. With seroconversion (acute-phase serum and convalescent serum obtained 14 to 21 days after the onset of clinical disease), one could serologically diagnose primary infection. The presence of an antibody titer in the initial specimen obtained at the onset of disease, strongly suggests recurrent infection. Results indicate that a one-strip rapid immunoblot assay and an indirect enzyme immunosorbent assay are useful and reliable for the detection of HSV-2–specific antibodies in sera.

TRANSMISSION

Sexual transfer to a susceptible partner is the most common mode of transmission of this viral STD. However, it must be reinforced that this virus is spread by direct contact from any body site or part to any site of the susceptible contact. Acute and recurrent herpes can be diagnosed in any part of the body, with the oral cavity and the genital tract infected most commonly. Genital-to-genital contact or contact of the genital tract with an area that is infected with HSV, such as oral-to-genital contact, can result in transmission.[2]

MANAGEMENT OF THE NONPREGNANT WOMAN

The use of antiviral medications in the management of genital herpes has been studied and found to be safe and highly effective in controlling this infection. Antiviral therapy is discussed in detail in another chapter. Additional management deals with the control of pain, the treatment and prevention of superimposed bacterial infections, and the determination and treatment of the other STDs. Patient education concerning genital herpes is mandatory, as well as education concerning safe sexual practices and the means of informing the partner and of preventing transmission of this virus.

HERPES DURING PREGNANCY

One of the major concerns of pregnant women infected with genital herpes is the risk of transmitting this virus to their fetus or newborn. Overall in the United States, infectious herpesvirus can be demonstrated in the genital tract of 3 per 1,000 gravid females at term. Subclinical shedding of HSV-2 from pregnant women with a history of recurrent genital herpes can be demonstrated in 0.65% to 3.03% of cultures.[18] With serial cultures, subclinical reactivation is detected in 2.3% to 14% of pregnant women with a history of genital herpes.[19] More frequent sampling in the antepartum period increases the detection of subclinical excretion.[17] The mean number of recurrences per trimester increased (from 0.01 to 1.26 to 1.63) in the first through the third trimesters. Transmission of HSV to the newborn is dependent on many factors. Subclinical versus symptomatic viral shedding determines the quantity of virus presented to the newborn. The duration of exposure to a given dose of virus and the presence of specific HSV-neutralizing antibodies play a role in viral transmission to the newborn. The risk of neonatal infection from a mother with primary herpetic vulvovaginitis is 30% to 50%.[18] With active recurrent herpes, the risk of neonatal infection at the time of delivery is estimated to be between 4% and 8%.[20, 21] With subclinical shedding, it is between 0.3% and 3%.[17, 18]

Patients presenting with their initial episode of genital herpes during pregnancy may have a severe recurrence—and not primary infection. It may be more difficult to distinguish cases of primary and re-current genital herpes during pregnancy.[22] Only 1 of 23 women with clinical illnesses consistent with primary genital HSV infections had serologically verified primary infection. Careful evaluation of all cases of a presumed first episode of genital herpes in pregnant women is needed. In the absence of HSV antibodies, the risk of congenital infection exists because of the possibility of blood-borne dissemination of the virus to the fetus.

Abortion rates following primary maternal genital HSV early in pregnancy have been reported[18]; however, this was not found in a more recent study.[23] Infection in the first trimester may produce a variety of anomalies.[24–26] Recurrent herpes is not associated with vertical transmission.

Brown and co-workers[27] demonstrated that 6 of the 15 gravidae with primary genital herpes but none of the 14 with nonprimary first episode infection had infants with serious perinatal morbidity. Therefore, circulating antibody to HSV-1 or HSV-2 is protective to the fetus developing in utero.

Primary genital HSV infection occurring during pregnancy increases the risk that this viral infection will have adverse consequences for the fetus and newborn. Antiviral therapy is recommended for this group of patients. Therapy is aimed at reducing viral shedding and enhancing lesion healing in the mother; the benefit on therapy to the fetus is not proven. Koelle and colleagues[8] reported on the potential of increased viral shedding from the cervix and vulva in nonpregnant women for 6 months following primary genital infection. The results of this study argue for the consideration of suppressive therapy for the duration of a pregnancy.[8]

Second- or third-trimester primary genital HSV infection increases the risk of preterm delivery, and there is a significant increased risk of herpesvirus transmission to the newborn.[18] Subclinical genital shedding of herpesvirus at the onset of labor because of a subclinical primary genital herpes infection is associated with preterm delivery.[23] This infection, which puts the newborn at greatest risk, is a significant diagnostic problem.

Obstetric Management

The use of antenatal viral cultures to predict whether the fetus will develop neonatal herpes has proved to be both costly and ineffective. A positive culture in a woman with subclinical viral shedding has a poor correlation with ensuing neonatally acquired disease. Negative cultures do not rule out the possibility of neonatal involvement. Current recommendations include the following: (1) do not use viral cultures in the gravida whose onset of disease antedated the pregnancy or in whom sexual consorts have had herpetic lesions[20]; and (2) do not culture asymptomatic patients who have a history of recurrent disease.[12]

Whether HSV antibody produced by the mother and transferred to the fetus will protect a neonate from infection is not well established. Reports describing neonatal infection in patients with high serum IgG antibody titers to HSV-2 show how complex the problem is. Preexisting HSV antibodies protect fully against congenital, but not neonatal, disease.[18] There is a risk to the neonate from any form of genital herpesvirus infection at term.[28] Of the newborns who develop neonatal herpes, as many as 70% of the mothers give no history of having genital HSV infection.

Clinical or subclinical primary genital herpes at or near the time of labor increases the risk of transmission to the newborn. In mothers who contracted primary herpes at or near the time of labor, neonatal herpes developed in 4 of 9 infants, but infection did not appear in any of the neonates of the 94 women who seroconverted prior to labor.[23]

The incidence of neonatal disease is low in cases of mothers with subclinical virus shedding at the time of labor. Treatment efforts need to be concentrated on (1) prevention of the maternal acquisition of HSV infection in the latter part of pregnancy[23] and (2) identification of pregnant women who are asymptomatic but infected with genital herpes.

In patients with only a history of genital HSV, there is no justification for cesarean delivery when there is no active disease during the last weeks of pregnancy or during labor.[29] With subclinical shedding, and the absence of lesions in the intrapartum period, the probability of neonatal disease appears to be exceedingly low. With symptomatic lesions at the time of parturition, the probability of neonatal infection is around 5% to 8%. In the presence of HSV lesions, cesarean section should be performed. Cesarean delivery with the increase in costs and increases in maternal morbidity and mortality should be performed only in well-defined clinical situations.

Special Clinical Problems and Presentations

Male Partner with Herpes. The male partner of the pregnant woman may be a potential source of genital HSV. A woman who is seronegative for HSV-2 may be infected during pregnancy from the male who may not know his HSV status. One in ten pregnant women were at risk for contracting primary HSV-2 infection from their HSV-2 seropositive husbands.[30] In nonpregnant populations, women acquire genital herpes from their male sexual partners with a greater frequency than that of female-to-male transmission. Much of the transmission and acquisition of genital herpes is asymptomatic.[31]

Invasive Fetal Monitoring in Labor. The fetal scalp electrode has the potential of producing local HSV infection and may be the portal of entry of HSV infection to the newborn.[32–34] If vesicular or vesiculopustular lesions develop at this site, it is important to make a quick and accurate diagnosis and start systemic antiviral therapy.

Breastfeeding. In one case, breast milk was the vehicle of dissemination of HSV-1 infection in the perinatal period.[35, 36] The mother was found to have HSV-1 in her breast milk. The death of an 8-day-old breastfed neonate with disseminated HSV-2, with the mother found to have bilateral herpetic nipple lesions, has been reported. Breast-feeding should be encouraged, with careful attention to inspection of the nipple and the breast.

Systemic Maternal Herpetic Infection. Disseminated herpes in pregnancy is life-threatening. The presentation is that of a fulminating hepatitis,[37, 38] with a maternal mortality rate of 43%. The presentation usually occurs in the third trimester, with a viral-like illness in association with genital or oral lesions.[39] Herpetic hepatitis should be included in the differential diagnosis of hepatic disease in the third trimester of pregnancy. Once the diagnosis has been made, intravenous acyclovir should be initiated to reduce maternal morbidity and mortality.[40, 41]

Acquisition of Neonatal Herpetic Infection Not from the Mother. Transmission of virus to the neonate may be mediated by individuals other than the mother and from sites other than the genital tract.[42, 43] Herpes acquired in this mode can be as lethal as that acquired by virtue of delivery through an infected birth canal. Oral or skin lesions can be an effective source of virus. HSV-1 is most commonly the cause of nosocomial neonatal disease. Direct contact (skin-to-skin or mouth-to-skin type of dissemination) is usually the mode of transmission. Screening of family contacts and visitors for the presence of herpetic skin and oral lesions is reasonable.

Premature Labor and Premature Rupture of Membranes (PROM) and HSV. When premature labor with or without PROM occurs in conjunction with a documented lesion of HSV, the question is how best to manage this rare patient. The use of antiviral therapy (parenteral acyclovir) and conservative management of the patient to achieve lung maturity has been reported, but this strategy should be considered carefully in the individual clinical situation.[44]

HIV and HSV. HIV-positive pregnant women have significantly higher rates of infection with HSV-2 than those of HIV-negative women.[45] The association of genital herpes and the acquisition of HIV has been demonstrated in varied populations. Women of child-bearing potential are at risk for all STDs, especially the viral STDs. The report by Hitti and colleagues[45] alerts the clinician to a group of women who may be at increased risk for transmitting HSV to their neonate.

REFERENCES

1. Fleming DT, McQuillan GM, Johnson RE, et al: Herpes simplex virus type 2 in the United States, 1976 to 1994. N Engl J Med 1997; 337:1105.
2. Mertz GL, Schmidt D, Jourden JL, et al: Frequency of acquisition of first-episode genital infection with herpes simplex virus from symptomatic and asymptomatic source contacts. Sex Transm Dis 1985; 12:33.
3. Mertz GJ, Benedetti J, Ashley R, et al: Risk factors for the sexual transmission of genital herpes. Ann Intern Med 1992; 116:197.
4. Benedetti J, Corey L, Ashley R: Recurrence rate in genital herpes after symptomatic first-episode infection. Ann Intern Med 1994; 121:847.
5. Prober C, Corey L, Brown ZA, et al: The management of pregnancies complicated by genital infections with herpes simplex virus. Clin Infect Dis 1992; 15:1031.
6. Frenkel LM, Garratty EM, Shen JP, et al: Clinical reactivation of herpes simplex virus type 2 infection in seropositive pregnant women with no history of genital herpes. Ann Intern Med 1993; 118:414.
7. Corey L, Spear PG: Infections with herpes simplex viruses. N Engl J Med 1986; 314:686, 749.
8. Koelle DM, Benedetti J, Langenberg A, Corey L: Asymptomatic reactivation of herpes simplex virus in women after the first episode of genital herpes. Ann Intem Med 1992; 116:433.
9. Mertz GL: Epidemiology of genital herpes infections. Infect Dis Clin North Am 1993; 7:825.
10. Hirsch MS: Herpes simplex virus. In: Mandell JE, Dolin R, et al (eds): Principles and Practice of Infectious Diseases, 4th ed. New York, Churchill Livingstone, 1995, pp 1336–1345.
11. Brock BV, Selke S, Benedetti J, et al: Frequency of asymptomatic shedding of herpes simplex virus in women with genital herpes. JAMA 1990; 263:418.
12. Prober C: Herpetic vaginitis in 1993. Clin Obstet Gynecol 1993; 36:177.
13. Wald A, Zeh J, Barnum G, et al: Suppression of subclinical shedding of herpes simplex virus type 2 with acyclovir. Ann Intern Med 1996; 124(1, pt 1):8.
14. Ashley RL: Laboratory techniques in the diagnosis of herpes simplex infection. Genitourin Med 1993; 69:174.
15. Woods GL: Update on laboratory diagnosis of sexually transmitted diseases. Clin Lab Med 1995; 15:665.
16. Slomka MJ, Emery L, Munday PE, et al: A comparison of PCR with viral isolation and direct antigen detection for diagnosis and typing of genital herpes. J Med Virol 1998; 55:177.
17. Scott LL, Hollier LM, Dias K: Perinatal herpesvirus infections. Infect Dis Clin North Am 1997; 11:27.
18. Brown ZA, Benedetti J, Ashley R, et al: Neonatal herpes simplex virus infection in relation to asymptomatic maternal infection at the time of labor. N Engl J Med 1991; 324:1247.
19. Cone RW, Hobson AC, Brown ZA, et al: Frequent reactivation of genital herpes simplex viruses among pregnant women. JAMA 1994; 272:792.
20. Arvin AM, Hensleigh PA, Prober CG, et al: Failure of antepartum maternal cultures to predict the infant's risk of exposure to herpes simplex virus at delivery. N Engl J Med 1986; 315:796.
21. Prober CG, Sullender WM, Yasukawa LL, et al: Low risk of herpes simplex virus infections in neonates exposed to the virus at the time of vaginal delivery to mothers with recurrent genital herpes simplex virus infections. N Engl J Med 1987; 316:240.
22. Hensleigh PA, Andrews WW, Brown Z, et al: Genital herpes during pregnancy: Inability to distinguish primary and recurrent infections clinically. Obstet Gynecol 1997; 89:891.
23. Brown ZA, Selke S, Zeh J, et al: The acquisition of herpes simplex virus during pregnancy. N Engl J Med 1997; 337:509.
24. Monif GRG, Kellner KR, Donnelly WH Jr: Congenital infection due to herpes simplex type II virus. Am J Obstet Gynecol 1985; 152:1000.
25. Altshuler G: Pathogenesis of congenital herpesvirus infection: Case report including a description of the placenta. Am J Dis Child 1984; 127:427.
26. Chalhub EG, Baenziger J, Feigen RD, et al: Congenital herpes simplex type 2 infection with extensive hepatic calcification, bone lesions and cataracts: Complete postmortem. Devel Med Child Neurol 1977; 19:527.
27. Brown ZA, Ashley R, Douglas J, et al: Neonatal herpes simplex virus infection: Relapse after initial therapy and transmission from a mother with an asymptomatic genital herpes infection and erythema multiforme. Pediatr Infect Dis J 1987; 6:1057.
28. Scott LL: Perinatal herpes: Current status and future management strategies. Adv Obstet Gynecol 1996; 3:47.
29. Roberts SW, Cox SM, Dax J, et al: Genital herpes during pregnancy: No lesions, no cesarean. Obstet Gynecol 1995; 85:261.
30. Kulhanjian JA, Soroush V, Au DS, et al: Identification of women at unsuspected risk of primary infection with herpes simplex virus type 2 during pregnancy. N Engl J Med 1992; 326:916.
31. Mertz GJ, Coombs RW, Ashley RI, et al: Transmission of genital herpes in couples with one symptomatic and one asymptomatic partner: A prospective study. J Infect Dis 1988; 157:169.
32. Amann ST, Fagnart RJ, Chartrand SA, Monif GRG: Herpes simplex infection with short-term use of a fetal scalp electrode. J Reprod Med 1992; 37:372.
33. Goldkrand JW: Intrapartum inoculation of herpes simplex virus by fetal scalp electrode. Obstet Gynecol 1982; 59:163.
34. Golden SM, Merenstein GB, Todd WA, Hill JM: Disseminated herpes simplex neonatorum: A complication of fetal monitoring. Am J Obstet Gynecol 1977; 129:917.
35. Dunkle LM, Schmidt RR, O'Connor DM: Neonatal herpes simplex infection possibly acquired via maternal breast milk. Pediatrics 1979; 63:250.
36. Kilbrick S: Herpes simplex virus in breast milk. Pediatrics 1979; 64:290.
37. Goyert GL, Bottoms SF, Sokol FJ: Anicteric presentation of fatal herpetic hepatitis in pregnancy. Obstet Gynecol 1985; 65:585.
38. Klein NA, Mabie WC, Shaver DC, et al: Herpes simplex virus hepatitis. Gastroenterology 1991; 100:239.
39. Chatelan S, Neumann DE, Alexander SM: Fatal herpetic hepatitis in pregnancy. Obstet Gynecol 1994; 1:236.
40. Grover L, Kane J, Kravitz J, et al: Systemic acyclovir in pregnancy: A case report. Obstet Gynecol 1985; 65:284.
41. Lagrew DC, Furlow TG, Hager D, et al: Disseminated herpes simplex virus infection in pregnancy: Successful treatment with acyclovir. JAMA 1984; 252:2058.
42. Hammerberg O, Watts J, Chernesky M, et al: An outbreak of herpes simplex virus type 1 in an intensive care nursery. Pediatr Infect Dis 1983; 2:290.
43. Douglas JM, Schmidt O, Corey L: Acquisition of neonatal HSV-1 infection from a paternal source contact. J Pediatr 1983; 103:908.
44. Major C, Towers C, Lewis D, Asrat T: Expectant management of patients with both preterm premature rupture of membranes and genital herpes. Am J Obstet Gynecol 1991; 164:248.
45. Hitti J, Watts H, Burchett SK, et al: Herpes simplex virus seropositivity and reactivation at delivery among pregnant women infected with human immunodeficiency virus-1. Am J Obstet Gynecol, 1997; 177:540.

39 Gonococcal Infections

SANJAY RAM ▶ PETER A. RICE

Gonorrhea, one of the "traditional" sexually transmitted diseases, remains a major public health problem worldwide. This disease has a significant impact on women, because of its devastating sequelae, infertility, ectopic pregnancy, and chronic pelvic pain. Although the incidence of gonorrhea has declined significantly in the United States, it remains a significant cause of morbidity in developing nations.

Gonorrhea is one of the oldest diseases known to humans, with references to this disease in the Old Testament and writings of the Chinese emperor Huang Ti (2637 BC), as well as in Hebrew, Egyptian, and Greek literature of antiquity. The term *gonorrhea* (*gonos*, meaning "seed"; *rhoea*, meaning "flow") was coined by Galen (AD 130). The organism was first identified by Albert Ludwig Siegmund Neisser in 1879 in stained smears of purulent exudates of urethritis, cervicitis, and ophthalmia neonatorum, and was subsequently cultivated in 1882 by Loeffler and Leistikow.

EPIDEMIOLOGY

Gonorrhea is one of the most commonly reported infectious disease in the United States. The number of reported cases probably represents half the true number of cases because of underreporting, self-treatment, and nonspecific treatment without culture-proven diagnosis. The number of reported cases of gonorrhea rose from approximately 250,000 in the early 1960s to a high of 1.01 million in 1978. The peak incidence of gonorrhea in modern times was 468 cases per 100,000 population, which occurred in 1975.[1] This was the result of the interaction between several variables, including improved accuracy of diagnosis, changes in patterns of contraceptive use, changes in sexual behavior (the "Sexual Revolution" of the 1960s). Following the availability of penicillin in the mid-1940s, the prevalence of gonorrhea declined. In 1957, however, the number of reported cases began increasing to its peak in 1978. The incidence of the disease has gradually declined since then except in 1985, when the total reported number of cases increased by 4% over the 1984 figure.

The highest incidence of gonorrhea is seen in developing countries. The exact incidence of sexually transmitted diseases (STDs) in developing countries is difficult to ascertain because of limited surveillance and variable diagnostic criteria. For example, in Kenya, it was estimated in 1987 that 10% of all live births were adversely affected by STDs, and gonococcal ophthalmia neonatorum affected 4% of all live births.[2] The median prevalence of gonorrhea in unselected populations of pregnant women has been estimated to be 10% in Africa, 5% in Latin America, and 4% in Asia.[2]

Gonorrhea predominantly affects young, nonwhite, unmarried, lesser educated, urban populations.[3] A recent study in inner London estimated the yearly incidence of gonorrhea at 138 cases per 100,000 women, with the highest incidence seen in young, ethnic minority groups. This rate was six times higher than the average incidence of the disease in England and Wales the preceding year.[4] In the United States, the highest attack rate occurs in the 20- to 24-year age group, which accounts for 75% of all cases.[1] When adjustment is made for the sexual experience of members of a population, the highest risk occurs in sexually active 15- to 19-year-old women.[5] Increasingly effective case-finding efforts in women have resulted in a decline in the male-to-female case ratio from 1.5 in 1981 to 1.3 in 1992.[1] The African-American–to–white incidence ratio rose from 12:1 in the early 1980s to 40:1 in the early 1990s.[1] The lowest rates have been observed in persons of Asian or Pacific Island ancestry.

Gonorrhea is more efficiently transmitted from males to females than the reverse, which may be because of anatomic factors. The risk that a male will acquire symptomatic infection during one act of intercourse with a chronically infected asymptomatic female is calculated to be about 20% per episode of vaginal intercourse, rising to 60% to 80% after four or more exposures.[6,7] The risk of male-to-female transmission has been less well studied; it is probably about 50% per contact, and reportedly rises to more than 90% after three exposures.[8] Oropharyngeal gonorrhea occurs in about 20% of women who practice fellatio with males with urethral infection. Transmission in either direction by cunnilingus is rare.[9]

The formula, $R_o = \beta cD$, describes the key parameters that influence the transmission of sexually transmitted diseases.[10] R_o represents the average number of secondary cases generated by one primary case in a susceptible population. R_o must be greater than 1 in order to sustain an epidemic within a population. β is the probability of transmitting infection; c is the mean rate of sexual partner change; and D is the duration of infectiousness. c is a measure of sexual behavior, while β and D depend on the biologic characteristics of the host and pathogen. There exists in any population a small minority of individuals who have high rates of new partner acquisition. They are termed *core-group members* or *high-frequency transmitters* and are vital in sustaining STD transmission at the population level. Although the concept of a core group has gained wide acceptance among STD epidemiology researchers, there is a lack of consensus on its precise definition. This term has been employed variously to refer to commercial sex workers,[11] persons who have very many sexual contacts,[12] census tracts that are sources of at least 50% of reported cases,[13] people repeatedly infected,[14] people who have high rates of acquisition of new partners,[15] smallest possible subpopulation so that removal of its members from the population would bring the basic reproductive rate of STD to less than 1.0,[16] people who, on average, generate more than one new case of infection,[17] drug-using prostitutes recurrently infected with STDs,[18] adolescent males in detention,[19] people with at least five sex partners per year,[20] and people with clusters of high-risk behaviors.[21] Based on all these definitions, a more effective definition has been developed, depending on whether the research perspective is mathematical, clinical-epidemiologic, or social-cultural.[22] An investigation into the geographic clustering of repeat cases of gonorrhea and chlamydial infection in San Francisco revealed that there were male and female core transmitters of gonococcal, but not chlamydial, infection.[23] Commercial sex workers and illicit intravenous drug users are often members of the core group. Another important factor that is instrumental in sustaining gonorrhea in the population is the large number of individuals who are asymptomatic, or have minor symptoms that are ignored.[24] These persons, unlike symptomatic individuals, do not cease sexual activity, and therefore continue to maintain transmission of the disease. This underscores the importance of contact-tracing and empirical treatment of sexual partners of index cases.

PATHOGENESIS

Neisseria gonorrhoeae is a gram-negative, nonmotile, non–spore-forming organism that grows in pairs (diplococci). Each individual organism is "coffee-bean" shaped, with concave sides facing each other. Gonococci, like all other *Neisseria* species, are oxidase positive. They are distinguished from other *Neisseria* by their ability to grow on selective media and to utilize only glucose, but not maltose, sucrose, or lactose.

The cell envelope of *N. gonorrhoeae* is similar to that of other gram-negative bacteria. The envelope is composed of three distinct layers: an inner cytoplasmic membrane, a middle peptidoglycan cell wall, and an outer membrane. The outer membrane is composed of phospholipid, lipo-oligosaccharide (LOS), and numerous proteins.

Fresh clinical isolates of *N. gonorrhoeae* initially form piliated colony types P^+ and P^{++} (formerly called T_1 and T_2), as seen during growth on translucent agar. P^- colonies (formerly T_3 and T_4) lack pili. Piliated strains show greater ability to adhere to cells derived from human mucosal surfaces[25] and increased virulence in organ culture models[26] and human inoculation experiments[27] when compared with nonpiliated variants. Pili are lost on repeated subcultures on nonselective media. Studies have shown that pili mediate gonococcal attachment to a variety of human cells, including spermatozoa, erythrocytes, buccal and vaginal epithelial cells, and amniotic cells, and also impede phagocytosis by polymorphonuclear leukocytes (PMNs).[28] In the fallopian tube model, pili mediate gonococcal attachment to nonciliated epithelial cells, which initiates phagocytosis and transport through these cells to intercellular spaces near the basement membrane or directly into the subepithelial tissue. This results in loss of cilia and sloughing of nearby ciliated cells.[26] Nonpiliated gonococci cause epithelial damage at a much slower rate. CD46 (membrane cofactor protein) has been determined to be the receptor for pilus.[29]

Another gonococcal surface protein that is important in adherence to epithelial cells is opacity protein (Opa) (formerly called protein II). Opa contributes to intergonococcal adhesion (which is responsible for the opaque nature of the colonies), and adherence to a variety of eukaryotic cells, including PMNs.[30–32] Certain Opa variants promote invasion of epithelial cells,[33, 34] and recently this has been linked with the ability of Opa to bind vitronectin.[35, 36] Opa proteins have also been shown to bind to several members of the carcinoembryonic antigen family (CD66).[30, 37, 38] Each strain of *N. gonorrhoeae* possesses as many as 11 different Opa genes, but usually only up to three types are expressed at any given time.[39] Isolates from normally sterile sites, such as fallopian tubes and synovial fluid, usually fail to express Opa, while isolates from other sites usually form opaque colonies.[40] Recently, it has been shown that female commercial sex workers with antibodies against Opa were less likely to develop pelvic inflammatory disease than were women without such antibodies.[41]

Porin (Por) (previously designated protein I) is the most abundant gonococcal surface protein, accounting for more than 50% of the total outer membrane protein. It provides anion aqueous channels through the otherwise hydrophobic outer membrane. Por shows stable interstrain antigenic variation and forms the basis for gonococcal serotyping.[42] Two main serotypes have been identified: Por 1A strains are often associated with disseminated gonococcal infection (DGI), while Por 1B strains usually cause local infections.[43, 44] DGI strains are usually resistant to the killing action of normal human serum, do not incite a significant inflammatory response, and therefore do not cause much genital symptomatology.

Another important gonococcal surface protein is Rmp (formerly called protein III), which is closely associated with Por and LOS. Rmp shows very little, if any, interstrain antigenic variation.[45] Antibody to Rmp ("blocking antibody") enhances susceptibility to gonococcal infection by reducing the bactericidal activity of normal human serum[46] and may potentiate re-infection after sexual exposure to an infected partner.[47]

Other outer membrane proteins include H.8, a lipoprotein present on all pathogenic neisserial species, the function of which has not been fully elucidated[48, 49]; transferrin-binding proteins (Tbp1 and Tbp2), which are required for scavenging iron from transferrin in vivo[50]; and IgA1 protease, which may protect the organism from the action of mucosal IgA.[51] Transferrin and iron have been shown to increase attachment of iron-deprived N. gonorrhoeae to human endometrial cells.[52]

Gonococcal LOS consists of a lipid A and a core oligosaccharide, which lacks the repeating O-antigenic side chain seen in other gram-negative bacteria.[53] LOS possesses marked endotoxic activity and contributes to the local cytotoxic effect in a fallopian tube explant model,[54] and to systemic manifestations of fever and toxicity in severe infections.[55] LOS core sugars undergo a high degree of antigenic variation in vitro and in vivo,[56] which may protect the organism from the bactericidal effect of naturally occurring anti-LOS antibodies in normal human serum. Many serum-sensitive strains of N. gonorrhoeae are capable of sialylating their LOS in vivo and in vitro, which converts them to a serum-resistant phenotype.[57–68] This may be explained by the ability of surface sialic acid to bind factor H and down-regulate the alternative complement pathway.[69] LOS sialylation may also mask bactericidal antibody-binding epitopes on LOS and Por,[70] as well as decrease opsonophagocytosis[71] and inhibit the oxidative burst in PMNs.[72]

ANTIMICROBIAL RESISTANCE IN *NEISSERIA GONORRHOEAE*

It is no surprise that *N. gonorrhoeae*, with its remarkable capacity to alter its antigenic structure and adapt to changes in the microenvironment, has become resistant to antibiotics that have been used to treat gonorrhea. The first effective treatment for gonorrhea was sulfonamides, which were introduced in the 1930s. Within a decade of their use, antibiotic resistance emerged, resulting in treatment failures in a third of patients. Penicillin was then employed as the drug of choice for the treatment of gonorrhea. By 1965, 42% of gonococcal isolates were resistant to penicillin G.[73] This resistance was because of an increase in the minimal inhibitory concentration (MIC) to penicillin, and led to the Centers for Disease Control and Prevention (CDC) recommendation of doubling the dose of penicillin for the treatment of gonorrhea from 1.2 million units of benzathine penicillin to 2.4 million units. Resistance due to the production of penicillinase arose later.

Gonococci become resistant to antibiotics either by (1) chromosomal mutations or (2) acquisition of R plasmids. Two types of chromosomal mutations have been described. The first, which is drug specific, is due to a single-step mutation leading to high-level resistance. The second type involves mutations at several chromosomal loci, the combination of which determines the level as well as the pattern of resistance. Strains with mutations in chromosomal genes were first observed in the late 1950s.[74]

Penicillinase-producing *N. gonorrhoeae* (PPNG) carrying plasmids with the Pc[r] determinant were seen almost simultaneously in the United States, England,[75, 76] as well as in western Africa and the Philippines.[77] Since then, PPNG has spread worldwide,[78–81] and it accounted for more than 50% of all gonococcal isolates in some parts of the developing world by the early 1980s. The average incidence of PPNG in the United States is on the order of 10%, with higher rates seen in certain areas.[1, 82]

Tetracycline-resistant *N. gonorrhoeae* (TRNG) was first reported in the United States in 1985.[83, 84] Within 2 years, TRNG had spread to virtually all parts of the United States[82, 85] as well as to parts of Europe.[86, 87] In 1992, about 6% of all gonococcal strains were reported to be resistant to tetracycline.[1]

The prevalence of gonococci with chromosome-mediated resistance has risen steadily in most parts of the world. Changes in the prevalence of chromosomally mediated resistance were associated with changes in treatment regimens,[88, 89] but not with changes in the rate of gonococcal disease.[90]

Spectinomycin resistance in *N. gonorrhoeae* was first reported in 1973,[91] and the first spectinomycin-resistant PPNG was seen in 1981.[92] Resistance to spectinomycin is usually not associated with resistance to other antibiotics; therefore, this drug can be reserved for treating multiresistant strains of *N. gonorrhoeae*. However, outbreaks caused by strains resistant to spectinomycin were observed in Korea[93] and England,[94] where the drug was used as the primary agent for treating gonorrhea.

Quinolone-resistant *N. gonorrhoeae* (QRNG) appeared soon after these agents were used to treat gonorrhea[95, 96] and have now been seen in the U.S. Even though the serum concentrations achieved by therapeutic dosages of these agents is about 100-fold more than the minimal inhibitory concentration (MIC) for *N. gonorrhoeae*, recent reports describe resistance to this class of antibiotics.[97–104] Alterations in DNA gyrase and topoisomerase IV have been implicated as mechanisms of fluoroquinolone resistance.[99] These reports underline the importance of constant monitoring for quinolone resistance in order to maximize the time during which quinolones may be used to treat gonorrhea. The CDC's Gonococcal Isolate Surveillance Project (GISP) detected quinolone resistance in only 0.05% of more than 4,500 isolates from 26 cities in the U.S. Quinolones may be used as therapy for gonorrhea as long as quinolone-resistant strains constitute less than 1% of all *N. gonorrhoeae*, in each of the cities.[105]

Resistance to azithromycin, which has recently been shown to be effective in the treatment of uncomplicated gonococcal infections,[106] has also been reported.[107, 108] Third-generation cephalosporins have remained highly effective as single-dose therapy for gonorrhea. Even though the MICs of ceftriaxone for certain strains may range as high as from 0.015 to 0.125 mg/L (higher than for fully susceptible strains [0.0001 to 0.008 mg/L]), nevertheless these levels are greatly exceeded in serum (and the urethra and cervix) by the routinely recommended ceftriaxone and cefixime regimens. These almost always result in an effective cure.[82, 109]

GONOCOCCAL CERVICITIS

Mucopurulent cervicitis is the most common STD diagnosis in U.S. women. Cervicitis may coexist with candidal or trichomonal vaginitis. In the absence of vaginitis, cervicitis is usually caused by *N. gonorrhoeae*, *Chlamydia trachomatis*, herpes simplex, or combinations of these microorganisms. In the U.S., *C. trachomatis* is the most common cause of cervicitis. Gonorrhea primarily infects mucosal surfaces lined with columnar or cuboidal epithelium, and therefore it does not infect the vaginal mucosa (which is lined by stratified squamous epithelium), except in rare instances (see later).

Clinical Features and Diagnosis

Most women infected with *N. gonorrhoeae* develop symptoms, but many remain asymptomatic or complain only of minor symptoms,[110] which may delay their seeking medical attention. Increased vaginal discharge and dysuria (often without urgency or frequency) are the most common symptoms. Although the incubation period of gonorrhea is less well defined in women than in men, symptoms usually develop within 10 days of infection[111] and are more acute and intense than those of chlamydial infection. In some cases, infection may extend deep enough to produce dyspareunia and lower abdominal or back pain. In such women, it is imperative to rule out pelvic inflammatory disease.

The physical examination often reveals a mucopurulent discharge (mucopus) from the cervical os. The examiner may check for mucopurulent discharge by swabbing a sample of mucus from the endocervix and observing its color against the white background of the swab; yellow or green mucus suggests mucopus. Edematous and friable cervical ectopy, and endocervical bleeding induced by gentle swabbing, are signs more often seen in chlamydial infection. Purulent discharge sometimes can be expressed from the urethra or Bartholin's glands. Only 35% of women with gonococcal cervicitis have a mucopurulent discharge according to the aforementioned criteria. Therefore, the diagnosis must be made by Gram stain and culture.

Samples should be collected with Dacron or rayon swabs. Cotton swabs may also be used, but some brands of cotton may contain fatty acids that may inhibit the growth of gonococci. Calcium alginate swabs should not be used, as they may be toxic to gonococci.[112] A thin film of mucus should be rolled onto a slide for a Gram stain examination of the PMNs. Instructions for performing a Gram stain are as follows: (1) flood the slide with gentian violet for 5 seconds and rinse thoroughly with cold water; (2) flood the slide with Gram's iodine for 5 seconds, and rinse with cold water; (3) flood the slide with 95% alcohol for about 10 seconds (or until the blue color begins to wash out), and rinse with cold water; and (4) flood the slide with basic fuchsin or safranin, allow to sit for 30 seconds, and rinse with cold water. Dry the slide completely by patting it with a paper towel or by letting it air-dry. The remaining sample should be transferred onto a modified Thayer-Martin plate for culture. This medium contains antibiotics (vancomycin, colistin, nystatin, and trimethoprim lactate) to prevent overgrowth of hardier and less fastidious saprophytes. Other selective media used include Martin-Lewis medium and GC-Lect medium. Non–choclate agar–based selective media, such as New York City medium, are also available but are not commonly used. Vancomycin may inhibit the growth of some gonococcal strains[113] and, in some cases, may impair the diagnosis of gonorrhea. It is important to process all patient samples immediately, because gonococci do not tolerate drying. If plates cannot be incubated immediately, they can be safely held for several hours at room temperature in candle extinction jars prior to incubation. If facilities for immediate inoculation into growth medium are not available, transport may be facilitated by the use of non-nutritive swab transport systems, such as Stuart's or Amie's medium, if processing is to occur within 6 hours. The recovery of *N. gonorrhoeae* from modified

Stuart's medium drops to 60% in 24 hours and to 27% after 48 hours. For longer holding periods, such as with specimen cultures that are to be mailed, culture media with self-contained CO_2-generating systems such as the JEMBEC or Gono-Pak systems may be used. Because proper preparation of the transport system cannot be guaranteed—resulting in the possibility that the appropriate concentration of CO_2 will not have been maintained—reincubation of the specimen for an additional 24 to 48 hours at 37°C in a 5% CO_2 incubator in the reference laboratory is obligatory. If *Chlamydia* diagnostic facilities are available, a second Dacron or cotton-tipped swab should be obtained, with the clinician being particularly careful to roll the swab against the walls of the endocervix to obtain sloughing cells that harbor chlamydiae.

PMNs are normally present in the endocervix,[114] but an abnormally increased number (20 or more PMNs per field in five 1000× oil-immersion fields) establishes the presence of an inflammatory discharge. Gram-negative intracelluar diplococci (GNID) are usually highly specific (100%), although not very sensitive (50%), in diagnosing gonococcal cervicitis. Gram-stained smears that show only extracellular gram-negative diplococci, or atypical gram-negative organisms, within PMNs are considered equivocal. Owing to the lack of sensitivity, it is advisable that only laboratories in STD clinics perform Gram stains of endocervical specimens. Nonpathogenic neisseriae, overdecolorized gram-positive cocci, anaerobic cocci, and gram-negative coccobacilli that are often found in the lower female genital tract may appear adherent or within leukocytes and may lead to a serious misdiagnosis of gonorrhea. Therefore, the diagnosis in females in this setting should be made by culture. The sensitivity of a single endocervical culture is about 80% to 90%, depending on the quality of the medium and the adequacy of the clinical specimen. The yield can be enhanced by taking a second cervical specimen for culture. If a history of rectal sex is elicited, a rectal specimen for culture should be obtained. The rectal swab should not be contaminated with fecal material, which will markedly diminish the yield of *N. gonorrhoeae*.

The nucleic acid probe test is now widely used for the direct detection of *N. gonorrhoeae* in urogenital specimens. The PACE (Probe Assay-Chemiluminescence Enhanced) System (Gen-Probe, San Diego, CA) for *N. gonorrhoeae* is a nonisotopic chemiluminescent DNA probe that hybridizes specifically with gonococcal 16s rRNA gene. Specimens are placed in a transport/lysing solution and then are mixed with the acridinium ester–linked probe. Hybridized probe is then separated from nonhybridized material. The acridinium ester–labeled probe–rRNA complex is then assayed in a semiautomated chemiluminometer by the addition of alkaline hydrogen peroxide solution, which causes a release of light resulting from disruption of the ester linkage of the probe label. In a study of 209 male urethral and 203 female endocervical specimens, this test had an overall sensitivity and specificity of 90% and 99.4%, respectively, when compared with culture.[115] In that study, the sensitivity was greater for male urethral specimens (95%) than for female endocervical specimens (86%). The predictive value of a positive PACE result was 98%, while the predictive value of a negative result was 97%. These predictive values may not be adequate in low prevalence populations. Recent studies assessing the utility of the PACE system in outpatients undergoing routine screening for STDs concluded that it was at least as sensitive as conventional culture techniques[116] and may provide a cost-effective alternative to culture, especially in high-risk males.[117] Although this test has not been approved for use in extragenital sites, a recent study found that the PACE assay performed as well as culture, when tested on pharyngeal and rectal specimens from homosexual men.[118] A possible disadvantage of the PACE assay is that specimens submitted in probe-transported fluids cannot be cultured subsequently. Therefore, a confirmatory test is not possible, and antimicrobial susceptibility testing, if needed, may be limited.

Other diagnostic methods include enzyme immunoassays (Gonozyme) with polyclonal antigonococcal antibodies, fluorescein-conjugated monoclonal antibodies for direct fluorescence microscopy, and DNA amplification tests. These tests are most useful when facilities for culture and rapid processing of clinical specimens are not readily available. The DNA amplification techniques may prove to be equivalent or more sensitive than culture methods. All other nonculture methods have sensitivities less than that of isolation, especially for endocervical specimens.

Treatment

Approximately 35% to 50% of women infected with *N. gonorrhoeae* are co-infected with *C. trachomatis*.[119–121] This has led to the recommendation that persons treated for gonococcal infection routinely should be treated with a regimen effective against genital *C. trachomatis* infection. Routine dual therapy can be cost-effective in areas where the rate of chlamydial co-infection exceeds 20% to 40%, because the cost of treating *C. trachomatis* infection is far less than the cost of testing. The recommended treatment regimens for uncomplicated gonococcal infections of the cervix, urethra, and rectum are listed in Table 39–1. The treatment regimen chosen should take into account patient preference, drug allergies, presumed patient compliance, and cost. Alternative treatment regimens for patients unable to tolerate the recommended regimens are also outlined in Table 39–1 and include (1) spectinomycin; (2) single-dose cephalosporins (other than ceftriaxone and

TABLE 39-1 ▶ TREATMENT REGIMENS FOR UNCOMPLICATED GONOCOCCAL INFECTION IN ADULTS

Recommended Regimens

Cefixime, 400 mg PO as a single dose, *OR* ceftriaxone, 125 mg IM as a single dose

Ciprofloxacin, 500 mg PO as a single dose, *OR* ofloxacin, 400 mg PO as a single dose

PLUS

Azithromycin, 1 g PO as a single dose, *OR* doxycycline, 100 mg PO twice daily for 7 days

Alternative Regimens

Spectinomycin, 2 g IM in a single dose

Single-dose cephalosporin regimens other than ceftriaxone and cefixime. These include the following:

    ceftizoxime, 500 mg IM

    cefotaxime, 500 mg IM

    cefotetan, 1 g IM

    cefoxitin, 2 g IM with probenecid 1 g PO

Single-dose oral quinolone regimens other than ciprofloxacin and ofloxacin. These include the following: enoxacin, 400 mg, lomefloxacin, 400 mg, and norfloxacin, 800 mg.

cefixime) administered intramuscularly; and (3) single-dose, oral quinolones other than ciprofloxacin and ofloxacin. Spectinomycin has demonstrated a cure rate of 98.2% in clinical trials, and it remains useful in patients who cannot tolerate cephalosporins or quinolones. None of the other alternative regimens have been extensively studied, and the data obtained thus far do not suggest any advantage over the recommended regimens. Azithromycin, as a single dose of 2 g PO, has proved to be efficacious in uncomplicated gonococcal infections, but it is expensive and is not well tolerated. About a third of patients treated with this regimen experience gastrointestinal side effects. Azithromycin, at a dose of 1 g PO, results in an unacceptably low cure rate (93% to 95%).[122–124]

Women with uncomplicated gonococcal infections, who have been treated with one of the recommended regimens, need not return for a test-of-cure. Persistent symptoms should be evaluated with a repeat culture for *N. gonorrhoeae*, and any organism isolated should be tested for antimicrobial susceptibility. Treatment failures with one of the established regimens are uncommon, and usually represent re-infection or infection caused by another organism distinct from *N. gonorrhoeae*.

Patients should be instructed to refer sex partners for evaluation and treatment. All sex partners of women who have been diagnosed with gonorrhea should be presumptively treated for gonorrhea and *Chlamydia* infection, if their last sexual contact with the patient was within 60 days of the onset of the patient's symptoms or diagnosis. If the patient's last sexual intercourse was more than 60 days prior to the onset of symptoms or diagnosis, the most recent sex partner should be treated. Patients should be advised to avoid sexual intercourse until therapy is completed, and un-

til the patient and her partner or partners are asymptomatic.

GONOCOCCAL VAGINITIS

Vulvovaginal candidiasis, bacterial vaginosis, and trichomonal vaginitis are the most common vaginal infections. Gonococcal vaginitis is a rare entity, except in children and postmenopausal women, because the stratified squamous vaginal epithelium in normal adults protects against infection by *N. gonorrhoeae*. During pregnancy, the vaginal epithelium is altered and may be susceptible to infection with *N. gonorrhoeae*, resulting in symptomatic vaginitis.

Clinical Features and Management

The intense inflammation of the vagina makes the physical (speculum and bimanual) examination extremely painful. The vaginal mucosa is red and edematous, and an abundant purulent discharge is present. The urethra and Skene's and Bartholin's glands are often involved. Inflamed cervical erosion or abscesses in nabothian cysts may occur. Coexisting cervicitis may result in pus in the cervical os. The diagnostic tests for, and treatment of, gonococcal vaginitis are the same as those described for cervicitis.

ANORECTAL GONORRHEA

Approximately 40% of women with uncomplicated cervical gonorrhea have positive rectal cultures for *N. gonorrhoeae*. The rectum is the sole site of infection in only 5% of women with gonorrhea. Most women are asymptomatic, but occasionally they may have acute proctitis manifested by anorectal pain or pruritus, tenesmus, purulent rectal discharge, and rectal bleeding. A mucopurulent exudate and inflammatory changes of the rectal mucosa may be seen on anoscopy. Gram smear of anorectal secretions often reveals PMNs. If any of these signs are present, the patient should be treated with ceftriaxone and doxycycline, as described for cervicitis, pending the results of further laboratory tests. Sexual contacts of the index case should be evaluated and treated.

PHARYNGEAL GONORRHEA

The incidence of gonococcal pharyngitis has increased over the past few years. Most cases of pharyngeal gonorrhea are mild or asymptomatic,[9] although the occasional case of symptomatic pharyngitis with cervical lymphadenitis is seen.[125] The mode of acquisition is orogenital sexual exposure, with fellatio being a more efficient means of transmission than cunnilingus.[9] About 10% to 20% of women with gonorrhea have pharyngeal infection, in contrast to only 3% to 7% of heterosexual men with gonorrhea.[9, 126] There is no concrete evidence that pharyngeal gonorrhea predisposes to disseminated infection.

Most cases resolve spontaneously, and transmission from the pharynx to other patients is rare. Pharyngeal infection almost always coexists with genital infection. Swabs from the pharynx should be plated directly onto gonococcal selective media. The diagnosis of pharyngeal gonorrhea is more expensive and difficult to make than anogenital gonorrhea, and the benign nature of the disease has led some experts to doubt the importance of documenting the diagnosis. In fact, most STD clinics with limited resources do not routinely perform throat cultures in patients with suspected pharyngeal gonorrhea, unless symptoms are present. Symptomatic gonococcal pharyngitis is more difficult to eradicate than is genital infection. Few regimens result in cure rates of more than 90%. Chlamydial coinfection of the pharynx is uncommon, but it may occur at other genital sites in conjunction with gonorrhea. Therefore, the treatment regimen should also include treatment for chlamydial infection. The recommended regimen is ceftriaxone, ciprofloxacin, or ofloxacin, plus either azithromycin, 1 g PO in a single dose, or doxycycline, 100 mg PO twice daily for 7 days. The dosages of the drugs are indicated in Table 39–1. Persons who cannot tolerate cephalosporins or quinolones can be treated with spectinomycin, but this results in a cure rate of only 52% or less.[127-131] Therefore, persons treated with this agent should have a pharyngeal culture performed 3 to 5 days after treatment as a test-of-cure.

OCULAR GONORRHEA IN THE ADULT

Ocular gonorrhea in the adult usually results from autoinoculation from an infected genital site. The manifestations range from severe disease to occasionally mild or asymptomatic disease, similar to that in genital infection. The variability in clinical manifestations may result from differences in the ability of the infecting strain to elicit an inflammatory response.[132]

Infection may result in a markedly swollen eyelid, severe hyperemia and chemosis, and a profuse purulent discharge. The massively inflamed conjunctiva may be draped over the cornea and limbus. Lytic enzymes from the infiltrating PMNs have been known to cause corneal ulceration, with subsequent perforation.

Prompt recognition and treatment of this condition is of paramount importance. Gram stain and culture of the purulent discharge establish the diagnosis. Genital cultures should also be performed. The treatment of this condition is based on the results of a single North American study that has been published in recent years.[133] In that study, all 13 patients responded favorably to a single dose of ceftriaxone, 1 g IM. Sex partners should be evaluated and treated as described previously.

PELVIC INFLAMMATORY DISEASE

Pelvic inflammatory disease and its sequelae, infertility, ectopic pregnancy, and chronic pelvic pain, is the most serious manifestation of gonorrhea in women. This disease has been discussed in a separate chapter.

DISSEMINATED GONOCOCCAL INFECTION

Disseminated gonococcal infection (DGI) results from gonococcal bacteremia and, in the 1970s, occurred in about 0.5% to 3% of persons with untreated mucosal infection.[134-138] However, the incidence at the present time seems to be falling, probably because of a decline in the prevalence of strains likely to disseminate.[139, 140] DGI occurs more commonly in women, probably because of the higher frequency of asymptomatic infection in this population.[134, 136] DGI has also been reported following asymptomatic infection of an intrauterine device (IUD).[141] Menstruation and pregnancy were associated with DGI in 22 of 31 (71%) of the women in one study.[136] In about half of the affected women, symptoms of DGI began within 7 days of the onset of menses.[134-137] Several factors may be responsible for this, including (1) maximal shedding of organisms during menstruation; (2) change in vaginal flora, particularly an increase in lactobacilli just prior to menses, which may stimulate the growth of gonococci; (3) increased alkalinity of secretions, which promotes growth of the normally acid-sensitive gonococci, as well as decreases the effectiveness of the peroxidase-mediated bactericidal system; and (4) diminished levels of progesterone (which inhibits gonococcal growth) during menses (this is, however, not applicable during pregnancy). Pharyngeal gonorrhea has been suggested as a risk factor for the development of DGI,[142] but this has not been substantiated. Complement deficiencies, especially the components involved in the assembly of the membrane attack complex (C5 through C9), predispose to neisserial bacteremia.[143-146] As many as 13% of patients with DGI have complement deficiencies, and persons with more than one episode of DGI should be screened with an assay for total hemolytic complement activity.

Certain organism characteristics are associated with the ability to cause disseminated disease. Strains that cause DGI often are resistant to the bactericidal action of nonimmune normal human serum, are usually of the transparent colony phenotype, require arginine, hypoxanthine, and uracil (AHU⁻ auxotype), belong to the Por 1A serogroup, and are markedly susceptible to penicillin.[139, 140] However, PPNG and strains with chromosomally mediated antibiotic resistance have also been reported to cause DGI.[140, 147–150] A decrease in the prevalence of Por 1A serotype/AHU⁻ auxotype strains has resulted in fewer cases of DGI overall and a greater proportion of DGI cases caused by other strains.[135, 140, 150, 151]

The clinical manifestations of DGI have sometimes been classified into two stages: an initial bacteremic phase, followed by a joint-localized stage of suppurative arthritis.[136, 152] Patients with the bacteremic phase may present earlier, and have higher temperatures than those of patients with the joint localized stage, accompanied more frequently by chills, tenosynovitis, and skin lesions. It has been proposed, therefore, that the bacteremic phase, when untreated, evolves into a joint-localized disease.[29, 136, 152] However, the utility and accuracy of clinical characterization of sequential stages of DGI has been questioned, because others have described similar features in patients with either positive blood or positive synovial fluid cultures.[153–155] Some authors have suggested that a transition state accounts for patients with clinical manifestations of both bacteremia and joint-localized disease.[156]

The early clinical manifestations of DGI include chills, fever, migratory polyarthralgias, metastatic skin lesions, and tenosynovitis. The joints primarily involved are the knees, elbows, and the more distal joints; the axial skeleton is usually spared. The skin lesions are seen in about 75% of patients and include papules and pustules, often with a hemorrhagic component. Rarely, hemorrhagic bullae and necrotic lesions resembling ecthyma gangrenosum are seen. These lesions are usually seen on the extremities, and number between 5 and 40.[134–137] If untreated, arthritis may subsequently develop in one or two joints and usually involves the knees, wrists, ankles, and elbows, in decreasing order of frequency. Other joints, such as the small joints of the hands and feet, and the sternoclavicular and temporomandibular joints, may be involved. This represents the septic joint phase of the disease. Some patients may develop septic arthritis without prior polyarthritis or dermatitis,[134–137] and in the absence of symptomatic genital infection cannot be distinguished from septic arthritis caused by other pathogens. However, the two phases of the disease may overlap. Rarely, osteomyelitis may complicate septic arthritis.[152, 157–161]

Although it has been postulated that the initial arthritis and skin lesions are due to direct tissue invasion by *N. gonorrhoeae*,[162] the organism has been recovered in fewer than 5% of skin lesions cultured.[134, 163, 164] This has been attributed to either a small inoculum of infecting organisms or to the fastidious growth requirement of *N. gonorrhoeae*.[162, 165] In one study, gonococcal antigens were identified in 14 of 16 "sterile" skin lesions by immunofluorescence staining techniques.[153] There is also evidence that immune-mediated or hypersensitivity phenomena caused by gonococcal antigens

may account for the skin lesions.[166, 167] Histopathologic descriptions of these skin lesions often reveal changes consistent with a polymorphonuclear vasculitis similar to that seen in a Shwartzman reaction,[168] or erythema nodosum.[134] Other manifestations of noninfectious dermatitis, such as urticaria and erythema multiforme, have also been described.[96, 163, 169] However, a study of immune complexes in patients with DGI failed to identify any circulating immune complexes in the pathogenesis of the arthritis-dermatitis syndrome.[170]

Until 1942, gonococcal endocarditis was relatively common, causing as many as 26% of reported cases of endocarditis.[171] Native pulmonary,[172] aortic,[173] and mitral[174] valve involvement has been described. Another unusual complication of DGI is meningitis. Only 20 cases were reported in the literature between 1922 and 1972,[136, 175] with two additional cases reported in Pennsylvania within a 1-month period in 1984.[176] An interesting case of gonococcal meningitis occurring 15 years after urethral infection, thought to be the result of chronic prostatitis, has also been reported.[177]

The CDC recommendations for the treatment of DGIs are outlined in Table 39–2.

GONORRHEA IN PREGNANT WOMEN AND THE NEWBORN

Gonorrhea in the pregnancy can have serious consequences for both the mother and the infant. Therefore, efforts to detect and eradicate the disease early in the mother are extremely important. The incidence of pregnant women with gonorrhea ranges from rare to about 10%, depending on the population surveyed. Two local factors may play a role in decreasing the risk of ascending gonococcal infection during pregnancy: the relatively impermeable cervical mucus under the

---

TABLE 39–2 ▶ TREATMENT OF DISSEMINATED GONOCOCCAL INFECTION

Recommended Initial Regimen
Ceftriaxone, 1 g IM or IV q24h

Alternative Initial Regimens
Cefotaxime, 1 g IV q8h, *OR* ceftizoxime, 1 g IV q8h, *OR*

For Persons Allergic to Beta-lactam Drugs
Ciprofloxacin, 500 mg IV q12h, *OR* ofloxacin, 400 mg IV q12h, *OR* spectinomycin, 2 g IM q12h

All regimens should be continued for 24–48 h after clinical improvement begins, at which time therapy may be switched to one of the following regimens to complete a full week of antimicrobial therapy:
Cefixime, 400 mg PO twice daily, *OR* ciprofloxacin, 500 mg PO twice daily, *OR* ofloxacin, 400 mg PO twice daily

Gonococcal meningitis and endocarditis should be treated with ceftriaxone, 1 to 2 g IV q12h. Therapy for meningitis should be continued for 10–14 days; therapy for endocarditis should be continued for at least 4 wk. Consultation with an expert should be considered.

influence of progesterone, that may provide a barrier against microorganisms,[178] and obliteration of the intrauterine cavity resulting from the attachment of the chorion to the endometrial decidua by around the twelfth week of gestation. Recognition of gonorrhea early in pregnancy identifies an at-risk population that should be followed closely throughout pregnancy.[179] The clinical spectrum of infection is similar to that seen in nonpregnant women. Pharyngeal infection may be more common during pregnancy because of altered sexual practices. One study reported that 39% of pregnant women with gonorrhea at any site had pharyngeal infection and 30% had pharyngeal involvement as the only disease manifestation.[180] Most women with pharyngeal infection tend to be asymptomatic.

Salpingitis and pelvic inflammatory disease that occurs during the first trimester is associated with a high rate of fetal loss.[181] Acquisition of infection later during the pregnancy can adversely affect labor and delivery as well as the well-being of the fetus. Prolonged rupture of the membranes, premature delivery, chorioamnionitis, funisitis, and sepsis in the infant with *N. gonorrhoeae* detected in the gastric aspirate during delivery all are complications that occur commonly with maternal gonococcal infection.[69, 182–185] Hazards to the fetus include abortion (2% to 35%), perinatal death (2% to 11%), prematurity (17% to 67%), perinatal distress (5% to 10%), and premature rupture of membranes (21% to 75%).[183, 184, 186–189] These studies provided little or no information on the role of potentially co-infecting microorganisms, such as *Mycoplasma hominis*, *Ureaplasma urealyticum*, *C. trachomatis*, and bacterial vaginosis, which have been associated with the same complications.[190–193]

The most common form of gonorrhea in infants is gonococcal ophthalmia neonatorum. This results from exposure to infected cervical secretions during parturition. Transmission rates of about 2% to 48% have been reported in exposed infants who had no ocular prophylaxis[194–196] and in 0% to 9.6% of exposed infants who received silver nitrate prophylaxis.[184, 197–199] An increased incidence of gonococcal ophthalmia has been observed in infants of mothers of lower socioeconomic status, unwed mothers, and mothers who had not had prenatal care.[200] Other risk factors for the acquisition of gonococcal ophthalmia include prior treatment of gonorrhea during pregnancy[179] and premature rupture of the membranes.

The clinical manifestations of ophthalmia neonatorum are acute and begin 2 to 5 days afte birth. In some cases, the initial course is indolent, and the incubation period can be longer than 5 days.[199, 201, 202] This may be related to a low inoculum of organisms, lower virulence of the infecting strain, or partial suppression by ophthalmic prophylaxis. Therefore, gonococcal infection must be ruled out in every case of conjunctivitis in infants. An initial nonspecific conjunctivitis with a serosanguineous discharge is followed by tense edema of both lids, chemosis, and a profuse, thick, purulent discharge. Corneal ulcerations that result in nebulae or perforation may lead to anterior synechiae, anterior staphyloma, panophthalmitis, and blindness. The diagnosis should be confirmed by culture, because other organisms that can cause conjunctivitis in the newborn, such as *Moraxella catarrhalis* and other *Neisseria* species, are indistinguishable by Gram stain alone. Infections at other mucosal sites in infants have been described and include vaginitis,[203–205] rhinitis,[206] and anorectal infection.[195] Most infants with infection at these sites are likely to be asymptomatic. Pharyngeal colonization has been demonstrated in 35% of cases of infants with gonococcal ophthalmia, and coughing was the most prominent symptom in these cases.[207] *Neisseria gonorrhoeae* has been recovered from orogastric fluid in 26% to 40% of infants born to infected mothers.[182, 184] Scalp abscesses have been reported in infants with intrauterine fetal monitoring.[208–211] Septic arthritis is the most common manifestation of systemic gonococcal infection in the newborn. The primary focus of infection in most of these cases in uncertain.[212] The onset is usually between 3 and 21 days of age, and polyarticular involvement is common.[213] Rarely, sepsis, meningitis,[214] and pneumonia may be seen.

Pregnant women should be treated with a recommended or alternative cephalosporin. Spectinomycin should be administered to women who cannot tolerate cephalosporins. Quinolones and tetracyclines are contraindicated during pregnancy. Prophylaxis for gonococcal ophthalmia is accomplished mainly through local instillation of 1% silver nitrate (the Credé procedure) or one of several antimicrobial agents (except bacitracin ointment, which is ineffective, and penicillin, which can lead to hypersensitivity reactions). The CDC recommend the use of silver nitrate (1%) aqueous solution, or erythromycin (0.5%) ophthalmic ointment, or tetracycline (1%) ophthalmic ointment, all as a single application.[105] Povidone-iodine (2.5%) was shown to be more effective, less toxic, and less expensive compared with silver nitrate and erythromycin.[215] The CDC recommendation[105] for the treatment of infants with gonococcal ophthalmia is ceftriaxone (Table 39–3). Topical antibiotic therapy alone is inadequate and unnecessary if systemic therapy is given. Disseminated infections in the newborn are treated with either ceftriaxone or cefotaxime. Infants born to mothers who have untreated gonococcal infection are at high risk for infection and should be prophylactically treated with ceftriaxone even in the absence of signs of infection. The CDC guidelines[105] for treatment of these conditions are outlined in Table 39–3. Concomitant chlamydial infection in the mother and the infant should be ruled out.

TABLE 39-3 ▶ TREATMENT OF GONOCOCCAL INFECTIONS IN INFANTS AND CHILDREN

Ophthalmia Neonatorum
Ceftriaxone, 25–50 mg/kg IV or IM, not to exceed 125 mg in a single dose
Disseminated Gonococcal Infection and Gonococcal Scalp Abscess in Newborns
Ceftriaxone, 25–50 mg/kg/day IV or IM in a single daily dose for 7 days, OR cefotaxime, 25 mg/kg IV or IM q12h for 7 days (or 10–14 days if meningitis is documented)
Prophylactic Treatment for Infants Whose Mothers Have Gonococcal Infection
Ceftriaxone, 25–50 mg/kg IV or IM, not to exceed 125 mg in a single dose
Uncomplicated Gonococcal Infections in Children
Recommended Regimen
Children who weigh ≥45 kg: treat as adults (see Table 39–1) (quinolones not approved for pediatric use)
Children who weigh <45 kg: ceftriaxone, 125 mg IM in a single dose
Alternative Regimen
Spectinomycin, 40 mg/kg (maximum dose: 2 g) IM in a single dose. Cefixime may be used orally, but no published data exist on safety and effectiveness for this purpose.
Bacteremia or Arthritis in Children
Children who weigh ≥45 kg: ceftriaxone, 50 mg/kg (maximum dose: 2 g) IM or IV in a single dose daily for 10–14 days
Children who weigh <45 kg: ceftriaxone, 50 mg/kg (maximum dose: 1 g) IM or IV in a single dose daily for 10–14 days

---

GONORRHEA IN CHILDREN AND ADOLESCENTS

Any STD in children beyond the neonatal period should always raise the possibility of sexual abuse, until proven otherwise. Rates of STDs in sexually abused children have been reported to be between 5% and 20%.[216–219] Gonorrhea was the most frequently recognized disease when that disease was highly prevalent in the general population. About 80% to 90% of abused children are female, with mean ages of 7 to 8 years.[220] Most have been abused by a male assailant known to the child. Vaginal penetration occurs in about half, and anal penetration in about a third of female victims.

Gonococcal vulvovaginitis is the commonest manifestation of gonococcal infection in children beyond infancy. The anestrogenic alkaline milieu of the vaginal mucosa of prepubertal females predisposes to colonization and infection by *N. gonorrhoeae*. Children usually are symptomatic, although mild or asymptomatic disease rarely may be seen. The acute phase of infection is characterized by inflammation and profuse purulent discharge. The child may complain of dysuria, vulvar discomfort, frequent urination, and pain on walking. Systemic symptoms are usually absent. Examination reveals an edematous and hyperemic vulvar tissue that is often covered by a profuse, thick, yellowish discharge from the vagina. The vaginal mucosa is also acutely inflamed, but the urethra and Bartholin's and Skene's glands are rarely involved. The upper genital tract is rarely, if ever, affected. Anorectal and pharyngeal infection are common and frequently asympto-

matic. If the infection goes untreated, the acute phase lasts for a few weeks, which then gives way to a chronic phase that is characterized by a scanty and seropurulent discharge. The vulvar and vaginal tissues may remain hyperemic and macerated.

The clinician must make the diagnosis of gonococcal infection in children using only standard culture systems because of the legal implications.[105] Nonculture tests for gonococcal infection, such as DNA probes, Gram stain, and enzyme immunoassays should not be used alone, and they have not been approved by the U.S. Food and Drug Administration (FDA) for use with specimens obtained from the genital tract, pharynx, and rectum of infected children. Cultures should be obtained from the pharynx and anus in both girls and boys. Cervical specimens are not recommended for prepubertal girls. Presumptive isolates of *N. gonorrhoeae* should be identified definitively by at least two independent methods (e.g., biochemical, enzyme substrate, or serologic). The CDC recommendations[105] for the treatment of gonococcal infections in children are outlined in Table 39–3. Quinolones are not approved for use in children because of concerns of toxicity in animal studies, but the use of ciprofloxacin in children with cystic fibrosis has not resulted in adverse effects. Follow-up cultures usually are not necessary if ceftriaxone is used. Spectinomycin is not as effective in treating gonococcal pharyngitis; thus, a follow-up would be indicated if this drug had been used. All children should also be evaluated for *Chlamydia* infection and syphilis. All cases of suspected and confirmed child abuse should be reported to the social services office of the county in which the child resides.

GONOCOCCAL INFECTION IN THE HIV-INFECTED FEMALE

The association between gonorrhea and the acquisition of HIV has been demonstrated in several well-controlled studies, mainly in Kenya and Zaire.[221–224] The nonulcerative STDs enhance the transmission of HIV by a factor of about 3 to 5. This may be because of increased viral shedding in persons with urethritis or cervicitis.[225–228] HIV has been detected by polymerase chain reaction (PCR) more commonly in urethral discharges of HIV-positive men with gonococcal urethritis than in discharges of those with nongonococcal urethritis. PCR positivity diminished two-fold following appropriate therapy for urethritis.[225] Not only does gonorrhea enhance the transmission of HIV, but also it may increase the risk of acquisition of HIV. A proposed mechanism is the significantly greater number of CD4 lymphocytes that can be infected by the virus in endocervical secretions of women with nonulcerative STDs compared with those of noninfected women.[229]

No data suggest that the course of uncomplicated gonococcal infection in women with HIV is any different from that in HIV-negative women. No difference in the microbiologic etiology of pelvic inflammatory disease between the two groups has been noted.[230–232] Some studies have shown that HIV-infected women with pelvic inflammatory disease had more severe symptoms,[233–235] were more likely to have tubo-ovarian abscesses,[236, 237] and required surgical intervention more often[238, 239] than did HIV-negative women. Severe sequelae from nongenital gonococcal infections in HIV-positive individuals have been reported.[240–242] The treatment of HIV-positive women with gonorrhea is similar to that of noninfected women. HIV-positive persons respond as well to therapy as do HIV-negative individuals.[232, 234] Some experts suggest that women with advanced HIV infection and pelvic inflammatory disease be hospitalized for treatment.[105] No data suggest an increase in treatment failures in women with HIV.

In conclusion, gonorrhea is an extremely important global health problem, especially in women. Screening of high-risk populations, early diagnosis, and prompt (and often empirical) therapy may reduce the incidence of the devastating sequelae of this disease. Proper diagnosis mandates appropriate specimen handling, because *N. gonorrhoeae* is a fastidious organism. The presence of concomitant STDs should be determined. Every person diagnosed with an STD should be offered HIV testing. Referral and treatment of all sexual contacts are critical in curbing the spread of this disease. Currently, third-generation cephalosporins and quinolones are the preferred therapeutic agents for gonorrhea. Antibiotic resistance patterns must be closely monitored in order to ensure that these agents remain effective in the treatment of this disease. Efforts to produce an effective vaccine against gonorrhea are underway. If they are successful, this vaccine could curtail the epidemic, which is especially prevalent in developing nations.

REFERENCES

1. Division of STD/HIV Prevention. Sexually Transmitted Diseases Surveillance, 1992. U.S. Department of Health and Human Services, Public Health Service. Atlanta, Centers for Disease Control and Prevention, 1993.
2. Brunham RC, C EJ: Sexually transmitted diseases: Current and future dimensions of the problem in the third world. In: Germain A, KKH, Piot PEA (eds): Reproductive Tract Infections: Global Impact and Priorities for Women's Reproductive Health. New York, Plenum Press, 1992, pp 35–58.
3. Dallabetta G, Hook EW 3d: Gonococcal infections. Infect Dis Clin North Am 1987; 1:25.
4. Low N, Daker-White G, Barlow D, Pozniak AL: Gonorrhoea in inner London: Results of a cross-sectional study. [See comments.] Br Med J 1997; 314:1719.
5. Rice RJ, Roberts PL, Handsfield HH, et al: Sociodemographic distribution of gonorrhea incidence: Implications for prevention and behavioral research. [See comments.] Am J Public Health 1991; 81:1252.
6. Holmes KK, Johnson DW, Trostle HJ: An estimate of the risk of men acquiring gonorrhea by sexual contact with infected females. Am J Epidemiol 1970; 91:170.

7. Hooper RR, Reynolds GH, Jones OG, et al: Cohort study of venereal disease. I. The risk of gonorrhea transmission from infected women to men. Am J Epidemiol 1978; 108:136.
8. Thin RNT, Williams IA, Nicol CS: Direct and delayed methods of immunofluorescent diagnosis of gonorrhea in women. Br J Vener Dis 1971; 47:27.
9. Wiesner PJ, Tronca E, Bonin P, et al: Clinical spectrum of pharyngeal gonococcal infection. N Engl J Med 1973; 288:181.
10. May RM, Anderson RM: Transmission dynamics of HIV infection. Nature 1987; 326:137.
11. Potterat JJ, Rothenberg R, Bross DC: Gonorrhea in street prostitutes: Epidemiologic and legal implications. Sex Transm Dis 1979; 6:58.
12. Anderson RM: Directly transmitted viral and bacterial infections of man. In: Anderson RM (ed): Population Dynamics of Infectious Diseases: Theory and Applications. London, Chapman & Hall, 1982, p 36.
13. Rothenberg RB: The geography of gonorrhea: Empirical demonstration of core group transmission. Am J Epidemiol 1983; 117:688.
14. McEvoy BF, Le Furgy WG: A 13-year longitudinal analysis of risk factors and clinic visitation patterns of patients with repeated gonorrhea. Sex Transm Dis 1988; 15:40.
15. Brunham RC, Plummer FA: A general model of sexually transmitted disease epidemiology and its implications for control. Med Clin North Am 1990; 74:1339.
16. Plummer FA, Nagelkerke NJ, Moses S, et al: The importance of core groups in the epidemiology and control of HIV-1 infection. AIDS 1991; 5(suppl 1):S169.
17. Garnett GP, Anderson RM: Contact tracing and the estimation of sexual mixing patterns: The epidemiology of gonococcal infections. Sex Transm Dis 1993; 20:181.
18. van Ameijden EJ, van den Hoek AJ, van Haastrecht HJ, et al: Trends in sexual behaviour and the incidence of sexually transmitted diseases and HIV among drug-using prostitutes, Amsterdam 1986–1992. AIDS 1994; 8:213.
19. Oh MK, Cloud GA, Wallace LS, et al: Sexual behavior and sexually transmitted diseases among male adolescents in detention. [See comments.] Sex Transm Dis 1994; 21:127.
20. Stigum H, Falck W, Magnus P: The core group revisited: The effect of partner mixing and migration on the spread of gonorrhea, *Chlamydia*, and HIV. Math Biosci 1994; 120:1.
21. Tanfer K: Sex and disease: Playing the odds in the 1990s. Sex Transm Dis 1994; 21:S65.
22. Thomas JC, Tucker MJ: The development and use of the concept of a sexually transmitted disease core. J Infect Dis 1996; 174(suppl 2):S134.
23. Ellen JM, Hessol NA, Kohn RP, et al: An investigation of geographic clustering of repeat cases of gonorrhea and chlamydial infection in San Francisco, 1989–1993: Evidence for core groups. J Infect Dis 1997; 175:1519.
24. Handsfield HH, Holmes KK, Wiesner PJ: Gonorrheal polyarthritis. N Engl J Med 1973; 288:218.
25. Schoolnik GK, Fernandez R, Tai JY, et al: Gonococcal pili: Primary structure and receptor binding domain. J Exp Med 1984; 159:1351.
26. McGee ZA, Johnson AP, Taylor-Robinson D: Pathogenic mechanisms of *Neisseria gonorrhoeae*: Observations on damage to human fallopian tubes in organ culture by gonococci of colony type 1 or type 4. J Infect Dis 1981; 143:413.
27. Kellogg DS Jr, Peacock WL Sr, Deacon WE, et al: *Neisseria gonorrhoeae*: I. Virulence genetically linked to clonal variation. J Bacteriol 1963; 85:1274.
28. Blake M, Swanson J: Studies on gonococcus infection. IX. In vitro decreased association of pilated gonococci with mouse peritoneal macrophages. Infect Immun 1975; 11:1402.
29. Kallstrom H, Liszewski MK, Atkinson JP, et al: Membrane cofactor protein (MCP or CD46) is a cellular pilus receptor for pathogenic *Neisseria*. Mol Microbiol 1997; 25:639.
30. Gray-Owen SD, Dehio C, Haude A, et al: CD66 carcinoembryonic antigens mediate interactions between Opa-expressing *Neisseria gonorrhoeae* and human polymorphonuclear phagocytes. EMBO J 1997; 16:3435.
31. Fischer SH, Rest RF: Gonococci possessing only certain P. II

outer membrane proteins interact with human neutrophils. Infect Immun 1988; 56:1574.

32. Virji M, Heckels JE: The effect of protein II and pili on the interaction of *Neisseria gonorrhoeae* with human polymorphonuclear leucocytes. J Gen Microbiol 1986; 132:503.

33. Chen T, Belland RJ, Wilson J, et al: Adherence of pilus-Opa+ gonococci to epithelial cells in vitro involves heparan sulfate. J Exp Med 1995; 182:511.

34. Makino S, van Putten JP, Meyer TF: Phase variation of the opacity outer membrane protein controls invasion by *Neisseria gonorrhoeae* into human epithelial cells. EMBO J 1991; 10:1307.

35. Duensing TD, van Putten JP: Vitronectin mediates internalization of *Neisseria gonorrhoeae* by Chinese hamster ovary cells. Infect Immun 1997; 65:964.

36. Gomez-Duarte OG, Dehio M, Guzman CA, et al: Binding of vitronectin to opa-expressing *Neisseria gonorrhoeae* mediates invasion of HeLa cells. Infect Immun 1997; 65:3857.

37. Chen T, Grunert F, Medina-Marino A, et al: Several carcinoembryonic antigens (CD66) serve as receptors for gonococcal opacity proteins. J Exp Med 1997; 185:1557.

38. Virji M, Watt SM, Barker S, et al: The N-domain of the human CD66a adhesion molecule is a target for Opa proteins of *Neisseria meningitidis* and *Neisseria gonorrhoeae*. Mol Microbiol 1996; 22:929.

39. Stern A, Brown M, Nickel P, et al: Opacity genes in *Neisseria gonorrhoeae*: Control of phase and antigenic variation. Cell 1986; 47:61.

40. Swanson J: Colony opacity and protein II compositions of gonococci. Infect Immun 1982; 37:359.

41. Plummer FA, Chubb H, Simonsen JN, et al: Antibodies to opacity proteins (Opa) correlate with a reduced risk of gonococcal salpingitis. J Clin Invest 1994; 93:1748.

42. Knapp JS, Tam MR, Nowinski RC, et al: Serological classification of *Neisseria gonorrhoeae* with use of monoclonal antibodies to gonococcal outer membrane protein I. J Infect Dis 1984; 150:44.

43. Hildebrandt JF, Mayer LW, Wang SP, et al: *Neisseria gonorrhoeae* acquire a new principal outer-membrane protein when transformed to resistance to serum bactericidal activity. Infect Immun 1978; 20:267.

44. Buchanan TM, Hildebrandt JF: Antigen-specific serotyping of *Neisseria gonorrhoeae*: Characterization based upon principal outer membrane protein. Infect Immun 1981; 32:985.

45. Blake MS, Gotschlich EC: Gonococcal membrane proteins: Speculation on their role in pathogenesis. Prog Allergy 1983; 33:298.

46. Rice PA, Vayo HE, Tam MR, et al: Immunoglobulin G antibodies directed against protein III block killing of serum-resistant *Neisseria gonorrhoeae* by immune serum. J Exp Med 1986; 164:1735.

47. Plummer FA, Chubb H, Simonsen JN, et al: Antibody to Rmp (outer membrane protein 3) increases susceptibility to gonococcal infection. J Clin Invest 1993; 91:339.

48. Black WJ, Cannon JG: Cloning of the gene for the common pathogenic *Neisseria* H.8 antigen from *Neisseria gonorrhoeae*. Infect Immun 1985; 47:322.

49. Hitchcock PJ, Hayes SF, Mayer LW, et al: Analyses of gonococcal H8 antigen: Surface location, inter- and intrastrain electrophoretic heterogeneity, and unusual two-dimensional electrophoretic characteristics. J Exp Med 1985; 162:2017.

50. Cornelissen CN, Biswas GD, Tsai J, et al: Gonococcal transferrin-binding protein 1 is required for transferrin utilization and is homologous to TonB-dependent outer membrane receptors. J Bacteriol 1992; 174:5788.

51. Mulks MH, Knapp JS: Immunoglobulin A1 protease types of *Neisseria gonorrhoeae* and their relationship to auxotype and serovar. Infect Immun 1987; 55:931.

52. Heine RP, Elkins C, Wyrick PB, et al: Transferrin increases adherence of iron-deprived *Neisseria gonorrhoeae* to human endometrial cells. Am J Obstet Gynecol 1996; 174:659.

53. Griffiss JM, Schneider H, Mandrell RE, et al: Lipooligosaccharides: The principal glycolipids of the neisserial outer membrane. Rev Infect Dis 1988; 10(suppl 2):S287.

54. Gregg CR, Melly MA, Hellerqvist CG, et al: Toxic activity of purified lipopolysaccharide of *Neisseria gonorrhoeae* for human fallopian tube mucosa. J Infect Dis 1981; 143:432.

55. Hook EWD, Holmes KK: Gonococcal infections. Ann Intern Med 1985; 102:229.

56. Apicella MA, Shero M, Jarvis GA, et al: Phenotypic variation in epitope expression of the *Neisseria gonorrhoeae* lipooligosaccharide. Infect Immun 1987; 55:1755.

57. Veale DR, Penn CW, Smith H: Factors affecting the induction of phenotypically determined serum resistance of *Neisseria gonorrhoeae* grown in media containing serum or its diffusible components. J Gen Microbiol 1981; 122:235.

58. Martin PM, Patel PV, Parsons NJ, et al: Induction of phenotypically determined resistance of *Neisseria gonorrhoeae* to human serum by factors in human serum. J Gen Microbiol 1981; 127:213.

59. Goldner M, Penn CW, Sanyal SC, et al: Phenotypically determined resistance of *Neisseria gonorrhoeae* to normal human serum: Environmental factors in subcutaneous chambers in guinea pigs. J Gen Microbiol 1979; 114:169.

60. Patel PV, Martin PM, Goldner M, et al: Red blood cells, a source of factors which induce *Neisseria gonorrhoeae* to resistance to complement-mediated killing by human serum. J Gen Microbiol 1984; 130:2767.

61. Patel PV, Veale DR, Fox JE, et al: Fractionation of guinea pig serum for an inducer of gonococcal resistance to killing by human serum: Active fractions containing glucopeptides similar to those from human red blood cells. J Gen Microbiol 1984; 130:2757.

62. Parsons NJ, Patel PV, Tan EL, et al: Cytidine 5′-monophospho-N-acetylneuraminic acid and a low molecular weight factor from human blood cells induce lipopolysaccharide alteration in gonococci when conferring resistance to killing by human serum. Microb Pathog 1988; 5:303.

63. Parsons NJ, Curry A, Fox AJ, et al: The serum resistance of gonococci in the majority of urethral exudates is due to sialylated lipopolysaccharide seen as a surface coat. FEMS Microbiol Lett 1992; 69:295.

64. Nairn CA, Cole JA, Patel PV, et al: Cytidine 5′-monophospho-N-acetylneuraminic acid or a related compound is the low Mr factor from human red blood cells which induces gonococcal resistance to killing by human serum. J Gen Microbiol 1988; 134:3295.

65. Tan EL, Patel PV, Parsons NJ, et al: Lipopolysaccharide alteration is associated with induced resistance of *Neisseria gonorrhoeae* to killing by human serum. J Gen Microbiol 1986; 132:1407.

66. Mandrell RE, Lesse AJ, Sugai JV, et al: In vitro and in vivo modification of *Neisseria gonorrhoeae* lipooligosaccharide epitope structure by sialylation. J Exp Med 1990; 171:1649.

67. Apicella MA, Mandrell RE, Shero M, et al: Modification by sialic acid of *Neisseria gonorrhoeae* lipooligosaccharide epitope expression in human urethral exudates: An immunoelectron microscopic analysis. J Infect Dis 1990; 162:506.

68. Fox AJ, Curry A, Jones DM, et al: The surface structure seen on gonococci after treatment with CMP-NANA is due to sialylation of surface lipopolysaccharide previously described as a 'capsule.' Microb Pathog 1991; 11:199.

69. Ram S, Sharma AK, Simpson SD, et al: A novel sialic acid binding site on factor H mediates serum resistance of sialylated *Neisseria gonorrhoeae*. J Exp Med 1998; 187:743.

70. Elkins C, Carbonetti NH, Varela VA, et al: Antibodies to N-terminal peptides of gonococcal porin are bactericidal when gonococcal lipopolysaccharide is not sialylated. Mol Microbiol 1992; 6:2617.

71. Wetzler LM, Barry K, Blake MS, et al: Gonococcal lipooligosaccharide sialylation prevents complement-dependent killing by immune sera. Infect Immun 1992; 60:39.

72. Rest RF, Frangipane JV: Growth of *Neisseria gonorrhoeae* in CMP-N-acetylneuraminic acid inhibits nonopsonic (opacity-associated outer membrane protein–mediated) interactions with human neutrophils. Infect Immun 1992; 60:989.

73. Martin JE Jr, Lester A, Price EV, et al: Comparative study of

gonococcal susceptibility to penicillin in the United States, 1955–1969. J Infect Dis 1970; 122:459.

74. Willcox RR: A survey of problems in the antibiotic treatment of gonorrhoea: With special reference to South-East Asia. Br J Vener Dis 1970; 46:217.

75. Phillips I: Beta-lactamase–producing, penicillin-resistant gonococcus. Lancet 1976; 2:656.

76. Ashford WA, Golash RG, Hemming VG: Penicillinase-producing *Neisseria gonorrhoeae*. Lancet 1976; 2:657.

77. Perine PL, Morton RS, Piot P, et al: Epidemiology and treatment of penicillinase-producing *Neisseria gonorrhoeae*. Sex Transm Dis 1979; 6:152.

78. Global distribution of penicillinase-producing *Neisseria gonorrhoeae* (PPNG). MMWR Morb Mortal Wkly Rep 1982; 31:1.

79. Chan RK, Thirumoorthy T: A decade of PPNG in Singapore. Ann Acad Med Singapore 1987; 16:639.

80. Ison CA, Easmon CS: Epidemiology of penicillin-resistant *Neisseria gonorrhoeae*. Genitourin Med 1991; 67:307.

81. Lind I, Arborio M, Bentzon MW, et al: The epidemiology of *Neisseria gonorrhoeae* isolates in Dakar, Senegal 1982–1986: Antimicrobial resistance, auxotypes and plasmid profiles. Genitourin Med 1991; 67:107.

82. Schwarcz SK, Zenilman JM, Schnell D, et al: National surveillance of antimicrobial resistance in *Neisseria gonorrhoeae*. The Gonococcal Isolate Surveillance Project. [See comments.] JAMA 1990; 264:1413.

83. Tetracycline-resistant *Neisseria gonorrhoeae*—Georgia, Pennsylvania, New Hampshire. MMWR Morb Mortal Wkly Rep 1985; 34:9.

84. Morse SA, Johnson SR, Biddle JW, et al: High-level tetracycline resistance in *Neisseria gonorrhoeae* is result of acquisition of streptococcal tetM determinant. Antimicrob Agents Chemother 1986; 30:664.

85. Knapp JS, Zenilman JM, Biddle JW, et al: Frequency and distribution in the United States of strains of *Neisseria gonorrhoeae* with plasmid-mediated, high-level resistance to tetracycline. J Infect Dis 1987; 155:819.

86. van Klingeren B, Dessens-Kroon M, Verheuvel M: Increased tetracycline resistance in gonococci in The Netherlands. [Letter.] Lancet 1989; 2:1278.

87. Ison CA, Bindayna K, Woodford N: *Neisseria gonorrhoeae* resistant to tetracycline. [Letter.] Br Med J 1988; 296:1471.

88. Evans AJ, Morrison GD, Price DJ: Prolonged use of the Greenland method of treatment of gonorrhoea. Br J Vener Dis 1980; 56:88.

89. Reichart CA, Neumann T, Foreman P, et al: Temporal trends in gonococcal antibiotic resistance in Baltimore. Sex Transm Dis 1992; 19:213.

90. Lind I: Epidemiology of antibiotic-resistant *Neisseria gonorrhoeae* in industrialized and developing countries. Scand J Infect Dis Suppl 1990; 69:77.

91. Reyn A, Schmidt H, Trier M, et al: Spectinomycin hydrochloride (Trobicin) in the treatment of gonorrhoea: Observation of resistant strains of *Neisseria gonorrhoeae*. Br J Vener Dis 1973; 49:54.

92. Ashford WA, Potts DW, Adams HJ, et al: Spectinomycin-resistant penicillinase-producing *Neisseria gonorrhoeae*. Lancet 1981; 2:1035.

93. Boslego JW, Tramont EC, Takafuji ET, et al: Effect of spectinomycin use on the prevalence of spectinomycin-resistant and of penicillinase-producing *Neisseria gonorrhoeae*. N Engl J Med 1987; 317:272.

94. Ison CA, Littleton K, Shannon KP, et al: Spectinomycin-resistant gonococci. Br Med J 1983; 287:1827.

95. Harrison WO, Wignall FS, Kerbs SB, et al: Oral rosoxacin for treatment of penicillin-resistant gonorrhoea. [Letter.] Lancet 1984; 1:566.

96. Wagenvoort JH, van der Willigen AH, van Vliet HJ, et al: Resistance of *Neisseria gonorrhoeae* to enoxacin. [Letter.] J Antimicrob Chemother 1986; 18:429.

97. Tzelepi E, Avgerinou H, Kyriakis KP, et al: Antimicrobial susceptibility and types of *Neisseria gonorrhoeae* in Greece: Data for the period 1990 to 1993. Sex Transm Dis 1997; 24:378.

98. Kam KM, Wong PW, Cheung MM, et al: Quinolone-resistant *Neisseria gonorrhoeae* in Hong Kong. Sex Transm Dis 1996; 23:103.

99. Deguchi T, Saito I, Tanaka M, et al: Fluoroquinolone treatment failure in gonorrhea: Emergence of a *Neisseria gonorrhoeae* strain with enhanced resistance to fluoroquinolones. Sex Transm Dis 1997; 24:247.

100. Tapsall J: Annual report of the Australian Gonococcal Surveillance Programme 1996. Commun Dis Intell 1997; 21:189.

101. Fox KK, Knapp JS, Holmes KK, et al: Antimicrobial resistance in *Neisseria gonorrhoeae* in the United States, 1988–1994: The emergence of decreased susceptibility to the fluoroquinolones. J Infect Dis 1997; 175:1396.

102. Knapp JS, Fox KK, Trees DL, et al: Fluoroquinolone resistance in *Neisseria gonorrhoeae* [published erratum appears in Emerg Infect Dis 1997 Oct–Dec; 3(4):584]. Emerg Infect Dis 1997; 3:33.

103. Knapp JS, Wongba C, Limpakarnjanarat K, et al: Antimicrobial susceptibilities of strains of *Neisseria gonorrhoeae* in Bangkok, Thailand: 1994–1995. Sex Transm Dis 1997; 24:142.

104. Gordon SM, Carlyn CJ, Doyle LJ, et al: The emergence of *Neisseria gonorrhoeae* with decreased susceptibility to ciprofloxacin in Cleveland, Ohio: Epidemiology and risk factors. [See comments.] Ann Intern Med 1996; 125:465.

105. 1998 Guidelines for treatment of sexually transmitted diseases. Centers for Disease Control and Prevention. MMWR Morb Mortal Wkly Rep 1998; 47:1.

106. Gruber F, Brajac I, Jonjic A, et al: Comparative trial of azithromycin and ciprofloxacin in the treatment of gonorrhea. J Chemother 1997; 9:263.

107. Young H, Moyes A, McMillan A: Azithromycin and erythromycin resistant *Neisseria gonorrhoeae* following treatment with azithromycin. Int J STD AIDS 1997; 8:299.

108. Ehret JM, Nims LJ, Judson FN: A clinical isolate of *Neisseria gonorrhoeae* with in vitro resistance to erythromycin and decreased susceptibility to azithromycin. Sex Transm Dis 1996; 23:270.

109. Handsfield HH, Hook EWD: Ceftriaxone for treatment of uncomplicated gonorrhea: Routine use of a single 125-mg dose in a sexually transmitted disease clinic. Sex Transm Dis 1987; 14:227.

110. McCormack WM, Stumacher RJ, Johnson K, et al: Clinical spectrum of gonococcal infection in women. Lancet 1977; 1:1182–5.

111. Platt R, Rice PA, McCormack WM: Risk of acquiring gonorrhea and prevalence of abnormal adnexal findings among women recently exposed to gonorrhea. JAMA 1983; 250:3205.

112. Lauer BA, Masters HB: Toxic effect of calcium alginate swabs on *Neisseria gonorrhoeae*. J Clin Microbiol 1988; 26:54.

113. Mirrett S, Reller LB, Knapp JS: *Neisseria gonorrhoeae* strains inhibited by vancomycin in selective media and correlation with auxotype. J Clin Microbiol 1981; 14:94.

114. Rees E, Tait IA, Hobson D, et al: Chlamydia in relation to cervical infection and pelvic inflammatory disease. In: Hobson D, Holmes KK (eds): Nongonococcal Urethritis and Related Infections. Lake Placid, NY, American Society for Microbiology, 1976, pp 67–76.

115. Granato PA, Franz MR: Use of the Gen-Probe PACE system for the detection of *Neisseria gonorrhoeae* in urogenital samples. Diagn Microbiol Infect Dis 1990; 13:217.

116. Sednaoui P, Malkin JE, Alonso JM: *Neisseria gonorrhoeae* RNA/DNA hybridization and culture for screening of gonococcal infections in a low-prevalence population. Eur J Epidemiol 1996; 12:651.

117. Ciemins EL, Borenstein LA, Dyer IE, et al: Comparisons of cost and accuracy of DNA probe test and culture for the detection of *Neisseria gonorrhoeae* in patients attending public sexually transmitted disease clinics in Los Angeles County. Sex Transm Dis 1997; 24:422.

118. Young H, Anderson J, Moyes A, et al: Non-cultural detection of rectal and pharyngeal gonorrhea by the Gen-Probe PACE 2 assay. Genitourin Med 1997; 73:59.

119. Jaschek G, Gaydos CA, Welsh LE, et al: Direct detection of *Chlamydia trachomatis* in urine specimens from symptomatic

and asymptomatic men by using a rapid polymerase chain reaction assay. J Clin Microbiol 1993; 31:1209.

120. Batteiger BE, Jones RB: Chlamydial infections. Infect Dis Clin North Am 1987; 1:55.

121. Handsfield HH, McCutchan JA, Corey L, et al: Evaluation of new anti-infective drugs for the treatment of uncomplicated gonorrhea in adults and adolescents. Infectious Diseases Society of America and the Food and Drug Administration. Clin Infect Dis 1992; 15(suppl 1):S123.

122. Odugbemi T, Oyewole F, Isichei CS, et al: Single oral dose of azithromycin for therapy of susceptible sexually transmitted diseases: A multicenter open evaluation. West Afr J Med 1993; 12:136.

123. Steingrimsson O, Olafsson JH, Thorarinsson H, et al: Azithromycin in the treatment of sexually transmitted disease. J Antimicrob Chemother 1990; 25(suppl A):109.

124. Waugh MA: Open study of the safety and efficacy of a single oral dose of azithromycin for the treatment of uncomplicated gonorrhoea in men and women. J Antimicrob Chemother 1993; 31(suppl E):193.

125. Tice AW Jr, Rodriguez VL: Pharyngeal gonorrhea. JAMA 1981; 246:2717.

126. Handsfield HH, Knapp JS, Diehr PK, Holmes KK: Correlation of auxotype and penicillin susceptibility of Neisseria gonorrhoeae with sexual preference and clinical manifestations of gonorrhea. Sex Transm Dis 1980; 7:1.

127. Collier AC, Judson FN, Murphy VL, et al: Comparative study of ceftriaxone and spectinomycin in the treatment of uncomplicated gonorrhea in women. Am J Med 1984; 77:68.

128. Hutt DM, Judson FN: Epidemiology and treatment of oropharyngeal gonorrhea. Ann Intern Med 1986; 104:655.

129. Lindberg M, Ringertz O, Sandstrom E: Treatment of pharyngeal gonorrhea due to beta-lactamase–producing gonococci. Br J Vener Dis 1982; 58:101.

130. Judson FN, Ehret JM, Handsfield HH: Comparative study of ceftriaxone and spectinomycin for treatment of pharyngeal and anorectal gonorrhea. JAMA 1985; 253:1417.

131. Holloway WJ: Spectinomycin. Med Clin North Am 1982; 66:169.

132. Podgore JK, Holmes KK: Ocular gonococcal infection with minimal or no inflammatory response. JAMA 1981; 246:242.

133. Haimovici R, Roussel TJ: Treatment of gonococcal conjunctivitis with single-dose intramuscular ceftriaxone. Am J Ophthalmol 1989; 107:511.

134. O'Brien JP, Goldenberg DL, Rice PA: Disseminated gonococcal infection: A prospective analysis of 49 patients and a review of pathophysiology and immune mechanisms. Medicine (Baltimore) 1983; 62:395.

135. Handsfield HH: Disseminated gonococcal infection. Clin Obstet Gynecol 1975; 18:131.

136. Holmes KK, Counts GW, Beaty HN: Disseminated gonococcal infection. Ann Intern Med 1971; 74:979.

137. Kerle KK, Mascola JR, Miller TA: Disseminated gonococcal infection. Am Fam Physician 1992; 45:209.

138. Mills J, Brook GF: Disseminated gonococcal infections. In: Holmes KK, Mardh PA, Sparling PF, et al (eds): Sexually Transmitted Diseases. New York, McGraw-Hill, 1984, p 229.

139. Bohnhoff M, Morello JA, Lerner SA: Auxotypes, penicillin susceptibility, and serogroups of Neisseria gonorrhoeae from disseminated and uncomplicated infections. J Infect Dis 1986; 154:225.

140. Tapsall JW, Phillips EA, Shultz TR, et al: Strain characteristics and antibiotic susceptibility of isolates of Neisseria gonorrhoeae causing disseminated gonococcal infection in Australia. Members of the Australian Gonococcal Surveillance Programme. Int J STD AIDS 1992; 3:273.

141. Colin MJ, Weissmann G: Disseminated gonococcal infection and tenosynovitis from an asymptomatically infected intrauterine contraceptive device. N Engl J Med 1976; 294:598.

142. Metzger AL: Gonococcal arthritis complicating gonorrheal pharyngitis. Ann Intern Med 1970; 73:267.

143. Petersen BH, Lee TJ, Snyderman R, et al: Neisseria meningitidis and Neisseria gonorrhoeae bacteremia associated with C6, C7, or C8 deficiency. Ann Intern Med 1979; 90:917.

144. Ellison RTD, Curd JG, Kohler PF, et al: Underlying complement deficiency in patients with disseminated gonococcal infection. Sex Transm Dis 1987; 14:201.

145. Lee TJ, Utsinger PD, Snyderman R, et al: Familial deficiency of the seventh component of complement associated with recurrent bacteremic infections due to Neisseria. J Infect Dis 1978; 138:359.

146. Petersen BH, Graham JA, Brooks GF: Human deficiency of the eighth component of complement: The requirement of C8 for serum Neisseria gonorrhoeae bactericidal activity. J Clin Invest 1976; 57:283.

147. Thompson J, Dunbar JM, van Gent A, et al: Disseminated gonococcal infection due to a beta-lactamase–producing strain of Neisseria gonorrhoeae: A case report. Br J Vener Dis 1981; 57:325.

148. Disseminated gonorrhea caused by penicillinase-producing Neisseria gonorrhoeae—Wisconsin, Pennsylvania. MMWR Morb Mortal Wkly Rep 1987; 36:161–162, 167.

149. Weiss PJ, Kennedy CA, McCann DF, et al: Fulminant endocarditis due to infection with penicillinase-producing Neisseria gonorrhoeae. Sex Transm Dis 1992; 19:288.

150. Rinaldi RZ, Harrison WO, Fan PT: Penicillin-resistant gonococcal arthritis: A report of four cases. Ann Intern Med 1982; 97:43.

151. Tabrizi SN, Paterson B, Fairley CK, et al: A self-administered technique for the detection of sexually transmitted diseases in remote communities. J Infect Dis 1997; 176:289.

152. Keiser H, Ruben FL, Wolinsky E, et al: Clinical forms of gonococcal arthritis. N Engl J Med 1968; 279:234.

153. Bayer AS: Gonococcal arthritis syndromes: An update on diagnosis and management. Postgrad Med 1980; 67:200–204, 207–208.

154. Brandt KD, Cathcart ES, Cohen AS: Gonococcal arthritis: Clinical features correlated with blood, synovial fluid and genitourinary cultures. Arthritis Rheum 1974; 17:503.

155. Brogadir SP, Schimmer BM, Myers AR: Spectrum of the gonococcal arthritis-dermatitis syndrome. Semin Arthritis Rheum 1979; 8:177.

156. Gelfand SG, Masi AT, Garcia-Kutzbach A: Spectrum of gonococcal arthritis: Evidence for sequential stages and clinical subgroups. J Rheumatol 1975; 2:83.

157. Wehrbein H: Gonococcal arthritis: A study of 610 cases. Surg Gynecol Obstet 1929; 49:105.

158. Angevine CD, Hall CB, Jacox RF: A case of gonococcal osteomyelitis: A complication of gonococcal arthritis. Am J Dis Child 1976; 130:1013.

159. Tindall EA, Regan-Smith MG: Gonococcal osteomyelitis complicating septic arthritis. JAMA 1983; 250:2671.

160. Magee G: Gonococcal arthritis. [Letter.] JAMA 1975; 234:1320.

161. Gantz NM, McCormack WM, Laughlin LW, et al: Gonococcal osteomyelitis: An unusual complication of gonococcal arthritis. JAMA 1976; 236:2431.

162. Holmes KK, Gutman LT, Belding ME, et al: Recovery of Neisseria gonorrhoeae from "sterile" synovial fluid in gonococcal arthritis. N Engl J Med 1971; 284:318.

163. Barr J, Danielsson D: Septic gonococcal dermatitis. Br Med J 1971; 1:482.

164. Wolff CB, Goodman HV, Vahrman J: Gonorrhoea with skin and joint manifestations. Br Med J 1970; 1:271.

165. Knapp JS, Holmes KK: Disseminated gonococcal infections caused by Neisseria gonorrhoeae with unique nutritional requirements. J Infect Dis 1975; 132:204.

166. Fleming TJ, Wallsmith DE, Rosenthal RS: Arthropathic properties of gonococcal peptidoglycan fragments: Implications for the pathogenesis of disseminated gonococcal disease. Infect Immun 1986; 52:600.

167. Manicourt DH, Orloff S: Gonococcal arthritis-dermatitis syndrome: Study of serum and synovial fluid immune complex levels. Arthritis Rheum 1982; 25:574.

168. Shapiro L, Teisch JA, Brownstein MH: Dermatohistopathology of chronic gonococcal sepsis. Arch Dermatol 1973; 107:403.

169. Wheeler JK, Heffron WA, Williams RC Jr: Migratory arthralgias and cutaneous lesions as confusing initial manifestations of gonorrhea. Am J Med Sci 1970; 260:150.

170. Ludivico CL, Myers AR: Survey for immune complexes in

disseminated gonococcal arthritis-dermatitis syndrome. Arthritis Rheum 1979; 22:19.

171. Cooke DB, Arensberg D, Felner JM, et al: Gonococcal endocarditis in the antibiotic era. Arch Intern Med 1979; 139:1247.

172. Rosoff MH, Cohen MV, Jacquette G: Pulmonary valve gonococcal endocarditis: A forgotten disease. Br Heart J 1983; 50:290.

173. Thompson EC, Brantley D: Gonoccocal endocarditis. J Natl Med Assoc 1996; 88:353.

174. Sugar AM, Utsinger PD, Santoro J: Gonococcal endocarditis in a patient with mitral valve prolapse: Study of host immunology and organism characteristics. Am J Med Sci 1982; 283:165.

175. Sayeed ZA, Bhaduri U, Howell E, et al: Gonococcal meningitis: A review. JAMA 1972; 219:1730.

176. Disseminated gonococcal infections and meningitis—Pennsylvania. MMWR Morb Mortal Wkly Rep 1984; 33:158–160, 165.

177. Stigler SL, McLester JS: Gonococcic meningitis fifteen years after urethritis. JAMA 1948; 136:919.

178. Moghissi KS: Composition and function of cervical secretion. In: Greep FL (ed): Female Reproductive System, part 2, vol. 2. Washington, DC, American Physiological Society, 1973, p 25.

179. Jones DE, Brame RG, Jones CP: Gonorrhea in obstetric patients. J Am Vener Dis Assoc 1976; 2:30.

180. Corman LC, Levison ME, Knight R, et al: The high frequency of pharyngeal gonococcal infection in a prenatal clinic population. JAMA 1974; 230:568.

181. Genadry RR, Thompson BH, Niebyl JR: Gonococcal salpingitis in pregnancy. Am J Obstet Gynecol 1976; 126:512.

182. Handsfield HH, Hodson WA, Holmes KK: Neonatal gonococcal infection. I. Orogastric contamination with Neisseria gonorrhoeae. JAMA 1973; 225:697.

183. Amstey MS, Steadman KT: Asymptomatic gonorrhea and pregnancy. J Am Vener Dis Assoc 1976; 3:14.

184. Edwards LE, Barrada MI, Hamann AA, et al: Gonorrhea in pregnancy. Am J Obstet Gynecol 1978; 132:637.

185. Rothbard MJ, Gregory T, Salerno LJ: Intrapartum gonococcal amnionitis. Am J Obstet Gynecol 1975; 121:565.

186. Charles AG, Cohen S, Kass MB, et al: Asymptomatic gonorrhea in prenatal patients. Am J Obstet Gynecol 1970; 108:595.

187. Sarrel PM, Pruett KA: Symptomatic gonorrhea during pregnancy. Obstet Gynecol 1968; 32:670.

188. Israel KS, Rissing KB, Brooks GF: Neonatal and childhood gonococcal infections. Clin Obstet Gynecol 1975; 18:143.

189. Handsfield HH, Holmes KK: Microepidemic of virulent gonococcal infection. J Am Vener Dis Assoc 1974; 1:20.

190. Kass EH, McCormack WM, Lin JS, et al: Genital mycoplasmas as a cause of excess premature delivery. Trans Assoc Am Physicians 1981; 94:261.

191. Kundsin RB, Driscoll SG, Monson RR, et al: Association of Ureaplasma urealyticum in the placenta with perinatal morbidity and mortality. N Engl J Med 1984; 310:941.

192. Gravett MG, Nelson HP, DeRouen T, et al: Independent associations of bacterial vaginosis and Chlamydia trachomatis infection with adverse pregnancy outcome. JAMA 1986; 256:1899.

193. Hillier SL, Nugent RP, Eschenbach DA, et al: Association between bacterial vaginosis and preterm delivery of a low-birth-weight infant. The Vaginal Infections and Prematurity Study Group. [See comments.] N Engl J Med 1995; 333:1737.

194. Rothenberg R: Ophthalmia neonatorum due to Neisseria gonorrhoeae: Prevention and treatment. Sex Transm Dis 1979; 6:187.

195. Fransen L, Nsanze H, Klauss V, et al: Ophthalmia neonatorum in Nairobi, Kenya: The roles of Neisseria gonorrhoeae and Chlamydia trachomatis. J Infect Dis 1986; 153:862.

196. Laga M, Plummer FA, Nzanze H, et al: Epidemiology of ophthalmia neonatorum in Kenya. Lancet 1986; 2:1145.

197. Laga M, Plummer FA, Piot P, et al: Prophylaxis of gonococcal and chlamydial ophthalmia neonatorum: A comparison of silver nitrate and tetracycline. N Engl J Med 1988; 318:653.

198. Allen JH BL: Prophylaxis of gonorrhea ophthalmia of the newborn. JAMA 1949; 141:522.

199. Armstrong JH, Zacarias F, Rein MF: Ophthalmia neonatorum: A chart review. Pediatrics 1976; 57:884.

200. Smith JA: Ophthalmia neonatorum in Glasgow. Scott Med J 1969; 14:272.

201. Valenton MJ, Abendanio R: Gonorrheal conjunctivitis: Complication after ocular contamination with urine. Can J Ophthalmol 1973; 8:421.

202. Fivush B, Woodward CL, Wald ER: Gonococcal conjunctivitis in a four-month-old infant. Sex Transm Dis 1980; 7:24.

203. Stark AR, Glode MP: Gonococcal vaginitis in a neonate. J Pediatr 1979; 94:298.

204. Barton LL, Shuja M: Neonatal gonococcal vaginitis. [Letter.] J Pediatr 1981; 98:171.

205. Benson RA WI: Gonococcal vaginitis in children. Am J Dis Child 1940; 59:1083.

206. Kirkland H SR: Gonococcal rhinitis in an infant. Br Med J 1931; 1:263.

207. Laga M, Naamara W, Brunham RC, et al: Single-dose therapy of gonococcal ophthalmia neonatorum with ceftriaxone. N Engl J Med 1986; 315:1382.

208. Thadepalli H, Rambhatla K, Maidman JE, et al: Gonococcal sepsis secondary to fetal monitoring. Am J Obstet Gynecol 1976; 126:510.

209. Plavidal FJ, Werch A: Gonococcal fetal scalp abscess: A case report. Am J Obstet Gynecol 1977; 127:437.

210. Reveri M, Krishnamurthy C: Gonococcal scalp abscess. J Pediatr 1979; 94:819.

211. Brook I, Rodriguez WJ, Controni G, Gold B: Gonococcal scalp abscess in a newborn. South Med J 1980; 73:396.

212. Copperman M: Gonococcus arthritis in infancy. Am J Dis Child 1927; 33:932.

213. Kohen DP: Neonatal gonococcal arthritis: Three cases and review of the literature. Pediatrics 1974; 53:436.

214. Bradford WL, Kelley HW: Gonococcic meningitis in a new born infant. Am J Dis Child 1933; 46:543.

215. Isenberg SJ, Apt L, Wood M: A controlled trial of povidone-iodine as prophylaxis against ophthalmia neonatorum. [See comments.] N Engl J Med 1995; 332:562.

216. Ingram DL, Runyan DK, Collins AD, et al: Vaginal Chlamydia trachomatis infection in children with sexual contact. Pediatr Infect Dis 1984; 3:97.

217. Ingram DL, Everett VD, Lyna PR, et al: Epidemiology of adult sexually transmitted disease agents in children being evaluated for sexual abuse. Pediatr Infect Dis J 1992; 11:945.

218. Rimsza ME, Niggemann EH: Medical evaluation of sexually abused children: A review of 311 cases. Pediatrics 1982; 69:8.

219. Wald ER, Woodward CL, Marston G, et al: Gonorrheal disease among children in a university hospital. Sex Transm Dis 1980; 7:41.

220. Glaser JB, Hammerschlag MR, McCormack WM: Epidemiology of sexually transmitted diseases in rape victims. Rev Infect Dis 1989; 11:246.

221. Laga M, Manoka A, Kivuvu M, et al: Non-ulcerative sexually transmitted diseases as risk factors for HIV-1 transmission in women: Results from a cohort study. [See comments.] AIDS 1993; 7:95.

222. Wasserheit JN: Epidemiological synergy: Interrelationships between human immunodeficiency virus infection and other sexually transmitted diseases. Sex Transm Dis 1992; 19:61.

223. Cameron DW, Simonsen JN, D'Costa LJ, et al: Female-to-male transmission of human immunodeficiency virus type 1: Risk factors for seroconversion in men. [See comments.] Lancet 1989; 2:403.

224. Laga M, Nzila N, Goeman J: The interrelationship of sexually transmitted diseases and HIV infection: Implications for the control of both epidemics in Africa. AIDS 1991; 5(suppl 1):S55.

225. Moss GB, Overbaugh J, Welch M, et al: Human immunodeficiency virus DNA in urethral secretions in men: Association with gonococcal urethritis and CD4 cell depletion. J Infect Dis 1995; 172:1469.

226. Clemetson DB, Moss GB, Willerford DM, et al: Detection of HIV DNA in cervical and vaginal secretions: Prevalence and

correlates among women in Nairobi, Kenya. JAMA 1993;
269:2860.

227. Cohen MS, Hoffman IF, Royce RA, et al: Reduction of
concentration of HIV-1 in semen after treatment of urethritis:
Implications for prevention of sexual transmission of HIV-1.
AIDSCAP Malawi Research Group. Lancet 1997; 349:1868.

228. Kreiss J, Willerford DM, Hensel M, et al: Association between
cervical inflammation and cervical shedding of human
immunodeficiency virus DNA. J Infect Dis 1994; 170:1597.

229. Levine WC, Pope V, Bhoomkar A, et al: Increase in
endocervical CD4 lymphocytes among women with
nonulcerative sexually transmitted diseases. J Infect Dis 1998;
177:167.

230. Moorman A, Rice R, Irwin K, et al: The microbiologic
etiology of pelvic inflammatory disease (PID) in HIV+ and
HIV− women: Preliminary findings of a multicenter study.
The Multicenter HIV and PID Study Group. Int Conf AIDS
1993; 9:458 (abstract no. PO-B23-1937).

231. Clarke L, Sierra M, Duerr A, et al: Prevalence of selected
organisms in HIV+ and HIV− women with pelvic
inflammatory disease (PID). Natl Conf Hum Retroviruses
Relat Infect (1st) 1993, p 98.

232. Moorman AC, Rice R, Irwin K, et al: The microbiologic
etiology of pelvic inflammatory disease (PID) in HIV+ and
HIV− women: Updated results from an ongoing multicenter
study. Natl Conf Hum Retroviruses Relat Infect (1st) 1993,
p 99.

233. Kamenga MC, De Cock KM, St. Louis ME, et al: The impact
of human immunodeficiency virus infection on pelvic
inflammatory disease: A case-control study in Abidjan, Ivory
Coast. Am J Obstet Gynecol 1995; 172:919.

234. Irwin K, Rice R, Sperling R, et al: Comparison of clinical
presentation and course of PID in HIV+ and HIV− women:
Updated results from an ongoing multicenter study. Natl
Conf Hum Retroviruses Relat Infect (1st) 1993, p 98.

235. Irwin K, Rice R, O'Sullivan M, et al: The clinical presentation
and course of pelvic inflammatory diseases in HIV+ and
HIV− women: Preliminary results of a multicenter study. The
Multicenter HIV and PID Study Group. Int Conf AIDS 1993;
9:50 (abstract no. WS-B07-1).

236. Bukusi E, Stevens C, Cohen C, et al: Impact of HIV on acute
pelvic inflammatory disease in a Nairobi outpatient clinic. Int
Conf AIDS 1996; 11:161 (abstract no. Mo.C.1618).

237. Cohen C, Sinei S, Reilly M, et al: HIV and acute pelvic
inflammatory disease: A laparoscopic study in Kenya. Int Conf
AIDS 1996; 11:219 (abstract no. Th.B.113).

238. Denenberg R: Pelvic inflammatory disease in HIV infection.
GMHC Treat Issues 1997; 11:19.

239. Hoegsberg B, Abulafia O, Sedlis A, et al: Sexually transmitted
diseases and human immunodeficiency virus infection among
women with pelvic inflammatory disease. Am J Obstet
Gynecol 1990; 163:1135.

240. Lau RK, Goh BT, Estreich S, et al: Adult gonococcal
keratoconjunctivitis with AIDS. Br J Ophthalmol 1990; 74:52.

241. Moyle G, Barton SE, Midgley J, et al: Gonococcal arthritis
caused by auxotype P in a man with HIV infection.
Genitourin Med 1990; 66:91.

242. Strongin IS, Kale SA, Raymond MK, et al: An unusual
presentation of gonococcal arthritis in an HIV-positive
patient. Ann Rheum Dis 1991; 50:572.

40 *Chlamydia trachomatis*

SEBASTIAN FARO

Chlamydia causes infection in humans, birds, and mammals.[1] *Chlamydia* is a true obligate prokaryotic parasite of eukaryotic cells. Chlamydiae are true bacteria, and not viruses, because they contain both RNA and DNA, have a cell wall that stains gram-negative and therefore are similar to gram-negative bacteria, reproduce by binary fission, are able to synthesize protein, contain ribosomes, and are susceptible to antibiotics. They are not capable of reproducing outside of an eukaryotic cell, however, and are considered true parasites because they can synthesize ATP.[2, 3] *Chlamydia* species belong to the Order Chlamydiales and the Family Chlamydiaceae, which contain a single genus, *Chlamydia*. Three species are known to infect humans; *Chlamydia psittaci*, *C. pneumoniae*, and *C. trachomatis*. *Chlamydia pecorum* is the one species that causes infection in pigs, ruminants, and marsupials.[4]

Chlamydia psittaci is an agent that causes infection primarily in nonprimate mammals. Humans become infected via zoonotic contact,[5] whereas *C. trachomatis* infects only humans, and the organism is spread via human-to-human contact.

Chlamydia pneumoniae is strictly a human pathogen, responsible for approximately 5% of the cases of community-acquired pneumonia. *Chlamydia pneumoniae* has also been associated with pharyngitis, bronchitis, and outbreaks of pneumonia in military personnel.[1, 6]

Chlamydia trachomatis is likely the most common bacterial sexually transmitted organism causing infection of the lower and upper genital tract of women. Together with *Neisseria gonorrhoeae*, these two bacteria are the most frequent causes of pelvic inflammatory disease (PID), found as either co-infection organisms or as individual causes of infection. It is estimated that among women of reproductive age, 10% to 15% will experience at least one episode of symptomatic or asymptomatic PID.[1] The disease PID is often insidious in onset and can remain asymptomatic even though it causes progressive damage to the reproductive system. PID can result in damage to the fallopian tubes that results in ectopic pregnancy, should the patient conceive, or infertility. The endstage of PID results in chronic pain or tubo-ovarian abscess formation, with either condition leading, ultimately, to hysterectomy.

MICROBIOLOGY

Chlamydiae are prokaryotic organisms that possess characteristics morphologically and structurally similar to gram-negative bacteria. They possess a trilaminar outer membrane consisting of lipopolysaccharide and proteins similar to that found in *Escherichia coli* (Fig. 40–1). Chlamydia seems to lack the typical peptidoglycan in the outer cell wall found in other bacteria. It does, however, contain the genetic material necessary for synthesizing peptidoglycan.[7–9] The elementary body (EB), or infectious particle, is the extracellular structure that forms disulfide cross-linkages between cysteine residues within and between proteins of the outer membrane.[10, 11] The EB resembles a spore-like struc-

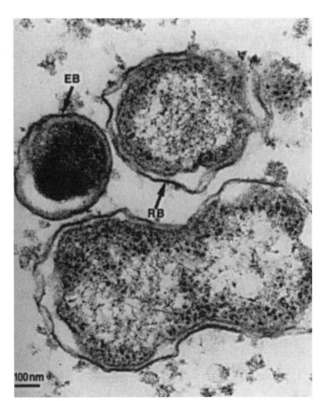

FIGURE 40–1 ▶ *Chlamydia* membrane. (From Mandell GL, Bennett JE, Dolin R [eds]: Bennett's Principles and Practice of Infectious Diseases, 5th ed. Philadelphia, Churchill Livingstone, 2000, p 1987.)

ture that is metabolically inert and enables the organism to exist outside the host.

The life cycle of *Chlamydia* is unique among bacteria in that it has two phases (Fig. 40–2). There are two stages in the organism's existence—the elementary body (EB), which is the infectious form and is metabolically inactive, and the reticulate body (RB), the metabolically active stage. The sole function of the EB is to adhere to susceptible host cells and gain entrance into them. The actual adhesions have not been identified, but apparently there are several adhesions and receptors.[9, 12] Once the EB becomes adherent to the host cell, it initiates entrance into the cell by way of receptor-mediated endocytosis via clathrin-coated pits.[13, 14] There appears to be an additional mechanism that allows the organism to gain entrance into the host cell, which includes pinocytosis via noncoated pits.[12] The EB becomes enveloped in the host cell membrane via the endocytic process and is absorbed into the host intracellular cytoplasm. This vacuole can be referred to as a phagosome, which is known as an inclusion. The EB does not fuse with a lysosome and therefore is protected from being attacked by the host cell at the molecular level. The inclusion prevents or inhibits lysosomal fusion through a mechanism that has not been defined. The EB is approximately 350 nm in diameter and is the smaller structural unit of *Chlamydia*. Once the EB has entered the cell in its protected vacuole, it undergoes a metamorphosis to become a reticulate body (RB).

The RB is a metabolically active stage and reproduces to form new EBs. The RB measures between 800 to 1,000 nm in diameter.[15] The mechanisms responsible for the metamorphosis of the EB to the RB are not known. However, there is synthesis of chlamydial proteins, reduction of a disulfide bond resulting in disruption of cross-linkage in the proteins within the cell membrane, and activation of adenosine triphosphate (ATP).[11, 13, 16] The parasitic properties are revealed during the metabolic phase of the life cycle as the organism derives high-energy phosphate compounds and amino acids from the host cells.[17] The RB is osmotically unstable, cannot exist outside the host cell, and is not able to infect host cells. The RBs are capable of reproducing via binary fission, thus increasing the size of the intracellular inclusion. The

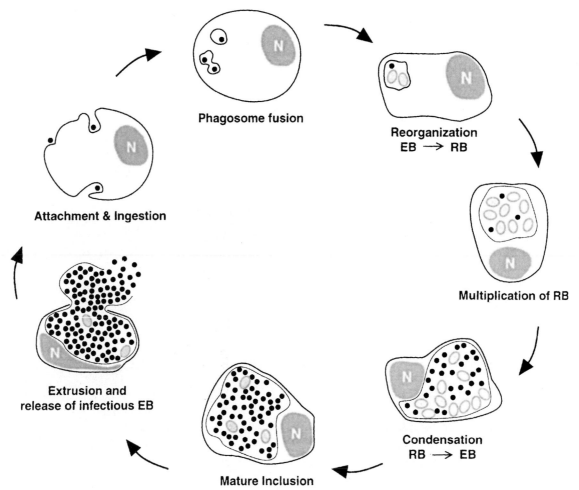

Phagosome fusion

Reorganization EB → RB

Multiplication of RB

Attachment & Ingestion

Extrusion and release of infectious EB

Condensation RB → EB

Mature Inclusion

FIGURE 40–2 ▶ Life cycle of *Chlamydia*. (From Mandell GL, Bennett JE, Dolin R [eds]: Bennett's Principles and Practice of Infectious Diseases, 5th ed. New York, Churchill Livingstone, 2000, p 1990.)

mechanism regulating the conversion of EBs to RBs and from RBs to EBs is also not known. The concentrations of cyclic adenosine monophosphate (cAMP) and cyclic guanine monophosphate (cGMP) appear to play a role in morphogenesis during the life cycle of *Chlamydia*.[18] Morphologic change of RBs to EBs results in a reduction in size, loss of membrane blebs containing lipopolysaccharide, and compaction of the chromatin into an electron-dense nucleoid.[19] This latter phase is mediated by a histone-like protein and signals the end of the metabolic phase.[20] The EBs are liberated from the host cells either as individual particles via lysis of the host cell or by exocytosis, a process by which an intact inclusion is extruded from the host cell.[21-23] Once the EBs or infectious particles are released, they can infect new host cells (see Fig. 40–2).

One interesting feature of the life cycle is that once the bacterium gains entrance into the host cell, it is protected from the host-cell lysozyme and prevents apoptosis of the host-cell via a variety of factors. This ensures that the host cell will survive until the life cycle is completed.[24] Therefore, when an endocervical columnar epithelial cell is infected, *Chlamydia* regulates the activity of the host epithelial cell in order to ensure that the infecting organism completes its life cycle to generate a new population of bacteria. This is accomplished through a variety of mechanisms, many of which have not been discovered; for example, preventing the epithelial cell lysozyme from attacking the inclusion body and host-cell apoptosis.

It has been demonstrated that *Chlamydia* does produce proteins that are localized in the cytoplasmic surface of the inclusion membrane, one of which is designated as Inc A.[25] This protein, Inc A, is believed to be involved in directing inclusions to the exocytic pathway to allow the inclusions to exit the host cell.[26] It is postulated that proteins such as Inc A direct or traffic host cell lipoproteins into chlamydial membranes and inhibit host apoptosis.[27, 28] It is theorized that these proteins enter the host cytoplasm from the inclusions via type III secretions.[29] Type III, or the contact-dependent secretion pathway, is a mechanism by which the bacterium alters or subverts the host cell to allow the pathogen to survive in the host cell.[30] Type II secretion systems have been described in several bacteria (e.g., *Salmonella*, *Shigella*, and *Yersinia*) that share structural and functional similarities and suggest a relationship to bacterial flagella.[31] The bacterium possesses a supramolecular structure that encompasses the entire cell wall and functions as a hypodermic syringe.[32] It is through this mechanism that the bacterium secretes effector proteins directly across host cell membranes. Type III systems are varied with regard to the tasks they accomplish—for example, some facilitate entry of the bacteria into the host cell, others initiate bacterial replication and nuclear transcriptase, stimulate mitogen-activated protein kinases, act as a virulence factor, act as an antiphagocytic factor, can induce apoptosis in activated macrophages, and can suppress synthesis of tumor necrosis factor.[33-38]

Chlamydial infections continue to pose many questions, as the natural history of these infections has not been completely described. Chlamydiae have the ability to cause chronic asymptomatic infection that can persist for prolonged periods of time. Intriguing data have appeared that, although controversial, implicate *C. pneumoniae* in the development of atherosclerosis and coronary artery disease.

CHLAMYDIA PSITTACI

Introduction

Chlamydia psittaci, the etiologic agent of psittacosis, is commonly found in birds and domestic animals. Ritter described an outbreak in Switzerland in 1879.[39] Morange was studying parrots with respiratory disease and applied the term *psittacosis*, which is derived from the Greek word for parrot.[40] The organism was identified in 1930 by independent investigators in several countries, by Bedson in the United Kingdom, by Kromede in the United States, and by Levinthal in Germany.[41]

Epidemiology

Chlamydia psittaci is not a common human pathogen, but it can be found to cause respiratory infections among individuals who have birds as pets, who work with birds or domestic animals, who raise chickens or turkeys (the latter appear to be more risky), and who process poultry for consumption by the public, and among veterinarians. Individuals working in abattoirs and processing plants are at greatest risk for contracting *C. psittaci* pneumonia.[42] However, Ni and colleagues[43] published the results of a seroepidemiologic study of *Chlamydia pneumoniae* in different populations on the mainland of China. These investigators reported that IgG antibodies to *C. pneumoniae*, *C. trachomatis*, and *C. psittaci* were present in 61.5%, 9.3%, and 3.5%, respectively.[43] Levels of IgG antibodies to *C. psittaci* in poultry workers were no higher than those in the general population study.[5] However, human psittacosis does occur sporadically as outbreaks among pet owners and those whose work puts them in close association with birds and domestic animals.[44-46]

Typically, patients with psittacosis have had contact with birds, specifically exotic birds, and this has been correlated with an increase in cases.[46] Contact with birds can be close, as seen with pets, or during a visit to an aviary, or during transport of birds such as parakeets, parrots, and pigeons. Acquisition of *C. psittaci* occus via aerosolization of the organism and inhalation of infected droplets.

TABLE 40-1 ▶ DIFFERENTIAL DIAGNOSIS ASSOCIATED WITH PSITTACOSIS[45,47]

Pneumonia	Fever of unknown origin
Meningitis	Pulmonary embolism
Gastroenteritis	Myocardial infarction
Vasculitis	Tonsillitis
Septicemia	Pancreatic carcinoma
Malaria	Polymyositis
Brucellosis	

Clinical Presentation

The incubation period for *C. psittaci* is 5 to 15 days, followed by a variety of symptoms. The disease process can be subacute or acute and can present as a nonspecific viral illness; a flu-like syndrome with fever and malaise; or a mononucleosis-like syndrome with fever, pharyngitis, hepatosplenomegaly, and lymphadenopathy. A more severe form of the disease can present as a typhoidal illness, with fever, bradycardia, malaise, and splenomegaly. The most common presentation is that of a clinical picture of atypical pneumonia with fever, headache, nonproductive cough, and an abnormal chest radiograph that appears more severe than the disease.

The nonspecific nature of the clinical presentation of psittacosis often initiates a rather extensive differential diagnosis (Table 40–1). Fever occurs in 50% to 100% of infected individuals.[44] In approximately 50% to 100% of the cases, a nonproductive cough develops late in the illness.[44] Headaches and myalgias, as well as chills, have been reported to occur in 30% to 70% of infected individuals.[44] A variety of signs and symptoms have been reported in association with psittacosis (Table 40–2).

Chlamydia psittaci is a rather common cause of abortion in sheep, as well as other mammals. Although psittacosis is relatively uncommon in humans, when it occurs in pregnancy it can present as a severe, progressive, febrile illness. The patient typically develops a headache, disseminated intravascular coagulation (DIC), abnormal liver enzymes, and impaired liver function.[52] In the United States, two cases of gestational psittacosis associated with psittacine birds had been previously reported. In 1997, Hyde and Benirschke[52] reported a case of ovine-related gestational

TABLE 40-2 ▶ SIGNS AND SYMPTOMS ASSOCIATED WITH PSITTACOSIS[45-51]

Diaphoresis	Vomiting	Epistaxis
Photophobia	Abdominal pain	Arthralgia
Tinnitus	Diarrhea	Rash
Ataxia	Constipation	Chest pain
Deafness	Pharyngitis	Hematuria
Anorexia	Dyspnea	Proteinuria
Nausea	Hemoptysis	Myelitis

psittacosis in the United States. In 1997, Jorgensen[53] reported a case of psittacosis in a pregnant Montana sheep rancher. Idu and co-workers[54] reported a case of psittacosis in a 33-year-old pregnant woman who presented with atypical pneumonia. This patient developed adult respiratory distress syndrome (ARDS), premature labor, and birth with perinatal mortality.[54] Pregnant women should be warned about the possibility of contracting psittacosis from birds and farm animals. This warning should not be taken lightly because the disease appears to become more severe in pregnant women, with atypical pneumonia, sepsis, multiorgan involvement, abortion, premature labor and delivery, and perinatal mortality.

Although *C. psittaci* commonly causes respiratory disease, manifestations of infection can be seen in other organs as well. Individuals can develop pericarditis, myositis, endocarditis, and valvular disease.[55, 56] Thus, psittacosis may appear to be a relatively minor respiratory infection causing atypical pneumonia, but it has the potential to be a severe disease, especially in the pregnant patient. Therefore, as part of the prenatal evaluation of patients, inquiries should be made as to the patient's potential risk of acquiring psittacosis. That is, does she have birds as pets, especially exotic birds (e.g., parakeets and parrots), or does she live on a ranch?

Diagnosis and Management

The diagnosis can be established by culturing the organism from blood and/or sputum. However, it is not recommended to attempt culturing the organism, since infection of laboratory personnel can easily occur. Infection can be established by the detection of complement-fixing or microimmunofluorescence antibodies in serum—a titer of at least 1:64 is indicative of acute infection.[40] There are false-positive and false-negative reactions. The complement-fixation test is genus specific and does not distinguish between species.[40]

Laboratory tests are nonspecific. The white blood cell (WBC) count is mildly elevated in most cases, with approximately 60% to 70% of the patients manifesting a left shift. A chest radiograph reveals a consolidation in a single lower lobe in 90% of the patients. Successful treatment results in resolution of the x-ray findings usually within 6 weeks, but resolution can take as long as 20 weeks.[40]

Treatment should be instituted when the diagnosis of atypical pneumonia is made. The failure to treat is associated with a 20% mortality rate, and with treatment there is a 1% mortality rate. Treatment is with tetracycline, 500 mg PO four times a day, or doxycycline, 100 mg PO twice a day for 10 to 21 days. Pregnant women should be treated with erythromycin, 500 mg four times a day for 10 to 21 days.

CHLAMYDIA PNEUMONIAE

Introduction

Chlamydia pneumoniae has a life cycle similar to that of *C. trachomatis* and *C. psittaci. Chlamydia pneumoniae* differs from the latter two species in that it is not sexually transmitted and is not found in birds or animals. *Chlamydia pneumoniae* is transmitted via respiratory secretions. There is only one strain that has thus far been identified, TWAR (Taiwan acute respiratory).

The organism was first isolated from a Taiwanese child with conjunctivitis in 1965, and designated as TW-183.[57] A second isolate was obtained from the conjunctiva of an Iranian child in 1968.[58] In 1977, an epidemic of mild pneumonia in Finland was linked to TW-183.[59] In 1983, a Seattle student with pharyngitis was infected with an organism designated as AR-39.[60] The strain name TWAR (TW + AR) was established from these conjunctival and respiratory isolates. The genus and species *Chlamydia pneumoniae* was established by DNA sequence analysis in 1989.[61]

Epidemiology

Chlamydia pneumoniae is a common cause of community-acquired acute pneumonia, with more than 50% of adults in the United States and throughout the world demonstrating antibodies to this bacterium.[62–64] *Chlamydia pneumoniae* accounts for 7% to 10% of the cases of community-acquired pneumonia.[65–69] Serum antibody levels are low among children 5 years of age or younger and rise rapidly among school-aged children.[65] Seropositivity rises rapidly with increasing age, and by age 20 years approximately 50% of the population are found to have antibodies to *C. pneumoniae* (Fig. 40–3). The antibody titers do not persist over time, and the persistent rates depicted in Figure 40–3 indicate that there has been re-infection.

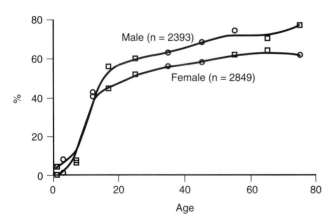

FIGURE 40–3 ▶ A seropositivity epidemiology study of 5,242 individuals. There is a noticeable increase in antibodies (IgG titer ≥8) to *Chlamydia pneumoniae* with increasing age. (From Grayson JT: Infections caused by *Chlamydia pneumoniae* strain TWAR. Clin Infect Dis 1992; 15:757–763.)

Since *C. pneumoniae* infection does not typically cause severe pneumonia, most patients do not require hospitalization. *Chlamydia pneumoniae* is responsible for approximately 5% of the cases of bronchitis and sinusitis.[70, 71] Thus, *C. pneumoniae* should be considered in patients in the reproductive and postmenopausal age group presenting with signs of upper and/or lower respiratory infection.

Clinical Signs and Symptoms

The most common infections caused by *C. pneumoniae* are bronchitis and pneumonia. Although patients can develop pharyngitis and sinusitis, these infrequently occur as isolated infections, but they can occur in conjunction with either bronchitis or pneumonia.

The incubation period is approximately 21 days, which is significantly longer than respiratory infection caused by other organisms.[72] Clinically nonapparent infection or asymptomatic carriage has also been documented, and these individuals can serve as vectors for transmission of the organism.[73–75]

Respiratory infection caused by *C. pneumoniae* typically begins with rhinitis and a sore throat. These initial signs do not persist for a prolonged period of time but, instead, last only a few days, and the patient then develops a cough. Cough is the characteristic feature of *C. pneumoniae* respiratory infection. Unlike patients with respiratory infection caused by organisms other than *C. pneumoniae,* patients with *C. pneumoniae* respiratory infection tend not to have a fever.[70, 71, 76] Symptoms are usually prolonged. The patients typically have a cough and malaise, which can persist for weeks to months even though the patient is receiving appropriate therapy.[71]

Diagnosis and Management

The diagnosis of respiratory infection caused by *C. pneumoniae* is established by serologic testing. The chest radiograph is nonspecific but is used to establish that the patient does indeed have a pneumonic process. *Chlamydia pneumoniae* can be grown in tissue culture, but this method is not useful for establishing a clinical diagnosis and is reserved mainly for research. Polymerase chain reaction (PCR) assay can also establish the presence of *C. pneumoniae,* but this method is also used mainly for research purposes. Although PCR is highly sensitive and has been used to isolate *C. pneumoniae* from specimens obtained via throat swab, sputum collection, and bronchial lavage, it is expensive and time-consuming.[77, 78]

The standard serologic test for the detection of *C. pneumoniae*–specific antibodies is the microimmunofluorescence test.[79] IgM antibodies appear within 2 to 4 weeks of the initial infection, with IgG antibodies appearing in 6 to 8 weeks.[58] Jackson and Grayson[58] recommend a delay in obtaining a second specimen for 3 to 4 weeks because of a possible delay in the rise in antibody titer following the initial or acute infection. The presence of circulating rheumatoid factor may give a false-positive IgM antibody finding for *C. pneumoniae*.[80] Individuals who become re-infected may not manifest IgM antibodies or if they do the antibody titer is very low. However, with re-infection, IgG antibodies are usually detectable in 1 to 3 weeks, and the titer is often high (≥512).[58]

Chlamydia pneumoniae pneumonia is effectively treated with erythromycin, tetracycline, doxycycline, azithromycin, or clarithromycin.[81–83] Combinations of azithromycin with ofloxacin, doxycycline, or rifampin were synergistic against *C. pneumoniae*.[84] Roblin and co-workers[85] tested grepafloxacin, levofloxacin, moxifloxacin, trovafloxacin, clarithromycin, and azithromycin activity against *C. pneumoniae*. They found that grepafloxacin was the most active quinolone, with a minimal bactericidal concentration (MBC_{90}) of 0.5 mg/L.[85]

Tetracycline and doxycycline should not be administered to pregnant or breast-feeding women. Although the quinolones (e.g., ofloxacin) have been shown to be active against *C. pneumoniae*, they are contraindicated in pregnant and breast-feeding women.

Associated Conditions

Chlamydia pneumoniae has been associated with several other conditions (Table 40–3). However, a direct cause-and-effect relationship has not been demonstrated. *Chlamydia pneumoniae* has also been linked to atherosclerotic cardiovascular disease via seroepidemiologic studies, isolation of the organism in atherosclerotic plaque specimens, experimental in vitro experiments, and the use of animal models, and by two clinical prevention studies.[58] However, the data still require much confirmation before a cause-and-effect relationship between *C. pneumoniae* and atherosclerotic cardiovascular disease can be established. Recently, Ridker and colleagues[86] studied whether previous exposures to *C. pneumoniae*, *Helicobacter pylori*, herpes simplex virus, or cytomegalovirus were associated with an increased risk of cardiovascular disease. These investigators performed a nested case control study among participants in the Women's Health Study that enrolled 39,876 postmenopausal women.[86] Case patients were participants who provided a baseline blood sample and subsequently reported a first cardiovascular event. Control subjects who remained free from cardiovascular disease during the course of the study were randomly selected.

There were 122 case-patients enrolled in the study, and 85 had experienced a myocardial infarction. Case-patients were more likely (statistically significant, $P = .001$) than were control subjects to have hyperlipi-

---

TABLE 40–3 ▶ RISK FACTORS ASSOCIATED WITH *CHLAMYDIA TRACHOMATIS* GENITAL TRACT INFECTION

Historical Factors
Sexual intercourse at an early age
Multiple sexual partners
A sexual partner who has multiple partners
Use of oral contraceptive pills for birth control
The presence of an intrauterine device (IUD)
Past history of a sexually transmitted disease (STD)
Partner known to have or suspected of having an STD
Previous treatment of PID
Frequency of sexual intercourse/month (≥10)[14]
History of cunnilingus[14]

Clinical Factors
Endocervical mucopus
Hypertrophy of the endocervical epithelium
Brisk bleeding when a Papanicolaou (Pap) smear is obtained or when the endocervix is gently touched with a cotton- or Dacron-tipped applicator
Acute onset of postcoital bleeding
Acute onset of dyspareunia
Development of lower abdominal discomfort or pain
Tenderness elicited when the cervix, uterus, or adnexa are palpated or mobilized
Irregular uterine bleeding
Presence of plasma cells in the endometrium
Purulent vaginal discharge in the absence of vaginitis

---

demia, hypertension, diabetes, and a family history of coronary artery disease.[84] These investigators did not find evidence of an association between infection based on seropositivity for antibodies against *C. pneumoniae* (rate ratio, 1.1; 95% confidence interval [CI], 0.7 to 1.8), *H. pylori* (relative risk, 0.9; CI, 0.6 to 1.4), and herpes simplex (rate ratio, 1.2; CI, 0.6 to 2.1).[86]

CHLAMYDIA TRACHOMATIS

Introduction

Chlamydia trachomatis is considered to be the most common sexually transmitted bacteria causing female pelvic infection. It is estimated that *C. trachomatis* causes 4 million genital infections each year.[87] *Chlamydia trachomatis* and *Neisseria gonorrhoeae* are the two types of bacteria that most frequently cause PID. Approximately 10% to 15% of women in the reproductive age group will experience at least one episode of PID.[88] *Chlamydia trachomatis* infection is asymptomatic in approximately 80% of the cases.[89] Therefore, *C. trachomatis* is particularly dangerous because it can progress to significant asymptomatic pelvic infection, resulting in the patient becoming infertile. Although women between the ages of 15 and 25 are at greatest risk, all sexually active women are at risk for contracting *C. trachomatis* infection.[91, 92] The prevalence rate of *C. trachomatis* pelvic infection among sexually active women is 5% to 20%.[89, 90] Once the organism has invaded the cervical columnar epithelium, it can evade the host immune system and remain in a latent state.

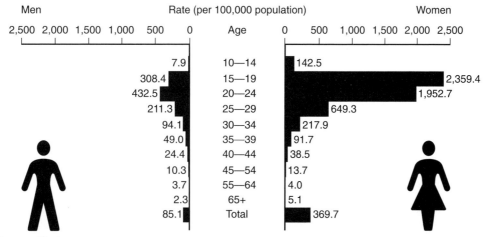

FIGURE 40-4 ▶ Incidence of *Chlamydia trachomatis* urogenital infection in the United States, 1998. (From Sexually Transmitted Disease Surveillance 1998. Centers for Disease Control and Prevention.)

Undetected *C. trachomatis* infection of the cervix, left untreated, can persist for months.[93, 94] It can also ascend to the upper genital tract without causing symptoms.[95] Infection of the fallopian tubes can result in infertility and ectopic pregnancy.[96] *Chlamydia trachomatis* is known to cause lymphogranuloma venereum, an STD not frequently seen in the United States. In addition, *C. trachomatis* can cause neonatal and adult ocular trachoma and neonatal pneumonia.

Clinical Manifestations

Pelvic Inflammatory Disease

The high incidence of asymptomatic chlamydial infection of the lower and upper genital tract led to the recommendation for universal screening of all sexually active women between the ages of 15 and 25 (Fig. 40–4). The distribution of *C. trachomatis* cases appears to be highest among the southern states from the east to the west coast, and the states bordering the Great Lakes, as well as Washington, Vermont, Massachusetts, Connecticut, New Jersey, Delaware, and Washington, DC (Fig. 40–5).

The high prevalence of *C. trachomatis* genital infections, especially among women (Fig. 40–6), would support the recommendation for universal screening of sexually active women who are at risk. It would, however, be more cost-effective to first determine who is at risk for acquiring an STD, and avoid screening women with an extremely low potential for contracting uro-

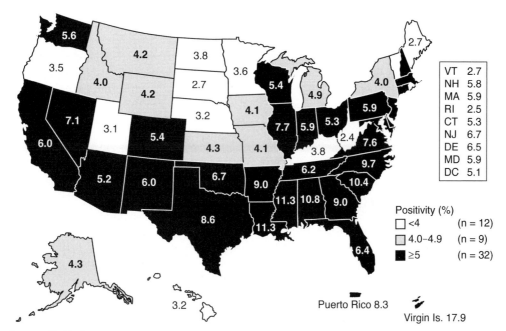

FIGURE 40-5 ▶ *Chlamydia trachomatis* rates among 15- to 24-year-old women tested in family planning clinics by state, 1998. (From Sexually Transmitted Disease Surveillance, 1998. Centers for Disease Control and Prevention.)

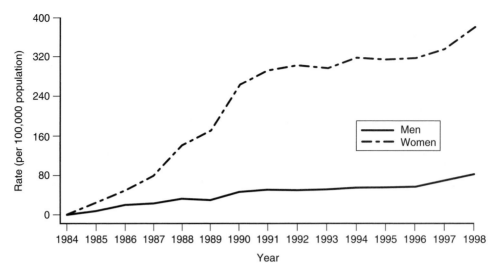

FIGURE 40–6 ▶ Rates of *Chlamydia trachomatis* infection by gender. Note the significant difference in infection rates between men and women. (From Sexually Transmitted Disease Surveillance, 1998. Centers for Disease Control and Prevention.)

genital infection caused by *C. trachomatis* or other sexually transmitted organisms.

The institution of screening programs has indicated that the incidence of PID can be reduced by 60%.[97] In a study by Scholes and co-workers,[97] 1,009 women were randomly assigned to *C. trachomatis* screening and 1,598 women were assigned to usual care (defined as the patients who saw their physicians or health care provider as needed). A total of 645 women in the screening group were tested for *C. trachomatis,* and 7% were positive and treated.[97] A total of 9 patients in the screening and treated group were diagnosed as having PID, compared to 33 women with PID in the usual care group (relative risk, 0.44; 95% confidence interval, 0.2 to 0.9).[97] The authors established that these patients had PID by reviewing the patients' medical records, by noting a discharge code of PID or cervicitis, by checking for a 10-course treatment of doxycycline, and by reviewing medical records of women suspected of having PID, and thus determining whether there was evidence of PID. Analysis of these data led to the conclusion that a universal screening program can reduce the incidence of PID.

However, this study does not establish that these patients actually had PID, since the diagnosis was based on a clinical impression by the patient's individual physician, not a laparoscopic diagnosis. Establishing a diagnosis of PID based solely on clinical findings is wrong in approximately 33% to 50% of the cases.[98, 99] Chaparro and colleagues[98] reported on 223 women who underwent laparoscopic examination because of a clinical diagnosis of PID. They found that 103 (46%) had PID, 31% had other pathologic conditions, and 23% had no evidence of disease.[98] Jacobson and Weström[99] reported a series of 814 cases of PID, in which the diagnosis was established by clinical signs and symptoms. However, they could confirm only 282 cases laparoscopically.[99] If this is true, then the actual number of PID cases in the group undergoing screening would be 3, and in the group not screened 11 could possibly have developed an upper genital tract infection.

Thus, it would appear that universal screening should be reserved for high-risk settings, such as a STD clinic, a family planning clinic, and a college student health clinic.[100] In these situations, the patients are more likely to fit the clinical criteria of high-risk sexual behavior. In the Scholes study only 7% of 645, or 45, patients receiving care in an HMO setting tested positive.[97] However, in a private practice setting or low-risk group, perhaps it would be more cost-effective to screen the individuals who were determined to be at risk by the history and clinical evaluation.

Patients with cervical infection, caused by any organism, are typically asymptomatic. Therefore, it is imperative that the health care provider obtain a detailed history, focusing on past pelvic infections. A history of repeated episodes of bacterial vaginosis might be a clue to the sexual behavioral practices of the patient. A history of repeated episodes of trichomoniasis, an STD, is also an indication that this individual is at risk for the acquisition of other STDs.

Pelvic examination begins with a careful inspection of the external genitalia (Fig. 40–7). The physician should closely inspect and palpate the urethra, and the orifices of Skene's glands (located at the three and nine o'clock positions adjacent to the urethra) and Bartholin's glands for the presence of erythema, purulent exudates, swelling, and pain. The rectum should also be examined for the presence of a purulent exudate. If any of these signs of inflammation are present, a specimen should be obtained for the detection of *C.*

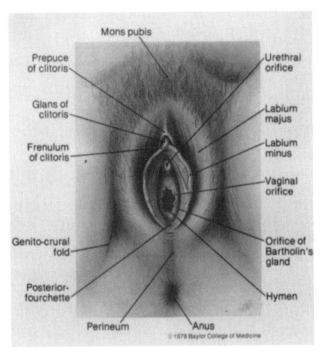

FIGURE **40-7** ▶ External genitalia. (From Kaufman R: Benign Diseases of the Vulva and Vagina, 4th ed. St Louis, Mosby–Year Book, 1994.)

trachomatis and *N. gonorrhoeae*. Patients with a Skene or Bartholin gland abscess can have inguinal lymphadenopathy on the ipsilateral side.

The vaginal ecosystem should be analyzed for the presence of bacterial vaginosis and trichomoniasis. This can be easily accomplished by examining the vaginal discharge microscopically, using either a wet preparation or a Gram stain. If the vaginal discharge contains numerous WBCs, and no detectable pathogen is seen (microscopically), the vaginal discharge should be cultured for *Trichomonas vaginalis,* and a specimen should be obtained from the vaginal walls for the detection of human papillomavirus, using PCR methodology.

The cervix is examined for the characteristics listed in Table 40–1. The patient with cervicitis caused by *C. trachomatis* or *N. gonorrhoeae* is typically asymptomatic. Therefore, the health care provider performing the examination must inspect the cervix very carefully to detect the presence of hypertrophy of the endocervical epithelium. Hypertrophy can be distinguished by eversion of the endocervical epithelium, and by the intense erythema and extreme friability of the hypertrophic epithelium. The hypertrophic epithelium bleeds easily and rather briskly when it is gently palpated with a cotton-tipped applicator. If a specimen is obtained for a Pap smear with the use of a brush, the bleeding can be profuse.

The presence of endocervical mucopus (Fig. 40–8*A* and *B*) is often difficult to detect. The initial step in determining whether the patient has endocervical mucopus is to gently wipe off the portio of the cervix to prevent bleeding, and remove as much of the vaginal discharge as possible. The anatomic position of the cervix constantly exposes it to the vaginal discharge, and if the cervix is located posterior it will sit in the vaginal discharge that collects in the posterior fornix. A Dacron-tipped applicator should be inserted into the endocervical canal, rotated 360 degrees for several seconds, and removed. If a yellow discharge is present, this is endocervical mucopus. The Dacron-tipped applicator should be placed in the appropriate transport medium for the detection of *C. trachomatis* and *N. gonorrhoeae*.

The test employed will determine only whether the *C. trachomatis* organism is present, and not the specific serovar. There are more than 15 serovars of *C. trachomatis:* A, B, and C are associated with trachoma; D through K are found in genital infections; and L1, L2, and L3 cause lymphogranuloma venereum.[101, 102] In one study, the distribution of serovars found in women with PID were as follows: B 1%, D 11%, E 14%, F 11%, G 2%, H 1%, Ia 5%, J 10%, and K 1%.[103] Workowski and co-workers[103] reported that women infected with serovars F and G had fewer signs of infection. These signs included cervical bleeding ($P = .04$), cervical

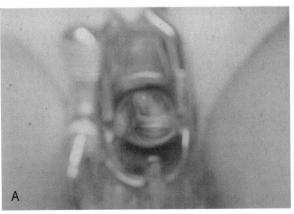

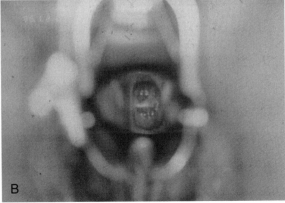

FIGURE **40-8** ▶ *A* and *B,* Endocervical mucopus.

edema ($P = .06$), grossly visible mucopus ($P = .03$), and mucopus documented colposcopically ($P = .007$).[103] The presence of a particular serovar does not impact or affect treatment outcomes. Thus, determining the specific serovar, at this particular time, is of research interest only.

There are several laboratory methods or tests for identifying *C. trachomatis* in clinical specimens. Although culturing the organism continues to be a method employed for identification, it is time-consuming and expensive, and is infrequently used. Culturing was considered the "gold standard" because the specificity in urogenital specimens is nearly 100%, but this test has a sensitivity of only 70% to 85% compared to DNA amplification techniques.[104–106] Several nonculture techniques rely on antibody-antigen reaction or analysis of DNA (Table 40–4).

CHLAMYDIAL INFECTION AND PREGNANCY

The asymptomatic nature of chlamydial infection makes this organism of particular concern for the pregnant patient, since it can cause abortion, interruption of the pregnancy resulting in premature rupture of amniotic membranes, premature labor and delivery, and postpartum endometritis. The prevalence of chlamydial infection in pregnancy has been reported between 2% and 21%.[126] Wager and colleagues[126] found that 41 of 1,447 (2.8%) patients developed postpartum febrile morbidity in those cases after excluding pneumonia, urinary tract infection, mastitis, or wound cellulitis. Thirty-six of the 41 (82%) were positive for *C. trachomatis*. Eight of the 36 (22%) of the *C. trachomatis*-positive women experienced febrile morbidity. The association between febrile morbidity and chlamydial cervicitis was significant ($P > .0001$; relative risk, 9.5; 95% CI, 4.5 to 20.1).[126]

Chlamydial cervicitis during pregnancy is more likely to result in postpartum endometritis if the patient delivers vaginally, rather than by cesarean section.[127–130]

Witkin and Ledger[131] demonstrated a relationship between a high titer of IgG antibodies to *C. trachomatis* and recurrent spontaneous abortion. They found 7 of 17 women with three abortions and 6 of 10 women

---

TABLE 40–4 ▶ NONCULTURE METHODS FOR THE DETECTION OF *CHLAMYDIA TRACHOMATIS*

Direct Cytologic Examination
This method is used to directly stain the organism in a clinical specimen using fluorescein-labeled antibodies. The use of stains containing monoclonal antibody specific for the MOMP of *C. trachomatis* has a sensitivity of 80% to 90% and a sensitivity of 98% to 99% when compared to culture.[107–109] Microtrak DFA (Behring Diagnostics, San Jose, CA) is a commercially available test kit containing anti-MOMP monoclonal antibody.

Immunohistochemical Detection of Antigen (EIAs)
There are basically two EIA test types: the direct and the indirect. Direct EIAs employ enzyme-labeled antibodies that bind to LPS extracted from elementary bodies from all species of *Chlamydia*. The indirect EIA test also employs LPS as the antigen that binds to a detector antibody (murine IgG) to LPS and a secondary antibody (antimurine IgG antibody). Commercially available tests are Chlamydiazyme (Abbott Diagnostics, North Chicago, IL) and Microtrak EIA (Behring), IDEIA (from Dako Diagnostics, Carpinteria, CA), Kallestad Pathfinder EIA (Sanofi Diagnostics Pasteur, Minneapolis, MN), Prima EIA (Baxter Diagnostics, McGaw Park, IL), and Pharmacia EIA (Pharmacia, Franklin, OH). In a comparison of Chlamydiazyme, Gen-Probe, Pathfinder EIA, Microtrak DFA, and Microtrak EIA, the sensitivities ranged from 62% to 75%, and the specificity was more than 99%.[110] The positive predictive value of each test ranged from 0.85 to 0.94.[110]

Rapid or "Point-of-Care" Tests
These tests employ EIA technology based on latex immunodiffusion using antibodies to LPS. The reported sensitivity for endocervical specimens is relatively low, 52% to 85%.[111–113] The low sensitivity does not make this methodology particularly useful in populations with a low prevalence of *Chlamydia* infection.

Nucleic Acid Detection Tests
The most commonly used test, the nucleic acid detection test is the DNA hybridization probe that is a chemoluminescent DNA probe. The test hybridizes to a species-specific sequence of chlamydial 16S rRNA and is available from Gen-Probe (San Diego, CA). The PACE 2C test has the ability to detect both *Chlamydia trachomatis* and *Neisseria gonorrhoeae* from a single specimen with a sensitivity of more than 89% and a specificity of more than 95%.[114]

Polymerase Chain Reaction Assay (PCR)
This test is extremely sensitive and highly specific and is able to detect a single gene copy.[115, 116] The commercially available PCR test Amplicor (Roche Diagnostics) has been modified to detect both *C. trachomatis* and *N. gonorrhoeae* from endocervical swab specimens, urethral swab specimens from men, and urine specimens from women and men, COBAS Amplicor PCR test.[117] Vincelette and colleagues[118] conducted a multicenter trial applying the COBAS Amplicor test compared to culture in 2,014 endocervical swab specimens and 1,278 urine specimens obtained from women. The sensitivity for the COBAS Amplicor PCR test was 96.5% for endocervical specimens and 95.1% for urine specimens obtained from women.[118] The results obtained with the COBAS Amplicor PCR test make this method applicable for screening of urine specimens. Thus, this test is noninvasive and can be collected by having the patient drop her specimen off or mail it to the laboratory, doctor's office, or health clinic. However, using urine to detect cervical chlamydial infection will detect 6% to 30% of women with cervical infection, but not urethral infection.[119–124]

Ligase Chain Reaction Test (LCR)
Abbott developed another nucleic acid test for the diagnosis of *C. trachomatis*, the ligase chain reaction test. LCR, like PCR, is highly sensitive and specific. Dean and co-workers[125] performed a comparative study examining DFA, LCR, and PCR as verification tests for EIA in cervical screening in a low- to moderate-prevalence population.[125] These investigators demonstrated that the tests that fell in the negative gray zone,[103] with the EIA screening test, were found to be positive by LCR and PCR.[125] There were 10 samples that tested positive by EIA/DFA but were negative by LCR and, therefore, were considered false positive.[125]

TABLE 40–5 ▶ OFFICE DIAGNOSTIC TEST FOR ASSESSING THE PATIENT FOR CHLAMYDIAL CERVICITIS

I. **Vaginal Assessment**
   A. Determine the pH of the vaginal discharge. Place pH indicator paper (or other material) against the lateral vaginal wall, at approximately the midregion of the vagina.
   B. Swab the lateral vaginal wall to obtain a specimen of discharge. Place a portion of this discharge on a glass slide and then immerse the swab in 2 mL of saline. Vigorously agitate the swab to dilute the vaginal discharge.
   C. Add a drop of 10% KOH on the glass slide with the drop of vaginal discharge and smell to determine whether a fishy odor is given off. If a fishy odor is emitted, this is highly suggestive of the presence of bacterial vaginosis (BV).
   D. Place 1 to 2 drops of the diluted vaginal discharge on a glass slide, place a coverslip on top of the specimen, and examine microscopically under 40× magnification.

II. **Interpretation**
   A. The absence of a fishy odor indicates that the vaginal discharge does not contain a significant number of anaerobic bacteria.
   B. Microscopic analysis:
      1. Squamous epithelial cells should be well estrogenized, and the gross cellular architecture should be easily identified. If the squamous cells are covered with bacteria, obscuring the cytoplasmic membrane, cytoplasm, and nucleus, this is a clue cell. This finding is characteristic of BV.
      2. There should be <5 WBC/hpf. The presence of >5 WBC/hpf is indicative of inflammation, and suggests the presence of infection.
      3. The dominant bacterial morphotype should be large bacillary forms, suggestive of *Lactobacillus*. There should be only one dominant morphotype, because the presence of more than one suggests that there is an imbalance in the microbial ecology of the vagina.

III. **Assessment of the Cervix**
   A. Cleanse the portio of the cervix with a saline-moistened swab to remove vaginal discharge. This should be done gently, in order to prevent bleeding secondary to trauma.
   B. Inspect the cervix for the presence of endocervical mucopus, hypertrophic endocervical columnar epithelium, petechial hemorrhages, and intense erythema. The presence of any one or all of these characteristics is suggestive of cervicitis and infection.
   C. Obtain a specimen of the endocervical discharge by placing a Dacron-tipped swab into the canal and rotating it 360 degrees several times. Withdraw the swab. If there is a yellow discharge on the end of the swab, this is consistent with mucopus.
   D. Place the swab in 2 mL of saline and agitate the swab vigorously.
   E. Take 1 to 2 drops of the diluted endocervical discharge and examine it microscopically under 40× magnification.
      1. If there are fewer than 5 squamous epithelial cells/40× magnification, this is considered a valid specimen not contaminated by vaginal discharge.
      2. The presence of WBCs is indicative of infection.
      3. The absence of trichomoniasis or yeast suggests the possibility of infection caused by *C. trachomatis* or *N. gonorrhoeae*, or both.
      4. If the specimen can be gram-stained and reveals WBCs, but not a pathogen, *C. trachomatis* may be present.

---

with four abortions, 6 of 47 with one abortion, and 4 of 33 with two abortions to have significant antibody titers to *C. trachomatis* ($P > .01$).[131] The incidence of three or more abortions among women with chlamydial antibody titers ($\geq 1{:}128$) was 32%, and among seronegative women the incidence of abortion was 7.5%.[131]

TREATMENT

Treatment of chlamydial genital infection should also incorporate treatment against *N. gonorrhoeae*. These two organisms are commonly found co-infecting the same individual. The Centers for Disease Control and Prevention (CDC) reports that *C. trachomatis* can be isolated in 20% to 40% of individuals with gonococcal infection.[132] The difficulty is in determining which patient should be treated, since there are no rapid tests that enable a physician or other health care provider to establish the diagnosis with a degree of certainty while the patient is in the office. However, physicians can rely on the history, signs and symptoms, and physical findings. Simple diagnostic tests performed in the office can be of assistance in establishing a significant degree of risk (Table 40–5). Although these tests will not confirm the diagnosis, they will allow institution of treatment while confirmatory test results are pending.

The cervix of all patients suspected of having an STD should be tested for the presence of *C. trachomatis* and *N. gonorrhoeae*. Treatment should be instituted prior to the return of confirmatory data (Table 40–6) to prevent damage to the fallopian tubes.

TABLE 40–6 ▶ TREATMENT OF CERVICITIS CAUSED BY *C. TRACHOMATIS* AND *N. GONORRHOEAE**

Nonpregnant Patients
   Azithromycin, 1 g PO in a single dose
   Doxycycline, 100 mg PO bid for 7 days
   Erythromycin base, 500 mg PO qid for 7 days
   Erythromycin ethylsuccinate, 800 mg PO qid for 7 days
   Ofloxacin, 300 mg PO bid for 7 days

Pregnant Patients
Combination Therapy
   Erythromycin base, 250 mg PO qid for 14 days,
   Erythromycin ethylsuccinate, 800 mg PO qid for 7 days OR
   Erythromycin ethylsuccinate, 400 mg qid for 14 days
   All of the above must be given with one of the following to provide activity against *N. gonorrhoeae*
   Ceftriaxone, 125 mg IM in a single dose,
   Cefixime, 400 mg PO in a single dose, OR
   Spectinomycin, 2 g IM in a single dose
Single Agent Therapy
   Azithromycin, 1 g PO in a single dose

*CDC: 1998 Guidelines for the treatment of sexually transmitted diseases. MMWR 1998; 47:52–62.

SEQUELAE OF CHLAMYDIAL INFECTION

Because of its propensity to cause asymptomatic infection, chlamydial infection is a particularly dangerous pelvic infection. Its insidious nature allows it to progress to involve the upper genital tract and cause significant tissue damage to the reproductive tract. Chlamydiae begin their ascent to the upper genital tract by infecting the endometrium. Infection of the endometrium may be asymptomatic or may present with vague symptoms that, at first, do not cause the physician to consider the possibility of chlamydial endometritis. The patient often presents with mild lower abdominal pain that may be confused with mittelschmerz, an ovarian cyst, cystitis, or dysmenorrhea. More intense pain increases the possibilities in the differential diagnosis to include endometritis, salpingitis, ectopic pregnancy, ruptured hemorrhagic ovarian cysts, torsion of adnexa, torsion of a hydatid of Morgagni, and endometriosis. Sexually active women presenting with lower abdominal pain, regardless of the severity, if accompanied by any symptom that suggests the presence of a significant disease process, should be screened for *C. trachomatis* and *N. gonorrhoeae*. In a study by Scott and co-workers,[133] 165 women with lower abdominal pain were screened for these two sexually transmitted bacteria. *Chlamydia trachomatis* was found as the single infecting organism of the endocervix in 21 patients, *N. gonorrhoeae* was isolated from 5 patients, and the two organisms were found together in 6 patients.[133] Thus, of the 32 (19%) patients harboring a sexually transmitted bacterium, 66% were infected with *C. trachomatis*, 16% had *N. gonorrhoeae*, and 18% had both *C. trachomatis* and *N. gonorrhoeae*.

Although it is not uncommon to find both *C. trachomatis* and *N. gonorrhoeae* simultaneously causing PID, endometritis is rarely detected in these patients because the diagnosis is not sought. However, the presence of irregular uterine bleeding or bloody discharge is often found in patients with a clinical syndrome of PID. Gump and colleagues[134] demonstrated the presence of *C. trachomatis* in a 23-year-old woman with endometritis. The endometrial biopsy revealed a severe inflammatory response with plasma cells, and *C. trachomatis* was cultured from a portion of the specimen. The biopsy was repeated following the completion of therapy and was negative for *C. trachomatis*, while histologic examination revealed a normal secretory endometrium void of an inflammatory response and plasma cells.[134] Jones and co-workers[135] studied 60 women who did not have symptoms or signs of infection but were at risk for chlamydial infection. These women underwent endometrial, endocervical, and urethral sampling for the detection of *C. trachomatis*. *Chlamydia* was isolated from the lower genitourinary tract in 26 (43%), and the endometrium in 12 (20%) of the women.[135] Krettek and co-workers[136] addressed the question of possible endometritis and chlamydial infection in a woman taking oral contraceptive pills and experiencing breakthrough uterine bleeding. These investigators studied three groups of women, with 65 in each group. They found that 19 (29%) women experiencing irregular uterine bleeding were positive for *C. trachomatis;* 7 (10.7%) matched control subjects not experiencing bleeding but taking oral contraceptive pills were also positive for *C. trachomatis;* and 4 (6%) who were screened prior to starting oral contraceptive therapy but had not experienced irregular bleeding were also positive for *C. trachomatis*.[136]

Thus, PID can be considered a spectrum of infection that begins with cervicitis and progresses up the genital tract to endometritis and salpingitis. The organism can exit the fallopian tubes and ascend the colonic gutters to cause a perihepatitis, known as the Fitz-Hugh-Curtis syndrome (Fig. 40–9). This syndrome, originally described in association with gonococcal infection, has been shown to be more frequently associated with chlamydial infection.[137, 138]

Most often patients with perihepatitis are asymptomatic. Symptomatic patients typically complain of pain in the upper right quadrant. The pain is accentuated when there is expansion of the thorax and abdomen, such as deep breathing, coughing, and significant movement of the abdominal wall. During the acute inflammatory phase, auscultation of the upper right quadrant during deep inspiration can reveal the presence of a friction rub. In addition, percussion and palpation of the upper right quadrant may elicit tenderness and guarding.

Infection of the fallopian tubes can result in damage to the ciliated columnar cells that line them. This

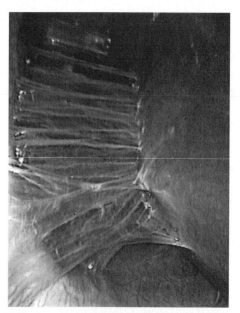

FIGURE 40–9 ▶ Fitz-Hugh-Curtis syndrome. Note the thin, delicate adhesive bands extending from the capsule of the liver to the anterior parietal peritoneum.

damage prohibits the movement of the cilia, which, in turn, prevents the ovum from migrating down the fallopian tube. In addition, the inflammatory response within the fallopian tube can result in the development of adhesions either blocking passage of the ovum or creating false passages. This, in turn, leads to the development of an ectopic pregnancy, since fertilization may not be inhibited, but the fertilized ovum cannot travel through the length of tube and exit into the uterine cavity for implantation.

Inflammation of the fallopian tube can result in formation of adhesions at the proximal and distal ends of the tube. The inflammatory response at the proximal end typically results in occlusion. The distal end, where the fimbriae are located, becomes agglutinated secondary to the inflammation accompanying infection. Once all the fimbriae become agglutinated, the distal end of the fallopian tube becomes agglutinated. This fallopian tube fills with purulent exudates, forming a pyosalpinx or abscess. The pyosalpinx can either resolve with treatment into a hydrosalpinx, undergo torsion, or, if closely pressed against the ovary, infect the ovary via pressure necrosis of the fallopian tube tissue and ovary, forming a tubo-ovarian abscess.

The patient often develops asymptomatic salpingitis. The result of infection becomes evident only if the patient subsequently develops an ectopic pregnancy or is infertile. During the infertility evaluation, either at the time of a hysterosalpingogram or diagnostic laparoscopy, the results of previous pelvic infection are uncovered.

Therefore, the physician must use the patient's history to determine whether upper genital tract infection may be present. This, combined with a careful examination of the abdomen and pelvis, may establish a clinical diagnosis of PID. The clinical parameters used to establish a diagnosis of PID have been published by the CDC and are practical but not definitive.[139]

Upper genital tract infection is diagnosed by the following criteria:

1. Lower abdominal pain
2. Purulent vaginal discharge
3. Purulent endocervical discharge
4. Cervical motion tenderness
5. Uterine tenderness to palpation or motion
6. Adnexal tenderness on pelvic examination
7. Presence of an adnexal mass that is cystic (possible tubo-ovarian complex or abscess)

An important consideration in diagnosing PID is treatment. One should remember that the two most common bacteria that cause PID are *C. trachomatis* and *N. gonorrhoeae*. Since confirmation of the presence of these bacteria cannot be established at the time of patient evaluation, treatment should be administered empirically against both of these bacteria. Instituting treatment based solely on clinical findings results in the treatment of a significant number of women who do not have PID. Judson and Tavelli[140] studied the clinical and epidemiologic characteristics of *C. trachomatis* and *N. gonorrhoeae* PID, and did not find any significant differences in disease caused by *C. trachomatis* and that caused by *N. gonorrhoeae*. These investigators found that *N. gonorrhoeae* was the sole infecting organism in 24 patients, *C. trachomatis* alone was isolated from 16 women, 14 patients had both organisms, and neither organism could be recovered from the endocervix of 35 women.[140] Although these investigators enrolled a total of 89 women who they believed had PID, laparoscopic studies suggest that one third to half of the patients did not have PID.

Chaparro and co-workers[141] studied 223 women who were clinically diagnosed with PID. They performed laparoscopy on all 223 patients and found that 103 (46.2%) had PID, 69 (30.9%) had other pathologies (e.g., ectopic pregnancy, hemorrhagic ovarian cyst, acute appendicitis, and ovarian cancer), and 51 (22.9%) had normal-appearing reproductive organs. Wølner-Hanssen and colleagues[142] performed laparoscopy on 104 patients with a clinical diagnosis of PID. They found that 76 (73%) had evidence of infection and 28 had normal-appearing reproductive organs.

TREATMENT OF PID

The basis of treating PID is the administration of antibiotic therapy that is effective against *C. trachomatis* and *N. gonorrhoeae*, as well as facultative and obligate anaerobic bacteria. The potential upward migration of bacteria from the lower genital tract, along with *C. trachomatis* and *N. gonorrhoeae*, must be considered, since the bacteria of the vaginal ecosystem tend to be destructive. Thus, early recognition or suspicion of the presence of PID is crucial in preventing tissue damage and destruction. Prior to initiating treatment, the clinician must decide whether the patient can be managed in an ambulatory setting or whether she must be hospitalized for treatment (Table 40–7).

TABLE 40-7 ▶ CRITERIA FOR OUTPATIENT TREATMENT
Does not have nausea.
Has not experienced vomiting.
Oral temperature <101°F.
Does not have any suggestion of appendicitis.
Ectopic pregnancy has been ruled out.
Able to tolerate oral liquids and solids.
The patient is known to be noncompliant.
The patient does not have any immunosuppressive therapy.
The patient is not receiving immunosuppressive therapy.
The patient can return for re-evaluation within 72 hours of starting therapy.
There is no evidence of a pelvic mass (i.e., pyosalpinx or tubo-ovarian abscess).

Patients who are treated in an outpatient setting must be able to return for re-evaluation within 72 hours to determine whether the therapy is effective. These patients should have early acute disease with no evidence of a tubo-ovarian complex or abscess. With appropriate treatment of uncomplicated PID, signs of resolution are typically seen within 48 hours of commencement of antibiotic therapy. Patients who do not demonstrate significant improvement are admitted to the hospital for evaluation (e.g., laparoscopy) and administered antibiotics intravenously.

The availability of newer broad-spectrum antibiotics allows for outpatient therapeutic agents that are the same as, or similar to, those that are administered intravenously. The following are regimens that are suitable for outpatient treatment of PID:

L-Ofloxacin (Levaquin) 500, mg PO once a day for 14 days,

Ofloxacin (Floxin), 400 mg PO twice a day for 14 days, *plus* metronidazole, (Flagyl), 500 mg PO twice a day for 14 days,*

Amoxicillin plus clavulanic acid (Augmentin), 500 mg PO three times a day for 14 days,

Ceftriaxone (Rocephin), 250 mg IM once, plus doxycycline, 100 mg PO twice a day for 14 days,* *or*

Cefoxitin (Mefoxin), 2 g IM, plus probenecid, 1 g PO in a single concurrent dose once, plus doxycycline, 100 mg PO twice a day for 14 days*

The author has concerns that the CDC's recommended regimens for using the cephalosporin component are not adequate for preventing tissue damage. Therefore, the administration of agents that provide better obligate anaerobic coverage than that of doxycycline appears to be more prudent and in the patient's best interest.

Treatment of the hospitalized patient should be directed at the same goal. However, if such patients truly have more advanced or complicated disease, broad-spectrum antibiotics should be administered (Table 40–8).

Parenterally administered antibiotics should be continued until the patient is afebrile for 24 hours, there is no evidence of peritonitis, the bimanual examination does not reveal significant tenderness on palpation and motion of the pelvic organs, and the WBC count has returned to normal. Oral antibiotics should be continued until the patient has received a total of 14 days worth of doses. The use of regimens such as L-ofloxacin (Levaquin) or metronidazole plus ofloxacin allows for switching to an oral regimen of the same drugs. When one uses other antibiotics parenterally, a change can be made to oral doxycycline or amoxicillin plus clavulanic acid or L-ofloxacin.

---

*CDC: 1998 Guidelines for the treatment of sexually transmitted diseases. MMWR 1998; 47:84.

TABLE 40–8 ▶	INTRAVENOUSLY ADMINISTERED ANTIBIOTIC REGIMENS FOR THE TREATMENT OF COMPLICATED PID

Piperacillin plus tazobactum (Zosyn), 3.375 g IV q6h,
Ampicillin plus sulbactum, 3 g IV q6h,
L-Ofloxacin (Levoquin), 500 mg IV q24h,
Cefotetan, 2 g IV q12h plus doxycycline, 100 mg IV q12h,*
Cefoxitin, 2 g IV q6h, plus doxycycline, 100 mg q12h*
Clindamycin, 900 mg IV q8h, plus gentamicin, IV, loading dose 2 mg/kg of body weight followed by a maintenance dose of 1.5 mg/kg q8h,* *or*
Ofloxacin, 400 mg IV q12h, plus metronidazole, 500 mg q8h*

*CDC: 1998 Guidelines for the treatment of sexually transmitted diseases. MMWR 1998; 47:82–83.

The key to successful treatment of PID is early recognition (e.g., cervicitis, endometritis, or early acute salpingitis), and institution of appropriate antibiotic therapy. The development of salpingitis, especially if a tubo-ovarian complex has formed, does not have a good prognosis with regard to tubal damage and infertility.

REFERENCES

1. Meyer KF: The host spectrum of psittacosis–lymphogranuloma venereum (PL) agents. Am J Ophthalmol 1967; 63:1225.
2. Moulder JW: The relation of the psittacosis group (Chlamydiae) to bacteria and viruses. Annu Rev Microbiol 1966; 20:107.
3. Moulder JW: The primer for chlamydiae. In: Mardh PA, Holmes KK, Oriel JD, et al (eds): Chlamydial Infections. Amsterdam, Elsevier Biomedical, 1982, pp 3–14.
4. Fukushi H, Hirai K: Proposal of *Chlamydia pecorum* sp. nov. for *Chlamydia* strains derived from ruminants. In J Syst Bacteriol 1992; 42:306.
5. Grayston JT, Kuo CC, Wang SP, Altman J: A new *Chlamydia psittaci* strain, TWAR, isolated in acute respiratory tract infections. N Engl J Med 1986; 315:161.
6. Storz J: *Chlamydia* and *Chlamydia*- Induced Diseases. Springfield, IL, Charles C Thomas, 1971.
7. Moulder JW: Looking at chlamydiae without looking at their hosts. Am Soc Microbiol News 1984; 50:353.
8. Fox A, Rogers JC, Gilbart J, et al: Muramic acid is not detectable in *Chlamydia psittaci* or *Chlamydia trachomatis* by gas chromatography–mass spectrometry. Infect Immun 1990; 58:835.
9. Stephens RS, Kalman S, Lammel C, et al: Genome sequence of an obligate intracellular pathogen of humans: *Chlamydia trachomatis*. Science 1998; 282:754.
10. Newhall WJ, Jones RB: Disulfide-linked oligomers of the major outer membrane protein of chlamydiae. J Bacteriol 1983; 154:998.
11. Hatch TP, Miceli M, Sublett JE: Synthesis of disulfide-bonded outer membrane proteins during the developmental cycle of *Chlamydia psittaci* and *Chlamydia trachomatis*. J Bacteriol 1986; 165:379.
12. Wyrick PB: Cell biology of chlamydial infections. In: Stephens RS, Byrne GI, Christiansen G, et al (eds): Chlamydial Infection. International Chlamydial Symposium, San Francisco, 1998; pp 69–78.
13. Moulder JW: Interaction of chlamydiae and host cells in vitro. Microbial Rev 1991; 55:143.
14. Wyrick PB, Choong J, Davis CH, et al: Entry of genital *Chlamydia trachomatis* into polarized human epithelial cells. Infect Immun 1989; 57:2378.
15. Schachter J, Caldwell HD: Chlamydiae. Annu Rev Microbiol 1980; 34:285.

16. Peeling RW, Peeling J, Brunham RC: High-resolution³¹P nuclear magnetic resonance study of *Chlamydia trachomatis:* Induction of ATPase activity in elementary bodies. Infect Immun 1989; 57:3338.

17. Hatch TP, Al-Hossainy E, Silverman JA: Adenine nucleotide and lysine transport in *Chlamydia psittaci.* J Bacteriol 1982; 150:662.

18. Kaul R, Wenman WM: Cyclic AMP inhibits developmental regulation of *Chlamydia trachomatis.* J Bacteriol 1986; 168:772.

19. Sterling P, Richmond SJ: Production of outer membrane blebs during chlamydial replication. FEMS Microbiol Lett 1980; 9:103.

20. Barry CE 3d, Hayes SF, Hackstadt T: Nucleoid condensation in *Escherichia coli* that express a chlamydial histone homolog. Science 1992; 256:377.

21. Todd WJ, Storz J: Ultrastructural cytochemical evidence for the activation of lysosomes in the cytocidal effect of *Chlamydia psittaci.* Infect Immun 1975; 12:638.

22. de la Maza LM, Peterson EM: Scanning electron microscopy of McCoy cells infected with *Chlamydia trachomatis.* Exp Mol Pathol 1982; 36:217.

23. Todd WJ, Caldwell HD: The interaction of *Chlamydia trachomatis* with host cells: Ultrastructural studies of the mechanism of release of a biovar II strain from HeLa 229 cells. J Infect Dis 1985; 151:1037.

24. Fan T, Lu H, Hu H, et al: Inhibition of apoptosis in *Chlamydia*-infected cells: Blockade of mitochondrial cytochrome c release and caspase activation. J Exp Med 1998; 187:487.

25. Rockey DD, Grosenbach D, Hruby DE, et al: *Chlamydia psittaci* IncA is phosphorylated by the host cell and is exposed on the cytoplasmic face of the developing inclusion. Mol Microbiol 1997; 24:217.

26. Hackstadt T, Scidmore MA, Rockey DD: Lipid metabolism in *Chlamydia trachomatis*–infected cells: Directed trafficking of Golgi-derived sphingolipids to the chlamydial inclusion. Proc Natl Acad Sci USA 1995; 92:4877.

27. Heinzen RA, Scidmore MA, Rockey DD, Hackstadt T: Differential interaction with endocytic and exocytic pathways distinguish parasitophorous vacuoles of *Coxiella burnetii* and *Chlamydia trachomatis.* Infect Immun 1996; 64:796.

28. Wylie JL, Hatch GM, McClarty G: Host cell phospholipids are trafficked to and then modified by *Chlamydia trachomatis.* J Bacterial 1997; 179:7233.

29. Hsia RC, Pannekoek Y, Ingerowski E, Bavoil PM: Type III secretion genes identify a putative virulence locus of *Chlamydia.* Mol Microbiol 1997; 25:351.

30. Hueck CJ: Type III protein secretion systems in bacterial pathogens of animals and plants. Microbiol Mol Biol Rev 1998; 62:379.

31. Relman DA, Falkow S: A molecular perspective of microbial pathogenicity. In: Mandell GL, Bennett JE, Dolin R (eds): Principles and Practice of Infections Diseases, 5th ed. Philadelphia, Churchill-Livingstone, 2000, p 2–12.

32. Kubori T, Matsushima Y, Nakamura D, et al: Supramolecular structure of the *Salmonella typhimurium* type III protein secretion system. Science 1998; 280:602.

33. Hardt WD, Chen LM, Schuebel KE, et al: *S. typhimurium* encodes an activator of Rho GTPases that induces membrane ruffling and nuclear responses in host cells. Cell 1998; 93:815.

34. Clemens JC, Guan K, Bliska JB, et al: Microbial pathogenesis and tyrosine dephosphorylation: Surprising 'bedfellows.' Mol Microbiol 1991; 5:2167.

35. Monack DM, Mecsas J, Bouley D, Falkow S: *Yersinia*-induced apoptosis in vivo aids in the establishment of a systemic infection of mice. J Exp Med 1998; 188:2127.

36. Schesser K, Spiik AK, Dukuzumuremyi JM, et al: The yopJ lucus is required for *Yersinia*-mediated inhibition of NF-kappaB activation and cytokine expression: YopJ contains a eukaryotic SH2-like domain that is essential for its repressive activity. Mol Microbiol 1998; 28:1067.

37. Zychlinsky A, Prevost MC, Sansonetti PJ: *Shigella flexneri* induces apoptosis in infected macrophages. Nature 1992; 358:167.

38. Zychlinsky A, Sansonetti PJ: Perspectives series: Host/ pathogen interactions: Apoptosis in bacterial pathogenesis. J Clin Invest 1997; 100:493.

39. Harris RL, Williams TW: Contributions to the Question of Pneumotyphus: A discussion of the original article by J. Ritter in 1880. Med Bull 1985; 7:119.

40. Schlossberg D: *Chlamydia psittaci* (psittacosis). In: Mandell GL, Bennett JE, Dolin R (eds): Principles and Practice of Infectious Diseases, 5th ed. Philadelphia, Churchill-Livingstone, 2000, pp 2004–2007.

41. Macfarlane JT, Macrae AD: Psittacosis. Med Bull 1983; 39:163.

42. Esposito AL: Pulmonary infections acquired in the workplace. Clin Chest Med 1992; 13:355.

43. Ni AP, Lin GY, Yang L, et al: A seroepidemiologic study of *Chlamydia pneumoniae, Chlamydia trachomatis,* and *Chlamydia psittaci* in different populations on the mainland of China. Scand J Infect Dis 1996; 28:553.

44. Crosse B: Psittacosis: A clinical review. J Infect Dis 1990; 21:251.

45. Schlossberg D, Delgado J, Moore MM, et al: An epidemic of avian and human psittacosis. Arch Intern Med 1993; 153:2594.

46. Reeve RVA, Carter LA, Taylor N, et al: Respiratory tract infections and importation of exotic birds. Lancet 1988; 2:829.

47. Yung AP, Grayson ML: Psittacosis—a review of 135 cases. Med J Aust 1988; 148:228.

48. Schaffner W, Drutz DJ, Duncan GW, et al: The clinical spectrum of endemic psittacosis. Arch Intern Med 1967; 119:433.

49. Chang KP, Veitch PC: Fever, hematuria, proteinuria, and a parrot. Lancet 1997; 350:1674.

50. Brewis C, McFerran DJ. 'Farmer's ear': Sudden sensorineural hearing loss due to *Chlamydia psittaci* infection. J Laryngol Otol 1997; 111:855.

51. Crook T, Bannister B: Acute transverse myelitis associated with *Chlamydia psittaci* infection. J Infect 1996; 32:151.

52. Hyde SR, Benirschke K: Gestational psittacosis: Case report and literature review. Mod Pathol 1997; 10:602.

53. Jorgensen DM: Gestational psittacosis in a Montana sheep rancher. Emerg Infect Dis 1997; 3:191.

54. Idu SR, Zimmerman C, Mulder L, Meis JF: A very serious course of psittacosis in pregnancy. Nederlands Tijdschrift Geneeskd 1998; 142:2586.

55. Shapiro DS, Kenney SC, Johnson M, et al: Brief report: *Chlamydia psittaci* endocarditis diagnosed by blood culture. N Engl J Med 1992; 326:1192.

56. Page SR, Stewart JT, Bernstein JJ: A progressive pericardial effusion caused by psittacosis. Br Heart J 1988; 60:87.

57. Kuo CC, Chen HH, Wang SP, Grayston JT: Identification of a new group of *Chlamydia psittaci* strains called TWAR. J Clin Microbiol 1986; 24:1034.

58. Jackson LA, Grayston JT: *Chlamydia pneumoniae.* In: Mandell GL, Bennett JE, Dolin R (eds): Principles and Practice of Infectious Diseases, 5th ed. Philadelphia, Churchill Livingstone, 2000, pp 2007–2014.

59. Saikku P, Wang SP, Kleemola M, et al: An epidemic of mild pneumonia due to an unusual strain of *Chlamydia psittaci.* J Infect Dis 1985; 151:832.

60. Grayston JT, Kuo CC, Wang SP, Altman J: A new *Chlamydia psittaci* strain, TWAR, isolated in acute respiratory tract infections. N Engl J Med 1986; 315:161.

61. Grayston JT, Kuo CC, Campbell LA, et al: *Chlamydia pneumoniae* sp. nov. for *Chlamydia* sp. strain TWAR. Int J Syst Bacteriol 1989; 39:88.

62. Forsey T, Darougar S, Treharne JD: Prevalence in human beings of antibodies to *Chlamydia* IOL-207, an atypical strain of chlamydia. J Infect 1986; 12:145.

63. Kanamoto Y, Ouchi K, Mizui M, et al: Prevalence of antibody to *Chlamydia pneumoniae* TWAR in Japan. J Clin Microbiol 1991; 29:816.

64. Marton A, Károlyi A, Szalka A: Prevalence of *Chlamydia pneumoniae* antibodies in Hungary. Eur J Clin Microbiol Infect Dis 1992; 11:139.

65. Grayston JT: Infections caused by *Chlamydia pneumoniae* strain TWAR. Clin Infect Dis 1992; 15:757.

66. Steinhoff D, Lode H, Ruckdeschel G, et al: *Chlamydia*

pneumoniae as a cause of community-acquired pneumonia in hospitalized patients in Berlin. Clin Infect Dis 1996; 22:958.

67. Fang GD, Fine M, Orloff J, et al: New and emerging etiologies for community-acquired pneumonia with implications for therapy: A prospective multicenter study of 359 cases. Medicine 1990; 69:307.

68. Marrie TJ, Durant H, Yates L: Community-acquired pneumonia requiring hospitalization: 5-year prospective study. Rev Infect Dis 1989; 11:586.

69. Porath A, Schalaeffer F, Lieberman D: The epidemiology of community-acquired pneumonia among hospitalized adults. J Infect 1997; 34:41.

70. Thom DH, Grayston JT, Wang SP, et al: *Chlamydia pneumoniae* strain TWAR, *Mycoplasma pneumoniae,* and viral infections in acute respiratory disease in a university student health clinic population. Am J Epidemiol 1990; 132:248.

71. Thom DH, Grayston JT, Campbell LA, et al: Respiratory infection with *Chlamydia pneumoniae* in middle-aged and older adult outpatients. Eur J Clin Microbiol Infect Dis 1994; 13:785.

72. Kishimoto T, Kimura M, Kubota Y, et al: An outbreak of *C. pneumoniae* infection in households and schools. In: Orfila J, Byrne GI, Chernesky MA, et al (eds): *Chlamydia* Infections—1994. Bologna, Italy, Societa Editrice Esculapio, 1994, pp 465–468.

73. Gnarpe J, Gnarpe H, Sundelöf B: Endemic prevalence of *Chlamydia pneumoniae* in subjectively healthy persons. Scand J Infect Dis 1991; 23:387.

74. Hyman CL, Roblin PM, Gaydos CA, et al: Prevalence of asymptomatic nasopharyngeal carriage of *Chlamydia pneumoniae* in subjectively healthy adults: Assessment by polymerase chain reaction–enzyme immunoassay and culture. Clin Infect Dis 1995; 20:1174.

75. Hyman CL, Augenbraun MH, Roblin PM, et al: Asymptomatic respiratory tract infection with *Chlamydia pneumoniae* TWAR. J Clin Microbiol 1991; 29:2082.

76. Grayston JT: *Chlamydia pneumoniae* (TWAR) infections in children. Pediatr Infect Dis J 1994; 13:675.

77. Campbell LA, Perez Melgosa M, Hamilton DJ, et al: Detection of *Chlamydia pneumoniae* by polymerase chain reaction. J Clin Microbiol 1992; 30:434.

78. Ramirez JA, Ahkee S, Tolentino A, et al: Diagnosis of *Legionella pneumophila, Mycoplasma pneumoniae,* or *Chlamydia pneumoniae* lower respiratory infection using the polymerase chain reaction on a single throat swab specimen. Diagn Microbiol Infect Dis 1996; 24:7.

79. Wang SP, Grayston JT: Immunologic relationship between genital TRIC, lymphogranuloma venereum, and related organisms in a new microtiter indirect immunofluorescence test. Am J Ophthalmol 1970; 70:367.

80. Verkooyen RP, Hazenberg MA, Van Haaren GH, et al: Age-related interference with *Chlamydia pneumoniae* microimmunofluorescence serology due to circulating rheumatoid factor. J Clin Microbiol 1992; 30:1287.

81. Kuo CC, Grayston JT: In vitro drug susceptibility of *Chlamydia* sp. strain TWAR. Antimicrob Agents Chemother 1988;32:257.

82. Kuo CC, Jackson LA, Lee A, Grayston JT: In vitro activities of azithromycin, clarithromycin, and other antibiotics against *C. pneumoniae.* Antimicrob Agents Chemother 1996; 40:2669.

83. Hammerschlag MR, Qumei KK, Robin PM: In vitro activities of azithromycin, clarithromycin, L-ofloxacin, and other antibiotics against *Chlamydia pneumoniae.* Antimicrob Agents Chemother 1992; 36:1573.

84. Freidank HM, Losch P, Vogele H, Wiedmann-Al-Ahmad M: In vitro susceptibilities of *Chlamydia pneumoniae* isolates from German patients and synergistic activity of antibiotic combinations. Antimicrob Agents Chemother 1999; 43:1808.

85. Roblin PM, Kutlin A, Reznik T, Hammerschlag MR: Activity of grepafloxacin and other fluoroquinolones and newer macrolides against recent clinical isolates of *Chlamydia pneumoniae.* Int J Antimicrob Agents 1999; 12:181.

86. Ridker PM, Hennekens CH, Buring JE, et al: Baseline IgG antibody titers to *Chlamydia pneumoniae, Helicobacter pylori,* herpes simplex virus, and cytomegalovirus and the risk for cardiovascular disease in women. Ann Intern Med 1999; 131:573.

87. Washington AE, Johnson RE, Sanders II Jr: *Chlamydia trachomatis* infections in the United States: What are they costing us? JAMA 1987; 257:2070.

88. Anonymous: Pelvic inflammatory disease: Research directions in the 1990s. Expert Committee on Pelvic Inflammatory Disease. Sex Transm Dis 1991; 18:46.

89. Anonymous: Recommendations for the prevention and management of *Chlamydia trachomatis* infections, 1993. Centers for Disease Control and Prevention. MMWR 1993; 42(RR-12):1.

90. Quinn TC, Gaydos C, Shepherd M, et al: Epidemiologic and microbiologic correlates of *Chlamydia trachomatis* in sexual partnerships. JAMA 1996; 276:1737.

91. Stamm WE, Holmes KK: *Chlamydia trachomatis* infections of the adult. In: Holmes KK, Märdh PA, Sparling PF, Wiesner PJ (eds): Sexually Transmitted Diseases, 2nd ed. New York, McGraw Hill, 1990, pp 181–193.

92. Stamm WE: Diagnosis of *Chlamydia trachomatis* genitourinary infections. Ann Intern Med 1988; 108:710.

93. Hanna L, Dawson CR, Briones O, et al: Latency in human infections with TRIC agents. J Immunol 1968; 101:43.

94. Oriel JD, Ridgeway GL: Studies on the epidemiology of chlamydial infections of the human genital tract. In: Mardh PA, Holmes KK, Oriel JD, et al (eds): Chlamydial Infection. Amsterdam, Elsevier, 1982, pp 425–454.

95. McCormack WM, Alpert S, McComb DE, et al: Fifteen-month follow-up study of a women infected with *Chlamydia trachomatis.* N Engl J Med 1979; 300:123.

96. Sweet RL: Chlamydial salpingitis and infertility. Fertil Steril 1982; 38:530.

97. Scholes D, Stergachis A, Heidrich FE, et al: Prevention of pelvic inflammatory disease by screening for cervical chlamydial infection. N Engl J Med 1996; 34:1362.

98. Chaparro MV, Ghosh S, Nashed A, Poliak A: Laparoscopy for the confirmation and prognostic evaluation of pelvic inflammatory disease. Int J Gynaecol Obstet 1978; 15:307.

99. Jacobson L, Weström L: Objectivized diagnosis of acute pelvic inflammatory disease: Diagnostic and prognostic value of routine laparoscopy. Am J Obstet Gynecol 1969; 105:1088.

100. Teisala K: Sexual behavior and risk for pelvic inflammatory disease. Arch Gyn Obstet 1988; 243:225.

101. Sexually Transmitted Disease Surveillance 1996. Centers for Disease Control and Prevention, 1997, p 9.

102. Washington AE, Johnson RE, Sanders LL, et al: Incidence of *Chlamydia trachomatis* infections in the United States: Using reported *Neisseria gonorrhoeae* as a surrogate. In: Oriel JD, Ridgeway GL, Schather J, et al (eds): *Chlamydia trachomatis* Infections. Proceedings Sixth International Symposium on Human Chlamydia Infections. New York, Cambridge University Press, 1986, pp 487–490.

103. Workowski KA, Stevens CE, Suchland RJ, et al: Clinical manifestations of genital infection due to *Chlamydia trachomatis* in women: Differences related to serovar. Clin Infect Dis 1994; 19:756.

104. Cherensky MA, Jang D, Lee H, et al: Diagnosis of *Chlamydia trachomatis* infections in men and women by testing first-void urine by ligase chain reaction. J Clin Microbiol 1994; 32:2682.

105. Cherensky MA, Jang D, Luinstra K, et al: Ability of ligase chain reaction and polymerase chain reaction to diagnose female lower genitourinary *Chlamydia trachomatis* infection by testing cervical swabs and first void urine. In: Orifila J, Byrne GI, Cherensky MA, et al (eds): Chlamydial infections. Proceedings of the Eighth International Symposium on Human Chlamydial Infections. Bologna, Italy, Societa Editrice Esculapio, 1994, pp 326–329.

106. Lee HH, Cherensky MA, Schachter J, et al: Diagnosis of *Chlamydia trachomatis* genitourinary infection in women by ligase chain reaction assay of urine. Lancet 1995; 345:213.

107. Chernesky MA, Mahony JB, Castriciano S, et al: Detection of *Chlamydia trachomatis* antigens by enzyme immunoassay and immunofluorescence in genital specimens from symptomatic and asymptomatic men and women. J Infect Dis 1986; 154:141.

108. Quinn TC, Gupta PK, Burkman RT, et al: Detection of *Chlamydia trachomatis* cervical infection: A comparison of

Papanicolaou and immunofluorescent staining with cell culture. Am J Obstet Gynecol 1987; 157:394.

109. Smith JW, Rogers RE, Katz BP, et al: Diagnosis of chlamydial infection in women attending antenatal and gynecologic clinics. J Clin Microbiol 1987; 25:868.

110. Newhall WJ, Johnson RE, DeLisle S, et al: Head-to-head evaluation of five chlamydia tests relative to a quality-assured culture standard. J Clin Microbiol 1999; 37:681.

111. Blanding J, Hirsch L, Stranton N, et al: Comparison of the Clearview Chlamydia, the PACE 2 assay, and culture for detection of *Chlamydia trachomatis* from cervical specimens in a low-prevalence population. J Clin Microbiol 1993; 31:1622.

112. Ferris DG, Martin WH: A comparison of three rapid chlamydial tests in pregnant and nonpregnant women. J Fam Pract 1992; 34:593.

113. Grossman JH 3d, Rivlin ME, Morrison JC: Diagnosis of chlamydial infection in pregnant women using the Testpack Chlamydia diagnostic kit. Obstet Gynecol 1991; 77:801.

114. Melton M, Hale Y, Pawlowicz M, et al: Evaluation of the Gen-Probe Pace 2C system for *Chlamydia trachomatis* and *Neisseria gonorrhoeae* in a high-prevalence population. In: Abstracts of the 95th General Meeting of the American Society for Microbiology 1995. Washington, DC, American Society for Microbiology, 1995, Abstr. C482, p 138.

115. Mullis KB, Faloona FA: Specific synthesis of DNA in vitro via a polymerase-catalyzed chain reaction. Methods Enzymol 1987; 155:335.

116. Saiki RK, Scharf SD, Faloona F, et al: Enzymatic amplification of β-globin genomic sequences and restriction site analysis for diagnosis of sickle cell anemia. Science 1985; 230:1350.

117. Crotchfelt KA, Welsh LE, DeBonville D, et al: Detection of *Neisseria gonorrhoeae* and *Chlamydia trachomatis* in genitourinary specimens from men and women by a co-amplification PCR assay. J Clin Microbiol 1997; 35:1536.

118. Vincelette J, Schrim J, Bogard M, et al: Multicenter evaluation of the fully automated COBAS AMPLICOR PCR test for detection of *Chlamydia trachomatis* in urogenital specimens. J Clin Microbiol 1999; 37:74.

119. Dille BJ, Butzen CC, Birkenmeyer LG: Amplification of *Chlamydia trachomatis* DNA by ligase chain reaction. J Clin Microbiol 1993; 31:729.

120. Johannisson G, Lowhagen GB, Lycke E: Genital *Chlamydia trachomatis* infection in women. Obstet Gynecol 1980; 56:671.

121. Lee HH, Chernesky MA, Schachter J, et al: Diagnosis of *Chlamydia trachomatis* genitourinary infection in women by ligase chain reaction assay of urine. Lancet 1995; 345:213.

122. Paavonen J, Vesterinen E: *Chlamydia trachomatis* in cervicitis and urethritis in women. Scand J Infect Dis 1982; 32(suppl):45.

123. Schachter J, Moncada J, Whidden R, et al: Noninvasive tests for the diagnosis of *Chlamydia trachomatis* infection: Application of ligase chain reaction to first-catch urine specimens of women. J Infect Dis 1995; 172:1411.

124. Sellors JW, Mahony JB, Jang D, et al: Comparison of cervical, urethral, and urine specimens for the detection of *Chlamydia trachomatis* in women. J Infect Dis 1991; 164:205.

125. Dean D, Ferrero D, McCarthy M: Comparison of performance and cost-effectiveness of direct fluorescent-antibody, ligase chain reaction, and PCR assays for verification of chlamydial enzyme immunoassay results for populations with a low to moderate prevalence of *Chlamydia trachomatis* infection. J Clin Microbiol 1998; 36:94.

126. Wager GP, Martin DH, Koutsky L, et al: Puerperal infectious morbidity: Relationship to route of delivery and to antepartum *Chlamydia trachomatis* infection. Am J Obstet Gynecol 1980; 138(7 pt, 2):1028.

127. Plummer FA, Laga M, Brunham RC, et al: Postpartum upper genital tract infections in Nairobi, Kenya: Epidemiology, etiology, and risk factors. J Infect Dis 1987; 156:92.

128. Eschenbach DA, Wager GP: Puerperal infections. Clin Obstet Gynecol 1980; 23:1003.

129. Faro S: *Chlamydia trachomatis* infection in women. J Reprod Med 1985; 30(3 suppl):273.

130. Watts DH, Eschenbach DA, Kenny GE: Early postpartum endometritis: The role of bacteria, genital mycoplasmas, and *Chlamydia trachomatis*. Obstet Gynecol 1989; 73:52.

131. Witkin SS, Ledger WJ: Antibodies to *Chlamydia trachomatis* in sera of women with recurrent spontaneous abortions. Am J Obstet Gynecol 1992; 167:135.

132. CDC, 1998 Guidelines for the treatment of sexually transmitted diseases. MMWR 1998; 47:59.

133. Scott GR, Thompson C, Smith IW, Young H: Infection with *Chlamydia trachomatis* and *Neisseria gonorrhoeae* in women with lower abdominal pain admitted to a gynecology unit. Br J Obstet Gynaecol 1989; 96:173.

134. Gump DW, Dickstein S, Gibson M: Endometritis related to *Chlamydia trachomatis* infection. Ann Intern Med 1981; 95:61.

135. Jones RB, Mammel JB, Shepard MK, Fischer RR: Recovery of *Chlamydia trachomatis* from endometrium of women at risk for chlamydial infection. Am J Obstet Gynecol 1986; 155:35.

136. Krettek JE, Arkin SI, Chaisilwattana, Monif GRG: *Chlamydia trachomatis* in patients who used oral contraceptives and had intermenstrual spotting. Obstet Gynecol 1993; 81:728.

137. Woølner-Hanssen P, Weström L, Mårdh P-A: Perihepatitis and chlamydial salpingitis. Lancet 1980; 1:901.

138. Wølner-Hanssen P, Svensson L, Mårdh P-A: Isolation of *Chlamydia trachomatis* from the liver capsule of a patient with Fitz-Hugh-Curtis syndrome. N Engl J Med 1982; 306:113.

139. CDC: 1998 Guidelines for the treatment of sexually transmitted diseases. MMWR 1998; 47:79.

140. Judson FN, Tavelli BG: Comparison of clinical and epidemiological characteristics of pelvic inflammatory disease by endocervical cultures of *Neisseria gonorrhoeae* and *Chlamydia trachomatis*. Genitourin Med 1986; 62:230.

141. Chaparro MV, Ghosh S, Nashed A, Poliak A: Laparoscopy for the confirmation and prognostic evaluation of pelvic inflammatory disease. Int J Gynecol Obstet 1978; 15:307.

142. Wølner-Hanssen P, Mårdh P-A, Svesson L, Weström L: Laparoscopy in women with *Chlamydia* infection and pelvic pain: A comparison of patients with and without salpingitis. Obstet Gynecol 1983; 61:299.

41

Human Papillomavirus

Stanley A. Gall

Genital warts have been recognized for centuries and were described in AD 25 by Celsus. Despite the early description of them and the ancient association between condylomas and the female genital tract, their true etiology has only recently been determined. As late as the 1960s, nonspecific material such as dirt and genital secretions were implicated in the development of genital warts. In 1907, skin warts were experimentally produced by inoculations of extracts of penile warts into nongenital epithelium, thereby strongly implicating an infectious etiology. In 1949, the viral etiology was demonstrated by the presence of viral particles in wart tissue by the use of the electron microscope. Sexual transmission of genital warts was affirmed in 1954, although the common viral etiology of skin and genital warts obscured the concept of genital warts as a sexually transmitted disease.[1] A critical step in our understanding of human papillomavirus (HPV) disease occurred with the demonstration by Zur Hausen and colleagues[2] that multiple HPVs exist and can be typed with recombinant DNA analysis. This discovery led to the determination that certain HPV DNA types have a predilection for certain anatomic sites.

The older concept that HPV manifests itself only in external genital warts has been broadened. It is now recognized that HPV functions as a co-carcinogen for many squamous carcinomas of the genital tract, including preinvasive as well as invasive cancers. Therefore, the spectrum of disease includes not only classic condyloma acuminata of the genital tract but also entities such as subclinical papillomavirus infection and intraepithelial and invasive neoplasia of the vulva, vagina, cervix, and anus. Recurrent respiratory papillomatosis (RRP) must also be included in the spectrum of disease.[3]

VIROLOGY

The papillomaviruses are members of the papovavirus family. They have a DNA genome associated with histones that are condensed into nucleosomes and surrounded by an icosahedral protein capsid.

The genetic information of the papillomaviruses is contained in a closed, circular, double-stranded DNA molecule of about 8,000 base pairs. The genomes of all papillomaviruses are organized similarly. A noncoding region with apparent regulatory function is located upstream from the first six open reading frames that are considered to be early genes; that is, E6, E7, E1, E2, E4, and E5. Two late genes, L2 and L1, complete the circle. The viral DNA molecules appear to replicate as episomes. The products of the early genes, when known, have been assigned functions that relate to the control of viral DNA replication, whereas the two late genes encode a major and minor capsid protein, respectively.[4] The HPV DNA is found to exist as plasmids in condyloma acuminata and in preinvasive lesions of the genital tract.[5] However, evidence has been presented that indicates that the viral DNA is integrated into cellular DNA in invasive cervical cancers.[6, 7]

HPVs have a molecular weight of 5×10^6 daltons, are highly host specific, and are characterized by their ability to transform epithelial cells. The existence of different HPV types was demonstrated through the finding of immunologically distinct strains as well as molecular hybridization. Originally, it was determined that a papillomavirus would be considered a new type if it had less than 50% DNA sequence homology with other papillomaviruses of the same species or if the virus was indistinguishable from known types but differed in its restriction cleavage pattern. Viruses with more than 50% DNA sequence homology to a known type were designated subtypes.[8] To date, more than 70 different types of HPV have been described, with about 40% associated with lesions in the anogenital tract.[9] The current standard of determining the similarity of HPV types is by DNA sequencing. The nucleotide sequence of the E6, L1, and noncoding region of a type must have less than 90% identity to any other type, whereas variants or subtypes typically differ by 0% to 10% in coding regions.[10, 11] Phylogenetic analyses of HPV genomes have suggested that the rate of mutation of the HPV genome is low. The finding that intratypic variation is very low suggests that a vaccine that uses a prototype strain would be effective against most variants of that strain.

Papillomaviruses can be divided into those that affect epithelial cutaneous tissues and those that affect mucosal tissues. Different HPV types have different biologic activity in tissues, whether it be association with neoplasia, effect on recurrence of cancer, or frequency or recurrence of condyloma acuminata. Several viral types have been studied more intensely to understand their association with genital tract neoplasia. HPV types 6, 11, 16, 18, 31, 33, and 35 have varying degrees of association with premalignant, malignant, and condylomatous lesions of the genital tract.

Human papillomavirus type 6 (HPV-6) and HPV-11 are almost always associated with benign lesions, such as condyloma acuminata, laryngeal papillomas, or low-grade squamous intraepithelial lesions (LGSIL), and very infrequently with squamous cell cancers of the genital tract. HPV-6 and HPV-11 have been found in as many as 40% of flat cervical lesions. They are rarely present in high-grade squamous intraepithelial lesions (HGSIL) or invasive cervical cancers.[12]

HPV-16 is the viral type most often detected in HGSIL[10–13] and invasive squamous cancers of the cervix and their metastases.[14] HPV-16 DNA sequences have been detected in all grades of cervical intraepithelial neoplasias as well. HPV-16 is thought to be a high-risk virus because of its prevalent association with high-grade lesions and invasive cancer of the cervix.

HPV-18 is also considered to be a high-risk type because it is frequently found in high-grade cervical lesions and invasive cancer. HPV-18 is found at a disproportionately low rate in LGSIL compared with its frequency in invasive cancer, suggesting that HPV-18 lesions may progress more rapidly or the DNA levels of HPV-18 are too low to detect.[15] HPV-18–associated cervical cancers tend to be associated with younger age, more frequent metastasis, a higher recurrence rate, and higher tumor grades; therefore, HPV-18–containing tumors are more clinically aggressive.[16]

HPV-31, HPV-33, and HPV-35 have been classified as an intermediate risk, as they are found in about 10% of the patients with cervical intraepithelial neoplasia and in about 5% of patients with invasive cancer.[17] The associations of other HPV types with benign, premalignant, and malignant lesions are less certain, mainly because of lower frequency of diagnosis and fewer samples having been studied. These viruses would include HPV types 30, 39, 40, 42 to 45, and 52 to 56.[18]

HPV types associated with risk of malignancy vary with geographic location. HPV-16 is found in 77% of cervical cancers in Germany, 71% of those in South America, and 59% of those in the United States, but in only 33% to 39% of cervical cancers in Japan.[3, 12, 17, 19] On the other hand, HPV-52 is found in 20% of invasive cervical cancers in Japan, but is rarely detected (2%) in cervical intraepithelial lesions or invasive cancer in the United States.[20] It is unknown whether these geographic differences represent mutated HPV genomes, simple distribution of HPV types, genetic selec-

tion in various populations, or some other unknown mechanism.

A major problem in HPV research is the inability to propagate HPV in culture. This is probably due to the fact that viral gene transcription and replication is tightly tied to the differentiated state of the epithelial cell. Conditions for achieving complete differentiation of cells in organotypic cultures with production of virion have been described; however, successive rounds of productive viral infections have not been achieved.[21] Other problems with the virus include (1) generally no sources of infectious virion and no assays for the ability to neutralize HPV infectivity in culture; (2) extremely low numbers of virions found in clinical lesions; and (3) no animal system in which HPV has been known to replicate or cause disease, since papillomaviruses are highly species specific. There is one exception. A xenograft system has been developed in which a particular strain of HPV-11 that is mixed with human epithelial cells and implanted under the renal capsule of a nude mouse is able to produce infectious virus.[22] The model has been used to assay for neutralizing antibodies that inhibit the infectivity of HPV-11 and HPV-6. The attempts at propagation of other HPV types in the model have been unsuccessful.

The cloning of HPV genes has been critical in the progress of identifying the functions of genes and has provided a source of viral proteins for agents in immunologic assays. As previously discussed, HPV consists of six early open reading frames (ORF) and two late open reading frames. L1 and L2 encode the major and minor capsid proteins, respectively. These are the only viral proteins present in the virion. The capsid is composed of 72 capsomeres, each of which is a pentamer of L1. The location of L2 is not known. The E6 and E7 genes are invariably expressed in tumors and are sufficient to induce proliferation and to immortalize cells in culture. Continuous expression of E6/E7 is required for maintaining the proliferative state of the cells.[23] The E2 protein represses transcription of the E6 and E7 genes, and elimination of E2 or dampening of its activity may be important in the development of malignancy. Both E1 and E2 are required for viral DNA replication. The function of E5 in HPVs is not known, but in bovine papillomavirus, the E5 gene is a membrane-associated protein that interacts with cellular growth factor receptors to trigger mitogenesis. The E5 gene is frequently lost in tumors. The E4 protein is abundantly expressed, interacts with the cytoskeleton, and may be involved in the maturation of the virion or its egress from the cell. The region between L1 and E6 does not encode any viral proteins but contains cis-acting elements that are required for regulation of transcription and replication and have been designated the noncoding region (NCR), upstream regulatory region (URR), or the long control region (LCR).

High-risk HPV E6 proteins can form complexes with the tumor suppressor protein p53.[24] In vitro studies demonstrate that on binding, high-risk HPV E6 proteins facilitate the rapid degradation of p53.[25] Since low-risk HPV E6 proteins do not specifically interact with p53, they have no direct effect on p53 stability. An additional cellular protein of 100 kDa, designated *E6-AP* (E6 associated protein), has been found to be necessary for the binding of E6 to p53 and the degradation of p53.[26]

The p53 tumor suppressor protein is a transcriptional activator that binds directly to its target DNA sequence. This results in markedly increased levels of intracellular p53 in response to DNA damage induced by radiation or chemical mutagens. The higher levels of p53 result in G1 growth arrest of the treated cells and allow for repair of damaged DNA (or for the cell to be eliminated by apoptosis) before DNA replication begins.[27] Elevated levels of p53 induce gene expression that encodes a protein designated p21 (WAF1 and CiP1), which acts as a potent inhibitor of several G1-specific cyclin-dependent kinases (cdks), leading to growth arrest.[28] E6-stimulated degradation of p53 nullifies the negative growth regulatory effect of p53 after DNA damage. Because HPV-E6 protein expression does not permit DNA repair after DNA damage, HPV immortalized cells or cell lines derived from cervical carcinomas often have abnormal karyotypes.

The HPV E7 genes encode zinc-binding nuclear phosphoproteins of approximately 100 amino acids. These proteins participate in the binding of several proteins, including the retinoblastoma tumor suppressor gene product pRB and structurally related proteins p107 and p130. The proteins p107 and p130 are structurally related to pRB and are identified as the binding pocket proteins for viral oncoproteins, including HPV E7.

In G_0, G_1, and late M phase of the cell cycle, pRB exists in a hypophosphorylated form whereas it exists in a hyperphosphorylated state during S, G_2, and early M phase. The interaction of HPV E7 with hypophosphorylated pRB may activate pRB and stimulate the cell cycle into S phase.[29] HPV E7 displaces cellular proteins that normally bind to pocket proteins and therefore interfere with the regulatory pathways that are present in noninfected cells. HPV E7 protein, in its intereaction with pocket proteins, actively disrupts the normal regulation of the E2F transcription factor. E2F complexes are markedly reduced in HPV E7–expressing cells.

Efficiency in the malignant transformation is determined by the amino terminal portion of E7, particularly the pRB binding site.[30] Sequence comparisons of high-risk and low-risk HPVs reveal amino-acid sequence differences at the pRB binding site. Additionally, E7 sequences with a single amino-acid variation are largely responsible for the different transforming capacity of low-risk and high risk E7 proteins.[31]

IMMUNOLOGY OF HPV INFECTIONS

The events occurring with regard to the immune biology of HPV infection remain incompletely elucidated. Because HPVs are epitheliotropic, they do not seem to induce an inflammatory response within the infected tissue. While keratinocytes, the natural target of papillomavirus infections, are not antigen-processing cells (APCs), Langerhans cells in the epithelium are APCs. Immune mechanisms clearly have a role in controlling HPV infections. This can be demonstrated clinically by the fact that many patients with external genital warts (EGWs) will clear their infection with time, and in the laboratory by the finding of mononuclear cells, mostly CD4 cells and macrophages, in regressing papillomas.[32] Another clinical example of the influence of the immune system is the increased frequency and severity of HPV infections in immunosuppressed individuals or in persons who have a temporary suppression of their immune system.[33, 34]

Information about the humoral immune response to HPV infections has been limited because there has been no experimental system for the large-scale production of papillomavirus. This has been circumvented by the use of papillomavirus proteins obtained by recombinant vectors, thus facilitating assays for antibodies directed against HPV types that could not be prepared from clinical lesions.[35, 36] Recombinant HPV proteins and synthetic peptides derived from seroreactive regions of the individual proteins have been used as antigens in several assays, the most common of which were enzyme-linked immunosorbent assay (ELISA) and Western blotting.[37, 38]

Another methodology for HPV serology, immunoprecipitation, is now available.[39] This method takes advantage of the immune precipitin curve, in which antigen-antibody complexes can be precipitated in solution by protein A–bound sepharose beads. Radioactive labeling of the antigen can be done, or a specific monoclonal antibody can be used.

A number of authors have addressed the question of whether a humoral response to HPV infections occurs. The questions to be answered are as follows: (1) what is the nature of the humoral immune response? (2) is the humoral response universal? and (3) does it protect the patient from re-infections?

Eisemann and co-workers[40] analyzed, by ELISA, a total of 478 human sera for the presence of antibodies to HPV-11 virus–like particles (VLPs). Sera was obtained from patients with condyloma acuminata, males with infertility disorders, blood donors, and general hospitalized patients. Antibody prevalence was 23.6% in the condyloma group, 18.2% in the blood-donor group, 16.6% in the hospitalized-patient group, and

TABLE 41–1 ▶ Prevalence of Antibodies Against HPV-16 E7 (6–35) in Sera of Patients with Cervical Intraepithelial Neoplasia (CIN), Cervical Cancer, and Control Subjects

Condition	N	Anti-E7 (6–35) Positive n	%
CIN	129	9*	7.0
Cervical cancer	424	75	17.7
Control subjects	218	24†	11.0

*P < .005 vs. cervical cancer patients.
†P < .05.
Adapted from Baar MF, Duk JM, Burger MM, et al: Antibodies to human papillomavirus type 16 E7 related to clinicopathological data in patients with cervical carcinoma. J Clin Pathol 1995; 48:410–414.

3.2% in the infertile-male group. This study demonstrated that an immune response was elicited in 23% of patients with condyloma acuminata, as measured by an HPV-11 VLP, which is an L1 protein. The lack of immune response is probably related to the method of testing, since most patients with EGWs are infected with HPV-6 that is closely related to HPV-11 in protein composition. The authors speculated that IgG antibodies to HPV-11 VLPs do not confer immunity to clinical HPV infection.

Baay and colleagues[41] investigated the correlation between antibodies to the transforming protein E7 of HPV-16 and several clinicopathologic indices in women with squamous cancer of the cervix. They used a synthetic peptide of HPV-16 E7 protein (amino acids 6–35) in an ELISA assay to test for the presence of HPV antigen-specific antibodies. Seroreactivity was significantly higher in patients with invasive carcinoma than in controls of women with cervical intraepithelial neoplasia (CIN; Table 41–1). Prevalence rates of antibodies in the different FIGO stages of disease are seen in Table 41–2. Although a statistically significant trend of increasing seropositivity with increasing stage was obtained, analysis of IgG content in patients' sera did not show any differences between the FIGO stages. No

TABLE 41–2 ▶ Prevalence of Antibodies Against HPV-16 E7 (6–35) in Sera from 424 Women According to Stage of Disease

FIGO Stage	N	Anti-E7 (6–35) Positive n	%
IB	203	30	14.6
II	163	30	18.4
III	39	5	12.8
IV	19	10	52.6

Adapted from Baar MF, Duk JM, Burger MM, et al: Antibodies to human papillomavirus type 16 E7 related to clinicopathological data in patients with cervical carcinoma. J Clin Pathol 1995; 48:410–414.

data concerning the presence of HPV DNA in the tumor tissues from patients in this study were available. The results of this study showed that the presence of antibodies against E7 (amino acids 6–35) in pretreatment sera correlated with the size of the lesion, lymph node involvement, and a worse prognosis. However, since antibodies were detected only in a minority of patients with cervical cancer, the clinical value of using these antibodies as a detection or progression marker is low.

Other investigators studied the prognostic significance of serum antibodies to HPV-16 E4 and E7 peptides in cervical cancer.[42] These authors studied 78 women with cervical cancer and 198 control subjects using an ELISA for reactivity with HPV-16 E4 (E401p) and E7 (E701p) synthetic peptides. Antibodies to E401p peptide were found in 5 of 198 (3%) control patients; 4 of 43 (9%) patients with FIGO stages Ia, Ib, and IIa; and 7 of 35 (20%) patients with FIGO stages IIb, III, and IVa. Antibodies to E701p were found in 25 (13%), 11 (26%), and 11 (31%), respectively. The differences between patients and control subjects are significant (P < .002). The authors concluded that the significance of serum antibodies against HPV-16 E4 and E7 in patients with cervical cancer is limited. The HPV DNA status of the patients was unknown, which limited the value of the study. Additionally, the clinical outcome was not predicted by serum antibody concentrations. Probably the major drawback of the studies using HPV peptides is that only reactivity with linear epitopes is measured.

A protein more closely resembling the conformational structure of the natural E7 protein might be more successful in detecting HPV antibodies. Bonnez and co-workers[43, 44] used HPV-11 viral particles grown in athymic mice as an antigen in an ELISA to compare the responses of 46 biopsy-proven condyloma acuminata and 44 controls. A total of 33% of the values in the sera from the condyloma acuminata group were higher than those of the controls, and the sera was significantly more reactive than those of controls. Unfortunately, the recombinant fusion proteins, when used in immunoassays, had difficulty in differentiating condyloma patient sera and control sera. The authors did demonstrate that some antibody reactive to HPV-11 protein was present.

In a follow-up study, the same authors evaluated the variation over time of seroreactivity of HPV-11 according to disease outcome. Pretreatment and posttreatment blood was obtained. In seven patients who cleared their condyloma acuminata with interferon therapy, the median optical density (OD) of the ELISA dropped 0.05% per day, whereas in a group of 11 who failed interferon therapy ODs increased by 0.07% per day (P < .006). The results suggest several conclusions: first, the dose of interferon (2 × 10^6 μ for 4 weeks) was too small; second, they did not treat their patients long enough; third, the group that failed therapy maintained a high level of virus; and fourth, the high levels of humoral antibodies did not control the disease.

Heim and co-workers[45] analyzed serum samples by ELISA for specific IgG and IgM antibodies, recognizing HPV types 6 and 11 L VLPs. Positive IgG and IgM reactivities were, respectively, 12% and 6% for 87 control subjects; 46% and 67% for 79 condyloma acuminata patients; 30% and 64% for 72 CIN patients; 16% and 19% for 63 pregnant women at the time of delivery; and 5% and 0% for their 63 newborns. IgA reactivities were low and not significant. In this study, 24% of patients were negative for both HPV-6 and HPV-11 L1. This study demonstrates immune reactivity as measured in this particular assay, but little more can be derived.

Dillner and colleagues[46] attempted to measure IgA antibodies in cervicovaginal secretions using purified bovine papillomavirus virions as antigens in an ELISA. A total of 8 of 9 patients with CIN had IgA antibodies, 3 of 9 with koilocytosis but no CIN were positive for IgA antibodies, but 6 of 24 women with normal Pap smears and negative colposcopy were also positive. The important finding is that the local immune response occurs, but the intensity, duration, and effect on the course of disease is unknown.

Studies for eliciting information regarding cell-mediated immunity (CMI) in women infected with HPV have been less frequent. Kadish and co-workers[47] studied 42 women with abnormal genital cytology and 13 normal control subjects for the presence of lymphocyte proliferation (LP), CMI responses, and serologic reactivity to E7 peptides of HPV-16. HPV was typed by Southern blot hybridization of exfoliated cell DNA. They found positive LP responses in 12 of 42 (28.6%) patients and 3 of 13 (23.1%) control subjects. Of the patients infected with HPV-16, -31, or -33, 7 of 11 (63.6%) showed a positive LP response, compared with only 2 of 14 (14.3%) infected with other HPV types (P < .02), 3 of 17 (17.6%) negative for HPV, and 3 of 13 (23.1%) control subjects. C-terminal peptide 109 (amino acids 72–97) elicited positive LP responses in 5 of 11 (45.4%) patients infected with HPV-16, -31, and -33, compared to 1 of 14 (7.1%) patients infected with other HPVs. ELISA reactivity occurred in 1 of 13 (7.7%) control subjects, 6 of 17 (35.3%) HPV-negative patients, 6 of 14 (42.9%) infected with other HPVs, and only 1 of 11 (9.1%) patients infected with HPV-16, -31, or -33. The authors demonstrated that CMI responses were related to ongoing cervical infections and were type-specific, whereas serologic reactivity to HPV-16 E7 peptides was not HPV type-specific.

Arany and colleagues[48] determined the pretreatment status of local CMI responses to HPV infection by reverse transcriptase–polymerase chain reaction (RT-PCR) in patients with condyloma acuminata who received interferon treatment and responded well or poorly to therapy. The authors found that biopsies from nonresponders were markedly depleted of Langerhans cells, leading to decreases in major histocompatibility complex class II expression and therefore diminished attraction of CD4[+] T cells. The mRNA levels of cytokines (interleukin-1α, interleukin-1β), granulocyte-macrophage colony-stimulating factor (GM-CSF), and tumor necrosis factor (TNF) that participated in the immune responses were low in nonresponders. In contrast, responders demonstrated high levels of macrophage–natural killer cells (CD16[+]) and activated CD4 (IL-2, interferon-γ–positive, T_H1 cells) T-cell recruitment against HPV-infected keratinocytes, which is consistent with the delayed-type, hypersensitivity-like cellular immune response. The lack of immune response in nonresponders appeared to correlate with high expression levels of the HPV E7 gene. The authors demonstrated that the responders' immune response to interferon therapy is characterized by an increase in activated CD4[+] T_H1 lymphocytes and macrophage–natural killer cells. The lack of immune response in nonresponders may be associated with an overexpression of the HPV E7 gene.

The previous studies would suggest that the humoral immune (HI) response occurs but is nonspecific, whereas the cell-mediated response is type-specific and is characterized by a definite sequence of cellular activity. The key element is the stimulation of the Langerhans cell, which attracts CD4[−] T cells. The increased levels of mRNA of IL-1α, IL-16, GM-CSF, and TNF indicate that a delayed-hypersensitivity–type reaction is present. The findings of high levels of CD16[+] and activated CD4[−] T-cell recruitment against HPV-infected keratinocytes support this thesis.

At this time, it seems that the association of serum antibodies to HPV proteins with HPV-related diseases is well established. Antibodies to some early viral proteins, but also to viral capsids (VLPs) and peptides, are found in many patients with benign and malignant forms of HPV-related disease. However, what is totally unclear is the role of humoral antibodies. The evidence, to date, would suggest that the role in protective immunity or in protection against recurrent infection has not been elucidated.

EPIDEMIOLOGY OF HPV-RELATED DISEASE

Since there is no compulsory notification system for HPV-related diseases, the true incidence can be obtained only from hospital series or physician-consultation statistics. There are strong indications that the incidence of HPV-related disease has substantially increased in Western countries and could well be the most common STD today.

One of the best available sources of data is the National Disease and Therapeutic Index (NDTI), which enumerates the initial consultations for diagnosis and treatment of genital warts in a stratified random sample of private practitioners. The true incidence rates cannot be computed because no denominators are given, cases admitted to STD clinics are not included, and the data are population based and do not include consultations for subclinical warts. Despite these shortcomings, the NDTI data have been widely used as a national surveillance indicator for genital warts[49] and have been featured in STD surveillance reports by the Centers for Disease Control and Prevention.[50] The NDTI data indicated a fourfold to fivefold increase in the number of initial office visits for HPV diseases from 1966 to 1990 by both sexes; an apparent decline, however, has occurred since 1990. A study conducted in Rochester, Minnesota, covering the period from 1950 to 1978 indicated an annual incidence of 107 cases per 100,000 population.[51] The authors found that the incidence of condyloma was 50% greater in women.

The risk factors for acquiring condyloma acuminata include multiple sexual partners, autoinoculation, and long-term use of oral contraceptives. Associated risks include cigarette smoking, alcohol beverage ingestion, and any lifestyle activity that is immunosuppressive.

The risk factors for squamous cancer of the cervix are strongly influenced by three measures of sexual activity: the number of sexual partners, age at first sexual intercourse, and the sexual behavior of the patient's consort.[52] Other important risk factors are tobacco smoking,[53] increasing parity, failure to have a Pap cancer test, and possible infection with herpes simplex virus type 2. Long-term oral contraceptive users are at risk for CIN, but not for invasive disease.[54]

It is now clear from the data accumulated over the past 25 years that a certain HPV type or types have been identified as the putative microbiologic agent or agents acting as a co-carcinogens for cervical cancer. Other co-carcinogens have been strongly implicated; namely, cigarette smoking and possibly HPV-2 or a lack of vitamin A. It seems to be well accepted that more than 95% of invasive squamous cancers of the cervix harbor certain HPV types that have been recognized as oncogenic. It is highly unlikely that squamous cancers of the cervix will be found in virginal women.[55, 56]

The epidemiologic studies for vaginal cancer and vulvar cancer have not allowed for meaningful conclusions, as the studies in cervical cancer have done. The data on clear cell adenocarcinoma of the vagina following in-utero exposure to diethylstilbestrol (DES) were identified with small numbers and are widely accepted. Squamous cell vaginal cancers are thought to be related etiologically to cervical cancer, on the basis that the epithelial lining of the female genital tract is the target for the same carcinogenic insults. Investigators have found a strong association among the risk of vaginal cancer and the number of lifetime sexual partners, a history of genital warts, and an antibody response to HSV-2 infection.[57] An ongoing case-control study of anogenital cancers in Washington state has found that 63% of vaginal tumors harbor HPV DNA by PCR.[57]

Epidemiologic studies of vulvar cancer indicate a profile similar to that of patients being treated for CIN or invasive cervical cancer. There is a strong relationship with the number of lifetime sexual partners and a strong association with a history of EGWs.[58, 59] The authors found that women who had a history of genital warts and who smoked had risks that were much greater than if these exposures were independent events. Vulvar cancer is increased in women in the highest percentile of body mass index and is not influenced by increasing parity or the use of oral contraceptives. The epidemiologic profiles suggest two exclusive pathogenetic mechanisms for vulvar cancer: one mediated by HPV with the characteristics of STD promoted by co-factors, such as smoking, and the other with later onset and associated with vulvar inflammatory disease and related lesions.[60–62]

PATHOGENESIS OF HPV INFECTIONS

The female genital tract contains highly specialized types of epithelium particularly susceptible to HPV infection. The cervical portio, vaginal walls, and vulvar vestibule are lined by a glycogenated, noncornified, stratified squamous epithelium. The labia minora, clitoris, and interlabial sulci are lined by thinly keratinized epithelium, but no hair follicles or sweat glands. The labia majora, mons pubis, and perianal areas are fully keratinized and contain hair follicles and sebaceous and sweat glands.

HPV infection is believed to begin with the entry of mature virions into the basal layer of the epithelium through microabrasions that occur at the time of coital activity. After infection, the viral DNA becomes stabilized as an independent, replicating episome within the nucleus of the epithelial cell. At this point, a number of events may occur in the papilloma cell cycle (Fig. 41–1). The virus may enter latency and never manifest itself as either condyloma acuminata or abnormal genital cytology. The events that determine whether the virus will enter latency directly are unknown, but the concept of latency is critical to the understanding of the life cycle of HPV and the events seen in clinical medicine. When the virus is in the latent phase, there are no clinical signs and no phenotypic changes in maturing cells. If the HPV infection becomes active, morphologic expression of early and late gene functions in differentiating squamous cells are present. Early gene functions are manifested histologically by an increase in the thickness of the stratum spinosum and the prickle cell layers (acanthosis). Late gene function is characterized by the expression of

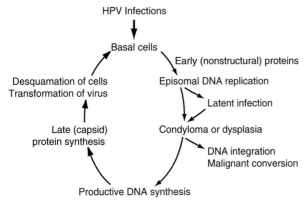

FIGURE 41-1 ▶ Papilloma cell cycle from infection to desquamation of cells.

intranuclear structural viral polypeptides in terminally differentiated keratinocytes. Viral capsid assembly follows, resulting in degenerative changes in epithelial cell cytoplasm (vacuolization) and nucleus (pyknosis, binucleation, and atypical sizes and shapes) referred to as koilocytotic atypia.[63] Viral capsid protein synthesis and virus assembly occur in koilocytes located in the terminally differentiating cells in the surface of the lesion.[64] The mature virus can cause other sites in the female genital tract to be infected or can act as an infecting agent at the time of viral activity.

Once an infection is established, a series of events in the papillomavirus life cycle may occur (Fig. 41–2). The flat condyloma that is established may remain in place, neither growing nor receding. This may represent a failure of the hosts' immune system to be appropriately stimulated because the majority of lesions (either EGWs or abnormal genital cytology) regress as CMI becomes activated. The average time from basal cell infection to overt condyloma is about 2 months. The average papillomavirus life cycle is 6 to 9 months. During that time, most overt condyloma and abnormal cytology will regress if the immunosuppressive conditions are removed. Since HPV infection is less well controlled in patients who are endogenously or exoge-

nously immunosuppressed, efforts should be made to eliminate these inciting factors. Immunosuppressive conditions could include unremitting stress, cigarette smoking, use of oral contraceptive agents, use of illegal illicit drugs, excessive alcohol intake, exogenous corticosteroids, uncontrolled diabetes mellitus, receiving an organ transplant, and human immunodeficiency virus (HIV) seropositivity. By removing the immunosuppressive cause when possible and attempting to control the problem when removal of the suppressor is not possible, control of the disease process will be greatly facilitated.

Overt condylomatous lesions can also increase in size, and changes in wart size during pregnancy are well known to clinicians. Although most genital warts do not significantly enlarge during pregnancy, some tend to become confluent over the vulva or to occlude the birth canal. At least one cause of these enlargements is hormonal. Studies with estradiol and/or levonorgestrol in the athymic mouse model seem to implicate levonorgestrol as the agent causing the increased wart growth. Most EGWs resolve by 6 weeks post partum.

The events that lead to malignant transformation are not totally clear. However, an oncogenic HPV must be present as well as another co-carcinogen or inciting factor. Once the HPV DNA is integrated into the genome, the transformation process is complete and malignant degeneration can occur.

In general, HPV-6 and -11 are most commonly found on the vulva and lower third of the vagina, whereas HPV-6 and -11 and a few HPV-16, -18, -31, -33, and -35 are found in LGSIL. HPV-16, -18, -31, -33, and -35 are usually found in HGSIL; few HPV-6 and -11 are found in HGSIL. HPV-16, -18, -31, -33, and -35 and other oncogenic strains are found in invasive cancer (Table 41–3).

Most HPV-associated lesions on the external genitalia and adjacent perineal body and perianal area are exophytic condylomas. Approximately 65% are HPV-6, and 20% HPV-11.[13, 17] They possess very little malignant potential unless they have mutated or are associated with potent co-factors.[65] Approximately 85% of newly acquired HPV infections are successfully treated with repeated physical or chemical agents. The remainder

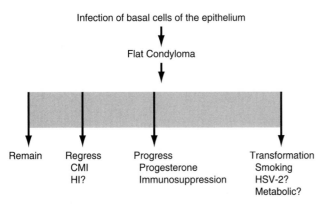

FIGURE 41-2 ▶ Papilloma cell cycle after infection is established. CMI, cell-mediated immune response; HI, humoral immunity.

TABLE 41-3 ▶	VARIATIONS IN DISEASE EXPRESSION BY VIRAL STATE
HPV Infectious State	**Disease Expression**
LATENT	NONE
Productive	Condyloma acuminata, most LGSIL; rare HGSIL
Nonproductive (transforming)	Rare LGSIL, most HGSIL; all invasive cancers

Adapted from Reid R, Greenberg M, Jenson AB, et al: Sexually transmitted papillomaviral infections. Am J Obstet Gynecol 1987; 156:212.

of patients develop resistant or persistent disease, which is defined as warts present for 6 months or longer despite 10 or more therapies. These patients may reflect an abnormality of their CMI in response to HPV infection.

HPV types 6 and 11 have been found to be present in patients with recurrent respiratory papillomatosis (RRP). These growths occur at various sites in the tracheobronchial tree and can cause hoarseness and compromise of the bronchi and trachea. Most cases are diagnosed prior to age 5 years. An association with maternal condyloma at the time of delivery has been suggested; although studies have found HPV to be present in some neonates, RRP is found significantly less often.

Tseng and colleagues[66] attempted to determine the rate of HPV in newborn infants of HPV-positive mothers and how the route of delivery affects transmission. They assessed the presence of HPV-16 and HPV-18 DNA sequences in buccal and genital swabs using PCR methodology.

The overall frequency of finding HPV-16 and HPV-18 particles was 68 of 301 (22.6%). The frequency of HPV transmission from positive mothers to newborns was 27 of 68 (39.7%). Vaginally delivered neonates were positive more frequently than neonates delivered by cesarean section; 18 of 35 (51.4%) versus 9 of 33 (27.3%; $P = .042$). Factors including the buccal site and the genital site as well as gender difference were not significant.

This report and others have documented the presence of HPV-16 and -18 DNA sequences in the neonate. It has not been established whether HPV DNA detected at birth necessarily causes a persistent infection later, rather than a transient, superficial presence. Other authors have calculated the risk of papillomatosis in a child born to a mother with condyloma to be between 1:400 to 1:1500.[67] Cesarean delivery is indicated in situations where the overt condylomas either occlude the birth canal or would make vaginal delivery dangerous, but not just for the presence of condylomas.

The prevalences of specific HPV types in neonates and children are significantly different and indicate that neonates harbor transient maternal HPV types, whereas HPV in children may be caused by factors other than perinatal transmission. Studies in neonates have shown the predominant HPV types to be 16 and 18.[66, 68] In children with or without proven sexual abuse, HPV types 6 and 11 followed by HPV types 2 and 3 are most common.[69] Although HPV types 16 and 18 are most commonly found in neonates, many studies have concluded that the presence of HPV-16 and -18 in children is strongly associated with sexual abuse and not maternal transmission.[70]

HPV-2 is the second most commonly found type of HPV in condylomatous lesions in the genital area in children.[69] The clinical presentation is similar to HPV types 6 and 11 and 16 and 18, but on histologic examination there is an absence of koilocytosis. Children who harbor HPV types 2 and 3 in the genital tract are more commonly found to have a relative who has body warts.[69]

Studies of HPV in cervical lesions of adolescents have shown a type of distribution similar to that in adults. HPV types 16 and 18 represent one third to one half of specific types identified.[71] In contrast to children, cutaneous HPV types are rarely, if ever, found in adolescents.

CERVICAL INTRAEPITHELIAL NEOPLASIA

Cervical intraepithelial neoplasia (CIN) has been studied extensively. The Bethesda system (TBS) provides uniform terminology and diagnostic criteria for reporting cervical smears[72] (Table 41–4). It is generally accepted that the majority of LGSILs will either regress or persist, whereas HGSILs are more likely to either persist or progress. LGSILs are a heterogenous group of lesions that are not necessarily premalignant.[73] Invasive carcinoma appears to develop from HGSIL in one third to two thirds of cases, with a transit time ranging from 10 to 15 years. The progression rate of LGSIL to HGSIL is thought to be approximately 15%, regardless of the cytologic pattern.[74]

Poor sample preparations have been implicated in false-negative cytologic interpretations. A new collection system has been developed in which the exfoliated cell samples are placed into fixative, rather than prepared as smears. The goals are to achieve consistent fixation and to reduce obscuring inflammation and blood (Cytic Corporation, Marlborough, MA.). Cells are placed in fixative and transported to the laboratory, where monolayer slides are prepared using a Thin-Prep processor. The cells are transfixed to a glass slide for Pap staining. The resultant slides contain approximately 50,000 cells. Comparisons using conven-

TABLE 41–4 ▶	THE BETHESDA SYSTEM CLASSIFICATION OF SQUAMOUS ABNORMALITIES COMPARED WITH OTHER NOMENCLATURE
Bethesda System	**Equivalent Terminology**
ASCUS	Squamous atypia; Pap class II
LGSIL	Mild dysplasia, CIN 1
	Koilocytotic atypia
	Condylomatous atypia
	HPV-related change
HGSIL	Moderate dysplasia, CIN 2
	Severe dysplasia, carcinoma in situ CIN 3

ASCUS = atypical squamous cells of undetermined significance; CIN = cervical intraepithelial neoplasia; HGSIL = high-grade squamous intraepithelial lesion; LSIL = low-grade squamous intraepithelial lesion.

tional techniques and Thin-Prep show agreement in 90% of cases.[75] In some studies, Thin-Preps have detected a greater number of SILs with fewer readings of atypical squamous cells of undetermined significance (ASCUS), and the number of slides classified as unsatisfactory for interpretation is less with Thin-Preps. Cytotechnicians must have additional training to properly interpret the Thin-Prep slides, but once that is accomplished, the better prepared slides are easier to interpret. A potential advantage of collecting cells in this manner is that the cells remaining in the vial may be used for ancillary studies, including HPV testing, immunochemistry, or computer-assisted review.

An additional testing technique now being evaluated is the hybrid capture assay (HCA). Nindl and co-workers[76] compared the Hybrid Capture assay to the PCR system to detect HGSIL. Comparison of PCR and HCA showed overall agreement in 84.2% (32 of 38) of cases and a significantly higher sensitivity of PCR (94.7% vs. 78.9%; $P \le .04$). No case positive by HCA was negative by PCR. The difference in sensitivity of the two tests could explain the differences obtained. At least 10,000 HPV copies have to be present to have a positive result with HCA, whereas PCR can detect as few as 1 to 10 copies of common HPVs.

Clinical Presentation

Exophytic condylomas usually appear first at the posterior fourchette and adjacent labia minora and may rapidly spread to other parts of the vulva. In more than 20% of patients, condylomas also appear on the perineum and perianal areas. Any part of the vagina may be involved, and in a few women the entire mucosal surface may be occupied by condylomatous tissue. Papular warts frequently are present on the labia majora and perineum.

The condyloma acuminata are pedunculated or broad-based, usually pink, when growing rapidly, to gray, soft, fleshy excrescences that occur singly or in clusters. The lesions vary in size from a pinhead to a large confluence of many smaller lesions that have a cauliflower appearance. Condyloma acuminata are usually asymptomatic, but they are friable and bleed easily. Their morphologic appearance is similar; however, the condylomas appearing in areas of epithelial cornification develop cornification with time. Lesions of the cervix tend to be flat and endophytic, but acuminata lesions are not uncommon. A high proportion of cervical lesions previously thought to be CIN 1 or CIN 2 are now thought to be a variant of HPV infection. The colposcopic findings of HPV infection of the cervix have been well described.[77]

HPV lesions have a raised, white appearance. Most exophytic condylomas present as aggregates of small papillae that encompass a vascular loop beneath the surface. HGSIL tend to be confined to the transforma-

tion zone, whereas papilloma infection can involve either the original squamous epithelium or the immature metaplastic tissue just proximal to the squamocolumnar junction.

Subclinical HPV infection of the vulva has been described. These lesions are described as flat vulvar lesions seen with the colposcope after application of acetic acid. Approximately 50% of women with vulvar warts have cervical HPV infection. Subclinical lesions can frequently be found in the vagina.

The diagnosis of EGWs is characteristic, and the diagnoses can usually be made on clinical grounds. This method of diagnosis has a 10% failure rate, so the clinician must be prepared to think of the differential diagnosis (Table 41–5). The most common error made in the diagnosis of condyloma acuminata is to confuse micropapillomatosis labialis with HPV disease. Micropapillomatosis labialis is characterized by small finger-like projections present on the medial aspect of the labia minora, usually located at the five to seven o'clock positions. Each papilloma has its own thinly walled projection, and each base is clearly seen. These papillomas are normal variants and are asymptomatic. Condylomata lata, caused by *T. pallidum* are broad based, smooth, usually multiple, moist, and heavily populated with spirochetes. Any ulcerated lesion other than classic herpes simplex virus infection requires biopsy.

Any patient presenting with the complaint of EGWs should have careful inspection of the entire genital tract and should have a cervical Pap smear done. In addition, the patient should be evaluated for the presence of bacterial vaginosis.[78] The authors used the Gram stain of vaginal secretions categorized as grade I, II, or III, according to Hillier and co-workers.[79] Grade I

TABLE 41–5 ▶ DIFFERENTIAL DIAGNOSIS OF GENITAL WARTS

Condition	Description
Micropapillomatosis labialis	Lesions on the epithelium of the labia minora
	Each projection has its own base
	Asymptomatic
Seborrheic keratoses	Hypertrophic lesions with rough surfaces
Nevus	Raised or pedunculated
Condyloma lata	Broad-based, smooth surface, moist
Herpes simplex virus	Painful vesicular eruption with red base and ulcerations
Molloscum contagiosum	Umbilicated yellowish papules with central core
Giant condyloma	Confluent, cauliflower-like mass of warts
Bowenoid papulosis	Rough papules 2 mm to 4 mm, flesh-colored to reddish brown, resist therapies
Squamous cell carcinoma	Red, firm nodule, forming shallow ulcer with indurated border
Malignant melanoma	Pigmented, flat or raised, with variable color or shape

was dominated by large, gram-positive rods suggestive of *Lactobacillus* species. The grade II pattern was characterized by gram-negative coccobacilli together with a few gram-positive rods. A grade III smear was dominated exclusively by gram-negative bacilli and long, filamentous gram-negative rods. Grades II and III are indicative of bacterial vaginosis. Grade I Gram smears were significantly associated with a negative HPV test ($P \le .001$), whereas the detection of HPV DNA was significantly associated with type II flora ($P \le .001$). Grade III flora was not observed in the study cohort. This would be consistent with a more transient flora, and one more likely to revert back to normal.

Ho and colleagues[80] followed 608 college women at 6-month intervals for 3 years to determine whether lifestyle and sexual behavior influenced the incidence of HPV on Pap smears. They obtained cervicovaginal lavage samples for the detection of HPV DNA by PCR. Pap smears were obtained annually. The cumulative, 36-month incidence of HPV infection was 43%. An increased risk of HPV infection was significantly associated with younger age, Hispanic ethnicity, black race, an increased number of vaginal-sex partners, high frequencies of vaginal sex and alcohol consumption, anal sex, and certain characteristics of partners (increased number of lifetime partners and not being in school). The median duration of infection was 8 months (range, 7 to 10 months). The persistence of HPV for more than 6 months was related to older age, HPV types associated with cervical cancer, and infection with multiple HPV types, but not with cigarette smoking. The risk of a persistently abnormal Pap smear increased with persistent HPV infection, particularly with high-risk types (rate ratio, 37.2; CI, 14.6 to 94.8). Other investigators have found similar variability in HPV infection. Evander and co-workers[81] found regression of HPV infection in 80% of the women in their study. A new HPV type-specific infection was detected in 7.2% of these women and was associated with a new sexual partner. Hildesheim and colleagues[82] found in their study that 41% of the women who were HPV positive had persistent HPV detection. Women 30 years of age or older had a higher persistence of infection than those 24 years or younger ($P = .01$). The percentage of persistence was greater among women infected with HPV types associated with cervical cancer (Table 41–6).

The course of HPV infection in some women who were HIV seropositive was compared with a group of women who were HIV seronegative by Sun and colleagues.[83] A total of 220 HIV seropositive and 231 seronegative control subjects were evaluated at two or more semiannual gynecologic examinations with Pap smears, a test for HPV DNA, and colposcopy. The cumulative prevalence of HPV infection after four examinations was 83% in the HIV-seropositive women and 62% in the HIV-seronegative women. Persistent

TABLE 41–6 ▶ ANOGENITAL HUMAN PAPILLOMAVIRUSES AND THEIR ONCOGENIC ASSOCIATION

HPV Type	Disease Association	Oncogenic Association
6	Condyloma acuminata LGSIL, laryngeal papillomas	Rarely malignant
11	Condyloma acuminata, LGSIL Laryngeal papillomas, conjunctival papillomas	Rarely malignant
16	Rare in LGSIL, frequent in HGSIL Bowenoid papulosis, Bowen's disease, invasive cervical, vulvar, anal cancers	Malignant
18	Rare in LGSIL, HGSIL, cervical cancers	Highly malignant
31	LGSIL, HGSIL, cancers	Malignant
33	LGSIL, HGSIL, cancers	Malignant
35	LGSIL, HGSIL, cancers	Malignant
39	Bowenoid papulosis	Rarely malignant
41	Condylomata, cutaneous flat warts	Benign
42	Flat condylomata, Bowenoid papulosis	Benign
43	LGSIL	Benign
44	Condyloma acuminata	Benign
45	Condylomata, LGSIL, HGSIL, cancers	?Highly malignant
51	LGSIL	Rarely malignant
52	Condylomata, LGSIL, HGSIL, cancers	Malignant
53	Condylomata	?
54	Condylomata	?
55	Condylomata	?
56	Condylomata, LGSIL, HGSIL, cancer	?Highly malignant
57	Condylomata	?
58	Condylomata, HGSIL, cancer	Malignant
59	Condylomata	?
61	Condylomata	Benign
66	Condylomata	Benign
68	Condylomata LGSIL, HGSIL, cancer	Malignant
73	Condylomata, LGSIL, HGSIL	?Malignant

HPV infections were found in 24% of the HIV-seropositive women, but in only 4% of the HIV-seronegative women ($P \le .001$). A total of 20% of HIV-seropositive women and 3% of HIV-seronegative women had persistent infections with HPV-16–associated types (16, 31, 33, 35, or 58) or HPV-18–associated types (18 or 45). These persistent infections may explain the increased incidence of HGSIL and invasive cancer in HIV-seropositive women. Chiasson and co-workers[84] studied the prevalence of HPV-associated vulvovaginal lesions in HIV-seropositive and HIV-seronegative women. Vulvar and/or vaginal condylomas were detected in 22 of 396 (5.6%) HIV-positive and 3 of 375 (0.8%) HIV-negative women ($P \le .001$). They also found that HPV-associated disease was more likely to be multicentric and involve the vulva, vagina, and cervix in HIV-seropositive women.

The diagnosis of subclinical infection is usually made with colposcopy following application of 3% to 5% acetic acid. Lesions appear to be shiny and white with irregular borders and the presence of satellite lesions. HPV lesions are not confined to the transformation zone of the cervix, as are CIN lesions. The colposcopy findings of subclinical HPV infection of the vagina may include (1) aspirates that are multiple, short spikes, representing small condyloma; and (2) reverse punctation, which is a diffuse pattern of slightly raised, white dots.[85]

Cytology is helpful in diagnosing subclinical HPV infection. The characteristic findings include koilocytosis, dyskaryosis, atypical basal cells, and multinucleation. The histologic findings include basal cell hyperplasia, acanthosis, papillomatosis, koiliocytosis, parakeratosis, and mild nuclear atypia.

DNA hybridization techniques are available for demonstrating HPV in tissues. Currently, the usefulness of typing technique in the clinical arena is debatable; therefore, until a clear need is demonstrated the technique will remain experimental.

TREATMENT OF HPV DISEASE: CONDYLOMA ACUMINATA

The goal of the treatment of condyloma acuminata is the removal of exophytic warts, amelioration of signs and symptoms, and induction of an immune response. Generally, genital warts are benign growths caused by HPV types 6 and 11 that cause only minor symptoms or no symptoms, aside from their cosmetic appearance. The treatment of condyloma acuminata is not likely to influence the development of cervical cancer. Clinical studies have demonstrated that currently available therapeutic methods are 22% to 94% effective in clearing exophytic genital warts and that recurrence rates are high. No evidence has been published indicating that currently available treatments eradicate, or affect the natural history of, HPV disease.

Therapeutic interventions for EGWs, as recommended by the Centers for Disease Control and Prevention (CDC), are listed in Table 41–7. The treatment of genital warts should be guided by the preference of

the patient, the available resources, and the experience of the health care provider. Most patients have 1 to 10 genital warts that are responsive to most treatment modalities. Factors that might influence the selection of treatment include wart size, wart number, anatomic site of the wart, wart morphology, patient preference, cost of the treatment, convenience, adverse effects, and provider experience. Having a detailed discussion with the patient regarding therapy and HPV is an important step in the formation of an enduring patient-health provider relationship. This communication leads to the development of a treatment plan, because many patients require a course of therapy, rather than a single treatment. In addition, it is important to discuss with the patient any medication or social activity that is immunosuppressive. Therefore, the patient should be advised to stop smoking cigarettes, to discontinue exogenous steroids, to stop using illicit drugs such as cocaine and heroin, and to avoid oral contraceptives if pregnancy can be prevented by other means, to bring insulin-dependent diabetes under tight control, and to relieve excessively stressful life situations. In general, warts located on moist surfaces and/or in intertriginous areas respond better to topical treatments, such as trichloroacetic acid (TCA) or imiquimod, than do warts on drier surfaces.

Podophyllin resin in tincture of Benzoin has been a popular treatment for genital warts. The major drawbacks to podophyllin are its unpredictable toxicity and efficacy, variation of which occurs from lot to lot. Podofilox is a purified form of podophyllin that can be self-applied and does not need to be washed off. The package insert reports a 50% per patient response rate and a 60% recurrence rate. Therapy is twice-daily application for 3 days, with the next 4 days treatment free. Podofilox is also available as a gel, but the response rates with this form are lower.[87]

Topical 5-fluorouracil (5-FU) cream (1% or 5%) has been used to treat vaginal warts and to prevent recurrence of vaginal and vulvar warts post ablation.[88] The usual dose of 5-FU cream is 2.5 g to 5.0 g (one half to one vaginal applicatorful) weekly for 10 weeks. There is an 8% vaginal ulceration rate, and patients complain of a watery discharge as the vaginal epithelium is denuded by the 5-FU. Success rates range from 50% to 70%, with recurrence rates of 13%.

The newest medication to be approved for treatment of condylomata acuminata is imiquimod. The drug is a biologic immune-response modifier and functions by stimulating Langerhans cells in the epithelium to produce interferon α, IL-1α, IL-1β, TNF, and IL-8. The medication has no antiviral properties but is effective through the formation of interferon and other cytokines following topical application. Imiquimod is applied three times a week for up to 16 weeks. It should be continued for 2 weeks after the last wart has disappeared. It does not induce any systemic response but

TABLE 41–7 ▶	THERAPY RECOMMENDATIONS FOR EXTERNAL GENITAL WARTS
Patient-administered	Podofilox 0.5% solution or gel applied to visible warts bid for 3 days, followed by 4 days of no therapy
	Imiquimod 5% cream—apply to warts T.I.W. for up to 16 wk.
Provider-administered	Cryotherapy with liquid nitrogen or cryoprobe; repeat every 1–2 wk.
	Podophyllin resin 10% to 25% in compound tincture of Benzoin; wash area thoroughly after 4 h; repeat weekly
	Trichloroacetic acid 80% to 90%—apply to warts and allow to dry; repeat weekly if necessary
	Surgical removal by scissor excision, shave excision, curettage, or electrosurgery
Alternative therapy	Intralesional interferon
	Laser surgery

From Centers for Disease Control and Prevention: 1998 Guidelines for treatment of sexually transmitted diseases. MMWR 1998; 47 (RR-1):88–98.

acts locally. There is no need to wash off the medication after application. It is important to show patients with a mirror the exact location of their warts, so that they apply the medication as precisely as possible. Patients frequently develop erythema in the area where the imiquimod is applied. This bothers the physician more than the patient and represents an intraepithelial reaction to the cytokines and is regarded as a favorable sign. The compound can weaken condoms and diaphragms (Table 41–8).

Trichloroacetic acid (TCA) is another popular physician-administered agent that is effective and relatively inexpensive. TCA is usually formulated in 20%, 50%, and 85% concentrations. Since its mechanism of action is coagulation of proteins, the higher the concentration, the greater the depth of coagulation and wart destruction. The application should be controlled so that excess TCA does not run onto adjacent normal skin and cause a reaction. If care is taken in applying TCA, it is unnecessary to coat the surrounding tissue with ointment. When one uses TCA 85%, it should not be administered more frequently than once every 3 weeks. After application, the patient experiences about 5 minutes of an intense burning sensation at the wart site. In 2 to 3 days, the wart peels away, leaving an ulcer that takes 2 to 3 weeks to heal. If one selects a less concentrated TCA solution, the frequency of administration can be increased. Efficacy data suggest a respone rate of 81%, with a recurrence rate of 36%.[87]

Cryotherapy, either with liquid nitrogen or cryoprobe, is usually limited to smaller warts and requires several office vistis. Transient pain, burning, and ulceration resolve in about 10 days and are usually tolerated well by patients. Efficacy rates range from 63% to 88%, with recurrence rates of 21% to 39%.[87]

Carbon dioxide laser ablation is a popular modality for treatment of condyloma acuminata. Laser therapy has been disappointing when evaluated in randomized clinical trials. Reid and co-workers[89] reported complete clearing of vulvar warts in only 8 of 20 (40%) women, whereas interferon alone cleared warts in 28 of 32 (87%). Laser therapy is expensive and painful and requires anesthesia. Clearance rates of 31% to 94% have been reported, and recurrences range between 3% and 95%.[87] This treatment method may pose a health risk to physicians, nurses, and patients because the laser smoke plumes can carry viral particles. Thus, good smoke evacuation methods and masks are essential during treatment.[90]

Standard surgical excision has been used, with a success rate of 93% and recurrence rates of 24% and 29%.[87] Excision requires local or general anesthesia, depending on the size of the warts. Excision is now used mainly for perianal warts. Scarring can be a major complication.

The loop electrosurgical excisional procedure (LEEP) has become popular in recent years. The procedure can be done in one sitting, provided that the number of warts is not too large. It can be used to treat vaginal as well as vulvar warts; its efficacy is similar to that of the CO_2 laser, but it is more cost-effective. The main complication is bleeding. Precautions regarding the smoke plume are similar to those regarding the CO_2 laser. The efficacy of LEEP is similar to that obtained with the CO_2 laser.

Successful treatment of condyloma acuminata requires that an immune response be induced. Therapy with interferons is a modality that addresses the issue. Interferons are a group of proteins made by human lymphoid cells in response to viral stimuli. Interferons constitute a subgroup of cytokines with antimicrobial, antitumor, and immunomodulatory properties. Two distinct classes exist. Interferons α and β, which are encoded by genes on the ninth chromosome, share a 25% nucleic acid homology, and use common membrane receptors. These interferons have antiviral, antiproliferative, and differentiation induction properties. The second class of interferons is interferon-γ, which is encoded on chromosome 11. This substance induces potent stimulation of macrophages and B lymphocytes, but lacks antiviral or antiproliferative activity. More than 20 subtypes of interferon-α are known. Pharmacologic preparations come from several sources: (1) natural interferon is obtained after viral stimulation of leukocytes and contains 19 kinds of interferon-α, and (2) recombinant interferon is obtained as a single interferon-α species. These compounds have been extensively used in the treatment of condyloma acuminata in the genital tract as well as in the tracheobronchial tree. Several studies have shown efficacy and absence of significant side effects in the treatment of condyloma acuminata. The widespread use of interferon is hampered by two problems. The first problem is that the U.S. Food and Drug Administration (FDA)

TABLE 41–8 ▶ IMIQUIMOD EFFECTS ON IMMUNOLOGICALLY COMPETENT CELLS

Cell Type	Effect Observed After Imiquimod
NK cell	Activation of NK cells to kill target cells
B lymphocyte	Stimulation of proliferation and differentiation
T lymphocyte	Augments IL-2 production in response to mitogens and antigens; enhances T_H1, responses such as DTH
Monocyte-macrophage	Activates these cells to secrete cytokines; i.e., interferon-α, TNF, IL-1, IL-6, IL-8, IL-10, and others
Neutrophil	No direct activation; indirectly, through IL-8 production, augments expression of MAC-1 surface expression and down-regulates expression of L-selectin
Human keratinocyte	Induces mRNA for interferon-α, IL-6, and IL-8

DTH = delayed-type hypersensitivity.
From data on file (1214-IMIQ), 3M Pharmaceuticals, St. Paul, MN.

approved interferon therapy by interlesional injection for condyloma. The technique is cumbersome and particularly inconvenient for the treatment of multiple warts. Intralesional interferon injections of condylomas are painful to the patient; and the clinician may resort to placing the interferon under the wart on subsequent injections, hence the term *regional subcutaneous*. Data suggest a similar efficacy when systemic therapy has been employed. This therapy involves patient self-administration of interferon sucutaneously into the anterior thigh. This route is more acceptable to the patient and is much more cost-effective. The second problem arises because a number of authors who have used interferons infrequently, or not at all, repeat myths regarding its efficacy and, in particular, its side effects.

The side effects of interferon are dose related. At doses of 5 million units (MU)/m² or higher, all patients exhibit an 8- to 12-hour elevation in temperature when the interferon is started; many exhibit a fatigue syndrome or malaise; and a few demonstrate a transient elevation of hepatic transaminases as well as diminution of the WBC count to as low as 3,000 cells/mm³ and of platelets to as low as 100,000/mm³. The levels of hepatic transaminases as well as the WBC and platelet counts return to normal while the interferon is being continued. At the doses used in current clinical medicine (2.5 to 3 MU three times per week), the number of side effects approaches zero. Interferon-α is very well tolerated at the doses described earlier.[91–93]

In reviewing published studies about interferon, one is struck by the observation that the authors who have reported no differences in response when comparing interferon to placebo have reported a length of interferon therapy usually of 4 weeks or less.[91–96] It is clear that although some condylomas resolve within 3 to 4 weeks, the course of therapy should be 6 to 8 weeks. Data from Eron and co-workers[94] are instructive in having demonstrated resolution of lesions during the 3 weeks of intralesional therapy, but with resumed wart growth when the interferon was discontinued. Prolonged therapy is more likely to result in sustained resolution. Interferon injections should be continued for 2 weeks after resolution of the warts.

A new strategy for treating condyloma acuminata involves an intralesional injection of 5-FU plus a gel containing epinephrine and bovine collagens.[97] This therapy does not have FDA approval. The agent is injected intralesionally once a week for 6 weeks. The complete response rate has been reported to be 77%, but the recurrence rate after 3 months follow-up was 50%. The drawbacks to this form of therapy are the intralesional approach, which requires that the patient come to the physician's office often; the high recurrence rate; the possiblity of induction of an immune response to bovine collagen, which could induce antibodies to react with natural human collagen; and the failure of the FDA to endorse the agent.

THERAPY FOR CONDYLOMA ACUMINATA IN PREGNANCY

The objectives of treating condylomas in the pregnant patient are different from those in the nonpregnant patient; they are to eliminate lesions that cause pain and/or discomfort, to induce an immune response, and to reduce warts in an attempt to decrease perinatal transmission. The increase in vascularity of the condylomas is well recognized by clinicians, so surgical excision is frequently accompanied by profuse bleeding. The following agents should not be used during pregnancy: (1) podophyllin, (2) podofilox, (3) 5-FU, and (4) interferon. Trichloroacetic acid (TCA) may be used both on the vulva and in the vagina. Imiquimod is listed as an FDA-class-B drug, but no studies in pregnancy have been reported. Imiquimod acts on the epithelial Langerhans cells to induce local interferons and cytokines, and no systemic response has been demonstrated. This information would lead one to believe that imiquimod could be safely used in pregnancy. Condylomas should not be allowed to grow to sizes that obstruct the birth canal. In addition, since bacterial vaginosis (BV) is almost always present with intravaginal condylomas and since BV may cause preterm birth, it is important to treat both conditions.

An association between maternal condyloma acuminata and the development of recurrent respiratory papillomatosis (RRP) in the neonate has been reported.[98] Kashima and Shah[67] calculate the risk to the neonate of developing RRP when born to a mother with condyloma to be between 1:400 and 1:1500. Sedlacek and co-workers[99] demonstrated HPV DNA in the oral cavity of 11 of 23 (47.8%) neonates born to mothers who had detectable HPV DNA in their cervical

---

TABLE 41-9 ▶ TRIAGE RULES

I. Exclude Invasive Cancer
   A. Colposcopist able to recognize invasive cancer
   B. Entire squamocolumnar junction seen
   C. Document endocervical canal status (colposcopy, cytobrush, endocervical curettage)
II. Restricted Indications for Conization
   A. Suspected microinvasive squamous carcinoma
   B. Adenocarcinoma in situ
   C. CIN 2–3 on portio, but squamocolumnar junction not definable
   D. Unexplained significant HGSIL
III. Most Conservative Therapy Compatible with Safety
   A. Cone biopsy = "therapeutic," not diagnostic
   B. Hysterectomy reserved for rare indications
   C. Remaining cases treated by transformation-zone ablation
   D. Treatment planned by topography, not histologic grade

Adapted from Reid R: The management of genital condylomas, intraepithelial neoplasia, and vulvodynia. Obstet Gynecol Clin North Am 1996; 23:924.

Method	Wart Volume* and/or Characteristics	Advantage	Disadvantage	Clinical Role
I. Traditional Office Methods for Lesion Eradication				
Scissor excision of isolated lesions	Vaginal, low volume	Obtain tissue for histology or viral typing	Cumbersome; local anesthesia, suture instruments needed; epithelial denudation and bleeding if done to excess	Baseline biopsy
TCA 85%	Low volume	Quick and easy method; can be used on mucosal surfaces (vagina, cervix, rectum, mouth); causes intense burning after application	Requires repeated office visits; more effective on mucosal warts; safe in pregnancy	Highly effective for localized disease
Podofilox	Low volume	Selective destruction of condylomatous areas; self-application; regimens more effective than single in-office therapy	Cannot be used on highly absorptive surfaces (vagina, cervix, rectum, mouth); contraindicated in pregnancy	Effective for cutaneous condylomas
Local physical destruction (hot cautery, liquid nitrogen, laser "spot" welding)	Vaginal, low volume	Immediate eradication of papillomas	Cumbersome; local anesthesia, special equipment needed; time-consuming for physicians; local infection and scarring more common	Destruction of refractory papillomas
5-Fluorouracil regimens	Vaginal, moderate volume	Nonsurgical method of lesion eradication; can reduce postoperative recurrences	Painful alternative; causes vaginal discharge and vaginal denudation; potentially teratogenic	Extensive external condyloma; vaginal condylomas
Alpha or gamma interferons primary therapy	Moderate or large; vaginal; perianal	Induction of immune response; documented antiviral and immunomodulatory; nonsurgical method of lesion eradication; systemic therapy is patient-controlled and treats all lesions at the same time; side effects low at standard doses	Intralesional routes are slow and painful; course must be at least 6–8 wk	Excellent for extensive warts or for resistant warts
II. Destruction Methods Requiring Operating Room				
Segmental excision and primary closure	Moderate to large	Tissue available for histology	Tissue removal is fundamentally undesirable	May be outmoded by CO_2 laser
Extensive diathermy ("Bovie")	Vaginal; moderate	Equipment available	Morbid recovery and unacceptable scarring	May be outmoded
Laser ablation	Vaginal; moderate to large volume	Can remove large areas of HPV	Requires extended training; highly developed skills not attained by all; frequently leaves scarring when extensive areas involved; not appropriate for simple cases; does not remove field of HPV expression, as recurrences are common; expensive	Use in extensive condylomas; high-grade intraepithelial neoplasia
III. Method for Controlling the Residual Viral Reservoir				
Noncytolytic 5-fluorouracil regimens	Vaginal, low volume	Relatively inexpensive; minimal systemic absorption; effective in immunosuppressed patients	Limited efficacy; poorly tolerated if fair complexion; distressing side effects	Useful in immunosuppressed patient
Prolonged interferon regimens, adjuvant regimens	Resistant and persistent warts	Biologic substance with antiviral and immunomodulatory actions; excellent effect in adjuvant trials; very few adverse effects	May not be effective in immunosuppressed	Resistant and persistent warts; vaginal warts

TCA = trichloroacetic acid.

*Low volume, ≤6 warts; moderate volume, 7–12 warts; large volume, 13 or more warts, or bulky warts.

Modified from Reid R, Dorsey J: Physical and surgical principles of carbon dioxide laser surgery in the lower genital tract. In: Koppelson (ed): Gynecologic Oncology, 2nd ed. London, Churchill Livingstone, 1992, p 1087.

cells. Tseng and colleagues[66] more recently reported a similar transmission and significantly more neonates who were HPV-DNA positive when born vaginally. However, in both reports, the authors are presenting data concerning material from the skin or mucosal surface, and this represents carriage but not infection. At the current time, cesarean delivery is indicated in situations in which the condylomas are so large that they obstruct the birth canal or place the patient at risk for significant hemorrhage.

MANAGEMENT OF INTRAEPITHELIAL DISEASE

The management of intraepithelial disease has been thoroughly reviewed in numerous publications.[100–102] It is mandatory that clinicians who deal with abnormal genital cytology and intraepithelial disease be experienced. Managing small, localized lesions by destruction of the physical transformation zone (TZ) with the use of cryosurgery, diathermy, or the CO_2 laser and understanding the need for conization prevent unnecessary hysterectomies. However, such modalities are safe, provided that a strict protocol is followed (Table 41–9).

Now that cervical excision biopsies can be done in an office setting using loop electrocautery excision procedure (LEEP) technology, some authors have advocated a "see-and-treat" protocol. The rationale for LEEP of the TZ allows the initial visit to be both diagnostic and therapeutic. This strategy is flawed because the indications for surgery are now based on a screening test (abnormal genital cytology), rather than on a diagnostic evaluation (directed biopsy). In clinical settings when follow-up is problematic, this policy is probably advantageous. However, with many inexperienced colposcopists evaluating many low-grade lesions in young and compliant patients, the see-and-treat strategy will lead to substantial overtreatment, additional morbidity, and unnecessary cost.

Traditional modalities for the treatment of mucosal and cutaneous condylomas are listed in Table 41–10. Information pertaining to the extent of warts has been added to guide the clinician (see Table 41–10).

Another promising avenue for the control of HPV disease is prophylactic vaccination. Studies with bovine papillomavirus (BPV) killed vaccine have shown protection against BPV disease following intramuscular administration. The prospects for an HPV vaccine are challenging because in order for the vaccine to be protective, it must stimulate CMI. Induction of human immunity does not seem to confer protection. Recombinant DNA technology has permitted expression of viral proteins in bacteria and eukaryotic cells and has allowed the preparation of a number of possible HPV vaccine antigens.[104] Expression of the major L1 capsid protein of HPV as recombinant protein in yeasts,[105]

insect cells,[106] or tissue culture[107] enables assembly of this protein into VLPs. These VLPs have been used successfully in cows, dogs, and cotton-tail rabbits. Although the prospects for a prophylactic vaccine are encouraging, significant trials are ahead.

CONCLUSION

Significant progress has been made in understanding HPV disease. The best therapeutic approaches are controversial, and the controversy should stimulate additional research. Newer immunomodulatory agents are available, and as clinicians understand the regimens and how to use them properly they will be rewarded with increased HPV control and greater patient satisfaction.

REFERENCES

1. Oriel J: Natural history of genital warts. Br J Vener Dis 1971; 47:1.
2. zur Hausen H, Meinhof W, Scheiber W, et al: Attempts to detect virus-specific DNA in human tumors. I. Nucleic acid hybridizations with complementary RNA of human wart virus. Int J Cancer 1974; 13:650.
3. Durst M, Gissmann L, Ikenberg H, et al: A papillomavirus DNA from a cervical carcinoma and its prevalence in cancer biopsy samples from different geographic regions. Proc Natl Acad Sci USA 1983; 80:3812.
4. Komly CA, Brietburd F, Croissant O, et al: The L2 open reading frame of human papillomavirus type 1a encodes a minor structural protein carrying type-specific antigens. J Virol 1986; 60:813.
5. Gissmann L, Boshart M, Durst M, et al: Presence of human papillomaviruses in genital tumors. J Invest Dermatol 1984; 83:26s.
6. Boshart M, Gissmann L, Ikenberg H, et al: A new type of papillomavirus DNA, its presence in genital cancer biopsies and in cell lines derived from cervical cancer. EMBO J 1984; 3:1151.
7. Matsukura T, Kanda T, Furuno A, et al: Cloning of monomeric human papillomavirus type 16 DNA integrated within cell DNA from a cervical carcinoma. J Virol 1986; 58:979.
8. Coggin JR, zur Hausen H: Workshop on papillomaviruses and cancer. Cancer Res 1979; 39:545.
9. zur Hausen H, de Villiers EM: Human papillomaviruses. Annu Rev Microbiol 1994; 48:427.
10. Chan SY, Bernard HU, Ong CK, et al: Phylogenetic analysis of 48 papillomavirus types and 28 subtypes and variants: A showcase for the molecular evolution of DNA viruses. J Virol 1992; 66:5714.
11. Van Ranst M, Kaplan JB, Burk RD, et al: Phylogenetic classification of human papillomaviruses: Correlation with clinical manifestations. J Gen Virol 1992; 73:2653.
12. Lorincz AT, Temple GF, Kurman RJ, et al: Oncogenic association of specific human papillomavirus types in cervical neoplasia. J Natl Cancer Inst 1987; 79:671.
13. McCance DJ, Campion MJ, Clarkson PK, et al: Prevalence of human papillomavirus type 16 DNA sequences in cervical intraepithelial neoplasia and invasive carcinoma of the cervix. Br J Obstet Gynaecol 1985; 92:1101.
14. Lancaster WD, Castellano C, Santos C, et al: Human papillomavirus deoxyribonucleic acid in cervical carcinoma from primary and metastatic sites. Am J Obstet Gynecol 1986; 154:115.
15. Kurman RJ, Schiffman MH, Lancaster WD, et al: Analysis of individual human papillomavirus types in cervical neoplasia: A possible role for type 18 in rapid progression. Am J Obstet Gynecol 1988; 159:293.
16. Walker J, Bloss JD, Liao S-Y, et al: Human papillomavirus

genotype as a prognostic indicator in carcinoma of the uterine cervix. Obstet Gynecol 1989; 74:781.

17. Reid R, Greenberg M, Jenson AB, et al: Sexually transmitted papillomaviral infections. I. The anatomic distribution and pathologic grade of neoplastic lesions associated with different viral types. Am J Obstet Gynecol 1987; 156:212.

18. de Villiers EM: Heterogeneity of the human papillomavirus group. J Virol 1989; 63:4898.

19. Yoshikawa H, Matsukura T, Yamamoto E, et al: Occurrence of human papillomavirus types 16 and 18 DNA in cervical carcinomas from Japan: Age of patients and histological type of carcinomas. Jpn J Cancer Res 1985; 76:667.

20. Yajima H, Noda T, de Villiers EM, et al: Isolation of a new type of human papillomavirus (HPV 52b) with a transforming activity from cervical cancer tissue. Cancer Res 1988; 48:7164.

21. Meyers C, Frattini MG, Hudson JB, et al: Biosynthesis of human papillomavirus from a continuous cell line upon epithelial differentiation. Science 1992; 257:971.

22. Kreider JW, Howett MK, Lill NL, et al: In vivo transformation of human skin with human papillomavirus type 11 from condylomata acuminata. J Virol 1986; 59:369.

23. von Knebel Doeberitz M, Rittmuller C, zur Hausen H, et al: Inhibition of tumorigenicity of cervical cancer cells in nude mice by HPV E6-E7 anti-sense RNA. [Letter.] Int J Cancer 1992; 51:831.

24. Werness BA, Levine AJ, Howley PM: Association of human papillomavirus types 16 and 18 E6 proteins with p53. Science 1990; 248:76.

25. Scheffner M, Werness BA, Huibregtse JM, et al: The E6 oncoprotein encoded by human papillomavirus types 16 and 18 promotes the degradation of p53. Cell 1990; 63:1129.

26. Huibregtse JM, Scheffner M, Howley PM: A cellular protein mediates association of p53 with the E6 oncoprotein of human papillomavirus types 16 or 18. EMBO J 1991; 10:4129.

27. Lane DP: Cancer p53, guardian of the genome [news comment]. Nature 1992; 358:15.

28. el-Deiry WS, Tokino T, Velculescu VE, et al: WAF1, a potential mediator of p53 tumor suppression. Cell 1993; 75:817.

29. Cobrinik D, Dowdy SF, Hinds PW, et al: The retinoblastoma protein and the regulation of cell cycling. Trends Biochem Sci 1992; 17:312.

30. Munger K, Phelps WC: The human papillomavirus E7 protein as a transforming and transactivating factor. Biochim Biophys Acta 1993; 1155:111.

31. Heck DV, Yee CL, Howley PM, et al: Efficiency of binding the retinobastoma protein correlates with the transforming capacity of the E7 oncoproteins of the human papillomaviruses. Proc Natl Acad Sci USA 1992; 89:4442.

32. Stanley MA, Coleman N, Chambers M: The host response to lesions induced by human papillomavirus. In: Mendel A (ed): Genital Warts and Human Papillomavirus Infection. London, Edward Arnold, 1994, pp 21–44.

33. Benton C, Shahidulah H, Hunter JAA: Human papillomaviruses in the immunosuppressed. Papillomavirus Rep 1992; 3:23.

34. Fisher SG, Gissmann L: Convergent infections: Human papillomavirus and human immunodeficiency virus. Antibiot Chemother 1994; 46:134.

35. Bream GL, Ohmstede CA, Phelps WC: Characterization of human papillomavirus type II E1 and E2 proteins expressed in insect cells. J Virol 1993; 67:2655.

36. Carter JJ, Yaegashi N, Jenison SA, et al: Expression of human papillomavirus proteins in yeast saccharomyces cerevisiae. Virology 1991; 182:513.

37. Bleul C, Müller M, Frank R, et al: Human papillomavirus type 18 E6 and E7 antibodies in human sera: Increased anti-E7 prevalence in cervical cancer patients. J Clin Microbiol 1991; 29:1579.

38. Dillner J: Antibodies to defined HPV epitopes in cervical neoplasia. Papillomavirus Rep 1994; 5:35.

39. Müller M, Viscidi RP, Sun Y, et al: Antibodies to HPV-16 E6 and E7 proteins as markers for HPV-16–associated invasive cervical cancer. Virology 1992; 187:508.

40. Eisemann C, Fisher SG, Gross G, et al: Antibodies to human papillomavirus type 11 virus–like particles in sera of patients with genital warts and in control groups. J Gen Virol 1996; 77:1799.

41. Baar MF, Duk JM, Burger MM, et al: Antibodies to human papillomavirus type 16 E7 related to clinicopathological data in patients with cervical carcinoma. J Clin Pathol 1995; 48:410.

42. Gaarenstroom KN, Kenter GG, Bonfrer J, et al: Prognostic significance of serum antibodies to human papillomavirus-16 E4 and E7 peptides in cervical cancer. Cancer 1994; 74:2307.

43. Bonnez W, Da Rin C, Rose RC, et al: Use of human papillomavirus type 11 virions in an ELISA to detect specific antibodies in humans with condylomata acuminata. J Gen Virol 1991; 72:1343.

44. Bonnez W, Da Rin C, Rose RC, et al: Evolution of the antibody response to human papillomavirus type 11 (HPV-11) in patients with condyloma acuminatum according to treatment response. J Med Virol 1993; 39:340.

45. Heim K, Christensen ND, Hoepfl R, et al: Serum IgG, IgM, and IgA reactivity to human papillomavirus types 11 and 6 virus–like particles in different gynecologic patient groups. J Infect Dis 1995; 172:395.

46. Dillner L, Bekassy Z, Jonsson N, et al: Detection of IgA antibodies against human papillomavirus in cervical secretions from patients with cervical intraepithelial neoplasia. Int J Cancer 1989; 43:36.

47. Kadish AS, Romney SL, Ledwidge R, et al: Cell-mediated immune responses to E7 peptides of human papillomavirus (HPV) type 16 are dependent on the HPV type infecting the cervix, whereas serological reactivity is not type-specific. J Gen Virol 1994; 75:2777.

48. Arany I, Tyring SK: Status of local cellular immunity in interferon-responsive and non-responsive human papillomavirus–associated lesions. Sex Transm Dis 1996; 23:475.

49. Beutner KR, Becker TM, Stone KM: Epidemiology of human papillomavirus infections. Dermatol Clin 1991; 9:211.

50. Division of STD Prevention: Sexually transmitted disease surveillance 1994. U.S. Department of Health and Human Services, Public Health Service, Atlanta, Centers for Disease Control and Prevention, 1995.

51. Chuang TY, Perry HO, Kurland LT, et al: Condyloma acuminatum in Rochester, Minn, 1950–1978. Arch Dermatol 1984; 120:469.

52. Brinton LA, Hamman RF, Huggins GR, et al: Sexual and reproductive risk factors for invasive squamous cell cervical cancer. J Natl Cancer Inst 1987; 79:23.

53. Naguib SM, Lundin FE Jr, Davis HJ: Relation of various epidemiologic factors to cervical cancer as determined by a screening program. Obstet Gynecol 1966; 28:451.

54. Irwin KL, Rosero-Bixby L, Oerle MW, et al: Oral contraceptives and cervical cancer risk in Costa Rica: Detection bias or casual association. JAMA 1988; 259:59.

55. Muñoz N, Bosch FX, de Sanjose S, et al: The causal link between human papillomavirus and invasive cervical cancer: A population-based case-control study in Colombia and Spain. Int J Cancer 1992; 52:743.

56. Bosch FX, Manos MM, Muñoz N, et al: Prevalence of human papillomavirus in cervical cancer: A worldwide perspective. International Biological Study on Cervical Cancer (IBSCC) Study Group. J Natl Cancer Inst 1995; 87:796.

57. Daling JR, Nadeline NN, Sherman KJ, et al: Anogenital tumors associated with human papillomavirus. In: Fortner JG, Rhoads JE (eds): Accomplishments in Cancer Research. Philadelphia, JB Lippincott, 1993, pp 280–287.

58. Brinton LA, Nasca PC, Mallin K, et al: Case-control study of cancer of the vulva. Obstet Gynecol 1990; 75:859.

59. Daling JR, Sherman KJ, Hislop TG, et al: Cigarette smoking and the risk of anogenital cancer. Am J Epidemiol 1992; 135:180.

60. Andersen WA, Franquemont DW, Williams J, et al: Vulvar squamous cell carcinoma and papillomaviruses: Two separate entities? Am J Obstet Gynecol 1991; 165:329.

61. Crum CP: Carcinoma of the vulva: Epidemiology and pathogenesis. Obstet Gynecol 1992; 79:448.

62. Hording U, Junge J, Daugaard D, et al: Vulvar squamous cell

carcinoma and papillomaviruses: Indications for two different etiologies. Gynecol Oncol 1994; 52:241.
63. Taichman LB, LaPorta RF: The expression of papillomaviruses in epithelial cells. In: Salzman NP, Howley PM (eds): The Papoviridae: The Papillomaviruses, vol 2. New York, Plenum Press, 1987, pp 109–139.
64. Olson C, Gordon DE, Robl MG, et al: Oncogenicity of bovine papilloma virus. Arch Environ Health 1969; 19:827.
65. zur Hausen H: Human genital cancer: Synergism between two virus infections or synergism between a virus infection and initiating events? Lancet 1982; 2:1370.
66. Tseng CJ, Liang CC, Soong YK, et al: Perinatal transmission of human papillomavirus in infants: Relationship between infection rate and mode of delivery. Obstet Gynecol 1998; 91:92.
67. Kashima HK, Shah K: Recurrent respiratory papillomatosis: Clinical overview and management principles. Obstet Gynecol Clin North Am 1987; 14:581.
68. Pakarian F, Kaye J, Cason J, et al: Cancer-associated papillomaviruses: Perinatal transmission and persistence. Br J Obstet Gynaecol 1994; 101:514.
69. Obalek S, Jablonska S, Favre M, et al: Condylomata acuminata in children: Frequent association with human papillomaviruses responsible for cutaneous warts. J Am Acad Dermatol 1990; 23:205.
70. Hanson RM, Glasson M, McCrossin I, et al: Anogenital warts in childhood. Child Abuse Negl 1989; 13:225.
71. Moscicki AB, Palefsky JM, Gonzales J, et al: The association between human papillomavirus deoxyribonucleic acid status and the results of cytologic screening tests in young sexually active women. Am J Obstet Gynecol 1991; 165:67.
72. Broder S: From the National Institutes of Health: The revised Bethesda system for reporting cervical/vaginal cytologic diagnoses: Report of the 1991 Bethesda Workshop. JAMA 1992; 267:1892.
73. Willett GD, Kurman RJ, Reid RR, et al: Correlation of the histologic appearance of intraepithelial neoplasia of the cervix with human papillomavirus types: Emphasis on low-grade lesions including so-called flat condyloma. Int J Gynecol Pathol 1989; 18:18.
74. Syrjanen K, Mantyjarvi R, Saarikoski S, et al: Factors associated with progression of cervical human papillomavirus (HPV) infections into carcinoma in situ during a long-term prospective follow-up. Br J Obstet Gynaecol 1988; 95:1096.
75. Bur M, Knowles K, Pekow P, et al: Comparison of ThinPrep preparations with conventional cervicovaginal smears: Practical considerations. Acta Cytol 1995; 39:631.
76. Nindl I, Zahm D, Meijer C, et al: Human papillomavirus detection in high-grade squamous intraepithelial lesions: Comparison of hybrid capture assay with a polymerase chain reaction system. Diagn Microbiol Infect Dis 1995; 23:161.
77. Meisels A, Fortin R, Roy M: Condylomatous lesions of the cervix. II. Cytologic, colposcopic and histopathologic study. Acta Cytol 1977; 21:379.
78. McNicol P, Paraskevas M, Guijon F: Variability of polymerase chain reaction–based detection of human papillomavirus DNA is associated with the composition of vaginal microbial flora. J Med Virol 1994; 43:194.
79. Hillier SL, Krohn MA, Nugent RP, et al: Characteristics of three vaginal flora pattern assessed by gram stain among pregnant women. Vaginal Infections and Prematurity Study Group. Am J Obstet Gynecol 1992; 166:938.
80. Ho GYF, Bierman R, Beardsley L, et al: Natural history of cervicovaginal papillomavirus infection in young women. N Engl J Med 1998; 338:423.
81. Evander M, Edlund K, Gustafsson A, et al: Human papillomavirus infection is transient in young women: A population-based cohort study. J Infect Dis 1995; 171:1026.
82. Hildesheim A, Schiffman MH, Gravitt PE, et al: Persistence of type-specific human papillomavirus infection among cytologically normal women. J Infect Dis 1994; 169:235.
83. Sun XW, Kuhn L, Ellerbrock TV, et al: Human papillomavirus infection in women infected with the human immunodeficiency virus. N Engl J Med 1997; 337:1343.
84. Chiasson MA, Ellerbrock TV, Bush TJ, et al: Increased prevalence of vulvovaginal condyloma and vulvar intraepithelial neoplasia in women infected with the human immunodeficiency virus. Obstet Gynecol 1997; 89:690.
85. Paavonen J: Colposcopic findings associated with human papillomavirus infection of the vagina and the cervix. Obstet Gynecol Surv 1985; 40:185.
86. Centers for Disease Control and Prevention: 1998 Guidelines for treatment of sexually transmitted diseases. MMWR 1998; 47(no.RR-1): 88.
87. Kraus SJ, Stone KM: Management of genital infection caused by human papillomavirus. Rev Infect Dis 1990; 12(suppl 6):S620.
88. Krebs HB: Treatment of genital condylomata with topical 5-fluorouracil. Dermatol Clin 1991; 9:333.
89. Reid R, Greenberg MD, Pizzuti DJ, et al: Superficial laser vulvectomy. V. Surgical debulking is enhanced by adjuvant systemic interferon. Am J Obstet Gynecol 92; 166:815.
90. Mayeaux EJ Jr, Harper MB, Barksdale W, et al: Noncervical human papillomavirus genital infections. Am Fam Physician 1995; 52:1137–1146, 1149–1150.
91. Friedman-Kien AE, Eron LJ, Conant M, et al: Natural interferon alfa for treatment of condylomata acuminata. JAMA 1988; 259:533.
92. Gall SA, Hughes CE, Mounts P, et al: Efficacy of human lymphoblastoid interferon in the therapy of resistant condyloma acuminata. Obstet Gynecol 1986; 67:643.
93. Rockley PF, Tyring SK: Interferons alpha, beta and gamma therapy of anogenital human papillomavirus infections. Pharmacol Ther 1995; 65:265.
94. Eron LJ, Judson F, Tucker S, et al: Interferon therapy for condylomata acuminata. N Engl J Med 1986; 315:1059.
95. Reichman RC, Oakes D, Bonnez W, et al: Treatment of condyloma acuminatum with three different interferons administered intralesionally. Ann Intern Med 1988; 108:675.
96. Reichman RC, Micha JP, Weck PK, et al: Interferon alpha-n1 (Wellferon) for refractory genital warts: Efficacy and tolerance of low-dose systemic therapy. Antiviral Res 1988; 10:41.
97. Swinehart JM, Sperling M, Phillips S, et al: Intralesional fluorouracil/epinephrine injectable gel for treatment of condylomata acuminata: A phase 3 clinical study. Arch Dermatol 1997; 133:67.
98. Cook TA, Cohn AM, Brunchwig JP, et al: Wart viruses and laryngeal papillomas. Lancet 1973; 1:782.
99. Sedlacek TV, Lindheim S, Eder C, et al: Mechanism for human papillomavirus transmission at birth. Am J Obstet Gynecol 1989; 161:55.
100. Reid R: The management of genital condylomas, intraepithelial neoplasia, and vulvodynia. Obstet Gynecol Clin North Am 1996; 23:917.
101. Richart RM: Causes and management of cervical intraepithelial neoplasia. Cancer 1987; 60:1951.
102. DiSaia PJ, Creasman WT: Preinvasive diseases of the cervix. In: DiSaia PJ, Creasman WT (eds): Clinical Gynecologic Oncology, 5th ed. St. Louis, Mosby–Year Book, 1997, pp 1–32.
103. Reid R, Dorsey J: Physical and surgical principles of carbon dioxide laser surgery in the lower genital tract. In: Koppelson (ed): Gynecologic Oncology, 2nd ed. London, Churchill Livingstone, 1992, p 1087.
104. Frazer IH: The role of vaccines in the control of STDs: HPV vaccines. Genitourin Med 1996; 72:398.
105. Hofman KJ, Cook JC, Joyce JG, et al: Sequence determination of human papillomavirus type 6a and assembly of virus-like particles in Saccharomyces cerevisiae. Virology 1995; 209:506.
106. Rose RC, Bonnez W, Reichman RC, et al: Expression of human papillomavirus type 11 L1 protein in insect cells: In vivo and in vitro assembly of viruslike particles. J Virol 1993; 67:1936.
107. Hagensee ME, Yaegashi N, Galloway DA: Self-assembly of human papilloma virus type 1 capsids by expression of L1 protein alone or by coexpression of L1 and L2 capsid proteins. J Virol 1993; 67:315.

42 Human Immunodeficiency Virus in Pregnancy

Daniel V. Landers ▶ Geraldo Duarte ▶ William R. Crombleholme

The World Health Organization (WHO) estimates over 34 million people are infected with the human immunodeficiency virus (HIV) worldwide and that 15,000 people are newly infected each day.[1] They further estimate that more than 15 million women are infected with the human immunodeficiency virus type 1 (HIV-1), the majority of whom are in their childbearing years. The number of cases of acquired immunodeficiency syndrome (AIDS) in females continues to rise each year, and the WHO had estimated that by the year 2000, 6 million pregnant women and 5 million infants and children would be infected.[2] Of the 119,810 AIDS cases in females reported in the United States by December 1999, more than 95% were in the reproductive-age group.[3] Currently, it is estimated that more than 6,000 to 7,000 HIV-infected women give birth annually in the United States.[4] Worldwide, more than 2 million HIV-infected women give birth each year. Of the 8,718 pediatric AIDS cases reported in the United States by December 1999, more than 90% are presumed to have acquired HIV infection perinatally.[3] Today, virtually all new HIV infections among children are acquired from their mothers during pregnancy or in the postpartum period.

The challenge presented to the providers of women's health care is effective management of the HIV-infected pregnant woman aimed at minimizing the risk of mother-to-infant transmission while providing optimal therapy for HIV disease. This requires an understanding of how pregnancy may affect HIV infection, how HIV affects pregnancy outcome, and the most effective methods of reducing the risk of vertical transmission. Two very important advances in HIV disease prevention and treatment have had a significant impact on the management of HIV infection in pregnant women. They are (1) the significant reduction in vertical transmission that can be achieved with antiretroviral treatment during pregnancy, and (2) the effectiveness of highly active antiretroviral therapy (HAART) in reducing plasma viral load and the onset of immunodeficiency. Our ability to monitor viral load in response to therapy and more effective therapy have improved the quality of life and survival among people infected with HIV. These current approaches in the management of HIV infection represent significant changes from the past, but it is important to be able to weigh the risks and benefits of HIV therapy during pregnancy. This chapter provides a review of how the application of HIV advances can improve the health of both HIV-infected pregnant women and their unborn babies.

COUNSELING AND TESTING

All the knowledge, drugs, and intervention strategies that we develop cannot help the HIV-infected woman whose infection status is unknown. In order for therapy to benefit all the infected women and to prevent vertical HIV transmission, it is necessary first to get women into a health care setting where counseling and testing can be provided, and second to offer these to them and obtain from them consent, and then to perform the testing. Current guidelines from the United States Department of Health and Human Services, Centers for Disease Control and Prevention (CDC), recommend HIV counseling and voluntary testing of all pregnant women.[5] Despite the burden of required comprehensive counseling of women who test positive, it is only the widespread screening of pregnant women that will make it possible to improve the outcome of these women and their unborn babies. Since many women do not consider themselves at risk for HIV or are not aware of their risk status (the woman who unknowingly is the partner of an injection drug user or a bisexual male), the screening of only those with identifiable risk factors will fall far short of identifying all infected women. In a study published in the Journal of the Canadian Medical Association, based on a review of articles and abstracts published from 1985 to 1997, it was recommended that only universal—and not targeted—counseling and offering of HIV testing be used because targeted testing fails to identify a substantial proportion of HIV-infected pregnant women.[6]

Since the CDC guidelines were published in 1995, 1

year after the first publication demonstrating a clear reduction in HIV vertical transmission by maternal zidovudine administration, progress toward the prevention of perinatal HIV transmission has been steady but considerably slower than we had hoped.[5, 7] There continues to be an immediate need to improve the number of women tested early in pregnancy (when the maximum benefit might be derived from available interventions) to both prevent vertical transmission and improve the overall outcome of maternal HIV infection. Despite the federal mandate of a 50% reduction in the number of perinatal HIV cases by the year 2000, a 95% testing rate among women seen at least twice by the 34th week of pregnancy, and the development of a program for the mandatory testing of newborns whose mothers' HIV status is unknown,[8] there continue to be untested, infected mothers giving birth and infecting babies with HIV both in the United States and worldwide.

Large, multicentered trials have demonstrated a dramatic reduction in mother-to-infant transmission with zidovudine use in pregnancy. The promise that newer, more potent regimens with rapid and durable reductions in viral load to undetectable levels will further reduce transmission, strengthens the need to screen all women for HIV infection during pregnancy to prevent mother-to-infant transmission. As other effective perinatal interventions are developed there is even greater need to screen and identify those who would benefit from the interventions.

The American College of Obstetrics and Gynecology also suggests counseling and testing of all pregnant women.[9] It recommended, in accordance with the CDC guidelines, that pretest counseling including information regarding the risk of HIV infection associated with sexual activity and intravenous drug use, the risk of transmission to an infected woman's infant, and the availability of zidovudine to reduce transmission risk. While legal requirements for HIV counseling and testing vary with geographic locations, counseling should include the potential social and psychological implications of testing and a description of testing procedures. When a woman declines to be tested, it should be documented in her medical record that she was offered testing and declined it.

The test offered for HIV screening is an enzyme-linked immunosorbent assay (EIA) with positive results confirmed by Western blot assay. In order to reduce the false-negative rate to nearly zero, EIA screening necessarily turns up a number of positive results that are not confirmed by Western blot, meaning that the HIV test is *NOT* positive. No EIA result should be considered positive until it is confirmed by Western blot. A negative Western blot is a negative HIV test. At times, the EIA may be positive but the Western blot is reported as "indeterminate." This indicates that the protein-binding pattern on the blot

was insufficient to make the diagnosis of HIV infection. These women should be counseled that the test needs to be repeated in 3 to 6 months. In the majority of patients, these indeterminate results do not indicate HIV infection, particularly when encountered in a patient without identifiable risk factors, but it is necessary to repeat the testing. If these patients consistently exhibit the same indeterminate banding on Western blot for more than 6 months, they are considered HIV negative.[10]

Following testing, post-test counseling involves informing the woman that false-negative results can occur owing to a prolonged latent phase of infection, in which case a person may test negative for HIV antibody and re-testing at a later date may be indicated. The actual rate of false-negative results depends on the interval from risk-related behavior to the time of testing. A pregnant woman with a positive test result should receive detailed counseling at the time the results are given and in follow-up sessions. Counseling should include a description of the early clinical manifestations of HIV disease, the current understanding of the prognosis of HIV disease, the risk of perinatal transmission to the fetus, and available interventions for preventing transmission. Such counseling may require a referral to a health care provider more knowledgeable in HIV disease. Additional counseling issues include responsible sexual behavior that will prevent further transmission, including the use of latex condoms, avoidance of injection-drug use, avoidance of donation of blood products and body organs, and avoidance of sharing toothbrushes, razors, and other instruments that could be contaminated with blood (e.g., tattooing devices and needles). Further counseling should include advising needle-sharing partners and sexual partners to seek testing. All individuals who test positive should receive appropriate referrals, including psychosocial support services.[10]

EFFECTS OF PREGNANCY ON HIV DISEASE

The protection of the antigenically distinct fetus from the maternal immune response has led some to describe pregnancy as a state of relative immunosuppression. Armed with data on severe clinical courses with some infections, such as poliomyelitis, hepatitis A, malaria, and coccidioidomycosis, proponents of immunosuppression in pregnancy have raised concerns regarding rapid progression of HIV disease and, in particular, immunodeficiency during pregnancy. Furthermore, altered numbers and ratios of CD4- and CD8-bearing T lymphocytes, decreased proliferative responses, and decreased immunoglobulin levels all have been reported in pregnancy.[11] Despite these findings, the normal pregnant woman is generally regarded as immunocompetent and capable of an appropriate and effective response to most infections. The problem with assessing immune responses in pregnancy is the difficulty in performing longitudinal studies during pregnancy. Biggar and colleagues[12] followed CD4 counts longitudinally in HIV-infected and noninfected gravidas through the postpartum period and found a decrease in the numbers of CD4+ T cells in both groups during pregnancy. Recovery was noted post partum, but only in the HIV-negative group. In another study, Dinsmoor and Christmas[13] evaluated lymphocyte counts among 23 HIV-infected pregnant women, 10 of whom received zidovudine. Both CD4 and CD8 counts decreased in those not taking zidovudine, but this finding may reflect the overall decrease in total lymphocyte numbers noted with advancing gestational age in that study.

In the largest and best controlled longitudinal study of T cells in pregnancy, Burns and colleagues[14] reported on 192 (HIV-positive) and 148 HIV-negative women followed longitudinally during, and for 2 years after, the index pregnancy. They used a mixed-effect model to compensate for repeated measurements and laboratory and calendar year effects. Using pairwise comparisons to determine significance, they found that CD4 T-cell percentage began to decrease during pregnancy and returned to normal post partum. However, among HIV-infected women, CD4 levels declined steadily during pregnancy and post partum among seropositive women. The percentage of CD8 cells increased at or near delivery and declined to baseline between 2 and 6 months post partum in both HIV-positive and HIV-negative women.

In an earlier study of 229 Malawian women in the third trimester and 128 women 6 weeks post partum, both HIV-positive and HIV-negative women demonstrated an increase in the absolute number of CD4 and CD8 T lymphocytes between late pregnancy and the early postpartum period, whereas percentages of CD4 and CD8 T cells remained unchanged.[15] Thus, the Malawian women were no more immunosuppressed, as determined by T-cell flow cytometric studies, in the third trimester of pregnancy than in the nonpregnant state.

Rich and co-workers[16] reported on T-cell phenotype and cell function in HIV-positive and HIV-negative pregnant and postpartum women and nonpregnant noninfected control subjects. All noninfected nonpregnant subjects, 74% of noninfected pregnant subjects, and 54% of HIV-infected pregnant women responded to all stimuli in terms of interleukin-2 (IL-2) production in vitro. All noninfected subjects had normal function 2 to 6 months post partum, compared with 27% of infected women. In addition, infected pregnant women had elevated levels of memory, reduced levels of naïve, and increased levels of activated lymphocytes as determined by three-color flow cytometry. These data suggest that CD4 T-cell function and phenotype

are altered in pregnancy and return to baseline post partum in noninfected, but not HIV-infected, women.

Data published in 1995 from the European Collaborative Study on CD4 counts in 867 HIV-positive women at 16 to 24 weeks of gestation, 28 to 32 weeks of gestation, and at delivery showed a 36% decline in the mean CD4 count over the study period.[17] Temmerman and colleagues[19] studied 416 HIV-positive and 407 HIV-negative women at enrollment, delivery, and 6 weeks post partum. They evaluated CD4 and CD8 cells, finding no significant differences in the course of pregnancy in either group.[19] Data from The Women and Infants Transmission Study (WITS) cohort showed very little change in percentages of CD4 and CD8 cells and no clinically significant changes during pregnancy or post partum among 226 HIV-positive women.[18]

Further data from the WITS cohort was analyzed to determine the influence of pregnancy on changes in HIV viral load.[20] They studied 160 HIV-positive women who had one or more serum plasma samples analyzed before and during the third trimester, and at 2, 12, and 24 months post partum. They found no significant change in HIV-1 viral load during pregnancy in these largely antiretroviral-untreated women. They concluded that changes in viral load during pregnancy appear to reflect slowly increasing viremia among a population of women with relatively advanced HIV disease. They further suggested that to detect any effect of pregnancy, labor, or delivery, a closely matched group of nonpregnant women would be necessary to serve as controls. Treatment with antiretroviral agents during pregnancy would, of course, further complicate the design of such a study.

Numerous other studies have shown conflicting results, leading to confusion as to whether or not pregnancy affects HIV disease status. If we accept the data from the largest, most-controlled longitudinal studies, we can conclude that women with HIV in pregnancy may experience some decline in CD4 T cells and their return to baseline may be slowed. Whether these findings lead to adverse long-term outcomes in these women is doubtful, and the consequences of pregnancy in women with HIV disease remain uncertain.

Some clinical data also exist from a longitudinal study[21] of cohorts of HIV-infected women regarding HIV disease progression among women who carried a pregnancy. In a report from the Italian Seroconversion Group, 94 women developed HIV-related disease and 47 developed AIDS. The results from a Cox proportional hazards model showed no difference in the rate of any endpoints measuring disease progression among pregnant women.[21] In another study[22] reporting on two Swiss cohorts that compared 32 women followed through pregnancy with 416 control subjects, no statistically significant differences were found for any AIDS-defining event except recurrent bacterial pneumonia (RR, 7.98;95% CI, 1.73 to 36.8). They concluded from their data that after taking into account the CD4 count before conception, accelerating disease progression is inconsistent among HIV-positive women who become pregnant.[22]

A meta-analysis of seven studies, all prospective cohorts, was published in 1998 to assess the effect of pregnancy on survival in HIV-positive women.[23] The summary odds ratios for the risk of an adverse maternal outcome related to HIV infection and pregnancy were as follows: death, 1.8 (95% CI, 0.99 to 3.3); HIV disease progression, 1.4 (95% CI, 0.85 to 2.33); progression to AIDS-defining illness, 1.63 (95% CI, 1.0 to 2.67); and decrease in CD4 cells to less than 200, 0.73 (95% CI, 0.17 to 3.06). Thus, there appears to be a weak association between adverse maternal outcomes and pregnancy among HIV-infected women, but this relationship may be due to confounding and study biases. The available data are not sufficient to clarify this issue at present.

PREGNANCY OUTCOME IN WOMEN INFECTED WITH HIV

A number of authors have reported data on pregnancy outcome in women with HIV infection. An early report on 50 women found that 35 (70%) had complicated prenatal courses, most commonly preterm labor or infectious complications.[24] In 1990, Minkoff and co-workers[25] reported that among 91 seropositive women, sexually transmitted diseases and medical complications during pregnancy were more common than among 126 seronegative control subjects. They did not find any association between HIV status and birth weight, gestational age at delivery, head circumference, or Apgar score after controlling for drug and tobacco use and maternal age.[25] In another report on 466 HIV-infected women in Zaire, their infants were more likely to be premature and to have lower birth weights and a higher neonatal death rate compared to the infants of 606 HIV-negative women.[26] This study differed from other reports in that the study population included a larger number of women with AIDS (18%). Temmerman and co-workers[27] reported an association between maternal HIV infection and low birth weight (mean weight 2,913 g vs. 3,072 g; $P = .003$), and prematurity (21.1% vs 9.4; $P \leq .0001$) in a Nairobi cohort of 315 HIV-seropositive and 311 HIV-seronegative women. They also found that in women with CD4 counts below 30% the preterm delivery rate was significantly higher (26.3% vs. 10.1%; $P = .001$). In that study, HIV-seropositive women also had higher rates of genital ulcer disease (4.7% vs. 2.0%; $P = .06$), genital warts (4.9% vs. 2.0%; $P = .03$), positive syphilis serology (7.9% vs. 3.2%), and postpartum endometritis (10.3% vs. 4.2%; $P = 0.01$). In 1990, Minkoff and colleagues[28] also reported an increased incidence of serious infections

in 9 of 16 HIV-seropositive pregnant women with CD4 counts less than 300 cells/mm^3. This included six women with *Pneumocystis carinii* pneumonia.

More recent studies have shed additional light on the impact of HIV infection on pregnancy outcome. In 1998, Leroy and colleagues[29] reported on pregnancy outcome, comparing 364 HIV-positive women with 365 HIV-negative women in Kigali, Rwanda, between 1992 and 1994. The adjusted estimated proportion of preterm births attributable to maternal HIV infection was 24% (95% CI, 2 to 38) among HIV-positive women.[29] When one considers the HIV prevalence of 34.4% in that population, the estimated proportion of preterm births attributable to maternal HIV in the Kigali population was 8.3%. The risk of intrauterine growth restriction among HIV-infected women, adjusted for confounding risk factors by multivariate logistic regression, was not significantly different from the risk among HIV-negative women (RR, 1.5; 95% CI, 0.7 to 2.9). In 1998, Brocklehurst and French[30] published a meta-analysis of the association between maternal HIV infection and perinatal outcome. They included 31 studies in their review. They found the summary odds ratios of adverse perinatal outcomes related to maternal HIV infection to be as follow: spontaneous abortion 4.05 (95% CI, 2.75 to 5.96); stillbirth, 3.91 (95% CI, 2.65 to 5.77); perinatal mortality, 1.79 (95% CI, 1.14 to 2.81); intrauterine growth retardation, 1.7 (95% CI, 1.43 to 2.03); low birth weight, 2.09 (95% CI, 1.86 to 2.35); preterm delivery, 1.83 (95% CI, 1.63 to 2.06); and infant mortality, 3.69 (95% CI, 3.03 to 4.49). Sensitivity analysis indicated that the association between infant mortality and maternal HIV infection was stronger in studies from developing countries, studies with higher methodologic quality, and those that controlled for confounding variables.

A report describes the WITS analysis of obstetric and newborn outcomes between 1989 and 1994.[31] The researchers reported on 634 women delivered after 24 weeks of gestation. The preterm birth, low birth weight, and small-for-gestational-age (SGA) rates were 20.5%, 18.9%, and 24%, respectively. Low CD4 counts (<14%) and a history of adverse pregnancy outcome were associated with preterm birth and low birth weight, and SGA was associated with maternal hard-drug use, trichomoniasis, hypertension, and a history of adverse outcome. Unfortunately, there was no matched HIV-negative control group reported to assess the relative risk of maternal HIV infection as an independent risk factor.

Overall, there is no definitive study that defines the effects of HIV on pregnancy outcome. Large cohorts of HIV-infected women followed through pregnancy still do not include enough patients with severely immunocompromised conditions to clarify effects that are diluted by including large numbers of women that are HIV-infected but do not exhibit immunocompromise. Nonetheless, there appears to be an association, although not strong, between maternal HIV infection and an adverse perinatal outcome, especially preterm delivery. However, this observation may be due to insufficient controls and residual confounding.

MANAGEMENT OF HIV DISEASE IN PREGNANCY

The majority of prenatal care providers do not have extensive experience with or knowledge of the management of HIV disease, but they will be faced with the challenge of integrating the management of HIV disease into that of pregnancy. The HIV-infected woman may already have a provider of HIV care or may need an appropriate and immediate referral. Whenever feasible, HIV disease in a pregnant woman is managed in the same manner as in the nonpregnant woman, with some important caveats regarding drug safety in pregnancy and reducing the risk of vertical transmission.

The report from the NIH Panel to Define Principles of Therapy of HIV Infection specifically states that women should receive optimal antiretroviral therapy regardless of pregnancy status.[32] This, of course, is tempered by the available fetal safety data on treatment strategies. Women who are first identified as being HIV-positive during the pregnancy or who are aware of their HIV positivity but are now faced with pregnancy must be presented with treatment options that consider the current and future health of the mother, perinatal transmission, and insuring the health of the fetus and neonate. The treatment recommendations for HIV-infected pregnant women are based on the premise that therapeutic modalities with known life-preserving benefits should not be withheld from HIV-infected women because of pregnancy unless there are known adverse effects on the mother, fetus, or infant that outweigh the potential benefit. In general, obstetricians tend to avoid therapeutic agents that have not been well established as safe in pregnancy. In reality, this decision is most often based on the risk-benefit ratio. A different disease or condition that is not life-threatening may be approached differently in items of avoiding agents with incomplete or unknown safety profiles in pregnancy.

Antiretroviral use in pregnancy has evolved over the past few years to the point that now the initially prescribed regimens are very similar for pregnant and nonpregnant women. While providers initiate mainly antiretroviral treatment in pregnancy to reduce HIV plasma RNA viral load, prolong clinical latency, and retard immunodeficiency, there are occasions when the purpose of antiretroviral therapy is solely to reduce the risk of perinatal HIV transmission. In this section we focus on antiretroviral use to treat maternal disease;

prevention of vertical transmission is discussed in a separate section of this chapter.

There are no good, long-term safety studies available on the use of antiretroviral agents during pregnancy. The most vulnerable period of fetal development is the first trimester; thus, when feasible, initiation of antiretroviral therapy should be withheld until after 14 weeks of gestation. When a woman is already receiving antiretroviral therapy at the time pregnancy is confirmed, therapy is continued unless the pregnancy is early in the first trimester (before 8 weeks). In that situation, some women will opt to stop therapy and to restart after 14 weeks. The NIH panel recommendations state that "although the effects of all antiretroviral drugs on the developing fetus during the first trimester are uncertain, most experts recommend continuation of a maximally suppressive regimen even during the first trimester."[32] Whenever antiretroviral therapy is discontinued for any reason during the pregnancy, all agents should be stopped and restarted simultaneously to avoid hastening drug resistance.

Choosing an antiretroviral treatment regimen should be done with the patient's full understanding of all the risks and benefits of treatment. Because compliance is crucial to success and to the avoidance of the rapid development of resistance, the patient must have an understanding of the complexity of combination antiretroviral therapy, the goals of treatment, and the consequences of noncompliance. The choice of which agents to use is complicated by the lack of safety data on drugs other than zidovudine. The regimen must be individualized, based on discussion with the patient and available data from preclinical and clinical testing of individual drugs. Table 42–1 summarizes the currently available antiretroviral agents and their pregnancy classification by the U.S. Food and Drug Administration (FDA).

Among the nucleoside reverse transcriptase inhibitors (NRTIs), the pharmacokinetics of zidovudine and lamivudine have been evaluated in HIV-infected pregnant women. These drugs are well tolerated at the usual adult doses and cross the placenta. Cord blood levels reach levels comparable to maternal serum. Both ddI and ddC show less placental transfer than do zidovudine, d4T, and 3TC.[33] All NRTIs except ddI have preclinical animal studies suggesting potential fetal risk and have been classified as FDA pregnancy category C. The one exception, ddI, has been classified as category B.[32]

The only pregnancy-related information on the nonnucleoside reverse transcriptase inhibitors (NNRTIs) is that for nevirapine administered once at the onset of labor. Neonatal blood concentrations reached maternal serum levels rapidly, and the mean half-life was prolonged (66 hours). As yet, there are no available data on multiple dosing during pregnancy.[32, 33]

Combination therapy including a protease inhibitor

TABLE 42-1 ▸ SUMMARY OF COMMONLY USED ANTIRETROVIRAL AGENTS FOR THE TREATMENT OF HIV-1 INFECTION

Class	Agent	Other Names	Brand Name	Dietary Cautions	FDA Pregnancy Category*
Nucleoside Reverse Transcriptase Inhibitors (NRTIs)	Zidovudine	AZT, ZDV	Retrovir	Empty stomach	(C)
	Lamivudine	3TC	Epivir	None	(C)
	Combination of AZT/3TC	AZT + 3TC	Combivir	None	(C)
	Didanosine	ddI	Videx	Take before meals	(B)
	Zalcitabine	ddC	Hivid	Empty stomach	(C)
	Stavudine	d4T	Zerit	None	(C)
	Abacavir	ABC	Ziagen	None	(C)
	Adefovir	ADV	Preveon	None	Pending
Non-Nucleoside Reverse Transcriptase Inhibitors (NNRTIs)	Nevirapine	NVP	Viramune	None	(C)
	Delavirdine	DLV	Rescriptor	None	(C)
	Efavirenz	EVZ	Sustiva	None	(C)
Protease Inhibitors	Ritonavir	RTV	Norvir	With meals	(B)
	Saquinavir	FTV	Fortovase	With fatty meals	(B)
	Indinavir	IDV	Crixivan	1 h before or 2 h after	(C)
	Nelfinavir	NFV	Viracept	With meals	(B)
	Amprenavir	AMV	Agenerase	None	(C)

*FDA ratings are based on the degree to which available information has ruled out risk to the fetus, balanced against the drug's potential benefit to the patient.
Category A: Controlled studies show no risk.
Category B: No evidence of risk in humans; animal studies negative or animal studies show risk but human studies do not.
Category C: Risk cannot be ruled out, studies lacking; however, potential benefit may justify potential risk.
Category D: Positive evidence of risk to fetus. Still, in some instances, benefit may outweigh risk.
Category X: Contraindicated in pregnancy. Fetal risk clearly outweighs potential benefit.

in pregnant HIV-infected women is now being used widely, and anecdotal reports and retrospective analyses are beginning to appear. HAART regimens, which generally include a protease inhibitor along with two NRTIs, have become fairly common at centers treating large numbers of HIV-infected pregnant women. In a recent report on protease inhibitor use in 89 pregnancies, no adverse fetal or maternal effects were noted.[34] In that study, 36 women received nelfinavir, 33 received saquinavir, 23 received indinavir, and 5 received ritonavir. The protease inhibitors were begun before pregnancy in 17 women, in the first trimester in 10, in the second trimester in 43, and in the third trimester in 13. The preterm delivery rate (<37 weeks of gestation) was 19.7% overall, and 21% for those receiving protease inhibitors from the first or second trimesters and onward. In another report, HAART therapy was used in 64 pregnant women.[35] Three drugs, including a protease inhibitor, were given to 27 women, nevirapine was given to 22, and combinations including both a protease inhibitor and nevirapine were given to 15. HIV RNA levels were undetectable (<400 copies/mL) in 67% of women on protease inhibitors, 78% of those on nevirapine, and 91% of those on both at the time of delivery. Birth weight and gestational age at delivery were not significantly different between groups.

Placental passage studies indicate that indinavir has substantial placental passage in mice, but little in rabbits. Indinavir is also associated with side effects, such as hyperbilirubinemia and renal stones, that could be problematic for the newborn if significant transplacental passage occurs. These concerns are theoretical, and

such effects have not been reported to date. Administration of protease inhibitors has been associated with new-onset diabetes, hyperglycemia, or exacerbation of pre-existing diabetes. Since pregnancy can lead to gestational diabetes or glucose intolerance, glucose levels should be closely monitored in HIV-infected pregnant women receiving protease inhibitor therapy. Glucose screening should be done early, and if normal, repeated at the usual time (26 to 28 weeks of gestation). Patients should be advised of early signs of hyperglycemia.

Pregnant women who are newly identified as being HIV-infected who are started on antiretroviral therapy usually receive Combivir, a combination of zidovudine and lamivudine (3TC) and a protease inhibitor, most often nelfinavir or indinavir at our institution. The exact choice of protease inhibitor varies, depending on the experience and preferences of local HIV providers. Women who are known to be HIV infected will often be on different regimens that may be the result of therapeutic changes necessitated by past viral resistance or drug toxicity. Most HIV-infected patients on therapy are on some sort of HAART regimen and occasionally Mega HAART (five or more antiretroviral agents), although Mega HAART is far less likely in the pregnant population of HIV-infected individuals.

MANAGEMENT OF PREGNANCY IN THE HIV-INFECTED WOMAN

The HIV-infected gravida must be provided with comprehensive care that takes into account the status of her pregnancy as well as her HIV disease. Newly diagnosed HIV-infected women require an approach different from that in an individual with long-standing HIV disease (Table 42–2). If a woman has a history of HIV infection, there should be some documentation of this in the form a Western blot result or detectable viral load data. Some effort should be made to determine the duration of infection, degree of immunocompromise, viral load status, and history of opportunistic infections, since continued treatment and the approach to prevention of vertical transmission are based on this history. Women newly identified as being HIV-infected require intensive counseling, and an assessment of disease status, the options for treatment of maternal disease, and the prevention of vertical transmission.

Whenever possible, the management of HIV disease in a pregnant woman is the same as that in a nonpregnant woman. There are certainly some precautions that must be taken into account concerning safety of the fetus whenever drugs are used in a pregnant woman. Attention must be afforded to the potential signs of HIV disease progression and the interactive sexually transmitted diseases and opportunistic infections. A comprehensive medical and obstetric-gynecologic history should be taken, particularly in the gravida who is not under medical care for her HIV disease. Particular attention should be given to conditions suggestive of HIV disease progression. The review of systems should focus on HIV-related signs of disease progression or opportunistic infections. The various nonspecific symptoms of pregnancy can cause providers to easily overlook early signs of opportunistic infections. The history should also include psychosocial factors that may adversely affect a patient's ability to maintain the pregnancy and her general health. Care should be taken in assessing the potential for continued or re-established substance abuse, including alcohol. Assessment should also be made of the patient's economic stability, any serious illness in family members, and the potential for or existence of domestic violence, all of which can potentially lead to a crisis

that interferes with a woman's ability to maintain her health and a healthy pregnancy and to comply with a regimen of multiple antiretroviral agents.

A detailed physical examination is performed at the initial prenatal visit, with attention to the systems most commonly affected by HIV disease. Each trimester, or whenever clinical suspicion arises, the physical examination is repeated. Laboratory evaluation must include the usual prenatal laboratory tests and additional testing to identify potentially problematic HIV-related disease. Papanicolaou (Pap) smears; sexually transmitted disease testing, including a serologic test for syphilis such as VDRL (Venereal Disease Research Laboratory); serologic testing for hepatitis B and C; screening for chlamydiosis, gonorrhea, and trichomoniasis; and bacterial vaginosis testing should be performed. A careful examination for genital lesions, particularly ulcerative lesions, should also be performed. A T-lymphocyte count, including CD3, CD4, CD8, and CD4/CD8 ratios, should be considered as well as viral load testing at the initial visit, and the viral load and CD4 counts should be repeated each trimester or as clinically indicated.

In accordance with the guidelines of the U.S. Public Health Service (USPHS)/Infectious Diseases Society of America (IDSA), baseline serologic evaluation for the opportunistic infections common in HIV-infected individuals that may pose additional risks to the fetus is performed.[10] All HIV-infected persons who lack IgG antibody to *Toxoplasma* should be counseled about the various sources of toxoplasmic infection. This warning includes avoiding raw or undercooked meat, especially pork, lamb, or venison. Meat should be cooked until no longer pink inside (internal temperature of 165°F). Hands should be washed after contact with raw meat and after gardening or other contact with soil. Fruits and vegetables should be washed well before they are eaten raw. Cat owners should have the litterbox changed daily, preferably by an HIV-negative, nonpregnant person, or the patient should wash the hands thoroughly after changing the litterbox. Cats should be kept inside, and stray cats should be avoided. Cats should further be fed only canned or dried commercial food or well-cooked table food, not raw or undercooked meats. HIV-infected women that are IgG seronegative for cytomegalovirus antibody should be advised about good hygienic practices, such as hand washing.

The initial visit should also include tuberculosis (TB) testing by purified protein derivative (PPD) skin testing for those without a history of a reactive PPD. Routine evaluation for anergy is not recommended; however, there are selected situations in which anergy testing may be helpful, particularly in women with very low CD4 counts.[9, 10] All HIV-infected women with a positive PPD should have a chest radiograph and clinical evaluation to exclude active TB. Among HIV-infected patients, induration of the PPD site of more

TABLE 42-2 ▶ MANAGEMENT APPROACHES TO HIV-1 INFECTED WOMEN IN PREGNANCY	
Known HIV-Positive	**Newly Identified HIV-Positive**
Verify Western blot results	Intensive counseling
Date of diagnosis	Diagnosis and prevention of
Estimate duration of	spread
infection	Natural history and prognosis
Initial CD4/viral load testing	Psychosocial needs
Hx opportunistic infections	assessment
Other signs of	Available treatments
immunodeficiency	Assessment of disease status
Antiretroviral Therapy	Treatment options
Current regimen	Options in pregnancy
Previous regimens	
Pregnancy options	

than 5 mm should be considered positive. Those with positive tests and no evidence of active disease or prior treatment should receive prophylaxis with isoniazid (INH) for 12 months, along with pyridoxine. A chest radiography with appropriate abdominal-pelvic lead apron shields should be performed to minimize radiation exposure to the embryo or fetus. Chemoprophylaxis, when indicated, should be administered during pregnancy. Some providers may choose to wait until after the first trimester because of theoretical concerns of possible teratogenicity associated with drug exposures during the early part of gestation. HIV-infected pregnant women who have a positive *Mycobacterium tuberculosis* culture or who are suspected of having TB disease should be treated without delay. Choices of TB treatment regimens should be made in consultation with a provider experienced in the area of TB treatment of HIV-infected patients. The CDC recommends that choices of TB treatment regimens for HIV-infected pregnant women include rifampin.[36] However, protease inhibitors and NNRTIs are not recommended for use in patients receiving rifampin. The routine use of pyrazinamide during pregnancy is recommended by international organizations, but not in the United States because of inadequate teratogenicity data. The benefits of a TB regimen that includes pyrazinamide may outweigh the potential risks to the fetus. Streptomycin and other aminoglycosides and capreomycin are contraindicated in all pregnant women.

A careful assessment of the pregnancy, including fetal growth and development, is important when one provides prenatal care to the HIV-infected pregnant woman. Ultrasound evaluation, nonstress testing, and biophysical profiles of the fetus are performed as clinically indicated. Women in whom prenatal genetic testing is indicated should be counseled regarding the added theoretical risk of infecting an otherwise noninfected fetus by amniocentesis, chorionic villus sampling, or cordocentesis. There are very few data on the magnitude of this risk in HIV-infected women. Women are generally given the option of amniocentesis if they desire; however, given the potential added risk, few women opt for the procedure. There is some evidence that amniocentesis is associated with an increased risk of vertical transmission.[37] Triple screening of the maternal serum for human chorionic gonadotropin, alpha-fetoprotein, and estriol can predict, to some degree, trisomy 21 as well as some neural tube defects without the risk of invasive procedures. Nuchal translucency on ultrasound can be assessed to further assist in noninvasive prediction of aneuploidy.[38] Amniocentesis, when performed, must be done with ultrasound guidance to assist in avoiding puncture of the fetal skin.

MOTHER-TO-INFANT (VERTICAL) TRANSMISSION

HIV transmission from a mother to her infant has been seen during pregnancy, and at the time of and following birth. In the United States and some other developed countries, the risk of vertical transmission has been greatly reduced in the last half decade. Research showing reduced transmission rates in women receiving antiretroviral therapy, along with widespread recommendations for HIV counseling and testing of all pregnant women and attention to obstetric practices aimed at reducing risks all have contributed to this reduction in vertical transmission. Following the early termination of the AIDS Clinical Trial Group (ACTG) protocol 076 in 1995 because of the proven efficacy of zidovudine therapy in preventing vertical transmission, the U.S. Public Health Service recommended routine HIV counseling and voluntary testing of all pregnant women.[5]

The ACTG 076 study, a randomized, controlled, interventional trial, clearly showed that mother-to-infant transmission could be reduced by as much as one third by administering oral zidovudine to the mother, following the first trimester and throughout pregnancy, along with intravenous zidovudine infusion during labor and oral zidovudine administered to the infant within 8 to 12 hours of birth, four times daily until 6 weeks of age.[7, 39] Table 42–3 lists the timing and doses of zidovudine necessary for reducing vertical transmission. Since that study, investigators have continued to generate important information on mother-to-infant transmission. The timing of transmission, the impact of viral load, CD4 counts, duration of fetal membrane rupture, mode of delivery, and maternal drug use all have been determined to be important factors in vertical transmission.

TABLE 42–3 ▶	ZIDOVUDINE ADMINISTRATION IN PREGNANCY FROM ACTG 076 PROTOCOL	
Mother	Oral zidovudine*	100 mg PO 5 times daily beginning after 14 weeks of gestation and continued throughout pregnancy
	Intravenous zidovudine	2 mg/kg body weight load over 1 h
		During the labor, intravenous administration of ZDV in a 1-h initial dose of, followed by a continuous infusion of, 1 mg/kg body weight/h until delivery
Infant	Oral zidovudine	Oral administration of ZDV to the newborn (ZDV syrup at 2 mg/kg body weight/dose q6h) for the first 6 wk of life, beginning at 8–12 h after birth
	Intravenous zidovudine	Intravenous dosage for infants who cannot tolerate oral intake is 1.5 mg/kg body weight IV q6h

*Many providers use alternative dosing of 200 mg PO tid or 300 mg bid to improve compliance.

Timing of Vertical Transmission

While the timing of HIV vertical transmission is associated with the route of transmission, there may be considerable overlap particularly with regard to intrapartum transmission. The relative proportion of HIV transmission that occurs ante partum versus intra partum remains unclear. Early evidence of HIV infection, such as AIDS in the first few months of life, strongly suggests that transmission may occur well before the intrapartum period. This finding, combined with the identification of HIV in fetal tissue, fetal blood samples, and amniotic fluid, and positive viral studies in 20% to 60% of infected infants at the time of birth all support the occurrence of HIV transmission in utero before the intrapartum period. This mode of transmission is thought to account for between 17% and 40% of vertical HIV transmission.[40, 41] Intrapartum transmission, as the term implies, is thought to occur at or near the time of labor and delivery. This mode of transmission accounts for roughly 40% to 80% of cases of vertically transmitted HIV. Intrapartum transmission has been the focus of many strategies for preventing vertical transmission because as many as 80% of cases of transmission occur in this short time period, making it more amenable to applied interventions.[42, 43]

Postpartum transmission can and does occur and may account for between 14% and 32% of cases, depending on the population and whether breastfeeding is feasible.[41, 42, 44] In industrialized countries where bottlefeeding is thought to be safe, all HIV-infected women are discouraged from breastfeeding as an adjunct to preventing vertical HIV transmission. Long-term breastfeeding increases vertical transmission of HIV.[45, 46] The mode and timing of vertical transmission is crucial to the development of interventional strategies aimed at preventing transmission. Strategies applied only to the intrapartum period (i.e., elective cesarean section at term) do not prevent early intrauterine transmission. Furthermore, strategies that can be applied throughout gestation, and include an intrapartum focus, have the greatest potential to prevent vertical transmission.

Risk Factors for Vertical Transmission

The risk factors associated with HIV vertical transmission are numerous and diverse and can be sorted out properly only when analysis is made of large cohorts with a large enough sample size to adjust for confounding variables. Factors that have been identified in univariate analyses include maternal factors, viral factors, fetal or infant factors, placental factors, and breast milk factors (Table 42–4).

One well-established risk factor for HIV vertical transmission is maternal viral load.[41, 47] Unfortunately, viral load is not the sole predictor. There is no viral

TABLE 42–4 ▶ HIV VERTICAL TRANSMISSION RISK FACTORS

Maternal Factors	Obstetric Factors
High maternal viral load	Duration of ruptured
Acute HIV infection	membranes
Advanced-stage disease	Amount of maternal-fetal
Low CD4 counts or percentage	transfusion
High CD8 counts or percentage	Blood exposure of fetus
Low levels of neutralizing	Invasive fetal testing:
antibodies	Internal electrodes
Maternal drug use	Scalp sampling
Unprotected intercourse during	Amniocentesis
pregnancy	Percutaneous umbilical blood
Vitamin A deficiency	sampling
Placental Factors	Mode of delivery
CD 4 expression among	
placental cells	**Fetal-Newborn Factors**
Loss of integrity of placental	Genetic susceptibility
barrier	Reduced-function immunity
Chorioamnionitis	Fetal cell susceptibility
Syphilis and other STDs	Skin integrity
Smoking	Low gastric acidity
	Prematurity
Virologic Factors	Low birth weight
Non-syncytium-induction	
Macrophage tropism	**Breast Milk Factors**
	Viral load in breast milk, cell
	free or cell associated
	HIV-specific antibody

load below which transmission does not occur, and conversely there is no viral load so high that transmission is ensured. This is not to say that transmission is not associated with plasma viral load. In a follow-up study of the ACTG 076 cohort, Sperling and co-workers[48] found that a high maternal viral load was a risk factor for the transmission of HIV from an untreated mother to her infant. The reduction in such transmission after zidovudine treatment was only partly explained by the reduction in plasma levels of viral RNA.[48] It is likely that in addition to viral load, administering zidovudine to the fetus prior to exposure (prophylaxis) served to further reduce the risk.

Along with viral load, acute maternal viral infection has been associated with an increased rate of vertical transmission, possibly related to viral burden and a lack of HIV antibody production early in the course of HIV infection. Advanced stage of HIV disease is a known risk factor for vertical transmission. Again, such women tend to have higher viral loads, lower CD4 counts, and higher CD8 counts, all known risk factors. Several studies have shown that the finding of low maternal CD4 T-lymphocyte counts is an independent risk factor in multivariate analyses.[49, 50]

Abnormally low maternal vitamin A levels during pregnancy have been associated with increased transmission.[51] A five-fold increased risk of transmission was reported in women with vitamin A levels less than 0.7 μmol/L (normal, >1.4 μmol/L). Vitamin A deficiency was also associated with vertical transmission in one U.S. cohort, independent of CD4 count and duration of membrane rupture[52, 53] In another U.S. study of 95

HIV-positive women, there was no association between vertical HIV transmission and serum retinol levels.[54]

Most women in the United States receive prenatal vitamin supplementation that includes vitamin A. There is no evidence that administering vitamin A to women with normal retinol levels further reduces the HIV transmission risk. Because vitamin A is potentially teratogenic in early gestation, supplementation over and above that received from prenatal vitamins should be discouraged.

Characteristics of the virus itself have been associated with increased risk of transmission. Quasispecies (multiple different strains of HIV-1) can exist in an infected woman, which may vary in several viral characteristics, including replication rate, syncytium-inducing capacity, and cellular tropism, which may cause differences in transmissibility. M-tropic strains of maternal isolates have been reported to be more likely to be transmitted than are T-cell tropic strains.[55] Neonatal macrophages have also been shown to be more susceptible than adult macrophages to infection in vitro by non–syncytium-inducing, M-tropic isolates.[56]

The risk factors related to obstetrics are listed in Table 42–4. Many of these are from univariate analyses of HIV-infected cohorts without enough numbers to control for confounding variables. The mechanisms by which these risk factors enhance transmission are usually obvious, but because they often appear together, it is difficult to determine their individual contribution to transmission risk. Among the obstetric components of this risk, duration of ruptured membranes and mode of delivery have received the most attention in recent years. In a large, prospective observational cohort study, The Women and Infants Transmission Study (WITS), 525 women delivering singleton infants with known HIV status were analyzed.[57] The rate of vertical transmission of HIV was 25% among mothers with membranes ruptured for longer than 4 hours before delivery, compared with 14% among mothers with membranes ruptured for less than 4 hours. In a multivariate analysis, membrane rupture of more than 4 hours nearly doubled the risk (odds ratio [OR], 1.83; 95% CI, 1.1 to 3.0; $P = .02$) regardless of mode of delivery. The other identified risk factors in this multivariate analysis included illicit-drug use during pregnancy (OR, 1.9; 95% CI, 1.14 to 3.16; $P = .01$), low antenatal CD4 count (OR, 2.82; 95% CI, 1.67 to 3.34; $P = .04$), and birth weight less than 2500 g (OR, 1.86; 95% CI, 1.03 to 3.34; $P = .04$). The cut-off of 4 hours was selected, based on the data from these patients, and does not imply that no increased risk occurs prior to 4 hours or that the risk stops rising after the 4-hour timepoint.

Data from several cohort studies suggest that infants delivered by elective cesarean section had a lower risk of HIV-1 infection than those delivered vaginally.[58–60] It has been suggested that this effect may be due to the short duration of ruptured membranes among the groups delivered by elective cesarean section. These observational studies led to the European Mode of Delivery Collaboration to carry out a prospective randomized, controlled trial comparing elective cesarean section at 38 weeks of gestation with vaginal delivery. The analysis of that data has been published.[61] Data were analyzed as intent-to-treat and actual mode of delivery. A total of 7 (3.4%) of 203 infants of women who actually gave birth by cesarean section were infected, compared with 15 (10.2%) of 167 infants born vaginally ($P = .009$). Among women undergoing cesarean section who were allocated to elective cesarean, 3 (1.8%) of 170 infants were infected, compared with 21 (10.5%) of 200 infants born to women assigned to vaginal delivery ($P < .001$). Among women receiving zidovudine who were allocated to cesarean section, 1 (0.8%) child was infected of 119, compared with 5 (4.3%) infants of those delivered vaginally. Thus, a clear association was established between mode of delivery and vertical transmission risk. This association may hold up even when zidovudine is administered during pregnancy.

Other obstetric risk factors, such as the use of internal fetal scalp electrodes, fetal scalp sampling, amniocentesis, and cordocentesis, very likely contribute to the vertical transmission rate. The sample size required for identifying these as independent risk factors is so high that it is unlikely these studies will ever be performed. In one study of 434 HIV-infected children, data were subjected to multivariate analysis, and it was found that the risk of infant infection was associated with advanced maternal HIV disease (OR, 4.5; 95% CI, 2.1 to 9.5), whether the infants were ever breastfed (OR, 2.2; 95% CI, 1.2 to 4.2), the child's negative Rh group (OR, 2.5; 95% CI, 1.2 to 5.5), and third-trimester amniocentesis (OR, 4.1; 95% CI, 1.2 to 13.5).[37]

Several risk factors have been attributed to the fetus or newborn. Certain fetal cells may be genetically more or less susceptible to infection by the HIV. For example, homozygous mutations in the gene for the CKR-5 co-receptor (β-chemokine receptor) have been associated with protection against HIV.[62] The newborn immune response may play a role in susceptibility to vertical transmission. A transient HIV-1–specific cellular immune response was observed in uninfected infants born to HIV-infected mothers.[63, 64]

The risk of postpartum HIV transmission associated with breastfeeding has been related to the amount of exposure, time of exposure, and infectivity of the milk. In an African cohort, breastfeeding beyond 15 months was associated with a nearly twofold increased risk of infection.[44] Using mathematical modeling, Nagelkerke and co-workers[45] estimated that the risk of HIV-1 transmission exceeded the potential benefits of breastfeeding after 3 to 7 months in such developing countries. Other studies have related HIV-1 by DNA polymerase chain reaction (PCR), and IgM antibodies to HIV-1, to HIV transmission via breast milk. Van de Perre and associates[65] reported their data from Rwanda showing that the combination of a positive HIV-1 DNA PCR in breast milk at 15 days post partum and a lack of persistent IgM response was a strong predictor of transmission.

The placenta itself is a barrier to vertical transmission, effectively separating the maternal and fetal circulations so as not to allow the passage of most organisms and large molecules, yet permitting the exchange of the gases and nutrients necessary for fetal growth and survival. HIV-1 has been isolated from the placenta and viral nucleic acids have been identified within placental cells, but these findings have not always correlated with infection of the infant.[41]

Placental risk factors for infection may involve a breakdown of the normal syncytiotrophoblast layer that separates maternal blood at the fetal interface. Disruption of this barrier could lead to virus entering the fetal space. Several conditions that are associated with placental disruption have been linked epidemiologically to vertical HIV transmission. These include chorioamnionitis, cigarette smoking, and illicit-drug use.[41, 66-70]

Finally, unprotected sexual intercourse before and during pregnancy has been associated with an increased perinatal transmission rate. This relationship has been borne out even after adjustment for multiple confounding variables.[69, 71, 72] The reason for this association remains unclear, although theories that immune activation may increase viral load, that exposure to different HIV-1 strains leads to the acquisition of a more fetotropic strain, and that disruption of placenta membranes due to trauma or inflammation all have been proposed.

PREVENTION STRATEGIES

Recommendations for the prevention of vertical transmission are based on the known risk factors and the available data on antiretroviral use and obstetric practices in reducing HIV-1 vertical transmission.

The current CDC recommendation for decreasing HIV-1 vertical transmission is the administration of zidovudine, as given in the ACTG 076 trial (see Table 42–3). As previously mentioned, this multicenter phase-3 (efficacy), randomized, placebo-controlled trial demonstrated that peripartum zidovudine treatment reduced the rate of transmission from 25.5% to 8.3%.[7] The women enrolled were not immunocompromised (all with >200 CD4 counts, and 59% with >500 CD4 counts) and were largely antiretroviral therapy naive. What remained unclear was how effective this regimen would be in women with CD4 counts of less than 200 and those who have been on long-term antiretroviral therapy. In addition, it was not clear how

much each of the three (antepartum, intrapartum, and postpartum) treatment components contributed to the reduced transmission rate. Frenkel and co-workers[73] reported on 188 zidovudine-treated mothers, in whom the median CD4 count closest to delivery was 339/μL and 21% had less than 200/μL. This population of 188 women includes 71 women who received antenatal oral and intrapartum intravenous zidovudine; 82 women who received oral, but not intravenous, zidovudine; and 20 who received only intrapartum, intravenous zidovudine. None of the infants were treated with zidovudine, since all these women delivered prior to February 1994. The overall transmission rate was 12.3% (95% CI, 7.9% to 18%). When the 38 women with fewer than 200 CD4 cells/μL were excluded, the vertical transmission rate was 8.3%. The transmission rate was similar whether or not the mothers received intravenous zidovudine during labor. Since this study was primarily observational, all three components of zidovudine treatment are recommended, based on the ACTG 076 results. In another report on abbreviated regimens of zidovudine prophylaxis, Wade and colleagues[74] reported transmission rates that varied with extent of prophylaxis. The transmission rate was 6.1% (26 of 423; CI, 4.1% to 8.9%), when treatment was begun in the prenatal period; 10% (5 of 50; CI, 3.3% to 21.8%) when treatment was begun intrapartum; 9.3% (8 of 86; CI, 4.1% to 17.5%) when therapy was begun within the first 48 hours of life; 18.4% (7 of 38; CI, 7.7% to 34.3%) when treatment was begun on day 3 of life or later; and 26.6% (63 of 237; CI, 21.1% to 32%) in the absence of zidovudine. Shaffer and co-workers[75] also showed that a short-course of zidovudine prophylaxis using oral treatment beginning at 36 weeks and every 3 hours in labor resulted in a reduction in vertical transmission (9.4% vs. 18.9%).

These results, although from retrospective, observational studies, suggest that the full zidovudine regimen may optimize reductions in transmission, but also that significant reductions may still be achieved if zidovudine is begun later, even when begun after delivery, but within 48 hours of life. Although it is often impossible to administer the full zidovudine regimen because of access of women to care, timely screening of pregnant women for HIV, or compliance with therapy or care, administration of the maximal therapy possible, even if only to the infant, is strongly suggested. Many HIV-infected women are treated with HAART, as previously discussed, and this may further reduce vertical transmission rates. Nonetheless, even if the women are receiving HAART, intrapartum zidovudine and oral zidovudine for the infant are recommended.[39]

Many major HIV centers now routinely treat HIV-infected pregnant women with HAART therapy, including a protease inhibitor. Some 142 patients have been reported in three series without a single reported mother-to-infant transmission. As more experience is reported and prevention trials that include HAART regimens are completed, we will probably see the lowest vertical transmission rates ever.[34, 35, 76]

Beyond antiretroviral therapy, other approaches to preventing vertical transmission are also under study. These strategies include adding passive immunization with hyperimmune HIV immune globulin to the antiretroviral regimen (ACTG protocol 185), and active immunization with recombinant vaccines as they become available.

The developing world continues to suffer the greatest toll of HIV disease, and mother-to-infant transmission is no exception. The aggressive use of antiretroviral agents, such as intravenous zidovudine, is not feasible in many of these developing countries, where access to prenatal care, expensive medications, and even prenatal vitamins is limited. Efforts are finally being made (perhaps too little, to late) to develop strategies of prevention that might be applicable to these impoverished communities. Biggar and co-workers[77] completed a controlled trial of cleansing the lower genital tract (vaginal and cervix) with chlorhexidine in 696 HIV-infected women, compared with 712 HIV-infected women without cleansing. There was no difference in the rate of mother-to-infant HIV transmission. Additional studies are underway in developing countries, one using chlorhexidine every 3 hours intra partum, and another benzalkonium chloride suppositories daily beginning at 36 to 38 weeks of gestation. To date, no data have been published to support the routine use of lavage or cleansing techniques to prevent transmission. Trials are also underway evaluating short-term oral antiretrovirals that may be feasible in the developing world. Various dosages of zidovudine beginning in the late third trimester (34 to 38 weeks of gestation), combined with an increased oral dosage in labor, and infant treatment have been incorporated into clinical trials. Another approach under investigation is combining zidovudine with another NRTI (3TC) or an NNRTI (nevirapine). Efforts to effect a reduction in vertical HIV transmission in the developing world must remain a focus of study if we are to decrease the rate of pediatric HIV infection worldwide.

INTRAPARTUM APPROACHES

The intrapartum management of an HIV-infected woman should be directed toward lowering the risk of transmission based on the knowledge of risk factors and the biologic plausibility that the strategy will reduce HIV infection. There should be a focus on reducing the direct contact of the fetus with maternal blood or genital secretions without adding undue morbidity to the mother. The mode of delivery has been shown to affect transmission risk and is discussed in detail later. If the vaginal route of delivery is deemed safe, then interventions such as artificial rupture of membranes or the placement of internal monitoring devices should be avoided unless the benefits of the procedure far outweigh the potential risk. Once the membranes do rupture, the course of labor and anticipated time of delivery should be assessed. Aggressive labor management to minimize the duration of ruptured membranes is appropriate. If prolonged rupture of membranes is anticipated, consideration of cesarean delivery must be balanced against the likelihood that this particular individual will transmit infection based on risk factors such as HIV disease status, viral load, and antiretrovirals. If the membranes rupture at an early gestational age, management depends on the risks of prematurity, which is also a risk factor for HIV transmission. In most cases of preterm, premature rupture of the membranes, particularly prior to 32 to 34 weeks of gestation, in the absence of intra-amniotic infection, the risks of prematurity outweigh the risks of transmission. These patients are managed by prolonging gestation, by administration of steroids for fetal lung maturity, and by continuing antiretroviral therapy. At any time in gestation, signs and symptoms of intra-amniotic infection (chorioamnionitis) should be immediately and aggressively treated with antibiotics.

MODE OF DELIVERY

Cesarean section has been associated with reduced vertical transmission rates in a number of observational studies.[59, 78–80] Several similar studies did not support this approach.[57, 81–84] In a meta-analysis of 15 prospective cohort studies, the International Perinatal HIV Group[85] found that elective cesarean section reduced the risk of mother-to-infant HIV transmission independent of the effects of zidovudine treatment. As Stringer and colleagues[86] pointed out in a recent commentary, this meta-analysis of observational studies poses an interesting hypothesis to be tested but one that, in and of itself, does not have the statistical quality to serve as the basis for broad clinical recommendations. A recently published, multicentered, randomized treatment trial compared elective cesarean delivery at 38 weeks with vaginal delivery.[85] Women randomized to cesarean delivery had a significantly lower rate of vertical transmission than those randomized to vaginal delivery (1.8% vs. 10.5%; $P < .001$). In those receiving zidovudine, the reduction was smaller but not statistically significant. Being the only randomized trial currently available, this presents insufficient evidence that prophylactic cesarean delivery substantially reduces vertical transmission in women on zidovudine monotherapy.

Currently, the evolving standards for antiretroviral therapy to combination therapy make the applicability of these studies somewhat limited. The information currently available on the effect of combination therapy on vertical transmission is limited to three presented abstracts, including a total of 142 women.[34, 35, 76] None of these women transmitted HIV to their infants. It has been estimated that the transmission risk among women on combination antiretroviral therapy is 2% or less. They further point out that if the rate of vertical transmission is 2% and could be reduced to 1% by elective cesarean, then each infection avoided would require 100 cesarean deliveries.[86] There is also substantial morbidity associated with cesarean section, particularly in the women most likely to transmit the virus; that is, those with high viral load and low CD4 counts. Semprini and co-workers[87] reported 6 cases of major postoperative complications (pneumonia, sepsis, hemorrhage requiring transfusion) in 156 HIV-infected women, compared with one such complication in 136 HIV-negative women (OR, 6.0; 95% CI, 0.9 to 38.5).

Thus, prophylactic cesarean delivery would most likely be beneficial in women not taking antiretroviral therapy or the rare woman who continues to have a high viral load despite antiretroviral therapy. There is no good evidence that cesarean delivery reduces the risk of vertical transmission in HIV-positive women with an undetectable viral load.

In summary, the field of HIV care is rapidly evolving, and these changes will influence the way women are managed in terms of their HIV disease and their pregnancies. Providing care in this climate presents a challenge to the clinician who must optimize the health of the woman while protecting a developing fetus. Decision-making is complex, and the pregnant woman is often willing to take on inappropriate risks for even the slightest chance of decreasing the odds of mother-to-infant transmission. Thus, the responsibility of objective, rational therapeutic guidance based on risks-benefits assessment often falls on the obstetric care providers.

REFERENCES

1. Joint United Nations Programme on HIV/AIDS (UNAIDS) and World Health Organization (WHO): Report on the global HIV/AIDS epidemic. UNAIDS/WHO, June 2000 (UNAIDS.org).
2. Mofenson LM; Mother-child HIV-1 transmission. Obstet Gynecol Clin North Am 1997; 24:759.
3. Centers for Disease Control and Prevention (CDC): HIV/AIDS Surveillance Rep 1999.
4. Davis SF, Byers RH, Lindegren ML, et al: Prevalence and incidence of vertically acquired HIV infection in the United States. JAMA 1995; 274:952.
5. Centers for Disease Control and Prevention (CDC): U.S. Public Health Service recommendations for human immunodeficiency virus counseling and voluntary testing for pregnant women. MMWR 1995; 44(RR-7):1.
6. Samson L, King S: Evidence-based guidelines for universal counseling and offering of HIV testing in pregnancy in Canada. Can Med Assoc J 1998; 158:1449.
7. Connor EM, Sperling RS, Gelber R, et al: Reduction of maternal-infant transmission of human immunodeficiency virus type-1 with zidovudine treatment. N Engl J Med 1994; 331:1173.
8. Wilfert CM: Beginning to make progress against HIV. N Engl J Med 1996; 23:438.
9. American College of Obstetricians and Gynecologists: Human immunodeficiency virus infections in pregnancy. ACOG Educational Bull 1997; 232:1.
10. U.S. Public Health Service (USPHS)/Infectious Diseases Society of America (IDSA): Members of the Prevention of Opportunistic Infections Working Group:1997 Guidelines for the prevention of opportunistic infections in persons infected with human immunodeficiency virus (HIV). Ann Intern Med 1997; 127:922.
11. Landers DV, Tejada BM, Coyne BA: Immunology of HIV and pregnancy. Obstet Gynecol Clin North Am 1997; 24:821.
12. Biggar RJ, Pahwa S, Minkoff H, et al: Immunosupression in pregnant women infected with human immunodeficiency virus. Am J Obstet Gynecol; 1989; 61:1239.
13. Dinsmoor MJ, Christmas JT: Changes in T lymphocyte subpopulations during pregnancy complicated by human immunodeficiency virus infection. Am J Obstet Gynecol 1992; 167:1575.
14. Burns DN, Nourjah P, Minkoff H, et al: Changes in CD4+ and CD8+ cell levels during pregnancy and postpartum in women seropositive and seronegative for human immunodeficiency virus type-1. Am J Obstet Gynecol 1996; 174:1461.
15. Miotti PG, Liomba G, Dallabetta GA, et al: T lymphocyte subsets during and after pregnancy: Analysis in HIV-1 infected and uninfected Malawian mothers. J Infect Dis 1992; 165:1116.
16. Rich KC, Siegel JN, Jennings C, et al: CD4+ lymphocytes in perinatal HIV infection: Evidence for pregnancy-induced immune depression in uninfected and HIV-infected women. J Infect Dis 1995: 172:1221.
17. Thorne C, Newell ML, Dunn D, et al: The European Collaborative Study: Clinical and immunological characteristics of HIV-infected pregnant women. Br J Obstet Gynaecol 1995; 102:869.
18. Tuomala RE, Kalish LA, Zorrilla C, et al: Changes in total, CD4+, and CD8+ lymphocytes during pregnancy and 1 year postpartum in human immunodeficiency virus–infected women. The Women and Infants Transmission Study. Obstet Gynecol 1997; 89:979.
19. Temmerman M, Nagelkerke N, Bwayo J, et al: HIV-1 and immunological changes during pregnancy: A comparison between HIV-1–seropositive and HIV-1–seronegative women in Nairobi, Kenya. AIDS 1995;9:1057.
20. Burns DN, Landesman S, Minkoff H, et al: The influence of pregnancy on human immunodeficiency virus type 1 infection: Antepartum and postpartum changes in human immunodeficiency virus type 1 viral load. Am J Obstet Gynecol 1998; 178:355.
21. Alliegro MB, Dorrucci MD, Phillips AN, et al: Incidence and consequences of pregnancy in women with known duration of HIV infection. Arch Intern Med 1997; 157:2585.
22. Weisser M, Rudin C, Battegay M, et al: Does pregnancy influence the course of HIV infection? Evidence from two large Swiss cohort studies. J Acquir Immune Defic Syndr Hum Retrovirol 1998; 17:404.
23. French R, Brocklehurst P: The effect of pregnancy on survival in women infected with HIV: A systematic review of the literature and meta-analysis. Br J Obstet Gynaecol 1998; 105:827.
24. Gloeb DJ, O'Sullivan MJ, Efantis J: Human immunodeficiency virus infection in women: The effect of HIV in pregnancy. Am J Obstet Gynecol 1988; 159:756.
25. Minkoff HL, Henderson C, Mendez H, et al: Pregnancy outcomes among mothers infected with HIV and uninfected control subjects. Am J Obstet Gynecol 1990; 163:1598.
26. Ryder RW, Nsa W, Hassig SE, et al: Perinatal transmission of the human immunodeficiency virus type 1 to infants of seropositive women in Zaire. N Engl J Med 1989; 320:1637.
27. Temmerman M, Chomba EN, Ndinya-Achola M, et al: Maternal human immunodeficiency virus-1 infection and pregnancy outcome. Obstet Gynecol 1994; 4:495.
28. Minkoff HL, Willoughby A, Mendez H, et al: Serious infections during pregnancy among women with advanced human

immunodeficiency virus infection. Am J Obstet Gynecol 1990; 162:30.

29. Leroy V, Ladner J, Nyiraziraje M, et al: Effect of HIV-1 infection on pregnancy outcome in women in Kigali, Rwanda, 1992–1994. AIDS 1998; 12:643.

30. Brocklehurst P, French R: The association between maternal HIV infection and perinatal outcome: A systematic review of the literature and meta-analysis. Br J Obstet Gynaecol 1998; 105:836.

31. Stratton P, Tuomala RE, Abboud R, et al: Obstetric and newborn outcomes in a cohort of HIV-infected pregnant women: A report of the women and infants transmission. J Acquir Immune Defic Syndr Hum Retrovirol 1999; 20:179.

32. Centers for Disease Control and Prevention (CDC): Report of the NIH Panel to Define Principles of Therapy of HIV Infection and Guidelines for the Use of Antiretroviral Agents in HIV-Infected Adults and Adolescents. MMWR 1998; 47(RR-5):1.

33. Sandberg JA, Slikker W: Developmental pharmacology and toxicology of anti-HIV therapeutic agents: Dideoxynucleosides. FASEB J 1995; 9:1157.

34. Morris A, Zorrilla C, Vajaranant M, et al: A review of protease inhibitor (PI) in 89 pregnancies. Abstract 686, 6th Conference on Retrovirus and Opportunistic Infections, Chicago, IL, 1999.

35. Stek A, Khoury M, Kramer F, et al: Maternal and infant outcomes with highly active antiretroviral therapy during pregnancy. Abstract 687, 6th Conference on Retrovirus and Opportunistic Infections, Chicago, IL, 1999.

36. Centers for Disease Control and Prevention (CDC): Prevention and treatment of tuberculosis among patients infected with human immunodeficiency virus: Principles of therapy and revised recommendations. MMWR 1998; 47(RR-20): 1.

37. Tess BH, Rodrigues LC, Newell ML, et al: Sao Paulo Collaborative Study for Vertical Transmission of HIV-1: Breastfeeding, genetic, obstetric and other risk factors associated with mother-to-child transmission of HIV-1 in Sao Paulo State, Brazil. AIDS 1998; 12:513.

38. Bahado-Singh RO, Goldstein I, Uerpairojkit B, et al: Normal nuchal thickness in the midtrimester indicates reduced risk of Down syndrome in pregnancies with abnormal triple-screen results. Am J Obstet Gynecol 1995; 173:1106.

39. Centers for Disease Control and Prevention (CDC): Public Health Service task force recommendations for the use of antiretroviral drugs in pregnant women infected with HIV-1 for maternal health and for reducing perinatal HIV-1 transmission in the United States. MMWR 1998; 47(RR-2):1.

40. Mayeux MJ, Burgard M, Teglas JP, et al: Neonatal characteristics in rapidly progressive perinatally acquired HIV-1 disease. JAMA 1996; 275:606.

41. Mofenson LM: Mother-child HIV-1 transmission: Timing and determinants. Obstet Gynecol Clin North Am 1997; 24:759.

42. Dunn DT, Brandt CD, Krivine A, et al: The sensitivity of HIV-1 DNA polymerase chain reaction in the neonatal period and the relative contributions of intrauterine and intrapartum transmission. AIDS 1995; 9:F7.

43. Tuomala RE: Prevention of transmission: Pharmaceutical and obstetric approaches. Obstet Gynecol Clin North Am 1997; 24:785.

44. Datta P, Embree JE, Kreiss JK, et al: Mother-to-child transmission of human immunodeficiency virus type 1: Report from the Nairobi study. J Infect Dis 1994; 170:1134.

45. Nagelkerke NJD, Moses S, Embree JE, et al: The duration of breastfeeding by HIV-1–infected mothers in developing countries: Balancing benefits and risks. J Acquir Immune Defic Syndr Hum Retrovirol 1995; 8:176.

46. Leroy V, Newell ML, Dabis F, et al: International multicentre pooled analysis of late postnatal mother-to-child transmission of HIV-1 infection. Ghent International Working Group on Mother-to-Child Transmission of HIV. Lancet 1998; 352:597.

47. Sperling RS, Shapiro DE, Coombs RW, et al: Maternal viral load, zidovudine treatment, and the risk of transmission of human immunodeficiency virus type 1 from mother to infant. Pediatric AIDS Clinical Trials Group Protocol 076 Study Group. N Engl J Med 1996; 335:1621.

48. Sperling RS, Shapiro DE, McSherry GD, et al: Safety of the maternal-infant zidovudine regimen utilized in the Pediatric AIDS Clinical Trial Group 076 Study. AIDS 1998; 12:1805.

49. Mayaux MJ, Blanche S, Rouzioux C, et al: Maternal factors associated with perinatal HIV-1 transmission. The French Cohort Study: 7 years of follow-up observation. J Acquir Immune Defic Syndr Hum Retrovirol 1995; 8:188.

50. European Collaborative Study: Vertical transmission of HIV-1: Maternal immune status and obstetric factors. AIDS 1996; 10:1675.

51. Semba RD: Vitamin A, immunity, and infection. Clin Infect Dis 1994; 19:489.

52. Greenberg BL, Semba RD, Vink PE, et al: Vitamin A deficiency and maternal-infant transmissions of HIV in two metropolitan areas in the United States. AIDS 1997; 11:325.

53. Semba RD, Miotti PG, Paolo G, et al: Maternal vitamin A deficiency and mother-to-child transmission of HIV-1. Lancet 1994; 343:1593.

54. Burger H, Kovacs A, Weiser B, et al: Maternal serum vitamin A levels are not associated with mother-to-child transmission of HIV-1 in the United States. J Acquir Immune Defic Syndr Hum Retrovirol 1997; 14:321.

55. Ometto L, Zanotto C, Maccabrini A, et al: Viral phenotype and host-cell susceptibility to HIV-1 infection as risk factors for mother-to-child HIV-1 transmission. AIDS 1995; 9:427.

56. Reinhardt PP, Reinhardt B, Lathey JL, Spector SA: Human cord blood mononuclear cells are preferentially infected by non–syncytium-inducing macrophage-tropic human immunodeficiency virus type 1 isolates. J Clin Microbial 1995; 33:392.

57. Landesman SH, Kalish LA, Burns DN, et al: Obstetrical factors and the transmission of human immunodeficiency virus type 1 from mother to child. The Women and Infants Transmission Study. N Engl J Med 1996; 334:1617.

58. Gabiano C, Tovo PA, de Martino M, et al: Mother-to-child transmission of human immunodeficiency virus type 1: Risk of infection and correlates of transmission. Pediatrics 1992; 90:369.

59. European Collaborative Study: Caesarean section and risk of vertical transmission of HIV infection. Lancet 1994; 343:1464.

60. Kind C, for The Paediatric AIDS Group of Switzerland: Mother-to-child transmission of human immunodeficiency virus type 1: Influence of parity and mode of delivery. Eur J Pediatr 1995; 154:542.

61. Parazzini F, for The European Mode of Delivery Collaboration: Elective cesarean section versus vaginal delivery in prevention of vertical HIV-1 transmission: A randomized clinical trial. The European Mode of Delivery Collaboration. Lancet 1999; 353:1035.

62. Liu R, Paxton W, Choe S, et al: Homozygous defect in HIV-1 coreceptor accounts for resistance of some multiply exposed individuals to HIV-1 infection. Cell 1996; 86:367.

63. Rowland-Jones SL, Nixon DF, Aldhous MC, et al: HIV-specific cytotoxic T-cell activity in an HIV-exposed but uninfected infant. Lancet 1993; 341:860.

64. De Maria A, Cirillo C, Moretta L: Occurrence of human immunodeficiency virus type 1 (HIV-1)–specific cytolytic T cell activity in apparently uninfected children born of HIV-1–infected mothers. J Infect Dis 1994; 170:1296.

65. Van de Perre P, Simonon A, Hitimana DG, et al: Infective and anti-infective properties of breastmilk from HIV-1–infected women. Lancet 1993; 341:914.

66. Burns DN, Landesman S, Mendez LR, et al: Cigarette smoking, premature rupture of membranes, and vertical transmission of HIV-1 among women with low CD4+ levels. J Acquir Immune Defic Syndr Hum Retrovirol 1994; 7:718.

67. Rodriguez EM, Mofenson LM, Chang BH, et al: Association of maternal drug use during pregnancy with maternal HIV culture positivity and perinatal HIV transmission. AIDS 1996; 10:273.

68. Saint Louis ME, Kamenga M, Brown C, et al: Risk for perinatal HIV-1 transmission according to maternal immunologic, virologic, and placental factors. JAMA 1993; 269:2853.

69. Burns DN, Landesman A, Wright DJ, et al: Influence of other maternal variables on the relationship between maternal virus load and mother-to-infant transmission of human immunodeficiency virus type 1. J Infect Dis 1997; 175:1206.

70. Bulterys M, Landesman S, Burns DN, et al: Sexual behavior and injection drug use during pregnancy and vertical transmission of HIV-1. J Acquir Immune Defic Syndr Hum Retrovirol 1997; 15:76.

71. Bulterys M, Chao A, Dushimimana A, et al: Multiple sexual partners and mother-to-child transmission of HIV-1. AIDS 1993; 7:1639.

72. Matheson PB, Thomas PA, Abrams EJ, et al: Heterosexual behavior during pregnancy and perinatal transmission of HIV-1. AIDS 1996; 10:1249.

73. Frenkel LM, Cowles MK, Shapiro DE, et al: Analysis of the maternal components of the AIDS Clinical Trial Group 076 zidovudine regimen in the prevention of mother-to-infant transmission of human immunodeficiency virus type 1. J infect Dis 1997; 175:971.

74. Wade NA, Birkhead GS, Warren BL, et al: Abbreviated regimens of zidovudine prophylaxis and perinatal transmission of the human immunodeficiency virus. N Engl J Med 1998; 339:1409.

75. Shaffer N, Chuachoowong R, Mock PA, et al: Short-course zidovudine for perinatal HIV-1 transmission in Bangkok, Thailand: A randomised controlled trial. Lancet 1999; 353:773.

76. Scott G, Shapiro D, Scott W, et al: Safety and tolerance of ritonavir in combination with lamivudine and zidovudine in HIV-1–infected pregnant women and their infants. Abstract 688, 6th Conference on Retrovirus and Opportunistic Infections. Chicago, IL, 1999.

77. Biggar RJ, Miotti PG, Taha TE, et al: Perinatal intervention trial in Africa: Effect of a birth canal cleansing intervention to prevent HIV transmission. Lancet 1996; 347:1647.

78. Mandelbrot L, Le Chenadec J, Berrebi A, et al: Perinatal HIV-1 transmission: Interaction between zidovudine prophylaxis and mode of delivery in the French Perinatal Cohort. JAMA 1998; 280:55.

79. Kind C, Brandle B, Wyler CA, et al: Epidemiology of vertically transmitted HIV-1 infection in Switzerland: Results of a nationwide prospective study. Swiss Neonatal HIV Study Group. Eur J Pediat 1992; 151:442.

80. Tovo PA, de Martino M, Gabiano C, et al: Mode of delivery and gestational age influence perinatal HIV-1 transmission. J Acquir Immune Defic Syndr Hum Retrovirol 1996; 11:88.

81. Mandelbrot L, Mayaux M-J, Bongain A, et al: Obstetric factors and mother-to-child transmission of human immunodeficiency virus type 1: The French Perinatal Cohort. Am J Obstet Gynecol 1996; 175:661.

82. Thomas PA, Weedon J, Krazinski K, et al: Maternal predictors of perinatal human immunodeficiency virus transmission. Pediatr Infect Dis J 1994; 13:489.

83. Simonds RJ, Steketee R, Nesheim S, et al: Impact of zidovudine use on risk and risk factors for perinatal transmission of HIV. Perinatal AIDS Collaborative Transmission Studies. AIDS 1998; 12:301.

84. Dunn DT, Newel ML, Mayaux MJ, et al: Mode of delivery and vertical transmission of HIV-1: A review of prospective studies. J Acquir Immune Defic Syndr Hum Retrovirol 1994; 7:1064.

85. The International Perinatal HIV Group: The mode of delivery and the risk of vertical transmission of human immunodeficiency virus type 1. N Engl J Med 1999; 340:977.

86. Stringer JSA, Rouse DJ, Goldenberg RL: Prophylactic cesarean delivery for the prevention of perinatal human immunodeficiency virus transmission: The case for restraint. JAMA 1999; 281:1946.

87. Semprini AE, Castagna C, Ravizza M, et al: The incidence of complications after caesarean section in 156 HIV-positive women. AIDS 1995; 9:913.

43

Ectoparasites

JOSEPH G. PASTOREK II

Bugs have been the vectors of human disease since the dawn of humankind. In historic times, for example, the "black death" spread by rat fleas is legendary. Mosquitoes and malaria, as detailed in a separate chapter, are familiar the world over. And ticks of various description may carry organisms of almost any type, from the rickettsia of Rocky Mountain spotted fever to the spirochete of borreliosis. Even so, most of these insects and arachnids only bite the human host and move on, satiated on blood or other body fluids. There are several such organisms, however, that live out their life cycle in, or on, the human host—true parasites. The most important of these ectoparasites are covered in this chapter.

SCABIES

Epidemiology

The so-called itch mite, *Sarcoptes scabies* var. *humanus*, is an arachnid that is an obligate parasite of humans. (The related dog parasite, *S. scabies* var. *canis*, is responsible for sarcoptic mange in man's best friend.) Fertilized females burrow into the skin of the human host and there live and lay their eggs. The young emerge from their cutaneous burrow in approximately 3 to 6 days to mate, and then to die (males), or to dig a new burrow (females) to start the process all over. The females may live for up to 6 weeks.[1]

These mites live out their life cycle in the human. Thus, the mites travel from human to human primarily by close human contact, even simple casual contact, and are found throughout the world. Fortunately, the itch mite does not carry any *other* diseases than itself. Epidemic outbreaks have been linked to wars, but this is probably simply because of the poverty, crowding, lack of hygiene, and promiscuous sexual activity that often accompanies military action, and the destruction and displacement caused by it.

Besides personal contact, fomites may play a role in the spread of scabies because live mites have been found in house dust.[2] Also, females have been demonstrated to survive for up to 48 hours away from the host, implying that mites can be picked up from the environment directly.[3]

Pathogenesis

After mating, the pregnant female mite burrows into the skin of the host down to the level of the base of the stratum corneum. The burrow is characteristically diagonal from the surface of the skin, producing linear furrows visible on the surface. In the burrow thus formed, she lays two to three eggs per day. The eggs hatch within a few days, and the larvae emerge from the skin to become adult in a little over 2 weeks, at which point they mate. Of course, all this time they live on the human host.[1]

Clinical Manifestations

Scabies mites are called "itch mites" for very good reason—the hallmark of the clinical disease scabies is intense itching, especially at night. There may be erythematous lesions, papules, macules, and occasionally vesicles, especially in intertriginous areas (e.g., folds of skin, between the fingers, scrotal folds).

Because of the initial break in the skin caused by the organism, as well as the scratching and excoriation due to the itching, secondary bacterial infection may complicate scabies infestations. It is not uncommon for impetigo to occur if *Staphylococcus aureus* is a factor in the contamination. If hypersensitivity develops to the mite or its excretions, an eczematous rash may be apparent.

In immunocompromised people, such as patients with acquired immunodeficiency syndrome, a severe form of scabies known as *Norwegian scabies* or *crusted scabies* may occur, consisting of hyperkeratotic, nodular lesions and plaques that appear almost like multiple keloids, spread about the body. Apparently the intact immune system does hold the mites in check ordinarily. In immunosuppressed patients, the mite density is extremely high, and the patient is extremely contagious from the sheer number of mites produced.[4]

Diagnosis

Although the clinical presentation of scabies can include highly pruritic lesions between the webs of the fingers, the presentation may be highly variable and sometimes confusing. Therefore, diagnosis is made by identifying the mite visually. This is accomplished by locating a burrow, coating it with mineral oil, and then scraping the superficial layers of skin over the burrow until the apex is reached, whereby the animal is scraped onto a slide for microscopic visualization (Fig. 43–1).

Treatment and Prevention

The long-standing treatment of choice for human scabies is 1% lindane (gamma benzene hexachloride, actually an insecticide as opposed to a human "drug") lotion. Lindane is applied to the entire body below the chin and left on for 8 to 12 hours.[5] Unfortunately, lindane is well absorbed through the skin and may occasionally prove neurotoxic, even causing seizures. Therefore, pregnant women and small children might be treated with 5% permethrin cream (a synthetic pyrethroid compound), which is also generally applied and left on for 8 to 10 hours, although experience is limited. A more odoriferous alternative is 6% to 10% precipitated sulfur in petroleum jelly daily for 3 days.[2]

Several other medications, including other insecticides, are used for treatment of scabies. Malathion preparations are rapidly cidal of both the mites and their eggs. Malathion is an organophosphate insecticide that is no longer available in the United States because of toxicity and the availability of other effective agents. Other agents that have been used for scabies include the antihelminthic thiabendazole (in a cream or suspension), crotamiton, dimethyldiphenylene di-

sulfide, dimethylthianthrene, dibenzoyl disulfide, tetraethylthiuram monosulfide soap, diethyxanthogene, and tripentyl antimony sulfide.[6, 7]

To give some perspective on use, a review of the Cochrane database on the subject indicates that permethrin is more effective than lindane and crotamiton. However, this advantage was not a consistent finding across all reported studies and was not statistically significant in the largest reported study. The choice of permethrin appeared to be based on potential safety compared with lindane, although this is not derived from actual study data. Cases of seizures and death have been reported with the treatment of scabies. There is little formal evaluatory evidence on the use of such drugs as malathion.[8]

Finally, if there is evidence of superimposed bacterial infection, it should be treated with the appropriate antimicrobials. Also, linen and clothing should be washed in hot, soapy water and dried in a hot dryer to kill mites and any eggs.

HEAD AND BODY LICE

Epidemiology

Members of the arachnid order Anoplura are bloodsucking lice that parasitize their hosts. The head louse, *Pediculus humanus capitis*, and the body louse, *Pediculus humanus corporis* (also termed *Pediculus humanus humanus*), are the human-parasitizing members of this order. These lice live in hairy areas of the human body and in clothing (*P. humanus corporis*) and are passed between victims by close personal contact and through fomites, such as clothing and bedding. Head lice are considered the most common human louse and lice accompany humans to all parts of the world, but they are particularly troublesome in times of inattention to hygiene (e.g., war and massive population migration).

Body lice are particularly important epidemiologically in that they are carriers of other, more serious human diseases, such as relapsing fever (borreliosis), typhus, and trench fever. Thus, eradication of lice is more profoundly important than, say, elimination of an infestation of scabies, which may simply be aggravating to the individual patient.

Pathogenesis

Lice feed on human blood by piercing the skin and injecting their saliva; they also defecate while feeding. The human host then acquires pruritic, papular lesions from hypersensitivity to antigens in these materials. Lice primarily locate in the hairy parts of the body so that their eggs, called *nits*, can be attached to the shafts of hair and gestate there. The head louse favors the hair on the scalp, particularly near the ears and occiput. Transmission of this subspecies is commonly

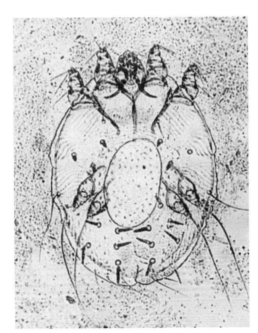

FIGURE 43-1 ▶ The human itch mite, *Sarcoptes scabies*, adult female. (From Markell EK, John DT, Krotoski WA: Markell and Voge's Medical Parasitology, 8th ed. Philadelphia, WB Saunders, 1999, p 358.)

through use of combs, brushes, and hats. The body louse may also place nits on articles of clothing and actually live off of the host, except to feed. Therefore, feeding is often on the trunk (especially the shoulders) and waist, and transmission to other victims is commonly through clothing and other fomites.

Eggs of the lice hatch within a week to 10 days, and the nymphal form of the louse feeds voraciously to mature, which it does in a few weeks. Thereafter, the female louse may lay several hundred eggs over her month-long life span.[7, 9]

Clinical Manifestations

Because the symptomatology attendant to lice bites is determined by the sensitivity of the host to antigens present in louse saliva and feces, the manifestations of those bites can lie anywhere along the spectrum from a small, pruritic papule to an impressive urticarial wheal or welt. These lesions are found in various parts of the body, depending on the subspecies of *Pediculus* involved. Body lice tend to feed under the clothes, especially on the waist and shoulders. Although head lice prefer the posterior and lateral scalp, they may descend into the beard area at times. Also, the nits are visible, cemented to hair shafts (or clothing in the case of *P. h. corporis*) after the female has laid her eggs.

After the infestation has been established and pruritus has occurred, excoriations due to scratching are evident. Secondary bacterial infection is a not-uncommon sequel to such cutaneous abrasion.

Diagnosis

The diagnosis of louse infestation is made by visualizing the organism either in the hair (*P. h. capitis*) or in the clothing (*P. h. corporis*; Fig. 43–2). Also, nits may be visualized in the hair (*P. h. capitis*) or in the clothing (*P. h. corporis*). Of course, the clinician must first *look* for the lice or their nits, which involves keeping the possibility of louse infestation in the clinical diagnosis attendant to any patient with pruritic lesions in the hair or body. If the physician (or patient) does not look for lice, they will not be found.

Treatment and Prevention

Because body lice do not actually live on the victim, eradication is achieved by treating the clothing and bed linen. Heat (as in hot laundering and hot ironing) kills the lice and their nits in clothing. Also, malathion or DDT powder may be used to dust the suspect material.

Body lice are amenable to treatment with lindane, permethrin, pyrethrin/piperonyl butoxide, and malathion, as well as other topical preparations. As stated

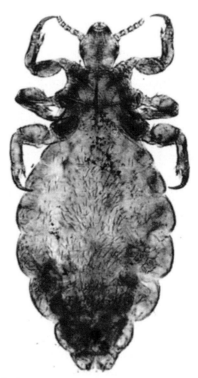

FIGURE 43–2 ▶ The head louse, *Pediculus humanus*. (From Markell EK, John DT, Krotoski WA: Markell and Voge's Medical Parasitology, 8th ed. Philadelphia, WB Saunders, 1999, p 363.)

previously, malathion is no longer available in the United States, although it is the most effective chemical against the intact nit.[10] For all these preparations, treatment is usually accomplished by shampooing the scalp or other affected area for 10 minutes and repeating the treatment in 1 week to finish off any newly hatched nymphs.

Secondary bacterial superinfection can be treated with the appropriate antimicrobial, with particular attention to the possibility of infection with *S. aureus*. Because much of the pruritus is due to hypersensitivity to louse antigens, antihistamines and antipruritics (e.g., hydroxyzine pamoate) and local steroids may be helpful in diminishing the inflammatory and irritant immunologic reaction to the infestation.

Nits should be combed or picked out of the hair as part of treatment. This may be facilitated by applying a 1:1 solution of vinegar and water and combing with a fine-toothed nit comb that has also been soaked in vinegar. The comb should then be treated with an insecticide.

PUBIC LICE

Epidemiology

The pubic louse, or crab louse, *Phthirus pubis*, is another member of Anoplura that affects humans. Pubic lice are transmitted by close contact, classically sexual

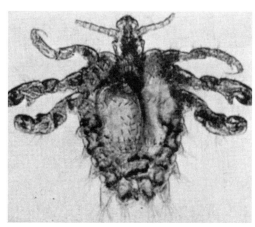

FIGURE 43-3 ▶ The pubic or "crab" louse, *Phthirus pubis.* (From Markell EK, John DT, Krotoski WA: Markell and Voge's Medical Parasitology, 8th ed. Philadelphia, WB Saunders, 1999, p 364.)

activity, and are common characters in literature and folklore. The organism is called the "crab" louse because of its crab-like appearance, as opposed to the more elongated appearance of the other species of louse (Fig. 43–3). Thus, in common parlance, venereal transmission of *P. pubis* results in a "case of the crabs."

Pathogenesis

The activities of the crab louse during reproduction and feeding on the human subject are similar to those of the body louse, although the host's hypersensitivity reaction is apparently less intense, leading to milder clinical symptoms.

Clinical Manifestations

As with body and head louse infestation, the patient with pubic lice complains mainly of itching in the involved areas. The crab louse classically affects the genital hair, although the armpits, trunk, and even the eyebrows may be infested. Although papular eruption is common, it is less severe than the rash from body and head lice. A particular finding, however, is maculae cerulae, small, blue spots on the trunk and extremities. These lesions are less than 1 cm in diameter and are said to represent small areas of hemorrhage due to the anticoagulant injected into the host's skin by the louse during feeding.[9]

Diagnosis

Diagnosis of pubic lice is made by direct visualization of the adult louse or its nits in the hair of the pubic region or other affected areas. As stated previously, if the physician or patient does not look, the infestation will go undiagnosed.

Treatment and Prevention

Therapy for crab lice is basically identical to that for body lice, as detailed earlier. All areas of the body should be treated except for the eyelids, where toxicity and irritation may occur. In that area, a thick coat of petroleum jelly may be placed over the eyelid margins twice weekly for 8 days, or mercuric oxide (1%) may be applied four times a day for 2 weeks.[11] In addition, antipruritics, antihistamines, and local steroid preparations may reduce the hypersensitivity reaction attendant to the louse bites.

REFERENCES

1. Wilson BB: Scabies. In: Mandell GL, Bennett JE, Dolin R (eds): Principles and Practice of Infectious Diseases, 4th ed. New York, Churchill Livingstone, 1995.
2. Hogan DF, Schachner L, Tanglertsampan C: Diagnosis and treatment of childhood scabies and pediculosis. Pediatr Dermatol 1991; 38:941.
3. Arlian LG, Estes SA, Vyszenski-Moher DL: Prevalence of sarcoptes scabies in the homes and nursing homes of scabietic patients. J Am Acad Dermatol 1988; 19:806.
4. Hall JC, Brewer HJ, Appl BA: Norwegian scabies in a patient with acquired immune deficiency syndrome. Cutis 1989; 43:325.
5. Juranek DD, Currier RW, Millikan LE: Scabies control in institutions. In: Orkin M, Maiback HI (eds): Cutaneous Infestations and Insect Bites. New York, Marcel Dekker, 1985.
6. Klaassen CD: Nonmetalic environmental toxicants. In: Hardman JG, Limbird LE, Molinoff PB, et al (eds): Goodman & Gillman's The Pharmacological Basis of Therapeutics, 9th ed. New York, McGraw-Hill, 1996.
7. Kimsey RB, Sanchez JL: Arthropods as sensitizing and pathogenic agents (arthropodiases); pentastomiasis; parasitism by leeches. In: Goldsmith R, Heyneman D (eds): Tropical Medicine and Parasitology. Norwalk, CT, Appleton & Lange, 1989.
8. Walker GJA, Johnstone PW: Interventions for treating scabies (Cochrane review). In: The Cochrane Library, Issue 1. Oxford: Update Software, 1999. (http://www.update-software.com/cochrane/cochrane-frame.html)
9. Wilson BB: Ectoparasites. In: Mandell GL, Bennett JE, Dolin R (eds): Principles and Practice of Infectious Diseases. 4th ed. New York, Churchill Livingstone, 1995.
10. Meinking TL, Taplin D, Kalter DC, et al: Comparative efficacy of treatments for pediculosis capitis infestations. Arch Dermatol 1986; 122:267.
11. Ashkenazi I, Desatnik HR, Abraham FA: Yellow mercuric oxide: A treatment of choice for phthiriasis palpebrarum. Br J Ophthalmol 1991; 75:356.

44 Genital Ulcer Disease

GEORGE P. SCHMID

Disruption of the skin in the genital area is an important complaint among patients seeking care for reproductive tract infections, and such disruption is frequently in the form of genital ulcers. The differential diagnosis of the causes of genital ulcers is fairly standard, but unfortunately the diagnostic steps in evaluating such lesions are not. As a result, the etiology of genital ulcers often remains unknown for many reasons. Clinicians may not be familiar with the possible diagnoses or with the diseases in their community that can cause ulcers. They may not take histories adequate for determining the likelihood of specific etiologies. All or some of the appropriate diagnostic tests may not be available, or the appropriate diagnostic tests may be available but not used. In some cases, the tests may be used but the lesions are too far advanced for accurate results. As a result, clinicians often make a clinical diagnosis, and clinical diagnoses are consistently incorrect in 40% of cases. Patients receive inappropriate diagnoses, which in turn lead to inappropriate treatment, inappropriate counseling (with resultant changes in life and partner choices), and inappropriate partner management. Accurate diagnosis is essential. It requires the consideration of not only clinical characteristics but also demographic and epidemiologic features. Most important, accurate diagnosis requires appropriate laboratory investigation of each case.

WHAT IS A GENITAL ULCER?

Stedman's Medical Dictionary defines an ulcer as "a lesion on the surface of the skin or a mucous surface, caused by superficial loss of tissue, usually with inflammation. A wound with superficial loss of tissue from trauma is not primarily an ulcer. . . ."[1] Despite this tidy distinction, it may be difficult to distinguish a genital ulcer from a wound due to trauma, particularly if a patient wishes not to admit to sexual misadventure. Patients often give a history of trauma preceding the appearance of the skin break. While these explanations may explain the skin break, all experienced clinicians have seen patients who have voiced such explanations who are found to have sexually transmitted infections (STIs) as etiologies. Thus, in practice, the clinician should consider any "genital lesion that (is) denuded of the normal epithelium" to be a genital ulcer.[2]

FREQUENCY OF EROSIONS AND GENITAL ULCERS

Erosions and ulcers of the genital tract are infrequent in clinical practice. In referral gynecologic practices, however, the number may be substantial. Young and colleagues,[3] in a referral vulvar disease clinic, found that ulcers or erosions were the reason for referral for 375 (43%) of 877 consecutive patients. These authors separated the erosions of trauma (excoriations from local or systemic pruritic, or psychogenic, disorders) from ulcers. Trauma was the most common etiology, constituting 183 (49%) of the 375 diagnoses. Neoplasms with associated erosions or ulcerations occurred in 11 (3%) of the patients. The remaining patients, 181 (48%), had genital ulcers. This substantial number shows the difficulty that primary care physicians who referred such patients have in diagnosing and managing women with genital ulcers.

Some of this difficulty arises from the fact that in the industrialized world genital ulcers are uncommon. Primary care physicians seldom see patients with genital ulcers, and even in STI clinics cases with genital ulcers make up only 1% to 2% of all clinical diagnoses.[4] In the developing world, however, individuals with genital ulcers are common in both primary care and STI clinics. In a primary care setting in South Africa, persons with STIs made up 10% of all persons seeking care, and, among these, ulcers were found in 10% to 20%.[5] In STI clinics in the developing world, the proportion of individuals with genital ulcers is 20% to 70% of patients, tremendously higher than that in similar clinics in the industrialized world.[4]

CAUSES OF GENITAL ULCERS

Genital ulcers may have infectious or noninfectious causes. It is very difficult to compare the relative frequencies of etiologies of genital ulcers among case series because of (1) the differing entry criteria for cases (e.g., were persons with trauma or vesicles excluded?), (2) location of the treatment facility (e.g., was the study at a primary health care site or a referral STI clinic?), (3) types of patients included (e.g., were one or two genders included, or were commercial sex workers excluded?), (4) diseases sought (e.g., were any other disorders besides common infectious causes of ulcers sought?), (5) use of self-medication with antibiotics by subjects (e.g., did the group of patients include those who took antimicrobials or who used topical self-treatment that would interfere with diagnosis?) or (6) use of inadequate diagnostic methods (e.g., were tests for herpes simplex virus (HSV) used and, if so, which?) Some general conclusions can, however, be made.

Common Causes

Five diseases—all STIs—are classically associated with genital ulcerations (Table 44–1). The distribution of these diseases between the developing and the industrialized worlds is distinctly different (Table 44–2). In the industrialized world, genital herpes is the most frequently encountered disease, with syphilis and chancroid being the next two most frequently diagnosed conditions. In the developing world, however, chancroid is the most commonly diagnosed disease, with syphilis second and genital herpes third. Recent evidence, however, suggests that genital herpes is far more common in the developing world than was formerly thought, as earlier studies did not include adequate tests for HSV (see section on undiagnosed ulcers). Lymphogranuloma venereum (LGV) is infrequent everywhere (in part, because an ulcer is not a

---

TABLE 44-1 ▶ DISEASES CHARACTERIZED BY GENITAL ULCERATIONS

Common Sexually Transmitted Infections
Genital herpes
Syphilis
Chancroid
Uncommon Sexually Transmitted Infections
Lymphogranuloma venereum
Donovanosis
Uncommon Diseases
Noninfectious
  Trauma
  Fixed drug eruption (most commonly, tetracycline or
    phenolphthalein)
  Foscarnet
  Aphthous ulcers
  Carcinoma
  Behçet's syndrome
  Nonoxynol-9 use
  Miscellaneous
Infectious
  Reiter's syndrome
  Infectious mononucleosis
  HIV infection
  Herpes zoster
  Cytomegalovirus
  Other microorganisms?

---

prominent part of its clinical course). Donovanosis (granuloma inguinale) occurs only in selected tropical geographic locales.

Uncommon Causes

Trauma. If individuals with trauma are not excluded from series of genital ulcers, a large number of cases seen in practice will be caused by trauma.[3] Such a diagnosis should be based only on a careful history and examination, with the clinician considering the likelihood that "trauma" brought a pre-existing, inapparent ulcer to the patient's attention.

Fixed Drug Eruptions. Fixed drug eruptions begin as sharply circumscribed erythematous plaques, but they may subsequently vesiculate or ulcerate. The lips and genitalia are the most frequently involved sites.[14, 15] Co-trimoxazole, tetracyclines, and phenolphthaleins are the most common drugs that cause genital ulcers.[14, 15]

Foscarnet. Foscarnet may be a more commonly encountered cause of ulcers, as it is increasingly used to treat herpesvirus infections in cases of infection with human immunodeficiency virus (HIV). The pathology of genital ulcers associated with the use of foscarnet differs from that of fixed drug eruptions.[16]

Behçet's Syndrome. Genital ulcers may be a prominent feature of Behçet's syndrome and occur in the majority of cases.[17] The ulcers are aphthous in nature and recurrent. Behçet's disease should be suspected in a patient having recurrent oral ulceration with recurrent genital ulcers, eye lesions (usually uveitis), or skin lesions (usually folliculitis or erythema nodosum).[17] The MAGIC syndrome (mouth and genital ulcers with inflamed cartilage) may be a variant.[18] Behçet's disease can be recognized in developing countries, if sought.[11]

Nonoxynol 9. Nonoxynol 9 (N-9) causes vulvar, vaginal, or cervical ulcers when used in high doses or with high frequency in sponge[19] or suppository vehicles.[20, 21] It appears likely that frequent use of N-9 (e.g., daily, *and* in high dose, such as ≥150 mg) may predispose to genital tract ulceration (particularly, cervical ulceration), whereas lower doses do not.[22]

Reiter's Syndrome. The characteristic signs of Reiter's syndrome include arthritis, usually with urethritis and conjunctivitis (or other mucocutaneous signs). This syndrome occurs in males far more commonly than in females. More than one half of all male cases have mucocutaneous signs, including circinate balanitis—shallow ulcerations with serpiginous, erythematous borders.

TABLE 44-2 ▶ COMPARISON OF ETIOLOGIES OF GENITAL ULCERS, MEN AND WOMEN

	Industrialized World								Developing World					
	Winnipeg (1984) (6)		New York City (1997) (7)		Jackson, MS (1998) (8)		United States (1998) (9)		Nairobi (1985) (2, 10)		South Africa (1991) (11, 12)		Rwanda (1998) (13)	
	Men (N = 73)	Women (N = 41)	Men (N = 35)	Women (N = 47)	Men** (N = 111)	Women (N = 32)	Men (N = 351)	Women (N = 165)	Men (N = 100)	Women (N = 89)	Men** (N = 100)	Women (N = 100)	Men (N = 247)	Women* (N = 148)
Chancroid	—	—	34%	32%	42%	28%	4%	1%	48%	48%	22%	12%	32%	25%
Total syphilis	36%	20%	34%	45%	18%	16%	15%	7%	10%	12%	42%	26%	23%	36%
Primary syphilis			All	All					10%	3%	All	11%		
Ulcerated condylomata lata			—	—					—	9%	—	15%		
Herpes simplex virus	38%	76%	23%	34%	26%	47%	59%	70%	6%	2%	10%	12%	21%	26%
Donovanosis	—	—	—	—	PNS	PNS	PNS	PNS	—	—	2%	10%	—	—
LGV	—	—	—	—	PNS	PNS	PNS	PNS	—	—	3%	5%	—	—
Mixed infection	—	—	14%	30%	9%	6%	NS	NS	6%	1%	9%	13%	10%	14%
Trauma	PNS	PNS	PNS	PNS	PNS	PNS	PNS	PNS	—	1%	PNS	PNS	PNS	PNS
Unknown	26%	5%	26%	17%	22%	16%	23%	22%	40%	44%	24%	18%	35%	27%

*Excluded persons with history of ulcers; women preferentially referred.
†Excluded persons with only vesicles.
‡Referral clinic.
NS = not stated; PNS = probably not sought.

Epstein-Barr virus. Epstein-Barr virus has been found in genital ulcers by culture[23] and polymerase chain reaction (PCR).[24] Almost all cases have been in young females.[25] The ulcers are few and painful, and may precede or accompany systemic illness. Whether the ulcers are the result of sexual transmission is unclear. Epstein-Barr virus has been found in cervical secretions,[26] and at least one case has occurred without vaginal intercourse.[24]

Aphthous Ulcers. Aphthous ulcers occur in the oral or genital region. Ulcers are painful, discrete, and sharply marginated. It has been estimated that 20% of the United States population has oral aphthous ulcers, and about 10% of these have genital aphthous ulcers.[27–29] Presumably, genital aphthous ulcers occur alone. Little is known of why the ulcers occur, but some experts believe they represent an incomplete form of Behçet's disease.

HIV Infection. Case reports of HIV-infected patients, almost all women, suggest that HIV infection characterized by low CD4 counts is associated with genital tract ulcers.[30, 31] The ulcers are vulvar or vaginal, solitary or few, and painful, and may be so large and deep as to result in fistulas. As many as one third are accompanied by oroesophageal ulcers. The term *aphthous ulcer* has been applied to the ulcers, but the etiology is unknown. Cases seem to respond to antiretroviral therapy, although systemic or topical steroids and possibly thalidomide may be beneficial.[30]

Miscellaneous. Illnesses that can uncommonly occur in the genital area include hidradenitis suppurativa, Crohn's disease, herpes zoster, and pemphigus, but these causes should be recognizable from the unusual nature of genital ulceration. Unusual microorganisms have been found in ulcers, and it is possible that they or yet-to-be-identified organisms are causes of ulcers.[32, 33]

Undiagnosed Ulcers

At least one quarter of the cases of genital ulcers have an unknown etiology. Most of these are probably cases of syphilis, genital herpes, or chancroid for which diagnostic tests are falsely negative, either through inadequacy of the tests or self-medication by patients (which, in one study, occurred in 28% of patients).[34] For example, PCR testing of ulcer exudate has recently shown that HSV culture, *Haemophilus ducreyi* culture, and dark-field microscopy are only 72%, 74%, and 81% sensitive, respectively.[35] HSV infection appears to be particularly underdiagnosed, most in the developing world. Studies published from 1995 to 1998 show that prevalences of HSV infection among patients with ul-

cers were 23% in Rwanda (13), 28% in Lesotho (36), 36% to 49% in Uganda,[37] and 82% in Thailand.[38]

Chlamydia trachomatis,[10, 31] *Neisseria gonorrhoeae,*[11, 12, 39–41] *Trichomonas vaginalis,*[2] *Mycoplasma hominis,*[39] *Gardnerella vaginalis,*[31] *Ureaplasma urealyticum,*[39, 42] and cytomegalovirus (CMV)[31, 43] have been found in genital ulcers. Their presence in the ulcer probably represents contamination from infection elsewhere in the genital tract, as opposed to a primary site of invasion and replication, although therapy directed solely at CMV has been curative.[31]

Genital Ulcers in Women

Genital ulcers are diseases of men (see Table 44–2). In all series, whether from the developing or industrialized world, men with ulcers outnumber women by two to six times (see Table 44–2; [44]). First, because of anatomic reasons, males notice ulcers more than do women. This is particularly so for diseases with ulcers that are minimally symptomatic, predominantly syphilis. In 1989, the male:female ratio for primary syphilis in the United States was 3.9:1, yet the ratio for secondary syphilis, in which men and women would have an equal chance of noting a rash, was 1:1.3 (unpublished CDC statistics). This ratio reversal indicates that many women do not notice the painless ulcers of primary syphilis. Second, some diseases, in particular syphilis and chancroid, are associated with prostitution, so a relatively few women infect many men. Third, in the developing world, men, who often have or control more economic resources than do women, may preferentially use the resources to seek health care for themselves (author's unpublished observations).

If the distribution of etiologies among men were different from that among women, such a finding would be diagnostically important. Data are limited, but do suggest two differences between men and women with genital ulcers in either the industrialized or the developing world (see Table 44–2). First, ulcerated condylomata lata occur almost exclusively in women, and make up about 10% of cases of genital ulcers among women in the developing world. Second, genital ulcers caused by HSV appear to be more common among women than men. This difference is clinically most pronounced in the industrialized world, but seroprevalence of antibody to HSV type 2 (HSV-2) has been found to be twice as common among women as among men attending an STD clinic in Tanzania,[45] suggesting results similar to those in the industrialized world.

EPIDEMIOLOGY
General Epidemiology

Knowing the frequency of diseases in a community is diagnostically helpful. First, infection with HSV is far more common than infection with the other classic causes of genital ulcers (see later). In a study of individuals with genital ulcers in 10 U.S. cities, infection with HSV was the cause in more than 50% of ulcers in each of the cities.[8] Second, whereas HSV infection is widespread throughout the U.S. population, infection with *Treponema pallidum* and *Haemophilus ducreyi* is not. In 1997, 80% of the 8,550 cases of primary and secondary syphilis that occurred in the United States did so in only 413 (13%) of the 3,115 U.S. counties[46]—2,324 (75%) counties reported no cases. The large majority of these counties (n = 376) are in the South where, compared to the rest of the country, syphilis is a common cause of genital ulcers. In the South, syphilis is also common in both urban and rural locations, unlike the remainder of the country, where syphilis is found basically only in urban locations. Thus, while syphilis should be considered as a cause of ulcers in all patients, the likelihood of *T. pallidum* being the cause in many communities is highly unlikely. Chancroid is an even more focally distributed disease. In 1997, 31 states reported no cases.[46] California, New York, South Carolina, and Texas reported 85% of the 243 cases reported in the United States. Even more focal, LGV occurs in only a few communities in the United States and donovanosis is not thought to be transmitted in the United States. Thus, knowing the relative frequencies of the diseases in a community provides powerful assistance in determining the initial likelihood of specific causes of disease. For example, in many communities, a genital ulcer is unlikely to be caused by anything but HSV. This observation also points out the importance of obtaining travel and sexual histories from patients, as either can provide information that the case was acquired, or linked closely to individuals, from geographic areas where other etiologies are more common.

Racial characteristics, whether representing socioeconomic status, possible genetic predisposition to certain diseases, or sexual activity patterns, are also diagnostically helpful. In the United States, syphilis and chancroid are highly associated with minority populations and, in particular, the black race. In 1997, 88% of primary or secondary syphilis cases occurred in blacks (82.4%) or Hispanics (5.3%). Although no national racial or ethnic data are kept on chancroid, experience with multiple outbreaks shows that minority populations are even more highly associated with this disease than with syphilis.[47] In contrast, HSV infection is widely spread among the U.S. population and *disease* caused by HSV is relatively more common among whites than blacks. This is despite seroprevalences of antibody to HSV-2 of 46% among U.S. blacks and 18% among U.S. whites 12 years of age or older.[48] This disparity between infection rates and those of clinical disease may be a consequence of higher prevalences of antibody to HSV-1 in blacks than in whites,

which offer cross-protection to the development of disease due to HSV-2, although they are not so effective at preventing infection. The seroprevalence of infection with HSV-1 of the U.S. population is 66%, three times higher than the seroprevalence of that with HSV-2, with rates higher in blacks than in whites.[49]

A history eliciting risk factors of either the patient or the partner is diagnostically helpful, as some risk factors are associated with specific diseases. Syphilis was, in the United States and in other industrialized countries, associated with male homosexual activity (particularly among white males) in the 1970s and 1980s. During that time period, male:female ratios of nationally reported primary or secondary cases were 2 to 3:1. With the widespread adoption of safe sex practices among male homosexuals due to the epidemic of acquired immunodeficiency syndrome (AIDS) that so largely affected them in the 1980s, this proportion dropped dramatically: in 1997, the male:female ratio was 1.2:1.[46] Nevertheless, homosexual males remain at increased risk for having syphilis, and there is concern that complacency among homosexual males about safe sex practices, particularly among young males who have not seen the effects of HIV infection, is now occurring.

Both syphilis and chancroid are highly associated with prostitution and, in urban areas, with crack cocaine use. Multiple epidemiologic studies have shown that male patients are likely to be using drugs or giving drugs to (relatively anonymous) women for sex; among female cases, the women are likely to be having sex for drugs or for the money to buy drugs. For example, one recent study in Mississippi found that more than half of the men with chancroid or syphilis had, in the month before diagnosis, used cocaine or exchanged money or drugs for sex.[8]

Syphilis

In the U.S., an epidemic of syphilis began in 1986, fueled by the introduction of crack cocaine. In multiple, successive cities, epidemics began weeks after crack cocaine made its appearance, with cases occurring as a result of prostitution for the drug. The number of cases peaked in 1990, when 135,043 cases (50,578 being cases of primary and secondary syphilis) occurred. The numbers have declined precipitously since, with 46,537 cases of all stages (the lowest number ever recorded) and 8,550 cases of primary and secondary syphilis reported in 1997.[46] The reasons for the decline are unknown but are thought to be due to a combination of events; for example, lessened crack use, increased rates of incarceration of individuals who practice high-risk sexual behavior, infected but untreated high-risk individuals (who therefore have latent syphilis but who will not transmit infection), enhanced control efforts, and increased general adoption of safe sex practices. As a result of the decline in case numbers, a national strategy is being developed for the elimination of syphilis in the United States.

Chancroid

Following many years in which chancroid was rare in the United States, outbreaks of chancroid occurred in the early 1980s in association with illegal immigration and related prostitution. Chancroid, like syphilis, then became highly associated with prostitution related to crack cocaine. The numbers of cases peaked in 1988, when 5,001 cases were reported, the most since 1949. Since then, the numbers of cases have declined precipitously for unknown reasons. In 1997, the number of cases reported was only 243, with one half (n = 119) being reported from New York City. Nevertheless, despite the distinctive clinical appearance of chancroid, cases go unrecognized and unreported.[9, 50] Cases of chancroid diagnosed in the United States may be acquired outside the country.[51]

Genital Herpes

In 1997, about 175,000 initial visits to private physicians for genital herpes were made in the United States, a marked increase from about 75,000 in 1978.[46] Whether this increase represents increasing health care–seeking behavior or a true increase in infection, or both, is unclear, but likely both are important. Despite the magnitude of these numbers, many more infections are acquired each year than result in visits to physicians' offices. In a random sample of the U.S. population that the National Health and Nutrition Examination Survey III (NHANES-III) conducted from 1988 to 1994, 22% of persons had serum antibody to HSV-2.[48] Seroprevalence was higher among blacks (46%) than among Hispanics (22%) or whites (18%). When statistically adjusted, the overall rate of 22% is 30% higher than that of a previous survey conducted from 1976 to 1980,[48] indicating that HSV-2 infection is increasing in frequency. It is estimated that 45 million Americans are infected. In the NHANES-III study, women were 1.4 times more likely than men to have HSV-2 antibody (26% vs. 18%, respectively), supporting the observed increased frequency of genital herpes among women compared to men in case series (see Table 44–2).

Studies similar to NHANES from other countries are lacking, but other data indicate that HSV-2 infection is common worldwide. In England, 23% of STD clinic attendees and 8% of blood donors had antibodies to HSV-2.[52] In Sweden, 33% of pregnant women in Stockholm in 1989 had antibodies to HSV-2 (vs. 17% in 1969).[53]

These figures, while high, modestly underestimate the number of people with genital herpes, because genital herpes can be caused by HSV-1 also. The pro-

portion varies by country but can be high, and as many as 40% of new cases in Great Britain may be caused by type 1.[54, 55] Type 2, however, rarely infects the oral cavity, and it is estimated that 99% of persons with type 2 antibody have genital tract infection.[56]

Lymphogranuloma Venereum

LGV is caused by any of the three L serotypes of *Chlamydia trachomatis*, which possess unique virulence characteristics compared to the non-L serotypes of *C. trachomatis*. In 1997, 113 cases of LGV were reported in the United States; the largest concentration of cases was in New York City.[46] The epidemiology of LGV in the United States is unknown. Our experience is that many cases are diagnosed on the basis of a complement fixation titer of at least 1:64, or high signals with enzyme-linked immunosorbent assays (ELISA) for *C. trachomatis*, in the absence of clinical features characteristic of LGV. These titers are likely generated by non-L serotype infections, perhaps persistent or repeated cases. Outside the United States, cases occur in tropical areas, although the epidemiology of LGV is little explored.

Donovanosis

Donovanosis is caused by *Calymmatobacterium granulomatis*, an elusive bacterium cultured on only 14 occasions through 1991[57] but recently isolated in cell culture.[58, 59] Donovanosis is found almost exclusively in Asia, principally in New Guinea and southern India. Cases also occur in southern Africa, the Caribbean, and parts of South America, particularly in the Guianas and Brazil.[57] In 1997, 8 cases were reported in the United States.

CLINICAL PRESENTATION

Syphilis

After a mean incubation period of 3 weeks (range, 90 days), most patients notice a brief papule or macule at the site where the ulcer will appear.[60] Classically, the ulcers (sometimes called chancres) of syphilis are thought of as being single and painless, with indurated margins (Fig. 44–1). While this is the single most common presentation, the presentation can be different. About one half of cases have more than one ulcer,[60] and so-called *kissing ulcers* occur in areas where skin surfaces contact one another (e.g., the labia or the foreskin). The ulcers are surprisingly painless, although there is usually tenderness (e.g., pain elicited by firm pressure during the taking of a specimen for dark-field microscopy). The borders are characteristically smooth and indurated; that is, with firm, palpable edges, while the base of the ulcer is smooth, with a

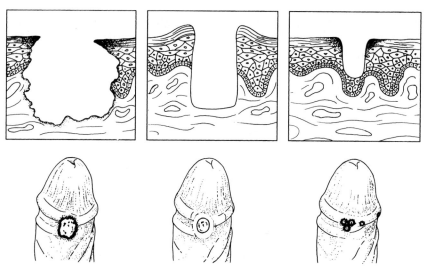

FIGURE 44-1 ▶ The appearance of the ulcers of chancroid, syphilis, and genital herpes *(from left to right)*. The ulcer of chancroid is inflamed *(shading)*, has irregular margins, and is deeply eroded with undermined edges (like an Erlenmeyer flask). The ulcer of syphilis has a smooth, indurated border and a smooth base. The genital herpes ulcer is superficial, with inflamed edges. (From Schmid GP, Schalla WO, De Witt WE: Chancroid. In: Morse SA, Moreland AA, Thompson SE [eds]: Atlas of Sexually Transmitted Diseases. Philadelphia: JB Lippincott, 1990.)

serous exudate. All experienced clinicians have seen cases that are atypical; for example, multiple ulcers, ulcers with nonindurated borders, and ulcers with purulent bases.

In men, one half of ulcers are on the foreskin (inner or outer surface) or coronal sulcus.[60, 61] In homosexual men, one third of cases have ulcers in the anorectal area that may require careful inspection for detection.[61]

In women, most ulcers occur on the external genitalia. Ulcers may also occur in the vagina, and in one series 21% of ulcers occured on the cervix.[61] It is likely that a greater proportion of ulcers than was thought occur on the cervix or vaginal walls. Because women have no way of noticing these painless lesions, women with them would not come to medical attention unless through partner notification efforts.

As many as 80% of cases have inguinal adenopathy, which is bilateral in most cases. The adenopathy is small, rubbery, and not painful, although tenderness can be elicited in one third of cases.[60]

Condylomata lata, the raised, fleshy lesions of secondary syphilis that occur in the genital tract, may ulcerate. Like the ulcers of primary syphilis, these ulcerations usually have smooth bases and regular borders. These occur far more commonly in women than in men (see Table 44–2).

Chancroid

After an incubation period of 3 to 7 days (range, 10 days), most patients note the appearance of a "sore," although an occasional patient may notice an initial papule. When lesions are seen by the clinician, there will be one, or a few that are "raw," deep, "beefy," ulcers with inflamed, often "undermined' margins (see Fig. 44–1). The bases of the ulcers are uneven, with a purulent exudate, and often bleed. Occasionally, ulcers are shallow but still have inflamed borders. The most characteristic feature of chancroid is the pain of the lesion. Patients are very reluctant to have the ulcers manipulated, and it is often difficult for them to remove underclothing. The ulcers are characteristically located on the coronal sulcus, or the foreskin of uncircumcised men. In women, the large female:male ratio suggests that many women may have asymptomatic colonization or ulcers of the vaginal walls or cervix. Such ulcers are uncommon, however, occurring in 7% to, at most, 14% of women with chancroid in one series.[2] A study of commercial sex workers in The Gambia found that 4 of 207 (2%) without ulcers had *H. ducreyi* detected by PCR from cervical secretions.[62]

About one half of men with chancroid have unilateral or bilateral painful inguinal lymphadenopathy. The lymphadenopathy can be fluctuant, forming buboes, with frank pus; patients sometimes limp because of the pain. Without therapy or occasionally even with therapy, the lymph nodes spontaneously drain. Women are less likely than are men to have inguinal lymphadenitis, presumably because of differing lymphatic drainage patterns. Nevertheless, inguinal lymphadenitis was present in at least 35% of Kenyan women with chancroid.[2]

Genital Herpes

Genital herpes is characterized by a prodrome of paresthesias in the genital area 24 to 48 hours prior to the appearance of blisters. The appearance of grouped blisters on erythematous bases is almost diagnostic of genital herpes. In the first few days, the blisters are filled with clear fluid (vesicles), and then they become filled with pus (pustules) and rupture, leaving multiple shallow, painful ulcers that may coalesce into fewer, larger ulcers. The severity of the initial clinically recognizable episode of genital herpes, *first-episode genital herpes,* varies considerably, in part depending on whether the person has been exposed to HSV in the past. If the first episode is a *primary infection,* that is, the first time the person has been exposed to either type 1 or 2 HSV, disease is more severe than if the first episode is a *nonprimary infection.* Determining whether a person has been exposed to HSV can be achieved by seeking a clinical history of genital or oral herpes (one study[63] found specificities of more than 90% for each) or, more accurately, obtaining HSV serology. With first-episode primary infection, blisters last 10 to 12 days before rupturing, with the ulcers remaining another 1 to 2 weeks until crusting and re-epithelialization occurs. With first-episode nonprimary infection, the duration of symptoms is about 10 days, and the symptoms are milder. Attacks of first-episode herpes tend to be in the midline or bilateral, while recurrent attacks tend to be unilateral.

First-episode genital herpes, particularly primary infection, is often severe, accompanied by manifestations outside the genital tract, and within the genital tract at places other than the site of the ulcers. Outside the genital tract, fever, headache, and myalgia are common with first episodes and aseptic meningitis may occur. In the genital tract, dysuria is frequent and some patients have difficulty in voiding; virus is often recovered from the urethra in these instances. The cervix of women is typically microbiologically involved in first-episode infection, with HSV being recovered from 88% of women with primary disease, 65% with nonprimary first-episode disease, and 12% to 20% with recurrent disease.[64] When HSV is recovered, the cervix is abnormal, with erythema and erosions; these are severe in first-episode primary disease, are less so in first-episode nonprimary infection, and may be subtle in recurrent episodes.[64]

The signs and symptoms of first-episode genital herpes presumably occur at the site of infection. During this episode, HSV travels along nerves to the dorsal root ganglia of the spinal cord, where infection remains for life. Following first-episode infection, recurrent attacks occur in the majority of persons. Periodically, virus travels peripherally to the genital area, resulting in recurrent clinical episodes or viral shedding. The number of attacks is highly variable.

Of the NHANES-III sample, only 2.6% had a history of genital herpes.[48] The overall seroprevalence of 22% obviously indicates a far greater prevalence of infection than is recognized or is admitted to by participants.

Considerable recent work has shown that many individuals with recurrent genital herpes have very mild symptoms and signs and do not recognize the outbreaks. With teaching using pictures or pamphlets, more than 50% of subclinically infected individuals can be trained to recognize the symptoms and signs of genital herpes.[56, 65]

Primary infection of the genital tract by HSV-1 results in illness similar to that caused by HSV-2, but recurrences are milder and less frequent than with infection with HSV-2, as is asymptomatic shedding; this difference in recurrence appears to be genetically determined.[54, 56]

Subclinical shedding of virus—that is, recovery of HSV from the genital tract in the absence of genital or perianal lesions noted by either the patient or the clinician—occurs regularly among infected individuals.[66] Among women with a history of recurrent genital herpes, shedding occurred in 36 of 65 women (55%) with HSV-2 infection and 4 of 14 women (29%) with HSV-1 infection over a median follow-up of 105 days (during which women self-collected genital specimens on 85% of all days).[67] Shedding occurred on a mean of 2% of days in women with HSV-2 infection and 0.7% of days in women with HSV-1 infection (range, 0% to 35%). Women who had acquired genital herpes within the past year and who had frequent episodes (>12/yr) were most likely to shed virus. Shedding was slightly more likely to occur from anal specimens than from vulvar or cervicovaginal specimens.

Unrecognized episodes of genital herpes and subclinical shedding are important, because most cases of genital herpes are acquired from individuals who have no history of genital herpes or who have no recognized lesions at the time of intercourse.[68] While persons with genital herpes are most infectious when lesions are apparent, most persons avoid sex at these times; hence, most transmission occurs from unrecognized lesions or subclinical shedding. Transmission rates among couples in which one partner has genital herpes and the other does not are substantial, about 10% per year.[69, 70] The risk is particularly high for women, who are several times more likely to acquire infection, and for persons without pre-existing antibody to HSV. In one study, after 1 year 32% of women without pre-existing HSV-1 antibody became infected, compared to 9% with antibody.[70]

The usual incubation period of first-episode disease is about 7 days. However, in one small study, the majority of persons experiencing first-episode disease had pre-existing HSV-2 antibody, suggesting previous asymptomatic or unrecognized infection that had become clinically apparent.[71] This observation has importance for counseling, as the individual's most recent sex partner may not have been the source of infection.

Lymphogranuloma Venereum. LGV is traditionally included in the differential diagnosis of genital ulcers, but an ulcer is a minor feature of this disease. The characteristic clinical presentation of LGV is enlarged, painful inguinal lymphadenopathy, often buboes. The lymphadenopathy is preceded, by 7 to 30 days, by a small, shallow painless ulcer in at least some cases, but at most 30% of men and fewer women have, or remember, the ulcer. The ulcer is rarely present when the patient sees the clinician, as the ulcer is seldom significant enought to lead the patient to seek medical attention and has healed in most cases by the time the lymphadenopathy appears.[72] Because of the prominence of painful, enlarged inguinal lymphadenopathy in both chancroid and LGV, the diseases may be confused with one another; the prominence of the ulcer in chancroid will readily differentiate the two.

Donovanosis. *Calymmatobacterium granulomatis* causes a slowly progressive disease of the genital area that is characterized as much by heaped-up granulomatous tissue as it is by genital ulceration. The tissue is fleshy, raw, nontender, and variable in appearance.[57, 73] Early lesions are likely to be ulcerative, and with progression induration and granulation tissue appear. Many cases appear not to be sexually transmitted, as sex partners usually are without symptoms; nevertheless, at least 80% of cases occur in the genital tract.[73] The incubation period is often difficult to determine, as the source is not necessarily clear, but the period is probably 3 to 40 days.[57] Without treatment, there is continued local destruction. Extragenital lesions may occur, presumably by autoinoculation.

DIAGNOSIS

Syphilis

Despite recent advances in the ability to culture *T. pallidum* in vitro, inoculation into rabbit testes remains the only means of recovering *T. pallidum* from clinical material. Thus, outside of the research setting, the only definitive means of diagnosing syphilis is by dark-field or fluorescence microscopy. Although dark-field microscopy takes only a few minutes to perform and detects 49% to 97% of cases,[8, 35, 74] it is used only in large clinics where patients with primary syphilis are likely to be seen. Fluorescence microscopy is available at many hospitals, fluorescein-tagged monoclonal antibodies are commercially available, and the methodology rivals dark-field microscopy[7] or even PCR in sensitivity.[74] Results generally cannot be obtained quickly enough to be used while the patient is present, however; thus, few medical care settings use this approach.

Serology remains the main diagnostic method for syphilis. Unfortunately, serology often provides only a presumptive diagnosis, as a single titer cannot distinguish present from past infection and serologic tests are not specific for syphilis. Two general types of syphilis serologic tests are available, "nontreponemal tests" and "treponemal tests." Nontreponemal tests do not measure specific treponemal antibody but, rather, detect antibody directed against cardiolipin, which makes up about 10% of the cell lipids of *T. pallidum* but which, unfortunately, is also found in mammalian tissue.[75] Such antibody is called "reaginic" antibody. The two nontreponemal tests most commonly used are the Venereal Disease Research Laboratory (VDRL) test, a microscopic agglutination test, and the rapid plasma reagin (RPR) test, a simple macroscopic agglutination test performed on cards and which takes only minutes to perform. These tests are positive in about 80% and 85%[76] of cases of primary syphilis at the first visit, respectively, with the RPR being slightly more sensitive than the VDRL. This proportion rises the longer the person has had the ulcer,[13] and the sensitivity of the tests approaches 100% in early latent and secondary syphilis. All positive nontreponemal tests should be confirmed by a treponemal test (e.g., the fluorescent treponemal antibody-absorption [FTA-ABS] or microhemagglutination assay–*Treponema pallidum* [MHA-TP] tests), because false-positive nontreponemal tests may occur, particularly with intravenous drug use (6% to 9%, compared to 1% in the general population[77]), acute viral infections (including genital herpes), some vaccinations, and autoimmune diseases.[76] Recently, automated treponemal tests with ELISA technology (using as antigen either sonicates of whole *T. pallidum* or 1 to 3 recombinant antigens) have been introduced into the U.S. and European markets. Some clinical laboratories have adopted them for screening and confirmation of positive reaginic tests. Evidence suggests that they perform with sensitivity and specificity similar to those of the traditional treponemal tests, thus having specificities of about 97% to 99%.[76, 78, 79]

Genital Herpes

Although some experts consider typical cases of genital herpes sufficiently characteristic to be diagnosed clinically, without a laboratory test, the author believes that it is important to confirm clinical suspicions with a laboratory test whenever possible, and always if there is clinical uncertainty. The diagnosis of genital herpes has, for many persons, a "profound emotional effect."[80] Having genital herpes alters self-image, and present and future sexual relations, may affect the management of pregnancies, and, for some women (incorrectly) affects their perceived ability to have children. Having a positive diagnostic test provides both patient and clinician with the surety of the diagnosis that is useful for counseling and for dealing with the future; in addition, typing of the isolate provides some indication of the future course of disease.

All tests are sensitive during the vesicle stage, when large quantities of virus are present in vesicle fluid.

Culture is the most sensitive and specific test, with a sensitivity approaching 100% in the vesicle stage and 89% in the pustular stage; this figure drops to as low as 33%, however, in patients presenting with ulcers.[81] Once ulcers have crusted, virus is difficult to detect. Nonculture tests are available, including immunofluorescence and ELISA. The sensitivity of the immunofluorescence and ELISA tests is about 80% compared to culture.[54, 64] A negative test, particularly during the ulcer stage, cannot be relied on to exclude the diagnosis of genital herpes. In cases suspected of being genital herpes but with a negative test, the patient should return at the first sign of a possible recurrence for a repeat test, which can then be performed at the vesicular stage.

PCR testing has received limited evaluation for genital herpes but appears more sensitive than culture, particularly for clinical situations in which viral titers are low; that is, later stages of illness (although not crusted lesions) or in detecting shedding of virus from asymptomatic individuals.[35, 54, 82, 83]

An easily performed but often overlooked test is the Tzanck smear. This test detects multinucleated giant cells that are formed as the result of infection with herpesviruses. The test is performed by scraping the bottom of the vesicle or ulcer with a swab or scalpel, placing the material on a slide, staining the slide (often with Wright's or Giemsa stain, which are commonly available), and looking for the characteristic cells by light microscopy. Solomon and co-workers[84] found the sensitivity of the Tzanck smear, compared to culture, to be 67% in the vesicle stage, 75% in the pustule stage, and 50% in the ulcer stage; the specificity was 94%. Others have found a lower sensitivity (21%) compared to culture but similarly high specificity.[7] Thus, this simple test, while certainly inferior to culture, is specific and readily available to all clinicians.

Serology may also be used to confirm a diagnosis of genital herpes. The serologic tests currently available commercially, despite sometimes claiming to be type-specific, are not. They are very good, however, at identifying species-specific antibody to HSV. Thus, an individual who has a negative serologic titer at the time of seeking care but who subsequently seroconverts has serologic confirmation of infection. Type-specific tests, both Western blot and ELISA, are available for research purposes and are truly type-specific. Type-specific tests are under development for commercial purposes, and the type-specificity of these tests appears to be quite good. One test was licensed in 1999. Although the role that type-specific serology will play in clinical practice is being explored, it was useful in the diagnosis, counseling, and partner management of 79% of patients with ulceration of unknown etiology in a genitourinary clinic in England.[85]

Chancroid

Because of uncertainty over the accuracy of Gram stain of ulcer secretions, and the unavailability of culture for *H. ducreyi*,[50] most cases are diagnosed on clinical grounds. Although the Gram stain is said to be insensitive and nonspecific,[40, 42] others have reported sensitivities of 62% and 89%, and specificities of 99% and 76%, for slides with gram-negative coccobacilli in parallel rows in a clustered, "school-of-fish" appearance.[7, 86] Many laboratories have difficulty in isolating *H. ducreyi*, and even experienced research laboratories recover *H. ducreyi* from at most 80% of clinically suspected cases[87]; such difficulty can have an impact on the perceived specificity of the Gram stain. To enhance yield, more than one type of culture medium should be used,[88] and incubation at 33°C produces more isolates than does incubation at 35°C.[89]

Haemophilus ducreyi can be cultured from lymph nodes, but recovery is less successful than that from ulcers. Gram-stained smears from lymph nodes show white blood cells, but organisms are infrequently seen, suggesting that organisms are fewer in number than in ulcers.

Research methods of confirming infection by *H. ducreyi* include immunofluorescence of ulcer or lymph node material using fluorescein-tagged monoclonal antibodies specific for *H. ducreyi*, nucleic acid amplification,[35] and, several methods of performing serology. It does not seem that any will be commercially available in the near future.

Lymphogranuloma Venereum

Diagnosis of LGV is almost always based on serologic evidence of infection, most commonly with a complement fixation titer of at least 1:64 (and preferably showing a four-fold rise in titer on paired sera). Although such titers support the diagnosis of LGV, particularly when present in a patient with clinical features compatible with LGV, titers of this magnitude occasionally occur as the result of infection with non-L serovars of *C. trachomatis* and are, thus, not specific for LGV. ELISA serology for *C. trachomatis* suffers from the same problem. Specific diagnosis of LGV requires recovery of the organism, with subsequent serotyping. Alternatively, microimmunofluorescence serology, to determine whether the infecting serovar is L$_{1-3}$, may be used, but such testing is available in only several laboratories in the United States.

Donovanosis

Because *C. granulomatis* cannot be cultured readily,[58, 59] diagnosis depends on visualizing it within cytology or biopsy specimens. This can be done by using a "crush preparation." A fragment of the friable tissue is removed, placed between two slides, and crushed. The slide is then stained (Wright's or Giemsa stain is satisfactory) and examined for typical "Donovan bodies", that is, bacillary organisms (*C. granulomatis*) within histiocytes. Alternatively, biopsy specimens, preferably deep specimens taken from the advancing margin of the lesion, can be examined; a silver stain is preferred.[73] Nucleic acid amplification to detect *C. granulomatis* in tissue has been described.[90] Indirect immunofluorescence serology is available for research purposes.[91]

ASSOCIATION OF GENITAL ULCERS WITH HIV INFECTION

Probably all STIs enhance the transmission of HIV infection, although to varying degrees, and there is sufficient evidence to show that HIV infection enhances the severity of some STIs. The evidence is strongest in both situations for STIs characterized by genital ulcers.

Genital Ulcers Enhance the Transmission of HIV. Computer modeling has estimated a powerful effect for ulcers in enhancing HIV transmission, with an increased transmission rate of as much as 300 times.[92] Evidence that genital ulcers enhance the transmission of HIV comes from three types of study.

Cross-Sectional Studies. Multiple cross-sectional studies from the United States, Africa, and Asia have shown that individuals with genital ulcers are more likely to be HIV-infected than persons without genital ulcers. In the United States, these prevalences can be high (18% in a recent national study of persons with syphilis[93]) and differ significantly from individuals without genital ulcers; for example, 10% in those with genital ulcers and 0% in those without in Jackson, Mississippi.[8] Chancroid and syphilis are the diseases most associated with HIV, but infection with HSV may also be associated.[94] These studies form the basis for the recommendation of testing all persons with genital ulcers, but certainly those with chancroid and syphilis, for HIV infection when seen.[95]

Such studies, however, are unsatisfying in trying to impute a causative role for ulcers in promoting HIV infection. Most HIV seroconversion occurs within 8 weeks. If the ulcer influenced transmission, either by being present in the index patient at the time of intercourse, or by being present in the transmitting partner with the index patient having acquired both the cause of the ulcer and HIV infection, the index patients must have had the ulcers for many weeks prior to seeking care. About three quarters of persons with an ulcer in the developing world seek care within 2 weeks of onset,[13, 96] a time period too short to be associated with significant rates of seroconversion, particularly with disease of short incubation (e.g., chancroid or genital herpes). An alternative explanation for at least some of the cases is that the presence of

an ulcer is a sign of previous ulcers, STIs, or other risky behavior that enhanced the previous acquisition of HIV infection, now discovered at the time the cross-sectional study is performed; data from Rwanda support this theory.[13] Nevertheless, despite this likelihood, the consistency of association among differing populations in many geographic areas suggests that the most likely explanation for the observed associations is a causative role for ulcers in enhancing the transmission of HIV. The relative risks or odds ratios reported in these studies are about 3 to 6, and many have been summarized.[97]

Cohort Studies. A better study design for showing causation is a type of cohort study, in which individuals with sexual exposure to HIV infection are followed to determine how many seroconvert. If it is known how many were exposed to an ulcer at the time of exposure or how many developed ulcers (thus inferring an ulcer in the partner), causation can be better determined. Cameron and co-workers[98] studied 73 HIV-seronegative men in Nairobi who had a single sexual exposure to a commercial sex worker, 85% of whom were known to be HIV infected. Twelve weeks later, 6 men (8.2%) had seroconverted. Ulcers played a powerful role in seroconversion and, if the man was uncircumcised and developed an ulcer, 43% seroconverted after this single exposure. This remarkable study shows a powerful, plausible effect on HIV transmission, a finding buttressed by another Nairobi study of 81 HIV-negative women with a genital ulcer, 10 (12%) of whom seroconverted.[99] In the United States, a seroconversion rate of 3% among seronegative men with a genital ulcer has been found in New York City,[100] a rate well worth detecting: in both the latter two studies, the proportion of "transmitting individuals" with HIV was unknown but was almost certainly less than the 85% in Nairobi commercial sex workers.

Biologic Studies. If ulcers promote HIV infection, then HIV should be found in ulcers. HIV has been found in high titers in exudate from the ulcers of both chancroid and genital herpes (Table 44–3). HIV appears particularly likely to be found in the ulcer exudate shortly after HIV infection is acquired and before the appearance of antibody,[104] a period characterized by very high levels of circulating HIV.[105] Nucleic acid amplification appears to identify far more infections of the ulcers than does culture (see Table 44–3). Data are too preliminary to tell whether ulcers of one disease harbor more virus than do ulcers of another.

Virus may be found free in ulcer exudate or within target cells for HIV, likely Langerhans cells, macrophages, and CD4 antigen-bearing cells. These cells are found in ulcer exudates caused by STIs.[106, 107] Chancroid, in particular, has abundant macrophages and CD4-bearing cells in the exudate.[107] Ulcers associated

TABLE 44-3 ▶ Presence of HIV in Ulcer Exudates

Disease	Culture for HIV (No. Positive/No. Tested)	PCR for HIV (No. Positive/No. Tested)
Chancroid[101]	4/35 (11%)	NT
Chancroid[102]	2/7 (30%)	6/7 (86%)
Chancroid[9]	NT	2/6 (33%)
Syphilis	NT	1/2 (50%)
Genital herpes	NT	1/3 (33%)
Unknown	NT	2/3 (67%)
Genital herpes episodes[103]	0/8 (0%)	25/26 (96%)

NT = not tested.

with N-9 were not associated with HIV acquisition.[22] Multiple explanations for this observation are possible, including the speculation of a lack of target cells within the ulcers associated with N-9 use.[22]

Lack of Male Circumcision Enhances Genital Ulcer and HIV Acquisition. The only recognized biologic risk factor for acquiring a genital ulcer is the absence of circumcision. While this association may be true in women and men, it has been studied only in men. Men who have not been circumcised are at increased risk for STIs characterized by genital ulcers, with a two- to three-fold increased risk.[108] This association has been hypothesized to be based on the foreskin being a tissue that is easily traumatized, and, indeed, ulcers often occur on the foreskin.[108, 109]

Since having a foreskin enhances the acquisition of genital ulcers, one might conclude that a foreskin predisposes to acquiring HIV infection. This appears true, yet the enhanced susceptibility to HIV infection among the uncircumcised may be due only in part to susceptibility to genital ulcers. One recent study provided an odds ratio of 2.2 for the acquisition of a genital ulcer among uncircumcised, compared to circumcised, individuals yet found an odds ratio of 4.7 for HIV infection.[109] It is not clear how much having a foreskin, as opposed to its presence's facilitating the acquisition of genital ulcers, contributes to the enhanced prevalences of HIV infection in uncircumcised men, but both appear important.[108, 109] Circumcision prior to the onset of sexual activity has been proposed as a means of controlling HIV infection in parts of the world where HIV and intact foreskin rates are high. The possible effect of a policy of circumcision on slowing the HIV epidemic in a population that might adopt such a policy has been likened to that of a modestly effective HIV vaccine.[109]

HIV Infection Enhances Occurrence of Genital Ulcers. It is possible that the immunosuppression of HIV infection predisposes infected individuals to acquiring or manifesting infections characterized by genital ulcers. Limited cross-sectional and cohort study evidence supports this hypothesis. Kaul and colleagues[110] fol-lowed 189 Kenyan sex workers for a mean of 24.3 months. A total of 541 new cases of genital ulcers were acquired, an incidence of 0.9 per woman. Using multivariate analysis, and controlling for the number of sexual partners and condom use, HIV seropositivity was highly associated with the development of a genital ulcer, with 82% of initially seropositive women developing an ulcer versus 48% of seronegative women (odds ratio [OR], 4.33; $P < .01$). This association was greatest among women with low CD4 counts (<200/mL) but was present even in women with higher counts. Ghys and co-workers,[111] in the Ivory Coast, found that the prevalence of genital ulcers among women with HIV infection increased as the CD4 count diminished, and the cohort study of Nasio and colleagues[109] also associated HIV seropositivity with the development of a genital ulcer (OR, 1.87; $P < .01$).

Why HIV infection, even without obvious immunosuppression, is a risk factor for ulcerations is unclear. One hypothesis is that overt or covert immunosuppression allows the expression of pre-existing HSV infection. Data from Africa suggest that HIV infection itself does not predispose to enhanced prevalences of genital herpes,[13, 34, 37] but as immunosuppression progresses there is an increased likelihood of individuals having genital herpes.[13] The latter observation suggests that as HIV infection progresses, whether in an individual or a community, genital herpes will make up a greater proportion of the diagnoses of genital ulcers. Another possibility is that HIV infection predisposes to unusual ulcers (e.g., aphthous ulcers). Kaul and colleagues, however, did not find an increased proportion of ulcers of unknown etiology among HIV-positive women compared to HIV-negative women, as one might expect if this were the case. These authors did note an unusually high frequency of genital ulcers shortly after seroconversion to HIV, when there is a rapid decline in the numbers of CD4 cells[105] and possible immunosuppression.[110]

HIV Infection May Alter the Clinical Course of Individuals with Genital Ulcers. Data showing that HIV-positive individuals have more extensive ulcerations or clinical courses different from those of HIV-negative individuals are limited. Bogaerts, in Rwanda, found that the accuracy of clinical diagnosis of ulcers did not vary between HIV-positive and HIV-negative individuals[13] and, in a separate study, that clinical disease did not.[34] These authors also found that the rate of ulcer healing was similar between HIV-positive and HIV-negative individuals.[13] Others, however, have found that HIV-positive individuals with chancroid are more likely to fail therapy clinically[112] or cases of syphilis are more likely to respond less favorably serologically but equally clinically,[93] than those without HIV infection. Kamya and co-workers showed that, among individuals with genital herpes, HIV-positive individuals are more likely to have large ulcers compared to HIV-negative individuals[37] and genital herpes in HIV-positive patients can be therapeutic problems. Thus, it is likely that differences exist in the clinical course and therapeutic response of individuals with genital ulcers; these alterations are minimal early in the course of HIV infection and become more marked as HIV infection progresses.

ACCURACY OF CLINICAL DIAGNOSIS

Evaluations of the accuracy of clinical diagnosis are generally either of two kinds: (1) how well do clinicians, using clinical experience, diagnose the etiology of a genital ulcer, or (2) how well do algorithms meant to standardize an approach to diagnosis, diagnose the etiology of a genital ulcer? The results show that clinical experience is inadequate for diagnosing the etiology of an ulcer, and that algorithms are useful but require overtreatment of some patients to be effective.

A series of 92 patients with one or more genital ulcers seen in Lesotho exemplifies both evaluations.[36] Clinical criteria, such as would be used by clinicians, were used to classify cases. Of the 92 patients, 76 were diagnosed as chancroid (54 confirmed by laboratory tests), 8 as genital herpes (7 confirmed), 6 as syphilis (5 confirmed), 2 as donovanosis (0 confirmed), and none as LGV; 17 patients (18%) had mixed infections. The authors determined that 57 patients (62%) would have received adequate treatment, while 35 patients (38%) would have received inadequate or inappropriate therapy. Multiple other studies have shown that clinical diagnosis is incorrect in about 40% of cases.[2, 10, 34, 60, 113]

Htun and colleagues[36] then examined the adequacy of two algorithms to manage cases. The algorithms used no laboratory tests and relied on history and clinical judgment. With algorithm A, 92% of patients would receive adequate treatment for chancroid, syphilis, or genital herpes, but overtreatment would have been provided for 63% of patients. With algorithm B, 90% of patients received adequate treatment but 57% received overtreatment. This study points out clearly the trade-offs in the use of clinical judgment—undertreatment versus overtreatment—and, most im-

portant, the need to use laboratory tests in managing patients with genital ulcers.

APPROACH TO THE PATIENT WITH A GENITAL ULCER

Diagnostic and therapeutic efforts are traditionally directed at detecting and managing syphilis because of the consequences of failure to detect and treat this disease, that is, the development of late syphilis or, in pregnant women, congenital syphilis in the fetus. Nevertheless, it is increasingly important in women to document a history of genital herpes because pregnant women should inform their obstetricians of a past history of genital herpes. Such women are at small, but increased, risk for delivering an infant with genital herpes. Management strategies for such women are different from treatment of those without such a history, and new strategies are under investigation, for example, the use of acyclovir around the time of delivery. Similarly, with the recent introduction of commercially available type-specific HSV serology, it is important to consider couples in which the man has a history of genital herpes, but the woman does not, as a unit. Probably, these serologic tests will be used to screen women in such partnerships who wish to become, or are, pregnant to determine whether they have been infected with HSV. If not, and because women who become infected with HSV during pregnancy have the greatest risk of delivering an infected neonate, counseling about the avoidance of sex or the adoption of safe sex procedures during pregnancy is increasingly being advocated. Last, diagnosis is important to the proper immediate treatment of patients with genital ulcers. It assists in shortening morbidity, partner notification (it is difficult to know how to treat and counsel the partner without knowing the disease the patient has), and, because many patients continue to have sex while symptomatic, in possibly preventing HIV acquisition or transmission.

Characteristic Features of Genital Ulcers. Despite the imprecision of clinical diagnosis in predicting the actual etiology of a genital ulcer, five presentations are highly suggestive of specific diagnoses:

1. The presence of grouped vesicles or pustules mixed with shallow ulcers, particularly if accompanied by a history of similar preceding episodes, is almost pathognomonic of genital herpes.
2. A single nonpainful and minimally tender ulcer, not accompanied by inguinal adenopathy or, if so, accompanied by small, rubbery nodes, is likely to be syphilis, particularly if the ulcer edge is indurated.
3. One to three extremely painful ulcers, accompanied by tender inguinal lymphadenopathy, is un-

likely to be anything but chancroid; if the lymph-adenopathy is fluctuant, that is, a bubo, the diagnosis is almost certain.

4. An inguinal bubo accompanied by one or several ulcers is most likely to be chancroid, but it could possibly be herpes; if the nodes are fluctuant, the diagnosis is chancroid.

5. An indurated ulcer is unlikely to be anything but syphilis or donovanosis.

Approach to Diagnosis. Because it is difficult in most cases to make a correct diagnosis on the basis of clinical features, epidemiologic features and laboratory testing are required for making an accurate diagnosis (Fig. 44–2). Even then, because laboratory tests for diagnosing all causes of genital ulcers are uncommonly available and few yield immediate results, the clinician must initially use clinical judgment in making a diagnosis. This judgment is based on (1) knowledge of diseases in the community; (2) individual risk factors; and (3) clinical appearance and relationship to systemic illness; for example, is the ulcer a manifestation of Epstein-Barr virus infection? In addition, clinicians should inquire about medications that the patient has used. These may be either the cause of the ulcer (e.g., a fixed drug eruption) or a reason for diagnostic difficulty, as many patients use oral or topical preparations in an attempt to treat the infection themselves.

All individuals should have a serologic test for syphilis and, ideally, a dark-field or immunofluorescence examination for syphilis and test for HSV performed on ulcer exudate. In areas where chancroid occurs, a Gram stain of the ulcer exudate may suggest that the diagnosis and culture should be performed, if possible. If initial dark-field (or immunofluorescence) and syphilis serologic tests are negative, the patient is reliable, and syphilis is thought to be likely, the patient can be asked to return the next day for repeat examination of ulcer exudate. The serum drawn for syphilis serology can be saved and convalescent serum obtained later to perform HSV serologic testing—if the initial sample is negative and the convalescent serum positive, this is excellent evidence of acute HSV infection. Because genital herpes is a devastating diagnosis for many persons and may affect pregnancy management, the author strongly believes that physicians should not make diagnoses of genital herpes on clinical grounds alone (because such diagnoses can be incorrect) and should liberally use tests to identify HSV in cases that would not otherwise be considered likely to be genital herpes.

If buboes are present, a diagnostic and therapeutic aspiration performed through intact skin (and not through inflamed skin, to prevent fistula formation) can be done. The exudate can be gram-stained, and cultures for *H. ducreyi* and *C. trachomatis* performed. Acute (and, later, convalescent sera) can be obtained for serology for lymphogranuloma venereum.

Management. If immediate clinical and laboratory evaluations are unrewarding, patients should be

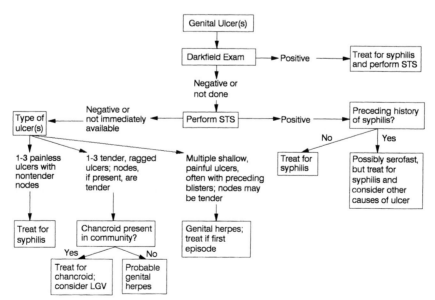

FIGURE 44–2 ▶ Algorithm for clinical approach to the diagnosis of genital ulcers, concentrating on common sexually transmitted causes. The history should initially separate traumatic from nontraumatic etiologies, and identify possible systemic diseases as possible causes. The clinician should seek risk factors for possible sexually transmitted causes, including knowledge of disease in the partner and the use of topical or systemic medications that might obscure a diagnosis. Laboratory testing should be done whenever possible (e.g., tests for herpes on ulcer exudate or serology). HIV testing should be encouraged for all patients, and for those with syphilis, chancroid, or an unknown cause testing should be repeated 3 months later. STS, serologic test for syphilis; LGV, lymphogranuloma venereum. (Modified from Schmid GP: Approach to the patient with genital ulcer disease. Med Clin North Am 1990; 74:1559.)

treated for the most likely diagnosis, or diagnoses, and seen again in a week, unless symptoms worsen. At that time, the patient should be re-evaluated. If symptoms worsen, and benzathine penicillin was not included in the original therapy, a repeat serologic test for syphilis should be obtained. In all patients not receiving adequate therapy for syphilis, and particularly those without a prompt response to clinical treatment, a serologic test for syphilis 1 to 3 months following therapy is prudent. Some clinicians, and particularly those practicing in areas where syphilis is prevalent, prefer to treat all cases of genital ulcers of unclear etiology with benzathine penicillin, in addition to therapy for other diseases as indicated.[95] Because of the association of genital ulcers with HIV infection, all persons with a genital ulcer of a sexually transmitted or unknown etiology should be offered an initial HIV test (those with genital herpes are at lowest risk and clinicians may use individual judgment based on the presence of other risk factors). If the tests are negative, those with chancroid, syphilis, or unknown causes should be offered a repeat test 3 months later. Sex partners may have histories or illnesses that strongly suggest the illness that the patient has. Sex partners of patients should be seen, examined, and treated for the same conditions for which the patient is receiving therapy.[95]

REFERENCES

1. Stedman's Medical Dictionary, 25th ed. Baltimore, Williams & Wilkins, 1990, p 1661.
2. Plummer FA, D'Costa LJ, Nsanze H, et al: Clinical and microbiologic studies of genital ulcers in Kenya women. Sex Transm Dis 1985; 12:193.
3. Young AW Jr, Tovell HMM, Sadri K: Erosions and ulcers of the vulva: Diagnosis, incidence and management. Obstet Gynecol 1977; 50:35.
4. Piot P, Meheus A: Genital ulcerations. In: Taylor-Robinson D (ed): Clinical Problems in Sexually Transmitted Diseases. Boston, Martinus Nijhoff Publishers, 1985.
5. Frame G, Ferrinho P de LGM, Phakathi G: Patients with sexually transmitted diseases at the Alexandra Health Centre and University Clinic. S Afr Med J 1991; 80:389.
6. Romanowski B, Blackwelder M, Draker JM: Etiology of genital ulceration. [Abstract.] In Programs and Abstracts of the Thirty-second General Assembly of the International Union Against Venereal Diseases and Treponematoses, Montreal, June 17–21, 1984.
7. Dillon SM, Cummings M, Rajagopalan S, McCormack WC: Prospective analysis of genital ulcer disease in Brooklyn, New York. Clin Infect Dis 1997; 24:945.
8. Mertz KJ, Weiss JB, Webb RM, et al: An investigation of genital ulcers in Jackson, Mississippi, with use of a multiplex polymerase chain reaction assay: High prevalence of chancroid and human immunodeficiency virus infection. J Infect Dis 1998; 178:1060.
9. Mertz KJ, Trees D, Levine WC, et al: Etiology of genital ulcers and prevalence of human immunodeficiency virus coinfection in 10 US cities. J Infect Dis 1998; 178:1795.
10. Fast M, D'Costa LJ, Nsanze H, et al: The clinical diagnosis of genital ulcer disease in men in the tropics. Sex Transm Dis 1984; 11:72.
11. O'Farrell N, Hoosen AA, Coetzee KD, van den Ende J: Genital ulcer disease in men in Durban, South Africa. Genitourin Med 1991; 67:327.
12. O'Farrell N, Hoosen AA, Coetzee KD, van den Ende J: Genital ulcer disease in women in Durban, South Africa. Genitourin Med 1991; 67:322.
13. Bogaerts J, Kestens L, van Dyck E, et al: Genital ulcers in a primary health clinic in Rwanda: Impact of HIV infection on diagnosis and ulcer healing (1986–1992). Int J STD AIDS 1998; 9:706.
14. Sehgal VH, Gangwani OP: Genital fixed drug eruptions. Genitourin Med 1986; 62:56.
15. Sharma VK, Dhar S, Gill AN: Drug-related involvement of specific sites in fixed eruptions: A statistical evaluation. J Dermatol 1996; 23:530.
16. Van der Piil JW, Frissen PH, Reiss P, et al: Foscarnet and penile ulceration. Lancet 1990; 335:286.
17. International Study Group for Behcet's Disease: Criteria for diagnosis of Behcet's disease. Lancet 1990; 335:1078.
18. Orme RL, Nordlund JJ, Barich L, Brown T: The MAGIC syndrome (mouth and genital ulcers with inflamed cartilage). Arch Dermatol 1990; 126:940.
19. Kreiss J, Ngugi E, Holmes K, et al: Efficacy of nonoxynol-9 contraceptive sponge use in preventing heterosexual acquisition of HIV in Nairobi prostitutes. JAMA 1992; 268:477.
20. Niruthisard S, Roddy RE, Chutivongse S: The effects of frequent nonoxynol-9 use on the vaginal and cervical mucosa. Sex Transm Dis 1991; 18:176.
21. Roddy RE, Cordero M, Cordero C, Fortney JA: A dosing study of nonoxynol-9 and genital irritation. Int J STD AIDS 1993; 4:165.
22. Weir SS, Roddy RE, Zekeng L, Feldblum PJ: Nonoxynol-9 use, genital ulcers, and HIV infection in a cohort of sex workers. Genitourin Med 1995; 71:78.
23. Portnoy J, Ahronheim GA, Ghibu F, et al: Recovery of Epstein-Barr virus from genital ulcers. N Engl J Med 1984; 311:966.
24. Taylor S, Drake SM, Dedicoat M, Wood MJ: Genital ulcers associated with acute Epstein-Barr virus infection. Sex Transm Dis 1998; 74:296.
25. Lampert A, Assier-Bonnet H, Chevallier B, et al: Lipschutz's genital ulceration: A manifestation of Epstein-Barr virus primary infection. Br J Dermatol 1996; 135:663.
26. Sixbey JW, Lemon SM, Pagano JS: A second site for Epstein-Barr virus shedding: The uterine cervix. Lancet 1986; 1:1122.
27. Graykowski E, Barile M, Lee W, Stanley H Jr: Recurrent aphthous stomatitis: Clinical, therapeutic, and histopathologic and hypersensitivity aspects. JAMA 1966; 196:637.
28. Ship H, Meritt AD, Stanley HR: Recurrent aphthous ulcers. Am J Med 1962; 22:32.
29. Sircus W, Church R, Kelleher J: Recurrent aphthous ulceration of the mouth: A study of the natural history, etiology and treatment. Q J Med 1957; 26:235.
30. Anderson J, Clark RA, Watts DH, et al: Idiopathic genital ulcers in women infected with human immunodeficiency virus. J Acquir Immun Defic Syndr 1996; 13:343.
31. LaGuardia KD, White M, Saigo PE, et al: Genital ulcer disease in women infected with human immunodeficiency virus infection. Am J Obstet Gynecol 1995; 172:553
32. Leibovitz A: An outbreak of pyogenic penile ulcers associated with a microaerophilic streptococcus resembling *Haemophilus ducreyi*. Am J Syph Neurol 1954; 38:203.
33. Ursi JP, Van Dyck E, Ballard RC: Characterization of an unusual bacterium isolated from genital ulcers. J Med Microbiol 1982; 15:97.
34. Bogaerts, J, Vuylsteke B, Martinez Tello W, et al: Simple algorithms for the management of genital ulcers: Evaluation in a primary health care centre in Kigali, Rwanda. Bull WHO 1995; 73:761.
35. Orle KA, Gates CA, Martin DH, et al: Simultaneous PCR detection of *Haemophilus ducreyi, Treponema pallidum,* and herpes simplex virus types 1 and 2 from genital ulcers. J Clin Microbiol 1996; 34:49.
36. Htun Y, Morse SA, Dangor Y, et al: Comparison of clinically directed, disease specific, and syndromic protocols for the management of genital ulcer disease in Lesotho. Sex Transm Infect 1998; 74(suppl):S23.
37. Kamya MR, Nsubuga P, Grant RM, Hellman N: The high

prevalence of genital herpes among patients with genital ulcer disease in Uganda. Sex Transm Dis 1995; 22:351.

38. Beyrer C, Jitwatcharanan K, Natpratan C, et al: Molecular methods for the diagnosis of genital ulcer disease in a sexually transmitted disease clinic population in northern Thailand: Predominance of herpes simplex virus infection. J Infect Dis 1998; 178:243.

39. Chapel TA, Brown WJ, Jeffries C, et al: The microbiological flora of penile ulcerations. J Infect Dis 1978; 137:50.

40. Coovadia YM, Kharsany A, Hoosen A: The microbial etiology of genital ulcers in black men in Durban, South Africa. Genitourin Med 1985; 61:266.

41. Nsanze H, Fast MV, D'Costa LJ, et al: Genital ulcers in Kenya: Clinical and laboratory study. Br J Vener Dis 1981; 57:378.

42. Sturm AW, Stolting GJ, Cormane RH, et al: Clinical and microbiological evaluation of 46 episodes of genital ulceration. Genitourin Med 1987; 63:98.

43. Friedmann W, Schafer A, Kretschmer R: CMV virus infection of the vulva and vagina. Geburtshilfe Frauenheilkd 1990; 50:729.

44. Brathwaite AR, Figueroa JP, Ward E: A comparison of prevalence rates of genital ulcers among persons attending a sexually transmitted disease clinic in Jamaica. W I Med J 1997; 46:67.

45. Langeland N, Haarr L, Mhalu F: Prevalence of HSV-2 antibodies among STD clinic patients in Tanzania. Int J STD AIDS 1998; 9:104.

46. Division of STD Prevention, Sexually Transmitted Diseases Surveillance, 1997. U.S. Department of Health and Human Services, Public Health Service. Atlanta, Centers for Disease Control and Prevention (CDC), September 1998.

47. Schmid GP, Sanders LL, Blount JH, et al: Chancroid in the United States: Reestablishment of an old disease. JAMA 1987; 258:3265.

48. Fleming DT, McQuillan GM, Johnson RE, et al: Herpes simplex virus type 2 in the United States, 1977–1994. N Engl J Med 1997; 337:1105.

49. Shillinger J, Johnson R, St. Louis M, et al: Trends in herpes simplex virus type 1 infection in the United States, 1976–1994. Abstract B2. 1998 National STD Prevention Conference, December 6–9, 1998.

50. Schulte JM, Martich FA, Schmid GP: Chancroid in the United States, 1981–1990: Evidence for underreporting of cases. MMWR 1992; 41(no. SS-3):57.

51. Flood JM, Sarafian SK, Bolan GA, et al: Multistrain outbreak of chancroid in San Francisco, 1989–91. J Infect Dis 1993; 167:1106.

52. Cowan F, Johnson A, Ashley R, et al: Antibody to herpes simplex virus type 2 as a serological marker of sexual lifestyle in populations. Br Med J 1994; 309:1325.

53. Fosgren M, Skoog E, Jeannsson S, et al: Prevalence of antibodies to herpes simplex virus in pregnant women in Stockholm in 1969, 1983, and 1989: Implications for STD epidemiology. Int J STD AIDS 1994; 5:113.

54. Slomka MJ, Emery L, Munday PE, et al: A comparison of PCR with virus isolation and direct antigen detection for diagnosis and typing of genital herpes. J Med Virol 1998; 55:177.

55. Ross JDC, Smith IW, Elton RA: The epidemiology of herpes simplex types 1 and 2 infection of the genital tract in Edinburgh 1978–1991. Genitourin Med 1993; 69:381.

56. Schomogyi M, Wald A, Corey L: Herpes simplex virus-2 infection. Infect Dis Clin North Am 1998; 12:47.

57. Richens J: The diagnosis and treatment of donovanosis (granuloma inguinale). Genitourin Med 1991; 67:441.

58. Carter J, Hutton S, Sriprakash KS, et al: Culture of the causative organism of donovanosis (Calymmatobacterium granulomatis) in Hep-2 cells. J Clin Microbiol 1997; 35:2915.

59. Kharsany AB, Hoosen AA, Kiepiela P, et al: Growth and cultural characteristics of Calymmatobacterium granulomatis—the aetiological agent of granuloma inguinale (Donovanosis). J Med Microbiol 1997; 46:579.

60. Chapel TA: The variability of syphilitic chancres. Sex Transm Dis 1978; 5:68.

61. Mindel A, Tovey SJ, Timmins DJ, et al: Primary and secondary syphilis, 20 years' experience. 2. Clinical features. Genitourin Med 1989; 65:1.

62. Hawkes S, West B, Wilson S, et al: Asymptomatic carriage of Haemophilus ducreyi confirmed by the polymerase chain reaction. Genitourin Med 1995; 71:224.

63. Cowan FM, Johnson AM, Ashley R, et al: Relationship between antibodies to herpes simplex virus (HSV) and symptoms of HSV infection. J Infect Dis 1996; 174:470.

64. Webb DH, Fife KH: Genital herpes simplex virus infection. Infect Dis Clin North Am 1987; 1:97.

65. Langenberg A, Benedetti J, Jenkins J, et al: Development of clinically recognizable genital lesions among women previously identified as having "asymptomatic" herpes simplex virus type 2 infection. Ann Intern Med 1989; 110:882.

66. Wald A, Zeh J, Barnum G, et al: Suppression of subclinical shedding of herpes simplex virus type 2 with acyclovir. Ann Intern Med 1996; 124:8.

67. Wald A, Zeh J, Selke S, et al: Virologic characteristics of subclinical and symptomatic genital herpes infections. N Engl J Med 1995; 333:770.

68. Mertz GH, Schmidt O, Jourden JL, et al: Frequency of acquisition of first-episode genital infection with herpes simplex virus from symptomatic and asymptomatic source contacts. Sex Transm Dis 1985; 12:33.

69. Bryson Y, Dillon M, Bernstein DI, et al: Risk of acquisition of genital herpes simplex virus type-2 in sex partners of persons with genital herpes: A prospective couple study. J Infect Dis 1993; 167:942.

70. Mertz GJ, Benedetti J, Ashley R, et al: Risk factors for the sexual transmission of genital herpes. Ann Intern Med 1992; 116:197.

71. Bernstein DI, Lovett MA, Bryson YJ: Serologic analysis of first-episode nonprimary genital herpes simplex virus infection: Presence of type 2 antibody in acute serum samples. Am J Med 1984; 77:1055.

72. U.S. Department of Health, Education and Welfare: Chancroid, donovanosis, lymphogranuloma venereum. DHEW Publication No. 75-8302, 1964.

73. Hart G: Donovanosis. Clin Infect Dis 1997; 25:24.

74. Jethwa HS, Schmitz JL, Dallabetta G, et al: Comparison of molecular and microscopic techniques for detection of Treponema pallidum in genital ulcers. J Clin Microbiol 1995; 33:180.

75. Musher D: Biology of Treponema pallidum. In: Holmes KK, Mardh PA, Sparling PF, et al (eds): Sexually Transmitted Diseases. New York, McGraw-Hill, 1990, pp 205–219.

76. Larsen SA, Steiner BM, Rudolph AH: Laboratory diagnosis and interpretation of tests for syphilis. Clin Microbiol Rev 1995; 8:1.

77. Kaufman RE, Weiss S, Moore JD, et al: Biological false-positive serological tests for syphilis among drug addicts. Br J Vener Dis 1974; 50:350.

78. Reisner BS, Mann LM, Tholcken CA, et al: Use of the Treponema pallidum–specific Captia syphilis IgG assay in conjunction with the rapid plasma reagin to test for syphilis. J Clin Microbiol 1997; 38:1141.

79. Nayar R, Campos JM: Evaluation of the DCL Syphilis-G enzyme immunoassay test kit for the serologic diagnosis of syphilis. Am J Clin Pathol 1993; 99:282.

80. Carney O, Ross E, Bunker C, et al: A prospective study of the psychological impact on patients with a first episode of genital herpes. Genitourin Med 1994; 70:40.

81. Mosley RC, Covey L, Benjamin D, et al: Comparison of viral isolation, direct immunofluorescence, and indirect immunoperoxidase techniques for detection of genital herpes simplex virus infection. J Clin Microbiol 1981; 13:913.

82. Cone RW, Hobson AC, Palmer J, et al: Extended duration of herpes simplex virus DNA in genital lesions detected by the polymerase chain reaction. J Infect Dis 1991; 164:757.

83. Wald A, Corey L, Cone R, et al: Frequent genital herpes simplex virus 2 shedding in immunocompetent women: Effect of acyclovir treatment. J Clin Invest 1997; 99:1092.

84. Solomon AR, Rasmussen JE, Varani J, et al: The Tzanck smear in the diagnosis of cutaneous herpes simplex. JAMA 1984; 251:633.

85. Munday PE, Vuddamalay J, Slomka MJ, Brown DW: Role of type-specific herpes simplex virus serology in the diagnosis

and management of genital herpes. Sex Transm Infect 1998; 74:175.

86. Taylor DN, Duangmani C, Suvongse C, et al: The role of *Haemophilus ducreyi* in penile ulcers in Bangkok, Thailand. Sex Transm Dis 1984; 11:148.

87. Ronald AR, Plummer FA: Chancroid and *Haemophilus ducreyi*. [Editorial.] Ann Intern Med 1985; 102:705.

88. Pillay A, Hoosen AA, Loykissoonlal D, et al: Comparison of culture media for the laboratory diagnosis of chancroid. J Med Microbiol 1998; 47:1023.

89. Schmid GP, Faur YC, Valu JA, et al: Enhanced recovery of *Haemophilus ducreyi* from clinical specimens by incubation at 33°C vs 35°C. J Clin Microbiol 1995; 33:3257.

90. Bastian I, Bowden FJ: Amplification of *Klebsiella*-like sequences from biopsy samples from patients with donovanosis. Clin Infect Dis 1996; 23:1328.

91. Freinkel AL, Dangor Y, Koornhof HJ, Ballard RC: A serological test for granuloma inguinale. Genitourin Med 1992; 68:269.

92. Hayes RJ, Schulz KF, Plummer FA: The cofactor effect of genital ulcers on the per-exposure risk of HIV transmission in sub-Saharan Africa. J Trop Med Hyg 1995; 98:1.

93. Rolfs RT, Joesoef MR, Hendershot EF, et al: A randomized trial of enhanced therapy for early syphilis in patients with and without human immunodeficiency virus infection. N Engl J Med 1997; 337:307.

94. Hook EW III, Cannon RO, Nahmias AJ, et al: Herpes simplex virus infection as a risk factor for human immunodeficiency virus infection in heterosexuals. J Infect Dis 1992; 165:251.

95. Centers for Disease Control and Prevention: 1998 Guidelines for treatment of sexually transmitted diseases. MMWR 1998; 47(no. RR-1):3.

96. Moses S, Ngugi EN, Bradley JE, et al: Health care–seeking behavior related to the transmission of sexually transmitted diseases in Kenya. Am J Public Health 1994; 84:1947.

97. Dickersin MC, Johnston J, Delea TE, et al: The causal role for genital ulcer disease as a risk factor for transmission of human immunodeficiency virus: An application of the Bradford Hill Criteria. Sex Transm Dis 1996; 23:429.

98. Cameron DW, Simonsen JN, D'Costa LJ, et al: Female-to-male transmission of human immunodeficiency virus type 1: Risk factors for seroconversion in men. Lancet 1989; 2:403.

99. Plourde PJ, Pepin J, Agoki E, et al: Human immunodeficiency virus type 1 seroconversion in women with genital ulcers. J Infect Dis 1994; 170:313.

100. Telzak EE, Chaisson MA, Bevier PJ, et al: HIV-1 seroconversion in patients with and without genital ulcer disease. Ann Intern Med 1993; 119:1181.

101. Kreiss J, Coombs R, Plummer F, et al: Isolation of human immunodeficiency virus from genital ulcers in Nairobi prostitutes. J Infect Dis 1989; 160:380.

102. Plummer FA, Wainberg MA, Plourde P, et al: Detection of human immunodeficiency virus type 1 (HIV-1) in genital ulcer exudate of HIV-1–infected men by culture and gene amplification. J Infect Dis 1990; 161:810.

103. Schacker T, Ryncarz AJ, Goddard J, et al: Frequent recovery of HIV-1 from genital herpes simplex virus lesions in HIV-infected men. JAMA 1998; 280:61.

104. Gadkari DA, Quinn TC, Gangakhedkar RR, et al: HIV-DNA shedding in genital ulcers and its associated risk factors in Pune, India. J Acquir Immune Defic Syndr Hum Retrovirol 1998; 18:277.

105. Schacker TW, Hughes JP, Shea T, et al: Biological and virologic characteristics of primary HIV infection. Ann Intern Med 1998; 128:613.

106. Koelle DM, Abbo H, Peck A, et al: Direct recovery of HSV-specific T-lymphocyte clones from recurrent genital HSV-2 lesions. J Infect Dis 1994; 169:956.

107. Spinola SM, Orazi A, Arno JN, et al: *Haemophilus ducreyi* elicits a cutaneous infiltrate of CD4 cells during experimental human infection. J Infect Dis 1996; 173:394.

108. Moses S, Plummer FA, Bradley JA, et al: The association between lack of male circumcision and risk for HIV infection: A review of the epidemiological data. Sex Transm Dis 1994; 21:201.

109. Nasio JM, Nagelkerke NJD, Mwatha A, et al: Genital ulcer disease among STD clinic attenders in Nairobi: Association with HIV-1 and circumcision status. Int J STD AIDS 1996; 7:410.

110. Kaul R, Kimani J, Nagelkerke NJD, et al: Risk factors for genital ulcerations in Kenyan sex workers: The role of human immunodeficiency virus type 1 infection. Sex Transm Dis 1997; 24:387.

111. Ghys PD, Diallo MO, Ettiegne-Traore V, et al: Genital ulcers associated with human immunodeficiency virus–related immunosuppression in female sex workers in Abdijan, Ivory Coast. J Infect Dis 1995; 172:1371.

112. Schmid GP: Treatment of chancroid, 1999. Clin Infect Dis 1999; (S)1:S29–36.

113. Chapel TA, Brown WJ, Jeffries C, Stewart JA: How reliable is the morphological diagnosis of penile ulcerations? Sex Transm Dis 1977; 4:150.

Antimicrobials

45

Penicillins

SEBASTIAN FARO

In 1928 while working at St. Mary's Hospital in London, Alexander Fleming observed that colonies of *Staphylococcus aureus* growing on a culture plate had been contaminated by *Penicillium notatum*. In the area where the two organisms were in close proximity, there was lysis of colonies of *S. aureus*. As the colonies were farther removed from the growing colony of *P. notatum*, lysis of the bacterial colonies diminished.[1, 2] At that time, Fleming did not truly appreciate these astounding observations. He did, however, test the substance, which he named penicillin, using filtrated broth from a culture of *P. notatum*. He demonstrated that this broth filtrate had selective antibacterial activity and was not toxic to rabbits. Twelve years later, Fleming wrote that the substance, when used as a topical antiseptic, yielded good results, but that "the trouble of making it seemed not worth while."[3]

In 1939, Floery and colleagues[3] proceeded to work out the isolation, structure, and chemical properties of penicillin. In the early 1940s, they demonstrated the effectiveness of penicillin in treating mice infected with streptococci. They also treated a few patients successfully.[3] World War II hastened large-scale production of penicillin. Production efforts led to the discovery that *Penicillium chrysogenum* yielded greater amounts of penicillin.

Thus, the discovery of penicillin opened the door to the development of antibiotics that continues today. Penicillin must be considered one of the greatest discoveries to benefit human beings around the world.

MECHANISM OF ACTION

The penicillin molecule consists of three components (Fig. 45–1), a thiazolidine ring, the beta-lactam ring, and a side chain.[4] The side chain is mainly responsible for the antibacterial spectrum and pharmacologic properties of the molecule; the beta-lactam nucleus provides antibacterial activity[4] (Table 45–1).

Penicillin's exact mechanism of action is not known. However, it is known that penicillin inhibits bacterial cell wall synthesis, binds with penicillin-binding proteins, and may be resistant to beta-lactamases. This latter ability is seen with the newer penicillins, such as piperacillin and ticarcillin, and their associated antibiotics, the beta-lactamase inhibitors (i.e., tazobactam and clavulanic acid).

The bacterial cell wall is a complex structure made up of alternating molecules of *N*-acetylglucosamine and *N*-acetylmuramic acid arranged linearly. The cell wall of gram-positive bacteria is thick, approximately 50 to 100 molecular layers. The cell wall of gram-negative bacteria is thin, only 1 to 2 layers in depth.[5, 6] The linear polymers are cross-linked by short peptides attached to *N*-acetylmuramic acid.[6] These peptides are cross-linked via amide linkage to D-alanine in gram-positive bacteria. In gram-negative bacteria, the cross-linkage is between diampimelic acid and the terminal alanine of an adjacent peptide.[6] It appears that penicillin inactivates transpeptidases, thus preventing the amide linkages between the short-chain peptides in the cell wall.[6]

Spratt[7, 8] discovered the presence of penicillin-binding proteins (PBPs) in the bacterial cell membrane and facilitated our understanding of their role in reproduction and morphology of the bacterial cell. The PBPs are found in the bacterial kingdom and, within a species, are numbered according to molecular weight, with the heaviest given number 1. The PBPs that are important in gram-negative bacteria appear to be 1, 2, and 3. If *Escherichia coli* is exposed to a low concentration of penicillin, the bacteria develop into filamentous forms, whereas high concentrations result

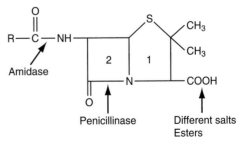

FIGURE 45–1 ▶ Chemical structure of penicillins. (From Andriole VT: Current Infectious Disease Drugs. Philadelphia, Current Medicine, 1996, p 62.)

TABLE 45-1 ▸ CLASSIFICATION OF THE PENICILLINS

Natural Penicillins
Penicillin G (oral, IM, IV)
Penicillin G potassium or sodium (IV)
Penicillin V (oral)
Phenethicillin (oral)
Penicillinase-Resistant Penicillins
Methicillin (IM, IV)
Nafcillin (IM, IV)
Isoxazolyl penicillins
   Cloxacillin (oral)
   Dicloxacillin (oral)
   Flucloxacillin (oral)
   Oxacillin (oral, IM, IV)
Aminopenicillins
Ampicillin (oral, IM, IV)
Amoxicillin (oral)
Bacampicillin (oral)
Cyclacillin (oral)
Epicillin (oral)
Hetacillin (oral)
Pivampicillin (oral)
Antipseudomonal Penicillins
Azlocillin (IM, IV)
Carbenicillin (IM, IV)
Indanylcarbenicillin (oral)
Ticarcillin (IM, IV)
Extended Penicillins
Mezlocillin (IM, IV)
Piperacillin (IM, IV)
Amidino Penicillins
Amdinocillin (IM, IV)
Pivamdinocillin (oral)
Stable Against Gram-Negative Beta-Lactamases
Temocillin (IM, IV)
Combination Penicillin + Beta-Lactamase Inhibitor
Ampicillin + sulbactam (IM, IV)
Piperacillin + tazobactam (IM, IV)
Ticarcillin + clavulanate (IM, IV)
Amoxicillin + clavulanate (oral)

Modified from Neu H: Penicillins. In: Mandell GL, Douglas RG, Bennett JE (eds): Principles and Practice of Infectious Diseases, 3rd ed. New York, Churchill Livingstone, 1985, pp 230–246.

in lysis of the bacteria.[8] Amdinocillin (mecillinam) binding to PBP 2 results in the development of spherical forms that initially are osmotically stable, but after several hours undergo lysis.[9] PBP 3 plays a role in cell division of members of the Enterobacteriaceae and pseudomonads.[10] The PBPs that are important in gram-positive bacteria are PBPs-1, -2, and -4.[11] The lack of activity of beta-lactam antibiotics against certain gram-positive and anaerobic bacteria results from the inability of these agents (e.g., aztreonam) to bind to PBPs.[12]

RESISTANCE

Resistance to penicillin can be achieved by a variety of mechanisms. Alteration in the structure of PBPs can prevent binding of penicillin. In the absence of binding to the PBPs, cell wall synthesis continues unabated. Bacteria that are resistant to penicillin have been found to have altered PBPs and produce an altered peptidoglycan[13] (Table 45–2).

In some instances, the penicillin may fail to reach its target. However, this mechanism is unlikely in gram-positive bacteria because the peptidoglycan is external to the cell membrane. Gram-negative bacteria have an outer membrane and an inner membrane between which lies the peptidoglycan.[14] Alterations in the cell membrane prohibit passage of the bacteria through the membrane.

The hydrolysis of the beta-lactam ring by bacterial beta-lactamases is probably the most important mechanism by which the bacteria are resistant to penicillin.[15] The beta-lactamases are classified according to whether they are chromosomal or plasmid derived (Table 45–3). Gram-positive bacteria can be induced to produce the enzyme and secrete it into the environment; it is an exoenzyme. In gram-negative bacteria, the beta-lactamases are confined within the periplasmic space, thereby prohibiting the antibiotic from reaching its target. The beta-lactamases of gram-negative bacteria are either constitutive or inducible, and are effective against both the penicillins and the cephalosporins.

PHARMACOLOGY

The penicillins are eliminated from the kidney mainly via tubular excretion. The isoxazolyl penicillins (e.g., nafcillin) and ureidopenicillins (e.g., piperacillin) have a dual method of excretion through tubular secretion from the kidney, and, for approximately 25% to 40%, via bleary secretion.[16, 17] The half-lives of the penicillins range from 30 to 60 minutes[16, 18]; therefore, they must be given every 6 hours. The pharmacologic characteristics are listed in Table 45–4.

CLINICAL USES OF PENICILLINS

The clinical use of penicillins covers a large spectrum of diseases—respiratory, skin, and skin related structures, bone, intra-abdominal, and pelvic—as well as prophylaxis. The development of the beta-lactamase inhibitors and their use in conjunction with broad-spectrum penicillins (e.g., ampicillin, piperacillin, and ticarcillin) have broadened the spectrum of antibacterial activity to include many beta-lactamase–producing facultative anaerobic bacteria as well as obligate anaerobic bacteria. Table 45–5 lists some of the clinical applications of the penicillins.

ADVERSE REACTIONS

The primary toxicity to penicillins is hypersensitivity allergic reaction. The first reported case of serious toxicity to penicillin was anaphylaxis in 1946.[21] The first reported death attributed to penicillin toxicity was reported in 1949.[22] The overall incidence of adverse reactions to penicillin is 0.7% to 4%.[23] There are basically five types of adverse (immunopathologic) reac-

TABLE 45-2 ▶ ANTIBACTERIAL SENSITIVITIES OF VARIOUS BETA-LACTAM ANTIBIOTICS

Organism	Amox	Amox + Clavul	MIC (µg/mL) Ticar	Ticar +	Amp Clavul	Amp + Sulbact	Pip	Pip + Tazob
*Staphylococcus aureus**	256	1	8	0.25–1	>200	6.25	>128	4
*S. epidermidis**	—	—	—	—	—	—	>25	1.56
Streptococcus pyogenes	0.01	0.01	—	—	0.025	0.025	—	—
Enterococcus faecalis	1.56	1.56	—	—	—	—	4	4
*Haemophilus influenzae**	64	0.5	1–8	.06–0.12	200	1.56	512	4
*Neisseria gonorrhoeae**	128	1	32	0.5	>10	0.31		
*Escherichia coli**	>512	8	>128	16	100	25	>128	8
*Klebsiella pneumoniae**	64	2	>128	4	50	6.25	>128	16
*Proteus mirabilis**	>512	4	0.25–64	0.25–1			2	2
Proteus vulgaris	—	—	—	—		>200	3.12	8	2
Yersinia enterocolitica	32	8	—	—	—	—	—	—
Enterobacter spp.	512	64	2–128	2–128	—	—	—	—
Enterobacter cloacae	—	—	—	—	200	50	—	—
Enterobacter aerogenes	—	—	—	—	—	—	32	8
Providencia rettgeri	64	32	1–128	1–64	—	—	—	—
Morganella morgagnii	64	64	0.5–1	0.50–.8	50	3.12	—	—
*Moraxella catarrhalis**	—	—	—	—	—	—	8	0.125
Serratia marcescens	64	64	>128	>128	200	12.5	—	—
Campylobacter jejuni	4	4	—	—	—	—	—	—
Pseudomonas aeruginosa	>512	512	8–1024	8–64	>400	1000	16	16
Stenotrophomonas maltophilia	—	—	512	128	—	—	>128	>128
Acinetobacter spp.	—	—	—	—	—	—	128	32
Bacteroides fragilis	32	0.5	4–1.024	0.008–8	200	3.12	128	4
Prevotella melaninogenica	16	0.1	—	—	—	—	—	—

*Beta-lactamase–producing strains resistant to amoxicillin, ampicillin, and piperacillin.
Data from Kucers A, Crowe ML, Grayson ML, Hoy J: The Use of Antibiotics: A Clinical Review of Antibacterial, Antifungal, and Antiviral Drugs, 5th ed. Oxford, Butterworth-Heinemann, 1997, pp 313, 211, 222.

TABLE 45-3 ▶ MICROBIAL BETA-LACTAMASES

GRAM-POSITIVE BACTERIA

Chromosomal	Plasmid
Bacillus species (penicillinase)	*S. aureus**
	*S. epidermidis**
	*S. haemolyticus**
Zn-stimulated	*E. faecalis** (TEM) (penicillinases primarily)
Enzyme hydrolyzes	
All beta-lactams	

GRAM-NEGATIVE BACTERIA

Chromosomal

Cephalosporinases
(Richmond Sykes type II)

Inducible	Constitutive	Broad-Spectrum	Cefuroxinases
Enterobacter	*Enterobacter*	*Klebsiella** (Richmond Sykes type IV)	*P. vulgaris**
C. freundii	*C. freundii*	*Bacteroides**	*P. cepacia*
S. marcescens	*Acinetobacter*	*Legionella**	
P. aeruginosa	*Bacteroides**		
M. morganii			
Providencia			
All Beta-Lactams			
Xanthomonas maltophilia			

Plasmid

Broad-Spectrum (Richmond Sykes type III)	Carbenicillinases	Oxacillinase	Cefotaximase
Tem-1*	Carb 1, 2, 3, 4*	Oxa 1, 2, 3, 4, 5, 6, 7*	TEM 3, 4, 5, 6, 7, 8*
TEM-2*	*Pseudomonas*	Enterobacteriaceae	Enterobacteriaceae (*Klebsiella*)
SHV-1*	*E. coli*		SHV-2, 3, 4, 5*
HMS-1*			
Enterobacteriaceae			
Neisseria gonorrhoeae			

*Inhibited by clavulanate, sulbactam, and tazobactam.
Adapted from Neu H: Penicillins. In: Mandell GL, Douglas RG, Bennett JE (eds): Principles and Practice of Infectious Diseases, 3rd ed. New York, Churchill Livingstone, 1985, pp 230–246.

TABLE 45–4 ▶ PHARMACOKINETIC CHARACTERISTICS OF THE PENICILLINS

Drug	Oral Bio-1 Availability (%)	Dose	Cmax, mg/L	Half-Life	Protein Binding (%)	Route of Excretion
Penicillin G	<20	2 g IV	120	0.5	60	R
Penicillin V	60	0.5 g	5	0.5	78	R
Methicillin	<5	2 g IV	100	0.5	37	R
Oxacillin	30	2 g IV	200	0.4	93	R + H
Cloxacillin	50	0.5 g PO	12	0.4	94	R + H
Dicloxacillin	50	0.5 g PO	15	0.7	97	R + H
Nafcillin	25	2 g IV	160	0.5	89	R + H
Ampicillin	40	2 g IV	100	1.0	18	R
Amoxicillin	80	0.5 g PO	8	0.9	17	R
Ticarcillin	<5	2 g IV	170	1.2	45	R
Mezlocillin	<5	2 g IV	200	1.0	35	R + H
Piperacillin	<5	2 g IV	200	1.0	50	R + H
Clavulanic acid	70	0.125 PO	3	0.8	<15	R
Sulbactam	<10	1 g IV	50	1.0	<15	R

H = hepatic; R = renal.
From Craig WA: Penicillins. In: Andriole VT (ed): Current Infectious Disease Drugs. Philadelphia, Current Medicine, 1996, pp 62–65.

tions that can occur secondary to penicillin administration (Table 45–6).[24] Although the risk of having a hypersensitivity reaction to penicillin is relatively low, if there is a prior history of an adverse reaction there is a 4- to 6-fold increased chance of a subsequent reaction if the patient is re-exposed to a penicillin.[25] It must be emphasized that most individuals who develop a serious and fatal allergic reaction to beta-lactam antibiotics are those with no prior history of an allergic reaction. It is theorized that these individuals may have been sensitized via their last exposure for treatment of an infection.[26] It has also been hypothesized that sensitization could occur via environmental factors, such as penicillin or other beta-lactam antibiotics being present in breast milk or in cows, steers, or pigs being treated with penicillins. Sensitization could also occur as the result of contact with the antibiotic during the manufacturing process.[22, 27–29] Penicillin allergy has

TABLE 45–5 ▶ CLINICAL APPLICATIONS AND PROPERTIES OF INDIVIDUAL PENICILLINS

Drug	Description
Natural Penicillins	
Penicillin G	Available in oral and parenteral (IM, IV, and intrathecal) forms.
	Oral form should be taken 1 hour prior to or 2 hours after meals.
	Used for gram-positive infections, e.g., *Streptococcus pneumoniae*, *S. pyogenes*, *S. agalactiae*, *S. viridans*, *S. moniliformis*, *Treponema pallidum*, *Erysipelothrix*, and *Pasteurella multocida*.
	Benzathine penicillin is administered IM (repository form) for slow release. Used for the treatment of primary and secondary syphilis.
Penicillin V	Available for oral use. Should be used instead of penicillin G.
	Available in dosages of 125, 250, and 500 mg.
	Use primarily in situations where Penicillin G is not needed; that is, the infection is not severe and can be treated with oral penicillin.
Penicillinase-Resistant Penicillins	
Methicillin	Available for parenteral use. Indicated for the treatment of non–methicillin–resistant *Staphylococcus aureus* and *S. epidermidis* strains. Methicillin is typically resistant to beta-lactamase–producing strains. Methicillin resistance is due to altered PBPs.
	Dosage is 4 to 12 g/day for adults, administered every 4 to 6 hours.
Nafcillin	Available for oral and parenteral use; however, the preferred route of administration is intravenous. Indications for use are the same as those for methicillin. Dosage is 4 to 9 g/day, administered every 4 to 6 hours.
Isoxazolyl Penicillins	
	Stable against staphylococcal beta-lactamases. Methicillin-resistant *S. aureus* and many strains of *S. epidermidis* are resistant to isoxazolyl penicillins. These antibiotics are not active against gram-negative bacteria. Bacterial resistance to the isoxazolyl penicillins is due primarily to alterations in the PBPs.
Oxacillin	Available for oral use in 250-mg and 500-mg capsules or suspension. Dosage: 1 to 4 g/day, taken 1 to 2 hours prior to meals. Intramuscular or intravenous administration is 2 to 12 g/day every 4 to 6 hours.
Cloxacillin	Available for oral use in capsules of 250 and 500 mg or suspension (125 mg/5 mL). Dosage is 1 to 4 g/day.
Dicloxacillin	Available for oral use in capsules of 125 and 250 mg and suspension (62.5 mg/5 mL). Dosage is 250 mg to 1 g/day every 6 hours.

also been related to receiving a transfusion of blood obtained from an individual recently treated with penicillin.[30]

SKIN TESTING FOR ALLERGY TO PENICILLIN

Patients with a suspected but undocumented allergy to penicillin may benefit from skin testing. However, testing may not be practical, and great care must be taken when one administers the test. Even when the penicillin determinants for skin testing have been used, anaphylactoid reactions have occurred. The penicilloyl-polylysine (PPL), a penicillin derivative, is termed the major antigenic determinant.[31] The minor determinants are also penicillin degradation products, for example, penicillinic acid and penillic acid.[32] Although skin testing with the major and minor determinants is safer than testing with native penicillin, the test does not detect all the individuals who are allergic to peni-

---

TABLE 45–5 ▸ **CLINICAL APPLICATIONS AND PROPERTIES OF INDIVIDUAL PENICILLINS** *Continued*

Drug	Description
Aminopenicillins	Not stable against beta-lactamases of gram-positive and gram-negative bacteria. In comparison to penicillin G, the aminopenicillins have variable activity against a variety of bacteria:

<**Penicillin G**	>**Penicillin G**	=**Penicillin G**
Streptococcus agalactiae	*Enterococcus faecalis*	*Clostridium*
Streptococcus pneumoniae	*Listeria monocytogenes*	
	Haemophilus influenzae	
	H. parainfluenzae	

Drug	Description
	Haemophilus sensitivity is variable and is dependent on whether the isolate produces beta-lactamase.
	E. coli sensitivity varies, with hospital strains tending to be resistant.
	The following bacteria tend to be resistant to the aminopenicillins because of beta-lactamase production: *Salmonella typhi, Shigella sonnei, Klebsiella, Serratia, Acinetobacter,* indole-positive *Proteus, Pseudomonas,* and *Bacteroides fragilis.*
Ampicillin	Available for oral use in capsules of 125, 250, and 500 mg; suspension of 125 and 250 mg/5 mL; drops of 100 mg/mL; and 125-mg chewable tablets.
	Suspension of 3.5 g of ampicillin trihydrate plus 1 g of probenecid.
	Ampicillin trihydrate for IM use. The sodium salt is available for intravenous use.
	Oral dose 2 to 4 g/day.
	Parenteral dose is 1 to 3 g/day every 4 hours.
Bacampicillin	Available for oral use, suspension 125 mg/mL or tablets 400 mg.
	The 400-mg dose is equivalent to 280 mg of ampicillin. Must be hydrolyzed to ampicillin.
	No advantage over ampicillin other than better absorption when taken with food than ampicillin.
Cyclacillin	No advantage over ampicillin.
Amoxicillin	Available for oral use, 250-mg capsules to be taken every 8 hours.
Carboxy Penicillins	Basically used as antipseudomonal agents.
Carbenicillin	Available for intravenous use. Dosage is 400 to 600 mg/kg/day every 4 hours. Patients with a creatinine clearance of <10 mL/min should not receive more than 2 g every 8 hours.
Ticarcillin	Available for intravenous use. Dosage is 1 to 6 g/day, depending on the severity of the infection and the renal status of the patient. In general, ticarcillin requires less dosing than carbenicillin; therefore, there is likely a reduced risk for platelet dysfunction.
Indanyl Carbenicillin	Available for oral use. Dosage is 500 mg (contains 382 mg of carbenicillin), to be taken every 6 hours. Primary use is as an alternative to quinolones for the treatment of *Pseudomonas* cystitis.
Ureidopenicillins	A broad-spectrum group of penicillins with enhanced antibacterial activity that includes gram-negative facultative anaerobes and obligate anaerobic bacteria. Available for parenteral use.
Azlocillin	More active against *Pseudomonas* than is carbenicillin. This agent is indicated primarily for *Pseudomonas.*
Mezlocillin	Available for intravenous use. Dosage 12 to 18 g/day. It is active against *Enterococcus faecalis, Klebsiella, Haemophilus influenzae,* and *Bacteroides fragilis.* It displays synergy with aminoglycosides against gram-negative facultative anaerobic bacteria.
Piperacillin	Probably the broadest spectrum of antibacterial activity of the class.
	Available for intravenous use. Dosage is 12 to 18 g/day. It is active against *Neisseria, Streptococcus* species, *Haemophilus,* and many gram-negative facultative anaerobes as well as gram-negative and gram-positive obligate anaerobic bacteria.
Beta-Lactamase Inhibitors	The beta-lactamase inhibitors, clavulanate, sulbactam, and tazobactam, act by competitively binding to beta-lactamase, causing destruction of the enzyme by forming an acyl enzyme intermediate.[19, 20] These agents have weak antibacterial activity but have much stronger anti–beta-lactamase activity than do the beta-lactam antibiotics.
	Combining a beta-lactamase inhibitor with a beta-lactam antibiotic increases the spectrum of antibacterial activity of the latter compound significantly. This is especially true for the gram-negative facultative anaerobic bacteria as well as the obligate anaerobic bacteria. Comparison of these agents (amoxicillin/clavulanic acid, ampicillin/sulbactam, piperacillin/tazobactam, and ticarcillin/clavulanic acid) is depicted in Table 46–2.

TABLE 45–6 ▶ IMMUNOPATHOLOGIC REACTIONS TO PENICILLIN

Type of Reaction	Description	Primary Effector Mechanism			Clinical Reaction
		Antibody	*Cells*	*Other*	
I	Anaphylactic (reaginic) Fatality, 1:50,000–100,000	IgE	Basophils Mast cells		Anaphylaxis occurs in 0.004%–0.015% of treatment courses. Urticaria, laryngeal edema, bronchospasm; cardiovascular collapse can occur. Clinical manifestations are due to the release of histamine, proteases, chemotactic factors, prostaglandins, leukotrienes, platelet-activating factor. Reaction occurs immediately within 1 hour of initial administration of antibiotic.
II	Cytotoxic or cytolytic damage	IgG, IgM	Any cell with isoantigen	C RES	Coombs-positive hemolytic anemia: drug-induced nephritis
III	Immune complex disease	Soluble immune complexes (Ag-Ab)	None directly	C	Serum sickness; drug fever
IV	Delayed or cell-mediated hypersensitivity	None known	Sensitized T lymphocytes		Contact dermatitis
V	Idiopathic	IgM? ?	? ? ? ?	? ? ? ?	Maculopapular eruptions Eosinophilia Stevens-Johnson syndrome Exfoliative dermatitis

Ag-Ab = antigen-antibody; C = complement; RES = reticuloendothelial system; ? = immunologic mechanism in doubt.

Data from Weiss ME, Adkinson NF: β-Lactam allergy. In: Mandell GL, Douglas RG Jr, Bennett JE (eds): Principles and Practice of Infectious Diseases, 3rd ed. New York, Churchill Livingstone, 1990, p 264; and Gell PGH, Coombs RRA: Classification of allergic reactions responsible for clinical hypersensitivity and disease. In: Gell PGH, Coombs RRA, Hachmann PJ (eds): Clinical Aspects of Immunology. Oxford, Blackwell Scientific Publications, 1975; pp 761–782.

cillin, especially those most likely to have an anaphylactoid reaction. The predictive value of penicillin skin testing can be enhanced if the test includes PPL minor determinants and some crystalline penicillin G.[33, 34] However, skin testing is still unsatisfactory for individuals with a history of penicillin allergy. Fortunately, there are other antibiotics for use in place of penicillin. The one area that still requires the use of penicillin, however, is the treatment of syphilis in the pregnant patient. Individuals who are pregnant and known to have syphilis, and are allergic to penicillin, should be desensitized.

Desensitization to penicillin should be performed in an intensive care unit, or at a place where all the equipment for resuscitation and necessary personnel are readily available in the event the patient develops an anaphylactoid reaction. Two protocols have been developed, one using oral penicillin and the other using parenteral penicillin (Tables 45–7 and 45–8).

If the patient develops a mild systemic reaction (e.g., pruritus, urticaria, rhinitis, or mild wheezing), the dose should be repeated until it is tolerated and there are no signs of systemic reaction.[26] If a serious reaction occurs, such as a significant decrease in blood pressure, laryngeal edema, or asthma, appropriate therapy should be instituted. A decision must be made to either discontinue desensitization or continue it. If the latter course is taken, the next dose should be decreased 10-fold and not administered until the patient

is stable.[36] At the time that desensitization has been accomplished, treatment must be completed. Allowing a lapse of time between desensitization and treatment places the patient at risk for an allergic reaction. If the patient requires treatment with a beta-lactam antibiotic in the future, desensitization will have to be repeated.[26]

JARISCH-HERXHEIMER REACTION

Patients infected with *Treponema* (e.g., *Treponema pallidum*) and treated with penicillin may experience a reaction characterized by fever, myalgia, hypotension, and tachycardia. This has been termed the *Jarisch-Herxheimer reaction*.[38] The Jarisch-Herxheimer reaction has also been seen when penicillin was used in the treatment of leptospirosis, yaws, rat-bite fever, and anthrax.[39] The reaction is secondary to the release of cytokines, which occurs within 6 to 8 hours of the administration of penicillin and lasts up to 24 hours.[40] Fekade and co-workers[41] found that the Jarisch-Herxheimer reaction was associated with the release of and increase in plasma tumor necrosis factor alpha, interleukin-6 (IL-6), and IL-8. These investigators demonstrated that the administration of antibody to tumor necrosis factor alpha could suppress the Jarisch-Herxheimer reaction. They conducted a double-blind, randomized, placebo-controlled trial in 49 patients known to have louse-borne relapsing fever.

The Jarisch-Herxheimer reaction is of particular im-

TABLE 45-7 ▶ ORAL DESENSITIZATION PROTOCOL FOR PENICILLIN ALLERGIC PATIENTS

Step*	Phenoxymethyl Penicillin (units/mL)	Amount (mL)	Dose (Units)	Cumulative Dosage (units)
1	1,000	0.1	100	100
2	1,000	0.2	200	300
3	1,000	0.4	400	700
4	1,000	0.8	800	1,500
5	1,000	1.6	1,600	3,100
6	1,000	3.2	3,200	6,300
7	1,000	6.4	6,400	12,700
8	10,000	1.2	12,000	24,700
9	10,000	2.4	24,000	48,700
10	10,000	4.8	48,000	96,700
11	80,000	1.0	80,000	176,000
12	80,000	2.0	160,000	336,700
13	80,000	4.0	320,000	656,700
14	80,000	8.0	640,000	1,296,700
		Observe patient for 30 minutes		
15	500,000	0.25	125,000	
16	500,000	0.50	250,000	
17	500,000	1.00	500,000	
18	500,000	2.25	1,125,000	

*Interval between steps, 15 min.
From Weiss ME, Adkinson NF: β-Lactam allergy. In: Mandell GL, Douglas RG Jr, Bennett JE (eds): Principles and Practice of Infectious Diseases, 3rd ed. New York, Churchill Livingstone, 1990, pp 264–269.

portance when it occurs in the pregnant patient. The pregnant patient diagnosed with syphilis and treated with penicillin may experience the Jarisch-Herxheimer reaction and develop premature labor with premature delivery.[42] Therefore, all pregnant patients with syphilis and treated with penicillin should be observed for approximately 12 hours for the development of the Jarisch-Herxheimer reaction. This includes monitoring the mother for uterine contractions and monitoring the fetus for evidence of distress. Wendel[42] reported that 78% of pregnant patients treated for primary or secondary syphilis in the second or third trimester experienced the Jarisch-Herxheimer reaction. Approximately 79% of these women develop fever and uterine contractions simultaneously. Some of the fetuses exhibit signs of distress; that is, tachycardia and decelerations in the fetal heart in association with uterine contractions. Uterine contractions and fetal tachycardia resolved within 24 hours after completion of therapy, as did the Jarisch-Herxheimer reaction.

TABLE 45-8 ▶ PARENTERAL PROTOCOL FOR DESENSITIZING PATIENTS ALLERGIC TO PENICILLIN

Injection No.	Benzylpenicillin Concentration (units/mL)	Volume and Route (CC)*
1†	100	0.1 ID
2	100	0.2 SC
3	100	0.4 SC
4	100	0.8 SC
5†	1000	0.1 ID
6	1000	0.3 SC
7	1000	0.6 SC
8†	10,000	0.1 ID
9	10,000	0.2 SC
10	10,000	0.4 SC
11	10,000	0.8 SC
12†	100,000	0.1 ID
13	100,000	0.3 SC
14	100,000	0.6 SC
15†	1,000,000	0.1 ID
16	1,000,000	0.2 SC
17	1,000,000	0.2 IM
18	1,000,000	0.4 IM
19	Continuous IV infusion (1,000,000 units/hr)	

*Administer progressive doses at intervals of not less than 20 minutes.
†Observe and record skin wheal and flare response to intradermal dose.
ID: intradermal; SC: subcutaneous; IM: intramuscular; IV: intravenous.
From Weiss ME, Adkinson NF: B-Lactam allergy. In: Mandell GL, Douglas RG Jr, Bennett JE (eds): Principles and Practice of Infectious Diseases, 3rd ed. New York, Churchill Livingstone, 1990, pp 264–269.

SUMMARY

The penicillins afford the practitioner a wide array of agents for the treatment of a variety of infections. The penicillins can be used for the treatment of infections caused by aerobic, facultative, and obligate anaerobic gram-positive and gram-negative bacteria. The combination of broad-spectrum penicillin and a beta-lactamase inhibitor permits the use of these agents for the treatment of infections caused by organisms resistant to the parent penicillin. The fact that the penicillins have proved safe for use in pregnant patients provides the obstetrician the same opportunity to use these agents with a significant margin of safety in the fetus. However, the physician must always be mindful of the serious adverse reactions that can result from treatment with beta-lactam antibiotics, especially anaphylaxis and, in the pregnant patient, the Jarisch-Herxheimer reaction.

REFERENCES

1. Fleming A: On the bacterial action of cultures of a penicillin, with special reference to their use in isolation of *B. influenzae*. Br J Exp Pathol 1929; 10:226.
2. Abraham EP: Fleming's discovery. Rev Infect Dis 1980; 2:140.
3. Morin RB, Gorman M: Chemistry and Biology of β-Lactam Antibiotics, vol. 1. Penicillins and Cephalosporins. New York, Academic Press, 1982, pp, xxi–xl.
4. Neu H: Penicillins. In: Mandell GL, Douglas RG, Bennett JE (eds): Principles and Practice of Infectious Diseases, 3rd ed. New York, Churchill Livingstone, 1985, pp 230–246.
5. Tipper DJ, Wright A: The structure and biosynthesis of bacterial walls. In: Shokatch JR, Ornstein LA (eds): The Bacteria, v. 7. New York, Academic Press, 1979, p 291.
6. Strominger JL: Penicillin-sensitive enzymatic reactions in bacterial cell wall synthesis. Harvey Lect 1968–69; 64:179.
7. Spratt BG: Distinct penicillin-binding proteins involved in the division, elongation, and shape of *Escherichia coli* K-12. Proc Natl Acad Sci USA 1975; 72:2999.
8. Spratt BG: Biochemical and genetical approaches to the mechanism of action of penicillin. Philos Trans R Soc Lond (Biol) 1980; 289:273.
9. Tamaki S, Nakajima S, Matsuhashi M: Thermosensitive mutation in *Escherichia coli* simultaneously causing defects in penicillin-binding protein-1 Bs and in enzyme activity for peptidoglycan synthesis in vitro. Proc Natl Acad Sci USA 1977; 74:5472.
10. Spratt BG, Bowler LB, Edelman A, et al: Membrane topography of PBPs 7B and 3 of *E. coli* and the production of water-soluble forms of high molecular weight PBPs. In: Shockman GD (ed): Antibiotic Inhibition of Bacterial Cell Surface Assembly and Function. Washington, DC, American Society for Microbiology, 1998, pp 292–300.
11. Yocum RR, Rasmussen JR, Strominger JL: The mechanism of action of penicillin: Penicillin acylates the active site of *Bacillus stearothermophilus* D-alanine carboxypeptidase. J Biol Chem 1980; 255:3977.
12. Georgopapadakou NH, Liu FY: Binding of β-lactam antibiotics to penicillin-binding proteins of *Staphylococcus aureus* and *Streptococcus faecalis*: Relation to antibacterial activity. Antimicrob Agents Chemother 1980; 18:834.
13. Garcia-Bustos JF, Chait BT, Tomasz A: Altered peptidoglycan structure in a pneumococcal transformant resistant to penicillin. J Bacteriol 1988; 170:2143.
14. Tomasz A: Penicillin tolerance and the control of murein hydrolases. In: Salton M, Stockman GD (eds): Beta-Lactam Antibiotics. New York, Academic Press, 1980, pp 227–247.
15. Sykes RB, Matthew M: The β-lactamases of gram-negative bacteria and their role in resistance to β-lactam antibiotics. J Antimicrob Chemother 1976; 2:115.
16. Craig WA: Penicillins. In: Andriole VT (ed): Current Infectious Disease Drugs. Philadelphia, Current Medicine, 1996, pp 62–65.
17. Eagle H, Newman E: Renal clearance of penicillin F, G, K, and X in rabbits and man. J Clin Invest 1947; 26:903.
18. Acocella G, Mattiussi R, Nicolis FB, et al: Biliary excretion of antibiotics in man. Gut 1968; 9:536.
19. Rolinson GN: History and mode of action of Augmentin. Postgraduate Medicine. Progress and Perspective on beta-lactamase Inhibition: A Review of Augmentin. New York, Custom Communications, 1984, p 23.
20. Payne DJ, Cramp R, Winstanley DJ, Knowles DJ: Comparative activities of clavulanic acid, sulbactam, and tazobactam against clinically important beta-lactamases. Antimicrob Agents Chemother 1994; 38:767.
21. Gorevic PD: Drug-induced autoimmune disease. In: Kaplan A (ed): Allergy. New York, Churchill Livingstone, 1985, p 480.
22. Schwartz HJ, Sher TH: Anaphylaxis to penicillin in a frozen dinner. Ann Allergy 1984; 52:342.
23. Parker CW: Drug allergy (first of three parts). N Engl J Med 1975; 292:511.
24. Gell PGH, Coombs RRA: Classification of allergic reactions responsible for clinical hypersensitivity and disease. In: Gell PGH, Coombs RRA, Hachmann PJ (eds): Clinical Aspects of Immunology. Oxford, Blackwell Scientific Publications, 1975, pp 761–782.
25. Sogn DD: Prevention of allergic reactions to penicillin. J Allergy Clin Immunol 1986; 78(5 pt. 2):1051.
26. Weiss ME, Adkinson NF: β-Lactam allergy. In: Mandell GL, Douglas RG Jr, Bennett JE (eds): Principles and Practice of Infectious Diseases, 3rd ed., New York, Churchill Livingstone, 1990, pp 264–269.
27. Wicher K, Reisman RE, Arbesman CE: Allergic reaction of penicillin present in milk. JAMA 1969; 208:143.
28. Wicher K, Reisman RE: Anaphylactic reaction to penicillin (or penicillin-like substance) in a soft drink. J Allergy Clin Immunol 1980; 66:155.
29. Shmunes E, Taylor JS, Petz LD, et al: Immunologic reactions in penicillin factory workers. Ann Allergy 1976; 36:313.
30. Michel J, Sharon R: Non-haemolytic adverse reaction after transfusion of a blood unit containing penicillin. Br Med J 1980; 280:152.
31. Cole M, Kenig MD, Hewitt VA: Metabolism of penicillins to penicilloic acids and 6-aminopenicillinic acid in man and its significance in assessing penicillin absorption. Antimicrob Agents Chemother 1973; 3:463.
32. Idsoe O, Guthe T, Willcox RR: Penicillin in the treatment of syphilis: The experience of three decades. Bull World Health Organ 1972; 47:1.
33. Levine BB, Zolov DM: Prediction of penicillin allergy by immunological tests. J Allergy 1969; 43:231.
34. Lin RY: A perspective on penicillin allergy. Arch Intern Med 1992; 152:930.
35. Sullivan TJ, Yecies LD, Shatz GS, et al: Desensitization of patients allergic to penicillin using orally administered beta-lactam antibiotics. J Allergy Clin Immunol 1982; 69:275.
36. Adkinson NF Jr: Penicillin allergy. In: Lichtenstein LM, Fauci A (eds): Current Therapy in Allergy, Immunology and Rheumatology. Ontario, Canada, BC Decker, 1983, pp 57–82.
37. Stark BJ, Earl HS, Gross GN, et al: Acute and chronic desensitization of penicillin-allergic patients using oral penicillin. J Allergy Clin Immunol 1987; 79:523.
38. Brown ST: Adverse reactions in syphilis therapy. J Am Vener Dis Assoc 1976; 3(2 pt. 2):172.
39. Kucera A, Crowe SM, Grayson ML, Hoy JF: Penicillin G. In: The Use of Antibiotics: A Clinical Review of Antibacterial, Antifungal and Antiviral Drugs, 5th ed. Oxford, Butterworth-Heinemann, 1997, pp 31–32.
40. Griffin GE: New insights into the pathophysiology of the Jarisch-Herxheimer reaction. J Antimicrobiol Chemother 1992; 29:613.
41. Fekade D, Knox K, Hussein K, et al: Prevention of the Jarisch-Herxheimer reactions by treatment with antibodies against tumor necrosis factor alpha. N Engl J Med 1996; 335:311.
42. Wendel GD: Gestational and congenital syphilis. Clin Perinatol 1988; 15:287.

46

Cephalosporins

Scott Roberts ▶ Sebastian Faro

The cephalosporins were discovered in the mid-1940s by Professor Giuseppe Brotzu at the University of Cagliari. Professor Brotzu noted that there was a periodic clearing of bacteria at a local sewage outlet in Cagliari. He isolated the fungus *Cephalosporium acremonium,* which produced a substance that had antibiotic properties.[1] Three substances that exhibited antibacterial properties were isolated: cephalosporin P, with activity against gram-positive bacteria; cephalosporin N, with activity against gram-negative bacteria; and cephalosporin C. The last compound was noted to be resistant to penicillinase. Cephalosporin C is the compound that became the foundation on which the current cephalosporins were developed.[2] The cephalosporins have become a main antibiotic used for prophylaxis in surgical patients and for treatment.

CHEMISTRY

The cephalosporin compounds consist of a four-membered ring fused to a six-membered dihydrothiazine ring, the cephem nucleus (Fig. 46–1). This is in contrast to the penicillins that have a beta-lactam ring fused to a five-membered thiazolidine ring. Substitution of different side chains at the 6-acylamino site of the 6-aminopenicillanic acid nucleus resulted in semisynthetic penicillins of increased potency. The chemical variations achieved with the penicillins allowed modifications of cephalosporin C, and thus enhanced its potency.[3] Acid hydrolysis of cephalosporin C resulted in a 7-aminocephalosporanic acid and the basic structure for the future development of cephalosporins.[4]

The modification of the basic cephem nucleus by substitutions at position 1, by the addition of substituents at position 3 or 7, or the addition of different acyl side chains at position 7 gave rise to the family of cephalosporin antibiotics. Modifications at position 7 alter antimicrobial activity, while substituents added at position 3 predominantly effect changes in metabolic and pharmacokinetic parameters.[5–7]

Cephalosporins, like all beta-lactam antibiotics, target penicillin-binding proteins (PBP) in bacterial cytoplasmic membranes. Cephalosporins, like penicillins, inhibit cell walls and, therefore, cause bacterial cell death (bactericidal agents). The first clinical cephalosporins that were active against gram-positive cocci, except for enterococci and methicillin-resistant staphylococci, were cephalothin and cephaloridine. The presence of a methoxy group at position 7 of the cephem nucleus resulted in increased activity against gram-negative bacteria.[8, 9] Two antibiotics commonly considered cephalosporins, which are actually cephamycins, are cefoxitin and cefotetan. These two antibiotics have enhanced activity against obligate anaerobic bacteria, but decreased gram-positive activity. The decrease in gram-positive activity is because of a reduction in their ability to bind to PBPs. Further modifications of the acyl side chain at position 7 by the addition of an aminotriazole group resulted in markedly enhanced activity of cephalosporins against many Enterobacteriaceae.[10, 11] The addition of an iminomethoxy group to the alpha-site of this side chain results in an aminothiazolymethoxy side chain that confers stability to many of the beta-lactamases of gram-negative bacteria. This occurs while cephalosporins retain activity against streptococci and, to a lesser degree, against methicillin-susceptible *Staphylococcus aureus.*[12–14] The addition of this side chain appears to enhance the penetration of the cephalosporin through the outer cell membrane of gram-negative bacteria and may also increase these compounds with PBP.

Modification of the cephalosporin basic unit to achieve a given pharmacokinetic effect can have unanticipated and undesirable consequences. The methylthiotetrazole (MTT) substituent, at position 3 in some cephalosporins and cephamycins, has been associated with prolongation of the prothrombin time and, in association with alcohol consumption, can result in a disulfiram-like reaction.

CLASSIFICATION

The most widely used, somewhat arbitrary system for classification of the cephalosporins combines parenteral and oral cephalosporins into generations based on their spectrum of microbiologic activity (Table 46–1). The first-generation cephalosporins have a rather

FIGURE 46-1 ▶ Penicillins and cephalosporins. Sources: F by fermentation; E by enzymic degradation of the corresponding fermentation product; S1 by chemical synthesis from 6-aminopenicillanic acid; S2 by chemical synthesis from 7-aminocephalosporanic acid; S3 semisynthetically from cephamycin C. (From Franklin TJ, Snow GA: Biochemistry of Antimicrobial Action, 3rd ed. New York, Chapman & Hall, 1981, p 44. With permission of Kluwer Academic Publishers.)

narrow spectrum of activity that is focused primarily on the gram-positive cocci but possesses significant activity against gram-negative facultative bacteria. The cephamycins are grouped into second-generation cephalosporins and have a broad spectrum of activity against gram-negative facultative and obligate anaerobic bacteria. The third-generation cephalosporins have marked activity against gram-negative facultative anaerobic bacteria and limited activity against gram-positive cocci, particularly methicillin-susceptible *S. aureus.*

Mechanism of Action

The antimicrobial activity of the cephalosporins, like that of other beta-lactam antibiotics, is due in part to inhibition of bacterial cell wall synthesis. Cephalosporins bind PBP in the cell walls of gram-negative and gram-positive bacteria. The PBPs of various bacteria do not have the same affinities for all cephalosporins and penicillins. The difference in the capacity for cephalosporins and penicillins to bind with PBPs is exemplified by *Enterococcus faecalis,* which is resistant to cephalosporins but is usually sensitive to penicillins.[15] The interaction between the cephalosporin and the PBP blocks cell wall synthesis at various stages. For example, PBP 3 that is involved in cell division and establishment of cross-wall synthesis in *Escherichia coli* can be blocked by beta-lactam antibiotics, resulting in the production of elongated, filamentous forms that eventually undergo cell lysis.[16, 17]

TABLE 46-1 ▶ CLASSIFICATIONS OF CEPHALOSPORINS

First-Generation Cephalosporins

Oral	Parenteral
Cefadroxil (Duricef)	Cefazolin (Ancef, Kezol)
Cephalexin (Biocef, Keflet, Keflex, Keftab)	Cephalothin (Keflin)
	Cephapirin (Cefadyl)
Cephradine	Cephradine

Second-Generation Cephalosporins

Oral	Parenteral
Cefprozil (Cefzil)	Cefamandole (Mandol)
Cefuroxime axetil (Ceftin)	Cefmetazole (Zefazone)
Loracarbef (Lorabid)	Cefonicid (Monocid)
	Cefotetan (Cefotan)
	Cefoxitin (Mefoxin)
	Cefuroxime (Kefurox, Zinacef)

Third-Generation Cephalosporins

Oral	Parenteral
Cefixime (Suprax)	Cefoperazone (Cefobid)
Cefpodoxime proxetil (Vantin)	Ceftazidime (Ceptaz, Fortaz, Tazicef, Tazidime)
	Ceftizoxime (Cefizox)
	Ceftriaxone (Rocephin)

Mechanisms of Resistance

Microbial resistance to cephalosporins is mediated through at least three mechanisms: alteration in PBPs, porin size, and the production of beta-lactamases. Alteration in the PBP decreases binding affinity between the PBP and the antibiotic, thus blocking penetration of the antibiotic. Beta-lactamases produced by the bacteria cleave the beta-lactam ring of the antibiotic. Furthermore, gram-negative bacteria have channels in the cell wall through which substances, antibiotics, enter the periplasmic space. Antibiotic passage through these porins is dependent on the size of the molecule as well as the charge.[18] Alteration of porin size inhibits penetration of the antibiotic through the cell wall and entrance into the periplasmic space.[19]

Pharmacology

The following cephalosporins are administered orally because significant absorption occurs from the gastrointestinal tract: cephalexin, cefaclor, cefuroxime axetil, loracarbef, cefixime, and cefpodoxime proxetil.[20] Other cephalosporins—e.g., cefotetan, cefoxitin, ceftizoxime, cefotaxime, ceftriaxone, cefpiramide, and cefoperazone—are administered either intramuscularly or intravenously. When administered intramuscularly, 1% Xylocaine (lidocaine) can be added to the diluent to relieve the discomfort associated with injection of the antibiotic. Following a 2-g intravenous dose of a cephalosporin, the peak serum concentration ranges between 100 and 150 µg/ml. Cephalosporins achieve good penetration into tissue and fluid compartments, including the female pelvic tissues.[21] Cefpiramide, cefoperazone, and ceftriaxone are excreted via the biliary system.[22] Cefuroxime, cefotaxime, ceftriaxone, and ceftazidime have significant penetration into the cerebrospinal fluid.[23] Most cephalosporins are excreted through the kidneys, achieve exceptionally high urine concentrations, and make good agents for the treatment of urinary tract infections. However, care should be taken when one uses cephalosporins or beta-lactam antibiotics for the treatment of cystitis because the uropathogens easily develop resistance to these antibiotics. Since the kidney excretes these antibiotics, dose adjustments are necessary for patients with kidney dysfunction.

Cephalosporins, in contrast to quinolones and aminoglycosides, do not exhibit concentration-dependent killing of bacteria. The bactericidal effect of cephalosporins reaches a maximum at four to five times the minimal inhibitory concentration (MIC) of the organism. Regrowth of the bacteria after exposure to the cephalosporins occurs promptly; therefore, continuous infusion therapy, shorter dose-to-dose intervals, or other strategies for delaying excretion may be necessary when one employs cephalosporin therapy.[23]

Adverse Reactions

Cephalosporins have a very favorable toxicity profile compared to other antimicrobials, such as vancomycin and the aminoglycosides. The adverse events are similar across the group (Table 46-2). Thrombophlebitis associated with intravenous administration occurs in 1% to 5% of recipients. Pain at the site of intramuscular injection can be decreased with the addition of 1% Xylocaine to the diluent.

Hypersensitivity reactions are the most common systemic adverse events that occur with cephalosporins. Skin rash with or without fever and eosinophilia occur in 1% to 3% of patients after variable periods of cepha-

TABLE 46-2 ▶ ADVERSE REACTIONS

Thrombophlebitis
Rash—occurs within 3 to 5 days of exposure to a cephalosporin
Serum sickness—rare (fever, lymphadenopathy, eosinophilia, eosinophiluria)
Immediate hypersensitivity (type 1) reaction—bronchospasm and hives
Positive Coombs' test
Hemolytic anemia
Bone marrow suppression—leukopenia, neutropenia, thrombocytopenia
Liver function abnormalities
Interstitial nephritis
Hypoprothrombinemia
Biliary sludging
Diarrhea
Urticaria
Angioedema
Stevens-Johnson syndrome (rare)

losporin therapy.[24] Immediate anaphylactic reactions are rare and occur in approximately 2 cases per 10,000.[25] Large surveys of patients with a history of penicillin allergy have demonstrated that 93% to 97% of patients do not react to cephalosporins.[26, 27] Although the risk of cross-sensitivity appears to be small, cephalosporins should not be administered to individuals who have experienced an anaphylactoid reaction to penicillin or other immediate-type hypersensitivity reaction.[28]

Allergy to a cephalosporin in the absence of a penicillin allergy does occur. In one study, 15 volunteers were administered 2 g of cephalothin intravenously four times a day for 2 to 4 weeks. They all developed a serum sickness-like illness, with malaise, weakness, arthralgia, myalgia, fever, lymphadenopathy, and skin rashes.[29]

Occasionally eosinophilia, and rarely neutropenia, are seen in association with the administration of cephalosporins. Hypoprothrombinemia has been associated with the competitive inhibition by the MTT group of vitamin K–dependent carboxylases responsible for converting clotting factors II, VII, IX, and X to their active forms.[30] The MTT group, which occupies position 3 in cefamandole, cefoperazone, cefotetan, and moxalactam, may also inhibit vitamin K 2,3-epoxide reductase, which converts inactive vitamin K to its active form.[31] This effect resembles the action of Coumadin. The frequency of hypoprothrombinemia in recipients is variable—4% to 68%—and is markedly enhanced by poor nutritional status, debilitation, recent gastrointestinal surgery, and renal failure.[32–34]

Cephalosporin therapy has been associated with pseudomembranous colitis or *Clostridium difficile* toxin-related colitis. The risk is not increased compared to other beta-lactam antibiotics and clindamycin. Cefoxitin can cause diarrhea, especially when high doses of the drug are administered.[35] Cefoxitin can alter the fecal flora as well as the vaginal flora, increasing colonization by *Enterococcus faecalis, Staphylococcus epidermidis, Clostridum difficile,* cefoxitin-resistant Enterobacteriaceae, and *Pseudomonas aeruginosa*.[36, 37] Cefuroxime axetil has been shown to cause nausea, vomiting, and diarrhea, but the incidence has been similar to that seen with other antibiotics. The incidence of colitis has been calculated to be 1:2,100 cases.[38]

Nephrotoxicity secondary to cefazolin, cefoxitin, cefuroxime, and cefotaxime, as with most cephalosporins, is uncommon.[39–41] Ingestion of alcohol by patients receiving cephalosporin therapy with the MTT group at position 3 has been associated with disulfiramlike reactions.[42]

FIRST-GENERATION CEPHALOSPORINS

The first-generation cephalosporins, except enterococci, are very active against gram-positive cocci and have moderate activity against community-acquired gram-negative rods.[42] Their weakness is against anaerobic gram-negative bacteria and beta-lactamase–positive Enterobacteriaceae.[43] They have poor activity against *H. influenzae* and methicillin-resistant staphylococci.[44]

Cefazolin is the most commonly used parenteral cephalosporin. It is a frequently used antibiotic for surgical prophylaxis and for the treatment of pyelonephritis in pregnant patients. Its spectrum of activity is very similar to that of cephalothin except that the former has slightly greater activity against *Escherichia coli* and *Klebsiella*.[45] Cefazolin has a longer half-life than that of cephalothin, 1.2 versus 0.6 hours; therefore, it requires less frequent dosing, 8-hour versus 6-hour dosing. Cephalothin is not as easily hydrolyzed by staphylococcal beta-lactamases and is well suited for the treatment of nonmeningeal staphylococcal infections.[46]

Cephalexin is well absorbed from the gastrointestinal tract and obtains good serum levels within 1 hour of administration. The half-life is 50 minutes. The drug is excreted unchanged in the urine.[47]

Pregnancy

The cephalosporins are class B antibiotics with no known adverse effects in pregnancy or in infants of breast-feeding mothers. Cephalosporins cross the placenta rapidly and obtain cord blood levels approximately half of the maternal peak level. The cephalosporins are frequently used agents for the treatment of pyelonephritis because of their activity against *E. coli* (*E. coli* is responsible for 90% to 95% of the cases) and their safety in the fetus. The emergence of beta-lactamase resistance in the Enterobacteriaceae is of concern because of the possibility of treatment failures. Their value lies in their ability to achieve excellent penetration into the kidney tissue. Significant blood levels have made first-generation parenteral cephalosporins excellent agents for the treatment of pyelonephritis (Tables 46–3 and 46–4).

SECOND-GENERATION CEPHALOSPORINS

The second-generation cephalosporins are made up of two groups: the true cephalosporins and the cephamycins. Compared to the first-generation cephalosporins, the second-generation cephalosporins have en-

TABLE 46–3 ▶ INDICATIONS

Respiratory tract	Gastrointestinal tract
Skin and Soft tissue	Bone and joint
Genitourinary tract	Perioperative prophylaxis
Septicemia	

TABLE 46-4 ▶	SPECTRUM OF BACTERIA

Staphylococcus aureus—penicillinase-producing and
    non–penicillinase-producing strains
Group A beta-hemolytic streptococci
Group B beta-hemolytic streptococci
Streptococcus pneumoniae
Streptococcus viridans
Escherichia coli
Klebsiella
Proteus mirabilis
Salmonella
Shigella

hanced activity against *H. influenzae, Moraxella catarrhalis, Neisseria meningitidis,* and *N. gonorrhoeae,* and in selected instances, in vitro and in vivo activity against many Enterobacteriaceae.[48] The cephamycins have lost some activity against staphylococci and streptococci but have significant activity against obligate anaerobic bacteria.[49] The cephamycins, because of their activity against obligate anaerobic bacteria, have become primary agents in the treatment of intra-abdominal and pelvic infections.

Cefamandole (Mandol), a parenteral cephalosporin, is excreted in the urine and has a serum half-life of 50 minutes. It has good activity against selected strains of *S. aureus* and coagulase-negative staphylococci. It also has significant activity against gram-negative facultative rods. Cefamandole does possess the MTT side chain at position 3, and thus bears the toxicities associated with increased bleeding tendencies seen with this moiety.

Cefuroxime (Zinacef) and cefuroxime axetil (Ceftin) have significantly-enhanced activity against *H. influenzae, N. gonorrhoeae,* and some members of the Enterobacteriaceae. It is more active against *S. pneumoniae* and *S. pyogenes* than are first-generation cephalosporins.[50] It has a long half-life, 1.3 to 1.5 hours, and can be administered intramuscularly, intravenously, or orally. Cefuroxime is the only second-generation cephalosporin to exhibit significant penetration into the cerebrospinal fluid. It has provided effective treatment for bacterial meningitis caused by *N. meningitidis, S. pneumoniae,* and *H. influenzae.*[51] However, in direct comparison to ceftriaxone, a third-generation cephalosporin, cefuroxime is associated with increased hearing loss and delayed sterilization of the cerebrospinal fluid in pediatric patients. Therefore, ceftriaxone is the preferred drug for the treatment of bacterial meningeal infections. Cefuroxime, because of its enhanced activity against *H. influenzae* and *S. pneumoniae,* is an excellent drug for the treatment of community-acquired pneumonia.

Cefuroxime axetil (Ceftin), an orally administered cephalosporin, has a bioavailability of 30% to 50%. Absorption is increased by food and diminished by antacids or H2 receptor antagonists. The long serum half-life allows for twice-a-day dosing.

Cefoxitin is notably resistant to beta-lactamases produced by gram-negative rods, yet it is an effective inducer of beta-lactamases in some members of the Enterobacteriaceae.[52] Its activity against staphylococci and streptococci is less than that of cefazolin, but it has excellent activity against obligate anaerobic bacteria. Among the second-generation cephalosporins and cephamycins, cefoxitin has the best activity against *Bacteroides fragilis* and the *B. fragilis* group. However, its efficacy against this group of pathogenic anaerobic bacteria is diminishing. Cefoxitin has good activity against *N. gonorrhoeae,* including the beta-lactamase–producing strains. It has a serum half-life of 40 to 45 minutes and requires a 4 to 6-hour dosing schedule to maintain bactericidal levels.

Cefotetan (Cefotan), a cephamycin, has an antibacterial spectrum of activity similar to that of cefoxitin. It does not have the same level of activity against *B. fragilis* and the *B. fragilis* group as that of cefoxitin. However, it has proved to be effective in the treatment of female pelvic infections. A major advance is its long half-life of 3.5 hours, thus allowing for twice-a-day dosing. Cefotetan also possesses the MTT side chain and has the same potential for bleeding as that of all cephalosporins with the MTT side chain; namely, bleeding and hypoprothrombinemia.

Cefaclor (Ceclor) has pharmacokinetic and biologic activities similar to those of cephalexin. It has a spectrum of activity similar to that of other second-generation cephalosporins, and has enhanced activity against *H. influenzae, P. mirabilis,* and *E. coli.* It has a half-life of 0.8 hours and, therefore, is administered every 8 hours.

Loracarbef (Lorabid) is an orally administered carbacephem with a spectrum of activity similar to that of Cefaclor. It has modestly increased activity against *H. influenzae, Moraxella catarrhalis,* and some Enterobacteriaceae. Virtually the entire oral dose is absorbed and excreted in the urine. It has a serum half-life of 1.1 hours, and is more stable in plasma than is cefaclor. The prolonged half-life permits twice-a-day dosing. (Tables 46–5 and 46–6).

THIRD-GENERATION CEPHALOSPORINS

The third-generation cephalosporins are the most potent of the class against gram-negative facultative an-

TABLE 46-5 ▶	MICROBIAL SPECTRUM

Staphylococcus aureus	*Morganella morganii*
Streptococcus (beta-hemolytic)	*Neisseria gonorrhoeae*
Streptococcus pneumoniae	*Neisseria meningitidis*
Escherichia coli	*Proteus mirabilis*
Haemophilus influenzae	*Providencia* spp.
Klebsiella spp.	*Salmonella* spp.
Moraxella catarrhalis	*Shigella* spp.

TABLE 46–6 ▶	INFECTIONS
Pharyngitis	Urinary tract
Tonsillitis	Skin and skin structures
Otitis media	Gonorrhea
Lower respiratory tract	

TABLE 46–7 ▶	MICROBIAL SPECTRUM
Staphylococci—penicillinase-producing, coagulase-positive, coagulase-negative strains	
Streptococci—beta-hemolytic	
Streptococcus pneumoniae	
Streptococcus viridans	
Enterobacter spp.	
Escherichia coli	
Haemophilus influenzae—penicillinase-producing and non–penicillinase-producing strains	
Klebsiella spp.	
Morganella morganii	
Neisseria gonorrhoeae—penicillinase-producing and non–penicillinase-producing strains	
Neisseria meningitidis	
Proteus mirabilis	
Proteus vulgaris	
Serratia marcescens	
Acinetobacter calcoaceticus	
Bacteroides spp.	
Peptostreptococcus	

aerobic bacteria. They have superior activity against *S. pneumoniae* and *S. pyogenes*. With the exception of ceftazidime, they have moderate activity against *S. aureus*. They have excellent activity against *H. influenzae, N. meningitidis, N. gonorrhoeae,* and *M. catarrhalis.*

In general, the third-generation cephalosporins do not have good activity against obligate anaerobic bacteria. Third-generation cephalosporins are segregated by whether they have good activity against *Pseudomonas* spp., the two best being cefoperazone and ceftazidime.

Cefotaxime (Claforan) is a parenteral agent with good activity against streptococci. However, it is not superior to, or preferred over, penicillin and first-generation cephalosporins. Cefotaxime is not particularly suited for the treatment of infections caused by *Pseudomonas*. Although first-generation cephalosporins are usually adequate for the treatment of uncomplicated cystitis and pyelonephritis, complicated urinary tract infections, particularly during pregnancy, may benefit from cefotaxime treatment. It has an excellent spectrum of activity against gram-negative facultative bacilli, the major cause of pyelonephritis in pregnancy. Cefotaxime also achieves good levels in the cerebrospinal fluid when given at 2 g every 4 hours.

Ceftizoxime (Cefizox) has a spectrum of activity that is similar to that of cefotaxime but differs because the former has better activity against obligate anaerobic bacteria, particularly *B. fragilis*. Ceftizoxime has a half-life of 1.7 hours and, therefore, is given every 8 hours. This agent can achieve effective levels in the cerebrospinal fluid.

Ceftriaxone (Rocephin) has activity similar to that of cefotaxime and ceftizoxime. It is the most potent cephalosporin against *N. gonorrhoeae, N. meningitidis,* and *H. influenzae*. Ceftriaxone is 90% protein bound and excreted to a small extent by the kidney, but mainly via the biliary tract. It has a serum half-life of 8 hours; therefore, it can be administered either every 12 or 24 hours, depending on the severity of the infection.

Cefoperazone (Cefobid) has moderate antipseudomonal activity, but it is not typically used to treat pseudomonal infections. It is highly protein bound and, therefore, does not achieve significant levels in the cerebrospinal fluid. Cefoperazone does possess the MTT side chain at position 3, and disulfiram-like reactions and hypoprothrombinemia have been reported.

Ceftazidime (Fortaz) is a unique third-generation cephalosporin with affinity for beta-lactamases, but it

is not a particularly good inducer of beta-lactamase. It does have excellent activity against gram-negative facultative anaerobic bacteria, including *P. aeruginosa*. However, it has poor activity against obligate anaerobes and staphylococci. It is used in the treatment of penicillin-sensitive pseudomonal infections, but it is ineffective against penicillin-resistant *Pseudomonas*.

Cefixime (Suprax), an oral third-generation cephalosporin, has a prolonged half-life, 3 to 4 hours, thus allowing single-daily dosing. It is active against *S. pneumoniae, H. influenzae, N. gonorrhoeae,* and *M. catarrhalis*. It has been approved by the Centers for Disease Control and Prevention (CDC) for one treatment of uncomplicated gonorrheal cervicitis (Tables 46–7 and 46–8).

SUMMARY

The cephalosporins offer suitable alternatives to antibiotics and cover a broad spectrum of bacteria. The three generations of cephalosporins differ from one another significantly. The first-generation agents are similar to the penicillins, perhaps with an increased spectrum against gram-negative facultative anaerobic bacteria. The second-generation agents maintain some of the gram-positive activity that is found with the first-generation cephalosporins; and, in addition, the cephamycins have added obligate anaerobic bacterial

TABLE 46–8 ▶	INFECTIONS	
Lower respiratory tract	Intra-abdominal
Skin and skin structures	Pelvic inflammatory disease
Urinary tract	Bacterial septicemia
Gonorrhea	Perioperative prophylaxis
Bone and joint	

activity. The third-generation agents have increased activity against the gram-negative facultative anaerobic bacteria, including *Pseudomonas,* but have virtually relinquished obligate anaerobic activity.

Hypersensitivity reactions are the most common adverse reactions observed with the cephalosporins. Diarrhea is seen in 1% to 7% of patients being treated with cephalosporins. Two special adverse effects have been seen with some cephalosporins: bleeding and a disulfiram-like reaction. Hypoprothrombinemia and bleeding have been associated with the use of moxalactam, cefoperazone, cefotetan, and cefamandole. Hypoprothrombinemia occurs because of the presence of the methyltetrathiazole (MTT) side chain. This inhibits the gamma carboxylation of glutamic acid, which is the vitamin K–dependent step in the synthesis of prothrombin. Clinically important bleeding normally develops in individuals with risk factors; for example, renal or liver disease, poor nutrition, use of anticoagulants or aspirin, or thrombocytopenia. The MTT side chain is also responsible for disulfiram-type reactions when taken prior to consuming alcohol-containing liquids.

REFERENCES

1. Abraham EP: Cephalosporins 1945–1986. In Williams JD (ed): The Cephalosporin Antibiotics. Auckland, Adis Press, 1987, pp 1–14.
2. Abraham EP, Loder PB: Cephalosporin C. In Flynn EH (ed): Cephalosporins and Penicillins: Chemistry and Biology. New York, Academic Press, 1972, pp 2–26.
3. Robinson GN: The Garrod lecture: The influence of 6-aminopenicillanic acid on antibiotic development. J Antimicrob Chemother 1988; 22:5.
4. Huber FM, Chauvette RR, Jackson BG: Preparative methods for 7-aminocephalosporanic acid and aminopenicillanic acid. In Flynn EH (ed): Cephalosporins and Penicillins. New York, Academic Press, 1972, p 27.
5. Neu HC: Structure-activity relations of new beta-lactam compounds and in vivo activity against common bacteria. Rev Infect Dis 1983; (Suppl):S319.
6. Neu HC: Relation of structural properties of beta-lactam antibiotics to antibacterial activity. Am J Med 1985; 79:2.
7. Allan JD, Eliopoulos GM, Moellering RC Jr: Antibiotics: Future directions by understanding structure-function relationships. In Root RK, Trunkey DD, Sande MA (eds): Contemporary Issues in Infectious Diseases, vol 6. New York, Churchill Livingstone, 1987, pp 263–284.
8. Onishi HR, Daoust DR, Zimmerman SB, et al: Cefoxitin, a semisynthetic cephamycin antibiotic: Resistance to beta-lactamase inactivation. Antimicrob Agents Chemother 1974; 5:38.
9. Stapely EO, Birnbaum J: Chemistry and microbiological properties of the cephamycins. In: Salton MRJ, Stockman GD (eds): Beta-Lactam Antibiotics. New York, Academic Press, 1981, pp 327–351.
10. Dunn GL: Ceftizoxime and other third-generation cephalosporins: Structure-activity relationships. J Antimicrob Chemother 1982; 10(suppl C):1.
11. Bucourt R, Bormann D, Heymes R, Perronnet M: Chemistry of cefotaxime. J Antimicrob Chemother 1980; 6(suppl A):63.
12. Neu HC: Beta-lactam antibiotics: Structural relationships affecting in-vitro activity and pharmacologic properties. Rev Infect Dis 1986; 8(suppl 3):S237.
13. Nikaido H, Nakae T: The outer membrane of gram-negative bacteria. Adv Microb Physiol 1979; 20:163.
14. Neu HC: Oral beta-lactam antibiotics administration from 1960 to 1993. Infect Dis Clin Pract 1993; 6:394.
15. Georgopapadakou NH, Liu FY: Penicillin-binding proteins in bacteria. Antimicrob Agents Chemother 1980; 18:148.
16. Curtis NA, Orr D, Ross GW, Boulton MG: Affinities of penicillins and cephalosporins for the penicillin-binding proteins of *Escherichia coli* K-12 and their antibacterial activity. Antimicrobial Agents Chemother 1979; 16:533.
17. Curtis NA, Eisenstadt RL, Turner KA, White AJ: Inhibition of penicillin-binding protein 3 of *Escherichia coli* K-12: Effects upon growth, viability and outer membrane barrier function. J Antimicrob Chemother 1985; 16:287.
18. Nikaido H, Rosenberg EY, Foulds J: Porin channels in *Escherichia coli*: Studies with beta-lactams in intact cells. J Bacteriol 1983; 153:232.
19. Brogard JM, Comte F: Pharmacokinetics of the new cephalosporins. Antibiot Chemother 1982; 31:145.
20. Barriere SL, Flaherty JF: Third-generation cephalosporins: A critical evaluation. Clin Pharm 1984; 3:351.
21. Cherubin CE, Eng RH, Norrby R, et al: Penetration of newer cephalosporins into cerebrospinal fluid. Rev Infect Dis 1989; 11:526.
22. Leggett JE, Fantin B, Ebert S, et al: Comparative antibiotic dose-effect relations at several dosing intervals in murine pneumonitis and thigh-infection models. J Infect Dis 1989; 159:281.
23. Agnelli G, Del Favero A, Parise P, et al: Cephalosporin-induced hypoprothrombinemia: Is the *N*-methylthiotetrazole side chain the culprit? Antimicrob Agents Chemother 1986; 29:1108.
24. Ries K, Levison ME, Kaye D: Clinical and in vivo evaluation of cefazolin, a new cephalosporin antibiotic. Antimicrob Agents Chemother 1973; 3:168.
25. Anne S, Resiman RE: Risk of administering cephalosporin antibiotics to patients with histories of penicillin allergy. Ann Allergy Asthma Immunol 1995; 75:167.
26. Dash CH: Penicillin allergy and the cephalosporins. J Antimicrob Chemother 1975; 1(3 suppl):107.
27. Boguniewicz M, Leung DY: Hypersensitivity reactions to antibiotics commonly used in children. Pediatr Infect Dis J 1995; 14:221.
28. Petz LD: Immunologic cross-reactivity between penicillins and cephalosporins: A review. J Infect Dis 1978; 137(suppl):S74.
29. Sanders WE Jr, Johnson JE 3d, Taggart JG: Adverse reactions to cephalothin and cephapirin: Uniform occurrence on prolonged intravenous administration of high doses. N Engl J Med 1974; 290:424.
30. Bechtold H, Andrassy K, Jahnchen E, et al: Evidence for impaired hepatic vitamin K1 metabolism in patients treated with *N*-methyl-thiotetrazole cephalosporins. Thromb Haemost 1984; 51:358.
31. Sattler FR, Weitekamp MR, Ballard JO: Potential for bleeding with the new beta-lactam antibiotics. Ann Intern Med 1986; 105:924.
32. Sattler FR, Colao DJ, Caputo GM, Schoolwerth AC: Cefoperazone for empiric therapy in patients with impaired renal function. Am J Med 1986; 81:229.
33. Baxter JG, Marble DA, Whitfield LR, et al: Clinical risk factors for prolonged PT/TT in abdominal sepsis patients treated with moxalactam or tobramycin plus clindamycin. Ann Surg 1985; 201:96.
34. Foster TS, Raehl CL, Wilson HD: Disulfiram-like reaction associated with a parenteral cephalosporin. Am J Hosp Pharm 1980; 37:858.
35. Trollfors B, Alestig K, Norrby R: Local and gastrointestinal reactions to intravenously administered cefoxitin and cefuroxime. Scand J Infect Dis 1979; 11:315.
36. Mulligan ME, Citron D, Gabay E, et al: Alterations in human fecal flora, including growth of *Clostridium difficile,* related to cefoxitin therapy. Antimicrob Agents Chemother 1984; 26:343.
37. Barza M, Giuliano M, Jacobus NV, Gorbach SL: Effect of broad-spectrum parenteral antibiotics on "colonization resistance" of intestinal microflora of humans. Antimicrob Agents Chemother 1987; 31:723.
38. Emmerson AM: Cefuroxime axetil. J Antimicrobial Chemother 1988; 22:101.

39. Smith CR: Cefotaxime and cephalosporins: Adverse reactions in perspective. Rev Infect Dis 1982; 4(suppl):S481.

40. Kosmidis J, Hamilton-Miller JM, Gilchrist JNG, et al: Cefoxitin, a new semi-synthetic cephamycin: An in-vitro and in-vivo comparison with cephalothin. Br Med J 1973; 4:653.

41. Brumfitt W, Kosmidis J, Hamilton-Miller JMT, Gilchrist JNG: Cefoxitin and cephalothin: Antimicrobial activity, human pharmacokinetics and toxicology. Antimicrob Agents Chemother 1974; 6:290.

42. Gustaferro CA, Steckelberg JM: Cephalosporin antimicrobial agents and related compounds. Mayo Clinic Proc 1991; 66:1064.

43. Myers JP, Linnemann CC Jr: Bacteremia due to methicillin-resistant *Staphylococcus aureus*. J Infect Dis 1982; 145:532.

44. Sabath LD, Wilcox C, Garner C, Finland M: In vitro activity of cefazolin against recent clinical bacterial isolates. J Infect Dis 1973; 128(suppl):S320.

45. Quinn EL, Pohlod D, Madhavan T, et al: Clinical experience with cefazolin and other cephalosporins in bacterial endocarditis. J Infect Dis 1973; 128(suppl):S386.

46. Hartstein AI, Patrick KE, Jones SR, et al: Comparison of pharmacological and antimicrobial properties of cefadroxil and cephalexin. Antimicrob Agents Chemother 1977; 12:93.

47. Neiss ES: Cephradine: A summary of preclinical studies and clinical pharmacology. J Irish Med Assoc 1973; 66(suppl):1.

48. Fraser DG: Drug therapy reviews: Antimicrobial spectrum, pharmacology and therapeutic use of cefamandole and cefoxitin. Am J Hosp Pharm 1979; 36:1503.

49. Ayres LW, Jones RN, Barry AL, et al: Cefotetan, a new cephamycin. Antimicrob Agents Chemother 1982; 22:859.

50. Neu HC, Fu KP: Cefuroxime, a beta-lactamase–resistant cephalosporin with a broad spectrum of gram-positive and negative activity. Antimicrob Agents Chemother 1978; 13:657.

51. Tunkel AR, Wispelway B, Scheld WM: Bacterial meningitis: Recent advances in pathophysiology and treatment. Ann Intern Med 1990; 112:610.

52. Sanders WE Jr, Sanders CC: Inducible beta-lactamases: Clinical and epidemiologic implications for use of newer cephalosporins. Rev Infect Dis 1988; 10:830.

47 Carbapenems

SEBASTIAN FARO

The carbapenems are a group of bicyclic beta-lactam antibiotics that possess a carbapenem nucleus. Currently, there are three carbapenems available, imipenem-cilastatin, meropenem, and the monobactam aztreonam (Figs. 47–1 and 47–2). Because imipenem and meropenem are very similar, the discussion focuses on imipenem. An antibiotic, named thienamycin, was isolated from the fungus *Streptomyces cattleya*. It was noted to have activity against aerobic, facultative, and obligate anaerobic bacteria.[1] Thienamycin was unstable in solution but was stabilized by forming an *N*-formimdoyl derivative termed *imipenem*. The study of thienamycin in animals and humans revealed that the drug was metabolized in the kidney by dehydropeptidase (DHP-1), which is located at the brush border of the proximal tubular cells.[2–4] Cilastatin, a competitive inhibitor of dehydropeptidase-I, was developed to prevent hydrolysis of imipenem.[2] Meropenem is much more stable in the presence of dehydropeptidase-I, does not require an inhibitor, and, therefore, is not metabolized.[5, 6] Imipenem is combined with cilastatin in a ratio of 1:1. Imipenem-cilastatin has a very broad spectrum of activity, which includes bacteria that are resistant to aminoglycosides and cephalosporins. Bacteria that are resistant to penicillins and cephalosporins are typically sensitive to imipenem-cilastatin.[7–10]

MECHANISM OF ACTION

Imipenem, like other beta-lactam antibiotics, acts by binding to penicillin-binding proteins (PBPs). When imipenem binds to PBPs, it inhibits cross-linking of peptides in the synthesis of the bacterial cell wall. This results in a weakened cell wall; the osmotic pressure within the cell cannot be contained, and the cell ruptures. Imipenem is very stable against class I beta-lactamases and is able to bind to a variety of PBPs, thus making imipenem and meropenem active against a larger number of bacteria than are other beta-lactam antibiotics[10–12] (Table 47–1). Imipenem, for example, binds to all PBPs found in *Escherichia coli*. It has the greatest affinity for PBP 1 and PBP 2, which are the transpeptidases responsible for elongation of the bacterial cell wall.[13] Beta-lactam antibiotics, such as penicillins and cephalosporins, bind to PBP 3 to produce elongated filaments, whereas imipenems bind to PBP 2 to produce lemon-shaped cells.[14, 15]

The postantibiotic effect on bacteria is defined as the time between exposure of bacteria to an antibiotic and the time when bacterial growth resumes.[16, 17] This delay in growth following exposure of a bacterium to an antibiotic was first noted in 1944, when Bigger[18] added penicillinase to a culture of bacteria that had previously been exposed to penicillin. In 1946 and 1948, Parker and colleagues[19, 20] observed that exposing staphylococci to penicillin for 5 to 30 minutes and subsequently transferring the bacteria to a medium not containing an antibiotic did not result in the immediate resumption of growth. There was, in fact, a delay of 1 to 3 hours.[19, 20] The persistent effect of some antibiotics on bacterial growth, following elimination of the antibiotic, has been demonstrated in vitro and in vivo for both gram-positive and gram-negative bacteria with a variety of antibiotics.[21–24]

The clinical significance of the postantibiotic effect resides in antimicrobial dosing schedules. A drug-organism combination that does not exhibit a postantibiotic effect may necessitate more frequent dosing of the antibiotic to achieve elimination of the bacteria. Patient exposure to the antibiotic appears to affect leukocyte function. Bacteria in the postantibiotic phase appear to be more susceptible to the antibacterial activity of human leukocytes.[25–30] This phenomenon of enhanced leukocyte antibacterial activity occurs in the postantibiotic phase and has been termed the *postantibiotic leukocyte enhancement phase*.[25–30]

Imipenem is able to penetrate most gram-negative bacteria easily. This is likely because of its compact molecular structure.[31] Imipenem was found to enter bacterial cells through porins much faster than were the cephalosporins.[32] Imipenem enters *P. aeruginosa* through the porins in the outer membrane that are facilitated by protein "D2."[33] Loss of this outer membrane protein, "D2," results in organism resistance to imipenem.[34]

The toxicity of imipenem and meropenem resembles that of other beta-lactams (Table 47–2). Grand mal seizures, focal seizures, and myoclonus have been

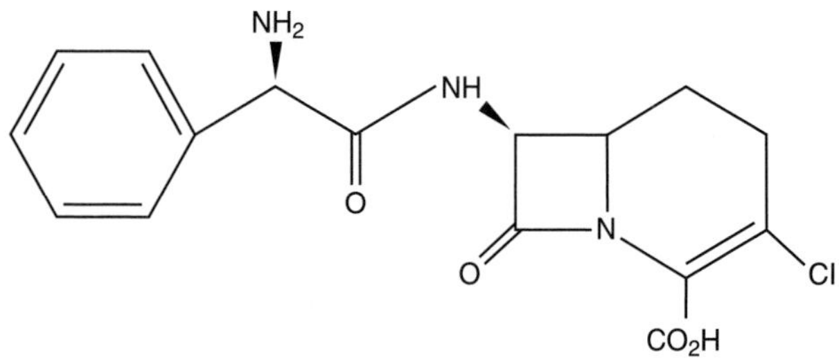

FIGURE 47-1 ▶ The structure of loracarbef. (From Andriole VT: Current Infectious Disease Drugs. Philadelphia, Current Medicine, 1996, p 62.)

reported with imipenem, but most patients had renal insufficiency and/or a history of prior seizure, brain tumor, brain abscess, or cerebral infarct.[38–40] Either reducing the dosage, or discontinuing therapy with imipenem, can prevent recurring seizure activity. Because there can be cross-allergy with penicillin, imipenem should not be administered to individuals known to have had a severe reaction to penicillin or a cephalosporin.

Microbial Spectrum of Activity

The antibacterial spectrum of activity for both imipenem and meropenem is very broad and includes gram-positive and gram-negative facultative and obligate anaerobes.[41–43] The activity of imipenem and meropenem against obligate anaerobic bacteria is equivalent to that of metronidazole. However, these agents do not have significant activity against *Xanthomonas maltophilia* and *Pseudomonas cepacia*.

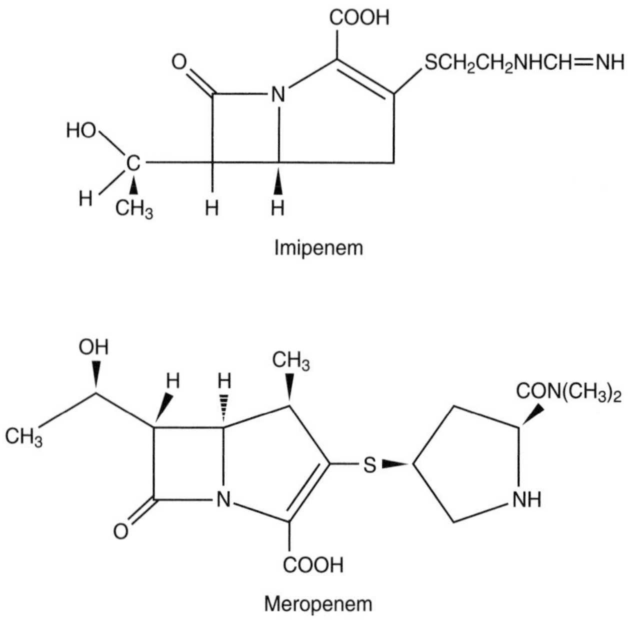

Imipenem

Meropenem

FIGURE 78-2 ▶ Carbapenem structures. (From Andriole VT: Current Infectious Disease Drugs. Philadelphia, Current Medicine, 1996, p 62.)

TABLE 47-1 ▶ **TOXICITY ASSOCIATED WITH IMIPENEM AND MEROPENEM**

Gastrointestinal	Nausea and vomiting 3%–4%
	Diarrhea
	Pseudomembranous colitis
	Change in colonic flora with an increase in yeast and enterococci, suppression of staphylococci, enterococci, enterobacteria, anaerobic cocci, eubacteria, lactobacilli, clostridia, fusobacteria, and bacteroides[35–38]
Central nervous system	Seizures
Hypersensitivity reactions	Rash
	Pruritus
	Urticaria
Hematologic	Neutropenia
	Eosinophilia
	Positive Coombs' test
Hepatotoxicity	Abnormalities in liver function test
	Jaundice
Nephrotoxicity	

AZTREONAM

Aztreonam, unlike imipenem and meropenem, has a narrow spectrum of activity that is limited mainly to gram-negative facultative anaerobic bacteria. Aztreonam does not have any significant activity against either gram-positive aerobic bacteria or obligate anaerobic bacteria. The limitations of this antibiotic require that it be used in combination with other agents that can provide coverage against gram-positive aerobic bacteria and obligate anaerobic bacteria. Some individuals consider it to be a substitute for aminoglycosides because of the similarity in the spectra of antibacterial activity. However, it must be pointed out that there is no synergy between aztreonam and the penicillins effective against the enterococci.

The half-life of aztreonam is longer (1.7 hours) than that of imipenem or meropenem (1 hour). The dosage for urinary tract infection is 500 mg every 8 to 12 hours. Treatment for moderately severe systemic infec-

TABLE 47-2 ▶ **CLINICAL USE OF IMIPENEM AND MEROPENEM**

Treatment of the neutropenic cancer patient
Intra-abdominal infections
Soft tissue pelvic infections
  Pelvic inflammatory disease
  Pelvic abscesses
  Pelvic cellulitis and peritonitis
Respiratory tract infections
  Postoperative nosocomial pneumonia
  Nosocomial pneumonia in patients in intensive care units
Osteomyelitis
Bacterial endocarditis—use imipenem or meropenem in conjunction with an aminoglycoside (not the regimen of choice; broad-spectrum penicillin + tobramycin would be preferable)
Bacterial meningitis
Urinary tract infections

tion is 1 to 2 g every 8 to 12 hours, and for severe infection 2 g every 6 to 8 hours. Patients with renal impairment should have their dosage calculated according to their renal clearance.

The adverse effects associated with aztreonam are those typically seen with antibiotic therapy. There does not appear to be any side effect that is unique to aztreonam.

REFERENCES

1. Albers-Schinberg G, Arison BH, Hensen OD, et al: Structure and absolute configuration of thienamycin. J Am Chem Soc 1978; 100:6491.
2. Kahan FM, Kropp H, Sundelof JG, Birnbaum J: Thienamycin: Development of imipenem/cilastatin. J Antimicrob Chemother 1983; 12(suppl D):1.
3. Kroop H, Sundelof JG, Hajdu R, Kahan FM: Metabolism of thienamycin and related carbapenem antibiotics by the renal dipeptidase, dehydropeptidase. Antimicrob Agents Chemother 1982; 22:62.
4. Gural R, Lin C, Chung M, et al: Oral absorption and tolerance in a man, of a new penem antibiotic Sch. 29428. J Antimicrob Chemother 1982; 9(suppl C):239.
5. Burman LA, Nilsson-Ehle I, Hutchison M, et al: Pharmacokinetics of meropenem and its metabolite ICI 213,689 in healthy subjects with known renal metabolism of imipenem. J Antimicrob Chemother 1991; 27:219.
6. Leroy A, Fillastri JP, Borsa-Lebas F, et al: Pharmacokinetics of meropenem (ICI 194,660) and its metabolite (ICI 213,689) in healthy subjects and in patients with renal impairment. Antimicrob Agents Chemother 1992; 36:2794.
7. Barry AL, Jones RN, Thornsberry C, et al: Imipenem (N-forminidoyl thienamycin): In vitro antimicrobial activity and beta-lactamase stability. Diagn Microbiol Infect Dis 1985; 3:93.
8. Geddes AM, Stille W: Imipenem: The first thienamycin antibiotic. Rev Infect Dis 1985; 7(suppl 3):353.
9. Kroop H, Gerkens L, Sundelof JG, Kahan FM: Antibacterial activity of imipenem: The first thienamycin antibiotic. Rev Infect Dis 1985; 7(suppl 3):389.
10. Buckley MM, Brogden RN, Barradell LB, Goa KL: Imipenem/cilastatin: A reappraisal of its antibacterial activity, pharmacokinetic properties and therapeutic efficacy. Drugs 1992; 44:408.
11. Sumita Y, Inoue M, Mitsuhashi S: In vitro antibacterial activity and beta-lactamase stability of the new carbapenem SM-7338. Eur J Clin Microbiol Infect Dis 1989; 8:908.
12. Yang YJ, Livermore DM: Interactions of meropenem with class I chromosomal beta-lactamases. J Antimicrob Chemother 1989; 24(suppl A):S207.
13. Kucera A, Crowe S, Grayson ML, Hoy J: Imipenem/cilastatin. In: Kucers LC (ed): Use of Antibiotics: A Clinical Review of Antibacterial, Antifungal and Antiviral Drugs, 5th ed. Oxford, Butterworth-Heinemann, 1997, pp 225–244.
14. Majcherczyk PA, Livermore DM. Penicillin-binding protein (PBP) 2 and the post-antibiotic effect of carbapenems. J Antimicrob Chemother 1990; 26:593.
15. Spratt BG, Jobanputra V, Zimmermann W: Binding of thienamycin and clavulanic acid to the penicillin-binding proteins of Escherichia coli K-12. Antimicrob Agents Chemother 1977; 12:406.
16. Fuursted K: Post-antibiotic effect and killing activity of ciprofloxacin against Staphylococcus aureus. Acta Pathol Microbiol Immun Scand 1987; 95:199.
17. Guan L, Blumenthal RM, Burnham JC: Analysis of macromolecular biosynthesis to define the quinolone-induced post-antibiotic effect in Escherichia coli. Antimicrob Agents Chemother 1992; 36:2118.
18. Bigger JW: The bactericidal action of penicillin on Staphylococcus pyogenes. Irish J Med Sci 1944; 227:533.
19. Parker RF, Marsh HC: The action of penicillin on Staphylococcus. J Bacteriol 1946; 51:181.
20. Parker RF, Luse S: The action of penicillin on Staphylococcus: Further observations on the effect of a short exposure. J Bacteriol 1948; 56:75.
21. Bodey GP, Pan T: Effect of cephalothin on growth patterns of microorganisms. J Antibiot 1976; 29:1092.
22. Bundtzen RW, Gerber AU, Cohn DL, Craig WA: Postantibiotic suppression of bacterial growth. Rev Infect Dis 1981; 3:28.
23. McDonald PJ, Craig WA, Kunin CM: Brief antibiotic exposure and effects on bacterial growth. In: Williams JD, Geddes AM (eds): Chemotherapy, vol 2. New York, Plenum, 1976, pp 95–102.
24. McDonald PJ, Craig WA, Kunin CM: Persistent effect of antibiotics on Staphylococcus aureus after exposure for limited periods of time. J Infect Dis 1977; 135:217.
25. McDonald PJ, Hskendorf P, Pruul H: Recovery period of bacteria after brief exposure to N-formimidoyl-thienamycin and other antibiotics. In: Periti P, Grassi GG (eds): Current Chemotherapy and Immunotherapy: Proceedings of the 12th International Congress of Chemotherapy—1981. Washington, DC, American Society for Microbiology, 1983, pp 741–743.
26. McDonald PJ, Wetherall BL, Pruul H: Postantibiotic leukocyte enhancement: Increased susceptibility of bacteria pretreated with antibiotics to activity of leukocytes. Rev Infect Dis 1981; 3:38.
27. Pruul H, McDonald PJ: Enhancement of leukocyte activity against Escherichia coli after brief exposure to chloramphenicol. Antimicrob Agents Chemother 1979; 16:695.
28. Pruul H, Wetherall BL, McDonald PJ: Enhanced susceptibility of Escherichia coli to intracellular killing by human polymorphonuclear leukocytes after in vitro incubation with chloramphenicol. Antimicrob Agents Chemother 1981; 19:945.
29. Pruul H, Hill N, McDonald PJ: Enoxacin-induced alteration of susceptibility of pneumococci and pseudomonas to phagocytosis by human polymorphonuclear leukocytes. J Antimicrob Chemother 1984; 14(suppl C):19.
30. Pruul H, Lewis G, McDonald PJ: Enhanced susceptibility of gram-negative bacteria to phagocytic killing by human polymorphonuclear leukocytes after brief exposure to aztreonam. J Antimicrob Chemother 1988; 22:675.
31. Yoshimura F, Nikaido H: Diffusion of beta-lactam antibiotics through the porin channels of Escherichia coli K-12. Antimicrob Agents Chemother 1985; 27:84.
32. Cornaglia G, Guan L, Fontana R, Satta G: Diffusion of meropenem and imipenem through the outer membrane of Escherichia coli K-12 and correlation with their antibacterial activities. Antimicrob Agents Chemother 1992; 36:1902.
33. Trtias J, Nikaido H: Outer membrane protein D2 catalyzes facilitated diffusion of carbapenems and penems through the outer membrane of Pseudomonas aeruginosa. Antimicrob Agents Chemother 1990; 34:52.
34. Trias J, Dufresne J, Levesque RC, Nikaido H: Decreased outer membrane permeability in imipenem-resistant mutants of Pseudomonas aeruginosa. Antimicrob Agents Chemother 1989; 33:1202.
35. Norrby SR, Finch RG, Glauser M: Monotherapy in serious hospital-acquired infections: A clinical trial of ceftazidime versus imipenem/cilastatin. J Antimicrob Chemother 1993; 31:927.
36. Kager L, Brismar B, Malmborg AS, Nord CE: Imipenem concentrations in colorectal surgery and impact on the colonic microflora. Antimicrob Agents Chemother 1989; 33:204.
37. Van der Leur JJ, Thunnissen PL, Clasener HA, et al: Effects of imipenem, cefotaxime and co-trimoxazole on aerobic microbial colonization of the digestive tract. Scand J Infect Dis 1993; 25:473.
38. Smith MD, Bielawska C, Kelsey MC, et al: Evaluation of imipenem/cilastatin for treatment of infection in an elderly population. J Antimicrob Chemother 1988; 21:481.
39. Calandra GB, Brown KR, Grad LC, et al: Review of adverse experiences and tolerability in the first 2,516 patients treated with imipenem/cilastin. Am J Med 1985; 78:73.
40. Barza M: Imipenem: First of a new class of beta-lactam antibiotics. Ann Intern Med 1985; 103:552.
41. Sheikh W, Pitkin DH, Nadler H: Antibacterial activity of

meropenem and selected comparative agents against anaerobic bacteria at seven North American centers. Clin Infect Dis 1993; 16(suppl 4):S361.

42. Hoban DJ, Jones RN, Yamane N, et al: In vitro activity of three carbapenem antibiotics: Comparative studies with biapenem (L-627), imipenem, and meropenem against aerobic pathogens isolated worldwide. Diagn Microbiol Infect Dis 1993; 17:299.

43. Lang C, Beuth J, Ko HL, et al: Antibacterial in vitro activity of meropenem against 200 clinical isolates in comparison to 11 selected antibiotics. Zentralbl Bakteriol 1992; 277:485.

48

Clindamycin

DAVID E. SOPER

Many pelvic infections in women are due to a polymicrobial flora in which anaerobic bacteria play a significant role. This reality became the stimulus for the initiation of combination antibiotic therapy utilizing an agent with excellent anaerobic bacterial coverage together with an agent with good aerobic bacterial coverage. Combination regimens with clindamycin have become the "gold standard" for the treatment of these infections.[1] Few agents have enjoyed as widespread a use as clindamycin in the treatment of obstetric and gynecologic infections.

STRUCTURE AND DERIVATION

Clindamycin is a semisynthetic derivative of lincomycin, a natural compound produced by an actinomycete, *Streptomyces lincolnensis*. It exceeds lincomycin in all desirable properties: absorption, serum concentration, and activity. Clindamycin is available in three forms for systemic administration: (1) clindamycin hydrochloride capsules, which contain 75, 150, or 300 mg of the drug; (2) clindamycin palmitate hydrochloride (75 mg of clindamycin per 5 mL), which is a water-soluble ester of clindamycin and palmitic acid and is used orally as a suspension because it does not have the objectionable taste of clindamycin hydrochloride; and (3) clindamycin phosphate (150 mg of clindamycin per 1 mL), which is a water-soluble ester of clindamycin and phosphoric acid and is used parenterally.[2] A 2% clindamycin phosphate cream is also available for a vaginal route of administration.

Studies demonstrate no inactivation or incompatibility when clindamycin phosphate is used in intravenous solutions containing sodium chloride, glucose, calcium, or potassium or in solutions containing vitamin B complex. No incompatibility has been demonstrated with the antibiotics cephalothin, kanamycin, gentamicin, or carbenicillin.[2]

MECHANISM OF ACTION

Clindamycin exerts its antibacterial activity through inhibition of the synthesis of proteins at the level of the 50S ribosome.[3] In addition, it facilitates opsonization, phagocytosis, and intracellular killing of bacteria, at drug concentrations below in vitro minimal inhibitory concentrations. Resistant strains do not break down or block the uptake of clindamycin. Clindamycin resistance results from an alteration of target site, possibly by ribosomal mutation. Plasmid-mediated transfer of resistance has been demonstrated.[4]

PHARMACOKINETICS

Clindamycin, as both the hydrochloride and the palmitate ester, is almost completely absorbed after oral administration, with the average peak serum levels reached in 45 to 60 minutes. Food taken concomitantly with clindamycin does not significantly reduce absorption. A single oral dose of 150 mg of clindamycin hydrochloride produces a mean peak serum level of 2.55 ± 0.92 µg/mL; a single oral dose of 300 mg produces a mean peak serum level of 3.44 ± 0.87 µg/mL. Clindamycin phosphate is well absorbed after intramuscular injection, with peak serum levels reached within 3 hours in adults. After an intramuscular injection of 300 mg of clindamycin phosphate, an average peak serum level of 5 µg/mL is reached. When clindamycin is given intravenously, peak serum levels are achieved at the end of the infusion, with levels ranging from 6 to 30 µg/mL after the infusion of 600 mg and 900 mg, and from 2.6 to 26 µg/mL after an infusion of 300 mg.

Clindamycin is widely distributed in many body fluids and tissues, and significant concentrations are reached in most tissues. Of special interest is the concentration of the drug in the fallopian tubes and uterus, shown in Table 48–1.[5]

Both clindamycin phosphate and clindamycin palmitate hydrochloride are hydrolyzed to active clindamycin within 1 to 2 hours. A state of equilibrium is reached in the serum after the third or fourth dose of clindamycin, and no accumulation has been reported after multiple doses. Most of the drug is metabolized by the liver and excreted into the bile, with the metabolites produced by the liver being biologically active. The normal half-life of clindamycin is 2 to 3 hours, and thus it can be given at 6-hour intervals. Comparative

TABLE 48-1 ▶ CLINDAMYCIN LEVELS IN TISSUES OF THE REPRODUCTIVE TRACT*

Tissue	Concentration (µg/g)
Cervix	2.63 ± 1.31
Endometrium	5.58 ± 4.58
Myometrium	2.40 ± 1.06
Fallopian tube	2.96 ± 1.55
Ovary	3.74 ± 3.12

*Following a single intravenous infusion of 600 mg of clindamycin phosphate. Mean serum level = 6.26 µg/mL.
Data from Johnson SR, Petzold CR, Galask RP: Clindamycin levels in reproductive tissues. Am J Reprod Immunol 1985; 8:67.

pharmacokinetic studies have been performed with 8-hour interval and 12-hour interval dosing. Higher concentrations of the antibiotic were found in the plasma of patients given a 900-mg dose every 8 hours compared to patients receiving the more standard 600 mg every 6 hours.[6] When the effectiveness of a 600-mg every 8 hour dosing regimen was compared with a 900-mg every 8 hour dosing regimen, cure and success rates were similar enough for both dosages to suggest that the routine use of 600 mg every 8 hours in women with mild to moderate pelvic infections is clinically acceptable. It is prudent, however, to use the 900-mg every 8 hour dose in patients with serious intra-abdominal infections or underlying conditions.[7] Mixing clindamycin with gentamicin (dosed by weight) may represent a more convenient and cost-effective means of delivery. About 10% to 30% of the drug is excreted by the kidneys, and the level of renal excretion may be increased in the presence of liver disease. Since most of the drug is excreted by the liver, no dose adjustment is necessary for most patients with renal failure, but it is recommended that modest dose decreases be made for patients with combined severe hepatic and renal diseases.

Clindamycin crosses the placental barrier. Cord concentrations were 46% of maternal levels after a single 600-mg intravenous dose.[8] Following multiple oral doses, fetal blood concentrations (mean, 0.7 µg/mL) were approximately 25% and amniotic fluid concentrations (mean, 0.82 to 1.07 µg/mL) were approximately 30% of maternal blood concentrations.[9] These concentrations in the majority of instances are within the therapeutic range for this antibiotic. Clindamycin is also transferred into human breast milk. There is marked interindividual variation in peak levels noted in breast milk following oral administration of the antibiotic. Levels ranged from 0.1 to several times the corresponding bioactivity in simultaneously collected plasma.[10]

Vaginal creams and suppositories are available for the treatment of a variety of vaginal conditions and are well accepted. With this in mind, clindamycin has been formulated into a vaginal cream. Possible advantages of this formulation include low cost compared

to systemic therapy, increased safety due to minimal systemic absorption, acceptability for use in pregnancy, and enhanced patient compliance. Systemic absorption following intravaginal application of a 1% clindamycin vaginal cream has been assessed in two trials involving both pregnant[11] and nonpregnant[12] women. The absolute bioavailabilities of the two intravaginal treatments were 6% and 13% for daily and twice-daily dosing, respectively.

Clindamycin is one of several antibiotics that possess a significant ability to concentrate within neutrophils. This characteristic may be important in the intracellular destruction of bacteria through either direct antibacterial activity or augmentation of neutrophil function.[13] The uptake of clindamycin by polymorphonuclear neutrophils is rapid, and the peak intracellular concentration is approximately 40 times greater than the extracellular concentration.[14] The intracellular drug appears to be lysosomotropic and is bioactive. These findings have implications for the treatment of abscesses in which transport of intracellular drug may be an important method of delivery or in the treatment of intracellular microorganisms, especially *Chlamydia trachomatis*. Clindamycin may also augment host immune response by enhancing opsonization of bacteria.[15]

SIDE EFFECTS

The most significant side effects of clindamycin develop in the gastrointestinal tract. Orally or parenterally administered clindamycin may cause anorexia, nausea, and vomiting. The most frequent side effect is the development of diarrhea, which occurs in as many as 20% of patients with varying degrees of severity.[2] Diarrhea is more common with oral administration. In general, the diarrhea is self-limited if the drug is promptly discontinued. Occasionally, pseudomembranous colitis (PMC) may occur, having been reported in 0.01% to 10% of clindamycin-treated patients.[16] PMC is produced by the release of exotoxins from *Clostridium difficile*, an organism usually resistant to clindamycin. PMC is rarely reported in studies of obstetric and gynecologic infections, probably because the patients usually do not have underlying debilitating conditions that may predispose to the development of PMC. Oral vancomycin or metronidazole is highly effective for the treatment of PMC.

Less severe side effects include rash (4%), neutropenia, eosinophilia, and an occasional increase in transaminase levels and alkaline phosphatase levels. Clindamycin is not ototoxic or nephrotoxic. When administered intravenously, it does not produce venous irritation.

No reports linking the use of clindamycin with congenital defects have been published. This agent is considered a category B drug. Animal-reproduction studies have not demonstrated a fetal risk, but there are no controlled studies in pregnant women.[17]

SPECTRUM OF ANTIBIOTIC ACTIVITY

Clindamycin is useful in the treatment of many bacterial infections caused by aerobic gram-positive bacteria and anaerobic bacteria. It is generally inactive against aerobic gram-negative bacteria. Additional activity is noted against *Chlamydia trachomatis* and *Toxoplasma gondii*. In vitro susceptibilities of selected microorganisms to clindamycin are listed in Table 48–2.[18, 19] Note that the commonly quoted "break point" for clindamycin is considered 4 μg/mL for parenteral therapy and 2 μg/mL for oral therapy. The break point of an antibiotic is the concentration of the drug that can be reliably obtained in the serum during therapy. Microorganisms sensitive to the antibiotic at this level or below are considered susceptible.

Gram-Positive Aerobic Microorganisms. The most important aerobic gram-positive pathogen encountered in obstetric and gynecologic infections is the group B streptococcus (GBS; *Streptococcus agalactiae*). In patients allergic to beta-lactam agents, clindamycin remains a good alternative agent for GBS infections.[20] In some patient populations, however, the in vitro resistance of GBS to clindamycin has been as high as 15%.[21] Clindamycin maintains excellent activity against other important streptococci, such as *Streptococcus pyogenes* (group A streptococcus), *Streptococcus pneumoniae* (the pneumococcus), and streptococci of the "viridans" group. In addition, this antibiotic has activity against most strains of *Staphylococcus aureus*, but it may not inhibit methicillin-resistant strains (MRSA). Other important resistant gram-positive aerobes are the enterococci (*Enterococcus faecalis, E. faecium, E. durans,* and *E. avium*). This observation is particularly important

in light of the common use of combination therapy (clindamycin plus an aminoglycoside) for the treatment of many obstetric and gynecologic infections, leaving the enterococci uncovered. The susceptibility of *Listeria monocytogenes* to clindamycin is unknown.

Gram-Negative Aerobic Microorganisms. These microorganisms are common causes of sepsis in obstetric and gynecologic patients. They include *E. coli, Klebsiella* sp., *Proteus* sp., and *Enterobacter* sp. These microorganisms, and, in fact, all the Enterobacteriaceae, are resistant to clindamycin. *Neisseria gonorrhoeae* is moderately sensitive (median MIC, 3.1 μg/mL) to clindamycin, but this agent cannot be used reliably for treatment of gonorrhea. *Gardnerella vaginalis* is very susceptible to clindamycin; on the other hand, clindamycin is generally inactive against *Haemophilus influenzae* at clinically achievable concentrations.

Gram-Positive Anaerobic Microorganisms. The commonly isolated anaerobic gram-positive cocci, *Peptococcus* sp. and *Peptostreptococcus* sp., are highly susceptible to clindamycin. In addition, this agent is active against *Clostridium perfringens*. The non-*perfringens* clostridia, particularly *C. difficile* and *C. ramosum*, are usually resistant. *Actinomyces israelii* and other *Actinomyces* species are also highly susceptible to clindamycin.

Gram-Negative Anaerobic Microorganisms. Clindamycin is highly active against gram-negative anaerobic bacteria.[22–24] Of particular importance are the *Bacteroides* species, which commonly elaborate a beta-lactamase that inactivates many penicillin and cephalosporin antibiotics. Members of the *Bacteroides fragilis* group of microorganisms, frequently recovered from pelvic infections, are commonly beta-lactamase positive; however, more than 90% of strains remain sensitive to clindamycin.[25] In addition, between 40% and 85% of the non-*fragilis Bacteroides* isolates and the fusobacteria are beta-lactamase positive and, therefore, resistant to penicillin. Beta-lactamase positive rates are highest for *Bacteroides bivius*.[19] Fewer than 5% of these isolates are resistant to clindamycin. *Mobiluncus*, a short, curved anaerobic gram-negative rod associated with bacterial vaginosis, is also highly sensitive to clindamycin.

Genital Mycoplasmas. *Mycoplasma hominis* is highly sensitive (median MIC, 0.12 μg/mL) to clindamycin, while *Ureaplasma urealyticum* is only moderately sensitive (median MIC, 4 μg/mL).[26] Clindamycin is generally considered an alternative to tetracycline for the treatment of *M. hominis* infections. It appears to have no effect on *U. urealyticum* colonization of the vagina in pregnant women.[27]

Chlamydia. Despite moderate antichlamydial activity (MIC range, 2 μg/mL to 4 μg/mL) in vitro, treat-

TABLE 48-2 ▶ IN VITRO SUSCEPTIBILITIES TO CLINDAMYCIN

Organism	Minimum Inhibitory Concentration (μg/mL)	
	Range	*Median*
Streptococcus agalactiae	<1–10	<1
Streptococcus pyogenes	0.02–0.1	0.04
Enterococcus spp.	12.5–>100	100
Staphylococcus aureus	0.04–>100	0.1
Clostridium perfringens	<0.1–8	0.8
Neisseria gonorrhoeae	0.01–6.3	3.1
Haemophilus influenzae	0.4–50	12.5
Bacteroides fragilis group	<0.125–>256	0.25
Non-*fragilis Bacteroides* spp.	—	≤0.5
Fusobacterium spp.	≤0.5	≤0.5
Peptostreptococcus spp.	≤0.1–0.8	≤0.5
Peptococcus spp.	≤0.1–>100	≤0.5
Mycoplasma hominis	—	0.12

ment failures appear common. In a trial of oral clinda- mycin for the treatment of nongonococcal urethritis, 30% of chlamydia-positive men were still infected after treatment.[28] The effectiveness of clindamycin in the treatment of uncomplicated *C. trachomatis* infection in women has not been determined. However, treatment with high-dose intravenous clindamycin has resulted in clinical evidence of cure and eradication of *C. tracho- matis* from the endometrium in a small series of pa- tients treated for pelvic inflammatory disease.[29, 30]

CLINICAL APPLICATION

Clindamycin is most commonly used to treat polymi- crobial intra-abdominal and gynecologic pelvic infec- tions, usually in combination with another antibiotic, such as an aminoglycoside. It is in these clinical scenar- ios that beta-lactamase–producing *Bacteroides* and *Prevo- tella* species are commonly found.

Postpartum Endomyometritis. Postpartum endo- myometritis remains the most common infection fol- lowing childbirth. Cesarean delivery continues to be the most significant predisposing factor. Anaerobic bacteria, particularly the beta-lactamase–producing *Bacteroides* and *Prevotella* species, play a prominent role in the pathophysiology of postpartum endomyometri- tis, being isolated in as many as 60% of women with this postpartum complication.[31, 32] Studies comparing the combination of penicillin plus an aminoglycoside with clindamycin combination therapy reveal a signifi- cantly lower cure rate with the former regimen (Table 48–3).[33, 34] Moreover, many patients failing initial ther- apy with the penicillin combination went on to develop serious sequelae, such as pelvic abscess formation or septic pelvic thrombophlebitis. Treatment with a com- bination regimen consisting of clindamycin resulted in the cure of more than 90% of infected patients, and fewer than 0.5% receiving this therapy developed seri- ous sequelae.[35] These data suggest that it is important to initiate therapy with an antibiotic with good activity against penicillin-resistant anaerobic bacteria. Now more than a dozen prospective, randomized compara- tive studies have been performed utilizing clinda- mycin, usually in combination with an aminoglycoside, such as gentamicin, for the treatment of postcesarean endomyometritis (see Table 48–3).[2, 36, 37] Treatment fail-

ures may be due to the presence of a resistant microor- ganism, usually *Enterococcus* species, and may respond promptly to the addition of ampicillin to the clinda- mycin-aminoglycoside regimen. Otherwise discontinu- ation of the initial antibiotic regimen is due to side effects, such as diarrhea. Patients responding to combi- nation antibiotic therapy with clindamycin do not re- quire further oral antibiotic therapy after discharge from the hospital.[38]

Postoperative Pelvic Cellulitis Following Hysterec- tomy. Pelvic cellulitis remains the most common seri- ous infection following hysterectomy. Postoperative cuff cellulitis or pelvic abscess, or both, occur in as many as 18% of women not receiving antibiotic pro- phylaxis.[39] The pathogenesis of this infection results from invasion of spaces superior and lateral to the vaginal cuff, including the parametrial tissue, by en- dogenous microorganisms found in the vagina. A polymicrobial etiology of this infection is common, with more than 90% of patients having more than one microorganism isolated. In addition, bacterial vag- inosis organisms (*G. vaginalis*, *Bacteroides* sp., or *Pepto- streptococcus* sp.) are isolated from the operative site in more than 50% of patients with cuff cellulitis or ab- scess. In studies evaluating the efficacy of clindamycin combination therapy in the treatment of pelvic infec- tions, some patients with postoperative cuff cellulitis have been included. Reports show a 100% success rate in the 42 patients who have been studied.[36, 40–42]

Pelvic Inflammatory Disease. Although the most common microbial etiology of pelvic inflammatory dis- ease (PID) remain *Neisseria gonorrhoeae* and *Chlamydia trachomatis*, a substantial proportion of patients hospi- talized with PID have a polymicrobial infection con- sisting of both aerobic and anaerobic microorgan- isms.[30, 43, 44] In addition, anaerobic bacteria are commonly isolated from the upper genital tract of women with tubo-ovarian abscesses, an important se- quelae of PID.[45] More than a dozen efficacy trials have been performed utilizing clindamycin in conjunction with an aminoglycoside in the therapy for PID. Overall success rates approach 93% (Table 48–4).[2] In addition, in patients with documented tubo-ovarian abscess, clin- damycin regimens were associated with a 72% response rate, suggesting that initially conservative treatment of

TABLE 48–3 ▶ TREATMENT OF POSTCESAREAN ENDOMYOMETRITIS

Drug Regimen	No. of Patients	Clinical Cure (Range %)	Weighted Mean Cure (%)
Penicillin/aminoglycoside	226	55–78	71
Clindamycin/aminoglycoside	829	76–100	91
Single-agent cephalosporin	346	78–96	85
Extended-spectrum penicillins	285	75–91	85

TABLE 48-4 ▶ TREATMENT OF PELVIC INFLAMMATORY DISEASE

Drug Regimen	No. of Patients	Clinical Cure (Range %)	Weighted Mean Cure (%)
Clindamycin-containing regimens	530	85–100	93
Cephalosporin ± doxycycline	268	84–96	92

tubo-ovarian abscesses is warranted.[46] Empirical broad-spectrum treatment remains the therapy of choice until better data concerning the microbiology of PID are available. The Centers for Disease Control and Prevention (CDC) continues to recommend a combination of clindamycin with an aminoglycoside for the treatment of PID.[47] Clinicians have extensive experience with this regimen, and it is associated with high rates of cure. In addition, owing to its excellent anaerobic spectrum and its ability to concentrate within polymorphonuclear leukocytes, clindamycin is an excellent choice for use in the treatment of pelvic abscesses.

Septic Abortion. *Septic abortion* most commonly refers to an infected incomplete abortion, although some patients present prior to the passage of any products of conception. Any threatened, inevitable, or incomplete abortion associated with fever should be considered a septic abortion. The most common microorganisms isolated from both the blood or the uterine cavity, or both, are anaerobes and microaerophilic bacteria. Anaerobic gram-positive cocci are the most common isolates, but *Bacteroides* species and *Clostridium* species can also play a major role. Early evacuation of the uterus is indicated in addition to broad-spectrum antibiotic therapy. Experience with clindamycin in the treatment of septic abortion has been limited, but a report from Panama noted that all 16 patients treated with a clindamycin-gentamicin combination responded to therapy.[48] Clindamycin-containing regimens can be expected to perform well in these clinical scenarios as well as in cases of postabortal endometritis.

Intra-amniotic infection. The most common microorganisms in patients with intra-amniotic infection (IAI) are anaerobes and group B streptococci.[49] *Mycoplasma hominis* is also commonly present in patients with IAI.[50] Most studies to date have evaluated a penicillin, usually ampicillin, in combination with an aminoglycoside for the treatment of IAI. Owing to good activity against the group B streptococci and excellent activity against anaerobes, a clindamycin-aminoglycoside regimen could be considered as alternative therapy for IAI in the penicillin-allergic patient. In addition, for patients with IAI who undergo cesarean delivery, it is prudent to add clindamycin postoperatively to avoid the high failure rates associated with ampicillin-aminoglycoside regimens alone.[51]

Necrotizing Fasciitis. Necrotizing fasciitis is an uncommon but life-threatening infection primarily involving the superficial fascia. It usually occurs in diabetics and involves most commonly the vulva, but less frequently it also involves the abdominal wall and subgluteal and retropsoal spaces. The microbiology of this disease consists of a polymicrobial flora involving both anaerobic and facultative aerobic bacteria. Surgical débridement is the mainstay of therapy for the patient with necrotizing fasciitis. In addition, broad-spectrum antibiotic therapy to cover both anaerobic and aerobic bacteria should be started. Clindamycin-containing regimens, usually in combination with an aminoglycoside and a penicillin, can be used for the treatment of this disease.

Bacterial Vaginosis. Bacterial vaginosis (BV) is a complex alteration of the vaginal flora resulting in a significant increase in the concentration of anaerobes and *Gardnerella vaginalis* in the vaginal fluid.[52] Anaerobic bacteria associated with this disease include *Bacteroides* sp., *Prevotella* sp., and *Peptostreptococcus* sp. In addition, the highly motile bacteria, *Mobiluncus*, has been associated with BV. The activity of clindamycin against anaerobes is well known. *Gardnerella vaginalis* is highly susceptible to clindamycin in vitro at an MIC of approximately 0.06 to 0.125 µg/mL.[53] *Mobiluncus* appears to be susceptible to clindamycin in vitro at an MIC of approximately 0.06 to 0.125 µg/mL.[54]

Therapeutic agents that are alternatives to metronidazole for the treatment of BV have been sought because of treatment failures, side effects, and the relative contraindication to metronidazole use in the first trimester of pregnancy. Clindamycin, 300 mg PO twice daily (failure rate, 4%), was as effective as metronidazole, 500 mg PO twice daily (failure rate, 6%), in the treatment of 143 nonpregnant women with BV. Three patients who received clindamycin developed nonbloody diarrhea, which was mild and did not necessitate discontinuing therapy.[55] Intravaginal clindamycin cream has also been evaluated. Five grams of 1.0% or 2.0% clindamycin cream administered intravaginally twice daily for 5 days was associated with clinical resolution of BV in 71% and 94% of women, respectively.[56] The intravaginal treatment effectively eradicated the microorganisms associated with BV and was associated with no significant side effects. In another study, 94% of patients with BV treated with clindamycin cream were cured, compared to only 25% who received placebos.[57] This 2% formulation is an acceptable alternative to oral or topical metronidazole in the treatment of BV.

Desquamative Inflammatory Vaginitis. Desquamative inflammatory vaginitis (DIV) is an uncommon disease characterized by a chronic purulent vaginal discharge. Microscopy of the vaginal secretions reveals a predominance of white blood cells accompanied by many parabasal cells, suggesting a desquamation of the vaginal epithelium. An overgrowth of streptococci and an absence of lactobacilli is noted microbiologically. Clindamycin vaginal cream is an effective first-line therapy for this disorder. Relapse can be prevented in many postmenopausal women by instituting hormonal replacement therapy.[58]

SUMMARY

Clindamycin has been extensively used in the treatment of obstetric and gynecologic infections for more than 20 years. This antibiotic is well known for it activity against anaerobic bacteria, particularly beta-lactamase–producing strains of the *Bacteroides* species. Clinicians should also recognize its very good activity against aerobic gram-positive cocci, such as the group B streptococcus, but should be aware of its absence of activity against aerobic gram-negative rods, such as *E. coli*. In combination with an aminoglycoside, clindamycin has become the "gold standard" by which other antimicrobials have been judged in the treatment of pelvic infections. A dose of 900 mg administered intravenously every 8 hours is recommended when one treats the serious infections discussed. Although concern about the potential side effect of pseudomembranous colitis is valid, in practice, this is an uncommon problem that responds well to discontinuation of the clindamycin and treatment of the *C. difficile*–induced condition with vancomycin or metronidazole.

REFERENCES

1. Hemsell DL, Solomkin JS, Sweet R, et al: Evaluation of new anti-infective drugs for treatment of acute pelvic infections in hospitalized women. Clin Infect Dis 1992; 15(suppl 1):543.
2. Zambrano D: Clindamycin in the treatment of obstetric and gynecologic infections: A review. Clin Ther 1991; 13:58.
3. Dhawan VK, Thadepalli H: Clindamycin: A review of fifteen years of experience. Rev Infect Dis 1982; 4:1133.
4. Tally FP, Cuchural GJ Jr, Malamy MH, et al: Mechanisms of resistance and resistance transfer in anaerobic bacteria: Factors influencing antimicrobial resistance. Rev Infect Dis 1984; 6:260.
5. Johnson SR, Petzold CR, Galask RP: Clindamycin levels in reproductive tissues. Am J Reprod Immunol 1985; 8:67.
6. Flaherty JF, Rodondi LC, Guglielmo BJ, et al: Comparative pharmacokinetics and serum inhibitory activity of clindamycin in different dosing regimens. Antimicrob Agents Chemother 1988; 32:1825.
7. Rovers JP, Ilersich AL, Einarson TR: Meta-analysis of parenteral clindamycin dosing regimens. Ann Pharmacother 1995; 29:852.
8. Weinstein AJ, Gibbs RS, Gallagher M: Placental transfer of clindamycin and gentamicin in term pregnancy. Am J Obstet Gynecol 1976; 124:688.
9. Philipson A, Sabath LD, Charles D: Transplacental passage of erythromycin and clindamycin. N Engl J Med 1973; 288:1219.
10. Steen B, Rane A: Clindamycin passage into human milk. Br J Clin Pharmacol 1982; 13:661.
11. Borin MT: Systemic absorption of clindamycin following intravaginal application of clindamycin phosphate 1% cream. J Clin Pharmacol 1990; 30:33.
12. Powley GW, Timm JA: Efficacy and systemic absorption of 1% clindamycin phosphate vaginal cream in pregnant women with bacterial vaginosis. UpJohn Technical Report 9156/88/021, August 1988.
13. Faden H, Hong JJ, Ogra PL: In-vivo effects of clindamycin on neutrophil function. J Antimicrob Chemother 1985; 16:649.
14. Klempner MS, Styrt B: Clindamycin uptake by human neutrophils. J Infect Dis 1981; 144:472.
15. Milatovic D, Braveny I, Verhoef J: Clindamycin enhances opsonization of *Staphylococcus aureus*. Antimicrob Agents Chemother 1983; 24:413.
16. Tedesco FJ: Clindamycin and colitis: A review. J Infect Dis 1977; 135(suppl):S95.
17. Briggs GG, Bodendorfer TW, Freeman RK, Yaffe SJ (eds): Drugs in Pregnancy and Lactation: A Reference Guide to Fetal and Neonatal Risk. Baltimore, Williams & Wilkins, 1984, p 79.
18. Steigbigel NH: Erythromycin, lincomycin, and clindamycin. In: Mandell GL, Douglas RG, Bennett JE (eds): Principles and Practice of Infectious Diseases, 3rd ed. New York, Churchill Livingstone, 1990, pp 312–315.
19. LeFrock JL, Molavi A, Prince RA: Clindamycin. Med Clin North Am 1982; 66:103.
20. Rouse DJ, Andrews WW, Lin F-Y, et al: Antibiotic susceptibility profile of group B *Streptococcus* acquired vertically. Obstet Gynecol 1998; 92:931.
21. Pearlman MD, Pierson CL, Faix RG: Frequent resistance of clinical group B streptococci isolates to clindamycin and erythromycin. Obstet Gynecol 1998; 92:258.
22. Cuchural GJ, Tally FP, Jacobus NV, et al: Susceptibility of the *Bacteroides fragilis* group in the United States: Analysis by site of isolation. Antimicrob Agents Chemother 1988; 32:717.
23. Appelbaum PC, Spangler SK, Jacobs MR: β-Lactamase production and susceptibilities to amoxicillin, amoxicillin-clavulanate, ticarcillin, ticarcillin-clavulanate, cefoxitin, imipenem, and metronidazole of 320 non–*Bacteroides fragilis Bacteroides* isolates and 129 fusobacteria from 28 US centers. Antimicrob Agents Chemother 1990; 34:1546.
24. Musial CE, Rosenblatt JE: Antimicrobial susceptibilities of anaerobic bacteria isolated at the Mayo Clinic during 1982 through 1987: Comparison with results from 1977 through 1981. Mayo Clin Proc 1989; 64:392.
25. Dalmau D, Cayouette M, Lamothe F, et al: Clindamycin resistance in the *Bacteroides fragilis* group: Association with hospital-acquired infections. Clin Infect Dis 1997; 24:874.
26. Harrison HR, Riggin RM, Alexander ER, Weinstein L: In vitro activity of clindamycin against strains of *Chlamydia trachomatis*, *Mycoplasma hominis*, and *Ureaplasma urealyticum* isolated from pregnant women. Am J Obstet Gynecol 1984; 149:477.
27. McCormack WM, Rosner B, Lee Y-H, et al: Effect on birth weight of erthromycin treatment of pregnant women. Obstet Gynecol 1987; 69:202.
28. Bowie WR, Yu JS, Jones HD: Partial efficacy of clindamycin against *Chlamydia trachomatis* in men with nongonococcal urethritis. Sex Transm Dis 1986; 13:76.
29. Walters MD, Gibbs RS: A randomized comparison of gentamicin-clindamycin and cefoxitin-doxycycline in the treatment of pelvic inflammatory disease. Obstet Gynecol 1990; 75:867.
30. Wasserheit JN, Bell TA, Kiviat NB, et al: Microbial causes of proven pelvic inflammatory disease and efficacy of clindamycin and tobramycin. Ann Intern Med 1986; 104:187.
31. Rosene K, Eschenbach DA, Tompkins LS, et al: Polymicrobial early postpartum endometritis with facultative and anaerobic bacteria, genital mycoplasmas, and *Chlamydia trachomatis*: Treatment with piperacillin or cefoxitin. J Infect Dis 1986; 153:1028.

32. Watts DH, Eschenbach DA, Kenny GE: Early postpartum endometritis: The role of bacteria, genital mycoplasmas, and *Chlamydia trachomatis.* Obstet Gynecol 1989; 73:60.

33. Gibbs RS, Jones PM, Wilder CJ: Antibiotic therapy of endometritis following cesarean section: Treatment successes and failures. Obstet Gynecol 1978; 52:31.

34. diZerega G, Yonekura L, Roy S, et al: A comparison of clindamycin-gentamicin and penicillin-gentamicin in the treatment of post-cesarean section endomyometritis. Am J Obstet Gynecol 1979; 134:238.

35. Duff P: Pathophysiology and management of postcesarean endomyometritis. Obstet Gynecol 1986; 67:269.

36. Hemsell DL, Martens MG, Faro S, et al: A multicenter study comparing intravenous meropenem with clindamycin plus gentamicin for the treatment of acute gynecologic and obstetrics pelvic infections in hospitalized women. Clin Infect Dis 1997; 24(suppl 2):S222.

37. Gall S, Koukol DH: Ampicillin/sulbactam vs. clindamycin/ gentamicin in the treatment of postpartum endometritis. J Reprod Med 1996; 41:575.

38. Soper DE, Kemmer CT, Conover WB: Abbreviated antibiotic therapy for the treatment of postpartum endometritis. Obstet Gynecol 1987; 69:127.

39. Hemsell DL, Reisch J, Nobles B, Hemsell PG: Prevention of major infection after elective abdominal hysterectomy: Individual determination required. Am J Obstet Gynecol 1983; 147:520.

40. Swenson RM, Michaelson TC, Daly MD, Spalding EH: Clindamycin in infections of the female genital tract. Obstet Gynecol 1974; 44:699.

41. Swenson RM, Lorber B: Clindamycin and carbenicillin in treatment of patients with intraabdominal and female genital tract infections. J Infect Dis 1977; 135(suppl):S40.

42. Gilstrap LC III, Maier RC, Gibbs RS, et al: Piperacillin versus clindamycin plus gentamicin for pelvic infections. Obstet Gynecol 1984; 64:762.

43. Sweet RL, Draper DL, Hadley WK: Etiology of acute salpingitis: Influence of episode number and duration of symptoms. Obstet Gynecol 1981; 58:62.

44. Brunham RC, Binns B, Guijon F, et al: Etiology and outcome of acute pelvic inflammatory disease. J Infect Dis 1988; 158:510.

45. Walker CK, Landers DV: Pelvic abscesses: New trends in management. Obstet Gynecol Surv 1991; 46:615.

46. Reed SD, Landers DV, Sweet RL: Antibiotic treatment of tubo-ovarian abscess: Comparison of broad-spectrum β-lactam agents versus clindamycin-containing regimens. Am J Obstet Gynecol 1991; 164:1556.

47. CDC: 1998 Guidelines for treatment of sexually transmitted diseases. MMWR 1997; 47:79.

48. Rodriguez-French A, Kennion G: Estudio comparativo abierto entre la asociacion clindamicina/gentamicina contra penicilina/gentamicina en aborto septico. Inv Med Int 1985; 11:211.

49. Gibbs RS, Blanco JD, St Clair PJ, Castaneda YS: Quantitative bacteriology of amniotic fluid from patients with clinical intraamniotic infection at term. J Infect Dis 1982; 145:1.

50. Blanco JD, Gibbs RS, Malherbe H, et al: A controlled study of genital mycoplasmas in amniotic fluid from patients with intraamniotic infection. J Infect Dis 1983; 147:650.

51. Gibbs RS, Duff P: Progress in pathogenesis and management of clinical intraamniotic infection. Am J Obstet Gynecol 1991; 164:1317.

52. Eschenbach DA, Hillier S, Critchlow C, et al: Diagnosis and clinical manifestations of bacterial vaginosis. Am J Obstet Gynecol 1988; 158:819.

53. McCarthy LR, Mickelsen PA, Smith EG: Antibiotic susceptibility of *Haemophilus vaginalis (Corynebacterium vaginale)* to 21 antibiotics. Antimicrob Agents Chemother 1979; 16:186.

54. Spiegel CA: Susceptibility of *Mobiluncus* species to 23 antimicrobial agents and 15 other compounds. Antimicrob Agents Chemother 1987; 31:249.

55. Greaves WL, Chungafung J, Morris B, et al: Clindamycin versus metronidazole in the treatment of bacterial vaginosis. Obstet Gynecol 1988; 72:799.

56. Hillier SL, Krohn MA, Watts H, et al: Microbiological efficacy of intravaginal clindamycin cream for the treatment of bacterial vaginosis. Obstet Gynecol 1990; 76:407.

57. Livengood CH III, Thomason JL, Hill GB: Bacterial vaginosis: Treatment with topical intravaginal clindamycin phosphate. Obstet Gynecol 1990; 76:118.

58. Sobel J: Desquamative inflammatory vaginitis: A new subgroup of purulent vaginitis responsive to topical 2% clindamycin therapy. Am J Obstet Gynecol 1994; 171:1215.

49

Metronidazole

JENNIFER GUNTER

STRUCTURE AND DERIVATION

Metronidazole is a nitroimidazole antibiotic that is bactericidal against most anaerobic bacteria and effective against a variety of protozoan infections. The first nitroimidazole, azomycin, was isolated from a *Streptomyces* species. Metronidazole is a synthetic nitroimidazole and was first introduced for clinical use in 1959 for the treatment of *Trichomonas vaginalis*. It is the most widely used nitroimidazole. The chemical formula of metronidazole is 1-(2-hydroxyethyl)-2-methyl-5-nitro-imidazole, with a molecular weight of 171.16. The chemical structure of metronidazole is shown in Figure 49–1.

MECHANISM OF ACTION

Metronidazole diffuses readily into both aerobic and anaerobic bacteria. Metronidazole is bactericidal, and the mechanism of action can be divided into four successive steps: (1) entry of metronidazole into the cell, (2) reductive activation, (3) toxic effects of the reduced products, and (4) release of inactive end products.[1, 2] Reductive activation of metronidazole is essential for cytotoxicity. During this process, the nitro group (see Fig. 49–1) is reduced in a series of one-electron steps by the pyruvate–ferredoxin oxidoreductase complex, also known as nitroreductase.[1–3] Cells with lower—that is, more negative—reduction potentials donate electrons to metronidazole; therefore, electrons are transferred from reduced ferredoxin to metronidazole, forming toxic intermediates including free radicals, a nitroso derivative, a nitroso-free radical, and a hydroxylamine derivative.[1, 2] These toxic intermediates damage DNA by inducing strand breakage and helix destabilization, which inhibits DNA synthesis and degrades existing DNA.[2, 4] These toxic intermediates are short-lived and are quickly inactivated and released by the cell.[1, 3]

Anaerobic conditions are required for the reductive activation of metronidazole. The lowest reduction potential of an aerobic cell is still more positive than that of metronidazole; thus, the electron transfer required for reduction of the nitro group cannot occur and the drug remains unchanged and is ineffective in an aerobic environment.[2] Cells undergoing anaerobic metabolism have a redox potential more negative than that of aerobic cells, and so in an anaerobic environment reductive activation of metronidazole occurs.[2] Some facultative bacteria are susceptible to metronidazole, but only under strict anaerobic conditions. Ongoing anaerobic conditions are required, as reduced metronidazole reoxidizes in the presence of oxygen to the original drug, reversing reductive activation.[1, 2] Metronidazole is active against both eukaryotic and prokaryotic cells, the common characteristic being anaerobic metabolism.[1, 5] Not only is reduction of the nitro group essential for cytotoxicity, but also it decreases the intracellular concentration of unchanged metronidazole, maintaining a diffusion gradient that favors further entry of the drug into anaerobic cells.[1, 2]

Resistance to metronidazole is not frequently encountered, although both resistant anaerobic bacteria and protozoa have been described.[6–8] The main mechanism of resistance to metronidazole appears to be decreased activity of the nitroreductase complex, which also results in decreased uptake of the antibiotic.[6, 8] Plasmid and chromosomally mediated resistances have been identified but are currently not believed to be a major concern in the emergence of metronidazole-resistant strains.[3, 7]

PHARMACOKINETICS

Metronidazole may be administered by a variety of routes: intravenous, oral, vaginal, and rectal. The half-life ranges from 6 to 10 hours; however, as metronidazole has dose-dependent pharmacokinetics, the half-life may be prolonged with larger doses.[9] The drug, therefore, has the potential to accumulate when administered in higher doses over a long period of use.

The standard intravenous administration of metronidazole has traditionally been 7.5 mg/kg (approximately 500 mg) every 6 hours, although the half-life would indicate that administration every 8 or 12 hours would be as effective.[3, 10] When metronidazole is administered at a dose of 500 mg intravenously every 6 hours, the mean plasma peak concentration is 25 µg/mL and the mean plasma trough concentration is 18

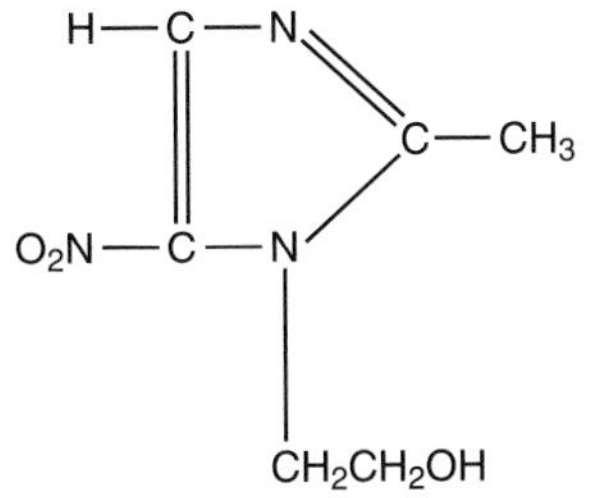

FIGURE 49-1 ▶ The chemical structure of metronidazole.

μg/mL.[3] If an equivalent dose is administered every 8 hours, the mean peak and trough drug concentrations at steady state are 26.7 μg/mL and 13.8 μg/mL; if 500 mg of metronidazole is given every 12 hours, the mean peak and trough concentrations are 23.6 μg/mL and 6.7 μg/mL, respectively.[9, 11] Based on these pharmacokinetics, dosing every 12 hours is now favored by many.[10]

Metronidazole is well absorbed after oral administration and has almost 100% oral bioavailability. As comparable serum levels are seen after equivalent intravenous and oral doses, when patients are able to tolerate and absorb oral medications there is little advantage to intravenous administration over oral.[9, 12] Oral administration of metronidazole results in rapid absorption, and peak serum levels are seen on average 1 hour after oral administration, with time to peak serum concentration ranging from 15 minutes to 4 hours.[13] Absorption is not affected significantly by food; however, the time to peak concentration may be delayed. The recommended oral dose for anaerobic infections is 1 to 2 g/day divided every 6 to 12 hours. After a single 2-g oral dose, the mean peak plasma concentration of metronidazole is 40.6 μg/mL.[14]

Metronidazole may be administered vaginally in a 0.75% gel formulation. A single 5-g dose of intravaginal gel (37.5 mg of metronidazole) produces only 2% of the mean peak serum concentration of a 500-mg oral dose.[15] Metronidazole has also been administered vaginally as a 500-mg tablet, with serum concentrations of 1.2 μg/mL approximately 8 hours after dosing.[13]

The volume of distribution of metronidazole is 80% of body weight, and less than 20% is bound to plasma proteins. Metronidazole is distributed well to almost all tissues, including vaginal secretions, saliva, seminal fluid, bone, unobstructed biliary tree, cerebrospinal fluid, and brain abscesses. The tissues of the upper genital tract achieve concentrations similar to serum levels.[3] Metronidazole crosses the placenta by simple diffusion, and levels in fetal serum and amniotic fluid approach maternal serum levels. Therapeutic levels of metronidazole are also found in breast milk, with maximal concentrations 2 to 4 hours after maternal dosing and a half-life of 8.7 to 9.9 hours, similar to the half-life in plasma.[16]

Metronidazole is metabolized by the liver to one of five end products. The major metabolite is the hydroxy derivative: 1-(2-hydroxyethyl)-2-hydroxymethyl-5-nitro-imidazole, which has antianaerobic activity against some bacteria.[7, 9] The other major metabolite is an acid derivative of metronidazole, acetylmetronidazole, which has weak antianaerobic properties.[1] The remaining three metabolites are metronidazole glucuronide, the glucuronide conjugate of hydroxymetronidazole, and a sulfate conjugate. Elimination of metronidazole is primarily renal, with 60% to 80% of the drug and metabolites excreted via the kidneys within 48 hours.[9] Most of the remaining drug and its metabolites are excreted via the biliary tree into the feces.

Hepatic dysfunction has a significant effect on the metabolism and on the elimination of metronidazole and its metabolites. In the presence of liver disease, decreased metabolism of metronidazole to its end products occurs, and the half-life may be prolonged up to 18 to 20 hours, depending on the degree of liver impairment.[9] The dose of metronidazole should be reduced by 50% in patients with significant hepatic dysfunction.[17] Renal dysfunction has less of an effect on the excretion of metronidazole, as only a small amount of unchanged drug is eliminated by this route; however, the hydroxy and acetic acid metabolites may accumulate when the creatinine clearance falls below 25 mL/min.[18] The effect of metabolite accumulation is unclear at this time. Lowering the dose in patients with renal impairment is usually not required unless the patient is receiving large doses, there is concomitant hepatic disease, or the creatinine clearance is less than 10 mL/min.[3] Hemodialysis removes metronidazole and its metabolites; therefore, metronidazole should be administered in the usual dose after dialysis. The pharmacokinetics of metronidazole are relatively unchanged in the patient receiving peritoneal dialysis, and a reduction in dose is usually not required, although some recommend reducing the dose by 50% in these patients.[9]

SIDE EFFECTS

Metronidazole is generally well tolerated, and major adverse reactions are rare, especially with standard doses. Most adverse reactions to metronidazole are minor and involve the gastrointestinal system; however, the potential for severe sequelae does exist (Table 49–1). Other important considerations regarding metronidazole therapy involve drug interactions and concerns over teratogenicity.

Minor gastrointestinal disturbances are the most frequent side effects with metronidazole therapy. The most common side effects seen after oral or intravenous administration are a metallic taste, nausea, and vomiting.[19] Diarrhea, glossitis, stomatitis, and dry mouth may also occur. Other more serious gastrointes-

TABLE 49-1 ▶ ADVERSE REACTIONS TO METRONIDAZOLE	
Neurologic	**Hypersensitivity**
Seizures	Anaphylaxis
Encephalopathy	Bronchospasm
Peripheral neuropathy	Urticaria, rash
Hallucinations, headache	Fixed drug eruption
Gastrointestinal	**Other**
Metallic taste, nausea	Reversible neutropenia
Vomiting	Discolored urine
Stomatitis, glossitis	Vaginal or urethral burning
Pseudomembranous colitis	Gynecomastia
Pancreatitis	

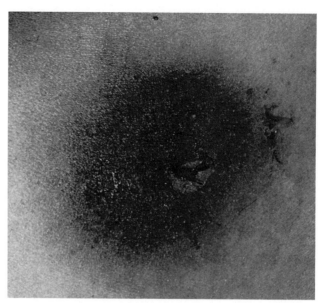

FIGURE 49-2 ▶ Fixed drug eruption from metronidazole therapy. (Copyright 1996, J. Gunter, MD.)

tinal side effects such as pancreatitis and pseudomembranous colitis, though rare, have been described. Less common minor side effects associated with metronidazole therapy include reversible neutropenia, headache, urethral or vaginal burning, discoloration of the urine, and gynecomastia.

Metronidazole may cause significant neurologic toxicity, such as hallucinations, mental status changes, ataxia, peripheral neuropathy, encephalopathy, and seizures. These side effects are rare when standard doses are used; however, metronidazole should be used with caution in individuals who have a seizure disorder or other neurologic condition. In one study with high doses of metronidazole (6 g/m^2) administered three times a week for 3 weeks, 6% of patients developed peripheral neuropathy and 25% experienced other significant neurologic toxicity.[20] The prevalence and severity of the peripheral neuropathy and the other central nervous system toxicities are related to the dose and length of therapy.[3, 20, 21] While the peripheral neuropathy is not transient, it is usually reversible and eventually subsides within 4 to 48 months off therapy.[22] Occasionally, however, it is irreversible.

Hypersensitivity reactions to metronidazole may occur, but they are relatively uncommon. Immediate hypersensitivity reactions ranging from urticaria and rash, to bronchospasm, vasodilation, and anaphylaxis have all been described.[23, 24] Safe and successful incremental dosing therapy for patients with documented immediate hypersensitivity reactions to metronidazole has been reported.[25, 26] Fixed drug eruptions may also occur and present as a variety of cutaneous lesions, including urticaria, bullous drug eruptions, maculopapular eruptions, and exanthems, or as contact dermatitis (Fig. 49-2). Transient myopia after metronidazole use has been reported and is hypothesized to be related to edema, secondary to an allergic reaction, causing displacement of the lens.[27]

Significant drug interactions have been described with metronidazole (Table 49-2). Perhaps the most clinically important interaction is the disulfiram effect of metronidazole with concurrent use of alcohol.[28] This disulfiram-like reaction can be severe and mani-

fests as nausea, vomiting, vasodilation, and tachycardia. Also of concern is the combination of disulfiram and metronidazole, which may result in acute psychotic reactions.[29] Metronidazole also interferes with the metabolism of oral anticoagulants and may potentiate the anticoagulant effect of warfarin, resulting in an elevated prothrombin time.[30] Metronidazole may increase the levels of lithium and phenytoin, although reports have been conflicting.[9, 31] Phenobarbital may accelerate hepatic metabolism of metronidazole; therefore, higher doses may be required when the two are administered concurrently.[9]

When one considers the adverse effects of metronidazole, special mention must be paid to concerns over carcinogenicity and teratogenicity. Concerns about mutagenicity were first raised when metronidazole and its metabolites were shown to induce mutations in *Salmonella typhimurium* (Ames test); however, studies supporting its mutagenicity in mammalian tissue are lacking.[4] Metronidazole itself is not believed to be mutagenic, but rather the concern has been with the toxic products of reductive activation, specifically free radicals and other cytotoxins.[4] While reductive activation occurs only under strict anaerobic conditions and the nitroreductase complex is present only in small

TABLE 49-2 ▶ MAJOR DRUG INTERACTIONS WITH METRONIDAZOLE	
Drug	**Interactions**
Alcohol	Disulfiram reaction
Disulfiram	Acute psychosis
Warfarin	Elevated prothrombin time
Lithium, phenytoin	Potential increase in drug levels

quantities in mammalian tissue, it has been postulated that some toxic products of reduction may escape and damage mammalian tissue.[3–5] This risk is theoretical, as these products of reduction either subsequently bond within the bacteria or are further reduced to nontoxic compounds.[1, 2] Concerns regarding carcinogenicity have been raised by several animal studies that have shown a tumorigenic potential of metronidazole in both rats and mice; however, in one study, the rats exposed to metronidazole actually had a longer life span.[32, 33] Other animal studies have shown no evidence of carcinogenicity.[4]

Few studies exist regarding the possible carcinogenicity of metronidazole in humans. Follow-up of a cohort of 771 women treated with metronidazole for trichomoniasis in the 1960s has revealed no increase in cancer.[34, 35] There are three case reports of carcinoma in patients with Crohn's disease who had long-term use of metronidazole, and while the diagnosis of Crohn's disease must be considered a confounding variable, few data exist regarding prolonged use of high-dose metronidazole.[36] There is, however, currently no evidence to support the carcinogenicity of metronidazole in humans with standard dosing practices.

Metronidazole easily crosses the placenta and rapidly achieves therapeutic levels in cord blood and amniotic fluid; therefore, potential fetal effects must be considered. Metronidazole is considered a category-B drug by the U.S. Food and Drug Administration (FDA); however, reports of possible teratogenicity have made its use in pregnancy somewhat controversial and the U.S. Centers for Disease Control and Prevention (CDC) recommends avoiding metronidazole in the first trimester. Studies in pregnant women have not revealed any increased teratogenetic effect after metronidazole use in pregnancy.[37, 38] Two recent meta-analyses, encompassing 30 years of data with more than 200,000 exposures to metronidazole during pregnancy, have been published and indicate no increased teratogenic risk after first-trimester exposure.[39, 40] Only one unusual cluster of three midline facial defects has been reported.[41] Approximately 25 cases of other anomalies after maternal metronidazole exposure have been reported and include limb defects, brain defects, craniosynostosis, peripheral neuropathy, and a ventricular septal defect.[38] Two cases of cancer diagnosed in the neonatal period after maternal metronidazole exposure have also been reported, one case of retinoblastoma and one case of adrenal neuroblastoma.[38, 42] Reports concerning the teratogenicity of metronidazole are at best anecdotal, and a growing body of literature supports the safety of metronidazole in pregnancy. Based on the available published data, metronidazole does not appear to be associated with an increased teratogenic risk.

The concentration of metronidazole in breast milk approaches the levels found in serum. During the first 24 hours after a single 2-g oral dose of metronidazole, a breastfed infant would receive approximately 21.8 mg of metronidazole and at 48 hours the total dose would be 25 mg. If breastfeeding is withheld for the first 24 hours, at 48 hours the neonate would be exposed only to approximately 3.5 mg of metronidazole.[16] The CDC recommends temporarily discontinuing breastfeeding after a 2.0-g dose of metronidazole.

SPECTRUM OF ANTIBIOTIC ACTIVITY

Metronidazole is very effective against a wide variety of anaerobes, some facultative anaerobes and certain protozoa. The breakpoint for anaerobic and facultative bacteria is considered to be 16 µg/mL or less.[43] Most clinically important anaerobes from the female genital tract are susceptible to metronidazole. Resistance of *Bacteroides fragilis* and other *Bacteroides* spp. to metronidazole is extremely rare, significantly less than 1%.[7, 8, 43, 44] Most anaerobic gram-negative bacilli are sensitive to metronidazole, including *Prevotella* spp., *Fusobacterium* spp., and *Campylobacter* spp. and more than 95% of anaerobic gram-positive cocci are susceptible to metronidazole at the breakpoint.[8, 43, 45] Anaerobic gram-positive bacilli susceptible to metronidazole include *Clostridium difficile*, *C. perfringens*, and other *Clostridium* spp.[45] The in vitro susceptibility of *Gardnerella vaginalis* and *Mobiluncus* spp. to metronidazole is variable, even though clinically metronidazole is effective against these organisms.[7] Interestingly, *Gardnerella vaginalis* is significantly more susceptible to the hydroxy metabolite of metronidazole than to metronidazole itself.[7] Bacteria considered resistant to metronidazole include anaerobic gram-positive nonsporulating bacilli, such as *Actinomyces*, *Propionibacterium*, and *Lactobacillus*.[3, 43, 45]

Metronidazole is also active against *Helicobacter pylori*, a microaerophilic, gram-negative rod, and several parasites, including *Trichomonas vaginalis*, *Entamoeba histolytica*, *Giardia lamblia*, and *Dracunculus medinensis*.

CLINICAL APPLICATIONS

Metronidazole is bactericidal for a number of anaerobic pathogens that cause diseases of the female reproductive tract and thereof has a variety of clinical applications in obstetrics and gynecology, including mixed pelvic infections, trichomoniasis, bacterial vaginosis, and antibiotic prophylaxis for pelvic surgery. Other important indications for metronidazole that may not be encountered as frequently in the practice of obstetrics and gynecology are *Clostridium difficile* enterocolitis, giardiasis, and amebic dysentery, and the treatment of peptic ulcer disease.

Pelvic Infections

Most pelvic infections are polymicrobial, involving both aerobic and anaerobic bacteria. Included in this category of infections are endometritis, postpartum infections, pelvic inflammatory disease, postoperative pelvic cellulitis, and pelvic abscesses. Most major pelvic infections involve several pathogens, including bacteria from the cervicovaginal flora and sexually transmitted organisms. Therefore, broad-spectrum antibiotics including anaerobic coverage are appropriate, especially when a pelvic abscess is suspected. Anaerobes commonly isolated from patients with severe pelvic infections or tubo-ovarian abscesses include *Bacteroides* spp., *Peptostreptococcus* spp., *Prevotella* spp., and *Fusobacterium* spp., all sensitive to metronidazole.[46] Metronidazole may be the superior anaerobic agent for pelvic abscesses, as in animals it has been shown to penetrate and remain active in the abscess cavity.[47] Metronidazole should be used in combination with an antibiotic that provides aerobic coverage in the treatment of mixed pelvic infections.[46] The standard dose of metronidazole for a polymicrobial pelvic infection is 500 mg intravenously every 8 to 12 hours; however, oral administration may be considered when appropriate. Some antibiotics commonly used in combination with metronidazole for these soft tissue infections include the following: ofloxacin, levofloxacin, ceftriaxone, or ampicillin and gentamicin. Other antibiotic combinations may also be used.

Trichomonas

Trichomonas vaginalis is a sexually transmitted, anaerobic, flagellated protozoan. It most commonly causes a vaginitis and cervicitis, but it has also been implicated in preterm labor and premature rupture of the membranes. The only agent that is currently effective against *Trichomonas* is systemic metronidazole. After oral administration of the drug, cell division and motility cease within 1 hour and cell death occurs within 8 hours.[48]

The recommended treatment of trichomoniasis is a single 2-g oral dose of metronidazole. Cure rates are 82% to 88% with this therapy, but they approach 95% when the partner of the patient is also treated.[49–51] Occasionally, patients may have significant gastrointestinal side effects from this dose and so may be treated with 500 mg twice daily for 7 days.[52] Metronidazole-resistant strains have been reported, although fortunately these are rare. Most cases of treatment failure are secondary to re-infection. Suspected metronidazole-resistant *Trichomonas* may respond to higher oral doses, or a combination of oral and vaginal metronidazole. Some resistant strains have been successfully treated with doses of 2 g per day for 5 days.[53] Caution should be exercised with higher doses, as peripheral neurotoxicity may occur when 3 g of metronidazole is given daily for more than 5 days.[6] There is no advantage to intravenous administration of metronidazole if the oral dose is well tolerated, owing to excellent absorption and bioavailability.

Bacterial Vaginosis

Bacterial vaginosis is the most common cause of vaginitis among women of reproductive age and is characterized by an increase in anaerobic bacteria. This infection is effectively treated with both oral and vaginal metronidazole. Oral metronidazole, 500 mg twice daily for 7 days, results in a cure rate of 82% to 92%.[54] A single 2-g oral dose of metronidazole may be used, and while it has a slightly lower cure rate and a higher relapse rate compliance may be higher for some populations.[54, 55] Treatment with vaginal metronidazole 0.75% gel, 5 g once or twice daily for 5 days, is also effective for bacterial vaginosis, with cure rates ranging from 78% to 87%.[56, 57] Vaginal metronidazole appears to be as effective as oral metronidazole for the treatment of bacterial vaginosis. As serum levels with vaginal administration are significantly lower compared to oral dosing, vaginal metronidazole is ideal for patients unable to tolerate oral metronidazole and when potential drug interactions are a concern. Some practitioners prefer to use vaginal metronidazole in the low-risk pregnant patient. Oral metronidazole for bacterial vaginosis has been shown to reduce the incidence of preterm delivery in certain high-risk populations.[58, 59]

Clostridium difficile Enterocolitis

Pseudomembranous colitis is due to intestinal infection with toxin-producing strains of *Clostridium difficile*, a gram-positive, anaerobic bacillus. Oral metronidazole at a dose of 250 mg four times daily for 10 days results in a 98% response rate.[60] Intravenous metronidazole may be used for patients unable to take oral medications. It is the only intravenous drug effective for pseudomembranous colitis, as it produces bactericidal levels in the gastrointestinal tract via excretion through the biliary tract and exudation from inflamed bowel.[60]

Antibiotic Prophylaxis

Metronidazole may be used as antibiotic prophylaxis for pelvic surgery. Metronidazole has been shown to be effective in preventing serious postoperative infectious morbidity after abdominal hysterectomy, vaginal hysterectomy, and cesarean section.[46, 61, 62] A single dose of metronidazole is usually well tolerated and has few systemic side effects, and major allergic reactions are rare. The dose for surgical prophylaxis is 500 mg given intravenously.

Other Indications

Metronidazole is indicated for other infections less frequently encountered by the obstetrician-gynecologist, including infections involving *Giardia lamblia, Entamoeba histolytica,* and *Helicobacter pylori.* Metronidazole is very effective for the treatment of giardiasis, a diarrheal illness due to intestinal infection with the protozoan *Giardia lamblia.* The recommended oral dose for adults is 250 mg three times a day for 5 to 7 days.[63] Metronidazole is also indicated for intestinal dysentery caused by *Entamoeba histolytica,* at a dose of 750 mg orally three times daily for 10 days, and oral antibiotic regimens for the treatment of duodenal or gastric ulcer due to *Helicobacter pylori* also include metronidazole.[64, 65]

COST

Not only is metronidazole a very effective antibiotic, but also it is very inexpensive in the generic form, with average wholesale prices for generic 250-mg and 500-mg tablets $0.08 and $0.17, respectively. An extended-release, 750-mg oral tablet for once-daily dosing, Flagyl ER, has an average wholesale price of $8.84 per tablet.[66] The average wholesale price of intravenous metronidazole is $10.61 for 500 mg.[66] A 0.75% vaginal gel preparation, MetroGel-Vaginal, is available in a 70-g tube, with an average wholesale price of $41.04.[67]

REFERENCES/BIBLIOGRAPHY

1. Muller M: Mode of action of metronidazole on anaerobic bacteria and protozoa. In: Rhone-Poulenc Pharma Inc, Montreal. Proceedings of the North American Metronidazole Symposium on Anaerobic Infections. Scottsdale, AZ, October 1981. Surgery 1983; 93:165.
2. Edwards DI: Nitroimidazole drugs—action and resistance mechanisms. I. Mechanisms of action. J Antimicrob Chemother 1993; 31:9.
3. Finegold SM, Mathisen GE: Metronidazole. In: Mandell GL, Bennet JE, Dolin R (eds): Principles and Practice of Infectious Disease, 4th ed. New York, Churchill Livingstone, 1995, pp 329–334.
4. Dobias L, Cerna M, Rossner P, et al: Genotoxicity and carcinogenicity of metronidazole. Mutation Res 1994; 317:177.
5. Hager WD, Rapp RP: Metronidazole. Obstet Gynecol Clinic North Am 1992; 19:497.
6. Edwards DI: Nitroimidazole drugs—action and resistance mechanisms. II. Mechanisms of resistance. J Antimicrob Chemother 1993; 31:201.
7. Jones BM, Geary I, Alawattegama AB, et al: *In-vitro* and *in-vivo* activity of metronidazole against *Gardnerella vaginalis, Bacteroides* spp., and *Mobiluncus* spp. in bacterial vaginosis. J Antimicrob Chemother 1985; 16:189.
8. Rasmussen BA, Bush K, Tally FP: Antimicrobial resistance in anaerobes. Clin Infect Dis 1997; 24(suppl 1):S110.
9. Lau AH, Lam NP, Piscitelli SC, et al: Clinical pharmacokinetics of metronidazole and other nitroimidazole anti-infectives. Clin Pharmacokinet 1992; 23:328.
10. Duff P: Antibiotic selection in obstetric patients. Infect Dis Clin North Am 1997; 11;1:1.
11. Earl P, Sisson PR, Ingham HR: Twelve-hourly dosage schedule for oral and intravenous metronidazole. J Antimicrob Chemother 1989; 23:619.
12. Houghton GW, Smith J, Thorne PS, Templeton R: The pharmacokinetics of oral and intravenous metronidazole administration in man. J Antimicrob Chemother 1979; 5:621.
13. Fredricsson B, Hagstrom B, Nord C-E, Templeton R: Systemic concentrations of metronidazole and its main metabolites after intravenous, oral and vaginal administration. Gynecol Obstet Invest 1987; 24:22.
14. Amon I, Amon K, Huller H: Pharmacokinetics and therapeutic efficacy of metronidazole at different dosages. Int J Clin Pharmacol Biopharm 1978; 16:384.
15. Cunningham FE, Kraus DM, Brubaker L, et al: Pharmacokinetics of intravaginal metronidazole gel. J Clin Pharmacol 1994; 34:1060.
16. Erickson SH, Oppenheim GL, Smith GH: Metronidazole in breast milk. Obstet Gynecol 1981; 57:48.
17. Falagas ME, Gorbach SL: Clindamycin and metronidazole. Med Clin North Am 1995; 75:845.
18. Bergan T, Thorsteinsson SB: Pharmacokinetics of metronidazole and its metabolites in reduced renal failure. Chemotherapy 1986; 32:305.
19. Greaves WL, Chungafung J, Morris B, et al: Clindamycin versus metronidazole in the treatment of bacterial vaginosis. Obstet Gynecol 1988; 72:799.
20. Urtasun RC, Rabin HR, Partington J: Human pharmacokinetics and toxicity of high-dose metronidazole administered orally and intravenously. Surgery 1983; 93:145.
21. Bernstein LH, Frank MS, Brandt LJ, Boley SJ: Healing of perineal Crohn's disease with metronidazole. Gastroenterology 1980; 79:357.
22. Learned-Coughlin S: Peripheral neuropathy induced by metronidazole. Ann Pharmacol 1994; 28:536.
23. Bochner BS, Lichtenstein LM: Anaphylaxis. N Engl J Med 1991; 324:1785.
24. Knowles S, Choudhury T, Shear N: Metronidazole hypersensitivity. Ann Pharmacol 1994; 28:325.
25. Pearlman MD, Yashar C, Ernst S, et al: An incremental dosing protocol for women with severe vaginal trichomoniasis and adverse reactions to metronidazole. Am J Obstet Gynecol 1996; 174:934.
26. Kurohara ML, Kwong FK, Lebherz TB, et al: Metronidazole sensitivity and oral desensitization. J Allergy Clin Immunol 1991; 88:279.
27. GrinBaum A, Ashkenazi I, Avni I, et al: Transient myopia following metronidazole treatment for *Trichomonas vaginalis.* JAMA 1992; 267:511.
28. Alexander I: Alcohol-antabuse syndrome in patients receiving metronidazole during gynecologic treatment. Br J Clin Pract 1985; 39:292.
29. Rothstein E, Clancey DD: Toxicity of disulfiram combined with metronidazole. N Engl J Med 1969; 280:1006.
30. Dean RP, Talbert RL: Bleeding associated with concurrent warfarin and metronidazole therapy. Drug Intel Clin Pharmacol 1980; 14:864.
31. Teicher MH, Altesman RI, Cole JO, et al: Possible nephrotoxic interaction of lithium and metronidazole. JAMA 1987; 257:3365.
32. Cohen SM, Erturk E, Van Esch AM, et al: Carcinogenicity of 5-nitrofurans, 5-nitroimidazoles, 4-nitrobenzenes, and related compounds. J Natl Cancer Inst 1973; 51:403.
33. Rustia M, Shubik P: Induction of lung tumors and malignant lymphomas in mice by metronidazole. J Natl Cancer Inst 1972; 48:721.
34. Beard CM, Noller KL, O'Fallon WM, et al: Lack of evidence for cancer due to metronidazole. N Engl J Med 1979; 301:519.
35. Beard CM, Noller KL, O'Fallon WM, et al: Cancer after exposure to metronidazole. Mayo Clin Proc 1988; 63:147.
36. Krause JR, Ayuyang HQ, Ellis LD: Occurrence of three cases of carcinoma in individuals with Crohn's disease treated with metronidazole. Am J Gastroenterol 1985; 80:978.
37. Piper JM, Mitchel EF, Ray WA: Prenatal use of metronidazole and birth defects: No association. Obstet Gynecol 1993; 82:348.
38. Rosa FW, Baum C, Shaw M: Pregnancy outcomes after first-trimester vaginitis drug therapy. Obstet Gynecol 1987; 69:751.
39. Caro-Paton T, Carvajal A, Martin de Diego I, et al: Is metronidazole teratogenic? A meta-analysis. Br J Clin Pharmacol 1997; 44:179.

40. Burtin P, Taddio A, Ariburnu O, et al: Safety of metronidazole in pregnancy: A meta-analysis. Obstet Gynecol 1995; 172:525.
41. Cantu JM, Garcia-Cruz D: Midline facial defects as a teratogenic effect of metronidazole. March Dimes Birth Defect Fdn 1982; 18:85.
42. Carvajal A, Sanchez A, Hurtarte G: Metronidazole during pregnancy. Int J Obstet Gynaecol 1995; 48:323.
43. Madinger NE, McGregor JA, McKinney PJ, et al: Comparative antibiotic susceptibilities of anaerobes associated with infections of the female genital tract. Clin Infect Dis 1993; 16(suppl 4):S349.
44. Pestana ACNR, Ribeiro RN, Diniz CG, et al: Resistance to metronidazole among *Bacteroides fragilis* group strains from humans and marmosets: Comparative study. Clin Infect Dis 1997; 259(suppl 2):S279.
45. Wexler HM, Molitoris E, Molitoris D: Susceptibility testing of anaerobes: Old problems, new options? Clin Infect Dis 1997; (suppl 2):S275.
46. ACOG Technical Bulletin: Antimicrobial Therapy for Gynecologic Infections. No. 153, March 1991.
47. Joiner KA, Lowe B, Dzink E, et al: Comparative efficacy of 10 antimicrobial agents in experimental *Bacteroides fragilis* infections. J Infect Dis 1982; 145:561.
48. Nelson MH: In vitro effects of metronidazole on the ultrastructure of *Trichomonas vaginalis*. Acta Pathol Microbiol Scand (B) 1976; 84:93.
49. Dykers JR: Single-dose metronidazole for trichomonal vaginitis. N Engl J Med 1975; 293:23.
50. Fleury FS, Van Bergen WS, Prentice RL, et al: A single dose of two grams of metronidazole for *Trichomonas vaginalis* vaginitis. Am J Obstet Gynecol 1977; 128:320.
51. Underhill RA, Peck JE: Causes of therapeutic failures after treatment of trichomonal vaginitis with metronidazole: Comparison of single-dose treatment with a standard regimen. Br J Clin Pract 1974; 28:134.
52. Hager WD, Brown ST, Kraus SJ, et al: Metronidazole for vaginal trichomoniasis: Seven-day vs. single-dose regimen. JAMA 1980; 244:1219.
53. Lossick JG, Muller M, Gorrell TE: In vitro drug susceptibility and dosages required for cure in metronidazole resistant vaginal trichomoniasis. J Infect Dis 1986; 153:948.
54. Losick JG: Treatment of sexually transmitted vaginosis/vaginitis. Rev Infect Dis 1990; 12(suppl 6):S547.
55. Swedberg J, Steiner JF, Deiss F, et al: Comparison of single-dose vs. one-week course of metronidazole for symptomatic bacterial vaginosis. JAMA 1985; 254:1046.
56. Hillier SL, Lipinski C, Briselden AM, et al: Efficacy of intravaginal 0.75% metronidazole gel for the treatment of bacterial vaginosis. Obstet Gynecol 1993; 81:963.
57. Livengood CH, McGregor JA, Soper DE, et al: Bacterial vaginosis: Efficacy and safety of intravaginal metronidazole treatment. Am J Obstet Gynecol 1994; 170:759.
58. Hauth JC, Goldenberg RL, Andrews WW, et al: Reduced incidence of preterm delivery with metronidazole and erythromycin in women with bacterial vaginosis. N Engl J Med 1995; 333:1732.
59. Morales WJ, Schorr S, Albritton J: Effect of metronidazole in patients with preterm birth in preceding pregnancy and bacterial vaginosis: A placebo-controlled double-blind study. Am J Obstet Gynecol 1994; 171:345.
60. Kelly CP, Pothoulakis C, LaMont JT: *Clostridium difficile* colitis. N Engl J Med 1994; 330:257.
61. Mittendorf R, Aronson MA, Berry RE, et al: Avoiding serious infections associated with abdominal hysterectomy: A meta-analysis of antibiotic prophylaxis. Am J Obstet Gynecol 1993; 169:1119.
62. Ruiz-Moreno JA, Garcia-Rojas JM, Lozada-Leon JD: Prevention of postcesarian morbidity with a single dose of intravenous metronidazole. Int J Gynecol Obstet 1991; 34:217.
63. Hill DR: Giardiasis: Issues in diagnosis and management. Infect Dis Clin North Am 1993; 7:503.
64. Ravdin JI, Petri WA: *Entamoeba histolytica*. In Mandell GL, Bennet JE, Dolin R (eds): Principles and Practice of Infectious Diseases, 4th ed. New York, Churchill Livingstone, 1995, pp 2395–2408.
65. Blaser M: *Helicobacter pylori* and related organisms. In Mandell GL, Bennet JE, Dolin R (eds): Principles and Practice of Infectious Diseases, 4th ed. New York, Churchill Livingstone, 1995, pp 1956–1964.
66. Drug Topics Red Book. Cardinale V (ed): Medical Economics, 2000, pp 411–412
67. Personal Communication, 3M Pharmaceuticals.

50 Aminoglycosides

DAVID GONZALEZ ▶ JOSEPH APUZZIO

The pharmacologic history of the aminoglycoside family began with the discovery of streptomycin in 1944.[1, 2] Although the use of streptomycin is limited today, its discovery led to the isolation of numerous other natural and semisynthetic aminoglycosides with greater potency and wider spectrums of antimicrobial activity. Today, there are more than 50 aminoglycosides known. However, only a few are available for use in clinical practice.[3]

STRUCTURE AND DERIVATION

The aminoglycosides are structurally related, natural or semisynthetic antimicrobials derived primarily from *Streptomyces* and *Micromonospora* species of bacteria, although *Bacillus* and *Pseudomonas* species have also been the progenitors of several aminoglycosides. Of the aminoglycosides available for clinical use, kanamycin, streptomycin, tobramycin, and neomycin are derived directly or indirectly from *Streptomyces* and are identified by the suffix -*mycin*. Gentamicin, amikacin, and netilmicin are derived from *Micromonospora* species and are identified by the suffix -*micin*.[3–5]

Structurally, the aminoglycosides are composed of two or more amino sugars glycosidically linked to an aminocyclitol ring. Except for streptomycin, which has a streptidine hexose nucleus, all of the aminoglycosides available for clinical use in the United States contain a 2-deoxystreptamine aminocyclitol ring. These include gentamicin, tobramycin, amikacin, netilmicin, kanamycin, paromomycin, and neomycin. The differences in bactericidal activity noted among the aminoglycosides can be attributed to the amino sugars that form the lateral chains of these molecules.[3, 6] These chains also are primarily responsible for differences in bacterial resistance to the different aminoglycosides.

MECHANISMS OF ACTION

The administration of an aminoglycoside is rapidly bactericidal to susceptible bacteria.[7] Although the aminoglycosides alter several aspects of bacterial cell function, the exact mechanism through which cell death occurs is not fully understood. There are two principal effects that are thought to explain why the aminoglycosides are rapidly bactericidal. The first effect involves disruption of normal protein synthesis. It is well established that once an aminoglycoside has penetrated the cell membrane of susceptible bacteria, the primary target is the ribosome. Aminoglycosides bind irreversibly to the 30S ribosomal subunits in the cell.[8, 9] There are also binding sites on the 50S subunit for some the aminoglycosides.[10] The ability of the aminoglycoside to bind to the ribosome and to cause misreading of DNA varies among the different antimicrobials; however, the consequences appear to be the same. The results are twofold: (1) a decline or inhibition of protein synthesis[11]; and (2) a misreading of messenger RNA, resulting in synthesis of nonfunctional proteins.[12, 13] Although the synthesis of abnormal proteins can be lethal to a bacterium, it is not enough to explain the rapidly bactericidal effects of the aminoglycosides. An additional mechanism through which the aminoglycosides are thought to exert a lethal effect may involve the incorporation of the abnormal proteins into the bacterial cell membrane. The result is a loss of membrane integrity that eventually kills the cell.[5, 14] The aminoglycosides can affect other cellular functions, but it is hypothesized that a combination of these two effects on the cell is primarily responsible for the bactericidal effects of the aminoglycosides.

RESISTANCE

As with other antibiotics, the use of aminoglycosides in clinical practice has resulted in the emergence of resistant bacterial strains. Fortunately, the development of resistance among bacteria to the aminoglycosides has remained low. The incidence of resistance is influenced by several factors, including the aminoglycoside being used, the type of organism, the patient population being treated, and the hospital and the patterns of antibiotic use.[15] The mechanisms of resistance, however are the same and can divided into three major categories: (1) decreased permeability of the bacterial cell wall, (2) mutations in the ribosomal binding site leading to changes in antibiotic affinity, and (3) enzyme-mediated inactivation of the drug.[15–17]

557

For the aminoglycoside to exert its effect, it must penetrate the bacterial cell wall into the cytoplasmic space. The diffusion of the aminoglycosides into susceptible bacteria involves two phases. The first phase involves passive diffusion of the aminoglycoside into the periplasmic space through aqueous channels located in the outer membrane of susceptible bacteria. The second phase involves energy-dependent transport across the inner bacterial membrane into the cytoplasmic space.[18, 19] The absence of or a mutation in the proteins involved in either phase can therefore result in resistance. Clinically, however, it is dysfunction of the second phase of transport that is most relevant.[18] Anaerobic bacteria have ribosomes that are sensitive to aminoglycosides in vitro. However, because the second phase of intracellular transport of the aminoglycosides is oxygen dependent, these antibiotics are excluded from the cytoplasm, making the organism resistant.[20] Facultative bacteria are also resistant to the aminoglycosides under anaerobic conditions because of the same mechanism. Mutations in the transport system may also occur de novo in organisms such as aerobic gram-negative bacteria and staphylococci that are in general susceptible to the aminoglycosides.[21, 22]

A second form of resistance occurs when bacteria acquire mutations at the aminoglycoside ribosomal binding sites. Ribosome mutations result in a decreased affinity for the aminoglycoside or inability to bind the drug. This type of resistance appears to be uncommon and has been reported primarily with streptomycin. Furthermore, changes in the ribosomal binding sites are antibiotic specific, with little cross-resistance exhibited among the aminoglycoside families when they do occur.[5, 23]

The third and most common mechanism of resistance noted among gram-negative bacteria results from plasmid-mediated enzymatic modification of the aminoglycosides. Enzymes coded by plasmid resistance transfer factors are widespread and are acquired by bacteria through conjugation.[17, 24] The production of these enzymes allows the resistant bacteria to inactivate the aminoglycosides through acetylation, adenylation, or phosphorylation before penetration in the cytoplasmic space.[3, 25] These resistance transfer factors can code for several enzymes that confer resistance to multiple aminoglycosides. The effectiveness of a specific aminoglycoside against a target organism demonstrating resistance therefore depends on its ability to resist enzymatic modification.

Resistance exhibited by certain bacteria, both natural and acquired, can be overcome with the use of combination antibiotic therapy. The addition of a cephalosporin or penicillin, which affects the structure of the bacterial cell wall, can increase the diffusion of the aminoglycoside into the cell, rendering the bacterium susceptible to the effects of the aminoglycosides.[26]

SPECTRUM OF ANTIBIOTIC ACTIVITY

The spectrum of activity of the various aminoglycosides is relatively wide and includes both gram-positive and gram-negative bacteria. However, as a group, the aminoglycosides are considered to be most effective in treating infections with aerobic and facultative gram-negative bacilli. Each aminoglycoside has its own unique spectrum of activity, which is in part determined by the resistance patterns of the target organism. Therefore, when choosing an antimicrobial regimen that includes an aminoglycoside, the susceptibility of the particular organism to the specific aminoglycoside must be taken into consideration. The following is a general discussion of the antibacterial activity of the aminoglycosides.[27-30]

Gram-negative bacteria susceptible to the aminoglycosides include *Enterobacter, Acinetobacter, Escherichia coli, Klebsiella, Citrobacter, Shigella, Salmonella, Serratia,* and *Haemophilus.*[23, 31-33] *Pseudomonas aeruginosa* is susceptible to aminoglycoside therapy, although other strains are often resistant.[34] *Neisseria gonorrhoeae* and meningococci are also susceptible.[35, 36]

The aminoglycosides also demonstrate activity against gram-positive bacteria, although usually limited. Staphylococci are in general susceptible to the aminoglycosides, but aminoglycosides are not considered as a first-line agent for monotherapy.[22] Staphylococci resistant to methicillin are also resistant to the aminoglycosides.[30] *Legionella* species are sensitive in vitro but have limited susceptibility in vivo because they are intracellular organisms.[37, 38] Diphtheroids are considered to be susceptible to the aminoglycosides. Streptococci, *Listeria,* and enterococci are in general resistant to the aminoglycosides when single-agent therapy is used.[39, 40]

Mycobacteria, including *Mycobacterium tuberculosis, Mycobacterium intracellulare,* and *Mycobacterium avium* are susceptible to aminoglycoside therapy. Streptomycin is the aminoglycoside that demonstrates the most activity in vivo against *M. tuberculosis,* whereas amikacin is used to treat infection with other mycobacteria. Intracellular infections, including brucellosis, yersiniosis, and tularemia, can also be treated with regimens that include an aminoglycoside.[28] The aminoglycosides are active in vitro against mycoplasmae[32]; however, no clinically significant activity against mycoplasmae is noted in vivo.

Anaerobic bacteria are resistant to the aminoglycosides[28] primarily because intracellular transport of the aminoglycosides is an energy-dependent process requiring oxygen. This property also makes the aminoglycosides poor choices for the treatment of abscesses.[16] Facultative bacteria under anaerobic conditions are resistant for the same reason. The aminoglycosides are also inactive against fungi and viruses.

Combination therapy, which includes an aminoglycoside and a beta-lactam antibiotic, has proven to be very effective against some of the organisms that demonstrate natural resistance against the aminoglycosides. Regimens that include a penicillin or a cephalosporin plus an aminoglycoside have been used successfully to treat infections secondary to staphylococci, streptococci, enterococci, and *Listeria*.[40, 41] In these cases, the cell wall–active antimicrobial permits penetration of the aminoglycoside, allowing the antibiotic to exert its effect. The result is enhanced bactericidal activity that surpasses the expected effect if the bactericidal activity of the two antibiotics were additive.[42]

CLINICAL APPLICATIONS

The clinical use of aminoglycosides can be divided into three general categories: empiric, specific, and prophylactic. An aminoglycoside should be considered for empiric therapy when there is suspicion of infection with a gram-negative organism causing sepsis, bone or joint infections, skin and soft tissue infections, respiratory tract infections, complicated urinary tract infections, postoperative infections, or intra-abdominal infections.[43–47] Traditionally, empiric therapy involves the combination of an aminoglycoside and a second antibiotic, usually a penicillin, cephalosporin, or clindamycin. Combination therapy using an aminoglycoside and a beta-lactam antibiotic not only provides broad-spectrum coverage but can yield effects that are considered additive or synergistic. Synergism is particularly desirable in the antibiotic coverage of the febrile, neutropenic patient in whom pseudomonal infection is suspected. In these cases, the aminoglycoside should be administered with a beta-lactam antibiotic that has antipseudomonal activity.

Specific therapy refers to the treatment of an infection where the organism has been cultured and the antibiotic susceptibilities are known. Monotherapy may be indicated when a susceptible gram-negative bacterium is isolated. Usually, however, an antibiotic that has less toxic potential is the antibiotic of choice.

Finally, the aminoglycosides have been used for prophylaxis during surgical procedures. Gentamicin in combination with ampicillin is recommended for the prophylaxis of subacute bacterial endocarditis in patients with risk factors undergoing surgical procedures. For those patients allergic to penicillin, vancomycin is used instead of ampicillin.[48] In patients undergoing intestinal surgery, neomycin, alone or in combination with erythromycin base, is administered orally for decontamination of the bowel before the procedure.[5, 49]

PHARMACOLOGY
Absorption and Distribution

Depending on the site of infection, the aminoglycosides can be administered orally, parenterally, or in creams or ointments.[50–52] Systemic therapy traditionally requires intravenous or intramuscular administration, given that aminoglycosides are not well absorbed from the gastrointestinal tract. This type of administration is preferred because it results in predictable serum levels. However, systemic absorption can also occur with other routes of administration. Topical application of an aminoglycoside in cases where the integrity of the skin has been compromised, such as administration to a patient with severe burns, can result in toxic serum levels of antibiotic. The aminoglycosides may also be absorbed from serosal surfaces, so intrapleural or intraperitoneal administration must be monitored carefully. This may occur when an aminoglycoside is used to irrigate the abdomen during laparotomy.[53]

The aminoglycosides are highly soluble in water. With the exception of streptomycin, no significant binding of the aminoglycosides to proteins has been demonstrated in studies. As a result, the aminoglycosides are readily distributed in the intravascular and interstitial spaces.[54, 55] These include ascitic, pericardial, peritoneal, pleural, synovial,[56] and abscess fluids. Aminoglycosides are also distributed into bile, saliva, sweat, tears, and sputum. The steady-state concentration of aminoglycoside in interstitial fluids is comparable to the plasma concentration. In contrast, the concentration of aminoglycoside in tissues is relatively low and varies with the tissue being studied.[57]

Suboptimal penetration into most tissues limits the spectrum of use of parenteral aminoglycoside therapy. Penetration across the blood–brain barrier into the cerebrospinal fluid is poor even in the presence of inflamed meninges.[58, 59] Levels achieved in the eye after intravenous or intramuscular administration are inadequate for therapy.[60] Penetration into the biliary tract and lungs is also poor.[61, 62] Therefore, when infection in these tissues is present or suspected, antibiotics with less toxicity and better penetration should be used.

Aminoglycosides can also accumulate in certain tissues, leading to the toxic effects attributed to this family of antimicrobial agents. In the kidney, selective uptake of the aminoglycosides by the proximal tubular cells results in concentrations that exceed plasma levels.[63, 64] This property can lead to high levels of aminoglycoside in the renal tubular cells, resulting in nephrotoxicity. In similar manner, ototoxicity can result from the accumulation of high levels of aminoglycoside in the inner ear. The half-life of aminoglycosides in the otic perilymph and endolymph is significantly higher than in plasma and contributes to the risk of toxicity. Furthermore, animal models have shown that the aminoglycosides are taken up by the cochlear hair cells in an energy-dependent transport mechanism that is dose dependent. Therefore, accumulation is greatest in those patients receiving prolonged courses of aminoglycosides administered by intermittent dosing.[65] Although the individual aminoglycosides differ in their affinity for renal and vestibulocochlear cells, all of the aminoglycosides can cause toxicity.

Elimination

Aminoglycosides that are administered parenterally are not metabolized and are eliminated almost entirely by glomerular filtration.[66–70] A small fraction is eliminated in feces and saliva. The liver contributes very little to the elimination of aminoglycosides. Aminoglycosides administered orally also are not metabolized and are eliminated in the feces. The plasma half-life of the aminoglycosides is approximately 2 to 4 hours in adults with normal renal function and in children older than 6 months of age.[71–73]

DOSING OF AMINOGLYCOSIDES

Aminoglycosides may be administered orally, parenterally, or topically. The route of administration depends on the target site. When systemic therapy is desired, aminoglycosides must be administered parenterally, given that absorption from the gastrointestinal tract is inadequate. Parenteral administration may be accomplished intravenously, intramuscularly, or through other routes, although the intravenous route is the one most commonly used. Traditionally, intravenous administration comprises an initial loading dose followed by maintenance doses, although more recently, single daily dosing has been advocated by some authors. The loading dose is different for each aminoglycoside and depends on the ideal body weight of the patient. The loading dose does not depend on clearance and so should be the same regardless of whether renal function is impaired. However, the volume of distribution affects peak levels. Calculation of maintenance dosing is slightly more complex in that in addition to the ideal body weight, the patient's renal function must be taken into consideration.[4, 5]

Aminoglycosides have a narrow therapeutic range. Serum levels of aminoglycosides are influenced by many factors, including weight, hydration, the patient's age, and pyrexia.[72] Determination of the plasma drug peak and trough levels during therapy is therefore essential. Peak levels should be determined approximately 30 minutes after the completion of the intravenous infusion or 1 hour after the initiation of the infusion. Trough levels should be obtained immediately before the next intravenous dose. Peak and trough levels after intramuscular injection are obtained 1 hour after administration and immediately before the next dose. Peak levels are important because they measure antimicrobial activity and should be high enough to be bactericidal. They are also necessary to avoid overdosage. Trough drug concentrations are indicative of renal clearance of the aminoglycoside

and should be low enough to avoid toxicity. High peak and trough serum aminoglycoside concentrations, either individually or in combination, may lead to ototoxicity or nephrotoxicity.[5, 74, 75]

Ultimately, the clinical situation and the adequacy of renal function should determine the frequency of testing. Patients with compromised renal function in whom aminoglycoside therapy is deemed necessary require a dosage of antibiotics determined by the degree of renal impairment. This may involve adjustments in the dose of aminoglycoside or the frequency of administration. Nomograms and formulas are available for calculation of appropriate dosages and dosage intervals.[76, 77] Peak and trough levels should also be used to maintain levels within established therapeutic ranges. In patients undergoing dialysis, aminoglycosides are removed during the procedure and therefore dosages must be adjusted accordingly.

Once-Daily Aminoglycoside Dosing

Once-daily aminoglycoside dosing has been proposed as an alternative to traditional multiple-dose administration. Advocates of once-daily dosing claim that in immunocompetent adults, this method provides better efficacy, equal or reduced toxicity, and lower cost compared with traditional regimens. There are two properties of the aminoglycosides that make once-daily dosing theoretically attractive. As noted previously, the aminoglycosides demonstrate concentration-dependent bactericidal activity, and therefore the administration of high doses of aminoglycoside is desirable. Also, because the transport of the aminoglycosides into the proximal renal tubules and hair cells in the ear is saturable, single-dose regimens can result in decreased accumulation of the drug in these tissues and therefore decreased risk of toxicity. Several meta-analyses support the use of single daily dosing regimens because of similar efficacy and equal or reduced toxicity.[78–82] Not all clinical situations are appropriate for once-daily dosing aminoglycoside therapy, however. Traditional dosing should be used in patients who are immunocompromised, those with complicated infections, elderly patients, in children, and in pregnant patients until conclusive evidence of efficacy is available in these groups.

ADVERSE EFFECTS

The aminoglycosides used in clinical practice have been associated with vestibular toxicity, cochlear toxicity, nephrotoxicity, and neuromuscular blockade.[83, 84] Ototoxicity and nephrotoxicity may be reversible or irreversible and represent the most serious adverse effects of aminoglycoside therapy. The patients most at risk are geriatric patients, dehydrated patients, patients with renal impairment, those receiving aminoglycosides in high doses or for prolonged periods, and those receiving other ototoxic or nephrotoxic drugs. Neuromuscular blockade does occur, but is rare.

Ototoxicity

Ototoxicity secondary to aminoglycoside therapy is usually irreversible and is the result of damage to the vestibular apparatus or cochlea.[85] The inner ear is particularly susceptible to damage because of the selective accumulation of the aminoglycosides in the hair cells of the organ of Corti, as well as the prolonged half-life of these antibiotics in the perilymph and endolymph of the inner ear.[65] The overall incidence of cochlear toxicity is difficult to ascertain, but is estimated to range from 3% to 25%.[86] It is manifested primarily by loss of high-frequency hearing, which can be detected only by audiometric testing.[87] Conversational hearing loss is also observed and usually occurs only after perception of high frequencies has been lost.[88] The patient with cochlear toxicity classically presents with complaints of tinnitus that is unilateral or bilateral. They may also complain of feeling a fullness in the ear. Therapy should be discontinued any time signs of toxicity present because the effects may be reversible early in the course. Some patients may not demonstrate any acute signs of toxicity. They experience progressive hearing loss resulting in deafness, which becomes evident only several weeks after the completion of therapy. The risk of cochlear toxicity is increased with the use amikacin, kanamycin, neomycin, or tobramycin, although it can occur with all members of the aminoglycoside family.[85]

Vestibular damage may occur in conjunction with or separately from cochlear toxicity. Acutely, the patient with vestibular toxicity complains of headaches, nausea, vomiting, and loss of equilibrium. Chronic manifestations primarily involve symptoms of labyrinthitis, which is manifested primarily by ataxia. Eventually the patient may be able to compensate visually for the effects of vestibular dysfunction, but residual effects are common. As with cochlear toxicity, any manifestation of vestibular dysfunction should prompt discontinuation of therapy, which may prevent permanent damage. The aminoglycosides most commonly associated with vestibular toxicity are streptomycin, gentamicin, and tobramycin.[5, 86]

The risk of toxicity is a function of the dose and duration of therapy; therefore, drug levels should be carefully monitored and the patient should be treated with the shortest course of therapy that is clinically appropriate.[85] Special attention should be paid to monitoring for signs of ototoxicity in patients receiving high doses of aminoglycosides or a prolonged course of therapy. Ototoxicity also can manifest after the completion of a single course of therapy or after several exposures that lead to cumulative damage.[84]

Nephrotoxicity

The incidence of nephrotoxicity with the use of aminoglycosides is approximately 5% to 25%.[70, 89, 90] The incidence is highly dependent on the characteristics of the patient receiving therapy. Risk is highest in older patients; patients with renal insufficiency, hypotension or volume depletion, frequent dosing intervals, or treatment for 72 hours or greater; and in patients on multiple antibiotics or those with multisystem disease.

Toxicity results from the accumulation of aminoglycosides in the proximal tubular cells.[64] Nephrotoxicity is most commonly manifested by a nonoliguric decrease in creatinine clearance and a mild rise in serum creatinine. The fall in glomerular filtration rate is usually small. Other laboratory abnormalities that may be observed include increased blood urea nitrogen, proteinuria, or the presence of hyaline or granular casts in the urine.[83] The tubular injury is usually reversible and dialysis rarely is needed. In general, when there is evidence of renal toxicity, therapy should be discontinued. Recovery in uncomplicated cases is usually achieved without intervention within a few days after discontinuation of the drug. Occasionally, it is clinically necessary to continue therapy even with evidence of renal toxicity. Renal function can be expected to return to baseline levels in some cases.[91]

The nephrotoxic potential of the aminoglycosides is variable. Neomycin is considered to be the most nephrotoxic of the aminoglycosides, whereas streptomycin, which is not concentrated in the renal cortex, has the lowest nephrotoxic potential. Again, serum levels of the aminoglycoside being used should be monitored and its use should be limited to the shortest duration that is clinically appropriate. Unfortunately, there is no proof that maintaining aminoglycoside levels within the established therapeutic range prevents nephrotoxicity. Studies do suggest that prolonged therapy increases the risk of nephrotoxicity. Specifically, there appears to be a direct correlation with the cumulative dose of aminoglycoside administered. Accidental overdosage has not been associated with acute renal injury.[92]

Neuromuscular Blockade

Neuromuscular blockade is a rare and unique adverse effect of aminoglycoside therapy. The aminoglycosides can inhibit the presynaptic release of acetylcholine, block acetylcholine receptors, and prevent the presynaptic absorption of calcium.[93] Neomycin and netilmicin are considered to be the most potent neuromuscular blocking agents.[94] Neuromuscular blockade can also occur with the use of kanamycin, amikacin, gentamicin, and tobramycin. Neuromuscular blockade is dose related and has been described with all forms of administration.[93] The highest incidence has been observed when administration is intrapleural or intra-peritoneal or with the concurrent administration of anesthetic agents or neuromuscular blocking agents. This complication is usually preventable by the slow infusion of the aminoglycoside over 20 to 30 minutes. If a blockade does occur, it is usually self-limited and rarely leads to respiratory paralysis. Neuromuscular blockade can be reversed by administering calcium gluconate intravenously.[95] Patients with myasthenia gravis should not receive aminoglycosides if other agents are available because these patients appear to be at increased risk for this complication.[96]

PREGNANCY AND LACTATION

Aminoglycosides administered to the pregnant patient readily cross the placenta. The use of streptomycin in pregnancy has been associated with congenital eighth nerve damage after long-term therapy in mothers with tuberculosis. Similar effects have not been reported with the use of the other aminoglycosides. Notwithstanding, the use of the aminoglycosides in pregnancy should be limited to those situations where less toxic antibiotics are ineffective. If aminoglycoside therapy is used, serum levels should be monitored.[97–100]

After administration, aminoglycosides are distributed into breast milk in very low concentrations. Absorption of aminoglycosides from the intestinal tracts is low; therefore, the risk of toxicity to the infant is low. According to the recommendations of the American Academy of Pediatrics, the administration of aminoglycosides to the nursing mother is compatible with breast feeding.[101]

REFERENCES

1. Waksman SA, Shatz AI: Present status of streptomycin therapy. Lancet 1946; 66:77.
2. Dubin DT, Hancock R, David BD: The sequence of effects of streptomycin in *Escherichia coli*. Biochim Biophys Acta 1963; 74:476.
3. Davies JE: Aminoglycoside–aminocyclitol antibiotics and their modifying enzymes. In: Lorian V (ed): Antibiotics in Laboratory Medicine, 3rd ed. Baltimore, Williams & Wilkins, 1991, pp 691–713.
4. Gilbert DN, Sanford JP: A clinical perspective of antibiotic therapy: Aminoglycosides vs. broad spectrum β-lactams. Rev Infect Dis 1983; 5(suppl 2):211.
5. Chambers HF, Sande MA: Antimicrobial agents: The aminoglycosides. In: Gilman AG, Goodman LS, Rall TW, et al (eds): Goodman and Gilman's the Pharmacological Basis of Therapeutics, 9th ed. New York, Macmillan, 1995, pp 1103–1121.
6. Rinehart KL Jr: Comparative chemistry of the aminoglycoside and aminocytosol antibiotics. J Infect Dis 1969; 119:345.
7. Shah RM, Heetderks G, Stille W: Bactericidal activity of amikacin and gentamicin. Chemotherapy 1977; 23:260.
8. Shannon, K, Phillips I: Mechanisms of resistance to aminoglycosides in clinical isolates. J Antimicrob Chemother 1982; 9:91.
9. Davies JE: Studies on the ribosomes of streptomycin-sensitive and resistant strains of *Escherichia coli*. Proc Natl Acad Sci U S A 1964; 51:659.
10. Davies J, Smith DI: Plasmid determined resistance to antimicrobial agents. Annu Rev Microbiol 1978; 32:469.
11. Kaji H, Kaji A: Specific binding of sRNA to ribosomes: Effect of streptomycin. Proc Natl Acad Sci U S A 1965; 54:213.
12. Gorini L: Streptomycin and misreading of the genetic code. In: Nomura M, Tissieres A, Lengyel P (eds): Ribosomes. Cold Spring Harbor, NY, Cold Spring Harbor Laboratory, 1974, pp 791–803.
13. Davies J, Gorini L, Davis BD: Misreading of RNA code words induced by aminoglycoside antibiotics. Mol Pharmacol 1965; 1:93.
14. Busse HJ, Wostmann C, Bakker EP: The bactericidal action of streptomycin: Membrane permeabilization caused by the insertion of mistranslated proteins into the cytoplasmic membrane of *Escherichia coli* and subsequent caging of the antibiotic inside the cells due to degradation of these proteins. J Gen Microbiol 1992; 138:551.
15. Murray BE, Moellering RC Jr: Patterns and mechanisms of antibiotic resistance. Med Clin North Am 1978; 62:899.
16. Bryan LE: General mechanisms of resistance to antibiotics. J Antimicrob Chemother 1988; 22(suppl):A1.
17. Davies J: Inactivation of antibiotics and the dissemination of resistance genes. Science 1994; 264:375.
18. Mates SM, Pael L, Kaback HR, et al: Membrane potential in anaerobically growing *Staphylococcus aureus* and its relationship to gentamycin uptake. Antimicrob Agents Chemother 1983; 23:526.
19. Bryan LE, Van Den Elzen HM: Effects of membrane energy mutations and cations on streptomycin and gentamicin accumulation in bacteria: A model for entry of streptomycin and gentamicin in susceptible and resistant bacteria. Antimicrob Agents Chemother 1977; 12:163.
20. Verklin RM Jr, Mandell GL: Alteration of effectiveness of antibiotics by anaerobiosis. J Lab Clin Med 1977; 89:65.
21. Buckel P, Buchberger A, Bock A, et al: Alteration of ribosomal protein L6 in mutants of *Escherichia coli* resistant to gentamicin. Mol Genet 1977; 158:47.
22. Michel J, Stessman J, Sacks T: Phenotypic variations in gentamicin resistant isolates of *Staphylococcus aureus*. Chemotherapy 1978; 24:314.
23. Lietman PS: Aminoglycosides and spectinomycin: Aminocyclitols. In: Mandell GL, Douglas RG Jr, Bennett JE (eds): Principles and Practice of Infectious Diseases, 3rd ed. New York, Churchill Livingstone, 1990, pp 269–284.
24. Benvenister R, Davies J: Mechanisms of antibiotic resistance in bacteria. Annu Rev Biochem 1973; 42:471.
25. Shaw KJ, Rather PN, Hare RS, et al: Molecular genetics of aminoglycoside resistance genes and familial relationships of the aminoglycoside-modifying enzymes. Microbiol Rev 1993; 57:138.
26. Gutschik E, Jepsen OB, Mortensen I: Effect of combinations of penicillin and aminoglycosides on *Streptococcus faecalis*: A comparative study of seven aminoglycoside antibiotics. J Infect Dis 1977; 135:832.
27. Moellering RC Jr: In vitro antibacterial activity of the aminoglycoside antibiotics. Rev Infect Dis 1983; 5(suppl): S212.
28. Moellering RC Jr: Clinical microbiology and the in vitro activity of aminoglycosides. In: Whelton A, Neu HC (eds): The Aminoglycosides: Microbiology, Clinical Use and Toxicology. New York, Marcel Dekker, 1982, pp 65–95.
29. Briedis DJ, Robson HG: Comparative activity of netilmicin, gentamicin, amikacin, and tobramycin against *Pseudomonas aeruginosa* and Enterobacteriaceae. Antimicrob Agents Chemother 1976; 10:592.
30. Young LS, Hewitt WL: Activity of the five aminoglycoside antibiotics in vitro against gram-negative bacilli and *Staphylococcus aureus*. Antimicrob Agents Chemother 1973; 4:617.
31. Thornsberry C, Kirvin LA: Antimicrobial susceptibility of *Haemophilus influenzae*. Antimicrob Agents Chemother 1974; 6:620.
32. Waitz JA, Weinstein MJ: Recent microbiologic studies with gentamicin. J Infect Dis 1969; 119:355.
33. Wiedeman B, Atkinson BA: Susceptibility to antibiotics: Species incidence and trends. In: Lorian V (ed): Antibiotics in laboratory medicine, 3rd ed. Baltimore, Williams & Wilkins, 1991, p 962–1062.

34. Uwaydah M, Taqi-Eddin AR: Susceptibility of nonfermentative gram-negative bacilli to tobramycin. J Infect Dis 1976; 134(suppl):S28.

35. Felarca AB, Laqui EM, Ibarra LM: Gentamicin in gonococcal urethritis in Filipino males. J Infect Dis 1971; 124(suppl): S287.

36. Greenstone G, Hammemberg S, Marks MI: In vitro activity of netilmicin (Sch 20569) against bacterial isolates from ill children. Chemotherapy 1978; 24:29.

37. Saravolatz LD, Pohlod DJ, Quinn EL: In vitro susceptibility of Legionella pneumophila, serogroups I–IV. J Infect Dis 1979; 140:251.

38. Thornsberry C, Baker CN, Kirven LA: In vitro activity of antimicrobial agents on Legionnaire's disease bacteria. Antimicrob Agents Chemother 1978; 13:78.

39. Moellering RC Jr, Medoff G, Leech I, et al: Antibiotic synergism against Listeria monocytogenes. Antimicrob Agents Chemother 1972; 1:30.

40. Moellering RC Jr, Weinberg AN: Studies on antibiotic synergism against enterococci. II: Effect of various antibiotics on the uptake of ^{14}C-labeled streptomycin by enterococci. J Clin Invest 1971; 50:2580.

41. Watanakunakorn C, Glotzbecker C: Enhancement of antistaphylococcal activity of nafcillin and oxacillin by sisomicin and netilmicin. Antimicrob Agents Chemother 1977; 12:346.

42. Eliopoulos GM, Moellering RC: Antimicrobial combinations. In: Loarian V (ed): Antibiotics in Laboratory Medicine, 3rd ed. Baltimore, Williams & Wilkins, 1991, pp 432–492.

43. Cox CE: Gentamicin, a new aminoglycoside antibiotic: Clinical and laboratory study in urinary tract infection. J Infect Dis 1969; 119:486.

44. Martin CM, Cuomo AJ, Geraghty MJ, et al: Gram negative rod bacteremia. J Infect Dis 1969; 119:506.

45. Fass RJ: Treatment of mixed bacterial infections with clindamycin and gentamicin. J Infect Dis 1977; 135(suppl):74.

46. Parry MF, Neu HC: A comparative study of ticarcillin plus tobramycin versus carbenicillin plus gentamicin for the treatment of serious infections due to gram-negative bacilli. Am J Med 1978; 64:961.

47. Goldenberg DL, Cohen AS: Acute infectious arthritis: A review of patients with nongonococcal joint infections. Am J Med 1976; 60:369.

48. Dajani AS, Taubert KA, Wilson W, et al: Prevention of bacterial endocarditis: Recommendations by the American Heart Association. JAMA 1997; 277:1794.

49. Gorbach SL: Antimicrobial prophylaxis for appendectomy and colorectal surgery. Rev Infect Dis 1991; 13(suppl 10):S815.

50. Breen KJ, Bryant RE, Levinson JD: Neomycin absorption in man. Ann Intern Med 1972; 76:211.

51. Kunin CM: Absorption, distribution, excretion, and fate of kanamycin. Ann NY Acad Sci 1966; 132:811.

52. Kunin CM, Chalmers TC, Leevy CM: Absorption of orally administered neomycin and kanamycin. N Engl J Med 1960; 262:380.

53. Davia JE, Siemsen AW, Anderson RW: Uremia, deafness, and paralysis due to irrigating antibiotic solutions. Arch Intern Med 1979; 125:135.

54. Carbon C, Contrepois A, Lamotte-Barrilson S: Comparative distribution of gentamicin, tobramycin, sisomicin, netilmicin, and amikacin in interstitial fluid in rabbits. Antimicrob Agents Chemother 1978; 13:368.

55. Craig WA, Suh B: Protein binding and antimicrobial effects: Methods for the determination of protein binding. In: Lorian V (ed): Antibiotics in Laboratory Medicine, 3rd ed. Baltimore, Williams & Wilkins, 1991, pp 367–402.

56. Dee TH, Kozin F: Gentamicin and tobramycin penetration into synovial fluid. Antimicrob Agents Chemother 1977; 12:548.

57. Chisolm GD, Waterworth PM, Calman JS, Garrod LP: Concentration of antibacterial agents in interstitial tissue fluid. BMJ 1973; 1:569.

58. Briedis DJ, Robson HG: Cerebrospinal penetration of amikacin. Antimicrob Agents Chemother 1978; 13:1042.

59. Kaiser AB, McGee ZA: Aminoglycoside therapy of gram-negative bacillary meningitis. N Engl J Med 1975; 293:1215.

60. Golden B, Coppel SP: Ocular tissue absorption of gentamicin. Arch Ophthalmol 1970; 84:792.

61. Pitt HA, Robert RB, Johnson WD Jr: Gentamicin levels in the human biliary tract. J Infect Dis 1973; 127:299.

62. Pennington JE, Reynolds HY: Pharmacokinetics of gentamicin sulfate in bronchial secretions. J Infect Dis 1975; 131:158.

63. Kunar MJ, Mak LL, Lietman PS: Localization of ^{3}H-gentamicin in the proximal renal tubule of the mouse. Antimicrob Agents Chemother 1979; 15:131.

64. Aronoff BR, Pottratz, ST, Brier ME, et al: Aminoglycoside accumulation kinetics in rat renal parenchyma. Antimicrob Agents Chemother 1983; 23:74.

65. Huy PTB, Meulemans A, Wassef M, et al: Gentamicin persistence in rat endolymph and perilymph after a two-day constant infusion. Antimicrob Agents Chemother 1983; 23:344.

66. Wilson TW, Mahon WA, Inaba T, et al: Elimination of tritiated gentamicin in normal human subjects and in patients with severely impaired renal function. Clin Pharmacol Ther 1973; 14:815.

67. Levy J, Klastersky J: Correlation of serum creatinine concentration and amikacin half-life. J Clin Pharmacol 1975; 15:705.

68. Riff LJ, Jackson GG: Pharmacology of gentamicin in man. J Infect Dis 1971; 124(suppl):98.

69. Wood MJ, Farrell W: Comparison of urinary excretion of tobramycin and gentamicin in adults. J Infect Dis 1976; 134(suppl):S133.

70. Kahlmeter G, Kammer G: Prolonged excretion of gentamicin in patients with unimpaired renal function. Lancet 1975; 1:286.

71. Gyselynck AM, Forrey A, Cutler R: Pharmacokinetics of gentamicin: Distribution in plasma and renal clearance. J Infect Dis 1971; 124(suppl):S70.

72. Barza M, Brown RB, Shen D, et al: Predictability of blood levels of gentamicin in man. J Infect Dis 1975; 132:165.

73. Clarke JT, Libke RD, Regamey C, et al: Comparative pharmacokinetics of amikacin and kanamycin. Clin Pharmacol Ther 1974; 15:610.

74. McCormack JP, Jewesson PJ: A critical reevaluation of the "therapeutic range" of aminoglycosides. Clin Infect Dis 1992; 14:320.

75. Edwards C, Bent AJ, Venables CW, et al: Sampling time for serum gentamicin levels. J Antimicrob Chemother 1992; 29:575.

76. Sarubbi FA, Hull H: Amikacin serum concentrations: Prediction of levels and dosage guidelines. Ann Intern Med 1978; 89:612.

77. Maderazo EG, Sun H, Jay GT: Simplification of antibiotic dose adjustments in renal insufficiency: The DREM system. Lancet 1992; 340:760.

78. Tulkens PM: Efficacy and safety of aminoglycosides once-a-day: Experimental and clinical data. Scand J Infect Dis 1991; 74(suppl):249.

79. Hatala R, Dinh T, Cook DJ: Once-daily aminoglycoside dosing in immunocompetent adults: A meta-analysis. Ann Intern Med 1996; 124:717.

80. Barza M, Ioannidis JPA, Cappelleri JC, et al: Single or multiple daily doses of aminoglycosides: A meta-analysis. BMJ 1996; 321:338.

81. Koo J, Tight R, Rajkumar V, et al: Comparison of once-daily versus pharmacokinetic dosing of aminoglycosides in elderly patients. Am J Med 1996; 101:177.

82. Avick MG, Whitten MK, Laurent SL, et al: A randomized, prospective study comparing once-daily dosing gentamicin versus thrice-daily gentamicin in the treatment of puerperal infection. Am J Obstet Gynecol 1997; 177:786.

83. Appel GB: Aminoglycoside nephrotoxicity. Am J Med 1990; 88(suppl C):16S.

84. Brummett RE, Fox KE: Aminoglycoside induced hearing loss in humans. Antimicrob Agents Chemother 1989; 33:797.

85. Brummet RE, Fox KE: Studies of aminoglycoside ototoxicity in animal models. In: Whelton A, Neu HC (eds): The

Aminoglycosides: Microbiology, Clinical Use and Toxicology. New York, Marcel Dekker, 1982, pp 419–451.

86. Moore RD, Lietman PS, Smith CR: Clinical response to aminoglycoside therapy: Importance of the ratio of peak concentration to minimal inhibitory concentrations. J Infect Dis 1987; 155:93.

87. Fausti SA, Henry JA, Schaffer HI, et al: High-frequency audiometric monitoring for early detection of aminoglycoside ototoxicity. J Infect Dis 1992; 165:1026.

88. Bendush CL: Ototoxicity: Clinical considerations and comparative information. In: Whelton A, Neu HC (eds): The Aminoglycosides: Microbiology, Clinical Use and Toxicology. New York, Marcel Dekker, 1982, pp 452–486.

89. Bertino JS, Booker LA, Franck PA, et al: Incidence of and significant risk factors for aminoglycoside-associated nephrotoxicity in patients dosed by using individualized pharmacokinetic monitoring. J Infect Dis 1993; 167:173.

90. Smith CR, Lipsky JJ, Laskin OL, et al: Double-blind comparison of the nephrotoxicity and auditory toxicity of gentamicin and tobramycin. N Engl J Med 1980; 302:1106.

91. Trollfors B: Gentamicin-associated changes in renal function reversible during continued treatment. J Antimicrob Chemother 1983; 12:285.

92. Ho PW, Pien FD, Kominami N: Massive amikacin "overdose." Ann Intern Med 1979; 91:227.

93. Snavely SR, Hodges GR: The neurotoxicity of antibacterial agents. Ann Intern Med 1984; 101:92.

94. Pittinger CB, Eryasa Y, Adamson R: Antibiotic-induced paralysis. Anesth Analg 1970; 49:487.

95. Singh YN, Harvey AL, Marshall IG: Antibiotic-induced paralysis of the mouse phrenic nerve-hemidiaphragms preparation, and reversibility by calcium and by neostigmine. Anesthesiology 1978; 48:418.

96. Sander DB, Kim YI, Howard JR Jr, et al: Intercostal nerve biopsy studies in myasthenia gravis: Clinical correlations and the direct effects of drugs and myasthenic serum. Ann NY Acd Sci 1981; 377:54.

97. Conway N, Birt DN: Streptomycin in pregnancy: Effect on the fetal ear. BMJ 1965; 2:260.

98. Gilstrap LC, Bawdon RE, Burris JS: Antibiotic concentration in maternal blood, cord blood, and placental membranes in chorioamnionitis. Obstet Gynecol 1988; 72:124.

99. Yoshioka H, Monma T, Matsuda S: Placental transfer of gentamicin. J Pediatr 1972; 80:121.

100. Fernandez H, Bourget P, Delouis C: Fetal levels of tobramycin following maternal administration. Obstet Gynecol 1990; 76:992.

101. American Academy of Pediatrics, Committee on Drugs: The transfer of drugs and other chemicals into human breast mile. Pediatrics 1994; 93:137.

51

Sulfonamides

PHILLIP PINELL

STRUCTURE AND DERIVATION

The clinically useful sulfonamides are derived from sulfanilamide (*para*-aminobenzenesulfonamide), which is very similar in structure to *para*-aminobenzoic acid (PABA). PABA is a factor required by bacteria for folic acid synthesis. Increased PABA inhibition is associated with substitutions at the sulfonyl radical, SO_2, attached to the number-one carbon, which provides increased antimicrobial activity. This is seen with sulfadiazine, sulfisoxazole, and sulfamethoxazole. These compounds are all more active than the parent compound, sulfanilamide. These substitutions are not only important in reference to activity of the antimicrobial agent, but determine other pharmacologic properties of the drug, including absorption, solubility, and gastrointestinal (GI) tolerance.[1]

The sulfonamide group may be classified as short- or medium-acting sulfonamides, long-acting sulfonamides, sulfonamides limited to the GI tract, and topical sulfonamides. The following drugs are examples of short- or medium-acting sulfonamides: sulfisoxazole (Gantrisin), sulfamethoxazole (Gantanol), sulfadiazine (Microsulfon), and sulfamethizole (Thiosulfil). Sulfisoxazole is a highly soluble drug that is particularly useful in treating urinary tract infections. Sulfamethoxazole is somewhat less soluble than sulfisoxazole and therefore yields higher blood levels. Sulfamethoxazole is the sulfonamide most frequently combined with trimethoprim. Sulfadiazine is highly active, achieving high blood and cerebrospinal fluid levels. Sulfadiazine has lower solubility than the aforementioned drugs and low protein binding. Sulfamethizole is used primarily to treat urinary tract infections.[2]

Some of the short-acting sulfonamides may be combined with phenazopyridine, which is a urinary analgesic; examples include Azo-Gantrisin and Azo-Gantanol.

Examples of long-acting sulfonamides include sulfamethoxytridazine, sulfadimethoxine, and sulfadoxine. Currently, only sulfadoxine is available in the United States for use. The long-acting sulfonamides have been associated with hypersensitivity reactions such as Stevens-Johnson syndrome. Sulfadoxine is a very long-acting sulfonamide and, when combined with pyrimethamine, is available in the United States as Fansi-dar. Fansidar is used in the treatment and prophylaxis of malaria due to chloroquine-resistant *Plasmodium falciparum*. Fansidar is not recommended for prophylaxis in pregnant patients secondary to the unknown teratogenic potential of pyrimethamine. Fansidar use has also been associated with the possibility of development of Stevens-Johnsons syndrome.[2]

Examples of sulfonamides that are limited to the GI tract include sulfaguanidine, sulfasuxidine, and sulfathalidine. These drugs are poorly absorbed from the GI tract and have been used in the past for bowel preparation before surgery to suppress susceptible bowel flora. Ulcerative colitis may be treated with salicylazosulfapyridine, a sulfonamide that is limited to the GI tract.[2–4]

Examples of topical sulfonamides include mafenide acetate, silver sulfadiazine (Silvadine cream), and sulfacetamide. Silvadine cream is used extensively for burns. Other combinations of sulfonamides are available as vaginal creams or suppositories, such as Sultrin vaginal cream. Sulfacetamide is available for use in treating conjunctivitis due to susceptible bacteria.[5]

MECHANISM OF ACTION

Sulfonamides are bacteriostatic. PABA is an essential component in folic acid synthesis. Microorganisms that endogenously synthesize folic acid are susceptible to the action of sulfonamides because sulfonamides competitively antagonize PABA. Sulfonamides competitively inhibit the incorporation of PABA into tetrahydropteroic acid.[6–8]

PHARMACOKINETICS

Oral sulfonamides are readily absorbed from the GI tract, with approximately 70% to 100% of an oral dose absorbed. Sulfonamides are distributed through all body tissues and readily enter the cerebrospinal fluid, synovial fluids, the eye, the pleura, the placenta, and the fetus. Sulfonamides are protein-bound in the plasma in varying degrees, depending on the sulfonamide. Free serum sulfonamide levels of 5 to 15 mg/dL may be therapeutic for most infections with susceptible organisms. Levels greater than 20 mg/dL should be avoided.[2, 9]

The sulfonamides readily cross the placenta to the fetus during all stages of gestation. Equilibrium with maternal blood is usually established after 2 to 3 hours, with fetal levels averaging 70% to 90% of maternal levels. When the sulfonamides are given near term, significant levels may persist in the newborn for several days after birth. The primary dangers of sulfonamide administration during pregnancy, including neonatal jaundice, hemolytic anemia, and kernicterus, are associated with administration of these agents close to delivery. Premature infants seem especially prone to the development of hyperbilirubinemia. Sulfonamides compete with bilirubin for binding to plasma albumin. In utero, the fetus clears free bilirubin by the placental circulation, but after birth this mechanism is no longer available. Therefore, unbound bilirubin is free to cross the blood–brain barrier in newborns. Although theoretically possible, kernicterus in the newborn after in utero exposure to sulfonamides has not been reported.[10–12]

Sulfonamide excretion into breast milk apparently does not pose a significant risk to the healthy, full-term newborn. Exposure to sulfonamides through the breast milk should be avoided in stressed, ill, or premature infants and in infants with hyperbilirubinemia or glucose-6-phosphate dehydrogenase (G6PD) deficiency.[13]

Metabolism of the sulfonamides occurs in the liver by conjugation, acetylation, and other metabolic pathways to inactive metabolites. The duration of antibacterial activity depends on the rate of metabolism and renal excretion. The acetylation of sulfonamides requires a coenzyme that is a pantothenic acid derivative. People who are deficient in this acid or acetylate slowly have an increased risk of toxicity from sulfonamide accumulation.

Renal excretion of sulfonamides is mainly by glomerular filtration. Renal tubular reabsorption occurs in varying degrees. Depending on the solubility of the acetylated metabolites, some of these metabolites may contribute to crystalluria and potential renal complications. When using the less soluble sulfonamides (i.e., sulfadiazine or sulfamerazine), increasing fluid intake and alkalinization of the urine decrease the possibility of crystalluria. Small amounts of drug and metabolites are eliminated in the feces, bile, breast milk, and other secretions.[2, 9]

SIDE EFFECTS

Common side effects of sulfonamide antibiotics as a class include nausea, diarrhea, vomiting, rash, fever, and headache. Hypersensitivity or allergic reactions that are common for sulfonamides include cutaneous reactions. Hematopoietic reactions associated with the sulfonamides include neutropenia, G6PD-associated hemolytic anemia, and thrombocytopenia. Hepatic reactions commonly associated with sulfonamides include increased levels of serum aminotransferases and cholestatic jaundice. Renal reactions commonly associated with sulfonamides include hypersensitivity nephritis and renal calculi.[14]

SPECTRUM OF ANTIBIOTIC ACTIVITY

Sulfonamides in general have a broad antibacterial spectrum that includes both gram-positive and gram-negative organisms. Sulfonamides also exhibits in vitro inhibitory activity against *Actinomyces,* chlamydiae, plasmodia, and *Toxoplasma.*

Resistance to sulfonamides develops in organisms that produce excessive amounts of PABA. Resistance may also occur secondary to destruction of the sulfonamide molecule. Cross-resistance between sulfonamides is common once resistance develops. In vitro sensitivity tests are not always reliable, and therefore careful observation of the clinical response is important.[2–4]

CLINICAL APPLICATIONS

Sulfonamides are primarily used in the treatment of acute urinary tract infections. Sulfisoxazole may be administered orally in a usual dosage of 1 g every 6 hours.

Sulfonamides may be effective in the prophylaxis of patients with recurrent attacks of rheumatic fever associated with group A beta-hemolytic streptococcal infections. They are not, however, effective therapy for an established streptococcal pharyngitis. Sulfonamide prophylaxis of close contacts of patients with meningitis secondary to *Neisseria meningitidis* is effective if the infecting organism is known to be sulfonamide sensitive. The usual adult dose for prophylaxis is sulfadiazine 1 g orally every 12 hours for 2 days.[1]

Sulfonamides also may be effective in therapy of infections secondary to *Nocardia asteroides,* as well as useful in combination with other antimycobacterial drugs for the management of infections secondary to rifampin-resistant *Mycobacterium kansasii.*[15]

Sulfonamides have also been used to treat toxoplasmosis in patients with and without acquired immunodeficiency syndrome (AIDS), or AIDS and chloroquine-sensitive and resistant *P. falciparum* malaria.[16, 17]

In summary, sulfonamides have a broad antibacterial spectrum with multiple major clinical uses. Diseases that may be treated with sulfonamides either as a primary or adjunct therapy include chancroid, colitis, inclusion conjunctivitis, malaria, meningococcal meningitis, nocardiosis, otitis media, rheumatic fever, toxoplasmosis, trachoma, and urinary tract infections.

Early in pregnancy, sulfonamides are categorized as

a Category B drug. It is only in the late third trimester or near birth that the sulfonamides carry risks, and are assigned Category D if administered near term. With regard to breast feeding, the American Academy of Pediatrics considers sulfonamides, including sulfapyridine, sulfisoxazole, and sulfamethoxazole, when combined with trimethoprim, to be compatible with breast feeding.

COST

Sulfonamides in general are relatively inexpensive antibiotics. Sulfisoxazole (Gantrisin) costs approximately 7 cents per 500-mg generic dose, and 0.41 cents per 500-mg brand name dose. Trimethoprim–sulfamethoxazole (Bactrim or Septra) costs approximately 9 cents per 160- to 800-mg dose for the generic brand, and approximately $1.25 per 160- to 800-mg brand name dose. An intravenous dose costs approximately $16.00.[18]

REFERENCES

1. Mandell G, Bennett J, Dolin R (eds): Mandell, Douglas, and Bennett's Principles and Practice of Infectious Disease, 4th ed. 1995, pp 354–364.
2. Garrod LP, Lambert HP, O'Grady F (eds): Antibiotic and Chemotherapy, 4th ed. London, Churchill Livingstone, 1973.
3. Bushby SRM: Trimethoprim-sulfamethoxazole: In vitro microbiologic aspects. J Infect Dis 1973; 128:S442.
4. Bach MC, Finland M, Gold W, et al: Susceptibility of recently isolated pathogenic bacteria to trimethoprim and sulfamethoxazole separately and combined. J Infect Dis 1973; 128:S508.
5. Ballin JC: Evaluation of a new topical agent for burn therapy: Silver sulfadiazine (Silvadene). JAMA 1974; 230:1184.
6. Brown GH: The biosynthesis of pteridines. Adv Enzymol 1971; 35:35.
7. Miller AK, Bruno P, Berglund RM: The effect of sulfathiazol on the in-vitro synthesis of certain vitamins by Escherichia coli. J Bacteriol 1947; 54:9.
8. Woods DD: Relation of p-aminobenzoic acid to mechanism of action of sulphanilamide. Br J Exp Pathol 1940; 1:955.
9. Amamd N: Sulfonamides and sulfones. In: Corcoran JW, Hahn FE (eds): Antibiotics III: Mechanism of Action of Antimicrobial and Antitumor Agents. Berlin, Springer-Verlag, 1975, p 668.
10. Richards IDG: A relationship inquiry into possible teratogenic effects of drugs in pregnancy. Adv Med Biol 1972; 27:441.
11. Nelson MM, Forfar JO: Association between drugs administered during pregnancy and congenital abnormalities of the fetus. BMJ 1971; 1:523.
12. Briggs GG, Freman RK, Yaffe SJ: Drugs in Pregnancy and Lactation: A Reference Guide to Fetal and Neonatal Risk, 5th ed. 1998.
13. Committee on Drugs, American Academy of Pediatrics: The transfer of drugs and other chemicals into the human milk. Pediatrics 1994; 93:137.
14. Gilbert DN: Aspects of safety profile of oral antibacterial agents. Infect Dis Clin Pract 1995; 4(suppl 2):S103.
15. Ahn CH, Wallace RJ Jr, Steel LC, et al: Sulfonamide-containing regimens for disease caused by rifampin-resistant Mycobacterium kansasii. Am Rev Respir Dis 1987; 135:10.
16. Peppercorn MA: Sulfasalazine: Pharmacology, clinical use, toxicity, and related new drug development. Ann Intern Med 1984; 3:377.
17. Pullar T, Hunter JA, Capell HA: Sulphasalazine in rheumatoid arthritis: A double-blind comparison of sulphasalazine with placebo and sodium aurothiomalate. BMJ 1983; 287:1102.
18. Gilbert D, Moellering R, Sande M: The Sanford Guide to Antimicrobial Therapy, 20th ed. 1998, p 70.

52

Vancomycin

PHILLIP PINELL

STRUCTURE AND DERIVATION

Vancomycin is a complex, soluble tricyclic glycopeptide antibiotic with a chemical formula of $C_{66}H_{75}C1_2N_9O_{24}$ and a molecular weight of 1449 daltons.[1, 2] Vancomycin is an antibiotic produced by *Streptomyces* (currently *Amycolatopsis*) *orientalis,* an actinomycete isolated from soil samples obtained in Indonesia and India. This antibiotic was purified and McCormick and colleagues[3] described its antimicrobial properties in 1956. Although vancomycin is similar to three other glycopeptide antimicrobial agents, teicoplanin, daptomycin, and ramoplanin, it is unrelated to other antibiotics. Vancomycin was introduced clinically in 1958, approximately 2 years before methicillin was introduced. It enjoyed widespread use in the treatment of infections caused by *Staphylococcus aureus* and other penicillin-resistant gram-positive bacteria.[4] After the introduction of other bactericidal antistaphylococcal penicillins and cephalosporins, vancomycin was used as an alternative therapy in patients allergic to beta-lactam antibiotics because of the perception of increased toxicity with vancomycin.[5] When vancomycin was first introduced, commercial preparations contained as much as 30% of another substance of unknown nature that possibly contributed to side effects. Current preparations are more pure, although not completely pure, and appear to be less toxic than earlier preparations.[1, 6] With the recent spread of methicillin-resistant *S. aureus* (MRSA) in the United States, vancomycin's popularity has markedly increased as the drug of choice for treating infections with these resistant organisms.[7-9] It has also been an effective agent for oral use in patients with severe antibiotic-associated pseudomembranous enterocolitis caused by *Clostridium difficile.*[7-9] Because of increasing concerns over enterococci resistant to vancomycin, metronidazole is being used more commonly to treat *C. difficile*-induced pseudomembranous enterocolitis.[2, 10, 11]

MECHANISMS OF ACTION

Vancomycin is a generally bactericidal antibiotic whose principal mode of action is to inhibit bacterial cell wall synthesis in dividing organisms.[2, 12] Vancomycin prevents polymerization of UDP-*N*-acetylmuramyl and pentapeptide and *N*-acetyglucosamine into peptidoglycan by tight binding of D-alanyl-D-alanine at the free carboxyl end of the cross-linking pentapeptide to the cleft in the chlorine-bearing phase of vancomycin. This prevents the binding of the peptide to the enzyme peptidoglycan synthetase. Vancomycin may also alter bacterial cell membrane permeability and RNA synthesis. The low frequency of development of resistance to vancomycin may be due in part to its multiple mechanisms of actions. Because of the large molecular size of vancomycin, it is unable to cross the outer cell membrane of gram-negative bacteria, thus limiting its effectiveness against gram-negative bacteria.[2] There is no known cross-resistance between vancomycin and the beta-lactams, probably because both the penicillins and cephalosporins inhibit the subsequent cross-linkage of the pentapeptide side chains of the peptidoglycan.

Enterococcal resistance to vancomycin is due to expression of an enzyme that modifies the cell wall precursor so that it no longer binds with vancomycin.[13, 14] The three types of resistance that have been described for vancomycin include the Van A phenotype, Van B phenotype, and Van C phenotype. Van A is the most common type of resistance, conferring resistance to both teicoplanin and vancomycin. This trait is inducible and has been identified in *Streptococcus faecium* and *Streptococcus faecalis.* The gene for Van A resistance has been cloned and has been found to be part of a cluster of plasma genes responsible for synthesis of peptidoglycan cell wall precursors containing a pentapeptide instead of the usual D-alanyl-D-alanine. Reduced affinity of the glycopeptides confers resistance to the aforementioned antibiotics. The Van B phenotype, which tends to confer a lower level of resistance, also has been identified in *S. faecium* and *S. faecalis.* The trait is inducible by vancomycin but not teicoplanin, and therefore many strains of bacteria remain susceptible to teicoplanin. The Van C phenotype confers resistance only to vancomycin, is constitutive, and is found in no enterococci other than *S. faecium* and *S. faecalis.*[15-17] Indiscriminate or prolonged use of these antibiotics when given orally or intravenously

568

(IV) may contribute to selective pressures for the elaboration of glycopeptide-resistant enterococci. Fortunately, there is no cross-resistance between vancomycin and unrelated antibiotics.[18, 19]

PHARMACOKINETICS

Absorption

Systemic absorption of oral vancomycin is in general poor, although there have been reports of clinically significant serum concentrations in patients with active *C. difficile*–induced enterocolitis and marked renal impairment. With 2-g daily oral doses, very high concentrations of vancomycin are found in the feces and very low concentrations found in the serum of patients with normal renal function who have pseudomembranous enterocolitis.[20–22] Intramuscular injection of vancomycin produces muscular necrosis and severe pain and is not used. Vancomycin may be given IV, but to minimize phlebitis and infusion-related reactions, it is recommended that the IV dose be reconstituted in 100 to 250 mL of dextrose or normal saline solution and infused at a rate not greater than 1 g/h. Rapid administration of the drug is dangerous because it may cause histamine release by basophils and mast cells. This in turn may lead to flushing or "red man" or "red neck" syndrome, hypotension, and anaphylactoid reactions and even cardiac arrest. Antihistamines or hydrocortisone may be added to the infusions to reduce these side effects, but these mixtures may precipitate at high concentrations.[23–28]

In patients with normal renal function, multiple IV dosing of 1 g infused over 1 hour produces mean plasma concentrations of approximately 63 μg/mL immediately after the completion of infusion. Two hours after infusion, the plasma concentration is approximately 23 μg/mL. Eleven hours after completion of infusion, the plasma concentration is approximately 8 μg/mL. The plasma concentrations during multiple dosing are similar to those after a single dose. IV vancomycin penetrates inflamed meninges at levels approximately 15% of those found in the serum. The drug also penetrates into the pleural, pericardial, ascitic, and synovial fluids in the presence of inflammatory reactions affecting these organs systems.[29–31]

The transplacental pharmacokinetics of vancomycin have been described. Accumulation of the antibiotic administered 1 g IV every 12 hours, equaling 15 mg/kg dosing, was demonstrated in the amniotic fluid at a level of 1.02 μg/mL on day 1 and 9.2 μg/mL on day 13 in a pregnant patient at 26.5 weeks' gestation. At delivery of a 28-week gestation, cord blood levels of vancomycin were 3.65 μg/mL 6 hours after the mother's maximum serum concentration was noted. This was equal to approximately 76% of the mother's serum level. The newborn serum level approximately 3 hours after birth was 2.45 μg/mL, indicating a half-life in the infant of approximately 10 hours.[32, 33]

Distribution and Excretion

Vancomycin is eliminated from the body mainly by glomerular filtration, although a very small amount may be metabolized by the liver and appear in the active form in the bile. The half-life of vancomycin in the serum is approximately 6 to 8 hours in people with normal renal function. Approximately 80% to 90% of the administered dose appears in the urine within 24 hours.[31] In renally compromised patients, the half-life may be prolonged up to 9 days, and the drug may be detected in the serum for as long as 21 days after a single 1-g dose. Serum protein binding of the drug is thought to have a negligible effect clinically. The creatinine clearance is linearly associated with vancomycin clearance. Vancomycin is not significantly removed by hemodialysis or continuous ambulatory peritoneal dialysis. There have been reports of increased clearance of vancomycin with hemoperfusion and hemofiltration.[31, 34]

SIDE EFFECTS

With the purified preparations of vancomycin currently available, adverse reactions appear to be much less frequent than when vancomycin was first introduced. Side effects include allergic reactions, infusion-related reactions, neurotoxicity, nephrotoxicity, and hematopoietic complications. The most frequent side effects consist of fever, chills, and phlebitis at the site of infusion. These are minimized if the drug is infused slowly and in a large volume of fluid. Hypersensitivity or allergic reactions with a typical erythematous and maculopapular rash have been noted in approximately 1% to 8% of patients receiving vancomycin. There has been one case reported of a systemic lupus erythematosus–like vasculitis syndrome.[35]

The "red man" or "red neck" syndrome is an infusion rate–dependent anaphylactoid reaction to vancomycin related to histamine release by plasma cells and mast cells.[36] It consists of pruritus and erythematous flushing of the head, face, neck, and upper torso, often associated with hypotension. These effects usually subside within minutes after the infusion is stopped. It may occur in 35% to 90% of patients receiving 1 g of vancomycin during 1 hour and in up to 10% of patients receiving 500 mg of vancomycin in 1 hour. Pretreatment with antihistamines may reduce the likelihood of this reaction. Concomitant administration of narcotics may potentiate the red man syndrome.[37, 38]

Neurotoxicity

Neurotoxicity, may occur with vancomycin, and is manifested primarily by auditory nerve damage and hearing loss. This is extremely uncommon, and most cases have been reported in patients receiving other ototoxic medications along with vancomycin, particularly aminoglycosides.[9, 39]

Nephrotoxicity

Nephrotoxic effects are occasionally associated with vancomycin. Clinical settings where this is most commonly seen include elderly patients, concomitant administration of an aminoglycoside, prolonged therapy, elevated serum vancomycin concentrations, high-grade bacteremia, and acute cardiovascular insufficiency. It has been noted that vancomycin and an aminoglycoside may significantly increase the risk of nephrotoxicity, from 5% with vancomycin alone to 35% with vancomycin and an aminoglycoside.[40, 41]

Hematopoietic Complications

Hematopoietic reactions, including thrombocytopenia, appear to be very uncommon with vancomycin. Vancomycin-associated neutropenia has been reported occasionally approximately 2 to 3 weeks into therapy and appears to be unrelated to drug serum levels. Periodic monitoring of the neutrophil count is recommended in patients receiving IV vancomycin therapy, especially when it is administered for longer than 2 weeks.[42]

SPECTRUM OF ANTIBIOTIC ACTIVITY

Vancomycin is a bactericidal agent and is highly active against most species of gram-positive cocci and bacilli. Practically all strains of *S. aureus*, including MRSA, are susceptible to vancomycin in low concentrations, with minimum inhibitory concentrations (MICs) lower than 5 mg/L. Vancomycin is also effective against most of the non-*aureus* staphylococci, including *Staphylococcus epidermidis*, *Staphylococcus saprophyticus*, *Staphylococcus haemolyticus*, and *Staphylococcus hominis*.[43–45]

Vancomycin is also effective against *Streptococcus pneumoniae*, including penicillin-resistant strains. It is bactericidal for all strains of *Streptococcus pyogenes* or group A streptococci, group C and group G streptococci, *Streptococcus viridans*, and *Streptococcus bovis*. Vancomycin is usually not bactericidal even for susceptible strains of enterococci at concentrations that can be achieved safely in humans.[46, 47] The minimum bactericidal concentrations (MBCs) are usually more than 32 times higher than the MICs. There are occasional isolates of group B streptococci that appear to be resistant to vancomycin. Most of these isolates, however, exhibit MICs lower than 4 mg/L. Most strains of *Listeria monocytogenes* are inhibited by clinically achievable levels of vancomycin. All strains of diphtheroids appear to be susceptible to vancomycin, with MICs lower than 1

mg/L. Some strains of *Lactobacillus* species are resistant to vancomycin.[48]

Vancomycin is also active against some anaerobes, including *Clostridium perfringens* and *C. difficile*, with MICs less than 1 mg/L. Only approximately half of the *Actinomyces* appear to be susceptible to vancomycin.[49, 50]

Vancomycin exhibits no significant activity against most gram-negative bacteria. Chlamydiae, rickettsiae, and mycobacteria are also resistant to vancomycin.[51]

Resistance

There has been a dramatic increase in the prevalence of vancomycin-resistant enterococci (VRE). From the late 1980s to the early 1990s, there has been a rise in VRE isolates from less than 0.5% to almost 8%. Clinical infections with VRE are associated with prolonged length of hospital stay, renal failure that requires peritoneal dialysis or hemodialysis, and prior antibiotic use.[48, 52–54]

Approximately two thirds of VRE isolates from hospitals in the United States have the Van A phenotype. This phenotype is characterized by high-level resistance to vancomycin, with MICs of 64 μg/mL or higher. Van A is a nine-gene complex located on a transposable genetic element, transposon 1546. It may be plasmid associated. Van A alters the usual target of vancomycin, which is the terminal D-alanyl-D-alanine of the muramyl pentapeptide, substituting instead D-alanyl-D-lactate. Van A has been found in *Streptococcus avium*, *S. faecium*, and *S. faecalis*. The Van B and Van C phenotypes have lower levels of resistance to vancomycin, with MICs of 16 to 1,024 μg/mL and 4 to 16 μg/mL, respectively. Van B phenotypes have been found in *S. faecium* and *S. faecalis*. Van C phenotypes have been found in *Streptococcus raffinosus*.[48, 52, 54–57]

Combined with certain antibiotics, vancomycin may provide synergy against certain strains of bacteria. Vancomycin and gentamicin are synergistic against most sensitive strains of enterococci, *Streptococcus viridans*, *Streptococcus bovis*, MRSA, methicillin-sensitive *S. aureus*, and approximately 33% to 50% of strains of *S. epidermidis*. The combination of vancomycin plus rifampin is not synergistic and may be antagonistic against enterococci.[58, 59] Vancomycin and rifampin have demonstrated synergy against approximately 20% to 33% of *S. aureus* isolates, although antagonism is also noted frequently here. The combination of vancomycin and rifampin has synergy against non-*aureus* staphylococci.[58, 59]

CLINICAL APPLICATIONS

Vancomycin is highly effective against *S. aureus*, coagulase-negative staphylococci, streptococci, and diphtheroids. It is the drug of choice for treatment of MRSA infections. Vancomycin is the treatment of choice in beta-lactam–intolerant patients who have serious infections secondary to *S. aureus,* including skin and soft tissue infections, pelvic infections, pneumonias, septic arthritis, endocarditis, and bacteremia. Vancomycin is also a drug of choice for treatment of infections due to diphtheroids, and is an effective agent against streptococci in patients who are allergic to beta-lactam antibiotics. Vancomycin is an option for penicillin-allergic patients with serious infections secondary to enterococci, but should be used in combination with an aminoglycoside for endocarditis to achieve bactericidal effects against enterococci in this setting. Vancomycin is also a mainstay of therapy for infections secondary to coagulase-negative staphylococci. Oral administration of vancomycin effectively treats pseudomembranous enterocolitis caused *C. difficile.* Because of the development of VRE, metronidazole is now the drug of choice to treat *C. difficile*–induced diarrhea. Intravenous administration of vancomycin is not effective in the treatment or prevention of antibiotic-associated colitis.[55, 60–64]

Vancomycin may be used for surgical prophylaxis in procedures involving placement of prostheses in beta-lactam–allergic patients, and is the drug of choice for endocarditis prophylaxis in beta-lactam–allergic patients.[63]

Vancomycin may be used in the pregnant patient and is a Category C drug. Vancomycin is excreted into the breast milk; it is poorly absorbed from the normal gastrointestinal tract, and therefore systemic absorption is not expected in the breast-feeding newborn. Because of the possibility of modification of bile flora, direct effects on the infant with regard to allergic response or sensitization, and interference with interpretation of culture results if a fever work-up is required, a decision should be made whether to discontinue nursing or discontinue the drug, taking into account the importance of the drug to the mother.[32, 33, 65–67]

COST

The usual dosage of vancomycin in a patient with normal renal function is 15 mg/kg IV every 12 hours or 125 mg orally every 6 hours. This is equivalent to 1 g IV every 12 hours in a 70-kg person. The cost of vancomycin 500 mg IV is $12.60. The cost of a "pulvule" of 125 mg is $5.35.

REFERENCES

1. Cooper GL, Given DB: Vancomycin: A Comprehensive Review of 30 Years of Clinical Experience. Indianapolis, Park Row Publishers, 1986.
2. Sheldrick GM, Jones PG, Kennard O, et al: Structure of vancomycin and its complex with acetyl-D-alanyl-D-alanine. Nature 1978; 271:223.
3. Griffith RS: Introduction to vancomycin. Rev Infect Dis 1981; 3:S200.
4. Ena J, Dick RW, Jones RN, Wenzel RP: The epidemiology of intravenous vancomycin usage in a university hospital: A 10-year study. JAMA 1993; 269:598.
5. Levine JF: Vancomycin: A review. Med Clin North Am 1987; 71:1135.
6. Moellering RC Jr, Krogstad DJ, Greenblatt DJ: Vancomycin therapy in patients impaired renal function: A nomogram for dosage. Ann Intern Med 1981; 94:343.
7. Cutler NR, Narang PK, Lesko LJ, et al: Vancomycin disposition: The importance of age. Clin Pharmacol Ther 1984; 36:803.
8. Freeman CD, Quintiliani R, Nightingale CH: Vancomycin therapeutic drug monitoring: Is it necessary? Ann Pharmacother 1993; 27:594.
9. Centers for Disease Control and Prevention: Preventing the spread of vancomycin resistance: A report from the Hospital Infection Control Practices Advisory Committee prepared by the Subcommittee on Prevention and Control of Antimicrobial-Resistant Microorganisms in Hospitals. Fed Reg 1994; 59:25758.
10. Green M, Binczewski B, Pasculle AW, et al: Constitutively vancomycin-resistant *Enterococcus faecium* resistant to synergistic β-lactam combinations. Antimicrob Agents Chemother 1993; 37:1238.
11. Perkins HR, Nieto M: The chemical basis for the action of the vancomycin group of antibiotics. Ann NY Acad Sci 1974; 235:348.
12. Swedberg G, Castenssos S, Skold O: Characterization of mutationally altered dihydropteroate synthase and its ability to form a sulfonamide-containing dihydrofolate analog. J Bacteriol 1979; 137:129.
13. Skold O: R-factor mediated resistance to sulfonamides by a plasmid-borne, resistant dihydropteroate synthase. Antimicrob Agents Chemother 1976; 9:49.
14. Radstrom P, Fermer C, Kirstiansen BE, et al: Transformational exchanges in the dihydropteroate synthase gene of *Neisseria meningitidis:* A novel mechanism for acquisition of sulfonamide resistance. J Bacteriol 1992; 174:6386.
15. Bissonnette L, Roy PH: Characterization of InO of *Pseudomonas aeruginosa* plasmid pVS1, an ancestor of intergrons of multiresistance plasmids and transposons of gram-negative bacteria. J Bacteriol 1992; 174:1248.
16. Then RL: Mechanisms of resistance to trimethoprim, the sulfonamides and trimethoprim-sulfamethoxazole. Rev Infect Dis 1982; 4:261.
17. Burman LG: Apparent absence of transferable resistance to nalidixic acid in pathogenic gram-negative bacteria. J Antimicrob Chemother 1977; 3:509.
18. Hansson HB, Walder M, Juhlin I: Susceptibility of shigellae to mecillinam, nalidixic acid, trimethoprim, and five other antimicrobial agents. Antimicrob Agents Chemother 1981; 19:271.
19. Bryan CS, White WL: Safety of oral vancomycin in functionally anephric patients. Antimicrob Agents Chemother 1978; 14:634.
20. Spitzer PG, Elipoulos GM: Systemic absorption of enteral vancomycin in a patient with pseudomembranous colitis. Ann Intern Med 1984; 100:533.
21. Pasic M, Carrel T, Opravil M, et al: Systemic absorption after local intracolonic vancomycin in pseudomembranous colitis. Lancet 1993; 342:443.
22. Brown GH: The biosynthesis of pteridines. Adv Enzymol 1971; 35:35.
23. Ryder RW, Blake PA, Murlin AC, et al: Increase in antibiotic resistance among isolates of salmonella in the United States, 1967–1975. J Infect Dis 1980; 142:485.
24. Albritton WL, Brunton JL, Slaney L, MacLean I: Plasmid-mediated sulfonamide resistance in *Haemophilus ducreyi.* Antimicrob Agents Chemother 1982; 21:159.
25. Garrod LP, Lambert HP, O'Grady F (eds): Antibiotic and Chemotherapy, 4th ed. London, Churchill Livingstone, 1973.
26. Bushby SRM: Trimethoprim-sulfamethoxazole: In vitro microbiologic aspects. J Infect Dis 1973; 128:S442.
27. Gordon RC, Thompson TR, Carlson W, et al: Antimicrobial resistance of shigellae isolated in Michigan. JAMA 1975; 231:1159.
28. Krontz DP, Strausbaugh LJ: Effect of meningitis and probenecid on the penetration of vancomycin into

cerebrospinal fluid in rabbits. Antimicrob Agents Chemother 1980; 18:882.

29. Viladrich PF, Gudiol F, Linares J, et al: Evaluation of vancomycin for therapy of adult pneumococcal meningitis. Antimicrob Agents Chemother 1991; 35:2467.

30. Moellering RC Jr: Pharmacokinetics of vancomycin. J Antimicrob Chemother 1984; 14:43.

31. Bourget P, Fernandez H, Delouis C, Ribou F: Transplacental passage of vancomycin during the second trimester of pregnancy. Obstet Gynecol 1991; 78:908.

32. Reyes MP, Ostrea EM Jr, Cabinian AE, et al: Vancomycin during pregnancy: Does it cause hearing loss or nephrotoxicity in the infant? Am J Obstet Gynecol 1989; 161:977.

33. Bryan CS, White WL: Safety of oral vancomycin in functionally anephric patients. Antimicrob Agents Chemother 1978; 14:634.

34. Markman M, Lim HW, Bluestein HG: Vancomycin-induced vasculitis. South Med J 1986; 79:382.

35. Polk RE, Healy DP, Schwartz LB, et al: Vancomycin and the red man syndrome: Pharmacodynamics of histamine release. J Infect Dis 1988; 157:502.

36. Wallace MR, Mascola JR, Oldfield EC: Red man syndrome: Incidence, etiology, and prophylaxis. J Infect Dis 1991; 164:1180.

37. Sahai J, Healy DP, Garris R, et al: Influence of antihistamine pretreatment on vancomycin-induced red man syndrome. J Infect Dis 1989; 160:876.

38. Bailie GR, Neal D: Vancomycin ototoxicity and nephrotoxicity: A review. Med Toxicol 1988; 3:376.

39. Farber BF, Moellering RC Jr: Retrospective study of the toxicity of preparations of vancomycin from 1974 to 1981. Antimicrob Agents Chemother 1983; 23:138.

40. Rybak MJ, Albrecht LM, Boike SC, Chandrasekar PH: Nephrotoxicity of vancomycin, alone and with an aminoglycoside. J Antimicrob Chemother 1990; 25:679.

41. Kesarwala HH, Rahill WJ, Amaram N. Vancomycin-induced neutropenia. [Letter.] Lancet 1981; 1:1423.

42. Lowy F, Wexler MA, Steigbigel NH: Therapy of methicillin-resistant *Staphylococcus epidermidis* experimental endocarditis. J Lab Clin Med 1982; 100:94.

43. Lowy FD, Hammer SM: *Staphylococcus epidermidis* infections. Ann Intern Med 1982; 97:503.

44. O'Brien TF, Acar JF, Altman G, et al: Laboratory surveillance of synergy between and resistance to trimethoprim and sulfonamides. Rev Infect Dis 1982; 4:351.

45. Friedland IR, McCracken GH Jr: Management of infections caused by antibiotic-resistant *Streptococcus pneumoniae*. N Engl J Med 1994; 331:377.

46. Kim MJ, Weiser M, Gottschall S, Randall EL: Identification of *Streptococcus faecalis* and *Streptococcus faecium* and susceptibility studies with newly developed antimicrobial agents. J Clin Microbiol 1987; 25:787.

47. Walsh CT: Vancomycin resistance: Decoding the molecular logic. Science 1993; 261:308.

48. Sapico FL, Kwok Y-Y, Sutter VI, Finegold SM: Standardized antimicrobial disc susceptibility testing of anaerobic bacteria:

In vitro susceptibility of *Clostridium perfringens* to nine antibiotics. Antimicrob Agents Chemother 1972; 2:320.

49. George WL, Sutter VL, Finegold SM: Toxigenicity and antimicrobial susceptibility of *Clostridium difficile*, a cause of antimicrobial agent-associated colitis. Curr Microbiol 1978; 1:55.

50. Cheung RPF, DiPiro JT: Vancomycin: An update. Pharmaco-therapy 1986; 6:153.

51. Uttley AH, Collins CH, Naidoo J, George RC: Vancomycin-resistant enterococci. [Letter.] Lancet 1988; 1:57.

52. Edmond MB, Ober JF, Weinbaum DL, et al: Vancomycin-resistant *Enterococcus faecium* bacteremia: Risk factors for infection. Clin Infect Dis 1995; 20:1126.

53. Herman DJ, Gerding DN: Minireview: Antimicrobial resistance among enterococci. Antimicrob Agents Chemother 1991; 35:1.

54. Quintilani R Jr, Evers S, Courvalin P: The vanB gene confers various levels of self-transferable resistance to vancomycin in enterococci. J Infect Dis 1993; 167:1220.

55. Fan C, Moews PC, Walsh CT, Knox JR: Vancomycin resistance: Structure of D-alanine: D-alanine ligase at 2.3 A resolution. Science 1994; 266:439.

56. Clark NC, Teixeira L, Facklam R, Tenover F: Detection and differentiation of Van C-1, Van C-2, and Van C-3 glycopeptide resistance genes in enterococci. J Clin Microbiol 1998; 36:2294.

57. Zinner SH, Lagast H, Klastersky J: Antistaphylococcal activity of rifampin with other antibiotics. J Infect Dis 1981; 144:365.

58. Watanakunakorn C, Tistone JC: Synergism between vancomycin and gentamicin or tobramycin for methicillin-susceptible and methicillin-resistant *Staphylococcus epidermidis*. Antimicrob Agents Chemother 1979; 16:655.

59. Tuazon CU, Shamsuddin D, Miller H: Antibiotic susceptibility and synergy of clinical isolates of *Listeria monocytogenes*. Antimicrob Agents Chemother 1982; 21:525.

60. Aber RC, Wennersten C, Moellering RC Jr: Antimicrobial susceptibility of flavobacteria. Antimicrob Agents Chemother 1978; 14:483.

61. Jaffe HW, Lewis JS, Wiesner PJ: Vancomycin-sensitive *Neisseria gonorrhoeae*. J Infect Dis 1981; 144:198.

62. Fekerty R: Vancomycin and teicoplanin. In: Mandell G, Bennett J, Dolin R (eds): Mandell, Douglas and Bennett's Principles and Practice of Infectious Disease, 4th ed. New York, Churchill Livingstone, 1995, pp 346–354.

63. Edberg SC, Hardalo CJ, Kontnick C, Campbell S: Rapid detection of vancomycin-resistant enterococci. J Clin Microbiol 1994; 32:2182.

64. Eli Lilly and Company: Product information: Vancocin. Indianapolis, Eli Lilly and Company, 1989.

65. Reyes MP, Ostrea EM Jr: Toxicity of vancomycin during pregnancy: Reply. Am J Obstet Gynecol 1990; 163:1376.

66. American Hospital Formulary Service: Drug Information 1997. Bethesda, MD, American Society of Health-System Pharmacists, 1997, pp 403–408.

67. Gilbert D, Moellering R, Sande M: Sanford Guide to Antimicrobial Therapy, 28th ed. Vienna, VA, Antimicrobial Therapy, Inc., 1998, pp 65–68.

53

Macrolides

SEBASTIAN FARO

The first macrolide was isolated from *Streptomyces* in 1950. It was named pikromycin because of its bitter taste.[1] The discovery of pikromycin led to the development of more than 90 compounds with a similar molecular structure—a macrocyclic lactone—and, subsequently, the discovery of macrolides.[1] Erythromycin was isolated from *Streptomyces erythraeus* in 1952[2] (Fig. 53–1). Erythromycin is the prototype of the macrolides, which include oleandomycin, josamycin, spiramycin, midecamycin, troleandomycin, clarithromycin, and azithromycin (an azalide). The only macrolides available in the United States are erythromycin, troleandomycin, clarithromycin, and azithromycin.

MECHANISM OF ACTION

Macrolides inactivate bacteria by binding to the 50S component of the 70S ribosome, thereby inhibiting protein synthesis. In addition, these agents cause the dissociation of peptidyl transfer RNA from ribosomes, blocking the utilization of amino acids for the synthesis of protein through elongation of the peptide chain.[3] Erythromycin is bacteriostatic for *Staphylococcus aureus* and bactericidal against *Streptococcus pyogenes* and *Streptococcus pneumoniae*.[4]

PHARMACOLOGY

Macrolides are lipophilic agents, and are classified according to the number of carbon atoms in the central lactone ring. The clinically useful macrolides have 14-membered rings, whereas the azolide, azithromycin, has a 15-membered ring. The erythromycin base is not readily absorbed from the gastric mucosa. It is inactivated by the acidity of the stomach and does not dissolve in aqueous solutions. Variations of erythromycin have been synthesized to avoid the destructive action of the stomach, such as enteric coating of the tablets and esters and ester salts to permit stability for liquid preparations. Some preparations, such as erythromycin base, are absorbed intact, whereas erythromycin state is absorbed as the base and erythromycin ethylsuccinate is absorbed as the intact ester and free base after hydrolysis in the small intestine.[5]

Erythromycin achieves peak serum levels 2 to 4 hours after oral administration. There does not appear to be significant differences between the available preparations of erythromycin. The distribution of erythromycin through the body tissue appears to be approximately 0.3 to no more than 4 µg/mL after a 500-mg oral dose.[5–7] Erythromycin distributed through total body water is 40% to 90% protein bound.[8, 9] The drug is concentrated by the liver and excreted in bile in rather high concentrations. During the first 8 hours of therapy, recovery of the drug in the bile is low. This is believed to be caused by reabsorption from the intestine.[10] Large amounts of the drug can be found in the feces after an oral dose, and this most likely represents unabsorbed drug. A small amount of drug can be found in the urine, 4.5% after oral administration and approximately 15% after intravenous infusion.[11, 12] The half-life of erythromycin is 1.4 hours and serum levels can be maintained for 6 hours.

Clarithromycin and azithromycin have greater bioavailability than erythromycin. The bioavailability of clarithromycin is 55%, and that for azithromycin, 37%. Although these drugs do not achieve particularly high serum levels (0.4 µg/mL), they do achieve high levels in the respiratory tract and prostate tissues. After a 500-mg oral dose, a concentration of 1 to 9 mg/kg of tissue is achieved.[13] These high doses are maintained

FIGURE 53-1 ▶ Erythromycin base is a 14-membered macrocyclic lactone ring with two sugar moieties, desosamine and cladinose. (From Mandell, Douglas, Bennett [eds]: Principles and Practice of Infectious Disease, 3rd ed. New York, Churchill Livingstone, 1990, p 308.)

573

for 4 to 8 days, thereby allowing azithromycin to be administered once a day for a short period, 5 days, and clarithromycin twice a day for 10 days.

CLINICAL INDICATIONS

The macrolides are indicated for the treatment of upper respiratory infections (i.e., pharyngitis, sinusitis, and otitis). Azithromycin and clarithromycin are indicated in the treatment of streptococcal pharyngitis and tonsillitis, sinusitis secondary to pneumococcal infection, chronic bronchitis caused by *Haemophilus influenzae, S. pneumoniae, Moraxella catarrhalis,* and pneumonia caused by *S. pneumoniae* and *Mycoplasma pneumoniae.* These two newer macrolides are also indicated in the treatment of *Mycobacterium avium* complex infection in patients with acquired immunodeficiency syndrome. Azithromycin 1 g orally in a single dose is indicated for the treatment of uncomplicated infection of the cervix, urethra, and rectum in nonpregnant and pregnant women caused by *Chlamydia trachomatis* and *Neisseria gonorrhoeae.*[14]

ADVERSE REACTIONS

The most common side effects are gastrointestinal disturbances. Approximately 20% of patients taking oral erythromycin experience cramps, diarrhea, nausea, and vomiting.[15] It appears that the gastrointestinal disturbances may be related to an increase in intestinal motility stimulated by the macrolides.[16] However, the incidence of gastrointestinal upset has been greatly reduced with the introduction of azithromycin and clarithromycin. Thrombophlebitis does occur with intravenous administration, especially with erythromycin. Diluting the drug in 250 to 500 mL of saline and infusing over 30 to 60 minutes can significantly reduce the occurrence of phlebitis.

A rare event is cholestatic hepatitis, and it appears to be associated mainly with erythromycin estolate, but has also been reported with the state salt and ethylsuccinate ester.[17–20] Hepatotoxicity caused by ingestion of erythromycin estolate has been reported in pregnancy.[19] The clinical syndrome usually occurs 10 days after the start of therapy, but may occur sooner in people previously treated with the antibiotic.[17, 18] Clinically, the patients have nausea, vomiting, abdominal pain, jaundice, and abnormal liver functions. These abnormalities usually resolve within days to a few weeks after discontinuing therapy. False elevation of serum glutamic oxalacetic transaminase (aspartate aminotransferase) has been reported after administration of erythromycin.[21]

Otic toxicity manifests as transient hearing loss secondary to administration of large doses of erythromycin lactobionate or oral erythromycin.[22, 23] This is more likely to occur in elderly patients with renal dysfunction.[22–26]

Other adverse side effects include skin rash, fever, and eosinophilia. Superinfection associated with macrolide therapy has been reported with *Candida* or gram-negative bacteria. Pseudomembranous colitis secondary to *Clostridium difficile* has been reported, although this is rare.[27, 28]

REFERENCES

1. Omura S, Tanaka H: Production and antimicrobial activity of macrolides. In: Omura S (ed): Macrolide Antibiotics: Chemistry, Biology, and Practice. New York, Academic Press, 1984, p 1.
2. Haight YM, Finland M: The antibacterial action of erythromycin. Proc Soc Exp Biol Med 1952; 81:175.
3. Mazzei T, Mini E, Novelli A, Periti P: Chemistry and mode of action of macrolides. J Antimicrob Chemother 1993; 31 (suppl C):1.
4. Neu HC: The development of macrolides: Clarithromycin in perspective. J Antimicrob Chemother 1991; 27(suppl A):1.
5. Malmborg AS: Effect of food on absorption of erythromycin: A study of two derivatives, the stearate and the base. J Antimicrob Chemother 1979; 5:591.
6. McDonald PJ, Mather LE, Story MJ: Studies on the absorption of a newly developed enteric-coated erythromycin base. J Clin Pharmacol 1977; 17:606.
7. DiSanto AR, Chodos DJ: Influence of study design in assessing food effects on absorption of erythromycin base and erythromycin stearate. Antimicrob Agents Chemother 1981; 20:190.
8. Osono T, Umezawa H: Pharmacokinetics of macrolides, lincosamides and streptogramins. J Antimicrob Chemother 1985; 16(suppl A):151.
9. Welling PG: The esters of erythromycin. J Antimicrob Chemother 1979; 5:633.
10. Hammond JB, Griffith RS: Factors affecting the absorption of and biliary excretion of erythromycin and two of its derivative in humans. Clin Pharmacol Ther 1961; 2:308.
11. Garrod LP, Lambert HP, O'Grady F: Antibiotic and Chemotherapy, 5th ed. Edinburgh, Churchill Livingstone, 1981, p 183.
12. Washington JA II, Wilson WR: Erythromycin: A microbial and clinical perspective after 30 years of clinical use. I. Mayo Clin Proc 1985; 60:189, II. 1985; 60:271.
13. Foulds G, Shepard RM, Johnson RB: The pharmacokinetics of azithromycin in human serum and tissues. J Antimicrob Chemother 1990; 25(suppl A):73.
14. Centers for Disease Control and Prevention: 1998 Guidelines for treatment of sexually transmitted diseases. MMWR Morb Mortal Wkly Rep 1998; 47:1.
15. Itoh Z, Suzuki T, Nakaya M, et al: Gastrointestinal motor-stimulating activity of macrolide antibiotics and their side effects on the canine gut. Antimicrob Agents Chemother 1984; 26:863.
16. Itoh Z, Suzuki T, Nakaya M, et al: Structure–activity relation among macrolide antibiotics in initiation of interdigestive migrating contractions in the canine gastrointestinal tract. Am J Physiol 1985; 248:G320.
17. Inman WH, Rawson NS: Erythromycin estolate and jaundice. BMJ 1983; 286:1954.
18. Braun P: Hepatotoxicity of erythromycin. J Infect Dis 1969; 119:300.
19. McCormick WM, George H, Donner A, et al: Hepatotoxicity of erythromycin estolate during pregnancy. Antimicrob Agents Chemother 1977; 12:630.
20. Sullivan D, Csuka ME, Blanchard B: Erythromycin ethylsuccinate hepatotoxicity. JAMA 1980; 243:1074.
21. Sabath LD, Gerstein DA, Finland M: Serum glutamic oxalacetic transaminase: False elevations during administration of erythromycin. N Engl J Med 1968; 279:1137.
22. Karmody CS, Weinstein I: Reversible sensorineural hearing loss

with intravenous erythromycin lactobionate. Ann Otol Rhinol Laryngol 1977; 86:9.

23. Eckman MR, Johnson T, Reiss R: Partial deafness after erythromycin. [Letter]. N Engl J Med 1975; 292:649.

24. Mery JP, Kanfer A: Ototoxicity of erythromycin in patients with renal insufficiency. [Letter.] N Engl J Med 1979; 301:944.

25. Taylor R, Schofield IS, Ramos JM, et al: Ototoxicity of erythromycin in peritoneal dialysis patients. [Letter.] Lancet 1981; 2:935.

26. Haydon RC, Thelin JW, Davis WE: Erythromycin ototoxicity: Analysis and conclusions based on 22 case reports. Otolaryngol Head Neck Surg 1984; 92:678.

27. Gantz NM, Zawacki JK, Dickerson WJ, Bartlett JG: Pseudomembranous colitis associated with erythromycin. Ann Intern Med 1979; 91:866.

28. Bartlett JG: Antimicrobial agents implicated in *Clostridium difficile* toxin-associated diarrhea or colitis. Johns Hopkins Med J 1981; 149:6.

54 Antifungal Agents

SEBASTIAN FARO

The emergence of human immunodeficiency disease resulted in a significant increase in opportunistic infections, especially fungal infections. Patients immunosuppressed for other reasons, such as organ and bone marrow transplantation, are also at risk for acquisition of fungal infections. These agents have always been present, but not to the degree that they are encountered today. In 1984, infections caused by *Candida* species represented 5.5% of all nosocomial infections, and these fungi were the eighth most common nosocomial pathogens.[1, 2] Nosocomial infections attributed to fungi other than *Candida* accounted for 1.7% of all infections.[2] For 30 years, the main agent for treatment of serious fungal infections was amphotericin B. It was not until the 1980s and 1990s that imidazoles and triazoles became available.

AGENTS THAT AFFECT STEROL SYNTHESIS

The most popular antifungal agents are the azoles, polyenes, and allylamine/carbonates. These agents either interfere with the synthesis of ergosterol or interact with it.[3] Ergosterol is a main component of the fungal cell membrane, and is synthesized from squalene (Fig. 54–1). Ergosterol imparts integrity to the fungal cell membrane.[4] Inhibition of the synthesis of ergosterol results in a cell membrane with an altered structure that cannot function. The imidazoles (i.e., miconazole, econazole, fluconazole, ketoconazole, and itraconazole) act on the heme protein that co-catalyzes cytochrome P-450–dependent 14α-demethylation of lanosterol.[5, 6] Inhibition of 14α-demethylase results in the inhibition and depletion of ergosterol. This in turn results in the accumulation of the metabolic intermediaries, lanosterol 4, 14-dimethylzymosterol, and 24-methylenedihydrolanosterol.[6] The triazoles (Fig. 54–2), fluconazole, itraconazole, and voriconazole (investigational drug), inhibit cytochrome P-450–dependent 14α-sterol demethylase.[7]

Resistance to azoles occurs through one of four mechanisms: alteration in 14α-demethylase, resulting in an inability of the azole to prevent synthesis of ergosterol; alteration in the cytochrome P-450 enzyme; reduction in the concentration of 14α-demethylase, which results in decreased transport of the azole across the cell membrane; and overexpression of 14α-demethylase, which results in an increase in synthesis of ergosterol.[6]

The polyenes (see Fig. 54–2) appear to interact directly with plasma membrane sterols. There are data supporting the hypothesis that amphotericin B binds hydrophobically to membrane sterols, forming aqueous pores[8, 9] (Fig. 54–3). This association creates a large pore in the cytoplasmic membrane, altering permeability and allowing for leakage of cytoplasmic contents, resulting in cell death.[10, 11] In an attempt to reduce the toxicity of the polyenes (i.e., amphotericin B and nystatin), these drugs have been formulated in liposomes.[12–14] The theory is that amphotericin B encased within a liposome and nystatin encased within a liposome (currently under investigation) allow the drugs to be delivered to the target site, the ergosterol-containing membrane.[12] This is accomplished via bonding of the liposome to the ergosterol moiety of the membrane.[12] This process is thought to be facilitated by fungal and host phospholipases.

Resistance to polyenes is rare and appears to occur among yeast that infrequently cause infection (e.g., *Candida lusitaniae, Candida glabrata,* and *Candida guillermondii*).[15] However, *C. glabrata* is more frequently found to cause yeast vaginitis in otherwise healthy women.[16] There are three theories regarding resistance. One theory is that there are, within any given population, small numbers of cells that are resistant to the polyenes. These cells contain sterols that have a lower affinity for the polyenes.[17] The other theory is that mutations confer resistance to the organism.[18] Hamilton-Miller[19] suggested that resistance develops secondary to changes in sterol content of the cell membrane. This results in a decrease in sterol quantity or quality, and therefore binding to the polyene is reduced. The decreased binding could be caused by (1) a reduction in the total ergosterol content in the cell membrane without significantly altering the overall steroid composition; (2) substitution of the polyene-binding sterols with sterols that do not bind polyenes as well (e.g., replacement of ergosterol, cholesterol, or

576

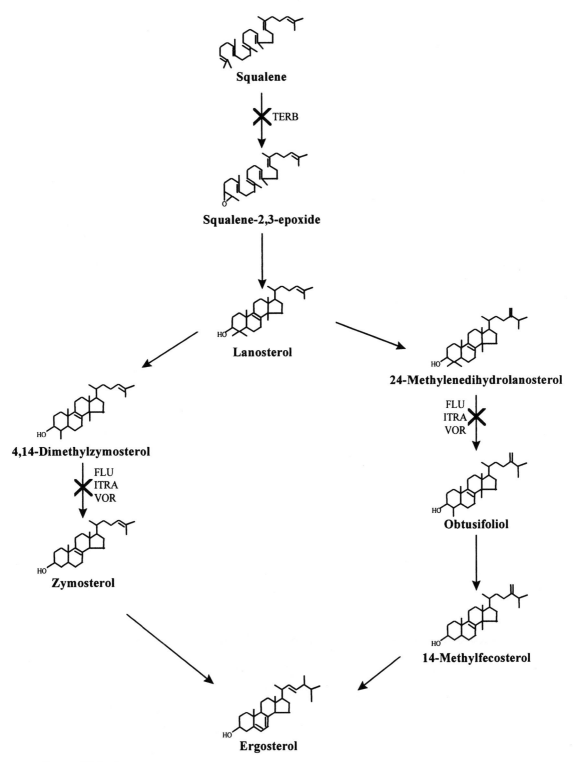

FIGURE 54-1 ▶ Ergosterol biosynthetic pathway. Steps at which various antifungal agents exert their inhibitory activities are shown. TERB = terbinafine; FLU = fluconazole; ITRA = itraconazole; VOR = voriconazole. (From Ghannoum MA, Rice LB: Antifungal agents: Mode of action, mechanisms of resistance, and correlation of these mechanisms with bacterial resistance. Clin Microbiol Rev 1999; 12:505, with permission.)

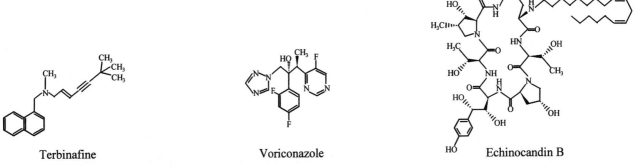

Amphotericin B

Fluconazole

Terbinafine

Voriconazole

Echinocandin B

FIGURE 54-2 ▶ Structures of representative antifungal agents. (From Ghannoum MA, Rice LB: Antifungal agents: Mode of action, mechanisms of resistance, and correlation of these mechanisms with bacterial resistance. Clin Microbiol Rev 1999; 12:502, with permission.)

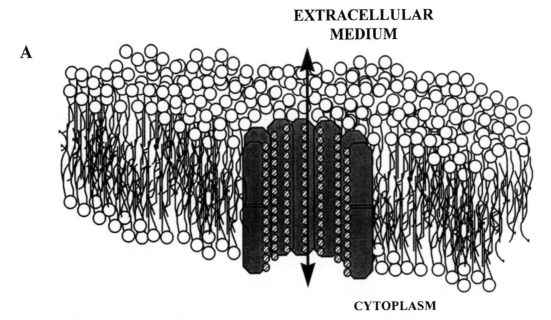

EXTRACELLULAR
MEDIUM

A

CYTOPLASM

FIGURE 54-3 ▶ Schematic representation of the interaction between amphotericin B and cholesterol in a phospholipid bilayer. The conducting pore is formed by the end-to-end union of two wells or half-pores. (From Ghannoum MA, Rice LB: Antifungal agents: Mode of action, mechanisms of resistance, and correlation of these mechanisms with bacterial resistance. Clin Microbiol Rev 1999; 12:510, with permission.)

stigmasterol by 3-hydroxy or 3-oxo sterol); or (3) altering ergosterol sterically or thermodynamically, thus reducing the affinity for polyenes.[2, 20, 21]

The allylamines (see Fig. 54–2), terbinafine and naftifine, are a newly developed class of drugs that inhibit ergosterol biosynthesis.[22, 23] It appears that the allylamines interfere with the enzyme squalene epoxidase, resulting in the accumulation of squalene and the prevention of ergosterol synthesis.[22, 24] Terbinafine appears to be highly effective against dermatophytes, azole-sensitive and azole-resistant *Candida albicans,* and *Cryptococcus neoformans.*[2, 22, 24] Resistance in clinical trails has not been documented, although failure to achieve a cure has been noted in patients receiving terbinafine.[2] Van den Bosche and colleagues[25] reported a strain of *C. glabrata* that was resistant to fluconazole and expressed cross-resistance to terbinafine. The drug efflux pump, CDR1, has been shown to use terbinafine as a substrate, thus demonstrating that a mechanism for resistance is already present in some fungi.[26]

AGENTS ACTIVE AGAINST CELL WALLS

The fungal cell wall is unique in that it consists of mannan, protein, chitin, and α- and β-glucans. The cell wall of yeast is a multilayered structure, with 80% consisting of β-glucan and mannoprotein.[27–29] The outer layers are made up of manna, mannoprotein, and β-(1,6)-glucan, and the inner layers consist mainly of β-(1,3)-glucan and chitin, with mannoprotein as a minor constituent.[30]

Numerous compounds have been discovered and described that interfere with the integrity of the fungal cell wall, but none has proven useful in the treatment of human disease.[31] A glucan synthesis inhibitor, MK-0991 (Merck & Co.), is under investigation and is being tested in clinical trials.[6] There are three groups of compounds that are specific inhibitors of fungal 3β-glucan synthetase: aculeacins, echinocandins, and papulacandins[6] (see Fig. 54–2). The only group that is being studied clinically is the echinocandins, which are lipopeptides that were shown to have activity against *Candida* and *Aspergillus* species.[32–34]

These compounds act as noncompetitive inhibitors of β-(1,3)-glucan synthetase.[31] The β-glucan synthetase inhibitors affect the structural integrity of the fungal cell wall without affecting nucleic acid or mannan synthesis.[35, 36] Pfaller and co-workers[37] have demonstrated that cilofungin, in addition to inhibiting β-(1,3)-glucan synthetase, interferes with carbohydrate, ergosterol, and lanosterol synthesis, reducing their content in the fungal cell membrane. Inhibition of cell wall synthesis and membrane structure results in cytologic changes in the cell wall, especially the growing tip of the hyphal cytoplasmic membrane. This results in lysis of the fungal cell because of its increased sensitivity to the osmotic pressure of the environment.[32, 38]

Because the β-(1,3)-glucan synthetase inhibitors have not been used clinically, resistance has not been demonstrated. Resistant strains have been induced in the laboratory in *Saccharomyces cerevisiae.*[39, 40] These laboratory experiments suggest that the mutations occurred in the genes that encode for glucan synthetase, and not for the entry mechanisms that allow the glucan synthetase inhibitors into the cell.

NUCLEIC ACID–INHIBITING AGENT

The agent in use is 5-fluorocytosine (5FC), which is a fluorinated pyrimidine. 5FC is active against yeasts, mainly *Candida* species, and *C. neoformans.* Although it is active against these two fungi, there is significant resistance. Approximately 58% of the *Candida* isolates tested were found to be sensitive, 36% were moderately resistant, and 5% were resistant.[41, 42] 5FC exerts its effect on the fungal cell by gaining entrance through a permease enzyme, after which it is converted to 5-fluorouracil (5FU) by cytosine deaminase.[6] Subsequently, 5FU is converted to 5-fluorouridylic acid (FUMP) by uridine monophosphate pyrophosphorylase. FUMP is then incorporated into RNA, causing disruption of protein synthesis.[41] 5FU is also converted into 5-fluorodeoxyuridine monophosphate.[42] This compound inhibits thymidine synthetase, the enzyme involved in the synthesis of DNA and in nuclear division.[6, 43, 44] 5FU inhibits fungi by interfering with pyrimidine metabolism and RNA, DNA, and protein synthesis.

Resistance to 5FC develops either by mutation in the permease enzyme, resulting in decreased uptake of 5FC by permease, or by loss of activity of uridine monophosphate pyrophosphorylase activity. The latter enzyme is responsible for the conversion of 5FU into FUMP. This mechanism is important in *C. glabrata* and *S. cerevisiae,* but not in *C. albicans* or *C. neoformans.*[45, 46] Formation of FUMP can be achieved by alternative mechanisms, referred to as the *salvage pathway,* either by cytosine deaminase or uracil phosphoribosyltransferase. Resistance to 5FC can result from loss of activity of either of these enzymes.[43, 47, 48]

REFERENCES

1. Centers for Disease Control: Nosocomial infection surveillance. MMWR Morb Mortal Wkly Rep 1984; 35:15SS.
2. Anaissie E, Bodey GP: Nosocomial fungal infections: Old problems and new challenges. Infect Dis Clin North Am 1988; 3:867.
3. Parks LW, Casey WM: Fungal sterols. In: Prasad R, Ghannoum M (eds): Lipids of Pathogenic Fungi. Boca Raton, FL, CRC Press, 1996, pp 63–82.
4. Nozawa Y, Morita T: Molecular mechanisms of antifungal agents associated with membrane ergosterol: Dysfunction of membrane ergosterol and inhibition of ergosterol biosynthesis. In: Iwata K, Vanden Bosche H (eds): In Vitro and In Vivo Evaluation of Antifungal Agents. Amsterdam, Elsevier, 1986, p 111.
5. Hitchcock CA, Dickinson K, Brown SB, et al: Interaction of azole antifungal antibiotics with cytochrome p-450-dependent

14α-sterol demethylase purified from *Candida albicans.* Biochem J 1990; 266:475.

6. Ghannoum MA, Rice LB: Antifungal agents: Mode of action, mechanisms of resistance, and correlation of these mechanisms with bacterial resistance. Clin Microbiol Rev 1999; 12:501.

7. Sanati H, Belanger P, Fratti R, Ghannoum M: A new triazole, voriconazole (UK-109,496), blocks sterol biosynthesis in *Candida albicans* and *Candida krusei.* Antimicrob Agents Chemother 1997; 41:2492.

8. Kruijff B de, Demel RA: Polyene antibiotic–sterol interactions in membranes of *Acholeplasma laidlawii* cells in lecithin liposomes. III: Molecular structure of the polyene antibiotic–cholesterol complexes. Biochim Biophys Acta 1974; 339:57.

9. Holz RW: The effects of polyene antibiotics nystatin and amphotericin B on thin lipid membranes. Ann NY Acad Sci 1974; 235:469.

10. Kerridge D: The plasma membrane of *Candida albicans* and its role in the action of antifungal drugs. In: Gooday GW, Lloyd D, Trinci APJ (eds): The Eukaryotic Microbial Cell. Cambridge, Cambridge University Press, 1980, p 103.

11. Kerridge D: The protoplast membrane and antifungal drugs. In: Perberdy JF, Ferenczy L (eds): Fungal Protoplasts: Applications in Biochemistry and Genetics. New York, Marcel Dekker, 1985, p 135.

12. Juliano R, Grant CW, Barber KR, Kalp MA: Mechanism of the selective toxicity of amphotericin B incorporated into liposomes. Mol Pharmacol 1987; 31:1.

13. Payne NI, Cosgrove RF, Green AP, Liu L: In-vivo studies of amphotericin B liposomes derived from proliposomes: Effect of formulation on toxicity and tissue disposition of the drug in mice. J Pharm Pharmacol 1987; 39:24.

14. Wallace TL, Paeznick V, Cassum PA, Anaisse: Nyotran (liposomal nystatin) against disseminated *Aspergillus fumigatus* in neutropenic mice. [Abstract.] In: Program and Abstracts of the 36th Interscience Conference on Antimicrobial Agents and Chemotherapy. Washington, DC, American Society for Microbiology, 19xx, p 31.

15. Martins MD, Rex JH: Resistance to antifungal agents in the critical care setting: Problems and perspectives. New Horiz 1996; 4:338.

16. Sobel JD, Faro S, Force RW, et al: Vulvovaginal candidiasis: Epidemiologic, diagnostic, and therapeutic considerations. Am J Obstet Gynecol 1998; 178:203.

17. Oehlschlager AC, Unrau AM, Fryberg M: Sterol biosynthesis in antibiotic-resistant yeast: Nystatin. Arch Biochem Biophys 1974; 160:83.

18. Athar MA, Winner HI: The development of resistance by *Candida* species to polyene antibiotics in vitro. J Med Microbiol 1971; 4:505.

19. Hamilton-Miller JM: Physiological properties of mutagen-induced variants of *Candida albicans* resistant to polyene antibiotics. J Mol Microbiol 1972; 5:425.

20. Hamilton-Miller JM: Chemistry and biology of the polyene macrolide antibiotics. Bacteriol Rev 1973; 37:166.

21. Michaelis S, Berkower C: Sequence comparison of yeast ATP-binding cassette proteins. Cold Spring Harb Symp Quant Biol 1995; 60:291.

22. Ryder NS, Favre B: Antifungal activity and mechanism of action of terbinafine. Rev Comtemp Pharmacother 1997; 8:275.

23. Ryder NS, Seidl SG, Troke PF: Effect of the antimycotic drug naftifine on growth and sterol biosynthesis in *Candida albicans.* Antimicrob Agents Chemother 1984; 25:483.

24. Jessup CJ, Ryder NS, Ghannoum MA: Evaluation of antifungal activity of terbinafine against a broad range of pathogenic fungi. [Abstract.] In: Program and Abstracts of the 36th Annual Meeting of the Infectious Diseases Society of America. 1998, p 122.

25. van den Bosche H, Marichal HP, Odds FC, et al: Characterization of an azole-resistant *Candida glabrata* isolate. Antimicrob Agents Chemother 1992; 36:2602.

26. Sanglard D, Kuchler K, Ischer F, et al: Mechanisms of resistance to azole antifungal agents in *Candida albicans* isolates

from AIDS patients involve specific multidrug transporters. Antimicrob Agents Chemother 1995; 39:2378.

27. Cassone A, Mason RE, Kerridge D: Lysis of growing yeast-form cells of *Candida albicans* following cessation of growth and their possible relationship to the development of polyene resistance. J Gen Microbiol 1979; 110:339.

28. Poulain D, Tronchin G, Dubremetz JF, Biguet J: Ultrastructure of the cell wall of *Candida albicans* blastospores: Study of the constitutive layers by the use of a cytochemical technique revealing polysaccharides. Ann Microbiol 1978; 129:141.

29. Sullivan PA, Yin CY, Molloy C, et al: An analysis of the metabolism and cell wall composition of *Candida albicans* during germ-tube formation. Can J Microbiol 1983; 29:1514.

30. Surarit R, Gopal PK, Shepherd MG: Evidence for a glycosidic linkage between chitin and glucan in the cell wall of *Candida albicans.* J Gen Microbiol 1988; 134:1723.

31. Hector RF: Compounds active against cell walls of medically important fungi. Clin Microbiol Rev 1993; 6:1.

32. Cassone A, Mason RE, Kerridge D: Lysis of growing yeast-form cells of *Candida albicans* by echinocandin: A cytological study. Sabouraudia 1981; 19:97.

33. Traxler P, Gruner J, Auden JA: Papulacandins, a new family of antibiotics with antifungal activity. I: Fermentation, isolation, chemical and biological characterization of papulacandins A, B, C, D, and E. J Antibiot 1977; 30:289.

34. Walsh TJ, Lee JW, Kelly P, et al: Antifungal effects of the nonlinear pharmacokinetics of cilofungin, a 1,3 β-glucan synthetase inhibitor, during continuous and intermittent intravenous infusions in treatment of experimental disseminated candidiasis. Antimicrob Agents Chemother 1991; 35:1321.

35. Mizoguchi J, Saito T, Mizuno K, Hayano K: On the mode of action of a new antifungal antibiotic, aculeacin A: Inhibition of cell wall synthesis in *Saccharomyces cerevisiae.* J Antibiot 1977; 30:308.

36. Titsworth E, Grunberg E: Chemotherapeutic activity of 5-fluorocytosine and amphotericin B against *Candida albicans* in mice. Antimicrob Agents Chemother 1973; 4:306.

37. Pfaller M, Riley J, Koerner T: Effects of cilofungin (LY121019) on carbohydrate and sterol composition of *Candida albicans.* Eur J Clin Microbiol Infect Dis 1989; 8:1067.

38. Bozzola JJ, Mehta RJ, Nisbet LJ, Valenta JR: The effect of aculeacin A and papulacandin B on morphology and cell wall ultrastructure in *Candida albicans.* Can J Microbiol 1984; 30:857.

39. Kurtz MB: New antifungal drug targets: A vision for the future. ASM News 1997; 64:31.

40. Kurtz MB, Douglas CM: Lipopeptide inhibitors of fungal glucan synthase. J Med Vet Mycol 1997; 35:79.

41. Defever KS, Whelan WL, Rogers AL, et al: *Candida albicans* resistance to 5-fluorocytosine: Frequency of partially resistant strains among clinical isolates. Antimicrob Agents Chemother 1982; 22:810.

42. Stiller RL, Bennett JE, Scholer HJ, et al: Susceptibility to 5-fluorocytosine and prevalence of serotype in 402 *Candida albicans* isolates from the United States. Antimicrob Agents Chemother 1982; 22:482.

43. Polak A, Scholer HJ: Mode of action of 5-fluorocytosine and mechanisms of resistance. Chemotherapy 1975; 21:113.

44. Diasio RB, Bennett JE, Myers CE: Mode of action of 5-fluorocytosine. Biochem Pharmacol 1978; 27:703.

45. Jund R, Lacroute F: Genetic and physiological aspects of resistance to 5-fluoropyrimidines in *Saccharomyces cerevisiae.* J Bacteriol 1970; 102:607.

46. Whelan WL: The genetic basis of resistance to 5-fluorocytosine in *Candida* species and *Cryptyococcus neoformans.* Crit Rev Microbiol 1987; 15:45.

47. Normark S, Schonebeck J: In vitro studies of 5-fluorocytosine resistance in *Candida albicans* and *Torulopsis glabrata.* Antimicrob Agents Chemother 1973; 2:114.

48. Whelan WL, Kerridge D: Decreased activity of UMP pyrophosphorylase associated with resistance to 5-fluorocytosine in *Candida albicans.* Antimicrob Agents Chemother 1984; 26:570.

55

Antivirals

DAVID A. BAKER ▶ SEBASTIAN FARO

Since the early 1980s, there has been a marked increase in the development, testing, and clinical availability of safe and highly effective antiviral compounds. These medications can treat and reduce the morbidity and mortality of many of the common viral infections seen in obstetrics and gynecology. The clinician must take into consideration the host immune response when treating the patient. In addition, the severity of the viral infection may influence the route of antiviral medication administration. Parenteral therapy may have greater and faster efficacy than oral administration of the same compound. Topical application of antiviral medications has very limited or no therapeutic benefit. Antiviral therapy in the intact host gives a far better therapeutic response with lower side effects and less risk of development of resistant virus.

The target of many of these compounds is viral nucleic acid synthesis. Most of the current antiviral agents require viral replication for them to function. These compounds are aimed at a specific event during viral attachment or replication to interrupt viral production and associated cell damage. Because of this, most of the current antiviral agents have a restricted spectrum of activity. Many of these antiviral agents prevent viral replication when they are present at therapeutic levels in the cell, but do not eliminate latent or dormant virus. When these medications are withdrawn, viral replication may recur or latent virus may be reactivated. The use of several antiviral medications taken together, as combination therapy, has been shown to be highly effective in the treatment of human immunodeficiency virus (HIV) infection.

Antiviral agents are not only recommended for treating and suppressing established infections, but have been shown to be highly effective in preventing acquisition of these viral infections. The major example of this approach to antiviral preventive therapy is the use of zidovudine in the pregnant, HIV-positive patient to prevent the transmission of HIV from mother to fetus and newborn. In the therapy of viral infections with antivirals, the use of adequate dosing and initiating medication as early as possible in the disease are important.

Research is developing new antiviral agents at an accelerated rate for the treatment of many other viral infections. This chapter deals mainly with the treatment of herpes virus infections. The chapters on HIV and human papilloma virus discuss therapy of these viral infections (see Chapters 42 and 43).

HERPES SIMPLEX VIRUS INFECTIONS

Extensive studies have been carried out in both men and women with genital herpes treated with acyclovir, valacyclovir, and famciclovir. The first compound to be developed and tested was acyclovir; the newer compounds, valacyclovir and famciclovir, have increased oral absorption, which gives higher serum levels with less frequent dosing. They all have a similar mechanism of action.

Varied treatments are available to the health care provider to manage patients with genital herpes.[1] Although there are extensive clinical data on the use of acyclovir in pregnancy, no antiherpes compounds have received approval for use in pregnancy by the Food and Drug Administration (FDA). The current FDA-approved antiherpes medications selectively inhibit viral replication and produce minimal effects on the cell. Acyclovir, a drug that serves as the prototype antiviral drug, was the first drug developed in this classification. Acyclovir was completely different from first-generation antiviral medications in that it showed a high safety profile while being selective against herpes virus–infected cells. The newer antiherpes medications are improvements on acyclovir, providing greater bioavailability and enhanced absorption, which translates into higher plasma levels of compound with fewer daily doses of medication.

Acyclovir

Acyclovir, 9-(2-hydroxyethoymethyl) guanine, is a deoxynucleoside analogue similar to idoxuridine and adenine arabinoside. For the drug to be active, it must first be phosphorylated to the triphosphate form. The initial phosphorylation is carried out by viral thymidine kinase. The second and third phosphorylations are carried out by the host thymidine kinase (Fig.

581

FIGURE 55-1 ▶ Acyclovir. (From Kucers A, Crowe, SM, Grayson ML, Hoy JF: The Use of Antibiotics: A Clinical Review of Antibacterial, Antifungal and Antiviral Drugs, 5th ed. Boston, Butterworth, Heinemann, [Elsevier Group], 1997, p 1518, with permission.)

55–1). Thus, acyclovir passes into host cells, and only in those cells that are infected with the herpes virus can acyclovir be phosphorylated and activated. The phosphorylated acyclovir then replaces deoxyguanosine during viral DNA synthesis.[2,3] When acyclovir is incorporated into the replicating DNA, it terminates growth of the DNA chain.

Acyclovir selectively inhibits viral DNA (i.e., herpes simplex types 1 and 2, and varicella-zoster virus). Although host cells can be affected, there is a 300- to 3,000-fold toxicity of acyclovir for herpes-infected compared with unaffected cells.[4]

Herpes simplex has evolved two mechanisms of resistance to acyclovir. One is through development of mutations that produce a truncated thymidine kinase because of the presence of insertions or deletions in the DNA chain, causing premature termination of the thymidine kinase gene.[5–9]

A second mechanism of resistance is caused by a mutation in the viral DNA polymerase.[10–12] Resistance to acyclovir has been associated with cross-resistance to foscarnet and penciclovir.[12,13] Although a given population of herpes simplex virus (HSV) resistant isolates can be detected within a population of predominantly acyclovir-sensitive strains. However, the emergence of acyclovir-resistant strains during the treatment of immunocompetent patients is rare.[14] Immunodeficient

patients appear more likely to elaborate resistant strains of HSV that do not respond to therapy.[15]

Oral administration of acyclovir gives a low bioavailability, with only approximately 20% of an oral dose absorbed.[16] Because plasma protein binding is less than 20%, acyclovir distributes widely in body fluids. Acyclovir is mainly excreted unchanged by the kidney.[17]

Renal and neurologic side effects of acyclovir parenteral therapy have been associated with high serum levels and are the major side effects reported with this route of administration.[18] The use of oral acyclovir in acute and long-term therapy has few side effects.[19,20]

Valacyclovir

By adding a valine ester to acyclovir (valacyclovir), bioavailability is increased three to five times compared with oral acyclovir.[21] Valacyclovir is for oral administration only because an intestinal enzyme cleaves valine. With oral administration of valacyclovir, intravenous levels of acyclovir can be obtained. Because valacyclovir becomes acyclovir in the circulation, its safety profile is that of acyclovir (Fig. 55–2).

Famciclovir

Famciclovir is a prodrug of penciclovir and is similar to acyclovir in its spectrum of antiviral activity[22] (Fig. 55–3). Like acyclovir, it is an acyclic nucleoside analogue that depends on viral thymidine kinase for initial phosphorylation, and a thymidine kinase–negative strain of HSV is resistant to all drugs in this class. Therefore, famciclovir is the oral form of penciclovir, and it is well absorbed and rapidly converted to the active drug. Because of its enhanced bioavailability, famciclovir requires less frequent dosing than acyclovir, but more frequent dosing than valacyclovir. There is

Valacyclovir

FIGURE 55-2 ▶ Valacyclovir. (From Weller S, Blum MR, Doucette M, et al: Pharmacogenetics of the acyclovir pro-drug valaciclovir after escalating single- and multiple-dose administration to normal volunteers. Clin Pharmacol Ther 1993; 54:595, with permission.)

FIGURE 55-3 ▶ Famciclovir. (From Vere Hodge RA, Sutton D, Boyd D, et al: Selection of an oral pro-drug (BRL 42810; famciclovir) for the antiherpesvirus agent BRL 39123 [9-(4-hydroxy-3-hydroxymethylbut-1-yl) guanine, penciclovir]. Antimicrob Agents Chemother 1989; 33:1765, with permission.)

less clinical short-term and long-term use of famciclovir than acyclovir.

HERPES ANTIVIRAL THERAPY IN THE NONPREGNANT PATIENT

The FDA has approved acyclovir, valacyclovir, and famciclovir for the treatment of primary genital herpes, recurrent episodes of genital herpes (episodic therapy), and daily suppressive therapy of this disease. The newer agents, valacyclovir and famciclovir, have greater bioavailability that requires a less frequent dosing schedule to get the same therapeutic benefit as with acyclovir, which may help with patient compliance.

Primary genital herpes requires prompt diagnosis, and all cases should be treated with antiviral medication. Antiviral therapy of primary genital herpes infections reduces viral shedding, reduces pain, and heals lesions statistically significantly faster than placebo.[23] Administration of antiviral medication as early in the course of the infection as possible gives the greatest therapeutic benefit. Antiviral therapy for the primary genital herpes infection does not alter the natural history of genital herpes or the frequency of recurrent disease. After primary genital herpes, there is increased symptomatic and asymptomatic shedding in the first 3 to 6 months after primary infection. In selected patients, continued therapy after acute therapy may be indicated.[24] The current Centers for Disease Control and Prevention (CDC) recommendations

for treatment of primary genital herpes is presented in Table 55–1.

Episodic or suppressive therapy to control genital herpes recurrences in immunocompetent patients can be selected. Starting episodic therapy as early as possible in the course of a recurrence gives the best result; this form of therapy limits each episode of recurrent disease, but does not prevent recurrences. Compared with placebo, famciclovir has been shown to be effective in treating genital herpes with episodic therapy.[25] Valacyclovir versus acyclovir has been tested in a larger number of patients with self-initiated episodic treatment for recurrent genital herpes. Valacyclovir is as effective as acyclovir in treating genital herpes episodically. Early in the prodromal phase, valacyclovir appears to prevent lesion development.[26]

Suppressive therapy is a management mode that may benefit many patients with frequent or severe recurrent genital herpes. Goldberg and colleagues[20] presented data from a long-term safety and efficacy study in which more than 1,140 immunocompetent patients with frequent recurrences of genital herpes (more than 12 episodes per year) were treated with acyclovir for the first 10 years of the study, and then with valacyclovir in the 11th year. Oral acyclovir used at 400 mg twice daily significantly reduced recurrent disease. Major insights and information concerning suppressive therapy were presented in this study. Of more than 1,140 patients, less than 2% reported a single side effect. Nausea, diarrhea, headache, and rash were seen during the study. A very small number of patients in this study (3%) required a higher dose of acyclovir to control recurrences.

More recent studies extend the information on the capability of valacyclovir and famciclovir to be used as suppressive therapy. Once-a-day valacyclovir therapy (500 mg) is effective in suppressing recurrent genital herpes. Patients on long-term suppressive therapy with oral acyclovir 400 mg twice a day can be changed to valacyclovir 500 mg once a day and maintain therapeutic safety and effectiveness.[27, 28] Two- or three-times-daily famciclovir therapy was tested in a large, randomized, placebo-controlled trial to suppress genital

TABLE 55–1 ▶ RECOMMENDED REGIMENS FOR FIRST CLINICAL EPISODE OF GENITAL HERPES INFECTION

Acyclovir	400 mg PO bid for 7–10 days OR
Acyclovir	200 mg PO five times a day for 7–10 days OR
Famciclovir	250 mg PO tid for 7–10 days OR
Valacyclovir	1 g PO bid for 7–10 days

From Centers for Disease Control and Prevention: 1998 Guidelines for the treatment of sexually transmitted diseases. MMWR Morb Mortal Wkly Rep 1998; 47:1.

TABLE 55–2 ▶	RECOMMENDED REGIMENS FOR EPISODIC RECURRENT GENITAL HERPES INFECTION
Acyclovir	400 mg PO tid for 5 days
	OR
Acyclovir	200 mg PO five times a day for 5 days
	OR
Acyclovir	800 mg PO bid for 5 days
	OR
Famciclovir	125 mg PO bid for 5 days
	OR
Valacyclovir	500 mg PO bid for 5 days

From Centers for Disease Control and Prevention: 1998 Guidelines for the treatment of sexually transmitted diseases. MMWR Morb Mortal Wkly Rep 1998; 47:1.

herpes. Famciclovir given once daily is ineffective in suppressing recurrent genital herpes; however, given two or three times daily, it is effective.[29, 30] Tables 55–2 and 55–3 give the most recent CDC recommendations for the episodic treatment of and suppressive regimens for genital herpes.

Daily oral acyclovir therapy has been shown markedly to reduce symptomatic recurrences of genital herpes. The appearance of a clinical lesion consistent with herpes is easy to recognize, and without the appearance of these lesions, recurrent disease is assumed to be suppressed by antiviral medication.[20] A different approach was taken by Wald and colleagues,[31] who reported that daily oral suppressive doses of acyclovir suppressed subclinical shedding of HSV-2 and that this therapy should be evaluated in an attempt to prevent transmission of this virus to a sexual partner.

With the use of any antimicrobial agent, the development of resistant organisms is of major concern. HSV isolates from patients naive of acyclovir contain acyclovir-resistant variants that account for approximately 1% of the total virus population.[32] This may explain why resistant virus is not a problem in the immunocompetent host but poses a significant problem when there is immune compromise.[33, 34] Deficient thymidine kinase activity in HSV isolates is the most common mechanism found for resistant HSV.[35] Fife

TABLE 55–3 ▶	RECOMMENDED REGIMENS FOR DAILY SUPPRESSIVE THERAPY OF GENITAL HERPES INFECTION
Acyclovir	400 mg PO bid
	OR
Famciclovir	250 mg PO bid
	OR
Valacyclovir	250 mg PO bid
	OR
Valacyclovir	500 mg PO qd
	OR
Valacyclovir	1,000 mg PO qd

From Centers for Disease Control and Prevention: 1998 Guidelines for the treatment of sexually transmitted diseases. MMWR Morb Mortal Wkly Rep 1998; 47:1.

and associates[19] showed that 6 years of continuous daily acyclovir suppressive therapy did not produce the emergence of acyclovir-resistant isolates in immunocompetent patients.

HERPES ANTIVIRAL THERAPY IN THE PREGNANT PATIENT

Safety of Acyclovir Used in Pregnancy

Of utmost importance when using antimicrobials in pregnancy is the safety profile of the medication. Reported studies have demonstrated the safety of acyclovir use in pregnancy.[36–38] Inadvertent administration of acyclovir or indicated use to treat severe HSV infection of the mother during all trimesters of pregnancy was not associated with any increased risk to the developing fetus.

A registry on acyclovir use in pregnancy, set up in 1984, published its data in 1993.[37] The data clearly demonstrated that with first-trimester acyclovir fetal exposure, there was no increase in fetal problems. The registry continues to accumulate this information.

Pharmacokinetics of Acyclovir in Mother, Fetus, and Newborn

Limited studies of acyclovir administration to pregnant women give data showing that acyclovir readily crosses the placenta and is concentrated in amniotic fluid and breast milk, but does not accumulate in the fetus.[39] Blood levels of acyclovir in the fetus are slightly higher than maternal blood levels after oral or intravenous dosing of the medication. The concentration of acyclovir in fetal cord blood is 1.3 times the maternal serum concentration.

Efficacy of Acyclovir Use in Pregnancy

Severe and life-threatening HSV infections in the mother have been successfully treated during pregnancy. Treatment of disseminated HSV infection, herpes pneumonitis, herpes hepatitis, and herpes encephalitis using acyclovir antiviral therapy has been reported and has been lifesaving to mother and fetus.[36, 40, 41]

Therapy to Prevent Herpes Simplex Virus Transmission to the Newborn at or Around the Time of Delivery

With the high risk of transmitting genital herpes from mothers to newborns, cesarean delivery in this group of patients has become a common clinical practice. As with the use of other antiviral medications to prevent newborn infection, investigators are looking at HSV antivirals to alter and enhance the management of these HSV-infected women. Relying on cesarean delivery to manage patients with genital HSV disease has many disadvantages.[42, 43] Prophylactic antiretroviral therapy has been shown to be safe and effective in reducing the spread of HIV from mother to newborn. With maternal genital herpes, the aim is to prevent maternal symptomatic and subclinical viral shedding during the intrapartum period.[44, 45] The use of antiviral therapy in the mother may achieve this goal.

More recent studies report the use of antiherpes medication in the last 4 weeks of pregnancy to suppress recurrent disease and allow for a vaginal delivery. Information on acyclovir use in pregnancy is the most complete. However, acyclovir is still categorized by the FDA as a Category C medication. Valacyclovir and famciclovir are categorized as FDA Category B medications.

An early study with only five pregnant women at term reported that acyclovir did not prevent subclinical viral shedding in one of the mothers or viral transmission to one of the newborns.[44] Brocklehurst and colleagues[46] reported from Europe a study of 63 pregnant women with recurrent genital herpes in a double-blind, placebo-controlled trial using acyclovir 200 mg four times a day, starting at 36 weeks' gestation. The data showed that the number of clinical recurrences was significantly reduced, but they were unable to demonstrate that acyclovir decreased the number of cesarean section deliveries.

Scott and co-workers[45] studied 46 pregnant women with a clinical diagnosis of first-episode genital herpes during pregnancy. The study design was a double-blind, placebo-controlled trial using acyclovir 400 mg three times a day starting at 36 weeks' gestation to see if this suppressive therapy could decrease the number of deliveries by cesarean section. The study showed a significant reduction in cesarean deliveries and there was no increase in subclinical shedding.

These studies mark a beginning in the investigation of the use of antiviral therapy to prevent cesarean sections and decrease viral shedding to prevent neonatal herpes. The limited number of patients, the different dosages of acyclovir, the differences in patient populations, and the differences in primary versus recurrent HSV disease make it impossible to arrive at definite conclusions at this time. If vaginal delivery can be increased in these patients, the use of antiviral medication in the last 4 weeks of pregnancy would be cost-effective.[47]

OTHER ANTIVIRAL AGENTS

Foscarnet

Foscarnet, an inorganic pyrophosphate (phosphofornate), is active against HSV types 1 and 2, cytomegalovirus, varicella-zoster virus, Epstein-Barr virus, and human herpes virus types 6 and 8.[48–50] Foscarnet appears to have a broad range of antiviral activity; it inhibits DNA polymerase of the hepatitis B virus, interferes with messenger RNA (mRNA) synthesis of the influenza viruses, and inhibits HIV reverse transcriptase.[51–55] Foscarnet inhibits viral polymerases directly and does not require phosphorylation to be activated.

Foscarnet is a second-line agent administered to immunosuppressed patients who cannot tolerate ganciclovir. It is also used to treat immunosuppressed patients infected with a virus found to be resistant to ganciclovir, and can be used in conjunction with ganciclovir for treatment of serious infection in those patients. Foscarnet can be used to treat HSV or varicella-zoster infection when resistance to acyclovir has been documented.

Foscarnet is not well absorbed when administered orally. This agent should be given intravenously, preferably in a central venous line, slowly, in a 1- to 2-hour infusion. Foscarnet is indicated for the treatment of cytomegalovirus retinitis in patients with acquired immunodeficiency syndrome (AIDS), the treatment of other cytomegalovirus infections in patients with AIDS, prevention and treatment of cytomegalovirus infection in bone marrow transplant recipients, and the treatment of acyclovir-resistant HSV and varicella-zoster infection, Kaposi's sarcoma, and hepatitis B.

The major adverse effect seen with foscarnet is nephrotoxicity. The earliest manifestations of impending renal toxicity are an elevation in serum creatinine and a decrease in creatinine clearance.[56] Rarely, patients have renal failure secondary to tubulointerstitial nephritis.[57] The risk of nephrotoxicity can be reduced when foscarnet is administered intermittently rather than by continuous intravenous infusion.[58] Patients receiving foscarnet therapy in whom renal impairment develops can have crystals of foscarnet in the glomerular capillaries, fever, and phosphaturia.[57, 59–61] Renal function returns to normal or prerenal function shortly after discontinuing foscarnet.[62] Another side effect associated with foscarnet therapy is a reduction in serum calcium, which can manifest as paresthesias, tremor, arrhythmias, and convulsions. Electrolyte disturbances have also been observed (i.e., hypocalcemia and hypercalcemia, hypophosphatemia and hyperphosphatemia, hypomagnesemia, and hypokalemia).

Foscarnet should not be administered simultaneously with any other drug. Co-therapy with ganciclovir and foscarnet does not result in alterations in plasma clearance or volume of either agent, but the two should not be given to a patient at the same time.[63] Foscarnet administered to patients receiving zidovudine does not alter plasma clearance or volume of either drug.[64]

Zidovudine

Zidovudine, (3'-azido-3'-deoxythymidine), also known as azidothymidine or AZT, is an analogue of thymidine and inhibits the HIV-encoded enzyme reverse transcriptase. Zidovudine, when used with other antiviral agents, such as lamivudine, saquinavir, nevirapine, or stavudine, has been shown to be additive or synergistic in effect.[65, 66] The combination of zidovudine and stavudine is synergistic against both zidovudine-sensitive and some zidovudine-resistant strains of HIV.[67] Zidovudine, or zidovudine administered with didanosine plus recombinant interferon, inhibits replication of HIV in peripheral mononuclear cells, monocytes, and bone marrow progenitor cells.[68–70] Recombinant interferon-alpha has been demonstrated to inhibit replication of HIV in chronically infected cells.[71] Combinations of antiviral agents, such as zidovudine, foscarnet, saquinavir, didanosine, and interferon-alpha, have demonstrated a greater degree of in vitro inhibition of viral replication, than single-drug therapy.[72]

Ribavirin, stavudine, and ganciclovir combined with zidovudine are anatagonistic.[66, 73, 74] Zidovudine is administered either orally or intravenously. The oral dose is 200 mg every 8 hours or 100 mg every 4 hours. Studies have demonstrated that zidovudine can be administered in a dose of 250 mg every 12 hours; compared with standard regimens, no difference in efficacy was found.[75] The dose of zidovudine for intravenous administration is 1.9 mg/kg of body weight every 4 hours. The drug should be administered over a 1-hour period.

The drug appears to be safe in pregnancy, but reduction in dosage is necessary.[76–78] Zidovudine levels in the mother and fetus are similar. Use of zidovudine during pregnancy has not been associated with any teratogenic effects, even among women who received the drug in the first trimester.[79] In one study of infants born to seven mothers who received zidovudine during pregnancy after 16 weeks' gestation, all infants had macrocystitis and anemia.[80]

Zidovudine enters host cells by simple diffusion, where cellular thymidine kinases initiate the first two phosphorylations and other cellular kinases complete the phosphorylation to produce the active triphosphate form of the drug.[81, 82] Thus, the initial phosphorylation of zidovudine is not like that of acyclovir, which requires viral thymidine kinase. Therefore, zidovudine is phosphorylated in both infected and uninfected cells.

Zidovudine can cause significant bone marrow suppression, resulting in anemia, neutropenia, and leukopenia. Myopathy can be induced by zidovudine and may be indistinguishable from that caused by HIV.[83, 84] Initially, the patient presents with fatigue and weakness. The proximal muscle groups are affected with weakness, wasting, and pain.[85, 86] Other potential adverse effects are hepatotoxicity, gastrointestinal disturbances, and neuropsychiatric toxicities such as mania, sleep disturbances, headache, focal seizures, somnolence, and coma.[87–90] A variety of mucocutaneous le-

sions have been reported due to zidovudine or drugs used in conjunction with it. Progressive pigmentation of the fingernails and toenails has been reported.[91–93] The nails begin to acquire a bluish color at the lunulae approximately 2 to 4 weeks after initiating therapy.[94] In patients with hepatic dysfunction receiving zidovudine, maculopapular eruptions have also been noted. The lesions have been described as erythematous, nonpruritic blisters.[95] Some patients recieving zidovudine and fluconazole have had cutaneous leukocytoclastic vasculitis.[96] The mucocutaneous lesions resolve with cessation of therapy. The mucocutaneous reactions appeared to be a hypersensitivity reaction to zidovudine because rechallenge with zidovudine after a 24- to 48-hour cessation of therapy results in recurrence of the lesions. Desensitization to zidovudine has been performed.[95]

Didanosine

Didanosine (2',3'-dideoxyinosine [ddI]) is the analogue of the purine inosine and inhibits HIV reverse transcriptase, thus preventing elongation of the newly synthesized HIV DNA.[97] Didanosine is derived from the conversion of 2',3'-dideoxyadenosine (ddA) through the action of adenosine deaminase. The prodrug ddA and didanosine can enter cells by passive diffusion. Once in the host cell, ddA is phosphorylated by one of two enzymes, deoxycytidine or adenosine kinase, to yield ddA monophosphate. The product ddA can be deaminated by adenosine deaminase to form didanosine, and subsequently phosphorylated by 5'-nuceotidase to form dideoxyinosine monophosphate (ddIMP). Adenylosuccinate synthetase converts ddIMP to dideoxyadenosine monophosphate (ddAMP).[98–101] ddAMP is subsequently phosphorylated in two steps to the triphosphate form (ddATP), which is the active form of the drug. The triphosphate form of dideoxyadenosine competes with adenosine for binding with HIV reverse transcriptase (main activity) and for cellular DNA polymerase. ddATP can also become incorporated into growing viral DNA, resulting in termination of the growing DNA molecule.[102]

Didanosine is synergistic with zidovudine against HIV-1 and HIV-2 in vitro.[103–105] Didanosine administered in combination with zidovudine and lamivudine has been shown to have greater antiviral activity than when only two of the drugs are given in tandem.[106]

The adverse effects of didanosine are pancreatitis, bilateral symmetric peripheral neuropathy, diarrhea, xerostomia, hepatitis, hepatic failure, increased serum uric acid, hypokalemia, electrolyte and acid–base abnormalities, and visual disturbances. The most serious of the adverse reactions is the development of pancreatitis, and this is most likely to occur in patients receiving doses greater than 9.6 mg/kg of body weight daily.[107] The incidence of pancreatitis in patients recieving 9.6 mg/kg daily is 0.9% to 2%, whereas in patients receiving 10 to 12 mg, the incidence is 23%.[108]

Zalcitabine

Zalcitabine (2′,3-dideoxycytidine [ddC]) is an analogue of the pyrimidine nucleoside deoxycytidine. For zalcitabine to be active, it must be phosphorylated to the triphosphate form.[109, 110] Zalcitabine enters infected and noninfected host cells by nonfacilitated and facilitated diffusion.[111, 112] The latter is accomplished by the nucleoside carrier.[111] Phosphorylation is accomplished equally in both uninfected and infected host T cells. The triphosphate form binds to HIV reverse transcriptase, preventing the conversion of HIV RNA to DNA and causing premature termination of viral DNA elongation.[112]

Zalcitabine and zidovudine act synergistically to inhibit replication of both zidovudine-sensitive and zidovudine-resistant isolates of HIV-1 in vitro.[102, 113, 114] Zalcitabine and recombinant interferon-alpha act synergistically against HIV-1 replication in vitro in tests against human leukocytes, T cells, and monocyte cell lines.[65, 115, 116]

Resistance to zalcitabine has been observed in patients receiving monotherapy for more than 1 year. Resistance was also found in patients receiving alternating therapy of zidovudine and zalcitabine.[117, 118]

Zalcitabine can cause peripheral neuropathy, pancreatitis, gastrointestinal distress, hepatic toxicity, thrombocytopenia, leukopenia, esophageal ulcerations, and aphthous stomatitis. The major toxicity is peripheral neuropathy, which reportedly occurs in 30% of patients.[119] The patient has pain because of the drug's effect on sensory nerves. Ototoxicity has also been reported in patients receiving zalcitabine therapy.[120]

Zalcitabine did not appear to have significant toxicity when administered to pregnant rats. However, there was minimal interference with embryonic development during blastocyst formation. Inhibition occurred at the two-cell stage at concentrations of 100 μmol/L or greater.[121]

Ganciclovir

Ganciclovir (9-[1-3-dihydroxy-2-propoxymethyl]guanine) is an analogue of guanine, and is active against the herpes viruses.[122] Ganciclovir and foscarnet are the drugs of choice for treatment of cytomegalovirus infection. Ganciclovir can be administered both intravenously and orally. Other viruses that are susceptible to ganciclovir are HSV, Epstein-Barr, varicella-zoster, human herpes virus type 6, adenovirus, hepatitis B, and Creutzfeldt-Jakob.

Ganciclovir must be triphosphorylated to achieve bioactivity. The initial phosphorylation is carried out in infected cells and requires viral thymidine kinase. The subsequent phosphorylations are performed by host cell thymidine kinase. Unlike HSV types 1 and 2, which possess a gene that encodes for thymidine kinase, it has not been demonstrated that cytomegalovirus possesses thymidine kinase. However, the UL97 region contains a gene that encodes for a protein with characteristics of thymidine kinase that is capable of phosphorylating ganciclovir in cytomegalovirus-infected cells.[123–125]

Ganciclovir inhibits replication of viral DNA by several mechanisms. Ganciclovir triphosphate competitively inhibits DNA polymerase by replacing deoxyguanine triphosphate. This results in ganciclovir triphosphate being incorporated into the DNA chain, limiting its replication. This action produces short fragments of DNA that accumulate in the infected cell but do not become incorporated into virions.[126–129] The main use of ganciclovir is the treatment and prevention of cytomegalovirus infection in patients with AIDS. The oral form of ganciclovir is approved for prophylaxis against cytomegalovirus infection in patients with AIDS and high-risk transplant recipients. Ganciclovir is also approved for the treatment of cytomegalovirus infection in immunosuppressed patients with disseminated disease, retinitis, pneumonia, and gastrointestinal involvement.

The principal toxicity of ganciclovir is bone marrow suppression and thrombocytopenia. The drug should not be administered to patients whose neutrophil count is less than 500/μL or whose platelet count is less than 25,000/μL. The development of neutropenia is independent of plasma drug level, duration of treatment, and the starting neutrophil count.[130, 131] Neutropenia is more likely to occur in patients receiving combination ganciclovir and foscarnet therapy.[132, 133] Patients in whom granulocytopenia develops are at risk for becoming bacteremic and contracting bacterial pneumonia and pulmonary aspergillosis.[134–136] Other adverse effects of ganciclovir therapy are listed in Table 55-4.

Because ganciclovir is mainly used to treat cytomegalovirus infection in patients with AIDS, care must be given when administering this agent because it is likely to interact with other antiviral agents being administered. Ganciclovir reduces the tolerance to zidovudine when administered with this drug because of the increased risk of bone marrow suppression.[137, 138] An interesting differential effect has been reported when ganciclovir and zidovudine are co-administered, depending on the route of administration. Ganciclovir given intravenously was found to increase the clearance of zidovudine and potentially decrease its plasma concentration.[139, 140] However, ganciclovir given orally was found to increase the plasma concentration of zidovudine by 14%.

Ganciclovir administered with didanosine results in

TABLE 55-4 ▸ ADVERSE EFFECTS OF GANCICLOVIR THERAPY

Event	Intravenous	Oral
Neutropenia	23%–37%	14%–15%
Thrombocytopenia	2%–7%	3%–9%
Anemia	24%–40%	15%–36%
Sepsis	8.5%–19%	3%–8%
Diarrhea	21%–54%	33%–50%
Rash	0%	10%
Nausea	29%	34%
Vomiting	15%	15%

Data from Drew WL, Anderson R, Lang W, et al: Failure of high-dose oral acyclovir to suppress GMV viruria or induced ganciclovir-resistant CMV in HIV antibody positive patients. J Acquir Immune Defic Syndr Hum Retrovirol 1995; 8:289; Drew WL, Ives D, King BD, et al: Oral ganciclovir as maintenance treatment for cytomegalovirus retinitis in patients with AIDS. N Engl J Med 1995; 333:615; and Ganciclovir. In: Kucers A, Crowe SM, Grayson ML, Hoy JF (eds): The Use of Antibiotics: A Clinical Review of Antibacterial, Antifungal and Antiviral Drugs, 5th ed. Oxford, Butterworth-Heinemann, 1997, pp 1557–1592. A division of Reed Educational and Professional Publishing Ltd. A member of the Reed Elsevier plc group.

a significant increase in the serum level of didanosine (>80%), and the serum level of ganciclovir is decreased by 23%.[141] This increase in the serum concentration of didanosine increases the risk of neutropenia.

REFERENCES

1. Lavoie SR, Kaplowitz LG: Management of genital herpes infections. Semin Dermatol 1994; 13:248.
2. Elion GB: Acyclovir: Discovery, mechanism of action, and selectivity. J Med Virol 1993; 1(suppl):2.
3. Balfour HH Jr: Resistance of herpes simplex to acyclovir. Ann Intern Med 1983; 98:404.
4. Elion GB: Mechanism of action and selectivity of acyclovir. Am J Med 1982; 73:7.
5. Ellis MN, Keller PM, Fyfe JA, et al: Clinical isolate of herpes simplex virus type 2 that induces thymidine kinase with altered substrate specificity. Antimicrob Agents Chemother 1987; 31:1117.
6. Kit S, Sheppard M, Ichimura H, et al: Nucleotide sequence changes in thymidine kinase gene of herpes simplex virus type 2 clones from an isolate of a patient treated with acyclovir. Antimicrob Agents Chemother 1982; 31:1483.
7. Chatis PA, Crumpacker CS: Analysis of the thymidine kinase gene from clinically isolated acyclovir resistant herpes simplex viruses. Virology 1991; 180:793.
8. Palu G, Gerna G, Bevilacqua F, Marcello A: A point mutation in the thymidine kinase gene is responsible for acyclovir resistance in herpes simplex virus type 2 sequential isolates. Virus Res 1992; 25:133.
9. Rechtin TM, Black ME, Mao F, et al: Purification and photoaffinity labeling of herpes simplex type-1 thymidine kinase. J Biol Chem 1995; 270:7055.
10. Collins P, Darby G: Laboratory studies of herpes simplex virus strains resistant to acyclovir. Rev Med Virol 1991; 1:19.
11. Crumpacker CS: Significance of resistance of herpes simplex virus to acyclovir. J Am Acad Dermatol 1988; 18:190.
12. Hwang CB, Ruffner KL, Coen DM: A point mutation within a distinct conserved region of the herpes simplex virus DNA polymerase gene confers drug resistance. J Virol 1992; 66:1774.
13. Safrin S, Phan L: In vitro activity of penciclovir against clinical isolates of acyclovir-resistant and foscarnet-resistant herpes simplex virus. Antimicrob Agents Chemother 1993; 37:2241.
14. Barry DW, Nusinoff-Lehrman S, Ellis NM, et al: Viral resistance, clinical experience. Scand J Infect Dis 1985; 47:155.
15. Collins P, Ellis MN: Sensitivity monitoring of clinical isolates of herpes simplex virus to acyclovir. J Med Virol 1993; 1(suppl):58.
16. Blum RM, Liao SH, de Miranda P: Overview of acyclovir pharmacokinetic disposition in adults and children. Am J Med 1982; 73:186.
17. de Miranda P, Good SS, Krasny HC, et al: Metabolic fate of radioactive acyclovir in humans. Am J Med 1982; 73:215.
18. Bean B, Aeppli D: Adverse effects of high-dose intravenous acyclovir in ambulatory patients with acute herpes zoster. J Infect Dis 1985; 151:362.
19. Fife KH, Crumpacker CS, Mertz GJ, et al: Recurrence and resistance patterns of herpes simplex virus following cessation of > or = 6 years of chronic suppression with acyclovir. J Infect Dis 1994; 169:1338.
20. Goldberg LH, Kaufman R, Kurtz TO, et al: Long-term suppression of recurrent genital herpes with acyclovir. Arch Dermatol 1993; 129:582.
21. Weller S, Blum MR, Doucette M, et al: Pharmacokinetics of the acyclovir pro-drug valacyclovir after escalating single- and multiple-dose administration to normal volunteers. Clin Pharmacol Ther 1993; 54:595.
22. Vere Hodge RA: Review: Antiviral portrait series. Number 3. Famciclovir and penciclovir: The mode of action of famciclovir including its conversion to penciclovir. Antiviral Chem Chemother 1993; 4:67.
23. Mertz GJ, Critchlow CW, Benedetti J, et al: Double-blind placebo-controlled trial of oral acyclovir in first-episode genital herpes simplex virus infection. JAMA 1984; 252:1147.
24. Koelle DM, Benedetti J, Langenberg A, Corey L: Asymptomatic reactivation of herpes simplex virus in women after the first episode of genital herpes. Ann Intern Med 1992; 116:433.
25. Sacks SL: Therapeutic use of newer antiviral agents. Int J Cell Clon 1986; 1(4 suppl):155.
26. Tyring SK, Douglas JM Jr, Corey L, et al: A randomized, placebo-controlled comparison of oral valacyclovir and acyclovir in immunocompetent patients with recurrent genital herpes infections: The Valacyclovir International Study Group. Arch Dermatol 1998; 134:185.
27. Baker DA, and the Valacyclovir Study Group: Once daily valacyclovir for suppression of recurrent genital herpes in patients previously receiving 10 years of twice daily acyclovir suppressive therapy. Annual Clinical Meeting, ACOG 1997.
28. Dracker JL, Miller JM, and The International Valacyclovir Study Group: Once-daily valacyclovir sustains the suppressive efficacy and safety record of acyclovir in recurrent genital herpes. [Abstract.] First European Congress of Chemotherapy, Glasgow, United Kingdom, 1996.
29. Diaz-Mitoma F, Sibbald RG, Shafran SD, et al: Oral famciclovir for the suppression of recurrent genital herpes: A randomized controlled trial. JAMA 1998; 280:887.
30. Mertz GL, Loveless MA, Kraus SJ, et al: Famciclovir for the suppression of recurrent genital herpes. [Abstract.] In: Proceedings of the 34th Interscience Conference on Antimicrobial Agents and Chemotherapy. Washington, DC, American Society for Microbiology, 1994.
31. Wald A, Zeh J, Barnum G, et al: Suppression of subclinical shedding of herpes simplex virus type 2 with acyclovir. Ann Intern Med 1996; 124:8.
32. Parris DS, Harrington JE: Herpes simplex virus variants restraint to high concentrations of acyclovir exist in clinical isolates. Antimicrob Agents Chemother 1982; 22:71.
33. Kost RG, Hill EL, Tigges M, Straus SE: Brief report: Recurrent acyclovir-resistant genital herpes in an immunocompetent patient. N Engl J Med 1993; 329:1777.
34. Erlich KS, Mills J, Chatis P, et al: Acyclovir-resistant herpes simplex virus infections in patients with acquired immunodeficiency syndrome. N Engl J Med 1989; 320:293.
35. De Clercq E: Virus-drug resistance: Thymidine kinase-deficient (TK−) mutants of herpes simplex virus. Therapeutic approaches. Ann Inst Sup Sanita 1987; 23:841.
36. Brown ZA, Baker DA: Acyclovir therapy during pregnancy. Obstet Gynecol 1989; 73:526.
37. Centers for Disease Control and Prevention: Pregnancy outcomes following systemic prenatal acyclovir exposure: June

1, 1984–June 30, 1993. MMWR Morb Mortal Wkly Rep 1993; 42:806.

38. Scott LL: Perinatal herpes: Current status and future management strategies. Adv Obstet Gynecol 1996; 3:47.

39. Frenkel LM, Brown ZA, Bryson YJ, et al: Pharmacokinetics of acyclovir in the term human pregnancy and neonate. Am J Obstet Gynecol 1991; 164:569.

40. Grover L, Kane J, Kravitz J, Cruz A: Systemic acyclovir in pregnancy: A case report. Obstet Gynecol 1985; 65:284.

41. Lagrew DC Jr, Furlow TG, Hager WD, Yarrish RL: Disseminated herpes simplex virus infection in pregnancy: Successful treatment with acyclovir. JAMA 1984; 252:2058.

42. Prober CG, Sullender WM, Yasukawa LL, et al: Low risk of herpes simplex virus infections in neonates exposed to the virus at the time of vaginal delivery to mothers with recurrent genital herpes simplex virus infections. N Engl J Med 1987; 316:240.

43. Brown ZA, Selke S, Zeh J, et al: The acquisition of herpes simplex virus during pregnancy. N Engl J Med 1997; 337:509.

44. Haddad J, Langer B, Astruc D, et al: Oral acyclovir and recurrent genital herpes during late pregnancy. Obstet Gynecol 1993; 82:102.

45. Scott LL, Sanchez PJ, Jackson GL, et al: Acyclovir suppression to prevent cesarean delivery after first episode genital herpes. Obstet Gynecol 1996; 87:69.

46. Brocklehurst P, Kinghorn G, Carney O, et al: A randomized placebo controlled trial of suppressive acyclovir in late pregnancy in women with recurrent genital herpes infection. Br J Obstet Gynaecol 1998; 105:275.

47. Randolph AG, Washington AE, Prober CG: Cesarean delivery for women presenting with genital herpes lesions: Efficacy, risks, and costs. JAMA 1993; 270:77.

48. Helgstrand E, Eriksson B, Johansson NG, et al: Trisodium phosphonoformate, a new antiviral compound. Science 1978; 201:819.

49. Mesri EA, Cesarman E, Arvanitakis L, et al: Human herpesvirus-8/Kaposi's sarcoma-associated herpesvirus is a new transmissible virus that infects B cells. J Exp Med 1996; 183:2385.

50. Wagstaff AJ, Bryson HM: Foscarnet: A reapprasial of its antiviral activity, pharmacokinetic properties and therapeutic use in immunocompromised patients with viral infections. Drugs 1994; 48:199.

51. Stridh S, Helgstrand E, Lannero B, et al: The effect of pyrophosphate analogues on influenza virus RNA polymerase and influenza virus multiplication. Arch Virol 1979; 61:245.

52. Oberg B: Antiviral effects of phosphonoformate (PFA, foscarnet sodium). Pharmacol Ther 1982; 19:387.

53. Strid S, Ekstrom C, Datema R: Comparison of foscarnet and foscarnet esters as anti-influenza virus agents. Chemotherapy 1989; 35:69.

54. Sandstrom EG, Kaplan JC, Byington RE, Hirsch MS: Inhibition of human T-cell lymphotrophic virus type III in vitro by phosphonoformate. Lancet 1985; 1:1480.

55. Sarin PS, Taguchi Y, Sun D, et al: Inhibition of HTLV-III/LAV replication by foscarnet. Biochem Pharmacol 1985; 34:4075.

56. Deray G, Martinez F, Katlama C, et al: Foscarnet nephrotoxicity mechanism, incidence, and prevention. Am J Nephrol 1989; 9:316.

57. Nyberg G, Svalander C, Blohme I, Persson H: Tubulointerstitial nephritis caused by the antiviral agent foscarnet. Transpl Int 1989; 2:223.

58. Chrisp P, Clissold SP: Foscarnet: A review of its antiviral activity, pharmacokinetic properties and therapeutic use in immunocompromised patients with cytomegalovirus retinitis. Drugs 1991; 41:104.

59. Beaufils H, Deray G, Katlama C, Dohin E, Henin D, Sazdovitch V, Jouanneau C. Foscarnet and crystals in glomerular capillary lumens. Lancet 1990; 336:755.

60. Trolliet P, Dijoud F, Cotte L, et al: Crescentic glomerulonephritis and crystals within glomerular capillaries in an AIDS patient treated with foscarnet. Am J Nephrol 1995; 15:256.

61. Loghman-Adham M, Levi M, Scherer SA, et al: Phosphonoformic acid blunts adaptive response of renal and intestinal Pi transport. Am J Physiol 1993; 265:756.

62. Seidel EA, Koenig S, Polis MA: A dose escalation study to determine the toxicity and maximally tolerated dose of foscarnet. AIDS 1993; 7:941.

63. Aweeka FT, Gambertoglio JG, Kramer F, et al: Foscarnet and ganciclovir pharmacokinetics during concomitant or alternating maintenance therapy for AIDS related cytomegalovirus retinitis. Clin Pharmacol Ther 1995; 57:403.

64. Aweeka FT, Gambertoglio JG, van der Horst C, et al: Pharmacokinetics of concomitantly administered foscarnet and zidovudine for treatment of human immunodeficiency virus infection (ACTG protocol 053). Antimicrob Agents Chemother 1992; 36:1773.

65. Mathez D, Schinazi RF, Liotta DC, Leibowitch J: Infectious amplification of wild-type human immunodeficiency virus from patients' lymphocytes and modulation by reverse transcriptase inhibitors in vitro. Antimicrob Agents Chemother 1993; 37:2206.

66. Merrill DP, Moonis M, Chou TC, Hirsch MS: Lamivudine or stavudine in two- and three-drug combinations against human immunodeficiency virus type 1 replication in vitro. J Infect Dis 1996; 173:355.

67. Sorensen AM, Nielsen C, Mathiesen LR, et al: Evaluation of the combination effect of different antiviral compounds against HIV in vitro. Scand J Infect Dis 1993; 25:365.

68. Hartshorn KL, Vogt MW, Chou TC, et al: Synergistic inhibition of human immunodeficiency virus in vitro by azidothymidine and recombinant alpha A interferon. Antimicrob Agents Chemother 1987; 31:168.

69. Berman E, Duigou-Osterndorf R, Krown SE: Synergistic cytotoxic effect of azidothymidine and recombinant interferon alpha on normal bone marrow progenitor cells. Blood 1989; 74:1281.

70. Johnson VA, Merrill DP, Videler JA, et al: Two-drug combinations of zidovudine, didanosine, and recombinant interferon-alpha A inhibit replication of zidovudine-resistant immunodeficiency virus type 1 synergistically in vitro. J Infect Dis 1991; 164:646.

71. Poli G, Orenstein JM, Kinter A, et al: Interferon-alpha but not AZT suppresses HIV expression in chronically infected cell lines. Science 1989; 244:575.

72. Mazzulli T, Rusconi S, Merrill DP, et al: Alternating versus continuous drug regimens in combination chemotherapy of human immunodeficiency virus type-1 infection in vitro. Antimicrob Agents Chemother 1994; 38:656.

73. Vogt MW, Hartshorn KL, Furman PA, et al: Ribavirin antagonizes the effect of azidothymidine on HIV replication. Science 1987; 235:1376.

74. Medina DJ, Hsiung GD, Mellors JW: Ganciclovir antagonizes the anti-human immunodeficiency virus type 1 activity of zidovudine and didanosine in vitro. Antimicrob Agents Chemother 1992; 36:1127.

75. Gill S, Tang A, Cordey M, et al: The effects of twice and four times daily zidovudine on p24 antigenaemia in CDC stage II/III patients. Genitourin Med 1991; 67:15.

76. Chavanet P, Diquet B, Waldner A, Portier H: Perinatal pharmacokinetics of zidovudine. [Letter.] N Engl J Med 1989; 321:1548.

77. Lopez-Anaya A, Unadkat JD, Schumann LA, Smith AL: Pharmacokinetics of zidovudine (azidothymidine): III. Effect in pregnancy. J AIDS 1991; 4(1):64–8.

78. Watts DH, Brown ZA, Tartaglione T, et al: Pharmacokinetic disposition of zidovudine during pregnancy. J Infect Dis 1991; 163:226.

79. Sperling RS, Stratton P: Treatment options for human immunodeficiency virus-infected pregnant women: Obstetric-Gynecologic Working Group of the AIDS Clinical Trials Group of the National Institute of Allergy and Infectious Diseases. Obstet Gynecol 1992; 79:443.

80. Ferrazin A, De Maria A, Gotta C, et al: Zidovudine therapy of HIV-1 infection during pregnancy: Assessment of the effect on the newborns. J AIDS 1993; 6:376.

81. Kong XB, Zhu QY, Vidal PM, et al: Comparisons of anti-human immunodeficiency virus activities, cellular transport, and plasma and intracellular pharmacokinetics of 3'-fluoro-3'-deoxythymidine and 3'-azido-3'-deoxythymidine. Antimicrob Agents Chemother 1992; 36:808.

82. Furman PA, Fyfe JA, St Clair MH, et al: Phosphorylation of 3'-

azido-3'-deoxythymidine and selective interaction of 5'-triphosphate with human immunodeficiency virus reverse transcriptase. Proc Natl Acad Sci U S A 1986; 83:8333.

83. Till M, MacDonell KB: Myopathy with human immunodeficiency virus type 1 (HIV-1) infection: HIV-1 or zidovudine? Ann Intern Med 1990; 113:492.

84. Espinoza LR, Aguilar JL, Espinoza CG, et al: Characteristics and pathogenesis of myositis in human immunodeficiency virus infection: Distinction from azidothymidine-induced myopathy. Rheum Dis Clin North Am 1991; 17:117.

85. Helbert M, Robinson D, Peddle B, et al: Acute meningoencephalitis on dose reduction of zidovudine. Lancet 1988; 1249.

86. Gertner E, Thurn JR, Williams DN, et al: Zidovudine-associated myopathy. Am J Med 1989; 86:814.

87. Wright JM, Sachdev PS, Perkins RJ, Rodriguez P: Zidovudine-related mania. Med J Aust 1989; 150:339.

88. Richman DD, Fischl MA, Grieco MH, et al: The toxicity of azidothymidine (AZT) in the treatment of patients with AIDS and AIDS-related complex: A double-blind, placebo-controlled trial. N Engl J Med 1987; 317:192.

89. Hagler DN, Frame PT: Azidothymidine neurotoxicity. Lancet 1986; 2:1392.

90. Riedel RR, Clarenbach P, Reetz KP: Coma during azidothymidine therapy for AIDS. J Neurol 1989; 236:185.

91. Furth PA, Kazakis AM: Nail pigmentation changes associated with azidothymidine (zidovudine). Ann Intern Med 1987; 107:350.

92. Grau-Massanes M, Millan F, Ferber MI, et al: Pigmented nail bands and mucocutaneous pigmentation in HIV-positive patients treated with zidovudine. J Am Acad Dermatol 1990; 22:687.

93. Rahav G, Maayan S: Nail pigmentation associated with zidovudine: A review and report of a case. Scand J Infect Dis 1992; 24:557.

94. Tosti A, Gaddoni G, Fanti PA, et al: Longitudinal melanonychia induced by 3'-azidodeoxythymidine: Report of 9 cases. Dermatologica 1990; 180:217.

95. Carr A, Penny R, Cooper DA: Allergy and desensitization to zidovudine in patients with acquired immunodeficiency syndrome (AIDS). J Allergy Clin Immunol 1993; 91:683.

96. Torres RA, Lin RY, Lee M, Barr MR: Zidovudine-induced leukocytoclastic vasculitis. Arch Intern Med 1992; 152:850.

97. Mitsuya H, Broder S: Strategies for antiviral therapy in AIDS. Nature 1987; 325:773.

98. McGowan JJ, Tomaszewski JE, Cradock J, et al: Overview of the preclinical development of an antiretroviral drug 2',3'-dideoxyinosine. Rev Infect Dis 1990; 12(suppl 5):S513.

99. Ahluwalia G, Cooney DA, Mitsuya H, et al: Initial studies on the cellular pharmacology of 2',3'-dideoxyinosine, an inhibitor of HIV infectivity. Biochem Pharmacol 1987; 36:3797.

100. Cooney DA, Ahluwalia G, Mitsuya H, et al: Initial studies on the cellular pharmacology of 2',3'-dideoxyadenosine, an inhibitor of HTLV-III infectivity. Biochem Pharmacol 1987; 36:1765.

101. Carson DA, Carrera CJ, Wasson DB, Iizasa T: Deoxyadenosine resistant human T lymphoblasts with elevated 5'-nucleoside activity. Biochim Biophys Acta 1991; 1091:22.

102. Mitsuya H, Jarrett RF, Matsukura M, et al: Long-term inhibition of human T-lymphotropic virus type III/lymphadenopathy-associated virus (human immunodeficiency virus) DNA synthesis and RNA expression in T cells protected by 2',3'-dideoxynucleoside in vitro. Proc Natl Acad Sci U S A 1987; 84:2033.

103. Dornsife RE, St Clair MH, Huang AT, et al: Anti-human immunodeficiency virus synergism by zidovudine (3'-azidothymidine) and didanosine (dideoxyinosine) contrasts with their additive inhibition of normal human marrow progenitor cells. Antimicrob Agents Chemother 1991; 35:322.

104. Johnson VA, Merrill DP, Videler JA, et al: Two-drug combinations of zidovudine, didanosine, and recombinant interferon-alpha A inhibit replication of zidovudine-resistant human immunodeficiency virus type I synergistically in vitro. J Infect Dis 1991; 164:646.

105. Cox SW, Aperia K, Albert J, Wahren B: Comparison of the sensitivities of primary isolates of HIV type 2 and HIV type 1 to antiviral drugs and drug combinations. AIDS Res Hum Retrovir 1994; 10:1725.

106. St Clair MH, Pennington KN, Rooney J, Barry DW: In vitro comparison of selected triple drug combinations for suppression of HIV-1 replication: The Inter-Company Collaboration Protocol. J AIDS 1995; 10(suppl 2):S83.

107. Yarchoan R, Mitsuya H, Pluda JM: The National Cancer Institute phase I study of 2',3'-dideoxyinosine administration in adults with AIDS or AIDS-related complex: Analysis of activity and toxicity profiles. Rev Infect Dis 1990; 12(suppl 5):S522.

108. Maxson CJ, Greenfield SM, Turner JL: Acute pancreatitis as a common complication of 2',3'-dideoxyinosine therapy in acquired immunodeficiency syndrome. Am J Gastroenterol 1992; 87:708.

109. Birnbaum GI, Lin TS, Prusoff WH: Unusual structural features of 2',3'-dideoxycytidine, an inhibitor of the HIV (AIDS) virus. Biochem Biophys Res Commun 1988; 151:608.

110. Silverton JV, Quinn FR, Haugwitz RD, Torado LJ: Structures of two dideoxynucleosides: 2',3'-Dideoxyadenosine and 2',3'-dideoxycytidine. Acta Crystallogr C 1988; 44:321.

111. Plagemann PG, Wohlhueter RM, Woffendin C: Nucleoside and nucleobase transport in animal cells. Biochim Biophys Acta 1988; 947:405.

112. Domin BA, Mahony WB, Zimmerman TP: Membrane permeation mechanisms of 2'3'-dideoxynucleosides. Biochem Pharmacol 1993; 46:725.

113. Balzarini J, Cooney DA, Dalal M, et al: 2',3'-Dideoxycytidine: Regulation of its metabolism and anti-retroviral potency by natural pyrimidine nucleosides and by inhibitors of pyrimidine nucleotide synthesis. Mol Pharamacol 1987; 32:798.

114. Eron JJ Jr, Johnson VA, Merrill DP, et al: Synergistic inhibition of replication of human immunodeficiency virus type 1, including that of a zidovudine-resistant isolate, by zidovudine and 2',3'-dideoxycytidine in vitro. Antimicrob Agents Chemother 1992; 36:1559.

115. Vogt MW, Durno AG, Chou TC, et al: Synergistic interaction of 2',3'-dideoxycytidine and recombinant interferon alpha-A on replication of human immunodeficiency virus type 1. J Infect Dis 1988; 158:378.

116. Degre M, Beck S: Anti-HIV activity of dideoxynucleosides, foscarnet and fisidic acid is potentiated by human leukocyte interferon in blood derived macrophages. Chemotherapy 1994; 40:201.

117. Shirasaka T, Yarchoan R, O'Brien MC, et al: Changes in drug sensitivity of human immunodeficiency virus type-1 during therapy with azidothymidine, dideoxycytidine, and dideoxyinosine: An in vitro comparative study. Proc Natl Acad Sci U S A 1993; 90:562.

118. Husson RN, Shirasaka T, Butler KM, et al: High-level resistance to zidovudine but not zalcitabine or didanosine in human immunodeficiency virus from children receiving antiretroviral therapy. J Pediatr 1993; 123:9.

119. Shelton MJ, O'Donnell AM, Morse GD: Zalcitabine. Ann Pharmacother 1993; 27:480.

120. Powderly WG, Klebert MK, Clifford DB: Ototoxicity associated with dideoxycytidine. Lancet 1990; 335:1106.

121. Toltzis P, Mourton T, Magnuson T: Comparative embryonic cytotoxicity of antiretroviral nucleosides. J Infect Dis 1994; 169:1100.

122. Martin JC, Dvorak CA, Smee DF, et al: 9-[(1,3-Dihydroxy-2-propoxy)methyl]guanine: A new potent and selective antiherpes agent. J Med Chem 1983; 26:759.

123. Littler E, Stuart AD, Chee MS: Human cytomegalovirus UL97 open reading frame encodes a protein that phosphorylases the antiviral nucleoside analogue ganciclovir. Nature 1992; 358:160.

124. Sullivan V, Talarico CL, Stanat SC, et al: A protein kinase homologue controls phosphorylation of ganciclovir in human cytomegalovirus-infected cells. Nature 1992; 358:162.

125. Sullivan V, Talarico CL, Stanat SC: A protein kinase homologue controls phosphorylation of ganciclovir in human cytomegalovirus-infected cells. Nature 1992; 359:85.

126. Frank KB, Chiou JF, Cheng YC: Interaction of herpes simplex

virus-induced DNA polymerase with 9-(1,3-dihydroxy-2-propoxymethyl) guanine triphosphate. J Biol Chem 1984; 259:1566.

127. St Clair MH, Lambe CU, Furman PA: Inhibition by ganciclovir of cell growth and DNA synthesis of cells biochemically transformed with herpesvirus genetic information. Antimicrob Agents Chemother 1987; 31:844.

128. Reardon JE: Herpes simplex virus type 1 and human DNA polymerase interactions with 2′-deoxyguanosine 5′-triphosphate analogues: Kinetics of incorporation into DNA and induction of inhibition. J Biol Chem 1989; 264:19039.

129. Hamzeh FM, Lietman PS: Intranuclear accumulation of subgenomic noninfectious human cytomegalovirus DNA in infected cells in the presence of ganciclovir. Antimicrob Agents Chemother 1991; 35:1818.

130. Reed EC, Shepp DH, Dandliker PS, Meyers JD: Ganciclovir treatment of cytomegalovirus infection of the gastrointestinal tract after marrow transplantation. Bone Marrow Transplant 1988; 3:199.

131. Reed EC, Bowden RA, Dandliker PS, et al: Treatment of cytomegalovirus pneumonia with ganciclovir and intravenous cytomegalovirus immunoglobulin in patients with bone marrow transplant. Ann Intern Med 1988; 109:783.

132. Dieterich DT, Poles MA, Lew EA, et al: Concurrent use of ganciclovir and foscarnet to treat cytomegalovirus infection in AIDS patients. J Infect Dis 1993; 167:1184.

133. Jacobson MA, Kramer F, Bassiakos Y, et al: Randomized phase 1 trial of two different combination foscarnet and ganciclovir chronic maintenance therapy regimens for AIDS patients with cytomegalovirus retinitis: AIDS Clinical Trials Group Protocol 151. J Infect Dis 1994; 170:189.

134. Miller WT Jr, Sais GJ, Frank I, et al: Pulmonary aspergillosis in patients with AIDS: Clinical and radiographic correlations. Chest 1994; 105:37.

135. Przepiorka D, Ippoliti C, Panina A, et al: Ganciclovir three times per week is not adequate to prevent cytomegalovirus reactivation after T cell-depleted marrow transplantation. Bone Marrow Transplant 1994; 13:461.

136. Shepp DH, Tang IT, Ramundo MB, Kaplan MK: Serious *Pseudomonas aeruginosa* infection in AIDS. J AIDS 1994; 7:823.

137. Hochster H, Dieterich D, Bozzette S, et al: Toxicity of combined ganciclovir and zidovudine for cytomegalovirus disease associated with AIDS: An AIDS Clinical Trials Group Study. Ann Intern Med 1990; 113:111.

138. Jacobson MA, Owen W, Campbell J, et al: Tolerability of combined ganciclovir and didanosine for the treatment of cytomegalovirus disease associated with AIDS. Clin Invest Dis 1993; 16(suppl 1):S69.

139. Burger DM, Meenhorst PL, ten Napel CH, et al: Pharmacokinetic variability of zidovudine in HIV-infected individuals: Subgroup analysis and drug interactions. AIDS 1994; 8:1683.

140. Jacobson MA, deMiranda P, Gordon SM, et al: Prolonged pancytopenia due to combined ganciclovir and zidovudine therapy. J Infect Dis 1988; 158:489.

141. Gaines K, Wong R, Jung D, et al: Pharmacokinetic interactions with oral ganciclovir: Zidovudine, didanosine, probenecid. Tenth International Conference on AIDS, Yokohama, Japan.

56

Quinolones

JENNIFER GUNTER

STRUCTURE AND DERIVATION

Quinolones encompass a rapidly expanding class of antibiotics with widespread clinical applications. Synthetic derivatives of nalidixic acid, quinolones have evolved from narrow-spectrum antibiotics with limited clinical applications to a class of antimicrobials with a broad spectrum of activity, including gram-positive and gram-negative aerobes, anaerobes, mycoplasmas, and mycobacteria.[2] The clinical usefulness of this class of antibiotics is further enhanced by high tissue and plasma levels, once-daily dosing regimens, good oral absorption, and relatively few side effects.[3, 4]

The core molecule for the quinolones is a dual-ring structure derived from naldixic acid, a 1,8-naphthyridine (Fig. 56–1). Most current quinolones have either a quinolone ring or a naphthyridine ring, defined by a carbon or a nitrogen atom at position 8, respectively.[3] Although nalidixic acid was discovered in the early 1960s, the therapeutic potential of quinolones remained largely untapped until the 1980s, when derivatives with improved potency and greater spectrum of activity were identified.[3, 4]

An understanding of the structure–activity relationships of the quinolones is important because some functional groups are essential for antibacterial activity and potency.[4, 5] No modifications may occur at position 3, a carboxyl group attached to the carbon, or at position 4, a carbonyl group. These sites control gyrase–DNA binding and may also play a role in bacterial transport; therefore, alterations at either of these positions would interfere with the basic mechanism of action.[4, 5] Position 2 also plays a role in gyrase–DNA binding, and for optimal antibacterial activity should be a hydrogen group. The addition of fluorine at position 6 greatly improves potency, up to 100-fold, and is integral for current quinolones.[3–5]

Substitutions at the remaining four positions affect potency, pharmacokinetics, toxicity, and spectrum of activity. Various substitutions at these four positions have produced over 10,000 quinolone analogues, although only a small percentage of these are of clinical importance[4, 5] (Table 56–1). Modifications at position 7 produce the greatest impact on the resulting quinolone, affecting potency, spectrum of activity,

and pharmacokinetics.[4] Substitutions at position 8 alter pharmacokinetics and can expand anaerobic activity; modifications at position 1 control potency; and substituents attached to C5 alter both potency and gram-positive activity.[4–6] Quinolones are classified into generations by these modifications. Second-generation quinolones have improved activity against gram-negative pathogens, and third-generation quinolones have enhanced pharmacokinetics and expanded spectrums of activity against gram-positive and anerobic bacteria.

MECHANISM OF ACTION

Quinolones target the topoisomerases, which are bacterial enzymes essential for DNA replication. Quinolones interact with two topoisomerases: DNA gyrase (topoisomerase II) and topoisomerase IV.[7, 8] DNA gyrase is the enzyme responsible for DNA supercoiling; topoisomerase IV removes links produced by bidirectional DNA replication.[7, 9] The topoisomerase target of quinolones differs between bacteria, with DNA gyrase primarily affected in gram-negative bacteria and topoisomerase IV targeted in gram-positive bacteria.[8] Some of the newer quinolones with expanded spectrums of activity interact equally with both enzymes.[8, 10]

An essential enzyme in DNA synthesis, DNA gyrase (topoisomerase II) is composed of four subunits, two A and two B monomers, encoded by the genes gyrA and gyrB.[7, 8] Bacterial DNA exists in a highly negatively supercoiled state, and DNA gyrase is the enzyme responsible for introducing negative supercoils into the double-stranded DNA helix. Breaks are introduced into the double-stranded DNA by the A subunit, allowing the B subunit to effect the negative supercoiling.[7] The A subunit then reseals the breaks. Gyrase control of negative supercoiling also aids with the process of replication and transcription, removes knots from DNA, and helps to bend and fold DNA.[7] Quinolones bind this gyrase–DNA complex, and there are two modes by which this interaction inhibits bacterial DNA replication and synthesis. Quinolone binding with the gyrase–DNA complex traps the enzyme on the DNA, which prevents the A subunit of gyrase from resealing the cleavage sites, thus inhibiting

592

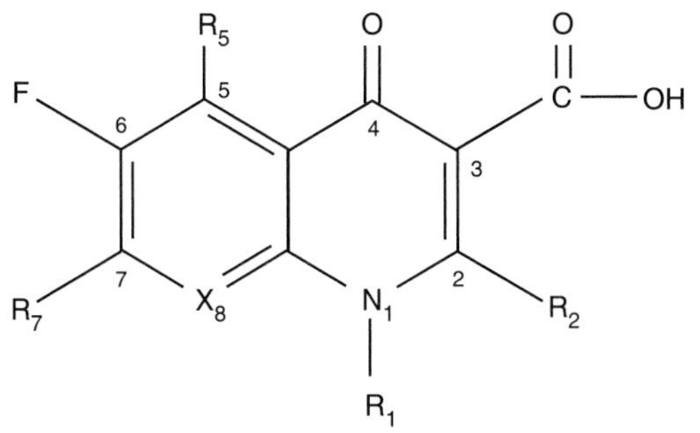

FIGURE 56-1 ▶ Quinolone core molecule.

DNA supercoiling.[7, 8] DNA replication forks also encounter these quinolone–gyrase–DNA complexes, halting their forward progress, which also inhibits DNA replication.[7, 8]

Topoisomerase IV is a tetramer composed of two subunits, C and E, products of the *parC* and *parE* genes.[7, 8] Like DNA gyrase, it is an essential enzyme, required for DNA replication and synthesis. Topoisomerase IV is a decatenating enzyme, recognizing DNA crossovers and resolving interlinked daughter chromosomes after DNA replication.[7] Quinolone binding to the topoisomerase IV–DNA complex interferes with the relaxing activity of topoisomerase IV, inhibiting DNA replication and synthesis.[6–8] DNA replication forks also collide with the quinolone–topoisomerase–DNA complex, inhibiting forward progression and thus DNA replication.[7, 8]

Although quinolones are bactericidal, some evidence suggests that this is not exclusively the result of inhibition of DNA synthesis by the effects of the quinolone–topoisomerase–DNA complex on DNA replication, as described earlier. First, the effects of quinolones on DNA synthesis can be reversed; however, quinolones are still lethal in this environment.[7, 11, 12] In addition, drugs such as chloramphenicol or rifampin that block the lethal action of quinolones have little effect on DNA replication. Finally, quinolones inhibit bacterial DNA synthesis at sublethal concentrations.[7, 12] Binding of the topoisomerase–DNA complex by quinolones is therefore essential for cell death, but it is the release of double-stranded DNA breaks from these complexes that is believed to be lethal.[7, 8]

TABLE 56-1 ▶ THE QUINOLONES		
First-Generation	**Second-Generation**	**Third-Generation**
Nalidixic acid	Norfloxacin	Levofloxacin
Cinoxacin	Ciprofloxacin	Trovofloxacin
Oxolinic acid	Ofloxacin	Grepafloxacin
	Lomefloxacin	Sparfloxacin
	Enoxacin	Clinafloxacin
	Fleroxacin	Sitafloxacin
	Pefloxacin	Gatifloxacin
	Tosufloxacin	Moxifloxacin

Resistance to quinolones occurs primarily by one of three methods: reduction in quinolone binding affinity for the topoisomerase–DNA complex; alterations in bacterial cell membrane permeability, which affects intracellular accumulation; and a quinolone efflux system that expels the drug from the cell.[6, 8, 13] Resistance to quinolones develops as the result of bacterial mutations. No bacterial enzyme has yet been identified that is capable of inactivating or modifying the quinolones to produce resistance.[13] Plasmid-mediated resistance to quinolones has been described in vitro, but no clinically resistant isolates have been identified.[3, 13]

Mutations that alter DNA gyrase or topoisomerase IV may induce resistance by affecting quinolone binding with the enzyme–DNA complex.[7, 13] Because there is much similarity between the genes and protein structures of these two enzymes, it is not surprising that mutations inducing resistance occur at the same region for both gyrase and topoisomerase IV. The main mutations for DNA gyrase and topoisomerase IV that produce quinolone resistance are found on the genes *gyrA* and *parC*, respectively, and specifically at the quinolone resistance determining region (QRDR), which extends between amino acids 67 and 106.[7, 13] Multiple mutations may occur in any gene. Whereas mutations in either *gyrA* or *parC* may confer resistance, bacteria with a double mutation (i.e., involving both genes) have a much higher level of resistance.[7] Mutations conferring resistance are less common in the *gyrB* and *parE* genes of gyrase and topoisomerase, and it is unknown what role, if any, these mutations have in the development of clinically apparent resistance.[7, 13]

Mutations affecting cell permeability may occur, reducing the intracellular concentration of antibiotic. This mechanism of resistance appears to occur primarily with gram-negative bacteria, which have a more complex cell envelope with outer membrane proteins that control diffusion through porin channels.[13] Mutations decreasing production of these outer membrane proteins confer a degree of low-level resistance, but it is unlikely that this is the primary mechanism of resistance for most bacteria.[3, 13]

Resistance to quinolones may also occur as the result of mutations that enhance the quinolone efflux system, which also reduces the intracellular concentration of antibiotic. This mechanism of altered accumulation exists for both gram-positive and gram-negative bacteria.[3, 5, 13] Membrane proteins that function as efflux pumps have been described for *Staphylococcus aureus*, *Streptococcus pneumoniae*, and *Pseudomonas aeruginosa*.[3, 12] Mutations in the corresponding genes enhance quinolone efflux from cells, which confers a high level of resistance. For some bacteria, such as *Escherichia coli*, this reduced efflux system may work in combination with decreased membrane permeability to confer resistance.[3, 13] A combination of mutations involving gyrase, topoisomerase IV, and the efflux system may produce bacteria that are highly resistant to quino-lones.

PHARMACOKINETICS

All quinolones have favorable pharmacokinetic pro-files, with the bioavailability of some of the newer third-generation compounds approaching 90% to 100%.[14–16] Quinolones are well absorbed and have large volumes of distribution and long half-lives, and therefore most of the newer quinolones may be dosed once daily, even for serious infections.

Quinolones are absorbed rapidly from the duode-num and jejunum, reaching peak serum concentra-tions within 2 hours after oral administration.[14, 15] Maxi-mum serum concentration of sparfloxacin occurs at 5 to 6 hours, possibly because of this drug's lower solubility.[14, 16] Administration of quinolones with food delays time to peak serum concentration by approxi-mately 1 hour, and absorption from the gastrointesti-nal tract is significantly reduced by multivalent cations such as aluminum, magnesium, calcium, and iron, and so quinolones should not be administered with ant-acids, certain medications, or dairy products.[14–16]

Quinolones have large volumes of distribution and relatively low protein binding. Volumes of distribution are approximately 1.5 to 3 L/kg, but may be as high as 7 to 8 L/kg for some of the newer third-generation drugs, such as grepafloxacin and sparfloxacin.[14–16] Pro-tein binding ranges from 10% to 50% for most clini-cally available quinolones, except trovafloxacin, which is 70% protein bound.[14–16] Quinolones penetrate well into tissues and body fluids, and tissue concentrations are often higher than the serum concentration. High concentrations of quinolones are found in the respira-tory tract, the kidney parenchyma, gallbladder tissue and bile, and the upper genital tract.[14, 16] The intracel-lular concentration of quinolones in neutrophils, mac-rophages, and lymphocytes may be three to nine times greater than in serum.[14–16] Consequently, high concen-trations of quinolones are found in blister fluid and inflamed tissues. This phenomenon explains how the relatively poor penetration of quinolones into cerebro-spinal fluid increases moderately in the presence of inflammation.[14, 16] Quinolones are also identified in human breast milk.[3, 17]

Quinolones are eliminated from the body by both renal and hepatic mechanisms, and they generally fall into one of two groups: primarily excreted by the kidney relatively unchanged into the urine, and pri-marily metabolized by the liver. The serum half-life of most of the quinolones is long. Most second-genera-tion quinolones have half-lives ranging from 3 to 5 hours after a single oral dose, and require twice-daily dosing. Elimination half-lives of the third-generation compounds varies from 4.6 to 21 hours, allowing for once-daily dosing.[14–16]

Drugs such as norfloxacin, ciprofloxacin, ofloxacin, levofloxacin, clinafloxacin, and sitafloxacin are primar-ily eliminated by the kidney, with over 60% of the drug excreted unchanged in the urine.[14–16] Clearance of these drugs may be reduced in patients with renal impairment and in the elderly because of decreased lean body mass, which decreases volume of distribu-tion. These age-related changes are minor, and dosage adjustments should be made on the basis of renal function, not age.[18]

Quinolones such as grepafloxacin, sparfloxacin, and trovafloxacin undergo significant hepatic metabolism, with less than 15% of these drugs cleared by the kid-ney.[14–16] Approximately 50% of an oral dose of these third-generation quinolones is excreted unchanged in the feces, representing a combination of transintestinal secretion and the unabsorbed fraction of drug. Some metabolites of these drugs have been identified, but they are relatively inactive compared with the parent compound.[14, 16] The pharmacokinetics of sparfloxacin appear unchanged for patients with liver disease, and therefore dose adjustments are not required.[19] This may be due to an increase in renal excretion. Paradoxi-cally, the elimination of sparfloxacin is significantly reduced for patients with moderate to severe renal disease, and dosing adjustments should be made accordingly.[15, 19] Dose adjustment of trovafloxacin is indicated in the presence of hepatic disease.

The pharmacodynamics of quinolones is based on dose-dependent killing. Optimal bactericidal activity occurs when the maximum plasma concentration is at least 10-fold greater than the minimum inhibitory concentration ($C_{max}/MIC > 10$), and the 24-hour area under the plasma concentration–time curve/minimum inhibitory concentration (AUC_{24}/MIC) ratio is greater than 125.[14, 15] Quinolones also have a significant post-antibiotic effect.

SPECTRUM OF ANTIMICROBIAL ACTIVITY

Quinolones have evolved from agents with a relatively narrow spectrum of activity, effective only against gram-negative aerobic bacilli, to broad-spectrum anti-microbials effective against gram-positive and gram-negative bacteria, anaerobes, mycoplasmas, and myco-bacteria.

Second- and third-generation quinolones have an expanded spectrum of activity against gram-negative bacteria compared with first-generation of drugs. Nor-floxacin and enoxacin, second-generation quinolones, have excellent activity against most Enterobacteria-ceae, but essentially no activity against other microor-ganisms.[3, 14, 16] All quinolones are active against *Hae-mophilus influenzae, Moraxella catarrhalis,* and *Neisseria* species. Ciprofloxacin and ofloxacin provide excellent coverage for almost all gram-negative pathogens, with the exception of *Stenotrophomonas maltophilia* and *Burkholderia cepacia*.[16, 20] Ciprofloxacin has the best activity against *Pseudomonas aeruginosa*, but ofloxacin provides no coverage against this pathogen. The third-generation quinolones such as levofloxacin, sparfloxacin, and trovofloxacin share this degree of activity against gram-negative bacteria, but are second to ciprofloxacin with regard to antipseudomonal activity.[16, 20–22] Clinafloxacin has, however, shown activity comparable with that of ciprofloxacin against *P. aeruginosa*.[23] Quinolones have also demonstrated excellent activity against *Haemophilus ducreyi*, with ciprofloxacin demonstrating the highest in vitro activity, followed by sparfloxacin and ofloxacin.[24, 25]

First-generation quinolones have no activity against gram-positive organisms, and second-generation quinolones such as norfloxacin, ciprofloxacin, and ofloxacin have limited gram-positive coverage. The newer third-generation drugs have significantly greater potency against gram-positive organisms than their predecessors, with excellent activity against most staphylococci and streptococci, including methicillin-sensitive *Staphylococcus aureus*, coagulase-negative staphylococci, *Streptococcus agalactiae*, *Streptococcus pyogenes*, and *Streptococcus viridans*.[20, 26] These antibiotics have varying activity against methicillin-resistant *S. aureus* (MRSA).[20–22] Third-generation quinolones are also highly effective against *Streptococcus pneumoniae,* and the MICs are the same for penicillin-sensitive and penicillin-resistant strains. Older quinolones, specifically ciprofloxacin and ofloxacin, are less active against pneumococci, and a higher degree of clinical failures has been reported with these drugs.[20, 21] Third-generation quinolones also have improved activity against *Enterococcus* species, although an increasing number of resistant *Enterococcus faecium* strains have been identified.[20, 21, 26] Ciprofloxacin and ofloxacin are the least active against the enterococci; sitafloxacin, clinafloxacin, and trovofloxacin are the most active.[20, 23, 26, 27] Current clinically available quinolones are ineffective against vancomycin-resistant enterococci.

Quinolones may be divided into three groups with regard to clinical effectiveness against anaerobic bacteria: inactive, intermediate activity, and highly active. Quinolones with minimal to no activity against anaerobes include norfloxacin, enoxacin, ciprofloxacin, ofloxacin, and lomefloxacin.[16, 28] Levofloxacin, sparfloxacin, and grepafloxacin have moderate antianaerobic activity, but in general are not clinically effective against these pathogens.[16, 21, 22, 28] Trovofloxacin, clinafloxacin, sitafloxacin, and moxifloxacin are some of the newer third-generation quinolones that have excellent activity against anaerobic bacteria. These quinolones possess low MICs for many anaerobes, including *Bacteroides fragilis*, other *Bacteroides* species, *Prevotella* species, *Fusobacterium* species, *Peptostreptococcus* species, and *Clostridium* species.[23, 27–30]

Second- and third-generation quinolones exhibit activity against a variety of other pathogens, including *Chlamydia* species, *Legionella pneumophila*, *Mycobacterium tuberculosis*, and mycoplasmas.[20–22, 30–33] *Chlamydia trachomatis* is sensitive to most of the quinolones, with the exception of norfloxacin, enoxacin, and ciprofloxacin. Quinolones are highly effective against *Chlamydia pneumoniae* and *L. pneumophila*.[20–22, 32, 33] The newer third-generation quinolones are active against *Mycoplasma pneumoniae* and the genital mycoplasmas.[20, 27, 33, 34] Some quinolones exhibit activity against mycobacteria, and may be used as part of combination therapy in multi-drug-resistant tuberculosis.[31]

ADVERSE EVENTS

The quinolones are usually well tolerated. The major toxicities attributed to these drugs involve gastrointestinal, central nervous system (CNS), cardiovascular, skin, and connective tissue effects, as well as teratogenicity and carcinogenicity. Drug interactions are also an important consideration for this class of antibiotics. Some side effects and drug interactions are functions of the drug class, but some are intimately associated with the varying substitutions and structural modifications of the different quinolones.[4, 5]

As with many other antibiotics, the most frequent side effects of the quinolones are gastrointestinal, including nausea, vomiting, abdominal pain, anorexia, gastritis, and diarrhea.[4, 5] Gastrointestinal side effects occur in 8% to 15% of patients; however, this side effect may be dose dependent, with an increased incidence reported at higher doses.[35–37] Discontinuation of quinolone therapy due to gastrointestinal side effects is uncommon.[36, 37] Serious liver injury in conjunction with trovofloxacin therapy has been described, prompting the U.S. Food and Drug Administration (FDA) to recommend that the use of this quinolone be limited to patients requiring in-hospital therapy for serious infections, including pneumonia, intra-abdominal infections, pelvic infections, and complicated skin and skin structure infections.[38] Trovofloxacin-associated liver toxicity is rare; however, liver failure necessitating transplantation and deaths have both been reported. Although liver toxicity from trovofloxacin is unpredictable, the risk increases significantly with more than 14 days of therapy.[38]

Central nervous system toxicity is associated with the use of quinolones, occurring in 4% to 10% of patients. CNS toxicity is dose dependent, with an increased incidence reported at higher doses. Most of these reactions are mild and include headache, dizziness, drowsiness, sleep disturbance, tremors, and restlessness.[4, 35, 36] Severe neurotoxicity, including psychotic reactions, convulsions, hallucinations, and depression, has been described. These serious reactions are rare, and are reported in less than 0.5% of patients.[36] Quinolones interact with gamma-aminobutyric acid (GABA) receptors, and various substitutions at position 7 affect GABA binding; however, CNS events cannot be predicted by the degree of GABA interaction, and so the mechanism of toxicity remains largely unknown.[4, 5, 35, 37]

Intravenous injection of quinolones can cause hypotension and tachycardia, and serious cardiac arrhythmias have been reported with the use of some oral agents. Grepafloxacin and sparfloxacin are associated with effects on cardiac repolarization, resulting in prolongation of the QT interval.[36, 39] Sparfloxacin should not be administered with drugs that induce bradycardia or prolong the QT interval; grepafloxacin has been voluntarily withdrawn from the market by the manufacturer because of a rare association with torsade de pointes.[36, 39]

Cutaneous reactions, both hypersensitivity reactions and phototoxicity, are well described in the literature. Exposure to ultraviolet A radiation causes a photochemical reaction that produces free radicals and singlet oxygen, resulting in tissue damage. All quinolones can induce a phototoxic reaction, but this response is most common with compounds that substitute a chlorine or a fluorine atom at position 8.[5, 35, 36] The quinolones with the highest phototoxic potential are norfloxacin, ciprofloxacin, ofloxacin, and sparfloxacin. Trovofloxacin and moxifloxacin have the lowest potential for phototoxicity.[5, 36]

The toxic effects of quinolones on joint cartilage and the epiphyseal growth plate have been described in juvenile animals.[3, 36] In humans, arthralgias, arthropathy, and arthritis have been reported with quinolone use. Although severe chondrotoxicity has not been described in the pediatric population, quinolone therapy usually is not recommended for children except for patients with cystic fibrosis or other patients for whom the benefits of quinolone therapy outweigh the potential risks.[3, 36, 40] Quinolone-induced tendinitis and tendon rupture have been well reported in the literature; tendon rupture is more common in populations older than 60 years of age, but may occur at any age, and may present several months after completion of quinolone therapy.[3, 35, 36]

Quinolones are considered class C drugs by the FDA because their safety in pregnancy has not yet been established. Some animal studies have indicated that ossification delays and skeletal variations are associated with quinolone exposure in utero; however, no teratogenic evidence exists for humans.[41] The evidence for quinolone-induced arthropathy in juvenile animals has limited the use of this class of drugs for pregnant and for pediatric patients. Quinolones have been used for younger patients with severe or resistant infections where antibiotic choice is limited, such as cystic fibrosis, complicated urinary tract infections, bacterial meningitis, and enteric infections.[40, 41] Quinolones are therefore not recommended during pregnancy or for pediatric use if an equivalent nonquinolone alternative is available; however, some conditions may exist where quinolones are the superior drug, and their use may be appropriate in these circumstances.

Quinolones may also inhibit mammalian topoisomerase II, potentially damaging DNA and producing chromosomal abnormalities.[4, 35] This genotoxicity is believed to occur at concentrations significantly higher than the bactericidal concentration.[4] Long-term studies have not uncovered any evidence of carcinogenicity.[4, 35]

Drug interactions with the quinolones vary with different substitutions, and therefore may not occur for all drugs in this class. The two most common drugs known to produce significant interactions with the quinolones are theophylline and nonsteroidal anti-inflammatory drugs (NSAIDs). Quinolones inhibit cytochrome P-450, which interferes with the metabolism of theophylline and related compounds, increasing the systemic levels of these drugs and resulting in CNS side effects, including seizures.[4, 35, 42] NSAIDs may potentiate quinolone binding to GABA receptors, increasing the risk of quinolone-associated neurotoxicity.[4, 38] As mentioned previously, administration of quinolones with multivalent cations must be avoided because these substances significantly reduce quinolone absorption.[14, 42]

CLINICAL APPLICATIONS

Quinolones have many applications in gynecology. Not only do these drugs have excellent pharmacokinetics, but they are generally well tolerated, with a spectrum of activity that makes them an excellent antibiotic choice for many infectious disorders encountered in gynecology. Quinolones have become important adjuvants in the management of many sexually transmitted diseases, pelvic infections, intra-abdominal infections, urinary tract infections, enteric infections, complicated upper respiratory tract infections, and pneumonia. Quinolones have also been used for surgical prophylaxis and febrile neutropenia. Quinolones are class C drugs with animal studies indicating that they have the potential to induce chondrotoxicity; therefore, the use of quinolones in pregnant patients should be limited to those situations where no other acceptable alternative agent exists.

Quinolones are now extensively used for treatment of a variety of sexually transmitted diseases due to the following bacteria: *Neisseria gonorrhoeae*, *Chlamydia trachomatis*, *Haemophilus ducreyi*, and *Calymmatobacterium gramulomatis*.[43] In the United States and Canada, quinolone resistance to *N. gonorrhoeae* is low, but the identification of quinolone-resistant gonorrhea is increasing in Asia.[44, 46] A variety of quinolones are effective as single-dose therapy for uncomplicated gonococcal cervicitis and gonococcal pharyngitis, including ciprofloxacin 500 mg and ofloxacin 400 mg.[43, 45, 47, 48] The newer third-generation quinolones are also effective against gonorrhea, but probably have no therapeutic advantage for single-dose therapy compared with ciprofloxacin and ofloxacin.

Chlamydia trachomatis is sensitive to most quinolones with the exception of ciprofloxacin.[33] Ofloxacin, 300 mg twice daily for 1 week, is effective treatment for chlamydial cervicitis.[43, 48–50] Regimens with other third-generation quinolones (e.g., levofloxacin, sparfloxacin, moxifloxacin, and clinafloxacin) would most likely also be effective for chlamydial infection and allow once-daily dosing; however, clinical information regarding their use for this indication is limited.[21, 27, 52] Trovofloxacin, 200 mg daily, is also effective for chlamydial cervicitis; however, oral trovofloxacin is no longer recommended for outpatient therapy because of toxicity concerns.[38, 51] Ciprofloxacin is not recommended for chlamydial infection, as it is ineffective against *C. trachomatis.*

Treatment regimens for genital ulcer disease due to *H. ducreyi* (chancroid) and *C. granulomatis* (granuloma inguinale) include ciprofloxacin. A recommended regimen for chancroid is ciprofloxacin, 500 mg twice daily for 3 days.[43] Ciprofloxacin, 750 mg twice daily for at least 3 weeks, is an alternative therapeutic option for granuloma inguinale.[43]

Recommended treatment regimens for pelvic inflammatory disease must include agents that are highly effective against both gonorrhea and chlamydial infection; therefore, many of the quinolones are suitable therapeutic options (Table 56–2). The Centers for Disease Control and Prevention (CDC) 1998 guidelines for both inpatient and outpatient treatment of pelvic inflammatory disease include quinolone-containing regimens.[43] Parenteral regimens include the following: ofloxacin, 400 mg every 12 hours, plus metronidazole, or ciprofloxacin, 200 mg every 12 hours, combined with doxycycline and metronidazole. Ofloxacin monotherapy has been described for outpatient management of acute salpingitis; however, the CDC-recommended quinolone oral therapy for pelvic inflammatory disease is ofloxacin, 400 mg twice daily, in combination with metronidazole.[43, 53, 54] Other quinolones may also be effective for pelvic inflammatory disease. Levofloxacin, 500 mg, may be substituted for ofloxacin in both parenteral and oral regimens. Not only does levofloxacin have a broader spectrum of activity, but the improved pharmacokinetics allow once-daily dosing. Other third-generation quinolones with broad-spectrum activity against gram-positive, gram-negative, anaerobic, and atypical organisms appear to be ideal agents for pelvic inflammatory disease, and trovofloxacin monotherapy has been described.[27, 55]

Quinolones are excellent antimicrobials for both pelvic and intra-abdominal infections, including postoperative and postpartum infections that require broad-spectrum antimicrobial coverage. Levofloxacin provides good gram-positive and gram-negative activity and may be administered for this indication in combination with metronidazole for anaerobic activity.[52] Trovofloxacin has been shown to be effective monotherapy for acute gynecologic infections and as effective as imipenem/cilastin for intra-abdominal infections.[56, 57] The other expanded-spectrum quinolones are under investigation for this indication.[27] Trovofloxacin has been studied as chemoprophylaxis for prevention of postoperative bacterial infection. Oral trovafloxacin and intravenous alatrofloxacin were found to be as effective as parenteral cefoxitin and cefotetan, respectively, for this indication.[58, 59] Currently, however, trovofloxacin is not recommended by the U.S. Food and Drug Administration for surgical prophylaxis, owing to the potential concern of hepatotoxicity.[38]

Quinolones are extremely active against most uropathogens, and are therefore very effective treatment for both lower and upper urinary tract infections. Uncomplicated lower urinary tract infections are effectively treated with an oral 3-day course of quinolones, whereas upper urinary tract infections usually require a 14-day course of therapy.[60] The expanded-spectrum quinolones do not appear to be more efficacious than ciprofloxacin, which has high levels in both the urine and renal parenchyma and excellent in vitro activity for Enterobacteriaceae and *P. aeruginosa*.[16, 61] Norfloxacin is not effective treatment for upper urinary tract infections because systemic levels are low and this drug has poor penetration into the renal parenchyma. Quinolones may also be used as chemoprophylaxis for patients with recurrent urinary tract infections.[62]

Nongynecologic indications for the newer broad-spectrum quinolones include treatment of community-acquired pneumonia, acute exacerbations of chronic bronchitis, sinusitis, and both uncomplicated and complicated skin infections.[3, 17, 63] Some quinolones may also be used as prevention and treatment of traveler's diarrhea and in multidrug regimens for tuberculosis.

TABLE 56-2 ▶	QUINOLONE-CONTAINING REGIMENS FOR PELVIC INFLAMMATORY DISEASE	
Parenteral	**Oral**
Ofloxacin, 400 mg q12h plus metronidazole	Ofloxacin, 400 mg q12h, plus metronidazole
Ciprofloxacin, 200 mg q12h, plus metronidazole and doxycycline	Outpatient oral ciprofloxacin therapy not recommended
Levofloxacin, 500 mg q24h, plus metronidazole	Levofloxacin, 500 mg q24h, plus metronidazole
Trovofloxacin, 200 mg q24h	Outpatient oral trovofloxacin therapy currently not recommended

REFERENCES

1. Lesher GY, Frielich ED, Gruet MD, et al: 1,8 Maphthyridine derivatives: A new class of chemotherapeutic agents. J Med Pharmacol Chem 1962; 5:1063.

2. Saravanos K, Duff P: The quinolone antibiotics. Obstet Gynecol Clin North Am 1992; 19:529.

3. Hooper DC: Quinolones. In: Mandell GL, Bennet JE, Dolin R (eds): Principles and Practice of Infectious Disease, 4th ed. New York, Churchill Livingstone, 1995, pp 364–376.

4. Domagala JM: Structure–activity and structure–effect relationships for the quinolone antibacterials. J Antimicrob Chemother 1994; 33:685.

5. Tillotson GS: Quinolones: Structure–activity relationships and future predictions. J Med Microbiol 1996; 44:320.

6. Boswell FJ, Wise R: Advances in the macrolides and quinolones. Infect Dis Clin North Am 1998; 12:647.

7. Drlica K, Zhao X: DNA gyrase, topoisomerase IV, and the 4-quinolones. Microbiol Mol Biol Rev 1997; 61:377.

8. Hooper DC: Mode of action of fluoroquinolones. Drugs 1999; 58(suppl 2):6.

9. Gelbert M, O'Dea MH, Mizuuchi K, Nash H: DNA gyrase: An enzyme that introduces superhelical turn into DNA. Proc Natl Acad Sci U S A 1976; 73:3872.

10. Pan XS, Fisher LM: DNA gyrase and topoisomerase IV are dual targets of clinafloxacin action in *Streptococcus pneumoniae.* Antimicrob Agents Chemother 1998; 42:2810.

11. Chen CR, Malik M, Snyder M, et al: DNA gyrase and topoisomerase IV on the bacterial chromosome-quinolone–induced DNA cleavage. J Mol Biol 1996; 258:627.

12. Goss W, Deitz W, Cook T: Mechanism of action of nalidixic acid on *Escherichia coli.* J Bacteriol 1965; 89:1068.

13. Piddock LJV: Mechanisms of fluoroquinolone resistance: An update 1994–1998. Drugs 1999; 58(suppl 2):11.

14. Stein GE: Pharmacokinetics and pharmacodynamics of newer fluoroquinolones. Clin Infect Dis 1996; 23(suppl 1):S19.

15. Turnidge J: Pharmacokinetics and pharmacodynamics of fluoroquinolones. Drugs 1999; 58(suppl 2):29.

16. Martin SJ, Meyer JM, Chuck SK, et al: Levofloxacin and sparfloxacin: New quinolone antibiotics. Ann Pharmacother 1998; 32:320.

17. Giamarellou H, Kilokythas E, Petrikkos G, et al: Pharmaco-kinetics of three newer quinolones in pregnant and lactating women. Am J Med 1989;87(suppl 5A):56S.

18. Nicole LE: Quinolones in the aged. Drugs 1999; 58(suppl 2):49.

19. Montay G: Pharmacokinetics of sparfloxacin in healthy volunteers and patients: A review. J Antimicrob Chemother 1996; 37(suppl A):27.

20. Blondeau JM: A review of the comparative in-vitro activities of 12 antimicrobial agents, with a focus on five new "respiratory quinolones." J Antimicrob Chemother 1999; 43(suppl B):1.

21. Abramowicz M (ed), Abeloff MD, Beaver WT, Goodman LS, et al (advisory board): Sparfloxacin and levofloxacin. Med Lett Drugs Ther 1997; 39:41.

22. Abramowicz M (ed), Abeloff MD, Beaver WT, Goodman LS, et al (advisory board): Grepafloxacin: A new fluoroquinolone. Med Lett Drugs Ther 1998; 40:17.

23. Bauerfeind A: Comparison of the antibacterial activities of the quinolones Bay 12-8039, gatifloxacin (AM 1155), trovafloxacin, clinafloxacin, levofloxacin and ciprofloxacin. J Antimicrob Chemother 1997; 40:639.

24. Schmid GP: Treatment of chancroid, 1997. Clin Infect Dis 1999; 28(suppl 1):S14.

25. Aldridge KE, Cammarata C, Martin DH: Comparison of the in vitro activities of various parenteral and oral antimicrobial agents against endemic *Haemophilus ducreyi.* Antimicrob Agents Chemother 1993; 37:1986.

26. Eliopoulos GM: Activity of newer fluoroquinolones *in vitro* against gram-positive bacteria. Drugs 1999; 58(suppl 2):23.

27. Blondeau JM: Expanded activity and utility of the new fluoroquinolones: A review. Clin Ther 1999; 21:3.

28. Appelbaum PC: Quinolone activity against anaerobes: Microbiologic aspects. Drugs 1995; 49(suppl 2):76.

29. Hect DW, Wexler HM: In vitro susceptibility of anaerobes to quinolones in the United States. Clin Infect Dis 1996; 23(suppl 1):S2.

30. Applebaum PC: Quinolone activity against anaerobes. Drugs 1999; 58(suppl 2):60.

31. Jacobs MR: Activity of quinolones against mycobacteria. Drugs 1999; 58(suppl 2):19.

32. Hammerschlag MR: Activity of quinolones against *Chlamydia pneumoniae.* Drugs 1999; 58(suppl 2):75.

33. Ridgway GL: Quinolones in sexually transmitted diseases. Drugs 1999; 58(suppl 2):92.

34. Bebear CM, Renaudin H, Boudjada A, et al: In vitro activity of Bay 12-8039, a new fluoroquinolone, against mycoplasmas. Antimicrob Agents Chemother 1998; 42:703.

35. Takayama S, Hirohashi M, Kato M, Shimada H: Toxicity of quinolone antimicrobial agents. J Toxicol Environ Health 1995; 45:1.

36. Stahlmann R, Lode H: Toxicity of quinolones. Drugs 1999; 58(suppl 2):37.

37. Chodosh S, Lakshminarayan S, Swarz H, et al: Efficacy and safety of a 10-day course of 400 or 600 milligrams of grepafloxacin once daily for treatment of acute bacterial exacerbations of chronic bronchitis: Comparison with a 10-day course of 500 milligrams of ciprofloxacin twice-daily. Antimicrob Agents Chemother 1998; 42:114.

38. U.S. Food and Drug Administration: Public health advisory: Trovan (trovafloxacin/alatrofloxacin mesylate). Washington, DC, FDA, June 9, 1999.

39. GlaxoWellcome, Inc.: Product withdrawal letter: Raxar (grepafloxacin HCL). Research Triangle Park, NC, GlaxoWellcome, Inc., October 28, 1999.

40. Schaad UB: Pediatric use of quinolones. Pediatr Infect Dis J 1999; 18:467.

41. Jafri HS, McCracken GH Jr: Fluoroquinolones in pediatrics. Drugs 1999; 58(suppl 2):43.

42. Munckhof WJ: Concurrent prescribing: Beware of drug interactions. Aust Fam Physician 1998; 27:895.

43. Centers for Disease Control and Prevention: 1998 Guidelines for treatment of sexually transmitted diseases. MMWR Morb Mortal Wkly Rep 1998; 47:18.

44. Harnett N, Brown S, Riley G, et al: Analysis of *Neisseria gonorrhoeae* in Ontario, Canada, with decreased susceptibility to quinolones by pulsed-field gel electrophoresis, auxotyping, serotyping and plasmid content. J Med Microbiol 1997; 46:383.

45. Centers for Disease Control and Prevention: Decreased susceptibility of *Neisseria gonorrhoeae* to fluoroquinolones—Ohio and Hawaii, 1992–1994. MMWR Morb Mortal Wkly Rep 1994; 43:325.

46. Moran JS, Levine WC: Drugs of choice for the treatment of uncomplicated gonococcal infections. Clin Infect Dis 1996; 20(suppl 1):S47.

47. Echols RM, Heyd A, O'Keefe BJ, Schacht P: Single-dose ciprofloxacin for the treatment of uncomplicated gonorrhea: A worldwide summary. Sex Transm Dis 1994; 21:345.

48. Corrado ML: The clinical experience with ofloxacin in the treatment of sexually transmitted diseases. Am J Obstet Gynecol 1991; 164:1396.

49. Hooton TM, Batteiger BE, Judson FN, et al: Ofloxacin versus doxycycline for treatment of cervical infection with *Chlamydia trachomatis.* Antimicrob Agents Chemother 1992; 36:1144.

50. Weber JT, Johnson RE: New treatments for *Chlamydia trachomatis* genital infection. Clin Infect Dis 1995; 20(suppl 1):S66.

51. Martin DH, Jones RB, Johnson RB: A phase-II study of trovafloxacin for the treatment of *Chlamydia trachomatis* infections. Sex Transm Dis 1999; 26:369.

52. Ernst ME, Ernst EJ, Klepser ME: Levofloxacin and trovafloxacin: The next generation of quinolones? Am J Health Syst Pharm 1997; 54:2569.

53. Wendl GD, Cox S, Bawdon RE, et al: A randomized trial of ofloxacin versus cefoxitin and doxycycline in the outpatient treatment of acute salpingitis. Am J Obstet Gynecol 1991; 164:1390.

54. Walker CK, Workowski KA, Washington AE, et al: Anaerobes in pelvic inflammatory disease: Implications for the Centers for Disease Control and Prevention's Guidelines for Treatment of Sexually Transmitted Diseases. Clin Infect Dis 1999; 28(suppl 1):S29.

55. Garey KW: Trovofloxacin: An overview. Pharmacotherapy 1999; 19:21.

56. Roy S, Kolton W, Chatwani A, et al: Treatment of acute gynecologic infections with trovofloxacin. Am J Surg 1998; 176(suppl 6A):67S.

57. Donahue PE, Smith DL, Yellin AE, et al: Trovofloxacin in the treatment of intra-abdominal infections: Results of a double-blind, multicenter comparison with imipenem/cilastin. Am J Surg 1998; 176(suppl 6A):53S.

58. Roy S, Hemsell D, Gordon S, et al: Oral trovafloxacin compared with intravenous cefoxitin in the prevention of bacterial infection after elective vaginal or abdominal hysterectomy for nonmalignant disease. Am J Surg 1998; 176(suppl 6A):62S.

59. Milsom JW, Smith DL, Corman ML, et al: Double-blind comparison of single-dose alatrofloxacin and cefotetan as prophylaxis of infection following elective colorectal surgery. Am J Surg 1998; 176(suppl 6A):46S.

60. Abramowicz M (ed): The choice of antimicrobial agents. Med Lett Drugs Ther 1998; 40:33.

61. Ronald A: The quinolones and renal infection. Drugs 1999; 58(suppl 2):96.

62. Krcméry S, Hromec J, Tvrdikova M, et al: Newer quinolones in the long term prophylaxis of recurrent urinary tract infections. Drugs 1999; 58(suppl 2):99.

63. Karchmer AW: Fluoroquinolone treatment of skin and skin structure infections. Drugs 1999; 58(suppl 2):82.

Laboratory Issues

57

Specimen Collection and Diagnostic Procedures for the Laboratory Diagnosis of Infections in Females

LouEllen Phillips-Smith ▶ Gerri S. Hall

A key role of clinical microbiology in the management of patients with an infectious disease is to identify the etiologic agent or agents of the disease, thereby supporting or allowing the correct differential diagnosis to be made in conjunction with clinical observation. This role is fulfilled by (1) direct visualization of the suspected pathogen by stained or unstained preparations of appropriate specimens, (2) detection of specific components of the agent, (3) cultivating the pathogen by appropriate culture techniques and subjecting the isolate to various identification tests, or (4) demonstrating a specific antibody response to the suspected agent. It is also the function of clinical microbiology to provide in vitro susceptibility information that will support or guide choices in the selection of appropriate antimicrobial therapy.

Many methodologies have been standardized for direct specimen examination, cultivation techniques, and antibody detection during the development of clinical microbiology. In some cases, the traditional procedures are still the preferred method. However, the field is experiencing a dramatic expansion of capabilities by the utilization of molecular techniques that may decrease the response time or allow more precise results to be obtained.

Regardless of the infectious disease involved or the procedures to be employed for laboratory diagnosis, essential components of the process are the proper collection of appropriate specimens and the delivery and maintenance of the specimen under suitable conditions until processing. Furthermore, it is imperative that adequate information be relayed to the laboratory concerning the source of the specimen and the test or tests requested. This information is usually conveyed in the form of a written or computer-generated laboratory requisition, which must be legible and contain all requested information. Laboratory requisitions for hospitalized patients now require a specific ICD-9*

code to be given by the ordering physician to facilitate Medicare reimbursement; laboratories may not be able to process requests that lack this code.

The first section of this chapter describes procedures utilized for collection and transport of clinical specimens for the detection and/or recovery of pathogens that cause infectious diseases common in women as well as those that have potential consequences for the fetus or newborn, infections of such a serious nature that their importance mandates their inclusion, or for newly recognized infections that may be of interest. Diagnostic tests employed for the detection and identification of pathogens, including some currently available nucleic acid–based methodologies, are briefly described in the second section of this chapter. Serologic procedures that are the primary method of laboratory diagnosis of certain infectious diseases are described in the third section. An overall summary of the diseases of interest, preferred specimens, and likely pathogens is presented in Table 57–1. Although some of the infectious agents described may not be limited to the female adult population, they have been included for the sake of completeness.

SECTION ONE: SPECIMEN COLLECTION BY BODY SITE OR TYPE OF INFECTION

The advent of increasing numbers of rapid detection systems (i.e., antigen detection, nucleic acid probes, and, more recently, amplification methods) may offer clinicians and microbiologists hope that the time-consuming and sometimes tedious process of cultivation will be replaced. To date, however, such reagents are not available for all potential pathogens. Consequently, in many cases, cultivation is still considered a primary or secondary approach to the laboratory diagnosis of infection, and recovery of the infectious agents may still be desirable for typing or susceptibility testing. Thus, it is often essential that after an appropriate specimen is collected it should be maintained under

---

*International Classification of Diseases, Ninth Revision.

602

TABLE 57–1 ▶ SUMMARY OF DISEASES, SPECIMENS, AND PATHOGENS OF INFECTIONS IN FEMALES

Site of Infection or Patient Population	Symptom or Disease	Preferred Specimen	Potential Pathogens
External genitalia (*see text for description of lesions*)	Bartholin's or Skene's gland abscess	Aspirate or swab	Mixed flora, *Neisseria gonorrhoeae*, *Chlamydia trachomatis*
	Herpes genitalis	Aspirate or swab of lesion or vesicle fluid	Herpes simplex virus type 1 or 2
	Condyloma acuminatum	Exfoliated cell sample, tissue biopsy	Human papillomavirus (HPV)
	Venereum molluscum	Expelled lesion material	Molluscum contagiosum virus
	Primary or secondary syphilis	Lesion or lymph node aspirate	*Treponema pallidum*
	Chancroid	Aspirate or swab of lesion material/biopsy	*Haemophilus ducreyi*
	Lymphogranuloma venereum (LGV)	Aspirate of lesion or purulence from inguinal node or biopsy	*C. trachomatis*, serotype LG1, LGV2, or LGV3
	Granuloma inguinale	Tissue prep and/or biopsy	*Calymmatobacterium granulomatis*
	Genital tuberculosis	Tissue biopsy	*Mycobacterium tuberculosis*
	Scabies	Skin scrapings from terminal part of burrow	*Sarcoptes scabiei*
	Pediculosis pubis	Plucked pubic hair	*Phthirus pubis*
Vagina	Vaginal discharge, itching, pain (vaginitis or vaginosis)	Vaginal swab Vaginal swab Vaginal swab	*Candida* spp., *Saccharomyces* *Trichomonas vaginalis* *Gardnerella vaginalis* Mixed anaerobes
	Lesions, as described for external genitalia	Aspirate or swab of ulcerative lesion or vesicle fluid	Herpes simplex *T. pallidum* (primary or secondary syphilis)
		Exfoliated cell sample from flat or fleshy lesion	HPV
Cervix	Cervical discharge, ulcerative lesions	Cervical swab of purulence Swab or cytobrush of cellular material	*N. gonorrhoeae* *C. trachomatis*
		Aspirate or swab of ulcerative lesion or vesicle fluid	Herpes simplex *T. pallidum* (primary or secondary syphilis)
	Flat or fleshy lesions (condylomata acuminata)	Exfoliated cell sample from flat or fleshy lesion	HPV
Upper genital tract: Nonpregnant patient	Pelvic inflammatory disease: salpingitis, tubo-ovarian abscess	Endometrial biopsy Culdocentesis Fallopian tube biopsy Peritoneal fluid Aspirate of abscess	*N. gonorrhoeae*, *C. trachomatis*, mixed anaerobes, *Mycoplasma* spp., *Ureaplasma urealyticum*, or *G. vaginalis*
	Granulomatous salpingitis	Endometrial biopsy, menstrual blood	*M. tuberculosis*
Antepartum	Premature labor or membrane rupture	Amniotic fluid, blood, placenta, postpartum	*Streptococcus agalactiae* (GBBS), *Escherichia coli*, *G. vaginalis*, anaerobes, *U. urealyticum*
		Endocervix	*N. gonorrhoeae*, *C. trachomatis*
		Urine	Gram-negatives, *N. gonorrhoeae*, *C. trachomatis*

Table continued on following page

TABLE 57–1 ▶ SUMMARY OF DISEASES, SPECIMENS, AND PATHOGENS OF INFECTIONS IN FEMALES *Continued*

Site of Infection or Patient Population	Symptom or Disease	Preferred Specimen	Potential Pathogens
Postpartum or postoperative	Aspiration pneumonia (not easily diagnosed)	Sputum	Enteric gram-negatives, *Staphylococcus aureus*
	UTI	Catheterized urine	Enteric gram-negatives
	Abdominal wound	Wound aspirate	**Early-Onset:** *Streptococcus pyogenes,* GBBS, *Clostridium perfringens, Mycoplasma hominis* **Late-Onset:** polymicrobial
	Endomyometritis	Endometrial aspirate	Indigenous vaginal flora, mixed aerobes, anaerobes, *C. trachomatis, N. gonorrhoeae*
	Peritonitis	Peritoneal fluid	**Primary:** *S. pneumoniae, Enterococcus, Streptococcus, N. gonorrhoeae, C. trachomatis, M. tuberculosis, Coccidioides immitis,* enteric gram-negatives **Secondary:** polymicrobial
	Pelvic cellulitis	Peritoneal fluid by culdocentesis	Endogenous vaginal flora
	Pelvic abscess	Aspirate of abscess	Endogenous vaginal flora
	Septic pelvic thrombophlebitis	Diagnosis made by defervescence of fever with heparin therapy	
Other postpartum infections	Mastitis, breast abscess	Aspirate of abscess, milk sample	*Staphylococcus aureus, Streptococcus pyogenes,* GBBS
	Episiotomy wound	Aspirate, tissue	*S. pyogenes,* anaerobes
	Vaginal cuff abscess	Aspirate	Polymicrobial
Urinary tract	Asymptomatic bacteriuria	Midstream urine, monitor during pregnancy	*E. coli,* other gram-negative rods, *Enterococcus,* GBBS
	Acute cystitis	Midstream urine	*E. coli,* other gram-negative rods, *Staphylococcus saprophyticus*
	Acute pyelonephritis	Midstream urine, catheterized specimen during pregnancy	*E. coli,* other gram-negative rods
	Urethritis	Endouretheral swab Clean-catch urine Endocervical swab	*N. gonorrhoeae, C. trachomatis*
	Acute urethral syndrome	Midstream urine, suprapubic aspiration Endocervical swab	*E. coli,* other gram-negative rods, *C. trachomatis*

Miscellaneous Infections by Body System and Disease

Body System	Disease	Preferred Specimen(s)	Potential Pathogens
Cardiovascular	Pericarditis	Pericardial fluid	Enteroviruses, enteric gram-negatives, *Neisseria meningitidis,* many others
Central nervous system	Brain abscess	Aspirate of abscess	Streptococci, anaerobes, enterics, polymicrobial
	Encephalitis	Brain biopsy, CSF	Several viral, bacterial, some fungal, parasitic agents
	Meningitis	CSF, blood	Several viral, bacterial, some fungal, parasitic agents
Circulatory	AIDS	Serum	HIV-1
	Sepsis	Blood	Gram-negative, some gram-positive bacteria
Eye infections	Conjunctivitis	Conjunctival swab	*N. gonorrhoeae, C. trachomatis,* several other bacterial, viral, fungal, and some parasitic agents
	Keratitis	Corneal scrapings	Several bacterial, viral, fungal, and parasitic agents

TABLE 57-1 ▶ SUMMARY OF DISEASES, SPECIMENS, AND PATHOGENS OF INFECTIONS IN FEMALES *Continued*

Body System	Disease	Preferred Specimen(s)	Potential Pathogens
Gastrointestinal (GI) tract	Diarrhea or other lower GI disturbances	Stool, duodenal contents, sigmoidoscopy	*Campylobacter jejuni, Shigella, Salmonella, E. coli, Clostridium difficile, Entamoeba histolytica, Giardia lamblia*
	Gastric ulcer disease	Expelled breath, sera, antral biopsy	*Helicobacter pylori*
	Hepatitis	Serum	Hepatitis virus A–E, Epstein-Barr virus (EBV), cytomegalovirus (CMV), other viral agents
	Mononucleosis	Serum	EBV
Intra-abdominal	Appendicitis	Appendix tissue	Polymicrobial
	Diverticulitis	Peritoneal fluid, blood	Polymicrobial
	Peritonitis	Peritoneal fluid	**Primary:** unimicrobial **Secondary:** polymicrobial, *see text*
Musculoskeletal	Acute infectious arthritis	Synovial fluid, blood; Paired sera	*S. aureus, Streptococcus* spp., gram-negative bacilli, *N. gonorrhoeae, N. meningitidis, Borrelia burgdorferi*
	Chronic arthritis	Synovial fluid, synovium, aspirate of draining sinus tract	*Brucella* spp., *Mycobacterium* spp., *Norcardia asteroides, Sporothrix schenckii, C. immitis, B. dermatidis, Candida albicans, Pseudoallescheria boydii*
Perinatal, congenital	Conjunctivitis	Conjunctival swab and/or scrapings	*C. trachomatis, N. gonorrhoeae, S. aureus, Streptococcus pneumoniae, Haemophilus influenzae,* HSV, enteroviruses
	Pneumonitis	Nasopharyngeal aspirates, washings, throat swab	CMV, HSV, rubella, enteroviruses, GBBS, *E. coli, C. trachomatis, Toxoplasma gondii, T. pallidum*
	Meningitis	CSF, blood, blood for serology	CMV, HSV, rubella, enteroviruses, GBBS, *E. coli, T. gondii, T. pallidum*
	Septicemia	Blood, buffy coat, urine, blood for serology	CMV, HSV, rubella, enteroviruses, GBBS, *E. coli, T. gondii, T. pallidum*
	Skin lesions: maculopapular exanthems	Throat swab, blood for serology	Enteroviruses, HIV, *T. gondii, T. pallidum*
	Petechiae, purpura	Scrapings, blood for serology	CMV, HSV, rubella, enteroviruses, GBBS, *E. coli, C. trachomatis, T. gondii, T. pallidum*
	Vesicles	Aspirate	CMV, HSV, *T. pallidum*
Respiratory, lower	Pneumonia (community-acquired)	Sputum, pleural fluid, BAL, blood	*S. pneumoniae, S. aureus, H. influenzae, Legionella, Mycobacterium,* influenza virus, *Pneumocystis carinii,* other bacteria, fungal, viral, parasitic agents
Respiratory, upper	Pharyngitis	Throat swab	*S. pyogenes,* viral agents
Urogenital	Toxic shock syndrome	Vaginal swab	*S. aureus, S. pyogenes*

Note: Skin is not included as body system because of the many dermatologic manifestations of several bacterial, viral, fungal, and parasitic diseases.
BAL = bronchoalveolar lavage; HSV = herpes simplex virus.

conditions that favor the viability of the suspected agents. In many cases, specimens collected for culture can also be used for other procedures, such as direct examination and some antigen testing. Suggested specimen types, transport devices, and favorable environmental conditions by body site and type of infection are listed in Table 57–2.

Specimens typically fall into four major categories. These are as follows:

1. Exudate, secretions, or cellular material collected by swab or brush

2. Body fluids or washings, i.e., cerebrospinal fluid (CSF), blood, amniotic fluid, bronchoalveolar lavage, collected by aspiration devices
3. Tissues collected by biopsy or at autopsy with surgical instruments
4. Passed or induced specimens, such as sputum, stool, and urine

Specimens collected on swabs should be placed in appropriate transport media (Table 57–3). Carey-Blair or similar media is often used for transport of specimens for cultivation of bacteria and 2SP may be used

Text continued on page 613

TABLE 57-2 ▶ SPECIMEN COLLECTION GUIDELINES

Specimen[a]	Collection and Transport		Delivery Storage Time and Temperature		Likely Agents/ Comments
	Procedures	Device and/or Minimum Vol	Bacterial, Fungal[b]	Viral	
General instructions. *See remainder of table and text for details*	Collect specimen as soon after onset as possible. Viral agents usually not recovered after 7 days of onset.	Calcium alginate swabs *not* recommended for collection of specimens for viral isolation. Some direct detection systems require special device and/or medium *See text.*	Most specimens submitted at RT.	Specimens usually submitted at 4°C and require viral transport medium	Most purulent infections due to bacteria or fungi. All can cause systemic illness.
Abscess:[a] Open	After disinfecting overlaying skin, aspirate if possible or pass swab deep into lesion. Firmly sample advancing edge.	Anaerobic transport system	<2 h at RT	Not routinely performed	Mixed aerobes, anaerobes, *Chlamydia trachomatis*, yeast, systemic fungi
Closed	Aspirate with needle/ syringe; *see text for brain abscess.*	Anaerobic transport system, >1 mL	<24 h at RT	Not routinely performed	Mixed aerobe, anaerobes, *C. trachomatis*, yeast, systemic fungi
Amniotic fluid[a]	Aspirate by amniocentesis, cesarean section, or intrauterine catheter.	Anaerobic transport tube or sterile tube, >1 mL	<15 min RT, optimal <24 h RT, maximum	<2 h 4°C optimal, 72 h 4°C maximum, 7 d −70°C if processing delayed	GBBS, *E. coli*, *Mycoplasma* spp., *Ureaplasma*, endogenous microflora, HSV, CMV
Anal crypts	Insert swab premoistened with saline or viral transport medium beyond anal ring, rotate for 5 sec and withdraw. Avoid fecal contamination.	Inoculate plates if possible. Otherwise use GC and/ or bacterial or viral transport system.	<30 min RT optimal (GC) <6 h at 4°C maximum (GBBS)	<2 h 4°C optimal, 72 h 4°C maximum, 7 d −70°C if processing delayed	GBBS, *N. gonorrhoeae*, HSV. *Also see Genital Tract Infections.*
Bartholin's duct[a]	Disinfect skin with 2% iodine tincture. Aspirate fluid or collect expressed exudate on swab.	Anaerobic transport system, 1 mL if possible *Chlamydia* transport tube, 1 mL if possible	<2 h at RT optimal 24 h RT maximum	Not routinely performed	*N. gonorrhoeae*, mixed anaerobes, *C. trachomatis*, *Ureaplasma*
Blood for culture	Disinfect blood culture bottle by applying 70% isopropyl alcohol to rubber stoppers and wait 1 min before inoculating. Disinfect venipuncture site by: cleansing site with 70% alcohol swabbing concentrically, starting at center, with iodophor allowing iodine to dry. Aspirate sample without palpating vein. Remove iodine from skin with alcohol.	*Bacteria:* Blood culture bottles. Adult, 10–20 mL/set; neonates 1–2 mL/set *Leptospires:* Sterile heparin tube *Brucella*/fungi: Biphasic culture, lysis, centrifugation *Viral:* Serum. *Also see Buffy Coat* *Borrelia:* Peripheral smear *Malaria:* Thick, thin smears *Filaria, Trypanosomes:* Sterile tube with citrate, oxalate, or heparin	<2 h, RT optimal 24 h RT maximum	<2 h, 4°C optimum; 48 h, 4°C maximum *Also see Buffy Coat.*	Depends on clinical situation; *see text.* *Viral:* Enterovirus from newborns
Blood for serology	Disinfect skin with 70% alcohol. Collect venous blood without anticoagulant. After clot forms, centrifuge tube at low speed. Aspirate serum, place in sterile tube.	6–8 mL venous blood	<24 h 4°C; 1 wk or longer −20° C	<24 h 4°C; 1 wk or longer −20° C	Depends on clinical situation; *see text.*
Breast abscess[a]	Disinfect skin with 70% alcohol. Aspirate with needle and syringe. May also collect milk; *see text.*	Anaerobic transport device	<2 h RT optimal, 24 h RT maximal	Not routinely performed	*Staphylococcus aureus*, *Streptococcus pyogenes*, GBBS

TABLE 57-2 ▶ SPECIMEN COLLECTION GUIDELINES *Continued*

Specimen[a]	Collection and Transport		Delivery Storage Time and Temperature		Likely Agents/ Comments
	Procedures	Device and/or Minimum Vol	Bacterial, Fungal[b]	Viral	
Buboes[a]	If nodes are fluctulant, disinfect overlaying skin; aspirate material with needle and syringe.	Inoculate chocolate plate directly and/or expel into *Chlamydia* transport medium	*Plates:* 15 min RT *Transport tube:* <2 h 4°C optimal, 24 h 4°C maximal	Not routinely performed	*C. trachomatis, Haemophilus ducreyi*
Buffy coat[a]	Disinfect venipuncture site as for blood culture. Collect in vacutainer tube with citrate, heparin, or EDTA. Fractionate in separatory medium to isolate white cells.	5–7 mL in vacutainer tube	<2 h RT optimal, 24 h maximal	<48 h 4°C	*Candida* spp., *Histoplasma*, HSV, CMV
Catheter: Central, CVP, Hickman, Broviac, etc. Not Foley	Cleanse surrounding skin with 70% ETOH. Aseptically remove catheter, clip 5-cm distal tip, place in sterile tube.	Sterile screw-cap tube or cup	<15 min RT to prevent drying	Not routinely performed	Skin flora. Use semiquantitative procedure for culture.
Cellulitis[a]:	Cleanse site with sterile saline or 70% ETOH.				
Dermal	Aspirate area of maximum inflammation, usually center, not leading edge. Aspirate small amount of sterile saline into syringe. Remove needle with protective device and cap; *see Cul-de-sac.*	Capped syringe or sterile tube, anaerobic transport device if gangrenous.	<15 min RT optimal	Not routinely performed	*S. pyogenes, S. aureus Gangrenous:* mixed with anaerobes or Enterobacteriaceae
Pelvic Cerebral spinal fluid (CSF)[a]	Disinfect site with 2% iodine tincture. Insert needle with stylet at L3–L4, L4–L5, or L5–S1 interspace. Remove stylet at subarachnoid space, collect 1–2 mL fluid into each of 3 tubes.	Sterile screw-cap tube: Bacterial, >1 mL Fungi, >2 mL AFB, >2 mL Viral, >1 mL	15 min RT, never refrigerate	On ice, <15 min optimal, 72 h 4°C, maximum	Depends on age group; *see text.*
Cervix[a]	Remove mucus and/or secretions with swab through unlubricated speculum. Discard swab. Press endocervical canal firmly with new swab or scrape with cytobrush. If lesions present, press base firmly with swab to collect fluid.	Bacterial or fungal, culturette or equivalent. *Chlamydia, Mycoplasma,* or viral: 2SP or specialized transport media. *Note:* Specific transport tubes required for Ag, probe, or amplification procedures.	<2 h, RT optimal, 24 h RT maximal	<2 h 4°C, optimal, 72 h maximal	*N. gonorrhoeae, C. trachomatis,* GBBS HSV, CMV; *see text for others.*
Conjunctiva[a]	Sample both eyes with separate swabs, premoistened with sterile saline, by rolling swab over each conjunctiva. Collect separate sample from infected site for viral culture. Make smears for staining.	*Bacteria:* Inoculate directly or place swab in transport medium. *Chlamydia,* viral: Place in transport medium.	*Inoculated plates:* <15 min RT optimal *Swabs:* <2 RT optimal, 24 h RT maximal	<2 h 4°C, optimal, 72 h maximal	Many agents, including *N. gonorrhoeae, C. trachomatis, S. pneumoniae, Haemophilus influenzae,* HSV, CMV, other viral agents

Table continued on following page

TABLE 57-2 ▶ **SPECIMEN COLLECTION GUIDELINES** *Continued*

Specimen[a]	Collection and Transport		Delivery Storage Time and Temperature		Likely Agents/ Comments
	Procedures	Device and/or Minimum Vol	Bacterial, Fungal[b]	Viral	
Corneal scrapings	Collect conjunctival swabs as described above. Instill 2 drops of local anesthetic. Scrape ulcers or lesion with sterile spatula. Inoculate scraping directly. Apply remaining material to 2 clean glass slides for staining.	*Bacteria:* Inoculate directly or place swab in transport medium. *Chlamydia,* viral: Place in transport medium.	*Inoculated plates:* <15 min RT optimal *Swabs:* <2 h RT optimal, 24 h RT maximal	<2 h 4°C, optimal, 72 h 4°C maximal	Large spectrum of etiologic agents; *see text.*
Cul-de-sac[a]	Cleanse vulva, vagina, and cervix with povidone-iodine. Insert sterile speculum, grasp anterior lip of cervix with tenaculum, pull forward to visualize vaginal fornix. Anesthetize posterior vaginal fornix. Aspirate fluid from cul-de-sac.	Place fluid in anaerobic transport device, >1 mL	<15 min RT optimal, 24 h RT maximal	Not routinely performed	Indigenous flora, mixed aerobes and anaerobes
Endometrium[a]	Collect transcervical aspirate via double-lumen catheter. Place entire specimen into anaerobic transport tube.	Anaerobic transport tube, >1 mL	<2 h RT optimal, 24 h RT maximal	Not routinely performed	Indigenous vaginal flora, mixed aerobes and anaerobes, *C. trachomatis, N. gonorrhoeae.* Also collect blood cultures.
Fluids,[a] other than amniotic, CSF, urine	Disinfect skin area with 2% iodine tincture. Collect specimen via percutaneous needle aspiration or at surgery.	Sterile screw-cap tube or anaerobic transport system, >1 mL	<15 min RT optimal, <24 h RT maximal *Except:* pericardial fluid and fungal cultures, 4°C <24 h	Not routinely performed; *see BAL.*	Wide spectrum of agents. Depends on clinical situation.
Gastrointestinal: gastric-antral biopsy[a]	After sedation, obtain biopsy with fiber-optic endoscopy instrument. Collect multiple samples for culture and smears.	Place in small volume, 0.5 mL, tryptic soy broth	<15 min RT optimal, 2 h 4°C maximal	Not routinely performed	*Helicobacter pylori* (urea rapid test or "breath test")
Duodenum	Use String Test (*see text*).	Mucus mixed with 0.5 mL sterile saline	<2 h or add formalin	Not routinely performed	*Giardia lamblia, Strongyloides stercoralis*
Gastric contents[a]	In AM, before patient eats, insert gastric tube orally or nasally to stomach. Instill 25–50 mL of chilled, sterile, distilled water. Aspirate sample and place in leakproof sterile container. Release suction and clamp tube before removing tube.	Sterile, leakproof container	<15 min RT optimal, neutralize within 1 h (*see text*); 24 h 4°C maximal	Not routinely performed	*Mycobacterium* spp.; *N. gonorrhoeae,* neonates
Sigmoidoscopy specimens	Insert lubricated sigmoidoscope into rectum. Pass to point of sigmoid colon. Aspirate material with serologic pipette or use curette to scrape suspect area.	Sterile culture tube	<15 min RT for wet preparation Do not refrigerate	Not routinely performed	*Entamoeba histolytica*

TABLE 57-2 ▶ SPECIMEN COLLECTION GUIDELINES *Continued*

| Specimen[a] | Collection and Transport | | Delivery Storage Time and Temperature | | Likely Agents/ Comments |
	Procedures	Device and/or Minimum Vol	Bacterial, Fungal[b]	Viral	
Rectal swabs	Insert swab beyond anal spincter, rotate for 3–5 sec. Withdraw swab and place in transport tube.	Enteric transport device Viral transport medium	Bacteria: <15 min RT optimal	<2 h 4°C optimal, 72 h maximal	Enteric pathogens, *Enterococcus* (vancomycin-resistant), viral agents
Stool	*Routine:* Specimen is passed into clean, dry container and transported immediately to lab or transferred to enteric transport pack. *Viral:* Specimen is collected into clean, dry container and viral transport medium added to prevent drying.	>2 g if formed; 2–5 mL if loose or liquid	*Unpreserved:* <1 h RT optimal, 24 h 4°C maximal *Preserved:* <48 h RT, 24–48 h −20°C for *Clostridium difficile*	Up to 24 h, 4°C after addition of 8–10 mL viral transport medium	*Enteric pathogens:* Adenoviruses, enteroviruses *Parasites: G. lamblia, E. histolytica,* etc., *C. difficile* toxin
Genital lesion: vesicles, ulcers[a]	Clean lesion with sterile saline. Aspirate if possible. If aspiration not possible, remove surface with sterile scalpel blade. Allow transudate to accumulate. Firmly sample exudate with sterile swab while pressing base of lesion. Collect multiple samples.	Bacterial transport tube *Chlamydia* or viral transport tube Touch clean glass slide to exudate if syphilis is suspected for dark-field examination	<2 h RT optimal, 12 h RT maximal	<1 h 4°C optimal, 72 h 4°C maximal, 7d −70°C	*Treponema pallidum, H. ducreyi,* HSV, *C. trachomatis, Calymmatobacterium granulomatis*
Intrauterine device[a]	Place entire device in sterile urine cup. Place urine container with cap partially closed in anaerobic generating bag.	Entire device, remove exudate and/or tissue for culture	<2 h RT optimal, 24 h maximal	Not routinely performed	*Actinomyces israelii*
Placenta[a]	Place entire placenta in sterile bag. See text for processing.	Sterile bag	Within 12 h from time of delivery	Not routinely performed	Indigenous vaginal flora
Products of conception[a]	If passed through vagina, place portion of tissue in sterile container. If collected at C section, transfer to anaerobic transport device.	Sterile tube or anaerobic transport system	2 h RT optimal, 24 h RT maximal	Not routinely performed	Mixed aerobes and anaerobes
Rash, maculo-papular	Cleanse area with sterile saline. Disrupt lesion surface by rubbing with sterile gauze. Sample lesion base with swab moistened with sterile saline *or* Inject sterile saline at edge and aspirate into syringe.	Viral transport tube	Not routinely performed	2 h 4°C optimal, 24 h 4°C maximal	Adenovirus, enterovirus, rubella virus, measles virus
Rash, vesicular	Cleanse area with sterile saline. Open vesicle with needle or scalpel. Aspirate if possible *or* Collect fluid and cellular material by vigorously sampling base of lesion with swab.	Viral transport tube	Not routinely performed	2 h 4°C optimal, 24 h 4°C maximal	HSV, VZV, coxsackievirus A, (some) echovirus

Table continued on following page

| TABLE 57–2 ▸ | SPECIMEN COLLECTION GUIDELINES *Continued* | | | | |

Specimen[a]	Collection and Transport		Delivery Storage Time and Temperature		Likely Agents/ Comments
	Procedures	Device and/or Minimum Vol	Bacterial, Fungal[b]	Viral	
Respiratory tract, lower	*Performed by Pulmonary Service:* Anesthesize by inhalation of 2% lidocaine. Lubricate both nares with xylocaine jelly. Insert lubricated bronchoscope transnasally. Attach 70-mL specimen trap to bronchoscope. Instill 100 mL nonbacteriostatic saline in 20-mL increments (aliquots?).	*See below* Sterile container, 10–20 mL	*See below* <2 h RT optimal, 24 h 4°C maximal	*See below* <2 h 4°C optimal, 72 h 4°C h maximal 7d −70°C if processing delayed	*See below* *Legionella, Mycobacterium, Nocardia*, other bacteria and fungi, viral agents, and *Pneumocystis carinii*
BAL[a]	After 3rd or 4th instillation, replace 70-mL trap with 40-mL trap. Aseptically remove 10 mL from each trap and place in sterile tube. Insert double-lumen cytology brush unit through channel opening of bronchoscope.	*Note:* Blood cultures should also be collected in cases of pneumonia *For mycobacteria:* Place material into 10 mL supplemented Middlebrook 7H9 broth (*see text*). *For other bacteria:* Place material in sterile saline or Ringer's lactate. *For viral agents:* 0.1 mL viral transport medium	<2 h RT optimal, 24 h 4°C maximal	<2 h 4°C optimal, 2 h 4°C h maximal 7d −70°C if processing delayed	*Legionella, Mycobacterium, Nocardia*, other bacteria and fungi, viral agents, and *P. carinii*
Bronchial brushings[a]	Advance the unit, push the brush out of its sheath, and obtain brushings. Retract brush into sheath and withdraw entire unit. Cut brush from unit and place into appropriate transport medium.				
Tracheal aspirate[a]	*Performed by Pulmonary Service:* Pass polyethylene catheter into trachea through a tracheostomy or endotracheal tube. Aspirate material with syringe or intermittent suction device. Remove catheter, disengage syringe or suction device.	Sterile container, 10–20 mL *Note:* Blood cultures should also be collected in cases of pneumonia.	<2 h RT optimal	<2 h 4°C optimal, 72 h 4°C maximal 7 d −70°C if processing delayed	*Legionella, Mycobacterium, Nocardia*, other bacterial fungal, viral agents, and *P. carinii*
Transtracheal aspirate[a]	*Surgical Procedure by Pulmonary Specialist:* Anesthetize skin over collection site and disinfect with 70% alcohol. Insert 14-gauge needle through the cricothyroid membrane. Pass 16-gauge polyethylene catheter through the needle into lower trachea. Remove needle. Aspirate secretions with 20-mL syringe of suction device. Inject 2–4 mL sterile saline to induce coughing if secretions are scant.	Syringe containing aspirate or the aspiration device with tubing attached, 3–5 mL	<2 h RT optimal, 24 h 4°C maximal	<2 h 4°C optimal, 72 h 4°C maximal 7 d −70°C if processing delayed.	*Legionella, Mycobacterium, Nocardia*, other bacterial fungal, viral agents, and *P. carinii*

TABLE 57-2 ▶ SPECIMEN COLLECTION GUIDELINES *Continued*

Specimen[a]	Collection and Transport		Delivery Storage Time and Temperature		Likely Agents/ Comments
	Procedures	*Device and/or Minimum Vol*	*Bacterial, Fungal[b]*	Viral	
Lung biopsy, by percutaneous, transbronchial, thoracoscopy, or open lung techniques[a]	A 3–4 cm specimen is removed during thoracotomy for open lung technique. Much smaller specimen is obtained with other methods.	Sterile container, divide specimen if possible. Several touch preps should be made.	<2 h RT optimal, 24 h 4°C maximal	<2 h 4°C optimal, 72 h 4°C maximal 7 d −70°C if processing delayed	*Legionella, Mycobacterium, Nocardia,* other bacterial fungal, viral agents, and *P. carinii*
Pleural fluid[a]	Overlaying skin is disinfected and anesthetized. Fluid is aspirated with 14-gauge needle on 50-mL syringe after insertion above lowest rib in area of effusion. Aspiration under fluoroscope or ultrasonic guidance may be required.	Anaerobic transport tube 10–40 mL may be withdrawn	<2 h RT optimal, 24 h 4°C maximal	<2 h 4°C optimal, 72 h 4°C maximal 7 d −70°C if processing delayed	*S. pyogenes,* gram-negative bacilli, *S. pneumoniae* (rare)
Sputum, expectorate[a]	Instruct patient to rinse or gargle with water. Instruct patient to cough deeply. Collect directly into sterile container.	Sterile screw-cap sputum collection cup >1 mL	<2 h RT optimal, 24 h 4°C maximal	Not routinely performed	*Legionella, Mycobacteria, Nocardia,* other bacterial fungal, viral agents, and *P. carinii*
Sputum, induced[a]	Instruct patient to brush teeth, gums, and tongue and rinse with water. Have patient inhale 25 mL of 3%–10% sterile saline with nebulizer. Collect induced specimen into sterile container.	Sterile screw-cap sputum collection cup >1 mL	<2 h RT optimal, 24 h 4°C maximal	Not routinely performed	*Legionella, Mycobacterium, Nocardia,* other bacterial fungal, viral agents, and *P. carinii*
Respiratory tract, upper NP aspirate, or wash[a]	Pass appropriate-sized tubing or catheter into the nasopharynx. Aspirate material with small?? syringe. If aspiration not possible, tilt patient's head back and instill 3–7 mL saline or viral transport medium until nostrils occluded. Reaspirate.	Sterile container and/or viral transport tube	<2 h RT optimal, 24 h RT maximal	<2 h 4°C optimal, 72 h 4°C maximal 7 d −70°C if processing delayed	*Bordetella pertussis,* parainfluenza virus, RSV, influenza virus, adenovirus
NP swab[a]	Pass flexible, fine-shafted swab into nasopharynx. Allow secretions to absorb for 5 sec. Carefully remove swab, inoculate directly or place in transport tube or device. With fresh swab, repeat for other nostril.	Inoculate plates directly and/or place in culturette tube or equivalent or viral transport tube.	*Plates:* <15 min, RT optimal Swabs: <2 h RT optimal, 24 h RT maximal	<2 h 4°C optimal, 72 h 4°C maximal 7 d −70°C if processing delayed	*Viral:* Influenza virus parainfluenza virus, rhinovirus, RSV, *C. trachomatis* (neonates) *Carrier: S. aureus, S. pyogenes, N. meningitidis, B. pertussis*
Nasal swab: viral/ carrier[a]	Pass flexible, fine-shafted swab into nostril. Rotate swab slowly for 5 sec to adsorb secretions. Remove swab and place in transport. With fresh swab, repeat in other nostril. Place both swabs in same transport tube.	Culturette or equivalent and/or viral transport tube	<2 h RT optimal, 24 h RT maximal	<2 h 4°C optimal, 72 h 4°C maximal 7 d −70°C if processing delayed	*Viral:* Influenza, parainfluenza, rhinovirus, RSV (see text). *Carrier: S. aureus, S. pyogenes, N. meningitidis, B. pertussis*

Table continued on following page

TABLE 57-2 ▶ SPECIMEN COLLECTION GUIDELINES *Continued*

Specimen[a]	Collection and Transport		Delivery Storage Time and Temperature		Likely Agents/ Comments
	Procedures	*Device and/or Minimum Vol*	*Bacterial, Fungal*[b]	*Viral*	
Throat[a]	Depress tongue with tongue depressor. Rub posterior pharynx, tonsils, and inflamed areas firmly with sterile swab. Place swab in transport tube.	Culturette or equivalent and/or viral transport tube.	<2 h RT optimal, 24 h RT maximal	<2 h 4°C optimal, 72 h 4°C maximal 7 d −70°C if processing delayed	*S. pyogenes, N. gonorrhoeae, M. pneumoniae, C. diphtheriae* (rare) Several viral agents
Skene gland Tissue[a]	See *Bartholin Gland.* Collect samples from areas directly adjacent to affected tissue. Add few drops of sterile saline to prevent drying and place specimen in anaerobic transport device. Use separate vial with viral transport medium if appropriate.	Anaerobic transport device and/or viral transport tube.	<15 min RT optimal, 24 h RT maximal	<2 h 4°C optimal, 72 h 4°C maximal 7 d −70°C if processing delayed	Depends on clinical situation. DO NOT ADD FORMALIN if cultivation attempts are desired.
Urinary tract: urine, midstream[a]	*Instruct patient to do the following:* Clean urethral area with soap and water. Wipe with wet gauze pads. While holding labia apart, begin voiding. After several mL have passed, collect midstream portion into sterile container, without stopping flow of urine.	Sterile, wide-mouth container >1 mL or urine transport kit.	*Unpreserved:* 2 h RT optimal, 24 h 4°C maximal *Preserved:* 24 h RT	Not routinely performed except in neonates	Enterobacteriaceae, other gram-negatives, *Staphylococcus saprophyticus,* CMV in neonates
Straight catheter[a]	Clean urethral area with soap and water. Wipe area with wet gauze pads. Aseptically insert catheter into bladder. Allow about 15 mL to pass and then collect specimen in sterile container.	Sterile, leakproof container >1 mL or urine transport kit.	*Unpreserved:* 2 h RT optimal, 24 h 4°C maximal *Preserved:* 24 h RT	Not routinely performed except in neonates	Enterobacteriaceae, other gram-negatives, *S. saprophyticus,* CMV in neonates
Indwelling catheter[a]	Disinfect catheter collection port with 70% ETOH. Aseptically collect 5–10 mL of urine with needle and syringe. Transfer specimen to sterile container.	Sterile, leakproof container >1 mL or urine transport kit.	*Unpreserved:* 2 h RT optimal, 24 h 4°C maximal *Preserved:* 24 h RT	Not routinely performed except in neonates	Enterobacteriaceae, other gram-negatives, *S. saprophyticus,* CMV in neonates
Suprapubic aspirate[a]	Disinfect skin area with povidone-iodine. Aspirate 10–15 mL bladder urine. Transfer to sterile, wide-mouth bottle or urine tube.	Sterile, leakproof container >10 mL of urine, >2 mL if neonate?	2 h RT optimal, 24 h 4°C maximal	Not routinely performed except in neonates	Enterobacteriaceae, other gram-negatives, *S. saprophyticus,* CMV in neonates

TABLE 57-2 ▶ SPECIMEN COLLECTION GUIDELINES Continued

Specimen[a]	Collection and Transport		Delivery Storage Time and Temperature		Likely Agents/ Comments
	Procedures	Device and/or Minimum Vol	Bacterial, Fungal[b]	Viral	
Urethral swab[a]	Clean urethral area with soap and water. Wipe area with wet gauze pads. Gently insert nasopharyngeal swab about 1 cm into orifice of urethra. Rotate for 5 sec and withdraw. Plate directly and then place tip of swab in *Chlamydia* transport medium.	*Neisseria* transport plates or tube and 2SP or other *Chlamydia* transport medium	*Plates:* <2 h RT optimal *Transport tubes:* <2 h RT optimal, 12 h maximal *Chlamydia tube:* <2 h 4°C optimal, 24 h 4°C maximal	Not routinely performed	*N. gonorrhoeae, C. trachomatis*
Vaginal cuff abscess[a]	Aspirate purulent material with needle and syringe, expel into anaerobic transport device.	Anaerobic transport system, 1 mL of aspirate if possible	15 min RT optimal, 24 h RT maximal	Not routinely performed	Mixed aerobes and anaerobes
Vaginal swab[a]	Remove excess discharge with a sterile swab. If vesicular lesions present, collect vesicle fluid as described above or Collect sample of vaginal pool or scrapping of plaque from vaginal wall on sterile swab. Mix with drop of saline on glass slide. Add coverslip and examine microscopically.	Clean glass slides. *See text for modifications of wet preparations. Also see "Lesions" above.*	Within 15 min RT	*See "Lesions" above.*	If lesions present, HSV, *T. pallidum*, *C. trachomatis* If only discharge present, *Candida*, *Trichomonas*, agents of BV
Wounds[a] Closed	Collect as for closed abscesses.	Anaerobic transport for closed wounds only.	<2 h RT optimal, 24 h RT maximal	Not routinely performed	*S. aureus, S. pyogenes, Clostridium*, mixed aerobes, anaerobes
Open	Collect as for open abscesses.	Aerobic transport for open wounds.			

[a]Gram stain should be performed.
[b]Parasitic agents indicated when appropriate.
GC = *Neisseria gonorrhoeae;* GBBS = *Streptococcus agalactiae* (group B beta-hemolytic streptococci). RT = room temperature.
Modified from Miller JM: A Guide to Specimen Management in Clinical Microbiology, 2nd ed. Washington, DC, ASM Press, 1999, pp 143–157, and 160–165; and Woods GL, Washington JA: The clinician and the microbiology laboratory. In: Mandell GL, Bennett JE, Dolin R (eds): Principles and Practice of Infectious Diseases, 4th ed. New York, Churchill Livingstone, 1995, pp 170–171.

as a transport medium for *Chlamydia, Mycoplasma,* and viral agents. Only cotton-tipped, Dacron or rayon swabs with aluminum or plastic shafts should be used if specimens will be cultured for viral agents. Calcium alginate swabs are not recommended.

Specimens in bacterial transport tubes should be processed within 24 hours. Transport medium for *Chlamydia, Mycoplasma,* or viral agents may be kept at 4°C for no longer than 3 days. If processing is delayed for longer periods, the specimens should be frozen at −70°C. However, anaerobic tubes or vials should be maintained at room temperature and processed as soon as possible, and blood culture bottles should be incubated within 2 hours if possible.

Specimens for *Neisseria gonorrhoeae* may be plated directly onto selective media and placed in a CO_2-generating transport system, available commercially.

Examples include JEMBEC and GONOPAK transport systems. These specimens should be delivered to the laboratory within 15 minutes for incubation.

For direct detection by immunoassay or nucleic acid techniques, special transport media and devices may be required, and these must be available at the time of specimen collection. Consultation with the microbiology laboratory is suggested to determine the availability of these procedures.

Following is a more detailed description of specimen collection. Additional information is provided in the tables that accompany the text.

Abscesses, Other than Brain, Pelvic, Tubo-Ovarian, and Vaginal Cuff

An abscess is a localized collection of pus that may occur anywhere in the body in response to the growth

TABLE 57–3 ▶ TRANSPORT MEDIA AND DEVICE GUIDELINES

Suspected Pathogen Type	Medium or Devices
Bacteria or Fungi	
Aerobes, facultatives from specimens collected by swab	Stuart's medium Amies medium Available commercially in ampules at bottom of plastic containers. Ampules must be broken to prevent drying of specimen
Anaerobic organisms from specimens collected by aspiration, biopsy or at surgery	Gassed out tubes or vials, with or without stabilizing medium Many available; devices should not be inverted to avoid escape of CO_2 and/or nitrogen gases within them
Enteric pathogens from stool or rectal swab	Carey-Blair medium Buffered glycerol
Neisseria gonorrhoeae from specimens usually collected on swabs of vagina, cervix, or throat, but may also be sought in aspirates and tissue	Amies medium with charcoal If immediate inoculation is performed, culture plates should be placed in CO_2-generating systems, which are commercially available
Parasites	
Specimens are usually stool but may be sputum, vaginal secretions	Polyvinyl alcohol (PVA) Sodium acetate–acetic acid formalin (SAF) Buffered formalin for ova, larvae, or concentration procedures 2–5 mL of sterile saline for wet mount
Others	
Chlamydia, Mycoplasma Ureaplasma, viral	0.2 M Sucrose in phosphate buffer (2SP) may be used for all Separate transport media are available
Special Procedures	
Antigen detection (ELISA), nucleic acid probes amplification	May require special transport formulations supplied by the manufacturer Consult microbiology laboratory

of bacteria or fungi. Since anaerobic organisms are frequently involved, it is essential that the specimens collected be maintained under anaerobic conditions. Depending on whether the specimen is fluid or tissue, commercially available anaerobic transport tubes or vials may be used (see Table 57–3). If a transport tube is opened to introduce the specimen, care should be taken to keep the device upright to prevent the loss of anaerobiosis by the escape of CO_2 and/or nitrogen gas, which are heavier than air.

Internal Abscesses

If the abscess is internal (e.g., hepatic abscess, pancreatic abscess, subphrenic abscess), specimens should be obtained for culture and gram-staining by percutaneous or surgical drainage after appropriate disinfection of the overlaying skin area. The specimen should be aspirated and immediately placed in an anaerobic transport device and delivered to the laboratory at room temperature for processing.

Internal abscesses of particular concern in females are those that occur within the female genital tract, such as tubo-ovarian abscess, vaginal cuff abscess, or pelvic abscess following childbirth or surgery. These

topics are discussed separately in a later section on upper genital tract infections.

Abscesses of Skin, Subcutaneous Tissue, and Mucous Membranes

Abscesses may also form in external surfaces, as follows:

1. If the abscess is closed, the area should be disinfected with povidone-iodine and/or 70% alcohol, and material aspirated with needle and syringe. If incision and drainage is performed, a portion of the abscess wall should be submitted for culture. An anaerobic transport device should be used to deliver the specimens to the laboratory at room temperature for processing.
2. If the abscess is open, the surface should be disinfected and material aspirated from within the abscess if possible. If aspiration is not possible, two swabs should be inserted into the abscess and pressed firmly to sample the edge of the abscess. Both swabs should be placed in an aerobic transport device; one is used for culture, the other for Gram stain. If exudate can be ex-

pressed, a sample should also be collected on a swab and transported aerobically. Anaerobic cultures are not recommended for specimens from open abscesses.

Following is a description of suggested specimen collection and transport methods for surface abscesses of particular concern in the female patient population. A summary of these procedures is given in Table 57–2.

Bartholin Gland Abscess, or Infection

EXUDATE

In the absence of a well-defined abscess, the mucocutaneous area surrounding the infected gland should be decontaminated with povidone-iodine and then be wiped with sterile saline. Alcohol is not recommended. Exudate may be collected on a swab following digital palpation. If possible, two swabs should be used, one for direct inoculation on selective medium for *N. gonorrheoae*, which is transported in a CO_2-enhanced environment, and the other for transport in *Chlamydia* transport medium. A smear for gram-staining should also be prepared.

If an abscess is present, an aspirate of material should be collected with needle and syringe. These specimens must be transported immediately to the laboratory for processing or must be expelled into anaerobic and *Chlamydia* transport tubes for delivery to the laboratory. A drop of the aspirate should be placed on slide, smeared into a thin layer, and stained by Gram stain. Anaerobic transport tubes should be kept at room temperature, and the *Chlamydia* transport tube should be kept on ice or refrigerated (4°C) until processing. These specimens collected by aspiration should be cultured for *N. gonorrhoeae*, facultatives, anaerobes, *Ureaplasma urealyticum*, and *Chlamydia trachomatis*.

ENDOCERVIX

Endocervical swabs should be collected and submitted for culture of *N. gonorrhoeae* and *C. trachomatis*. See the section on cervical infections below for collection techniques.

TISSUES AND OTHER SPECIMENS

In rare instances, toxic shock syndrome, septic shock, or necrotizing fasciitis may result from bartholinitis.[1-3] In these cases, blood cultures or débrided tissue, respectively, should be submitted for culture and gram-staining for detection of *Staphylococcus aureus* or other causative agents.

Breast Abscess and/or Mastitis

EXUDATE

The area to be sampled should be decontaminated with alcohol and povidone-iodine if skin is intact (with warm water and antimicrobial soap if lesions are present), and the specimen collected by aspiration with needle and syringe. The material should be expelled into an anaerobic transport device and delivered to the laboratory at room temperature. Samples from an open abscess should be collected as described previously for skin and subcutaneous open abscesses. Although *S. aureus* is the most frequent causative agent, *Streptococcus pyogenes* (group A *Streptococcus*), *S. agalactiae* (group B *Streptococcus*), *Haemophilus influenzae*, *H. parainfluenzae*, and other skin flora are also recovered.[4] Specimens should be submitted for gram-staining and culture of aerobes and facultative organisms, since microbes that are not susceptible to commonly used antimicrobial agents may be recovered in some cases.[5] Cultivation for anaerobes should be performed only if the specimen is taken from a closed abscess.

BREAST MILK

Although not routinely performed in most settings, Gram stain and culture of breast milk may be appropriate in sporadic cases of mastitis occurring from 2 to 3 weeks to several months after delivery.[4] To collect a sample of breast milk, the skin surrounding the nipple should be decontaminated and the milk expressed manually into a sterile container. If open lesions are present, the area should be washed gently with warm water and an antibacterial soap prior to collecting the specimen. The specimen should be submitted to the laboratory at room temperature. A quantitative culture of the milk specimen should be made with a 0.01-mL loop as well as inoculating routinely.

Lesions Such as Carbuncles, Hidradenitis, and Folliculitis

The same general guidelines described previously for abscesses should be followed; that is, material should be aspirated from a closed abscess, the advancing margin of the lesion should be pressed firmly with a swab, and a part of the wall of the abscess should be sampled. Aspirated specimens should be placed in an anaerobic transport media and cultured for aerobes and anaerobes. If the specimen is collected by swab, it should be cultured for aerobes and facultative organisms. *Staphylococcus aureus* is often involved, but other aerobic or facultative bacteria may also be recovered.

Skene Gland Abscess, or Infection

EXUDATE

A drop of purulent material may sometimes be expressed from this tiny gland that empties into the urethra.[6] If so, the pus should be collected on a sterile swab and cultured for *N. gonorrhoeae*. The role of other potential pathogens has not been determined.

ENDOCERVIX

Endocervical specimens should be collected by swab and cultured for *N. gonorrhoeae* as well.

Anal Specimens

Specimens taken by swab from the anal crypts just inside the anal ring may be submitted for recovery of *N. gonorrhoeae* and for screening for the presence of *S. agalactiae* (group B *Streptococcus*). Contamination with fecal material should be avoided. (See section on rectal swabs as well.)

1. For recovery of *N. gonorrhoeae*, direct inoculation onto selective media and incubation in a CO_2-enriched atmosphere is recommended.
2. Anal swabs may also be used for recovery of *S. agalactiae* (group B *Streptococcus*) when combined with collection of vaginal swabs. An appropriate bacterial transport tube or device should be used to prevent drying, and the specimen should be submitted at room temperature and refrigerated if a delay in processing is unavoidable. The specimen should be inoculated within 24 hours. Both anal and vaginal swabs may be placed in the same transport tube.

The anal area may serve as a site of infection by agents, discussed later in the section on genital tract specimens. Whenever lesions typical of these infections occur in the anal area, they should be sampled as described in that section and in Table 57–2.

Anal swabs are *not* usually acceptable specimens for recovery of agents of diarrhea.[7]

Blood

The blood stream can be invaded by several viral, bacterial, fungal, and some parasitic agents, and special considerations for collection of blood specimens may be necessary, depending on the suspected pathogen. Typical clinical situations in which blood specimens should be collected include postpartum bacteremia or septicemia, meningitis, osteomyelitis, arthritis, pneumonia, fever of unknown origin in adults, as well as suspected bacteremia or septicemia and meningitis of the newborn. Other clinical settings in which collection of blood is indicated include subacute or acute bacterial endocarditis, and low-grade intravascular infections or catheter-related bacteremia.[8]

Major factors that directly influence the results of testing of blood specimens include the volume of blood collected, timing of specimen collection, and method of skin disinfection. Suggested guidelines for the volume of blood that should be collected are given in Table 57–4. A summary of disinfection procedures is presented in Table 57–2.

For recovery of bacterial agents in adult patients, 10- to 20-mL samples (preferably 20 mL) are usually collected from each arm, and the samples are inoculated into aerobic and anaerobic blood culture bottles containing 100 mL of appropriate liquid culture medium. Alternatively, 5 to 10 mL may be inoculated into lysis centrifugation systems, or larger volumes of blood may be inoculated into bottles of a nonradiometeric automated blood culture system. Specimens should be transported at room temperature as soon as possible to the laboratory for incubation. The inoculated bottles or tubes are incubated at 35°C for 5 to 7 days with a preliminary report based on Gram staining of the broth being sent after 24 to 48 hours. One- to two-mL samples are collected from newborns. Pediatric blood culture systems are available commercially, but the 100-mL bottles have been used successfully.[9–11]

Additional notes on collection of specimens for blood culture are as follows:

Bacterial Detection

1. To prevent possible contamination of blood from patients who have indwelling catheters, specimens should *not* be withdrawn through an indwelling intravenous or intra-arterial catheter unless the specimen cannot be obtained by venipuncture. The specimen should be drawn *below* an existing intravenous line to prevent dilution of the blood with infusion fluid.[12]
2. If meningococcemia or gonococcemia is suspected or if the patient is post partum, has a history of bacterial vaginosis, and is febrile, blood culture medium without the anticoagulant sodium dodecyl sulfate (SDS) may be required for recovery of the pathogen.[13]
3. Patients with endocarditis and negative growth on subculture from positive growth in blood culture bottles, and the presence of gram-positive cocci in chains on Gram stain, may be harboring a nutritionally deficient strain of *Streptococcus*, which requires special subculturing procedures.[13]
4. In cases of suspected leptospirosis, fresh or anticoagulated blood from the patient collected within the first 10 days of illness should be inoculated into several tubes of semisolid culture medium, such as Fletcher's. Citrate is toxic to leptospires and should not be used as an anticoagulant.[14]

Fungal Detection

1. The same guidelines used for recovery of bacterial agents should be used for recovery of suspected fungal agents. Blood culture bottles or ly-

TABLE 57-4 ▶ GUIDELINES FOR COLLECTION OF BLOOD SPECIMENS

Clinical Setting	Collection Schedule	Comments
Adults and adolescents: severe septicemia, meningitis, osteomyelitis, arthritis, pneumonia	Two specimens over 24-h period prior to therapy	One 10- to 20-mL sample should be collected from each arm, or separate sticks from same arm
Fever of unknown origin (patients on therapy)	Four to six specimens within 48 h	Specimen should be collected just before administration of antibiotic
Febrile episodes	Up to three specimens within 24 h	Bacteremia may precede fever by 1 h
Subacute bacterial endocarditis	Three specimens within 24 h	Collect specimens at start of fever spikes throughout the 24-h period; collect three more if first set negative after 24 h
Acute bacterial endocarditis	Three specimens within 1–2 h prior to therapy	
Low-grade intravascular infection	Three specimens within 24 h	Collect specimens at least 1 h apart; collect two at start of febrile episode
Newborns and younger children	1- to 2-mL samples	Two specimens usually adequate for diagnosing bacteremia

Adapted from Miller JM: A Guide to Specimen Management in Clinical Microbiology, 2nd ed. Washington, DC, ASM Press, 1999, p 53.

sis centrifugation tubes may be used as well as biphasic systems that are commercially available.

2. Fungemia due to *Malassezia furfur* (i.e., in patients receiving intravenous lipids via hyperalimentation) may not be detected by the lysis centrifugation system unless sterile olive or coconut oil or another source of lipid is added to the agar medium onto which the blood culture sediment is inoculated.[13]

Viral Detection

1. Serum samples may be used for recovery of enteroviruses from newborns.[15] In that case, a 1- to 2-mL sample of blood should be collected without anticoagulants, and the serum (0.2 mL) should be inoculated into appropriate cell culture tubes or vials.

2. Leukocyte fractions or buffy coat may also be used to isolate some viruses, such as members of the Herpesvirus group, primarily Cytomegalovirus (CMV). Approximately 5 to 8 mL or 1 to 2 mL of blood should be collected from adults or newborns, respectively, into tubes containing either sodium citrate or heparin anticoagulant and thoroughly mixed before transport to the laboratory. The leukocyte fractions are prepared using Ficoll-Hypaque/Macrodix centrifugation or other separation methods.[15] The leukocyte fraction is then inoculated into conventional cell culture tubes and/or shell vials for isolation attempts of the suspected viral agent. Immunofluorescence staining within 24 to 48 hours of the shell vial culture may provide an early identification. A drop of the cellular preparation may also be placed on a microscope slide, fixed, and stained with fluorescence antibody reagents and examined for the presence of viral inclusions. Alternatively, a nucleic acid probe available commercially may be used. Additional information on these and other diagnostic techniques is presented in section two of this chapter.

Parasite Detection

1. Systemic parasites, such as *Plasmodium* spp., *Babesia* spp., *Trypanosoma* spp., *Leishmania* spp., microfilariae, and *Toxoplasma gondii*, may be detected in whole blood, buffy coat preparations or by several concentration methods. Identification is made by examination of stained thick and thin blood films. See reference 16 for a more detailed description of these techniques.

Central Nervous System Infections

Brain Abscess

This relatively rare form of central nervous system infection is a focal suppurative process within the brain parenchyma, which typically develops in four clinical settings: (1) in association with a contiguous suppurative focus, for example, otitis media and mastoiditis, and splenoidal sinusitis; (2) after hematogenous spread from a distant focus, for example, lung or other internal abscess or congenital heart disease; (3) following trauma; and (4) cryptogenic, that is, no known source. As many as 72% of cases are associated with (1) and (2), 15% with (4), with the remainder associated with nonsurgical forms of trauma.[17]

The presence of a brain abscess is usually diagnosed by magnetic resonance imaging (MRI), computed tomography (CT) scan, or technetium 99m (^{99m}Tc) scan. If specimens are required for culture or other testing procedures, they should be collected at the time of surgical management; that is, by aspiration of abscess material after burr hole placement, or complete excision following craniotomy. Aspirates and abscess material should be placed into an anaerobic transport device. Smears should be made for gram-staining, and the specimen inoculated for recovery of aerobes, anaerobes, and fungi. Lumbar puncture for collection of spinal fluid is contraindicated for patients with suspected or proven cranial abscess, since the diagnostic yield is poor and the procedure is dangerous.[17]

Although the likely organisms are related to the source of infection, the organisms most commonly associated with brain abscesses overall are listed in Table 57–5. As many as 60% of these pyogenic infections are of mixed etiology.[17]

Encephalitis

BRAIN BIOPSY

Specimens of brain tissue collected in suspected cases of encephalitis will be quite small. The specimen should be placed in a sterile container, and part of it used to prepare impression smears for immunofluorescence staining. A small amount of tissue may be placed between two slides, which are slid apart lengthwise to produce a pair of thin smears in the centers of the two slides.[15] The remainder of the specimen and the air-dried slides should be taken to the laboratory as soon as possible after collection.

CEREBROSPINAL FLUID (CSF)

Specimens of CSF should be collected and examined as described later for meningitis. Potential etiologic agents include several viral and bacterial agents as well as some parasitic pathogens.[18] Diagnostic tests include electron microscopy, immunofluorescence staining, and nucleic acid amplification of specimens (especially for herpes simplex virus [HSV]), cultivation of the agents, and/or serologic testing.

Meningitis

The meninges may be the primary focus of infection by several pathogens; however, positive CSF findings may be obtained as a secondary manifestation of other central nervous system conditions; that is, trauma, infectious complications of surgery, cranial and spinal epidural abscesses, subdural abscess, septic thrombophlebitis of the venous sinuses, brain abscess, and encephalitis.[19] Table 57–6 lists some of the agents isolated most frequently from cases of *acute* meningitis by age group. In addition to the agents in Table 57–6, rickettsial agents, spirochetes, acid-fast organisms, fungi, and various noninfectious causes of acute meningitis have been identified.[20]

Agents such as systemic fungi, *Brucella* spp., acid-fast organisms, spirochetes, and some viral and parasitic agents may also be responsible for the clinical syndrome of *chronic meningitis*. These cases are associated with a high morbidity and mortality and can be successfully managed only by administration of specific forms of therapy.[21] Hence, early, correct diagnosis is essential.

CEREBROSPINAL FLUID SPECIMENS

Regardless of suspected etiology, specimens of CSF should be obtained, as summarized in Table 57–2, by a properly trained physician. In addition, the patient should be informed that although Novocain (procaine HCl) will be used, she may experience some pain at the time of needle insertion.[22]

The specimens should be placed in a sterile tube for transport to the laboratory. If bacterial, fungal, or parasitic etiology is suspected, the fluid should be transported at *room temperature* in a sterile tube. The specimen must be processed as soon as possible, that is, within 24 hours from the time of collection. If viral etiology is suspected, the specimen should be transported *on ice* or kept at $-4°C$ and be processed as soon as possible but within 72 hours. It may be necessary to divide the specimen for microbiologic testing. If more than one tube is obtained, the second or third tube, whichever is less bloody, should be sent for microbiologic testing. If only one tube is obtained, it should be sent to the microbiology laboratory first.

Diagnostic procedures include wet preparation (if free-living amebae are suspected), Gram stain, acid-fast stain, India ink preparation, antigen detection, amplification, and cultivation of the suspected agent.

BLOOD CULTURES

Blood cultures should also be collected in cases of suspected meningitis prior to the initiation of therapy.

TABLE 57–5 ▶	ORGANISMS ISOLATED FROM BRAIN ABSCESSES
Organism	**Relative Frequency (%)**
Streptococcus (*S. milleri* group)	60–70
Bacteroides and *Prevotella* spp.	20–40
Enterobacteriaceae	23–33
Staphylococcus aureus	10–15
Fungi	10–15
Others	
Haemophilus influenzae	<1
S. pneumoniae	<1
Protozoa, helminths	<1

Modified from Mandell GL, Bennett JE, Dolin R (eds): Principles and Practice of Infectious Diseases, 4th ed. New York, Churchill Livingstone, 1995, p 889.

TABLE 57-6 ▶ SUSPECTED AGENTS OF ACUTE MENINGITIS BY PATIENT POPULATION	
Patient Population	**Likely Etiologic Agents**
Neonates 0–4 weeks	*Streptococcus agalactiae* (GBBS), *Escherichia coli, Listeria monocytogenes, Klebsiella pneumoniae, Enterococcus* spp., *Salmonella* spp. Viral: CMV, rubella, enterovirus, HSV
Infants 4–12 weeks	GBBS, *E. coli, L. monocytogenes,* plus *Haemophilus influenzae, S. pneumoniae, Neisseria meningitidis*
Children 3 months–18 years	*Haemophilus influenzae* serotype B,[a] *N. meningitidis, Streptococcus pneumoniae* Viral: Mumps and others Parasites: *Acanthamoeba, Naegleria* (rare)
Adults 18–50 years	*Streptococcus pneumoniae, N. meningitidis* Viral: Enteroviruses, arbovirus Parasites: *Acanthamoeba, Naegleria* (rare)
Adults >50 years	*Streptococcus pneumoniae, N. meningitidis, L. monocytogenes,* Gram-negative bacilli, including *Pseudomonas aeruginosa*
Immunocompromised	As in adults >50 years plus *Cryptococcus neoformans, Toxoplasma gondii*

[a]Vaccine has reduced incidence.
Modified from Mandell GL, Bennett JE, Dolin R (eds): Principles and Practice of Infectious Diseases, 4th ed. New York, Churchill Livingstone, 1995, p 834.

SEROLOGIC TESTING

In cases of suspected neurosyphilis or congenital syphilis, specimens of CSF may be tested with the Venereal Disease Research Laboratory (VDRL)–CSF test for antibody detection. A comparison of antibody levels in CSF versus those in serum may be useful for diagnosing infection with *Borrelia burgdorferi, Histoplasma capsulatum, Coccidioides immitis, Taenia solium,* and measles virus.[21] Antibody detection in acute and convalescent sera is often required for the diagnosis of meningitis caused by viral and parasitic agents.

Dermatologic Conditions

Owing to the immunosuppressive effects of pregnancy, some agents capable of causing dermatologic manifestations may initially appear, recur more frequently, or become more severe during pregnancy. Some of these may have serious adverse effects on the fetus, as discussed in Chapter 35.

Bacterial and Fungal Agents

BORRELIA BURGDORFERI (LYME DISEASE)

Borrelia burgdorferi is a spirochete organism that is transmitted to humans by the bite of a tick of the *Ixodes ricinus* complex. The first stage of disease consists of erythema chronicum migrans (ECM), which often occurs following the bite of the tick. Diagnosis may be made by observing a typical clinical picture following exposure to a tick bite in an endemic area and by detecting antibodies to *B. burgdorferi.* However, the serologic response is slow, and only 30% to 40% of patients with ECM are reported as having positive serologic tests in acute specimens and 60% to 70% of patients are positive by convalescence sera.[23]

CANDIDA SPP.

In addition to infections of the external genitalia, *Candida* spp., primarily *C. albicans,* is also capable of causing infection of the skin, nails, or oral mucosa. The most common form of skin involvement, intertrigo, may affect any area where skin surfaces are in close contact and a moist, warm environment is provided. The skin lesions begin as vesicopustules, which may enlarge and rupture, causing a maceration and fissuring. The affected skin area usually has a scalloped border with a white rim composed of necrotic epidermis. Both the area surrounding the nail and the nail bed itself may become infected with *Candida* spp. The infection surrounding the nail usually appears as a localized area of inflammation that becomes warm, glistening, and tense and may extend extensively under the nail. Infection of the oral mucosa (thrush) is characterized by creamy white, curd-like patches on the tongue and other oral mucosal surfaces.

Although the incidence of vaginal candidiasis is reported to be elevated during pregnancy, it is not known whether the same is true for these other infections. Skin scrapings, nail cuttings, subungual debris, and scrapings of infected mucous membranes should be collected for examination with a KOH wet preparation, as described in the second section of this chapter. The specimens should be placed in a small volume (1 mL) of sterile saline for delivery to the laboratory at room temperature. The specimen may also be cultured for recovery of the organism on mycology media.

COCCIDIOIDES IMMITIS

Although rashes (erythema nodosum, erythema multiforme) may be seen with primary disease, these are allergic reactions and the organism is not recovered or detected within them. Of greater concern is the appearance of papules, pustules, plaques, nodules, ulcers, abscesses, or large proliferative lesions that may develop in the skin as a sign of disseminated disease. The likelihood of dissemination is greatly increased in pregnant patients who contract the disease after conception (see Chapter 35). In such cases, expectorated or induced sputum samples or aspirated specimens of purulent material from the skin lesions, superficial soft tissue lesions, or joint fluid may be examined for typical spherule morphology by lactophenol cotton blue preparation as described in the second section of this chapter. Cultures of these specimens may be attempted, but recovery of *C. immitis* does pose an additional health hazard to laboratory personnel. Serologic tests may be used to detect the presence of specific IgM, which appears 1 to 3 weeks after infection, as well as an increase in titer of IgG. See the third section of this chapter for a description of the tests used.

Viral Agents

HUMAN SIMPLEX VIRUS

Herpetic lesions not only may occur in the lower genital tract but also may be found in the mouth, on the thigh or buttock, and in the rectal mucosa. Specimens from these lesions should be collected and tested as described later in the section on the lower genitalia.

HUMAN IMMUNODEFICIENCY VIRUS

Among the dermatologic manifestations of human immunodeficiency virus (HIV) infection associated with significant morbidity or life-threatening illness for the pregnant patient are bacillary angiomatosis, disseminated protozoal and systemic fungal infections, disseminated herpes zoster, and Kaposi's sarcoma. In addition, the immunosuppressive effect of the HIV infection itself is associated with infection by a broad range of other potential pathogens that may cause dermatologic manifestations with unusual presentations.

Vesicular or ulcerative lesions, if present, may be sampled and analyzed as described later in the section on lower genital tract infections. However, because of the large number of probable pathogens and the potential abnormal presentation that may occur in immunocompromised patients, laboratory diagnosis of cutaneous lesions in the HIV-infected pregnant patient may require biopsy specimens (see section on collection of tissue specimens later in this section). The

specimen should be divided into two portions: one should be processed histologically and stained with routine and special stains to detect fungi, mycobacteria, and other bacteria; the other portion should be submitted for cultivation of aerobes, anaerobes, mycobacteria, and fungi. Viral cultures should be performed if herpesviruses are suspected. Touch preparations should be stained with Gram stain and acid-fast stains as well as immunofluorescent reagents for detection of HSV, varicella-zoster virus (VZV), and CMV.[24] Cutaneous forms of the diseases that are often diagnosed by serologic methods may be more likely diagnosed by biopsy in immunocompromised patients owing to the unreliability of their immune response.

HUMAN PAPILLOMAVIRUS (HPV)

Lesions due to HPV (condylomata acuminata) may occur not only on areas of the lower genital area, as described later, but also in the perineum and anus. These lesions should be sampled, as described in the section on the lower genital tract, and submitted for hybridization or amplification procedures to differentiate them from lesions of secondary syphilis (condyloma lata).

HUMAN PARVOVIRUS B19

Human parovovirus B19 infection may be asymptomatic or cause an acute illness with rash and/or arthropathy. It has been associated with fetal hydrops and demise. Definitive diagnosis of infection with human parvovirus B19 may be made by serologic tests that detect the presence of specific IgM. The specimen should be collected early in the disease, since IgM is usually detectable within 3 days after onset and begins to decline within 1 month. Testing for rubella should also be performed in pregnant patients owing to the overlap in symptoms and potential consequences to the fetus of rubella infection.[25] Other diagnostic procedures include antigen detection, hybridization, and amplification by polymerase chain reaction (PCR) in respiratory secretions, amniotic fluid, and other specimens.

MEASLES VIRUS

Although measles is not known to cause congenital abnormalities in the fetus, it has been associated with serious respiratory complications in pregnant patients.[26] The diagnosis is usually made by serologic testing, as described in the third section of this chapter.

RUBELLA

Rubella is a mild, exanthemous disease when acquired postnatally, but primary infection during pregnancy can have serious consequences for the fetus. The fact that as many as 20% of the younger population may not have received rubella vaccine and are thus susceptible to primary infection during pregnancy emphasizes the importance of its recognition.[27] Laboratory diagnosis is usually made by serologic tests, as described in the third section of this chapter.

VARICELLA-ZOSTER VIRUS

Diagnosis of infection with VZV is usually made by history taking and physical examination; however, laboratory diagnosis can be achieved by antigen detection with immunofluorescence staining of lesion material. Other infections that may have a presentation similar to that of VZV infection include impetigo, infection with HSV, or disseminated enterococcal infection, particularly group A coxsackieviruses. Impetigo may be recognized by gram-staining lesion material and detecting gram-positive cocci. The other viral infections may be diagnosed by antigen detection and/or viral culture of lesion material.[28]

Eye Infections

Conjunctivitis

In adults, conjunctivitis may be caused by *N. gonorrhoeae* or *C. trachomatis* or may be a sequela of bacterial or viral upper respiratory infections. Neonatal conjunctivitis may be caused by *N. gonorrhoeae, C. trachomatis* (serotypes D to K), CMV, or HSV. Trachoma, a chronic conjunctivitis that may lead to blindness, is caused by *C. trachomatis,* serotypes L_1, L_2, and L_3. Although usually considered to be endemic to Asia and Africa, cases have also occurred in the southwestern United States.

CONJUNCTIVAL SWABS

Conjunctival specimens are obtained by swabbing the infected area (see Table 57–2). Multiple specimens should be collected for cultivation and staining. Smears should be made for staining with Gram stain to detect *N. gonorrhoeae* and other bacteria, direct fluorescent antibody staining for *N. gonorrhoeae* and *C. trachomatis,* and/or direct immunofluorescence staining for HSV or CMV. DNA probes are available for the detection of *N. gonorrhoeae* and/or *C. trachomatis* on eye specimens in suspected cases of trachoma. The specimens should be placed in the probe collection tube for transport to the laboratory.

For recovery of bacteria, a swab should be used to inoculate blood agar and chocolate agar plates directly after specimen collection. The plates should then be placed in a CO_2-generating environment. If direct inoculation is not possible, the swab must be placed in a transport tube or device (see Table 57–3) containing appropriate transport media (i.e., Carey-Blair) to prevent drying of the specimen, or, preferably, special transport tubes designed for enhancement of recovery of *N. gonorrhoeae.* For recovery of *C. trachomatis* and/or viral agents, the swab must be placed in appropriate transport media (i.e., 2SP or M-4).

Inoculated plates should be transported to the laboratory within 15 minutes. Swabs in transport tubes should be delivered at room temperature for inoculation within 24 hours. Swabs in viral transport medium should be delivered on ice and/or held at 4°C for no longer than 72 hours prior to processing.

Keratitis

This inflammation of the cornea is a potentially sight-threatening condition caused by a variety of bacterial, fungal, parasitic, and viral agents. Some of the same agents that cause conjunctivitis are also involved in keratitis.

CORNEAL SCRAPINGS

Laboratory diagnosis is based on the collection of corneal scrapings for culture and staining. See Table 57–2 for a summary of collection procedures, which should be performed by an ophthalmologist.

Gastrointestinal Tract Infections

Infections may occur at different sites throughout the length of the gastrointestinal (GI) tract. The specimens to be collected depend on which segment is thought to be involved.

Duodenal Contents

The duodenum is the site of infection primarily by two parasites, *Giardia lamblia* and *Strongyloides stercoralis.* If the diagnosis cannot be made from stool specimens, or if the patient is unable to pass a specimen, duodenal contents may be obtained by the string test (Enterotest), available commercially. The system consists of a capsule containing a weighted, coiled length of nylon yarn or string. The patient swallows the capsule, the gelatin dissolves, and the weighted string is carried by peristalsis into the duodenum. After 4 hours, the string is withdrawn through the oral cavity and the string portion with bile mucus attached is sent for analysis.[29]

The string must be delivered immediately to the laboratory, where the mucus specimen is expressed from the string, mixed with a small volume of saline, and examined microscopically for motile organisms. If examination cannot be made within 2 hours, the specimen should *not* be refrigerated but should be preserved in formalin and stained with iodine or trichrome.

Feces

See section on stool specimens.

Gastric-Antral Biopsy

Cases of duodenal or gastric ulcers due to *Helicobacter pylori* may be diagnosed by either invasive or noninvasive techniques. The invasive technique involves collection of specimens by endoscopic biopsy of the gastric antral mucosa. The specimen should be obtained by a gastroenterologist or other appropriately trained medical staff member. The procedure involves sedating the patient and obtaining the specimen with a fiberoptic endoscopy instrument. Multiple samples should be taken and submitted for histopathologic staining and microbiologic testing.

Specimens for microbiologic testing should be placed in transport medium, such as tryptic soy broth, and delivered to the laboratory immediately. The samples may be refrigerated for up to 1 hour if processing will be delayed.[30] Diagnostic tests include a screening test in which a small portion of the sample is placed on or in a urea slant or broth, respectively. Some authorities recommend cultivation for confirmation; however, culture may not be as sensitive as histopathology or the urease test.[31] If specimens are cultured, the samples should be minced or ground to release the organisms from tissue. The specimen should then be gram-stained and inoculated onto bacteriologic media for detection and recovery of the organism.

Less invasive techniques include a urea breath test and serology. In addition, a test for the detection of *H. pylori* antigens has recently become available. Studies are in progress to demonstrate its utility in the clinical laboratory.

Gastric Contents

These specimens are usually collected in cases in which *Mycobacterium tuberculosis* is suspected and sputum specimens are not available. This approach is most often used in children younger than 7 years of age. The procedure should be performed on 3 consecutive days in the early morning before the patient has had anything to eat or drink.

A number 14 or 16 Levin tube is used for nasal insertion, or a Rehfuss-type tube is used for oral insertion. Fluoroscopy is used to guide the tube to the tip of the antrum, if patient is sitting, or the middle of the greater curvature, if the patient is lying on the left side. Material is aspirated by syringe or mechanically and is placed in a sterile transport tube without preservatives. Sterile saline (20 to 30 mL) may then be introduced into the stomach and aspirated as lavage fluid. The gastric contents and lavage fluid may be combined in a sterile container. The specimen should be neutralized with 100 mg of sodium carbonate, preferably immediately after collection but within 4 hours if transport is delayed. The specimen should be delivered to the laboratory as soon as possible and refrigerated if not processed immediately.[32]

In newborns, this specimen is sometimes collected for gram-staining in an attempt to detect gram-positive cocci in suspected cases of invasive disease due to *S.*

agalactiae.[33] The potential usefulness of this approach, as well as problems associated with the nonspecificity of Gram stain results, have been documented.[34] Culturing of this specimen from newborns is not recommended, owing to the potential misleading results from the mixed flora recovered.[35]

Sigmoidoscopy Specimens

Specimens obtained by sigmoidoscopy are obtained in cases of suspected amebiasis in which stool specimens are negative. A lubricated sigmoidoscope should be gently inserted into the rectum and passed to the point where the sigmoid colon can be seen. Material is aspirated with a serologic pipette from visible lesions and the mucosal surface. A curette may also be used to gently scrape suspicious areas.

The specimen should be placed in a sterile culture tube and delivered immediately to the laboratory for wet preparation examination and staining. The specimen should *not* be refrigerated.[36]

Rectal Swabs

Rectal swabs are acceptable for culture of enteric pathogens only from infants or patients who are acutely ill with a diarrheal illness. The swab should be gently inserted beyond the anal sphincter and rotated for 3 to 5 seconds. The swab is withdrawn and placed in an appropriate transport medium. Some fecal material should be seen on the tip of the swab.[37]

Routine culture for agents of diarrhea usually includes attempts at recovery of *Shigella* spp., *Salmonella* spp., and *Campylobacter* spp. If other agents are suspected, that is, *Vibrio* spp., *Aeromonas* spp., *Plesiomonas* spp., or *Escherichia coli* O157:H7, the laboratory must be notified in advance. Diagnostic procedures include cultivation of the organism on appropriate culture medium, followed by serologic or biochemical identification procedures.

Although not a good substitute for stool specimens, rectal swabs may be used for viral isolation if stool is not available. The likelihood of obtaining an adequate specimen is relative to the amount of fecal material adhering to the swab. The swab should be placed in viral transport medium, and the shaft of the swab cut at a length shorter than the tube. The tube should be transported on ice, and material extracted from the swab by vortexing. The specimen is centrifuged prior to inoculation into appropriate tissue culture tubes.[15]

The rectum may serve as a site of infection for the diseases discussed in the section on genital tract specimens. Whenever lesions typical of these infections occur in the rectum, they should be sampled as described in that section and in Table 57–2. Cultivation of specimens from the rectum (in addition to vaginal cultures) have been reported to enhance recovery of *S. agalactiae* in screening cultures for pregnant patients.

Note: Rectal swabs should *not* be submitted for the detection of parasites or for direct-detection procedures (i.e., enzyme immunoassay [EIA] tests for rotavirus), since they do not provide sufficient material for these tests. Rectal swabs are also unacceptable for testing for the detection of *Clostridium difficile* toxin.[37]

Stool Specimens for Enteric Pathogen Detection

For recovery of bacterial pathogens, three specimens submitted on 3 consecutive days is optimal. For recovery of parasites, three specimens collected every 2 to 3 days may be necessary. These should not be submitted if collected less than 5 days from the date the patient received barium oil, magnesium, or crystalline compounds.[37] For viral agents, a single specimen may be adequate. Specimens should not be collected for a routine diarrhea work-up if the patient has been hospitalized for 3 days or more.

Specimens should be collected as soon after onset of diarrhea as possible. They may be submitted in a clean, cardboard container for immediate transport to the laboratory, or they may be placed in appropriate transport medium if a delay is unavoidable (see Table 57–3). Specimens for viral detection should be submitted without fixation. If culture attempts are to be made, a 2- to 3-g sample of the stool specimen may be placed in a viral transport tube and delivered on ice.

Diagnostic testing includes cultivation for bacterial pathogens, wet and fixed preparations for direct examination for parasitic pathogens, and cultivation attempts for certain viral pathogens. For viral agents that cannot be cultivated, electron microscopy (EM), immunoelectron microscopy (IEM), enzyme-linked immunosorbent assay (ELISA), or other antigen detection methods may be used.

Stool Specimens for Clostridium difficile and/or Toxin Detection

Specimens for these tests may be submitted for patients who have been hospitalized, have received systemic antimicrobial or antineoplastic agents, and who are passing five or more liquid stools per day. The specimen should be collected in a sterile, leak-proof container and submitted to the laboratory within 1 hour. If delay in processing is unavoidable, the specimen should be refrigerated.

Diagnostic tests available include latex agglutination for toxin A, and EIAs for toxin A or B, or both. An extract of the stool sample may also be inoculated into tissue culture for detection of cytopathic effects that are neutralized by antibody to *C. difficile* or *C. sordellii*. A selective agar containing cycloserine, cefoxitin, and fructose (CCFA) is available for the isolation of the organism. However, isolates should be tested for toxin production, since not all isolates are positive.

Genital Tract Infections, External and Lower

A variety of lesion types may be encountered in the vulva, vagina, perineum, and perianal area, and adjacent cutaneous areas such as the buttocks and thighs. A diagnosis may be suggested by the morphology of the lesion. However, variation in the appearance of lesions and overlap among the diseases occurs. These areas are heavily contaminated by normal flora, and collection of a diagnostic specimen is challenging. In general, lesions that can be aspirated or biopsied provide more reliable specimens than those collected on swabs. Since mixed infections are not infrequent, multiple samples should be taken whenever possible to screen for multiple likely agents.

External Genitalia

GENITAL ULCERS

Herpes genitalis, Chancroid, Lymphogranuloma venereum (LGV), Syphilis, Tularemia, Candidiasis

The lesion should be cleansed with sterile saline, and the surface removed with a sterile scalpel blade. If syphilis is suspected, a glass slide should be touched to the fluid, a coverslip added, and the preparation delivered to the laboratory in a humid chamber for dark-field examination. Alternatively, the edges of the coverslip can be sealed with petroleum jelly to minimize evaporation, since *Treponema pallidum* is very sensitive to desiccation. The slides must be read as soon as possible in either event. Air-dried smears may also be submitted for staining with a fluorescent antibody. Specimen should be collected on 3 successive days before the lesions are considered to be negative.[38]

In addition, transudate should be allowed to accumulate, and the base of the lesion pressed firmly with sterile swabs to collect multiple samples, if possible, for the following:

1. One swab should be used to inoculate plates of selective media if chancroid is suspected, since *Haemophilus ducreyi* does not survive well in transport media.
2. A second swab should be used to prepare smears for staining with immunofluorescence or immunoperoxidase reagents for HSV and *C. trachomatis.*
3. The same or additional swab should then be placed in a *Chlamydia* transport tube. This specimen may then be cultured for viruses and *C. trachomatis.*

4. If ELISA or nucleic acid probes are to be used, special transport tubes may be required.

5. A wet mount of a scraping from the lesion may reveal the presence of *Candida* spp.

6. The laboratory requires prior notification in the unlikely event that *Francisella tularensis* is suspected (flea, tick, mosquito bite, or association with animals by patient), since specialized media and additional safety precautions are necessary.

Granuloma Inguinale

If the lesion has a beefy red, velvety, ulcerative appearance, a biopsy should be taken from the edge of the lesion and stained with Wright or Giemsa stain to look for typical Donovan bodies. These appear as large, darkly staining bacilli in the cytoplasm of large mononuclear cells and are typical of infections due to *Calymmatobacterium granulomatis*. Alternatively, scrapings taken from the edge of the lesion or granulation tissue collected by a scalpel and crushed between two microscope slides may be stained to detect the typical structures.[38]

Inguinal Adenopathy

Infections of the external genitalia caused by some of the aforementioned agents (HSV, *C. trachomatis* [LGV], *H. ducreyi*, *T. pallidum*) may be accompanied by inguinal adenopathy or by the formation of a granuloma (*C. granulomatis*) leading to the appearance of inguinal buboes ("pseudobuboes" in the case of *C. granulomatis*). If fluctuant, the buboes of suspected cases of chancroid and LGV may be aspirated, and the material submitted for culture. Part of the specimen should be inoculated directly for isolation of *H. ducreyi* and submitted at room temperature. The other portion should be placed in *Chlamydia* transport media and kept on ice or refrigerated if immediate inoculation is not possible. (*Note:* If LGV is suspected, paired serum specimens should be submitted for serologic testing.)

Other conditions that may exhibit genital ulcers include amebiasis, histoplasmosis, mycobacteriosis, trichomoniasis, Behçet's syndrome, malignancy, trauma, or fixed drug eruptions.[39]

VESICLES AND BULLAE

Herpes Genitalis, Varicella, Scabies

The surface of the lesion should be cleansed with sterile saline. If possible, fluid should be aspirated with a 26- or 27-gauge needle into a tuberculin syringe. If aspiration is nonproductive or is not possible, the surface of lesion should be removed with a sterile scalpel blade. The transudate should be allowed to accumulate, and the base of lesion pressed firmly with a sterile swab. The swab should be placed in viral transport medium and delivered to the laboratory at 4°C.

Vesicles appearing on the buttocks and other perigenital areas may be due to VZV. The correct etiology may be made by shell vial or conventional cell culture of specimens collected as described earlier.

Scabies may occasionally cause vesicles or bullous lesions, but more typical lesions are described later.

Genital Tuberculosis

In rare instances, ulcers or vesicles caused by *Mycobacterium tuberculosis* may be found in the vulva[40] and regions adjacent to the external genitalia (in cases of cutaneous tuberculosis). The area should be cleansed with 70% alcohol, and, if possible, material should be aspirated from under the margin of a lesion. The aspirate should be placed in a small volume (0.5 mL) of 7H9 broth or Amies or Stuart's media for transport to the laboratory.[41] Alternatively, a biopsy can be taken from the periphery of the lesion, which is then placed in a sterile container for immediate transport to the laboratory. Specimens should be stained with an acid-fast stain and inoculated for culture.

SIMPLE PAPULES

These red, elevated areas that are solid and circumscribed are often the transient state of several genital infections, including primary or secondary syphilis, scabies, LGV, chancroid, herpes, human papillomavirus (HPV) infection, candidiasis, and molluscum contagiosum.[39] If more typical lesions are not present, the papules should be scraped with a scalpel after disinfecting with 70% alcohol, pain level permitting, or washed with an antibacterial soap. A clean glass slide should be used to touch any exudate that accumulates and the specimen examined by dark-field illumination for *T. pallidum*. The scrapings should be inoculated directly for *H. ducreyi* and/or placed in *Chlamydia* transport medium for cultivation of *C. trachomatis*. A biopsy of the papule may be processed for HPV detection, and microscopic examination will reveal the mite, eggs, and/or fecal pellets of *Sarcoptes scabiei*.

VERRUCOUS PAPULES

Condyloma Acuminatum

Small, fleshy vascular growths resembling cauliflowers may be found on the external genitalia (as well as the vaginal wall, cervix, and anus). These growths, condylomata acuminata or genital warts, should be biopsied. If possible, the specimen should be bisected, and one half fixed and embedded in paraffin for a permanent record; the other half should be placed in a transport medium appropriate for hybridization tests for detection of HPV.

Flat lesions due to HPV may also be present in the vulva region (as well as the cervix). These may be visualized by culdoscopic examination after application of acetic acid.[42] These areas should be biopsied and submitted for hybridization tests.

UMBILICATED LESIONS

Venereum Molluscum

Firm, umbilicated nodules that are pearly and flesh-colored may be found on the labia majora as well as on the thighs and buttocks. To confirm a diagnosis of venereum molluscum, caused by *Molluscum contagiosum virus* (MCV), the lesion should be squeezed to express white caseous material which is collected on a swab, or the lesion may be removed by curettage. The specimen should be crushed on a slide and stained with Wright's, Giemsa, or Gram stains. Microscopic examination reveals the presence of large intracytoplasmic "molluscum bodies" within the cells.[39] Electron microscopy of negatively stained preparations may also be used to visualize the virus.

DIFFUSE ERYTHEMA

Infection with *Candida* spp. may sometimes cause diffuse reddening in the vulvovaginal area. A scraping of the area with a scalpel blade examined by wet mount demonstrates typical yeast cells and/or pseudohyphae if present. Other causes of diffuse erythema include contact dermatitis, fixed drug eruption, or trauma.[39]

CUTANEOUS BURROWS, PRURITIC PAPULAR RASH, AND NODULES

Scabies

The presence of burrows that are 5 to 10 mm in length in the skin and are accompanied by an intensely pruritic rash and nodules is pathognomonic for the presence of *Sarcoptes scabiei*, the agent of scabies. To confirm the diagnosis, visualization of the skin burrows may be accomplished with the use of a hand lens. Visualization may be enhanced by applying mineral oil to the skin. Saturating the skin area with liquid ink will also demonstrate areas of burrowing. Covering the skin area with a solution of tetracycline in alcohol and viewing the area under a Wood's light will detect fluorescent yellow or green lines, indicating the burrows in which the solution was retained. Alternatively, skin scrapings may be taken in the area of the burrows, placed on a microscope slide, and examined with 25× or 50× magnification to detect the mites, eggs, and/or fecal pellets.[43]

ABRASION-LIKE RASH WITH PALE BLUE-GRAY MACULAE

Pediculosis Pubis

Intense itching in the pubic area should suggest infestation with *Phthirus pubis*, the crab louse. The clinical diagnosis is confirmed by examination of the affected area with a magnifying glass to observe the louse, larvae, and nits in the pubic area. Alternatively, a pubic hair may be plucked and examined for the organism.[43]

CRUSTED LESIONS

A dry scab may be observed in older, healing lesions of herpesvirus. These do not contain viable agents and should not be cultured. Crusts or scabs are also typical of scabies but may be accompanied by moist papules or burrows.[39] These specimens should be collected and examined as described earlier.

Vaginal Infections and Syndromes

Active Infection Due to HSV, T. pallidum, HPV, Trichomonas, Candida, Bacterial Vaginosis, C. trachomatis, or the Presence of Atrophic Vaginitis

LESIONS

Lesions typical of HSV, *T. pallidum*, and HPV that appear in the vulvar area may also appear on the walls of the vagina, as well as the cervix, and should be sampled as described earlier. In addition, the presence of a mucopurulent or watery discharge within the vagina suggests a diagnosis of vaginitis, due to *T. vaginalis* or *Candida* spp., or bacterial vaginosis (BV) due to an overgrowth of anaerobic, pleiomorphic gram-negative organisms and a decrease in the levels of *Lactobacillus* spp.

EXUDATE OR VAGINAL SECRETIONS

Excess discharge should be removed with a sterile swab. An aliquot of the vaginal pool or scraping of a white plaque from the vaginal wall, if present, should be mixed with a drop of sterile saline. A cover slip should be added, and the wet preparation examined microscopically. Findings depend on the causative agent and may include (1) motile trophozoites of *Trichomonas vaginalis*; (2) hyphal forms interspersed with epithelial cells, suggestive of *Candida* vaginitis; (3) epithelial cells covered with small rod-shaped bacteria and relatively few gram-positive bacilli *(Lactobacillus)*, suggestive of BV.

A second preparation should be prepared and a drop of 10% KOH added. If the preparation emits a definite "fishy" amine odor, bacterial vaginosis is suggested and should be confirmed by Gram stain (separate preparation) in which the relative numbers of *Lactobacillus*-appearing organisms and pleomorphic gram-negative rods attached to epithelial cells are evaluated. A coverslip should be added, and the preparation examined after approximately 5 minutes. This procedure will clarify the epithelial cells and allow fungal cells to be more easily visualized, if present. Culture may be more sensitive than wet mount for the detection of *T. vaginalis*, and commercial formulations of media are available. In addition, fluorescent, immunofluorescent, and EIAs as well as a nucleic acid probe may be used. See the second section of this chapter.

ENDOCERVIX

Other causes of purulent discharge to be observed in the vagina include cervicitis due to *C. trachomatis*, first-episode HSV cervicitis, or atrophic vaginitis. If the patient is otherwise asymptomatic, an endocervical specimen should be collected with a swab or cytobrush for analysis for the presence of *C. trachomatis* or HSV. Atrophic vaginitis should be considered if the patient complains of spotting, burning, or pruritus.

Screening Cultures for Group B Beta-Hemolytic Streptococcus in Pregnancy

VAGINAL WALL, ENDOCERVIX, ANAL SWAB

Specimens of the vaginal wall, cervix, and anal orifice should be taken from expectant mothers of infants who are at high risk for developing group B streptococcal sepsis; that is, premature labor, premature rupture of membranes over 12 hours at any gestational age, and fever during labor. The swabs should be used to inoculate a colistin–nalidixic acid (CNA) blood agar plate and then be placed in Todd-Hewitt broth with sheep blood and antibiotics. The swab containing broth is incubated until turbidity develops or for 24 hours. The broth is then used to inoculate a CNA plate for recovery of the organism or for testing with commercially available antigen detection systems (EIA, latex agglutination) or nucleic acid probe.[38]

EXUDATE

Group B streptococci can occasionally cause a purulent vaginitis, in which case a Gram stain smear of vaginal secretions revealing numerous polymorphonuclear cells and a predominance of gram-positive cocci in chains may lead to an early presumptive diagnosis.[38] Culture confirmation is recommended.

Screening Cultures for Listeria moncytogenes

VAGINA, ENDOCERVIX

In suspected cases of listeriosis in a prepartum or postpartum patient, a sterile swab should be used to sample the epithelial surface of the vaginal wall, as well as the endocervix. The swabs should be placed in transport medium, such as Stuart's modified medium, and cultured aerobically. A cold enrichment procedure may be performed, in which case the specimen is placed in the refrigerator (4°C) for at least 4 weeks and inoculated weekly.

BLOOD, PRODUCTS OF CONCEPTION, PLACENTA

Better specimens for the recovery of *L. moncytogenes* include blood cultures of symptomatic mothers or newborns, products of conception, or placenta.[38] See the sections on tissues and chorioamnionitis later.

Screening Cultures for HSV in Pregnancy

LESIONS, VAGINAL SWABS

Specimens of lesions should be sampled as described previously anytime a pregnant patient is noted to have developed them and at 3- to 5-day intervals if present near the time of delivery; that is, after 36 weeks of gestation. In pregnant patients with a history of HSV for herself or partner and with no visible lesions during the pregnancy or at the time of birth, vaginal specimens should be obtained at delivery and cultured for HSV.[44]

NEONATAL SPECIMENS

Neonatal specimens of conjunctiva, throat, and urine should be collected and cultured for HSV if the newborn is asymptomatic, and skin lesions and CSF should be collected and cultured if the newborn is symptomatic. The infant's blood may also be tested for the presence of anti-HSV IgM antibody.

Screening Cultures for Staphylococcus aureus and Streptococcus pyogenes in Toxic Shock Syndrome

Patients at risk for toxic shock syndrome due to *S. aureus* include females using tampons during menstruation, and postpartum and postsurgical patients with wound infections. Cases of toxic shock–like syndrome due to *Streptococcus pyogenes* (group A *Streptococcus*) have been observed in patients with bartholinitis, septic abortion, cervicitis, postpartum endometritis, and intrauterine device (IUD)–related infections.[38]

VAGINAL SWAB

Specimens of the epithelial wall of the vagina should be collected with a swab and placed in appropriate transport medium (i.e., modified Stuart's) and cultured for *S. aureus* and *S. pyogenes*. The swab should be transported to the laboratory for immediate inoculation. Isolates of *S. aureus* may be sent to reference laboratories for toxin testing if desired.[38]

Cervical Infections

As suggested earlier, the presence of a purulent discharge in the vagina may indicate an infection of the cervix. On the other hand, the cervix may be infected in the absence of lesions or symptomatology in the vagina or external genitalia.

Neisseria gonorrhoeae, Chlamydia trachomatis

ENDOCERVICAL SWAB, SCRAPINGS OR BRUSHINGS

The most common causes of cervicitis accompanied with a discharge are *N. gonorrhoeae* and *C. trachomatis*.

Specimens should be collected to detect both organisms, since they commonly occur together. Excess discharge should be removed from the cervix with a large cotton-tipped applicator. Separate swabs or cytobrush specimens should be obtained by inserting the collection device into the cervical os and rubbing vigorously the cervical transition zone and endocervical canal to obtain cells and secretions.

The specimen for detection of *N. gonorrhoeae* should be used for direct inoculation onto Thayer-Martin or other GC medium, placed in a transport bag designed for providing an atmosphere enriched with CO_2, and delivered to the laboratory. The specimen for detection of *C. trachomatis* should be placed in *Chlamydia* transport media and transported on ice. Smears may also be made for immunofluorescence staining. Special transport media may be required if EIA, hybridization, or amplification studies are to be performed.

Herpes Simplex Virus

Cervicitis due to HSV may be asymptomatic or accompanied by a copious, clear discharge. The cervix should always be examined for typical herpes lesions whether or not external lesions are present when one screens for agents responsible for a vaginal discharge. *Lidocaine gel or ointment should be placed on the vulva prior to inserting a vaginal speculum to decrease the level of discomfort from any external lesions that may be present.*[45]

Specimens for HSV should be obtained after removing the top of the lesion, if possible, firmly rubbing the base of the lesion, and collecting the fluid on a swab. One swab should be placed in viral transport medium and delivered to the laboratory on ice. A second swab should be used to prepare smears for immunofluorescence staining.

Cytomegalovirus, Calymmatobacterium granulomatis, Human Papillomavirus

Other causes of asymptomatic cervicitis include CMV, *C. granulomatis*, and HPV. Examination may reveal absent or minimal clinical findings or extensive cervical erosion with CMV infection. The greatest risk of serious infection and sequelae in newborns from CMV infection is in those born to mothers who experience a primary infection early during pregnancy. Since most of these infections are asymptomatic, many will not be diagnosed.

ENDOCERVIX, URINE, SERUM, AMNIOTIC FLUID FOR CMV

In the cases in which screening for CMV is desired, the simplest approach is to collect endocervical and urine specimens for viral isolation. These should be delivered to the laboratory on ice and kept at 4°C for no longer than 72 hours before inoculation into tissue

culture. A serum sample may also be collected and tested for the presence of anti-CMV IgM antibodies. Alternatively, amniocentesis may be performed, and the amniotic fluid cultured for the virus. Samples of fetal blood obtained by fetoscopy or cordocentesis may be collected in an effort to detect elevated levels of anti-CMV IgM.[46]

Calymmatobacterium granulomatis

BIOPSY

If a beefy red ulcer typical of donovanosis is seen, a biopsy specimen should be taken and stained with Wright's or Giemsa staining as described previously for external genitalia.

Human Papillomavirus

BIOPSY OR EPITHELIAL SCRAPINGS

If wart-like lesions typical of HPV are seen, a biopsy should be obtained that is at least 5 mm in cross-section. If flat lesions are suspected, scrapings of the cervix should be obtained. Both specimens should be placed in appropriate transport media and submitted for liquid hybridization studies, if available. The manufacturer's instructions for storage and shipping must be followed. The specimens may also be prepared routinely for histologic examination and/or in situ hybridization. The laboratory diagnosis of HPV is important not only as detection of a sexually transmitted disease but also for obtaining prognostic information on the development of cervical intraepithelial hyperplasia, which appears to be associated with specific subtypes of the virus and which can be identified by some available reagents.

Genital Tract Infections: Upper

The endogenous microflora of the lower genital tract may spread to regions of the upper genital tract, causing infection in this internal site. The upward migration is also possible for exogenous pathogens that may intermittently be introduced into the lower genital tract. A summary of upper genital tract infections, risk factors involved, and probable pathogens is presented in Table 57–7.

Intra-amniotic Infection (Chorioamnionitis)

Pregnant patients may develop clinical signs of chorioamnionitis (e.g., fever, leukocytosis, tachycardia) with or without ruptured membranes or preterm labor. However, patients who present with premature rupture of membranes or preterm labor in the absence of those symptoms should be suspected of having a sub-

TABLE 57-7 ▶	SUMMARY OF PELVIC (AND RELATED) INFECTIONS, RISK FACTORS, AND LIKELY PATHOGENS		
Type of Infection	**Risk Factors**	**Specimens**	**Likely Pathogens[a]**
Chorioamniotis	Premature rupture of membranes Premature labor	Amniotic fluid Placenta (optional) Endocervical swab Blood, urine	*Streptococcus agalactiae, Escherichia coli, Gardnerella vaginalis, Mycoplasma hominis, Ureaplasma urealyticum,* other indigenous microflora, HSV, CMV
Endomyometritis	Sexually transmitted disease Pelvic inflammatory disease Cesarean section Bacterial vaginosis (BV)	Endometrial aspirate	*Chlamydia trachomatis, Neisseria gonorrhoeae, S. agalactiae, G. vaginalis,* enterococci, *E. coli,* anaerobes, other indigenous flora
Pelvic cellulitis	Hysterectomy (with BV)	Peritoneal fluid via culdocentesis	Indigenous microflora
Peritonitis	Hysterectomy or other surgery Abortion or abdominal focus of infection	Peritoneal fluid via paracentesis	*N. gonorrhoeae, C. trachomatis, Mycobacterium tuberculosis,* indigenous microflora
Pelvic abscess other than TOA	Cesarean section Hysterectomy or other surgery Abdominal focus of infection	Percutaneous aspirate of abscess Aspirate of abscess at surgery Abscess wall collected at surgery	Indigenous flora, frequently including *Bacteroides fragilis*
Abdominal wound infection	Cesarean section, hysterectomy, other abdominal surgery	Aspirate of closed wound; swab and advancing edge of open wound	*Streptococcus* spp., *Clostridium* spp., indigenous microflora
Necrotizing fasciitis	Abdominal wound	Débrided tissue	*Streptococcus* spp., *Clostridium* spp., other indigenous microflora
Septic pelvic thrombophlebitis	Cesarean section, hysterectomy, other surgery ? (SF)	Serum for hematology and PTT testing Blood, urine Endometrial aspirate	*Note:* Usually diagnosed by CT scan and sonography in patients with previous pelvic infection
Pelvic inflammatory disease	Sexually transmitted disease Abortion Vaginal delivery	Endocervical swab Endometrial aspirate Peritoneal fluid via culdocentesis Fallopian tube at surgery	*N. gonorrhoeae, C. trachomatis,* indigenous microflora
Tubo-ovarian abscess	Pelvic inflammatory disease	Percutaneous aspirate of abscess Aspirate of abscess at surgery Abscess wall collected at surgery	*N. gonorrhoeae, C. trachomatis,* indigenous microflora

[a]Indigenous microflora = *Enterococcus, S. aureus, S. epidermidis, Klebsiella, Proteus mirabilis, Peptostreptococcus, Bacteroides fragilis* group, *Prevotella (Bacteroides) bivius, Prevotella (Bacteroides) disiens, Fusobacterum.*

clinical infection of the uterine cavity. The specimens that should be collected include the following:

AMNIOTIC FLUID

In any suspected case of intra-amniotic infection, specimens of amniotic fluid should be collected via amniocentesis, from an intrauterine catheter, or at the time of delivery by cesarean section. Specimens of the placenta and maternal-fetal membranes may be examined as well. Multiple agents have been associated with chorioamnionitis, such as various anaerobic and aerobic bacterial species, including genital *Mycoplasma* spp., *S. agalactiae* (group B *Streptococcus*), and *E. coli* (see Table 57–7).

Amniocentesis. The abdomen is disinfected with the same technique described for collecting blood specimens. At least 1 mL of fluid should be aspirated.

Intrauterine Catheter. If not already placed, a catheter should be passed through the endocervical canal and into the uterus. The first 7 mL aspirated with needle and syringe is discarded in an effort to prevent contamination from vaginal flora. One milliliter of fluid should be withdrawn with a new needle and syringe.[47]

Cesarean Section. One milliliter of fluid should be collected by aspiration at the time of delivery by cesarean section.

One drop of unspun fluid should be placed on a microscope slide for staining, and the remainder should be expelled into an anaerobic transport device for delivery to the laboratory at room temperature. If viral or chlamydial etiology is suspected, a 1-mL specimen should be placed in a sterile, conical centrifuge tube and taken to the laboratory on ice. If isolation attempts for *Mycoplasma* spp. are to be made, the specimen should be inoculated within 1 hour after collection. Otherwise, the fluid should be diluted 1:10 in transport medium and kept at 4°C until inoculation. Suitable transport media for *Mycoplasma* include 2SP, Shepard's 10B or SP4 media supplemented with antibiotics, or trypticase soy broth with 0.5% bovine serum albumin.[38]

Note: Quantitative inoculation, as with a 0.01-mL loop, may be useful in differentiating a predominant pathogen from contaminating organisms.[47]

PLACENTA

The placenta is a difficult tissue to analyze because of its size and extent of contamination, especially if delivered vaginally. However, for instances in which it is desirable to ascertain the presence and extent of infection within the placenta, the following approach has been successfully used as a research tool.[48] The complete placenta should be placed in a sterile bag and transported to the laboratory for processing within 12 hours of delivery. Both microbiologic and histologic studies should be performed:

1. For microbiologic examination, the placenta should be placed on a clean surface and the chorion and amnion separated and peeled apart. Care should be taken to prevent contamination of the exposed surfaces by the placenta or the environment. Multiple sterile swabs should be used to sample the exposed surface of the extraplacental membrane at least 4 cm from the site of rupture. Two swabs should be placed in anaerobic transport devices and used for preparation of smears for gram staining and cultivation of aerobes, facultatives, and anaerobes. Other swabs should be placed in appropriate transport medium and kept at 4°C for delivery to the laboratory and isolation attempts for *Mycoplasma hominis, U. urealyticum,* and *C. trachomatis* (see Table 57-3). For enhanced recovery of *M. hominis* and *U. urealyticum,* some practitioners recommend vigorously agitating the swab in transport medium, expressing excess liquid, and discarding the swab.[38]

2. For histologic examination, the chorioamnion should be grasped with forceps and a sample that is 2 to 3 cm wide should be cut from the point of rupture to the placental margin. With the site of rupture at the center, a "membrane roll" should be made by rolling the fetal membranes into a 1-mm wooden dowel. The membrane should then be fixed in 10% neutral buffered formalin, embedded in paraffin, and stained with hematoxylin and eosin. A suggested interpretation of histologically confirmed chorioamnionitis is observation of at least 10 polymorphonuclear leukocytes per field in 10 nonadjacent 400× power fields.

ENDOCERVIX

Endocervical swabs should be collected to screen for *S. agalactiae* (group B *Streptococcus*), *N. gonorrhoeae, C. trachomatis,* HSV, or CMV, and vaginal specimens should be examined for *T. vaginalis* if patient's history or clinical presentation is suggestive of these organisms. See previous section on external genitalia for collection and handling of these specimens.

BLOOD

Two to three specimens of blood should be collected over a 24-hour period, especially in the presence of fever, to rule out bacteremia or septicemia.

URINE

A urine specimen should be obtained for Gram stain and culture to rule out urinary tract infection, particularly pyelonephritis. Specimens of urine can also be submitted for amplification for detection of *N. gonorrhoeae* and *C. trachomatis.*

OTHER MARKERS OF INFECTION

The detection of leukocyte esterase, by either a dip stick or spectrophotometric method, and decreased levels of amniotic fluid glucose levels may be helpful in supporting the diagnosis of intra-amniotic infection.[47]

Postpartum and/or Postoperative Infections

Infections in the pelvic area not associated with consequences of a sexually transmitted disease are generally associated with obstetric or gynecologic procedures (e.g., cesarean section, hysterectomy). Furthermore, patients subjected to obstetric or gynecologic surgical procedures are at risk for developing the same complications as those of other postsurgical patients. These include bacteremia or septicemia, aspiration pneumonia, urinary tract infections, and wound infections. See the sections on blood infections, respiratory tract infections, urinary tract infections, and wound infections for descriptions of appropriate specimens for collection. In addition, pelvic abscesses and peritonitis may be secondary to nongynecologic or obstetric conditions, such as appendicitis and diverticulitis.

ENDOMYOMETRITIS

1. **Endometrial Biopsy.** Obtaining an uncontaminated specimen of the endometrium while passing through the heavily contaminated vagina and cervix requires special care. Protected swabs, suction-curettes, or other protected devices should be used in an effort to collect an adequate specimen. One such double-lumen collection device has been reported to provide an

adequate sample from the endometrium.[49] The specimen should be placed in an anaerobic transport tube for delivery to the laboratory at room temperature. The etiologic agents of endometritis are usually polymicrobial mixtures of endogenous flora that include aerobic, facultative, and anaerobic bacteria. However, isolates of *M. hominis* and *U. urealyticum* have also been recovered, either in mixed or pure cultures,[38] but their significance is difficult to ascertain. The specimen should be placed in appropriate transport medium and transported on ice if these organisms are suspected.

2. **Cervical Swab.** In addition to the endometrial culture, cervical specimens may be collected with a swab to screen for *S. pyogenes, S. agalactiae,* and *N. gonorrhoeae,* owing to the implication that the presence of these organisms may have on isolation procedures for the mother, in the case of *S. pyogenes,* as well as implications for examination of the newborn, in the case of *S. agalactiae* and *N. gonorrhoeae.* Specimens should be collected as described for cervicitis.

3. **Blood Cultures.** Since many cases of endometritis are accompanied by bacteremia, two sets of blood cultures should be obtained during a 24-hour period. A correlation between endometrial culture results and organisms isolated from the blood must be made to determine what significance the blood isolate has on the infectious process and to the management of the patient.

4. **Cul-de-sac Aspirate.** A specimen of fluid from the cul-de-sac may be aspirated in cases of postpartum endometritis, in which case information obtained from the Gram stain and/or culture of that specimen could significantly affect the management of the patient. See description of pelvic cellulitis, below. This procedure should not be performed in posthysterectomy patients who have an adynamic ileus.[50]

PELVIC CELLULITIS

Peritoneal Fluid via Culdocentesis
The appropriate specimen for detecting the causative agent or agents for pelvic cellulitis is peritoneal fluid obtained via culdocentesis.[51] Prior to the procedure, the methods to be used and the reasons for performing them should be explained to the patient. The patient should be placed in the lithotomy position with her head elevated. A bimanual examination should be performed to determine whether the uterus is retroverted, retroflexed, or antiverted. The bimanual examination also determines whether the uterus is tender, whether there are any adnexal masses, and whether the cul-de-sac is clear.

A sterile speculum is placed in the vagina after cleansing the vulva with an antiseptic solution. The vagina and cervix are also thoroughly cleansed with an antiseptic, such as povidone-iodine solution. The anterior lip of the cervix should be grasped with a single-tooth tenaculum and pulled forward and upward to allow the posterior vaginal fornix to come into full view. Any excess povidone-iodine should be allowed to dry. Local infiltration with an agent such as 1% lidocaine should be used to anesthetize an area in the posterior vaginal fornix. An 18-gauge spinal needle may then be used to aspirate fluid from the cul-de-sac.[50] The fluid should be expelled into an anaerobic transport device and delivered to the laboratory at room temperature for gram-staining and cultivation of facultative and anaerobic organisms.

PELVIC ABSCESS, OTHER THAN TUBO-OVARIAN ABSCESS

If possible, material from the abscess may be aspirated percutaneously with an 18-gauge spinal syringe under sonographic direction after the overlaying skin area has been disinfected. The material should be placed in an anaerobic transport device and sent to the laboratory for gram-staining and cultivation of facultative and anaerobic organisms.

If laparoscopy is required, not only should material be aspirated from the abscess but also tissue from the abscess wall should be submitted in an anaerobic transport device for gram-staining and cultivation attempts for facultative and anaerobic organisms.

PERITONITIS

See previous section on pelvic cellulitis and subsequent section on intra-abdominal infections.

SEPTIC PELVIC THROMBOPHLEBITIS

This condition should be suspected whenever a patient has experienced a prior pelvic infection, continues to have fever spikes despite appropriate antibiotic therapy, and signs of pelvic mass or abscess or other obvious causes of fever are lacking. The diagnosis is usually one of exclusion, but computerized axial topography and sonography may be helpful in visualizing the thrombosis.[52, 53] The diagnosis is "confirmed" by a relatively rapid clinical response to heparin. If the patient remains febrile at 36 hours following heparin therapy, pelvic abscess may be suspected.[54] Specimens for culture should be collected at laparoscopy, as described previously for pelvic abscess.

VAGINAL CUFF ABSCESS

Exudate. Purulent material should be aspirated. The specimen should be expelled into an anaerobic transport device and delivered to the laboratory for gram-staining and cultivation of facultative and anaerobic organisms.

Blood. In addition, two blood cultures should be collected over a 24-hour period.

PELVIC INFLAMMATORY DISEASE (PID)

The clinical diagnosis of PID is challenging. The same is true for the laboratory diagnosis. The most definitive procedures involve laparoscopy or laparotomy for visualization and collection of specimens, but they are expensive and logistically difficult for the large number of patients who present with clinical symptoms suggestive of PID. On the other hand, the clinical scenarios that are considered to be part of the differential diagnosis (i.e., ectopic pregnancy and acute appendicitis) may be life-threatening situations and require accuracy of diagnosis. The laboratory procedures that are used, then, will be mandated by the severity of the presentation and the patient's history.

Specimens that may be collected are as follows:

▶ **Fimbrial or Fallopian Tube Biopsy Taken at Laparoscopy.** The specimen should be divided, and one half placed in anaerobic transport, the other half in *Chlamydia* transport medium.

▶ **Specimens from the Tubal Lumen.** A urogenital Dacron or calcium alginate swab or bronchoscopy cytologic brush should be inserted into the tube, pressed against the wall of the tube, and withdrawn. If blocked, the contents of the tube may be aspirated with needle and syringe. Specimens should be placed in anaerobic transport medium and *Chlamydia* transport medium.

▶ **Peritoneal Fluid Taken at Laparoscopy.** Fluid should be aspirated with needle and syringe. Part of the specimen should be expelled into an anaerobic transport device and the other part into *Chlamydia* transport medium.

▶ **Endometrial Biopsy.** A double-lumen catheter should be used as described under the section on endomyometritis earlier. Part of the specimen should be placed in a sterile container for histopathology (to look for plasma cell endometritis), one part in anaerobic transport and one part in *Chlamydia* transport medium. If granulomatous salpingitis is suspected, the specimen should be collected just prior to menses, at which time the most common causative organism *(M. tuberculosis)* is at the maximal stage of growth and may be more easily seen in acid-fast stained smears.[55]

▶ **Peritoneal Fluid Collected by Culdocentesis.** See section on pelvic cellulitis earlier. Part of the specimen should be placed in an anaerobic transport device and the other part in *Chlamydia* transport medium.

▶ **Endocervical Specimen.** See section on cervical infections earlier. The specimen should be submitted for detection of *N. gonorrhoeae* and *C. trachomatis* only. Cultivation for anaerobes from this specimen is not recommended.

▶ **Intrauterine Device.** The entire device plus associated exudate should be placed in a sterile urine cup, which is then placed in a self-contained anaerobic atmosphere–generating bag for delivery to the laboratory for processing.

▶ **Menstrual Blood.** In cases of granulomatous salpingitis, a sterile, disposable, plastic pipette should be used to aspirate as much menstrual blood as possible for processing and cultivation attempts for *M. tuberculosis.*

▶ **Other Tests.** Other diagnostic tests or approaches include C-reactive protein (CRP) and erythrocyte sedimentation rate (ESR), both of which have been reported to be elevated in cases of PID, but these are certainly not specific tests for PID.[56] Transabdominal ultrasound and/or transvaginal sonography have also been used to facilitate the diagnosis of PID.[57, 58]

Microorganisms typically associated with PID include exogenous organisms such as *N. gonorrhoeae* and *C. trachomatis*, as well as endogenous mixed aerobic and anaerobic flora. *Actinomyces israelii*, an anaerobic gram-positive rod not considered to be part of the normal flora of the genital tract, is associated with cases of PID in patients who have had an intrauterine device in place.[59, 60]

TUBO-OVARIAN ABSCESS (TOA)

A TOA is a potential consequence of previous episodes of PID but can also be found in patients who have recently experienced postpartum endometritis or who have undergone a hysterectomy or other surgical procedures of the female genital tract. Diagnosis may be clinically aided by sonography and CT scanning.[57] These techniques are usually employed in patients who cannot be examined because of tenderness and pain or who do not respond to antibiotics within 48 to 72 hours. Specimens should be collected from the endocervix and cul-de-sac if possible and transported in an anaerobic transport device.

If surgical intervention is required, the abscess should be sampled with a needle and syringe, and the specimen expelled into an anaerobic transport device. A portion of the abscess wall should also be collected and placed in an anaerobic transport device. The microorganisms usually involved are those associated with PID (see Table 57–7).

Postabortion Infections

Endometritis, salpingitis, and peritonitis may develop following induced abortions owing to uterine perforation, the presence of necrotic debris, and retained placental products. Specimens for laboratory evaluation should be taken from the cervix, endometrium, fallopian tube, and peritoneal fluid, and two sets of blood cultures obtained as described in earlier sections. Infections may be due to a single organism or may be polymicrobial. Bacteremia, when present, may also be polymicrobial. Clostridial sepsis and myometrial necrosis are potentially lethal complications.[38]

Intra-abdominal Infections

Appendicitis

Appendicitis is usually diagnosed clinically and requires surgical removal of the inflamed organ. When the identity of the specific etiologic agent or agents is required, part of the appendix should be placed in an anaerobic transport device and transported to the laboratory at room temperature for culture. If the appendix ruptures prior to surgery, spreading peritonitis may result. This infection is most often polymicrobial and is due to anaerobes, primarily *Bacteroides fragilis*, *Prevotella melaninogenica*, anaerobic gram-positive cocci, and Enterobacteriaceae.[61] See the description of peritonitis that follows.

Diverticulitis

Inflammation of herniations of the colon through the muscular layer of abdominal organs is the most frequent complication of diverticulosis. Further complications include perforation with pericolic abscess to which adjacent viscera and omentum become adherent, fistula formation, or, infrequently, free perforation with spreading peritonitis. The passage of flatus or fecal material through the vagina indicates fistulas into the uterus or vagina. Since the causative organisms are those found in feces, cultivation attempts with peritoneal fluid would be labor-intensive and possibly unrewarding.[61] Blood cultures may be of greater value.

Peritonitis

In adults, primary peritonitis is most often associated with cirrhosis and ascites. In women, however, it is often associated with a gonococcal perihepatitis (Fitz-Hugh–Curtis syndrome), in which case the infecting organism has presumably migrated from the infected fallopian tube into the peritoneum. Secondary peritonitis follows one of many possible diseases of the GI tract, such as perforation of a peptic ulcer, traumatic perforation of the uterus, appendicitis, diverticulitis, infections of the female genital tract such as septic abortion, and postpartum and postsurgical conditions, described earlier.[61]

PERITONEAL FLUID VIA PARACENTESIS

In cases in which infection of the upper peritoneum is suspected, paracentesis should be performed. While the patient is in a sitting position, an area of the abdomen 3 to 5 cm below the umbilicus should be decontaminated with tincture of iodine. After administering a local anesthetic, the skin is opened with a scalpel and a dialysis catheter is placed into the pouch of Douglas. This procedure may be guided by ultrasound. Fluid is aspirated, if possible, with a needle and syringe through the catheter. If no fluid can be aspirated, washings with sterile saline should be performed and the fluid collected in a sterile container.[62] If gross blood or intestinal contents are recovered, a laparotomy should be performed.

In either case, an aliquot of the fluid should be cytocentrifuged and a drop of the sediment used for gram-staining. The remainder should be used to inoculate media for recovery of likely agents. Organisms associated with primary peritonitis include *S. pneumoniae*, *Enterococcus*, other *Streptococcus* spp., *N. gonorrhoeae*, *C. trachomatis*, *M. tuberculosis*, *C. immitis*, and enteric organisms. Organisms associated with secondary peritonitis include a polymicrobial mixture of anaerobes and facultative organisms.[61] It should be noted, however, that peritoneal fluid cultures may be unrewarding owing to perforation of the gut and fecal contamination.

BLOOD

Bacteremia occurs in up to 75% of cases of primary peritonitis and usually consists of aerobic organisms only. Bacteremia occurs in 20% to 30% of cases of secondary peritonitis and consists of anaerobic or facultative organisms. Hence, at least two blood cultures should also be collected in a 24-hour period in suspected cases of peritonitis.[61]

Perinatal and Congenital Infections

The major clinical symptoms, preferred specimens, and probable pathogens or perinatal or congenital infections are listed in Table 57–1. Appropriate specimens for the laboratory diagnosis of these infections should be obtained by a neonatologist or pediatrician using the guidelines that follow.

CONJUNCTIVITIS

Swabs of Exudate. Two swabs should be used to collect samples of purulent exudate from the infected eye or eyes. One should be used to inoculate plates directly for *N. gonorrhoeae* and other aerobic and facultative organisms or should be placed in a transport device that provides an atmosphere enriched in CO_2 for delivery to the laboratory. The second swab should be used to make smears for gram-staining.

Conjunctival Scrapings. After removing exudate with a swab, the clinician should use a new swab to press against the conjunctiva in an effort to recover cellular material. At least two specimens should be taken: one to be used to prepare smears for immunofluorescence staining for *C. trachomatis* or viral agents, the other to be placed in a *Chlamydia* transport medium for culture attempts for *C. trachomatis* or viral agents.

Skin Lesions

Vesicles. The area should be cleansed with a gauze square moistened with sterile saline. Fluid should be aspirated with a needle and syringe, or the base of the lesion may be rubbed firmly with a swab. The specimens should be placed in 1 mL of viral transport medium and delivered on ice for viral isolation attempts. If syphilis is suspected, fluid may be collected with a capillary tube and a drop placed on a clean glass slide for dark-field examination.

Maculopapular Exanthems, Petechiae, or Purpura. The surface of the lesion should be cleansed, as previously described for vesicles. The surface of the lesion should be disrupted by the gauze pad, and the base of the lesion should be firmly sampled with a swab premoistened with viral transport medium. The swab should be placed in viral transport medium and delivered to the laboratory on ice for viral isolation attempts.

Respiratory

Nasopharyngeal Aspirates or Washings (Preferred Specimen). An aspirate can be collected with a No. 8 French 16-inch suction catheter. A washing may be obtained with a rubber suction bulb used to instill and withdraw 3 to 7 mL of buffered saline. Part of the aspirate or washings should be placed in a viral transport media and delivered to the laboratory on ice, and the other portion should be submitted for bacterial culture.

Nasopharyngeal Swabs. If nasopharyngeal aspirates or washings are not possible, a small swab may be placed into the nose after mucus from the nasal passages has been removed. The swab should be moved along the nasal septum to the posterior pharynx and rotated against the mucosa. The swab should then be transported to the laboratory in viral transport medium.

Throat Swabs. Swabs premoistened with viral transport medium should be used to collect cellular material from the oropharynx. The swab may be placed in the same viral transport tube as the nasopharyngeal swab if cultivation attempts are to be made. These specimens may be useful in the detection of HSV and CMV, particularly as part of surveillance cultures.

Meningitis

CSF. Two milliliters of CSF may be removed from a premature infant and up to 10 mL from a 10-kg infant with no deleterious effects. Fluid should be al-lowed to drip from the collection needle hub into test tubes for cytologic, chemical, and microbiologic analysis. A separate tube should be used if virus culture is required. One to two drops may also be dropped onto culture medium directly. Specimens should be transported as for specimens from adult patients.

In addition to cultivation for suspected pathogens, the specimen may be tested with antigen detection or amplification procedures.

Blood. A 1- to 2-mL sample should be collected in a sterile tube with anticoagulant from a peripheral vein, if possible, after disinfection of the venipuncture site. The specimens are collected, delivered, and processed as described for specimens from adult patients.

Septicemia

Blood. Collect specimen as previously described for meningitis.

Buffy Coat. Approximately 1 mL of blood should be collected for leukocyte smears by capillary heel stick, from peripheral vessels, or from vascular catheters into a sterile tube containing EDTA. After processing, slides are prepared from the buffy coat preparation, air-dried, and stained with acridine orange or Gram stain. Smears stained with acridine orange can subsequently be stained with Gram stain. If viral agents are suspected, the smears should be stained with immunofluorescent reagents for CMV or HSV.

Urine. Neonates with sepsis may also have a urinary tract infection. Specimens should be obtained by percutaneous needle aspiration of bladder urine after disinfection of the skin. At least 1 mL should be collected. If bladder aspiration is not possible, the specimen should be obtained by catheterization. This specimen should be cultured for bacteria as well as viral agents.

Autopsy Specimens. In fatal cases, appropriate tissues should be collected, placed in separate sterile jars, and submitted to the laboratory for staining and culture. See the section on tissues that follows.

Respiratory Tract Infections, Lower

Aspiration or Community-Acquired Pneumonia

Although obtained through the heavily contaminated area of the mouth and upper respiratory tract, sputum specimens remain the mainstay of laboratory evaluation of cases of pneumonia.[63] Patients who are unable to give an adequate sputum sample, who do not respond to therapy, or who may demonstrate a life-threatening condition pose some of the situations in which more invasive techniques may be needed to obtain a diagnostic specimen. These specimens are usually collected from hospitalized patients by physicians or other staff in the pulmonary service specifically trained to perform these techniques. The collection of sputum and some of the more invasive collection procedures are briefly described in Table 57–2. The relative merits of each are described as follows.

Sputum

A specimen is most likely to be of diagnostic value when it is taken before the administration of an antimicrobial, when it is taken under the supervision of a physician or other health-care professional, and the specimen is processed within 1 to 2 hours after collection. A gram-stained smear should reveal 25 or more neutrophils and fewer than 10 epithelial cells per low power field (LPF) if taken from an immunocompetent patient.[64] Only the specimens that meet these criteria should be inoculated for bacterial culture. Up to three specimens are recommended if *M. tuberculosis* is suspected. Evaluating gram-stained smears for specimen adequacy is controversial in these cases. Any isolation of *M. tuberculosis* is considered important, and therefore all samples are generally accepted. However, as in the case of routine cultivation for respiratory pathogens, the better the quality of the specimen, the more likely the pathogen will be recovered.

Pleural Fluid

Cases of pneumonia associated with a pleural effusion provide a specimen uncontaminated with upper respiratory flora. A positive culture may have important therapeutic implications. Either the patient should lie on her side in a semirecumbent position with her arm held above the head, or she can lean forward from a sitting position, or lean on a bedside table. The skin should be disinfected at the puncture site, which may be located by radiograph and/or percussion sounds. After anesthetizing the puncture site with Novocain (procaine HCl), a needle should be inserted between the ribs during inspiration to avoid the intercostal blood vessels which lie along the inferior margins of the ribs. The patient should be instructed to avoid coughing. Air can be prevented from entering the cavity by placing a three-way stopcock on the needle.

A syringe or tubing from a vacuum bottle should be attached to the needle, the stopcock opened, and fluid drained into a small, sterile, screw-cap jar. The specimen should be transported immediately to the laboratory at room temperature and cultured for suspected agents of pneumonia.[65]

Bronchoscopy Specimens

Bronchial Brushings. The use of a protected brush catheter through a fiberoptic bronchoscope in combination with quantitative culture techniques has been successfully used to obtain adequate specimens and diagnostic information in some cases of pneumonia. However, the specimens are still contaminated with upper-airway flora, it is an expensive procedure requiring technical expertise, and complications have been observed. The procedure has proven benefit for the collection of specimens for *Pneumocystis carinii* and other opportunistic fungi (other than *Candida* spp.), CMV, HSV, *Legionella* spp., and mycobacteria. Its utility for the recovery of other pathogens is considered to be no better than an adequately collected sputum specimen.[65]

Bronchoalveolar Lavage (BAL). This procedure involves washing a segment of the lung that is thought to be infected. Approximately 15 mL of BAL fluid should be used to directly inoculate media for aerobic bacteria, *Legionella* spp., *Norcardia* spp., fungi, and mycobacteria and tissue culture for viruses. Cytocentrifugation for smear preparation for gram-staining and immunofluorescence staining as well as inoculation of shell vials for viral culture is also recommended.[65]

Transtracheal Aspirate (TTA). Owing to risks involved with this procedure, it should be reserved for patients whose severity of illness justifies these risks, in whom there are no contraindications (bleeding disorders, severe hypoxemia, inability to cooperate, recent antimicrobial use), whose results from alternative, less-invasive specimens are inconclusive, and for whom laboratory resources are available to process the specimen expeditiously. This method has been shown to be useful for the recovery of bacterial pathogens, including *Legionella* spp., and is the only respiratory specimen other than lung biopsy that should be cultured for anaerobes. This procedure may also be used for the detection of *Norcardia* spp., *Mycobacterium* spp., *P. carinii*, and other fungi excluding *Candida* spp.[65]

Lung Biopsy. As indicated in Table 57–2, lung tissue may be obtained via a bronchoscope, percutaneously through the thoracic wall, via a thoroscope or by open lung biopsy. All specimens except those obtained by open lung biopsy will be exceedingly small, and great care must be made to handle them efficiently. Impression smears should be made on sterile slides for staining as for a BAL specimen. The lung tissue should be divided for multiple testing procedures, which include staining procedures and inoculation for recovery of aerobes, facultatives, and anaerobes, *Legionella* spp., *Mycobacterium*, fungi, and viral agents.

Respiratory Tract Infections, Upper

Upper respiratory specimens ideally should be collected within the first 3 days of illness, and no later than 5 days after onset. In general, these specimens consist of swabs, washes, or aspirates collected for isolation attempts or direct antigen detection.

NASAL SWABS

These specimens are collected by inserting a dry swab into the nostril parallel with the palate and rotating the swab gently. After the swab is withdrawn, it is placed in a bacterial transport tube. The second nostril should also be sampled using a fresh swab. These specimens are used solely to detect a carrier state for methicillin-resistant *S. aureus* (MRSA) and beta-hemolytic streptococci.[66] Other specimens are preferred for laboratory detection of respiratory pathogens.

NASOPHARYNGEAL WASHINGS

These specimens are collected by instilling several milliliters of sterile saline into each nostril while the patient's head is tilted slightly backward and then collecting the fluid in a small sterile container as the patient leans forward. Gelatin or bovine serum albumin (1%) may be added to the washings to stabilize any viral agent present if the specimen is to be submitted for culture. This step should be *omitted*, however, if the washings are to be submitted for antigen detection by immunofluorescence or EIA or if the specimen is to be submitted for bacterial culture.[67] Cellular material may be concentrated by centrifugation prior to testing.

NASOPHARYNGEAL ASPIRATES OF SECRETIONS

These specimens are collected by gentle suction with a polyethylene catheter of appropriate size and mucus trap. Three milliliters of Hanks' BSS may be passed through the tube and into the trap after collection to retrieve the specimen. These specimens are suitable for culture as well as direct antigen detection but require dilution of mucus and centrifugation for concentration of cellular material.[68, 69]

NASOPHARYNGEAL SWABS

These specimens are collected by passing a flexible, thin-shafted swab into the nasopharynx and allowing the secretions to absorb for at least 5 seconds. The swab is then removed and placed in 2 to 3 mL of bacterial or viral transport medium if isolation is to be attempted. A second specimen is collected through the other nostril, and the swab is placed in the same transport tube as the first. Alternatively, the swab may be discarded after pressing against the side of the transport medium tube. The tube should then be centrifuged to collect cellular material for analysis.

If immunofluorescence or EIA procedures are to be performed, the specimen should be used to make smears on glass slides before being placed in transport medium.

Nasopharyngeal specimens may be used to detect a carrier state for *S. pyognenes* (group A *Streptococcus*), *Neisseria meningitidis, Corynebacterium diphtheriae,* and *B. pertussis* as well as the laboratory diagnosis of several viral infections, including measles and pneumonia caused by *C. trachomatis* in newborns.[13]

THROAT SWABS

The tongue should be depressed with a tongue depressor, and the posterior pharynx, tonsils, exudation, ulceration, capsule formation, and inflamed areas should be sampled with a swab.[70] Rapid screening tests for group A *Streptococcus* may require special transport medium. If *N. gonorrhoeae, C. diphtheriae,* or *Mycoplasma pneumoniae* is suspected, the laboratory should be notified in advance. Nonroutine or special media may be required.

For viral cultures (adenovirus, enterovirus, HSV, and CMV), specimens should be collected by using a swab premoistened with viral transport medium and by rubbing the pharynx vigorously. The tip of the swab should be broken or cut off and placed in the same transport medium as that for a nasal swab, if cultivation attempts are to be made.

Sepsis, Septic Shock

Specimens of urine, sputum, if present, blood, and operative site wound or abscess cavity, if present, should be collected to confirm the diagnosis of septic shock and to determine the origin of infection.[71] Organisms typically involved include enteric gram-negatives and *S. aureus.* For patients receiving parenteral hyperalimentation and/or immunosuppressive drugs, the specimens of blood and sputum should be examined for fungi as well as cultured routinely. See the appropriate section of this chapter for specimen collection information.

Tissues from Autopsy and Biopsy

Autopsy Specimens. Autopsy specimens for isolation attempts should be collected as soon after death as possible, preferably within 24 hours. Samples consisting of 1.0- to 2.5-cm cubes of tissue from probable sites of pathology, each being collected with separate, sterile instruments, should be placed in separate sterile containers, such as 1-oz. screw-capped jars, containing a small volume of transport medium.

Biopsy Specimens. Biopsy specimens, many of which are collected by needle, may be of small size but are still collected separately and placed in separate containers. The tissues should be submitted as soon as possible at room temperature for bacterial isolation or on ice for viral isolation. Specimens for bacterial or fungal culture may be kept up to 24 hours at room temperature if processing is delayed, but they should be frozen at −70°C if they cannot be processed within 72 hours for viral recovery.

The tissue specimens that are usually sampled for cases of suspected infectious etiology include *brain, lung, heart muscle, lymph node,* and *kidney.* Tissue specimens are usually homogenized into suspension for inoculation into appropriate cultivation systems. Since liver tissue may be toxic to cell cultures, the suspension should be diluted before inoculation. Tissues for electron microscopy analysis should be fixed immediately in 2% glutaraldehyde in 0.1 M PBS, pH 7.2, and may be transported in ambient air.

Smears of tissues for immunofluorescence staining are prepared by cutting three or four pieces of tissue, approximately 10 to 15 mm², and gently pressing the freshly cut surface to clean, dry microscope slides while holding the tissue with forceps. A series of impressions should be made over an area that is 30 to 40 mm in length on each of three to four slides.

If the tissue is soft, such as brain, slip smears can be prepared by crushing a small piece of tissue between two slides and sliding them apart to create thin smears in the center of the opposing surfaces of the slides. In all cases, the slides must be clearly labeled with nonsmudging pencil on the frosted end of the slide. The smears should be air-dried and transported to the laboratory at ambient temperature.[72]

Urinary Tract Infections and Urine Specimens

Urinary tract infections occur in most females at some point in their lifetime and are the most common medical complication of pregnancy. The risk of pyelonephritis exists for untreated urinary tract infections in both pregnant and nonpregnant patients, but pregnant patients are more likely to have an asymptomatic bacteriuria, placing them at greater risk than the nonpregnant patient.[73] The specimens that are usually collected and the indication for each is described as follows:

Bacterial or Fungal Agents

MIDSTREAM, CLEAN-CATCH URINE

The patient should be instructed to thoroughly cleanse the urethral area with soap and water or pads that have been impregnated with a cleansing solution, and then to remove the soap with wet gauze pads. She should be told to hold the labia apart and begin voiding into the comode and after several milliters have been passed to collect at least 1 mL of urine into a sterile container without interrupting the flow of urine. The specimen should be delivered to the laboratory within 2 hours at room temperature or kept at 4°C if delivery will be delayed.

This specimen is usually collected in cases of symptomatic cases of urinary tract infection and may be tested with a leukocyte esterase dipstick or examined microscopically. Cultures are not indicated unless pyuria accompanies symptoms suggestive of acute cystitis, or there are signs and symptoms of pyelonephritis.

STRAIGHT CATHETER

The urethral area should be thoroughly cleansed with soap and water and then rinsed with wet gauze pads. The catheter should be inserted aseptically into the bladder, and the first 15 mL allowed to pass. The following 2- to 5-mL sample should be collected in a sterile container and handled as described previously. Quantitative cultures and gram-staining should be performed on these specimens.

This specimen should be collected only when the patient is unable to give a clean-catch specimen owing to the small risk of contaminating the bladder with urethral flora.

INDWELLING CATHETER

For collecting specimens from patients with an indwelling catheter in place, the port of the catheter should be disinfected with 70% alcohol. A needle and syringe is then used to collect 5 to 10 mL from the catheter. The specimen should be transferred to a sterile tube or other container and handled as previously described. Quantitative cultures and gram-staining should be performed on these specimens.

SUPRAPUBIC ASPIRATE

The skin over the bladder should be disinfected and anesthetized. A 22-gauge needle should be inserted into the full bladder at the midline between the symphysis pubis and the umbilicus, 2 cm above the symphysis. Approximately 20 mL of urine is aspirated and transferred to a sterile tube or container. The specimen should be handled as described previously. Quantitative cultures and gram-staining should be performed on these specimens.

This method is often used in pediatric patients, patients with spinal cord injury, and patients for whom a definitive culture has not been obtained, and in rare cases of suspected anaerobic urinary tract infection.

Escherichia coli is the most common urinary tract pathogen in nonhospitalized patients. *Staphylococcus saprophyticus* is reported to be a major pathogen in young females. Hospitalized patients are more likely to suffer from urinary tract infections due to *Proteus* spp., *Pseudomonas* spp., *Klebsiella* spp., *Enterobacter* spp., *Enterococcus* spp., *Staphylococcus* spp., or yeast.[74]

Viral Agents

Urine specimens are particularly useful in the detection of CMV in cases of congenital CMV and other viral infections. The specimen should be collected as soon as possible after the onset of illness or as soon as congenital disease is suspected. For newborns, the specimen is usually collected by catheterization.

For adults, clean-voided specimens, 10 to 15 mL in volume, are collected in sterile containers and transported to the laboratory on ice. The chance of recovery is improved if two to three specimens are collected. The specimen should be diluted with five volumes of 2SP and processed immediately or frozen at −70°C. The specimen should be centrifuged at 500× G and antibiotics added to the supernatant before inoculation into cell culture.[15]

Wounds

Abdominal Wounds (Postpartum, Postsurgical)

CLOSED WOUND

Whenever possible, material should be aspirated from a closed wound after disinfecting the skin. If the area to be sampled is intact (i.e., no open sores), the area should be disinfected with alcohol followed by an iodophor such as Betadine (povidone-iodine). If open sores, abrasions, or other disturbances are present, external exudate, crusts, or other debris should be removed by wiping the area with a sterile 4 × 4 inch gauze pad that has been moistened with sterile saline. After aspirating material from the wound, the specimen should be expelled into an anaerobic transport device and delivered to the laboratory at room temperature for gram-staining and culture. If incision and drainage is performed, a specimen of the advancing edge of the infected area should be placed in an anaerobic transport vial and submitted for Gram stain and culture as well.[75]

OPEN WOUND

If the wound is open, the area should be cleansed of external exudate, crusts, or other surface debris by wiping the area with a sterile 4 × 4 inch gauze pad that has been moistened with sterile saline. Any exudate that may be present can be sampled by passing a swab deep within the wound. More importantly, the margin of the lesion should be sampled by firmly pressing it with a swab. The swabs should then be placed in an aerobic transport device and delivered to the laboratory for Gram stain and culture. Anaerobic culture of open wounds is not suggested. For patients who have normal immunologic status, the Gram stain should reveal many neutrophils and none or few squamous epithelial cells in a properly collected specimen.

Early-onset simple wounds are often unimicrobial and are typically due to *S. pyogenes* (group A *Streptococcus*), *S. agalactiae* (group B *Streptococcus*), or *Clostridium perfringens*. A Gram stain of material aspirated from the advancing margin of the wound can be diagnostic; for example, gram-positive cocci in pairs and chains suggest *Streptococcus* spp., while plump, gram-positive rods suggest *Clostridium* sp. Late-onset wounds are more likely to be polymicrobial in nature and respond to incision and drainage.[76] However, a specimen of the wound should be taken for Gram stain and culture, as described for early wounds, in case the patient does not respond to incision and drainage and antibiotics need to be added. The Gram stain and/or culture results may be useful in guiding the choice of antibiotics in that situation.

Mycoplasma hominis has also been recovered from these wounds. For recovery of this organism, the specimen may be transported in 2SP if specific *Mycoplasma* transport tubes are not available (see Table 57–3). The organisms can be detected on anaerobically incubated blood agar plates, but preferably they should be inoculated onto specific *Mycoplasma* medium.

Serious sequelae of abdominal wound infection include necrotizing fasciitis, progressive synergistic bacterial gangrene, and clostridial gas gangrene (clostridial anaerobic myonecrosis). The first two are polymicrobial in nature, while the third, as the name implies, is due primarily to the presence of a single species of *Clostridium*.[76]

The diagnosis of necrotizing fasciitis may be made at surgery, at which time a frozen-section biopsy of infected tissue is submitted for examination. The biopsy specimen should include infected subcutaneous tissue, fascia, and muscle beneath the involved dermis and should be at least 10 × 7 × 7 mm. A portion of the biopsy specimen should also be submitted for culture and Gram stain.

Since surgical débridement may be necessary in the management of bacterial gangrene and myonecrosis, tissue specimens should be submitted for Gram stain and culture. Specimens should be placed in an anaerobic transport device and sent to the laboratory at room temperature.

EPISIOTOMY WOUNDS

Although rare, these infections are similar in type and potential consequences (necrotizing fasciitis, myonecrosis) to abdominal wound infections. Specimens of exudate and/or tissue samples should be transported in anaerobic transport devices for Gram stain and culture for aerobes and anaerobes. *S. pyogenes* and anaerobic organisms are most often recovered.[76]

SECTION TWO: DIAGNOSTIC PROCEDURES FOR THE LABORATORY DIAGNOSIS OF INFECTIONS IN WOMEN
Evaluations of Laboratory Diagnostic Test Procedures

The value of any diagnostic test depends on the reliability of the test in providing correct results; that is, results that reflect the true disease state of the patient. A general approach to the evaluation of the reliability of a test is to determine at least four performance characteristics[77]:

1. **Sensitivity.** Sensitivity, the frequency of a positive test in patients who have the disease that the test is designed to detect, is expressed mathematically as follows:

$$\frac{\text{True-positives}}{\text{True-positives} + \text{False-negatives}}$$

2. **Specificity.** Specificity, the frequency of a negative test result in patients who do not have the disease, is expressed mathematically as follows:

$$\frac{\text{True-negatives}}{\text{True-negatives} + \text{False-positives}}$$

3. **Positive Predictive Value (PPV).** PPV, the probability that a patient with a positive test result is truly infected, is expressed thus:

$$\frac{(\text{prevalence})\,(\text{sensitivity})}{(\text{prevalence})\,(\text{sensitivity}) + (1 - \text{prevalence})\,(1 - \text{specificity})}$$

4. **Negative Predictive Value (NPV).** NPV, the probability that a patient with a negative test result truly does not have the disease, is expressed thus:

$$\frac{(1 - \text{prevalence})\,(\text{specificity})}{(1 - \text{prevalence})\,(\text{specificity}) + (\text{prevalence})\,(1 - \text{sensitivity})}$$

Traditionally, the aforementioned performance characteristics have been determined by comparing new test procedures to standard methodology, and in many cases the comparator, or "gold standard," has been the results of cultivation attempts of the suspected agent. Since detection of suspected pathogens by culture techniques depends on the presence of viable agents, tests that are able to detect nonviable components will, in fact, be more sensitive than the standard test, true-positives will be identified as "false-positives," and the specificity of the test will be decreased.

The development of techniques that are more sensitive than culture, such as those that use monoclonal antibodies to detect antigenic components and nucleic acid detection reagents, has led to an attempt to identify truly positive patients who are missed with cell culture by using a discrepant analysis. Discrepant analysis involves subjecting apparent false-positive samples;

that is, those that give positive results with the test under evaluation but negative culture results, to additional testing with alternative procedures. If any of the additional tests yield a positive result, the original positive result by the new test procedure is considered a true-positive and the original negative culture result is considered a false-negative. Although results may be biased in favor of the new test,[78] true-positive and true-negative results currently are usually determined by the combination of test results and may include correlation with clinical findings as well.

The PPV and NPV may be used to rule in or rule out the presence of the disease. As seen in equations 3 and 4 earlier, both PPV and NPV are influenced not only by the sensitivity and specificity of the test procedure but also by the disease prevalence within the population being tested. In a low-prevalence population, both the PPV and the NPV increase with increasing sensitivity. The PPV increases to a much greater extent, however, with increasing specificity. Furthermore, although decreased specificity in a low-prevalence population results in a reduced PPV, the NPV will still be high. Hence, the NPV value is most predictive of the accuracy of the test in a low-prevalence population. In a high-prevalence population, the PPV increases slightly with increasing sensitivity, and greater increases in NPV are seen with increasing specificity. In general, tests with a high PPV are useful as diagnostic tools, especially in situations in which a false diagnosis results in therapy that is potentially harmful or has economic, social, or psychological consequences. Tests with a high NPV are useful as screening tests when the goal is to detect all positive patients.[77, 79] Many current published reports of comparative studies include PPV and NPV calculations. When calculations of these parameters are not included, perhaps particular attention should be paid to the specificity of the test system in low-prevalence populations and the sensitivity in high-prevalence populations.

To ensure that an adequate sample size has been tested when one evaluates a new test procedure, it has been suggested that the confidence intervals (CIs) be calculated for the aforementioned parameters. CIs would give an estimate of the precision or imprecision of the parameter for the test method and vary with sample size and level of confidence (e.g., 90%, 95%, or 99%). The larger the CI, the less precise the estimate of sensitivity, specificity, and predictive value will be.[79] However, these calculations have not always been included in published reports of comparative studies.

The remainder of this section briefly summarizes the principles underlying the various techniques used for detection of pathogens, presents a general description of how the procedures are performed, and indicates which agents are likely to be detected or identified by each technique. However, the tests that are available in any particular setting will be determined not only by the performance characteristics of the test but also by economic factors. Communication with the clinical laboratory is necessary for determining which techniques are available and for providing input on the needs of the medical staff.

Descriptions of Laboratory Diagnostic Test Procedures

Wet (Unfixed) Preparations

Wet preparations are simple and allow direct examination of the specimen in a short period of time. A summary of microscopic techniques used with wet preparations is presented in Table 57–8.

PREPARATIONS FOR DARK-FIELD EXAMINATION OF SPIROCHETES

Treponema pallidum

Exudate from lesions of primary, secondary, or congenital syphilis is collected as described in the first section of this chapter; that is, a sterile slide is touched to lesion exudate and a cover slip is added immediately. The slide should be examined at 40× to 45× magnification as soon as possible for the presence of motile spiral organisms. When an organism is observed, a drop of immersion oil should be added and the field examined at 90× to 100× magnification.

▶ Organisms that are 6 to 15 μm in length and that have 5 to 20 rigid, regular spirals and a motility typically described as "corkscrew" are reported as "organisms found that have characteristic morphology and motility of *T. pallidum.*"[80]

▶ This procedure is relatively insensitive, since a concentration of 10^3 organisms/mL may require examination of up to a 1,000 HPFs for detection.[81] Hence, the recommendation is for the clinician to submit at least three preparations before considering the ulcer negative for spirochetes. Some authors have successfully used fluorescent antibody stains to detect *T. pallidum,*[82] but this procedure is currently not widely used.

Leptospira

Specimens of blood, urine, or CSF may also be examined by dark-field illumination in suspected cases of leptospirosis. Anticoagulated blood should be examined only within the first week of illness, and urine and CSF during the second week.

TABLE 57–8 ▶ MICROSCOPIC TECHNIQUES AND NONIMMUNOLOGIC STAINS USED TO DETECT MICROORGANISMS IN SPECIMENS		
Method or Stain	**Typical Agents Detected**	**Description**
Wet Preparations		
Dark-field examination	*Treponema pallidum,* other spirochetes	White, spiral organisms against black background Negative result does not rule out disease
Saline preparations	Motile parasites, fungal elements, clue cells	Unstained structures against a clear background Lactophenol cotton blue (LPCB) may be added for contrast
KOH preparation	Fungal elements	Unstained structures against a clear background LPCB may be added for contrast
India ink	*Cryptococcus neoformans*	Capsule excludes ink, giving white-halo appearance against a gray to black background
Lugol's iodine	Parasites (ova, cysts, etc.)	Light brown structures differentiated from nonstaining WBCs
Fluorescent Stains		
Acridine orange	Many microorganisms, including *Cryptosporidium*	Bacterial and fungal DNA fluoresce orange; mammalian DNA fluoresces green More sensitive than Gram stain for blood culture, buffy coat, CSF Gram stain can be performed on same slide
Auramine-rhodamine	*Mycobacterium, Cryptosporidium*	Acid-fast organisms fluoresce orange-yellow against black background More sensitive than nonfluorochrome stains, but positive result needs confirmation
Calcofluor white	Fungi, *Pneumocystis carinii* (cysts)	Organisms appear green or blue against dark background

Table continued on following page

TABLE 57–8 ▶	MICROSCOPIC TECHNIQUES AND NONIMMUNOLOGIC STAINS USED TO DETECT MICROORGANISMS IN SPECIMENS *Continued*	
Method or Stain	**Typical Agents Detected**	**Relative Sensitivity/Comments**
Colorimetric Stains		
Gram Stain	Bacteria, yeasts	Gram-positive bacteria, yeasts stain blue; gram-negative organisms stain red. Used to evaluate adequacy of specimen, especially from respiratory tract
Toluidine blue	*Pneumocystis carinii* (cysts)	*P. carinii* cysts and fungi stain lavender against a blue background
Ziehl-Neelsen, Kinyoun	*Mycobacterium*	Acid-fast organisms stain red against a blue background
Modified Kinyoun	*Nocardia, Cryptosporidium, Isospora, Cyclospora*	Acid-fast organisms stain red against a blue background. As sensitive as FA for cryptosporidia in diarrhea stools
Trichrome	Parasites (cysts and trophozoites)	Cytoplasm of cysts and trophozoites stain blue-green, tinged with purple; nuclear chromatic, chromatoid bodies, ingested RBCs stain red or red purple; background is green
Blood or Histologic Stains		
Giemsa/Wright's	*Plasmodium,* trypanosomes, leishmania, *Toxoplasma gondii, Histoplasma capsulatum, Pneumocystis carinii* (trophozoites), *Borrelia* spp., viral and chlamydial inclusions	Stains basophilic material blue, acidophilic material red, but does not determine bacterial Gram reaction
Gomori's methenamine silver	*Pneumocystis carinii,* fungi	Cell walls of *P. carinii* and fungi stain black against a green background
Dieterle	*Legionella* spp., spirochetes, *Bartonella*	Organisms stain black against yellowish background
Mucicarmine	*Cryptococcus neoformans*	Encapsulated yeasts stain dark red against a pink background; halo sometimes seen
Periodic acid–Schiff	Fungal elements	Organisms stain pink-magenta against a pink background
Electron Microscopy (usually by negative staining with uranyl acetate and phosphotungstic acid [PTA])	Many viral agents	Agents and internal structures are outlined against a grayish-white background. Has limited sensitivity and specificity but can be augmented by immunoelectron microscopy

Modified from Mandell GL, Bennett JE, Dolin R (eds): Principles and Practice of Infectious Diseases, 4th ed. New York, Churchill Livingstone, 1995, p 184.

▶ Organisms that are 6 to 10 μm in length, have 18 or more tight coils, and have one or both ends hooked or bent may be presumptively identified as *Leptospira* sp. Cultivation in Fletcher's or another special medium is probably the preferred method of laboratory diagnosis in most settings.

Saline Wet Mounts for Parasites and Fungi

This procedure involves simply adding a drop of 0.85% warm (37°C) aqueous NaCl to a clean, glass microscope slide, adding a drop of specimen to the slide, and mixing. Specimens usually are vaginal discharge or stool. The mixture is overlaid with a coverslip and examined at 100× to 1,000× magnification.

▶ This method detects motility and gross morphology of protozoan trophozoites (e.g., *Trichomonas vaginalis, Giardia lamblia*) as well as morphology of fungal hyphal forms, endospores, and helminth eggs and larvae. It is reported to have a sensitivity of 49% to 80% for detection of *T. vaginalis*, while culture is reported to have a sensitivity of 85% to 95%.[83]

Modified Saline Wet Mount with 10% KOH for Fungal Elements

A drop of the specimen is mixed with a drop of 10% KOH, rather than saline. A coverslip is added, and the slide is allowed to sit a room temperature for 5 to 30 minutes to allow digestion of proteinaceous components of the host cell. A drop of 40% dimethyl sulfoxide may be added, or the slide may be heated gently to enhance the digestive process.

▶ This method is useful in identifying fungal elements in mucoid or keratinous specimens, such as sputum, skin, hair, and nails. It is reported to have a sensitivity of 50% to 70%, compared to diagnosis by clinical features and microscopy negative for other pathogens, for detection of *Candida* spp. in cases of vulvovaginitis.[6]

KOH Preparation with Lactophenol Cotton Blue (LPCB) for Fungal Elements
A drop of the specimen is mixed with a drop of 10% KOH and a drop of LPCB. The LPCB enhances the visibility of fungal elements, since the lactic acid serves as a clearing agent and the aniline blue stains the outer cell wall of the fungus.

▶ This method is also useful in distinguishing fungal elements in mucoid or keratinous specimens, such as sputum, skin, hair, and nails.

Colloidal Carbon Wet Mounts, India Ink, Nigrosin for Cryptococcus
A drop of spinal fluid is added to and mixed with a drop of either Pelikan India Ink or nigrosin on a clean microscope slide. A coverslip is added, and the preparation is examined at $100\times$ to $1,000\times$ magnification.

▶ This method is used to visualize the polysaccharide capsules of *Cryptococcus neoformans*, which appear as clear haloes around the organisms on a semiopaque background. India ink preparations usually have a sensitivity of only 50%. Antigen detection tests, however, have a reported sensitivity of more than 90% and can also be performed on serum.[13] There are at least two commercially available sources (Table 57–9).

Lugol's Iodine
A drop of Lugol's iodine is added to a mixture of saline and a drop of fecal material.

▶ This method is useful in visualizing intestinal protozoa and helminth ova or larvae, since the iodine stains the nuclei and intracytoplasmic organelles brown, making them more easily seen on microscopic examination.

Fixed and Stained Preparations

Fixed and stained preparations are more permanent than wet preparations and allow greater detail to be observed. A summary of the more frequently used microscopic techniques is presented in Table 57–8.

TABLE 57–9 ▶ ANTIGEN DETECTION PROCEDURES			
Agent	**Specimen(s)**	**Procedure/Product Name**	**Source**
Bacteria *Chlamydia trachomatis*	Cervical or conjunctival swab	Direct FA/MicroTrak Indirect FA ELISA or EIA/MicroTrak Chlamydiazyme, TestPack, Sanofi EIA, Quick Vue Chlamydia Test	Syva, Diasorin, Hemagen Inc. Syva, Abbott Laboratories, Sanofi Diagnostics, Quidel
Clostridium difficile	Stool for toxin testing	EIA/Premier, others Agglutination/Culturette CDT *Clostridium difficile* Rapid, test	Meridian, Alexon, Bartels, Becton-Dickinson, Biosite, BioWhittaker, Tech-Lab Becton-Dickinson
Haemophilus influenzae type b, *Neisseria meningitidis*, *Streptococcus agalactiae, S. pneumoniae*	CSF	Agglutination/Bactigen, Directogen, Wellcogen	Wampole HWD Wellcome
Escherichia coli (enterohemorrhagic)	Stool for toxin testing	EIA/Premier EHEC	Meridian
S. agalactiae	Vaginal swab	Agglutination/Wellcogen EIA/ICON STREP B, Group B Strep Test Optical EIA/Strep B OIA	Wellcome Hybritech Quidel Biostar
Helicobacter pylori	Stool	EIA/Premier Platinum HpSA	Meridian
Legionella pneumophila serotype 1	Respiratory or urine	Direct FA ELISA Legionella Urinary Ag (LUA)	Sanofi, Zeus Scientific, MarDX Diagnostics Binax
N. gonorrhoeae	Urogenital	ELISA/Gonozyme	Abbott Laboratories
Streptococcus pyogenes	Throat swab	Agglutination Detect A Strep EIA/Signify Strept Quick Vue BioStar Strep AOIA Test Others	Murex Abbott Laboratories Quidel Biostar Meridian, Binax, Wyntek

Table continued on following page

TABLE 57-9 ▶   ANTIGEN DETECTION PROCEDURES *Continued*

Agent	Specimen(s)	Procedure/Product Name	Source
Fungi			
Cryptococcus neoformans	CSF, serum	Agglutination/CALAS, Pasteur Cryptococcus EIA/Premier	Meridian Sanofi Meridian
Histoplasma capsulatum	Urine, serum	EIA	HRL*
Candida spp.	Urine, serum	Agglutination/Cand-TEC	Ramco Labs
Pneumocystis carinii	Respiratory	Direct FA	Chemicon, Sanofi, Meridian
Parasites			
Cryptosporidium and/or *Giardia lamblia*	Stool	Direct FA/Merifluor Giardia/ Crypto IF Kit EIA/ProSpecT Others	Meridian TechLab Alexon Cambridge Biotech
Entamoeba histolytica	Stool	EIA	Wampole, Alexon
Trichomonas vaginalis	Vaginal swab	Direct FA	Integrated Diagnostics,
Viruses			
Adenovirus	Stool, urine, conjunctiva respiratory	EIA/Adenoclone, others Indirect FA Agglutination	Cambridge Biotech, Biotrin Chemicon, Sanofi Chemicon
CMV	Respiratory, buffy coat	Direct, Indirect FA Antigenemia/CMV-vue CMV Brite	Bartels, Chemicon, Dupont, Hemagen, Virgo Diasorin Biotest
EBV	Serum	Indirect FA for EBNA	Organon Teknika, Hemagen, Virgo, Granbio, Inc.
HSV	Vesicle fluid, brain biopsy	Direct/indirect FA EIA/Premier HSV	Bartels, Chemicon, Sanofi, Diasorin Meridian
HBV	Serum	EIA for HBe, HBs/TestPack Others	Abbott Laboratories Sanofi, Ortho Diagnostics, Diasorin
HIV	Serum	Indirect EIA, p24 Ag HIV-1 Ag Test, Vironstika HIV-1 Ag Test, others	Ortho Diagnostics Organon Teknika Abbott, Genetic Systems, Cellular Products, Dupont, Coulter
Influenza A/B	Respiratory	Direct, indirect FA EIA/ZstatFlu Agglutination	Sanofi, Chemicon Zymetrix Chemicon
Measles	Nasopharyngeal swab, aspirate	Indirect FA	Hemagen, Virgo
Mumps	Nasopharyngeal swab, aspirate	Indirect FA	Hemagen, Virgo
Parainfluenza	Nasopharyngeal aspirates	Direct FA/ViraSTAT Others EIA Agglutination	Zymetrix Sanofi, Chemicon Chemicon Chemicon
Rabies	Brain tissue	Direct FA	Chemicon
Rotavirus	Stool	Direct, Indirect FA EIA/VIDAS Rotazyme, TestPack Others Agglutination	Chemicon, Diasorin BioMerieux Vitek Abbott Hemagen, Virgo, Diasorin Meridian
RSV	Nasopharyngeal swab, aspirate	Direct, indirect FA ELISA/VIDAS, TestPack Others	Bartels, Chemicon BioMerieux Vitek, Abbott, Diasorin, Hemagen, Virgo
Rubella	Throat swab	Indirect FA	Hemagen, Virgo
VZV	Vesicle fluid	Direct, indirect FA	Chemicon, Meridian, Hemagen, Virgo
Viral respiratory panel	Respiratory	Indirect FA EIA/Simufluor FluA/B; RSV/A; CMV/Adeno Others	Bartels Chemicon Biotrin

*HRL = Histoplasmosis Reference Laboratory, 1001 W. 10th Street, OPW #30, Indianapolis, IN 46202.

GRAM STAIN FOR DIRECT SPECIMEN EXAMINATION

A drop of specimen is placed on a clean, microscope slide and spread into a thin smear. The material is fixed to the slide either with heat or by placing a drop of 95% methanol on the mixture and allowing it to stand for 2 minutes. The slide is flooded sequentially with crystal violet, Gram's iodine, decolorizer, and safranin. The slide is then rinsed with water and allowed to dry before it is examined at 100× to 1000× magnification (under oil immersion).

▶ This procedure allows assessment of the adequacy of the specimen and also allows visualization of microorganisms in clinical specimens. The stain identifies organisms into two broad categories, gram-positive, which retain the crystal violet stain and appear blue, and gram-negative, which are decolorized and take up the safranin counterstain and appear red. Rapid presumptive diagnosis can sometimes be made for agents of urinary tract infections, bacterial meningitis, or pneumonia. Gram stain has also been shown to be a reliable method for diagnosing bacterial vaginosis.[84, 85]

ZIEHL-NEELSEN AND KINYOUN ACID-FAST STAINS FOR MYCOBACTERIA: MODIFIED KINYOUN FOR *NOCARDIA* AND SOME PARASITES

A thin smear of unconcentrated or concentrated specimen is made on a clean, glass microscope slide, and the smear is heat-fixed for 2 hours. The slide is flooded with basic carbol fuchsin and either the slide is allowed to steam for 2 to 5 minutes (Ziehl-Neelsen) or the slide is flooded with phenol (Kinyoun). The slide is decolorized with 3% H_2SO_4 in 95% alcohol and counterstained with methylene blue. In the modified Kinyoun stain, a more dilute decolorizer (0.5% to 1.0% H_2SO_4) is used. These staining procedures allow the identification of red-staining, acid-fast bacilli, notably *Mycobacterium* spp., *Nocardia* spp., and the oocyts of *Cryptosporidium* spp., *Isospora belli*, *Cryptospora* spp., and *Sarcocystis* spp. The walls of these organisms are impervious to crystal violet and other basic dyes, and heat or detergent must be used to allow penetration of the primary dye into the cell.[84]

TOLUIDINE BLUE-O FOR *PNEUMOCYSTIS CARINII*

A thin smear of bronchoalveolar lavage specimen or a lung biopsy touch preparation that has been allowed to air-dry is flooded with a sulfation reagent, followed by the toluidine blue-O stain. The smear is fixed in absolute ethanol and examined at 100× to 1,000× magnification.

▶ This is a rapid, reliable stain for detecting the cysts of *P. carinii* in respiratory tract material. The cysts stain reddish blue or dark purple against a light blue background. The cysts may be clumped and have a crescent-shaped appearance. Trophozoites of the organism are not visualized by this method.[84]

Note: Sputum is not a recommended specimen for this or other stains for P. carinii unless it is induced sputum from an HIV-positive patient, in which the load of organisms is usually very high.

TRICHROME STAIN

This rather complex staining procedure may be used on fresh stool or specimens fixed in PVA, SAF, or MIF to provide a permanent record and confirmatory identification of intestinal parasites. See reference 86 for details.

WRIGHT'S AND GIEMSA STAINS FOR INTRACELLULAR PARASITES

These hematology stains are used for demonstrating differences in nuclei and cytoplasmic features of blood cell components. Both, however, detect certain pathogens that may be located within the blood. Both stains consist of a combination of methylene blue and eosin.

▶ These stains can detect blood parasites, such as *Plasmodium* spp., *Leishmania* spp., *Babesia* spp., and microfilaria, which demonstrate a red nucleus and gray-blue cytoplasm. They also detect blue-staining intracellular yeast cells of *Histoplasma capsulatum* in peripheral blood or bone marrow smears, purple-staining elementary bodies of *Chlamydia* spp., and intracystic bodies and trophozoites of *P. carinii* and bluish-purple–staining *Rickettsia* spp.[84]

Fluorescent-Staining Procedures

Some stains that fluoresce when exposed to ultraviolet radiation have the ability to bind to various sites on microorganisms and can be used as an aid in visualizing organisms in patient specimens.

ACRIDINE ORANGE

Acridine-orange staining is a rapid, sensitive technique that allows visual differentiation of bacterial and fungal DNA from that of mammalian cells. A thin smear of the specimen is fixed to a microscope slide with methanol. The acridine-orange solution is added, and the smear is examined without a coverslip with an ultraviolet microscope after excess stain has been washed off the slide.

▶ This stain is useful in locating small numbers of organisms, such as in spinal fluid or blood culture medium, as well as buffy coat preparations from neonates. This stain may also be helpful in thick or purulent specimens, the Gram stain of which is not easily read. The DNA of bacteria and fungi fluoresce orange, and mammalian DNA fluoresces green under ultraviolet light.[84]

AURAMINE-RHODAMINE STAINING FOR MYCOBACTERIA

A thin smear is heat-fixed to a clean microscope slide, and the slide is flooded with the auramine-rhodamine primary stain. The specimen is decolorized with acid alcohol, and the slide is flooded with potassium permanganate. The slide is then examined without a coverslip at 100× to 400× magnification.

▶ This is a relatively rapid method for screening specimens for the presence of acid-fast bacilli. The auramine and rhodamine reagents are non-specific fluorochromes that bind to mycolic acids and resist decolorization with acid alcohol. Acid-fast organisms (e.g., *Mycobacterium* spp.) fluoresce orange-yellow against a black background. This procedure is reported to have a sensitivity of up to 96% when more than one appropriately collected specimen is submitted.[87] It has been shown to be more sensitive than the colorimetric Kinyoun stain described previously, owing to decreased difficulty in finding fluorescing organisms against a black background. However, positive auramine-rhodamine smears are often confirmed by the Ziehl-Neelsen or Kinyoun acid-fast stain.

CALCOFLUOR WHITE FOR YEASTS AND *PNEUMOCYSTIS CARINII*

This reagent is a nonspecific fluorochrome that binds to the β1,3-linked polysaccharides, specifically cellulose and chitin, in the cell walls of fungi. A drop of the calcofluor white reagent is added to a thin smear of specimen on a clean microscope slide, followed by a drop of 10% KOH. A coverslip is added, and the preparation is examined at 100× to 400× magnification.

▶ Fungal elements (yeast cells, hyphae, pseudohyphae, spherules) and cysts of *P. carinii* appear bright green or blue against a dark background. The cysts of *P. carinii* are generally 5 to 7 μm in diameter and exhibit a characteristic peripheral cyst wall staining with an intense internal "double parenthesis–like" structure. Yeast cells are differentiated from *P. carinii* by the presence of budding and intense internal staining.[84]

Histologic Tissue Staining

Tissue specimens should be submitted for histologic staining in addition to other diagnostic procedures.

▶ Stains commonly used on paraffin-embedded specimens include Gomori's methenamine silver (GMS) for detection of cysts of *P. carinii*, *Actinomy-ces* spp., and yeasts and hyphal forms; mucicarmine for detecting *C. neoformans;* periodic acid–Schiff (PAS) for detecting fungal forms; and Dieterle stain for detecting *Legionella* spp., spirochetes, and *Bartonella* spp.[13]

Electron Microscopy

Examination by EM of specimens stained with uranyl acetate or phosphotungstic acid (PTA) is typically used for direct observation of viral particles. Such staining identifies an agent only as a member of a virus family but may provide an early presumptive diagnosis. EM examination can be performed on cellular specimens and thin sections of tissues embedded in epoxy resin. Specimens may include samples of tissue, stools, urine, cellular scrapings, vesicular fluids, nasopharyngeal secretions, and tissue smears on glass slides.

▶ EM may be used to detect a wide variety of viral agents in patient specimens. The main usefulness of the technique, however, is the detection of viruses in the stools of patients with gastroenteritis, the detection of CMV in the urine of infected neonates, and the differentiation of poxviruses (e.g., molluscum contagiosum) from herpesviruses in skin or genital lesions. See reference 88 for a more complete listing.

Antigen Detection by Antibody-Staining Techniques

These techniques have combined the specificity of antibodies formed to antigenic determinants on the target agent with the ability to visualize resulting antigen-antibody complexes. The most commonly used antibody-staining procedures for detecting antigen in fresh clinical specimens, in fixed tissue preparations, or for culture confirmation after isolation (bacteria) or amplification by growth in tissue culture (viral agents) are *immunofluorescence, enzyme immunoassay,* or *radioimmunoassay.* These procedures utilize *direct* or *indirect staining*[89, 90]:

▶ **Direct:** A separate antibody is produced for each target antigen, labeled with an immunofluorescent substance, enzyme, or radiolabel, and allowed to react with specimen. The enzyme substrate must be added if the antibody is enzyme-labeled, to allow formation of a colored product. Direct antibody tests are simple to perform and are generally considered to be very specific.

▶ **Indirect:** Unlabeled antibody is allowed to react with antigen in the sample, followed by a second labeled antibody produced in a separate species from the first antibody and which is directed at the Fc fragment of the first antibody. If the second antibody is enzyme labeled, a substrate is added and a colored product is produced and detected in a spectrophotometer. Indirect tests may be more sensitive than direct tests but may lack specificity.

IMMUNOFLUORESCENCE STAINING

Labeled antibody is added to a specimen fixed to a glass slide, and the direct format is most often used. The most commonly employed fluorescent label is fluorescein isothiocyanate (FITC). These tests are particularly useful for laboratory diagnosis of respiratory infections (due to viral agents, *Legionella pneumophila*, and *P. carinii*), infections due to *C. trachomatis*, and for the detection of some parasitic agents. They are also used to confirm the identification of several viruses in tissue culture, and the direct immunofluorescent antibody test is often used to confirm positive results for *C. trachomatis* obtained with EIA systems. A list of immunofluorescent staining reagents commonly used for laboratory diagnosis is presented in Table 57–9.

ENZYME IMMUNOASSAYS

The indicator antibodies used in EIAs are linked to a fluorescent dye or an enzyme. The antigen-antibody reaction is visualized by the addition of substrate for the enzyme. The most commonly used enzymes include horseradish peroxidase (HRP), alkaline phosphatase (AP), glucose oxidase (GO), and β-D-galactosidase (β-Gal). These tests are useful for the in situ detection of antigens within infected cells of patient specimens, within liquid-phase reaction mixtures, and in infected tissue culture cells. Since HRP is very often used as the enzyme label, these tests are sometimes referred to as immunoperoxidase staining.

A modification of the immunoenzyme staining methodology uses immobilization of antibodies on a solid surface to separate antigen-antibody complexes from the reaction mixture. Surfaces used to immobilize antibody for antigen detection include polystyrene beads, tubes, and wells of microtiter plates, including polyvinyl chloride plates. Such techniques utilizing solid surfaces and staining with enzyme-labeled reagents have historically been termed *enzyme-linked immunosorbent assays* (ELISAs) to distinguish them from assays performed as cytostaining or in liquid phase (homogeneous assays), which require no separation of the antigen-antibody complexes.

The solid-phase procedures also can be performed in a direct or an indirect format. In the direct assays, an unlabeled antibody is adsorbed to the solid surface, and the specimen is added, incubated, and washed a number of times. A second antibody, directed against the antigen that has been *"captured"* by the first antibody, is added. After the incubation and washing steps, the substrate is added, and the resultant color changes may be read in a spectrophotometer. For the indirect assay, the antigen is adsorbed to an unlabeled antibody on the solid phase, a second unlabeled antibody directed against the antigen is added, and the antigen is thus "sandwiched" between two unlabeled antibodies. A third antibody, which is labeled and directed against the second antibody, is added, followed by substrate for detection of antigen-antibody complexes. The main advantage of indirect assays is a reduction in background interference and thus a reduction in the number of false-positive reactions.

Enzyme immunoassays are available for the detection of several infectious disease agents (see Table 57–9). They have become popular as a result of their ability to automate the testing procedures, allowing many specimens to be tested at one time. One disadvantage of these tests, however, is their inability to evaluate the adequacy of clinical specimens, since they are not examined microscopically, as is done with immunofluorescence tests.

RADIOIMMUNOASSAYS

Radioimmunoassay (RIA) procedures are similar to immunofluorescence and immunoenzymatic assays in that antibodies labeled with a radioisotope do not lose immunologic specificity and can be used as indicator molecules for detecting homologous antigen. Procedures may be direct or indirect, as described for fluorescence and enzymatic staining. Solid-phase procedures have been developed that utilize direct and indirect formats as well as sandwich, or antibody-capture, techniques.

Radioimmunoassay procedures have often been replaced by other procedures, owing to concerns over safe handling, storage, and disposal of radiolabeled substances, coupled with the increasing availability of enzyme-labeled reagents that are of sensitivity and specificity equivalent to that of RIA reagents. In most clinical laboratory settings, RIA procedures are currently used primarily for the detection of HBsAg in serum.

AVIDIN-BIOTIN MODIFICATIONS

Biotin, a component of the vitamin B_2 complex, has a high affinity for avidin, a glycoprotein obtained from egg white. This affinity has been utilized in fluorescence, enzyme immunostaining, and RIA by linking biotin to the antibody, which is reacted with specimen, and the reaction is then detected with labeled avidin. Streptavidin, a protein obtained from *Streptomyces avidinii*, has binding properties similar to those of avidin and is sometimes used as a substitute for the egg white avidin.

Other Antigen Detection Techniques

AGGLUTINATION AND CO-AGGLUTINATION TESTS

In many agglutination tests, polystyrene beads of uniform size are coated with antibody and mixed with test specimen. In co-agglutination tests, protein A–enriched cells of *S. aureus* sensitized with monoclonal antibodies against specific microorganisms are mixed with the specimen (e.g., CSF, urine, other body fluids). The suspension is examined for visible evidence of clumping. These tests originally found wide application in testing for soluble antigens in fluid specimens from patients with infection due to *H. influenzae, S. pneumoniae*, group B streptococci, and *N. meningitidis*. However, one large retrospective analysis of 1,268 clinical samples revealed that all CSF specimens positive by latex agglutination were also positive by Gram stain. Furthermore, among the 57 specimens positive by latex agglutination, only 22 (38%) were true-positives, 31 (54%) were false-positives, and 4 (7%) were indeterminate.[91] On the other hand, another retrospective study of 146 consecutive patients with bacterial meningitis revealed a much higher detection rate with bacterial antigen tests than with culture if patients had received treatment prior to lumbar puncture.[92] Hence, clinical laboratories may reserve these tests for specimens from previously treated patients.

Both LA and co-agglutination have been used to detect pneumococcal antigen in sputum from patients with suspected pneumococcal pneumonia. The sensitivity of each of these tests is reported to be approximately 80% in confirmed cases compared to Gram stain, which has a reported sensitivity of 50%. The specificities of these tests are reported to be only about 70%, owing to false-positive results in patients with chronic bronchitis.[13]

Latex tests for group A streptococci from throat specimens are reported to be highly specific but may lack sensitivity, and negative results should be confirmed by culture.[13] The sensitivity of *Cryptococcus* antigen tests for CSF or serum, or both, has been reported to be up to 90% for patients with confirmed cryptococcal meningitis.[93]

A summary of agents typically identified by antigen detection tests, described previously, is presented in Table 57–9. Some these have recently been compared with nucleic acid techniques, and comparative performance characteristics of agents of particular interest are presented later in the chapter.

Nucleic Acid Analysis

The previously described immunoassays detect protein antigenic components of viral agents or microorganisms. Since about 1985, procedures have been developed that allow detection of the nucleic acid components of suspected pathogens. Several molecularly based techniques are currently at different stages of investigation for application in the clinical laboratory, for either diagnostic or research purposes. This section of the chapter describes the methods that are currently marketed and those that may become available in the

near future. Owing to the rapid rate of change and advancement in this area, however, the discussion may not be inclusive of all reagents approved by the U.S. Food and Drug Administration (FDA) that are available for detection of pathogens or of all method-organism combinations under investigation. The different nucleic acid–based technologies are, for the most part, manufacturer specific, and the commercial developers are identified in the following text. Each method may require specific transport devices and/or media, as well as time and temperature conditions, before processing. Each method may also require sample preparation (extraction) before testing, but these aspects of the procedures are not described.

Hybridization Procedures

In hybridization procedures, specific segments of the nucleic acid (DNA or RNA) of the agents react (hybridize) with labeled complementary oligonucleotide sequences (probes). The labels used include radioisotopes (^{32}S, ^{35}P, ^{125}I) or, more commonly in clinical laboratory settings, enzymatic moieties (biotin, digoxigenin, and HRP) or a fluorescent label. Hybridization with labeled probes is detected by autoradiography, scintillation counting, chromogenically or by chemiluminescence. Probes can be used to detect native DNA, or RNA, in fresh clinical specimens, in fixed tissue specimens, or in infected tissue culture cells, or to detect segments of DNA or RNA that have been amplified exponentially and to identify infectious agents that have been isolated by cultivation.[94, 95]

Hybridization Reactions with Native DNA/RNA (Probes) Solution-Phase Hybridization
Many of the commercially available DNA probe assays utilize solution-phase hybridization in which both the target nucleic acid and the probe are free to interact in an aqueous reaction mixture, which shortens the time required for hybridization to occur. Applications of this procedure are listed in Table 57–10 and include the following:

1. *Pace 2* (Gen-Probe). For detection of *C. trachomatis* and *N. gonorrhoeae* from a single endocervical swab. These tests use a chemiluminescent (acridinium ester)-labeled, single-strand DNA probe complementary to ribosomal RNA of the target organism. The ribosomal RNA is released from the target organism and combines with the labeled probe, forming a stable DNA-RNA hybrid. The labeled hybrid is separated from nonhybridized probe, and the amount of chemiluminescence is measured in a luminometer.
2. *GP-ST test* (Gen-Probe). GP-ST is used for the detection of *S. pyogenes* in throat swabs and also uses an acridinium ester–labeled, single-strand DNA probe complementary to the ribosomal RNA of the group A streptococcus.

TABLE 57-10 ▶ NUCLEIC ACID PROBE REAGENTS FOR DIRECT DETECTION IN CLINICAL SPECIMENS

Source	Product Name	Agents Detected
Abbott Laboratories	HBV Hybridization Test	Hepatitis B virus
Becton-Dickinson	Affirm	*Gardnerella vaginalis*
BioGenex	ISH	*Trichomonas vaginalis*
		Candida albicans
		Human papillomavirus
Digene	HC II CT-ID Test	*Chlamydia trachomatis*
	HC II GC-ID Test	*Neisseria gonorrhoeae*
	CMV DNA Assay*	Cytomegalovirus
	EBV DNA Assay*	Epstein-Barr virus
	HBV DNA Assay*	Hepatitis B virus
	HPV DNA Assay*	Human papillomavirus
	HSV DNA Assay*	Herpes simplex virus
Enzo	Pathotech	Human papillomavirus
Gen-Probe	Pace 2	*C. trachomatis*
	Pace 2	*N. gonorrhoeae*
	GP-ST	*Streptococcus pyogenes*

*Available for research purposes only.

3. ***Hybrid Capture*** (Digene) products. For detection of CMV, HBV, and HPV in appropriate specimens. These tests employ RNA probes to hybridize with target single-stranded DNA. This method is also being evaluated as a diagnostic test for detection of *C. trachomatis* and *N. gonorrhoeae* from the same endocervical swab. The hybrid molecules are captured onto the surface of a plastic tube by immobilized antibodies specific for RNA-DNA hybrids. Unreacted single-stranded RNA and nonspecifically bound material are eliminated by washing steps. The captured hybrids are detected by reaction with an AP-conjugated antibody to RNA-DNA hybrids followed by a chemiluminescent substrate. The enzyme cleaves the substrate, resulting in the emission of light that is measured in a luminometer and is directly proportional to the quantity of hybrid captured. The presence of multiple AP molecules on each antibody and the binding of each captured target by several antibodies result in substantial, specific signal amplification.[96]

4. ***Affirm*** (Becton-Dickinson) hybridization products. For detection of *Gardnerella vaginalis*, *Trichomonas vaginalis*, and *C. albicans* from a single vaginal swab. The technique uses a capture bead containing the probe molecules complementary to the ribosomal RNA target. The hybridized molecules are detected by the formation of a complex structure composed of signal polymers that bind to the hybridized rRNA captured on the bead as well as to color development probes, which are subsequently added to the reaction mixture. The color development probes are bound by a streptavidin-HRP enzyme conjugate. After addition of substrate, the precipitated blue-colored products are detected spectrophotometrically.

In Situ Hybridization

In situ hybridization (ISH) allows the detection of target agent as well as the cytologic characterization of cells in sections of biopsy material. Currently, three systems are available that utilize a probe technique for identification of HPV. All three systems use RNA probes labeled with biotin, and all three systems employ the same *NBT/BCIP* substrate, which produces a bluish-black color at the site of the probe-target complex, owing to the action of AP.[97] The systems are as follows:

1. ***PathoGene*** (Enzo) and ***ISH*** (BioGenex) employ an anti-biotin antibody that binds to the hybridized probe, followed by an alkaline phosphatase–streptavidin for in situ examination of cervical biopsy material for the presence of HPV.

2. The ***Hybrid Capture*** system, described previously for HPV DNA detection, can also be used for in situ studies. It is a one-step procedure in which a streptavidin–AP conjugate is added and binds to the hybridized biotin probe.

AMPLIFICATION TECHNIQUES

The limit of detection of the procedures described previously in this section is dictated by the number of viral agents or microorganisms present in the specimen. The ability to increase the number of target sequences or some other component of a detection reaction mixture would be advantageous in cases in which there is a limited amount of target within a specimen. Procedures in which sequences of known nucleic acid components are amplified have been developed with the goal of greatly increasing sensitivity.

The amplified product is detected by hybridization with specific probes and detected by the generation of a colorimetric signal. Other methods have been developed that increase the number of probe molecules after they have hybridized with a specific nucleic acid sequence in the target. Another approach has been amplification of the signal generated to detect hybridization reactions.[94, 98, 99]

The use of different enzymes and/or varying reaction conditions have allowed the development of these different amplification procedures. To date, the amplification techniques that are available or under development for diagnostic testing include *amplification of target sequence* (polymerase chain reaction [PCR], nucleic acid sequence–based amplification [NASBA], transcription-mediated amplification (TMA), strand displacement amplification [SDA]), *probe amplification* (ligase chain reaction [LCR], Q-beta replicase amplification), and *signal amplification* (branched DNA [bDNA]). These techniques are summarized in Table 57–11.

Amplification of Target Sequences

Polymerase Chain Reaction (PCR) (Roche Molecular Systems). The most widely used amplification strategy is the DNA-dependent PCR. The target DNA sequence to be amplified is approximately 100 to 1,000 base pairs in length and may be located in the cell genome or plasmid. Two oligonucleotide primer sequences typically containing 18 to 20 bases are synthesized that are complementary to the ends of the sequence to be amplified.

The procedure is based on the repetition of three successive reactions, which consist of (1) denaturing double-stranded DNA into single strands at high temperature, (2) hybridizing specific primers to each of the DNA strands, and (3) extension of the primers from the 3′ to the 5′ direction by enzymatic action of a heat-stable DNA polymerase (Taq) on the abundant nucleotides present in the reaction mixture to synthesize new complementary DNA (cDNA) strands. During subsequent cycles, the DNA target and newly synthesized DNA strands act as templates for amplification, and repeated cycles result in the exponential accumulation of specific DNA fragments. With commercially available procedures, the amplified products (amplicons) are detected by the addition of avidin-HRP–labeled probe followed by substrate. Color development is read in a spectrophotometer.

Reverse Transcriptase PCR (RT-PCR). Modifications of the PCR procedure allow amplification of RNA molecules, rather than DNA. The procedure consists of four basic steps. Initially, a heat-stable reverse transcriptase isolated from *Thermus thermophilus* is used to convert RNA to DNA (cDNA) at 72°C in the presence of Mn^{2+}. The addition of other reagents to the reac-

tion mixture chelates the Mn^{2+} and brings about a switch in the template specificity of the *T. thermophilus* polymerase from RNA to DNA, and additional DNA strands are formed and detected as described in the preceding paragraph. By the addition of an RNA quantitation standard of known copy number that is co-amplified with the target sequence, a copy level can be assigned to the specimen and the number of target sequences present in the original specimen can be determined. Hence, successive changes in the patient's viral load can be monitored for prognostic evaluations.

Currently, the PCR reagents are manufactured by Roche Molecular Systems and include the following qualitative detection reagents:

1. **Amplicor *Chlamydia* PCR Test.** Amplifies a cryptic plasmid DNA sequence in endocervical specimens in females and urethral and urine samples in males.
2. **Amplicor *Neisseria gonorrhoeae* PCR Test.** Amplifies a genomic DNA sequence, the cytosine methyltransferase gene, M.Ngo P11, unique to *N. gonorrhoeae*, in endocervical specimens in females and urethral specimens in males. Commercial availability is pending FDA approval.
3. **Amplicor *Mycobacterium tuberculosis* PCR Test.** Amplifies a genomic DNA sequence that codes for 16s rRNA in specimens of bronchoalveolar lavage and sputum that are positive by acid-fast staining.
4. **Amplicor CMV PCR Test.** Amplifies a region of the CMV DNA polymerase gene (UL54) in specimens of CSF.

The aforementioned tests can be performed manually in a microwell system or in an automated COBAS system, the latter of which is pending FDA approval.

1. **Amplicor Hepatitis C.** Amplifies a segment of RNA genome after reverse transcription in plasma samples.
2. **Amplicor HIV-1.** Amplifies a highly conserved segment of the gag gene in the RNA genome after reverse transcription in plasma samples.
3. **Amplicor HBV.** Amplifies a segment of the genomic DNA.

Quantitative levels of hepatitis C virus, HIV-1, and HBV can be determined with the *Amplicor HCV Monitor* and *Amplicor HIV-1 Monitor* and *Amplicor HBV Monitor kits*. These reagents are useful in monitoring disease progression and/or response to therapy.

An advantage of the aforementioned amplification techniques is that they can be performed relatively rapidly, and results can be available within the same day that a patient's specimen is received in the laboratory. However, the success of amplification relies on utilizing tightly controlled procedures to prevent cross-contamination of amplified sequences and to avoid

TABLE 57-11 ▶ DESCRIPTIVE SUMMARY OF NUCLEIC ACID AMPLIFICATION PROCEDURES

Procedure (Source)	Agent/Target	Description	Enzymes Used	Detection Method
PCR [Amplicor (Roche)]	*Chlamydia trachomatis/* plasmid DNA *Neisseria gonorrhoeae/* genomic DNA *Mycobacterium tuberculosis/* genomic DNA CMV/genomic DNA HBV/genomic DNA*	Heat-dependent method of **target** amplification by repeated cycles of denaturation–primer annealing–primer extension; amplicon captured by probes immobilized to wells of microtiter plate	Thermophilic DNA polymerase	Avidin-HRP–labeled probe binds to DNA amplicon; reaction with substrate read in spectrophotometer
RT-PCR [Amplicor/ Monitor (Roche)]	HIV-1 HCV	Modification of PCR, reverse transcriptase converts RNA into complementary DNA (cDNA), which then serves as template for thermophilic DNA polymerase	Reverse transcriptase, thermophilic DNA polymerase	Avidin-HRP–labeled probe binds to RNA amplicon; reaction with substrate read in spectrophotometer
NASBA* [Nuclisense, Organon Teknika)]	HIV/genomic RNA CMV pp667/mRNA *C. trachomatis/*16s rRNA	Isothermal **target** amplification in which DNA intermediate is transcribed from RNA, and large amounts of RNA are subsequently produced with cDNA as template	Reverse transcriptase, RNase H, RNA polymerase	Labeled probe and electrochemilumi-nescence
TMA [Amp (Gen-Probe)]	*C. trachomatis/*23s rRNA *M. tuberculosis/*rRNA *N. gonorrhoeae* HIV-1* HCV*	Isothermal **target** amplification in which primers anneal to specific RNA target sequences, and DNA intermediates are produced that serve as templates for large amount of RNA	Reverse transcriptase, RNA polymerase	RNA amplicon binds with chemiluminescent ssDNA probe, and emitted light is measured in luminometer after hybrid protection reaction
SDA [Probe-Tec, Becton-Dickinson]	*M. tuberculosis/* genomic DNA* *N. gonorrhoeae/* genomic DNA *C. trachomatis/* plasmid DNA	Isothermal **target** amplification in which site-specific nicks in one DNA strand are made by restriction endonuclease followed by DNA synthesis at the nick and displacement of the nicked strand	Restriction endonucleases, DNA polymerase	Chemiluminescent probe binds to amplicon; emitted light measured in luminometer
LCR [LCX, (Abbott)]	*C. trachomatis/* plasmid DNA *N. gonorrhoeae/* genomic DNA *M. tuberculosis/* genomic DNA*	Heat-dependent **probe** amplification in which product is formed by ligation of two probes after their binding to adjacent complementary target sequences; new strand then serves as target for additional cycle	Thermostable DNA ligase	Microparticle EIA
Q-beta* (Vysis)	*C. trachomatis/ plasmid DNA* *M. tuberculosis/*23s rRNA *M. avium* complex/ 23s rRNA *M. pneumoniae/*16s rRNA *Pneumocystis carinii/* 18s rRNA *Legionella pneumophila/*16s rRNA	Detector **probes** are geometrically amplified by Q-beta replicase following hybridization to specific DNA or RNA target	Q-beta replicase	RNA detector probe and binding of free propidium iodide resulting in fluorescent signal
bDNA [Quantiplex (Chiron)]	HCV/genomic RNA HIV-1/genomic RNA HBV/genomic DNA	**Signal** amplification in which target nucleic acid is captured by probes immobilized to a solid phase; the bDNA amplifier is added, followed by enzyme-labeled probes specific for the bDNA	None	Chemiluminescent substrate is added, and emitted light is measured in luminometer

*Under development or pending FDA approval.

primer artifact formation and nonspecific hybridization of primers. In addition, the presence of inhibitors in some specimens may diminish the sensitivity of these tests. Furthermore, some of the other amplification methods involve isothermal reactions and do not require the use of thermocoupling devices.

Nucleic Acid Sequence–Based Amplification (NASBA) (Organon-Teknika) (previously known as Amplification by Self-Sustaining Sequence Replication [3SR]). This procedure is an outgrowth of an earlier technique called transcription-based amplification system or (TAS) and is a non-PCR nucleic acid amplification technique. The 3SR procedure utilizes the collective activities of three enzymes. These are an avian myeloblastosis virus reverse transcriptase, an RNase H, and a bacteriophage T7 DNA-dependent RNA polymerase.

The initial step of this procedure involves the formation of cDNA from the target RNA sequence by using oligonucleotide primers containing a T7 polymerase binding site. The initial strands of target RNA in the RNA-DNA hybrids are degraded by the RNase H after they have served as templates for the first primer. The newly formed cDNA is bound by the second primer and is extended, resulting in the formation of double-stranded cDNAs with one or both strands capable of serving as transcription templates for T7 RNA polymerase. The amplified product is detected by hybridization with a labeled probe followed by electrochemiluminescence.

Currently the NASBA reagents, available for research use only, include the following products:

1. **Nuclisense HIV-1 QT.** For the detection after amplification of genomic HIV RNA in a wide range of specimens, from CSF to feces. By including internal calibrators of known RNA levels and utilization of computerized data analysis, the level of HIV RNA present in the original sample can be quantified.
2. **Nuclisense CMV pp67.** To detect messenger RNA coding for the matrix tegument protein pp67 of CMV, which indicates viral replication and active infection in specimens of whole blood.

This procedure is also being evaluated for the detection of the 16S ribosomal RNA of *C. trachomatis* in cervical scrapings and urine.[100]

Transcription-Medicated Amplification (TMA) and Hybrid Protection Assay (Gen-Probe). This procedure is another isothermal technique in which primers anneal to specific RNA target sequences that are amplified via DNA intermediates (cDNA). A chemiluminescent DNA probe that is complementary to the amplicon hybridizes to the amplicon to form a stable RNA-DNA complex. A selection reagent is added that hydrolyzes the chemiluminescent label on any unhybridized probe in the mixture. Thus, the label on the hybridized probe is "protected" and is detected in a luminometer. Currently, the TMA reagents that are available include the following products:

Amplified *Chlamydia trachomatis* Assay (AMP CT). To detect ribosomal RNA in endocervical and male urethral swab specimens and in female and male urine specimens. During the procedure, the 23s rRNA target is amplified via cDNA intermediates and detected by hybridization with a chemiluminescent single-stranded DNA probe.

Amplified *Mycobacterium tuberculosis* Detection Test (AMTDT). To detect ribosomal RNA in respiratory specimens that are positive by acid-fast staining. Reagents for detecting *N. gonorrhoeae* have recently been FDA-approved. In addition, TMA procedures for detection of HIV-1, hepatitis C, and other agents are currently under development or awaiting FDA approval.

Strand Displacement Amplification (SDA) (Becton-Dickinson). This rather recent addition to the target amplification systems is based on the ability of DNA polymerase to initiate DNA synthesis at a single-stranded nick within a DNA target molecule and to displace the nicked strand during DNA synthesis. Modifications involving reverse transcriptase and amplification via cDNA intermediates are also possible. This procedure is being developed by Becton-Dickinson and includes the following products:

BDProbeTec MTB Test. For detection and quantitation of *M. tuberculosis* complex in respiratory specimens. Reagents for detection of *N. gonorrhoeae* and *C. trachomatis* have recently been FDA-approved. These tests utilize a double-dye–labeled hairpin probe, which reduces the overall test performance time.

Probe Amplification

DNA Amplification by Ligase Chain Reaction (LCR) (Abbott Laboratories). This technique is based on sequential rounds of template-dependent ligation of two juxtaposed oligonucleotide probes. In the LCR procedure, two sets of oligonucleotide probes that are complementary to opposite strands of the target DNA are used. The probe pair anneals to the target DNA sequence at 65°C in a head-to-tail fashion, with the 3'-end of one probe abutting the 5'-end of the second. DNA ligase joins the adjacent end to form a duplicate of one strand of the target. A modification of the procedure utilizes probes that are staggered in their alignment, so that there is a gap of one or more nucleotides between adjacent probes. The short gap is then filled by the action of DNA polymerase before the ligation step. Repetition of this process results in a logarithmic increase in ligation products that can be detected by the functional groups attached to the oligonucleotide primers.

The commercial source of LCR reagents is Abbott Laboratories, and the products include the following:

LCX* Chlamydia trachomatis *Assay. For detection of plasmid DNA of *C. trachomatis* in endocervical and male urethral swab specimens and in female and male urine specimens.

LCX* Neisseria gonorrhoeae *Assay. For detection of genomic DNA of *N. gonorrhoeae* in endocervical and male urethral swab specimens and in female and male urine specimens.

LCX* Mycobacterium tuberculosis *Assay. For detection of genomic DNA of *M. tuberculosis* in respiratory specimens. This test is currently not FDA approved.

Qβ Replication Amplification of RNA Probe Molecules (Vysis). This procedure utilizes an RNA-dependent RNA polymerase enzyme, Q-beta replicase, which is derived from the Q-beta RNA bacteriophage. This enzyme brings about the replication of a naturally occurring 221-base RNA (MDV-1), producing full-length complementary plus and minus strands of MDV-1 RNA, each of which can serve as templates for additional rounds of replication. The MDV-1 RNA can be used solely as an amplifiable reporter group that is attached by a biotin-avidin linkage to a specific targe probe. Alternatively, recombinant MDV-1 RNA probes can be constructed that contain complementary sequences to a specific target and that can hybridize to the target and become exponentially amplified by the Q-beta replicase.

Currently, no products are commercially available that utilize this technique. However, there have been published evaluations of a system designed to detect specific regions of 23S ribosomal RNA of *M. tuberculosis*,[101] the 23s ribosomal RNA of *C. trachomatis*,[102] and the 23S, 16S, 18S, and 16S ribosomal RNAs of *M. avium* complex, *M. pneumoniae*, *P. carinii*, and *L. pneumophila*, respectively.[103] These evaluations were conducted by GENETRAK, but the commercial development of these products is now being conducted by Vysis.

Signal Amplification
Branched DNA (bDNA) (Chiron Corporation). Signal amplification procedures are designed to increase the signal generated by the probe hybridized to a specific sequence of target DNA or RNA, rather than increasing the nucleic acid target itself. The bDNA probe system has been developed commercially for research use and utilizes multiple probes together with complex reporter molecules (see Table 57–11).

This procedure involves the denaturation of the specimen DNA or RNA in a microtiter well containing specific target-capture probes adsorbed to the solid surface. Capture of the target is facilitated by soluble target probes with regions complementary to the target as well as the immobilized capture probe. A second set of target probes is added that bind to a different region of the target molecule and that are complementary to the amplification multimer that is added to the reaction mixture after overnight incubation. During incubation, the probes hybridizes with and isolate the nucleic acid sequence of interest.

The multimer is chemically synthesized as an oligonucleotide that has nucleoside analogs attached along its length, forming a "branched" or comb-shaped structure. After addition of the multimer and incubation, enzyme-labeled oligonucleotide probes are added that bind to the multimer (bDNA) by homologous base pairing. Substrate is added, and the enzyme-probe complex is measured by detection of chemiluminescence. The mean relative luminescence value for duplicate determinations is compared with a four-point standard curve that has been run in the same assay to obtain a quantitation of the amount of target present in the original specimen.[104]

The manufacturer of bDNA reagents, available for research purposes, is Chiron Corporation, and the products include the following:

1. **Quantiplex HCV-RNA Assay, Quantiplex HIV-1.** For detection of HCV and HIV-1 RNA respectively in serum.
2. **Quantiplex HBV-DNA Assay.** For detection of HBV DNA in serum.

Performance Characteristics of Diagnostic Tests for Detection of Agents of Particular Interest

Chlamydia trachomatis

The development of antigen detection methods expanded the capability of detection of *C. trachomatis* to settings other than full-scale virology laboratories and decreased the burden of detection inherent in the complex cultivation procedures. The most widely used antigen detection techniques have been the Syva Microtrak Direct Fluorescent Assay (MT-DFA), the Syva Microtrak Enzyme Immunoassay (MT-EIA), and Abbott's EIA, Chlamydiazyme (CZ). These products are not the only such tests on the market (see Table 57–9), but they are probably the most thoroughly investigated.

Initial investigations consisted of comparisons of results from endocervical swabs submitted to antigen detection systems with results of culture. However, when the specimens that yielded positive results from the antigen tests and negative culture results were

TABLE 57–12 ▶ PERFORMANCE OF MICROTRAK DFA AND CHLAMYDIAZYME FOR DETECTION OF *CHLAMYDIA TRACHOMATIS*[a] COMPARED TO CULTURE OR TRUE-POSITIVES IN DIFFERENT PATIENT POPULATIONS

			Sensitivity[a]		
Reference	N	Percentage of Prevalence (Population)	Culture	MicroTrak DFA[b]	Chlamydiazyme (%)[c]
Chernesky et al[105]	619	27.7 (STD clinic) 16.3 (Planned Parenthood) 3.4 (OB/GYN)	Not done	87.9	98.3
Lefebvre et al[107]	715	6.7 (asymptomatic)	Not done	81.1	79.4
	827	9.1 (nonpregnant)	*88*	*65.5*	*60*
	231	12.1 (pregnant)	*82.1*	*84.6*	*85.7*
Baselski et al[106]	20.1	20.1 (OB/GYN)	*84.4*	*95.2*	*95.3*

[a]Numbers in italics reflect results after discrepant analysis.
[b]Specificity >96%.
[c]Specificity >92.9%.

subjected to additional testing—that is, reculturing, repeat antigen testing, or use of an alternative test procedure (discrepant analysis)—it was recognized that culture is not 100% sensitive and that the gold standard should be expanded. Selected examples of published evaluations are presented in Tables 57–12 and 57–13.

A wide range of results have been obtained from the many evaluations conducted with these test systems. The sensitivity of the antigen detection systems approached the sensitivity and specificity of culture in some settings,[105, 106] while it fell short in other settings.[107–109] Olsen and coworkers[110] found the MT-EIA system to be significantly more sensitive than CZ (see Table 57–13). Some investigations with MT-DFA found it to be of nearly equivalent sensitivity to that of CZ[106, 107, 111] (see Table 57–12), while Thomas and colleagues[112] have found the MT-DFA to be more sensitive than either of the EIA systems (see Table 57–13).

A similar range of results have been obtained in comparisons of probe-type test procedures with culture and antigen detection systems for detection of *C. trachomatis.* Selected published works are presented in Table 57–14. The Pace 2 system has been found to be less sensitive than culture,[113] more sensitive than

culture,[114] and of nearly equivalent sensitivity.[115] The Pace 2 was found to be more sensitive than the MT-DFA[116] and CZ,[114] and of nearly equivalent sensitivity to that of MT-EIA.[109] Two recent evaluations of the Digene Hybrid Capture system found it to be more sensitive than culture.[117, 118]

A listing of selected published evaluations of other recently developed nucleic acid techniques is presented in Table 57–15. Comparisons were made to the total number of true-positives as determined by discrepant analysis, as described previously. Overall, the PCR, TMA, and LCR assays performed with specimens of urine or endocervical swabs appear to have similar sensitivities,[115, 119–121] and results with urine specimens were usually equivalent to or better than that with the endocervical specimens. However, statistically significant higher sensitivity was noted for PCR compared to LCR[122] and for PCR COBAS compared to LCR[123] with urine specimens. The LCR assay was found to be more sensitive than TMA with urine specimens[124] (9/98). The sensitivity of detection with vulval specimens compared well with detection from endocervical swabs with both TMA and LCR.[124] In addition, the LCR assay performed on patient-collected vulval swabs and vaginal swabs compared favorably with the LCR assay

TABLE 57–13 ▶ COMPARATIVE SENSITIVITIES OF MICROTRAK EIA AND CHLAMYDIAZYME FOR DETECTION OF *CHLAMYDIA TRACHOMATIS*

			Sensitivity (%)[c]		
Reference	Prevalence	N	MicroTrak EIA	Chlamydiazyme	Comparator
Olsen[a] et al[110]	5.6	550	95[b]	79[b]	MicroTrack DFA
Thomas et al[112]	24.5	151	87.5	75	MicroTrack DFA
Skulnick et al[108]	1.1	993	61.1	Not tested	Culture (72.2)[d]
Clarke et al[109]	22.1	217	80	Not tested	Culture

[a]Discrepant results resolved by DFA.
[b]$P = .49$.
[c]Specificity of MicroTrak EIA >98.2%, specificity of Chlamydiazyme >92.9%.
[d]Results after discrepant analysis.

TABLE 57-14 ▶	COMPARISON OF PROBE-TYPE ASSAYS FOR DETECTION OF *CHLAMYDIA TRACHOMATIS*[a, b]					
Reference	N	Prevalence (%)	Test	Sensitivity (%)	Comparator	Sensitivity (%)
Blanding et al[113]	940	3.9	Pace 2	75.5	Culture	97.3
Warren et al[114]	1037	5.9	Pace 2	96.7	CZ	79.5
					Culture	80
Pasternack et al[115]	666	5.9	Pace 2	79.5	Culture	84.6
Iwen et al[116]	318	9.4	Pace 2	93	MT DFA	81
Clarke et al[109]	217	22.1	Pace 2	78	MT EIA	80
Williams et al[117]	415	5.1	Digene HC	100	Culture	71.4
Girdner et al[118]	587	11.1	Digene HC	95.4	Culture	81.5

[a]Specificity of all tests >97%.
[b]When reported, positive predictive values varied from 91.3 to 92.5 for Digene HC, and from 85 to 93.6 for Pace 2. Negative predictive values >99 for both Digene HC and Pace 2.

conducted on urine[124, 125] and/or physician-collected endocervical swabs.[126] The sensitivity of cultures performed on endocervical, urethral, or vulval swabs varied from a low of 22%[125] to a high of 88%.[119] (Data not shown.)

Neisseria gonorrhoeae

An antigen detection system for *N. gonorrhoeae* was developed by Abbott Laboratories using an ELISA format (Gonozyme) similar to that used for the detection of *C. trachomatis* (CZ). In some settings, however, the sensitivity of Gonozyme did not approach that of culture techniques.[127, 128] Other attempts at developing techniques for rapid and specific identification of *N. gonorrhoeae* have included nucleic acid probes for specimens collected on swab, and PCR and LCR testing of urine as well as endocervical and urethral swabs. Results of selected published comparisons are presented in Table 57–16. Except for the results with Gonozyme,

TABLE 57-15 ▶	COMPARATIVE PERFORMANCE CHARACTERISTICS OF TARGET AMPLIFICATION SYSTEMS FOR THE DETECTION OF *CHLAMYDIA TRACHOMATIS* IN DIFFERENT PATIENT POPULATIONS							
Test	Specimen	N	Prevalence	Sens	Spec	PPV	NPV	Ref
PCR (micro-well)	Urine	1,005	4	95[a]	99.9	97.4	99.8	Schepetiuk et al[122]
		666	5.9	82	99.7	Not given		Pasternack et al[115]
		442	11.3	100	99.7	98	100	Pasternack et al[119]
	Endocervix	666	5.9	82	99.8	Not given		Pasternack et al[115]
		442	6.3	96.4	99.8	96.4	99.8	Puolakkainen et al[121]
PCR COBAS	Urine	1,000	7.7	92.7[b]	99.4	Not given		Goessens et al[123]
		442	11.3	94	99.2	92.2	99.2	Pasternack et al[119]
	Endocervix	447	6.3	78.6	98.8	81.5	98.6	Puolakkainen et al[121]
TMA	Urine	1,000	7.7	85.4	99	Not given		Goessens et al[123]
		308	8.1	76[c]	99.3	90.5	97.9	Stary et al[124]
	Endocervix	308	8.1	88	99.6	95.7	99.9	Stary et al[124]
	Vulva	308		92	99.6	95.8	99.3	Stary et al[124]
LCR	Urine	1,005	4	75[a]	100	100	99	Schepetiuk et al[122]
		443	5.6	92.6	100	100	99.5	Puolakkainen et al[121]
		312	7.7	92.3	100	Not given		Stary et al[125]
		1,000	7.7	83.7[b]	99	Not given		Goessens et al[123]
		308	8.1	96[c]	100	100	99.6	Stary et al[124]
		602	10.1	78.8	99.4	94.5	97.4	Buimer et al[135]
		442	11.3	94	100	100	99.2	Pasternack et al[119]
	Endocervix	448	4.9	81.5	100	100	98.8	Puolakkainen et al[121]
		308	8.1	92	99.6	95.8	99.3	Stary et al[124]
		602	9.6	87.9	100	100	98.5	Buimer et al[135]
		309[c]	14.9	89.8	100	100	98.1	Hook et al[126]
	Vulva	312	7.4	85.2	100	100	97.3	Stary et al[125]
		308	8.1	92	100	100	99.3	Stary et al[124]
	Vagina	309[d]	14.9	91.8	99.6	97.8	98.5	Hook et al[126]

Compared to true-positives after discrepant analysis.
[a]Microwell PCR more sensitive than LCR with urine specimens; $P < .0001$.
[b]Automated COBAS PCR more sensitive than LCR with urine specimens; $P = .047$.
[c]LCR more sensitive than TMA with urine specimens; $P = .0253$.
[d]Vaginal specimen collected by patient; endocervical specimen collected by physician.

TABLE 57-16 ▶	COMPARISONS OF *NEISSERIA GONORRHOEAE* DETECTION ASSAYS							
Test	Specimen	N	Prevalence	Sensitivity[a]	Specificity	PPV	NPV	Ref
Gonozyme	Endocervix	866	4.5	50	97.1	40	98	Donders et al[128]
Pace 2	Endocervix	1,750[b]	8.7	97.1	99.1	90.6	99.8	Vlaspoder et al[130]
		436[c]	33.5	99.4	99.6	99.4	99.6	Hale et al[129]
HC II	Endocervix	415[d]	2.4	90	99.8	90	99.8	Williams et al[117]
		477	17	90.8	99.3	95.2	98.6	Cullen et al[131]
	Urine	477	17	87.7	96.6	80.3	98	Cullen et al[131]
PCR	Endocervix	100	7.8	100	99.4	Not given		Crotchfelt et al[132]
	Urine	90	7.8	90	95.9	Not given		Crotchfelt et al[132]
LCR	Endocervix	383	5.5	95.4	100	100	99.7	Buimer et al[135]
		125	8.8	89.5	99.1	94.4	98.1	Stary et al[134]
		309[e]	17.5	84.6	99.2	95.7	98	Hook et al[136]
	Vagina	309[e]	17.5	100	99.6	98.1	100	Hook et al[136]
	Urine	383	5.5	50	100	100	97	Buimer et al[135]
		125	8.8	94.7	100	100	99.1	Stary et al[134]
	Urethra	125	8.8	84.2	100	100	97.2	Stary et al[134]

[a]When reported, sensitivity of culture after discrepant analysis varied from 50% (Buimer et al[135]) to 92.3% (Cullen et al[131]) with endocervical specimens, and was 63.2% for urethral swabs (Stary et al[97]) and 57.7% for vaginal specimens (Hook et al[136]).
[b]496 females, [c]623 males, [d]271 females, 165 males specimens also used for *C. trachomatis* testing.
[e]Vaginal specimens collected by patient, endocervical specimens collected by physician.

the performance characteristics are compared to true-positives as determined by additional and/or alternative testing of specimens giving discordant results.

The results presented indicate that the sensitivity of the probes tested approach that of culture,[117, 129–131] with a slightly reduced PPV being observed with both the Pace 2 and the Hybrid Capture systems in some cases.[117, 130] The Roche Amplicor System for *N. gonorrhoeae* has not yet been approved for commercial use, and published comparisons are limited. Results of a small study conducted by Crotchfelt and colleagues[132] suggested that the PCR test was much more sensitive than culture when either endocervical swabs or urine was compared to culture of the endocervix. The LCR procedure, which is available commercially, has been more thoroughly studied. Investigators have found that the sensitivity of LCR conducted with urine or endocervical swabs exceeds or is nearly equivalent to that of culture.[131, 133–135] A slightly decreased PPV was observed by Cullen[131] and Stary[134] and their colleagues. Hook and co-workers[136] found greater sensitivity with specimens of the vagina collected by the patients compared with physician-collected specimens of the endocervix.

Streptococcus agalactiae (Group B Streptococcus)

Several attempts have been made by commercial suppliers to provide an assay for rapid detection of group B streptococci in vaginal specimens of pregnant patients. To date, the results have been generally disappointing (Table 57–17).

Adraanse and colleagues[137] conducted a rather large study comparing the sensitivity of two EIA assays (Quidel Group B Strep Test and Hybritech ICON Strep B)

and two agglutination assays (Wellcogen and Slidex) to culture. Although the EIA assays were found to be statistically more sensitive than the agglutination assays ($P < .05$), the investigators concluded that none of the tests studied were sensitive enough for general screening of the pregnant population.

Similar conclusions have been drawn from other investigators who have compared rapid screening tests for group B *Streptococcus* to culture results.[138–142] One especially interesting finding has been that routine culture of vaginal specimens on blood agar plates is not as sensitive a method of recovery of *S. agalactiae* as is cultivation in broth (see Table 57–17). Thus, cultivation in broth culture remains the most reliable method of detecting the presence of group B streptococci in the vagina of pregnant females. Platt and colleagues[143] found recovery to be increased when both vaginal and rectal swabs are collected and incubated overnight in an enrichment broth.

The restricted utility of antigen detection systems for identification of group B streptococci in CSF of neonates has been described earlier in the chapter. Greenberg and coworkers,[144] however, found that Directigen and Bactogen LA tests detected 98% and 92% of newborns with group B streptococcal sepsis, respectively, by using concentrated specimens of urine. The Wellcogen latex test and ICON EIA test did not perform as well on concentrated urine samples, and none of the tests performed well with unconcentrated urines.

Human Papillomavirus

Evaluations of the performance characteristics of tests for HPV have included not only the detection of the presence of the virus as the end point but also resolu-

| TABLE 57-17 ▶ ANTIGEN DETECTION SYSTEMS FOR *STREPTOCOCCUS AGALACTIAE* COMPARED TO CULTURE ||||||

Reference	Prevalence[a]	N	Specimen	Test[c]	Sensitivity[a, b]
Simpson et al[138]	14.3 (9.8)	266	Vaginal swab	Wellcogen[d]	78.9 (100)
	13.7 (8.5)	117		ICON	68.8
Hordnes et al[139]	13.5 (4)	200	Uterine cervix	ICON	7.4 (100)
Park et al[140]	18.8	531	Vaginal swab	ICON	39
				Biostar	72
				Culture, TSA	68
				Culture, EB	100
Baker et al[141]	25.1	502	Distal vagina	ICON	15
				Quidel	12
				Culture, SB	100
				ICON	21 (46)
				Quidel	16 (36)
				Biostar	53 (100)
				Culture, BAP	69
		305		Biostar	37 (100)
Andreu et al[142]	11.2	192	Vaginal exudate	ICON	35
		133		Equate	47
		88		Phadebact[c]	38

[a]Numbers in parenthesis indicate heavy colonization.
[b]When reported, specificity of ICON ≥ 96.5%, Equate = 91%, others > 98%.
[c]Culture, TSA = direct plating on trypticase soy agar; Culture, EB = enhancement in broth prior to plating; Culture, SB = cultivation in selective broth; Culture, BAP = cultivation on blood agar plates.
[d]4-Hour incubation before testing.

tion of abnormalities seen on Papanicolaou's (Pap) smear as correlated with high-risk serotypes of HPV. The Pap smear is a valuable screening method for the detection of HPV and cervical abnormalities, but it is rather insensitive. Other tests available include Southern blot, dot blot, ISH, hybrid capture, and PCR. Margiotta and coworkers[145] compared the performance of three commercially available in situ assays for HPV and found similar sensitivities among them. Among the other DNA detection methods, PCR, currently under development by Roche, is the most sensitive, and the Hybrid Capture (HCT, Digene) assay is among the least labor-intensive test. HCT has been shown to be nearly as sensitive as Southern blotting,[146] which has been considered to be the gold standard for detection of HPV.

A comparison of PCR and HCT in 596 females, 499 of whom had normal cytology and 97 or whom had abnormal cytology, was conducted by Cope and coworkers.[147] Overall, the two methods agreed 93% of the time on the positivity or negativity of endocervical lavage specimens for 1 of the 14 HPV types detectable by both methods. When PCR was used as the reference method, HCT was found to be only 46.7% sensitive among women with normal cytology but 81% sensitive among women with abnormal cytology (79.5% in those with LSIL, and 84.2% in those with HSIL). Uberti-Foppa and colleagues[148] found that cytologic evaluation alone underestimated the presence of histologic alterations in nearly 43% of HIV-positive women. Conflicting results have been reported by Clavel and coworkers[149] who found that classic cytologic screening was a more sensitive method for detecting HSIL than

testing for HPV with HCT. Recio and coworkers[150] found an increase in sensitivity in detecting moderate to severe dysplasia in specimens referred because of abnormal cervical cytology results when Pap smear was combined with testing with HCT. Cox and coworkers[151] found that HCT was 86% sensitive in detecting HPV in any CIN in specimens with ASCUS Pap smear interpretation and 93% sensitive in detecting HPV in CIN (2/3) in specimens with ASCUS Pap result. Repeat Pap smear, on the other hand, was found to be only 60% and 73% sensitive in detecting any CIN or CIN (2/3), respectively, in the same patients.

An evaluation of a second-generation hybrid capture assay (HCT II) compared to the first-generation hybrid capture system (HCT I) was conducted by Ferris and colleagues[152] in endocervical specimens from 242 women with ASCUS or LSIL Pap smear reports. The results demonstrated an increase in sensitivity of detection of HPV in CIN (2/3) from 61.9% with the HCT I to 90.5% in patients with LSIL or ASCUS and to 88.9% in patients with only ASCUS Pap smear interpretations. Additional testing with the new formulation may increase the sensitivity and positive predictive value of the hybrid capture methodology, making the test more useful for screening purposes.

HIV

Methods for the diagnosis of HIV infection include those that not only detect the presence of HIV-1 but also can quantitate the levels of HIV-1 in blood. Commercially available assays for the detection of the p24 HIV antigen have been available for the past several years and have been used successfully to monitor levels of this antigen in infected individuals as well as to monitor the effects of therapy.[153] The detection or quantitative systems based on nucleic acid methodology include RT-PCR (Amplicor and Monitor, respectively). Other systems currently available that allow quantitation of HIV are NASBA (Nuclisense), and bDNA (Quantiplex). Detection and quantitation by TMA and SDA are under investigation. The tests currently available have been evaluated individually or in comparison to each other for monitoring response to therapy or predicting fetal transmission from infected mothers.

Uvin and coworkers[154] compared the HIV RNA levels detected by NASBA in paired plasma and cervicovaginal lavage specimens from 72 HIV-infected women. HIV RNA was detected in 61 (85%) of the paired plasma samples at levels of 330 to 1,600,000 copies/mL and 28 (39%) of the cervicolavage specimens were positive at levels of 320 to 440,000 copies/mL. There was a positive correlation between the levels detected in the lavage specimens with the levels in plasma, and a negative correlation between levels in lavage specimens and CD4+ cell counts.

Thea and colleagues[155] and O'Shea and co-workers[156] evaluated the level of HIV RNA detected by NASBA in infants born to HIV-infected mothers. Both observed that the level of viral load detected in the mother is a strong predictor of transmission. Lambert and coworkers[157] studied a cohort of 152 infants perinatally infected with HIV-1 and correlated infant outcome with maternal CD4+ count and the presence of maternal AIDS near delivery. They also correlated infant outcome with maternal viral burden measured by NASBA in a subset of 50 infants. A low maternal CD4+ count and high viral burden were associated with decreased time to category C disease or death in infants infected with HIV-1. Furthermore, high viral load in pregnant women, independent of the advanced maternal disease, appears to increase the risk of rapidly progressive disease in the infected offspring. Delamare and coworkers[158] compared the levels of HIV RNA detected by NASBA and PCR in infants born to HIV-1–infected and noninfected mothers. HIV RNA was detected by NASBA in plasma collected during the first 10 days of life from 12 (25%) and by RT-PCR in peripheral blood mononuclear cells in 11 (22.9%) of the 48 infants born to HIV-1–infected mothers. Both test systems detected HIV RNA in the 39 specimens collected before the age of 3 months, suggesting equivalent sensitivity and specificity of NASBA and RT-PCR in the newborn population.

Alaeus and colleagues[159] evaluated the detection of HIV RNA by NASBA and RT-PCR in plasma samples from 95 patients infected with different genetic subtypes of HIV-1. There was good correlation between the two test systems for detection of types B, C, and D,

but not for type A. A total of 15 (56%) of the 27 subtype A samples were negative by RT-PCR, and 12 (44%) were negative by the NASBA assay. Hence, these assays may not be able to accurately quantify HIV-1 RNA levels in samples from many subtype A–infected patients. Coste and coworkers[160] evaluated the detection of HIV RNA in 60 patients infected with different subtypes of HIV and found that 56 (93.3%) were detected by RT-PCR, 41 (68.3%) were detected by NASBA, and all 60 (100%) were detected by bDNA. When different HIV-1 subtype strains were tested, differences in detection and levels were observed according to strain in some cases. Only bDNA was able to detect all subtypes A to H, while RT-PCR did not detect all group A subtypes and NASBA did not detect all group G subtypes. In addition, the copy number detected by RT-PCR was much lower than the copy number detected by bDNA in one subtype E and one subtype F strain. The specificity of all three tests was 100%.

Different test methods used to diagnose AIDS were evaluated in 199 patients with CD4 counts less than 200. The serum from all patients was positive for HIV antibody by EIA and Western blotting. Of the 125 PMCB pellets tested by RT-PCR, 117 (93.6%) were positive. All eight specimens initially negative by PCR were positive on retesting. The authors concluded that Western blot testing for HIV antibody is the most reliable test for diagnosis of advanced AIDS.[161]

An evaluation of one newly developed ELISA compared to NASBA demonstrated nearly equivalent sensitivity between the two test systems.[162] Considering the potential sensitivity of ELISA systems, and their low cost, simplicity, and potential for full automation, ELISA techniques may remain valuable tools for determining viral load, especially in areas with few resources where it may not be feasible to implement the procedures based on molecular techniques. Consultation with the microbiology laboratory is encouraged, to obtain current information on which tests are utilized in any particular setting.

Hepatitis B Virus

Several commercially available test kits are available for the detection of HBsAg and HBeAg that use either an RIA or ELISA approach (see Table 57–9). These tests are widely used because of their relative simplicity, low cost, and sensitivity and specificity, which approach those of the nucleic acid–based procedures that are under development.[163]

Molecular methods currently used for detecting HBV in serum include hybrid capture, radiologic liquid hybridization, PCR, and bDNA. Comparisons between the bDNA and liquid hybridization tests in serum samples from patients with hepatitis have indicated a strong linear relationship between the two methodologies, but the bDNA is more sensitive and specific.[164, 165] The bDNA test detected HBV DNA in 107 (94%) of 114 serum samples, while the liquid hybridization assay detected HBV DNA in 85 (95%) of 89 specimens with a known high HBV DNA level but only 3 (17%) of 18 specimens with a low HBV DNA level.[164]

The sensitivity and reproducibility of the PCR test was compared with hybrid capture by 10-fold dilution series of two HBV reference plasma specimens and 196 sera from 14 children with chronic HBV infection. The detection limit of the two assays was 10^3 copies/mL and 10^6 to 10^7 copies/mL for PCR and hybrid capture, respectively. However, 26.2% of the HBV DNA–positive clinical samples were found between 10^3 copies/mL and 10^7 copies/mL, and all were below the detection limit of the hybridization assay.[166] When hybrid capture was compared to bDNA in 300 sera of patients suspected of having hepatitis, the latter detected 15% more positive specimens than the former, all of which contained low levels of viral DNA but were associated with clinically significant liver disease.[167]

Trichomonas vaginalis

The testing approaches that have been used for detection of *T. vaginalis* are listed in Table 57–18, which presents the results of some comparative testing of these methods. Cultivation in Diamond's modified medium has been considered the gold standard and the most sensitive method for detection of *T. vaginalis*. However, this cultivation procedure is not undertaken in all laboratories. A newer diagnostic culture system is the InPouch (Biomed, San Jose, CA), which consists of a plastic bag culture system with an upper chamber that allows immediate examination of the specimen plus a lower chamber for *Trichomonas* culture. Some studies have shown that the rate of recovery of *T. vaginalis* with this product approaches that obtained with conventional culture on Diamond's medium.[168–171] Furthermore, Schwebke and colleagues[171] found that the sensitivity of recovery of *T. vaginalis* from patient-collected vaginal swabs was nearly equivalent to physician-collected vaginal swabs when each was inoculated into the InPouch (see Table 57–18).

Although microscopic examination of a wet preparation is commonly used, it appears to be the least sensitive method of other methods available. Pap smear and acridine-orange staining appear to be only slightly more sensitive than wet mount examination.[172, 173] A direct fluorescent antibody test (Integrated Diagnostics) was found to be nearly as sensitive as culture.[172] The Affirm VP DNA probe was found to be nearly as sensitive as culture in a large study reported by DeMeo and coworkers,[174] conducted in a high-prevalence population. A lower sensitivity was reported in a smaller study conducted in a lower-prevalence population.[175] One study found PCR to be more sensitive than culture[176] after resolution of discrepancies in a high-prevalence population.

Cultivation Procedures

In cases in which there are no rapid techniques available or when the performance characteristics of the available reagents do not allow a definitive laboratory diagnosis to be made, it is necessary to attempt to recover the suspected etiologic agent or agents by cultivation techniques. It may also be desirable to isolate the organisms, particularly bacterial agents, to be able to test their susceptibility to commonly used antimicrobial agents.

TABLE 57–18 ▶ RELATIVE SENSITIVITIES OF LABORATORY DIAGNOSTIC TESTS FOR TRICHOMONAS VAGINALIS

Reference	N	Prevalence	Specimen	Test	Sensitivity
Bickley et al[172]	104	37	Vaginal wash	Direct FA	96
				Acridine orange	67
				Wet mount	53
				Culture	95
Ohlemeyer et al[173]	268	15.6	Vaginal swab	InPouch	81
				Wet mount	36
				PAP smear	56
Schwebke et al[171]	100	26	Patient-collected vaginal swab	Culture*	84.6
			Physician-collected vaginal swab		88.5
Briselden et al[175]	176	8.5	Vaginal swab	Probe	80
				Wet mount	80
				Culture	100
DeMeo et al[174]	615	15.4	Vaginal swab	Probe	90.5
				Wet mount	80
				Culture	98
Heine et al[176]	300	20.3	Distal vagina	PCR	91.8
			Post vaginal fornix	Wet mount	80.3
			Post vaginal fornix	Culture	80.3

*InPouch used.

The cultivation techniques employed are dependent on the source of the specimen and the suspected agents. A brief summary of the techniques used for recovery of bacteria, fungi, viral agents, and parasites follows.

Bacteria and Fungi

Many bacterial or fungal agents can be isolated by using a relatively small number of medium types. Several specialized media have been developed for recovery of the organisms that have particular nutritional needs. A summary of the media used commonly to recover bacteria from clinical specimens is presented in Table 57–19 as well as an indication of typical staining procedures and instances in which specialized media may be required. Once isolated, the organisms are identified by observing characteristic morphology, metabolic activity, or serotyping by immunologic reagents or by direct antigen or nuclei acid detection tests, as described previously. Although *C. trachomatis* is classified as a gram-negative bacterium, its growth requirements are similar to those of viruses, and hence

cultivation techniques are similar to those used for recovery of viral agents.

Parasitic Agents

The routine method of detection of *T. vaginalis* as a cause of vaginitis is the examination of a wet preparation for detection of the motile trophozoites, but cultivation of the organism is still considered to be the gold standard for detection. Earlier evaluation of commercially available media demonstrated that Diamond's medium gave the highest recovery rate. But, as mentioned previously, the InPouch may offer a more convenient method of cultivation than that of routine inoculation into Diamond's medium.

Acanthamoeba spp. and *Naegleria* spp. may be responsible for keratitis or primary amebic meningoencephalitis, respectively. Specimens of corneal scrapings and/or biopsies or CSF may be cultured for these organisms. Specialized transport devices are commercially available. The specimens are inoculated onto nutrient agar surfaces on which *E. coli* has been inoculated. As the amebae consume the *E. coli*, they move outward in

---

TABLE 57–19 ▶ RECOMMENDED STAINING AND INOCULATION MEDIA FOR DETECTION AND RECOVERY OF BACTERIAL PATHOGENS FROM CLINICAL SPECIMENS

Specimen	Stains	Blood Agar	Chocolate	MacConkey	Anaerobic	Broth	AFB/ Fungal	Additional
Abscess	Gram	√	√		√ (closed)	√		
Biopsy/tissue	Gram	√	√	√	√	√		GC selective for endometrium
Body fluid	Gram	√	√	√	√	√		GC selective for culdocentesis
Devices:								
IUD		√			√			GC selective, semiquantitative culture useful
Catheter tip		√						Semiquantitative inoculation useful
Eye		√	√			√		GC selective, *Chlamydia*
Genital	Gram	√	√					GC selective; Todd-Hewitt for GBBS
Intestinal		√		√				SS and XLD for *Shigella* and *Salmonella*; CIN for *Yersinia*, TCBS for *Vibrio*; CCFA for *Clostridium difficile*
Urine	Gram	√		√	√ (suprapubic aspirate)			Quantitative culture
Wounds	Gram	√	√	√	√ (aspirates)	√ (aspirates)		
Throat		√						GC selective, Löffler, Tinsdale for *C. diphtheriae*
Nasopharynx		√	√					Löffler, Tinsdale for *C. diphtheriae*, Bordet-Gengou for *Bordetella*
Sputum	Gram, AFB	√	√	√			√	
Bronchoalveolar lavage	Gram, AFB	√	√	√			√	
Tracheal aspirate	Gram	√	√	√			√	CYE for *Legionella*
Transtracheal aspirate	Gram	√	√	√	√	√	√	
Lung biopsy	Gram, AFB	√	√	√	√	√	√	

AFB = acid-fast bacillus; GBBS = group B streptococci; CYE = charcoal yeast extract agar; CCFA = cycloserine-cefoxitin-fructose agar; GC = gonococcus; SS = *Salmonella-Shigella* agar; XLD = xylosine-lysine-deoxycholate agar.

the plate from the area where the specimen was inoculed. Plates are examined for up to 7 days by 10× and 40× illumination for the presence of ameba, which is indicated by areas lacking *E. coli.*

Viral Agents

Viral agents require a living substrate in which to propagate. Many of the agents pathogenic to humans can be recovered by inoculating specimens into susceptible tissue culture cells. In general, a specimen is inoculated into two or more different types of tissue culture cell types, which are suggested by the source of the specimen, in an effort to maximize recovery. The tissue culture cells are typically grown in monolayers on the surface of tubes, vials, or microtiter plates.

Traditionally, the presence of the virus has been confirmed by the detection of (1) cytopathic effects in the tissue culture cells, (2) hemabsorption, (3) hemagglutination, or (4) neutralization of viral propagation by specific antibody. A shell vial cultivation technique combines virus isolation and rapid specific identification using monoclonal antibodies to detect the virus before cytopathic effect develops.[177]

SECTION THREE: SEROLOGIC TESTING FOR LABORATORY DIAGNOSIS OF INFECTION

Since most infectious disease agents elicit the formation of detectable levels of specific antibodies following a primary infection and may induce an increase in levels of antibody following re-exposure, tests designed for detecting the appearance of or increase in antibody titers may be useful in establishing a diagnosis. In general, two specimens of serum are required for testing, the first or acute-phase specimen being collected as soon after the onset of illness as possible but no later than 7 days post onset, and the second, or convalescent, phase specimen being collected 2 to 4 weeks after the acute-phase specimen has been collected. Both specimens must be tested at the same time to ensure that differences in titer are not due to factors involved with the procedure.

In cases in which antibody production is rapid, as in rubella, specimens collected 2 to 3 days after onset and the second collected 2 to 3 days later may be diagnostic. In other cases, as with anti–HBsAg, antibody production is slower and the convalescent specimen should be collected several weeks after onset.

To establish a diagnosis serologically, it is usually necessary to do the following:

▶ Demonstrate the absence of antibody in the acute-phase specimen and the presence of antibody in the convalescent specimen (seroconversion)

▶ Demonstrate a four-fold or greater rise in antibody titer between the acute and the convalescent specimens, *or*
▶ Demonstrate the presence of specific IgM class antibody in a single early specimen

In cases of suspected congenital infections, the first specimen should be collected at birth, or soon thereafter, and subsequent specimens should be collected for a period of weeks to months to demonstrate a decline (if antibody was from mother) or increase (if antibody has been made by the newborn). The detection of IgM antibodies may be particularly useful in cases of congenital infections, since mother's IgM does not cross the placenta. The presence of IgM antibody at birth suggests congenital infection, while the absence of IgM at birth and the presence of IgM in a later specimen suggest postnatal infection.

In addition to the use of serologic testing for detection of IgG and/or IgM for the diagnosis of disease, the detection of IgG has more recently been widely used to determine immune status and hence presumed protection from infection by certain agents (i.e., rubella, CMV, and VZV). Such screening tests have also been used for screening blood and blood products for the presence of antibodies to HIV, hepatitis, and CMV in an effort to prevent transmission of these agents in infected blood or transplanted organs.

The traditional methods of serologic testing for diagnostic purposes are many. Several of the immunoassay procedures developed for detection of antigens (i.e., fluorescence, EIA, and RIA) are applicable for the detection of antibody. A listing of the clinical situations that may depend heavily on serology for diagnosis is presented in Table 57–20. A brief description of each of the techniques used for this purpose follows.

Anti-DNase B

This test is a quantitative determination of the presence of antibodies to deoxyribonuclease activity (anti–DNase-B) produced by *S. pyogenes.* The enzymatic activity of DNase-B is to depolymerize its substrate, DNA. However, if antibodies are present, they neutralize the enzyme activity and inhibit the depolymerization of DNA. The inclusion of a color indicator that changes from blue to pink when the DNA is depolymerized allows the determination of the degree of inhibition by dilution of patient sera. This test may be useful in suspected cases of either rheumatic fever following streptococcal pharyngitis or glomerulonephritis following streptococcal pyoderma.

Anti–Streptolysin O (ASO)

Streptolysin O is one of several toxic immunogenic exoenzymes produced by *S. pyogenes* and an elevated

TABLE 57–20 ▶ INFECTIOUS DISEASE AGENTS THAT MAY BE DIAGNOSED BY SEROLOGIC TESTING

Agents[a]	Tests Typically Used[b]	Interpretation or Comments
Bacterial		
Bartonella henselae	FA, EIA	Reagents not commercially available; reference laboratory may be required
Bordetella pertussis	EIA	Titers develop slowly, paired sera required; IgA detection useful for detection of acute illness
Borrelia burgdorferi	Immunofluorescence EIA Western blot (WB)	Positive or indeterminate reactions by FA or EIA should be tested by Western Blot
Brucella	Tube or microagglutination	Titer of 1:60 consistent with disease but may be common in endemic areas, cross-reactions common; culture should also be performed
Chlamydia trachomatis, Pneumonitis in newborn LGV	Microimmunoflurescence (micro-IF) test	Antigen is type specific; IgM titers of >1:32 and IgG titers >1:2,000 suggestive of current disease
		Positive IgM titers suggest congenital infection
Chlamydia pneumoniae	Micro-IF test	Four-fold increase in IgG titer; single IgG titer >1:512 or IgM titer >1:16 consistent with acute infection
Chlamydia psittaci	CF	Titer of 1:128 suggestive of disease; antigen is genus specific
Coxiella	CF, immunofluorescence	Four-fold rise in titer between acute and convalescent sera diagnostic; no cross-reactions
Ehrlichia	Immunofluorescence	Four-fold rise in titer or convalescent titer of 1:64 suggestive of infection but needs confirmation with immunoblot due to cross-reactivity with other agents
Francisella tularensis	Tube or microagglutination (MAT) EIA	Titer ≥1:160 supports presumptive diagnosis EIA, microtest more sensitive; usually requires four-fold rise in titer
Legionella pneumophila	FA	Four-fold rise in titer to 1:128 indicative of recent infection; titers of 1:256 or more may occur in asymptomatic population; not primary method of diagnosis
Leptospira	Microagglutination EIA	Four-fold rise in titer or titer of 1:800 considered diagnostic Sensitive and specific test, less cumbersome than MAT
Mycoplasma pneumoniae	CF EIA	Four-fold rise in titer indicative of recent infection High IgG titers may persist for up to 1 year Positive IgM titer consistent with acute infection
Rickettsia	Indirect FA	Four-fold rise consistent with active or recent infection; titers of >1:64 indicative of exposure
Streptococcus pyogenes	Neutralization (ASO) Anti–DNase B	Four-fold rise in titers seen in 45% of children with pharyngitis and positive throat cultures; used as aid in diagnosing sequelae, not primary infection
Treponema pallidum	Nonspecific: VDRL, RPR	Reactive samples should be confirmed with specific test; titers can be used to evaluate efficacy of therapy; also see Table 57–21
Yersinia pestis	Specific: FTA-ABS, MHA-TP	Titers not as useful as RPR for following disease; also see Table 57–21
	EIA	Testing available at CDC; titer of 1:10 presumptive evidence of infection

ASO titer is usually an indcation of a recent infection with *S. pyogenes*. This test may be useful in the diagnosis of suspected cases of rheumatic fever in which a throat culture was not obtained or was negative at the time of the preceding pharyngitis. One version of the test involves adding patient serum to highly purified recombinant streptolysin O and testing for an increase in light scatter, which is converted into a peak rate signal in an automated protein analyzer. The peak rate signal is a function of the ASO concentration and is automatically converted into concentration units by the analyzer.

Complement Fixation (CF)

Complement is a component of human blood and consists of a series of heat-labile serum proteins that function in sequence to produce several biologic ef-

| TABLE 57–20 ▶ | INFECTIOUS DISEASE AGENTS THAT MAY BE DIAGNOSED BY SEROLOGIC TESTING *Continued* |

Agents[a]	Tests Typically Used[b]	Interpretation or Comments
Viruses		
Alpha virus: EEE, WEE, VEE	HI, CF FA (IgG, IgM) EIA (IgM)	Acute and convalescent sera required for HI and CF; usually performed in reference labs; IFA test can be used on CSF; single specimen for IgM tests adequate if specimen obtained early
Arena viruses: LCM, Lassa fever Others: AHF, BHF, VHF	FA, EIA (IgG, IgM) CF	Arenaviruses readily invade the fetus; Lassa fever associated with abortion, maternal mortality; LCM detected in 5% adults in U.S. cities; congenital infection due to this virus may be underestimated
Bunyavirus: CEE Hanta	EIA (IgG, IgM) FA	Serum and CSF may be tested in suspected cases of CEE Four-fold rise suggestive of infection
EBV	Heterophile agglutination EB-associated antigens	Nonspecific test is positive in 90% of cases of infectious mononucleosis Titers of ≥1:5 of IgG VCA, IgM VCA, and IgA VCA suggest primary infection
Filoviruses: Marburg Ebola hemorrhagic fevers	FA, EIA (IgG, IgM)	EIA method should be used to confirm IFA results
Flavivirus Yellow fever Dengue SLE	EIA (IgM), CF FA (IgG, IgM) EIA (IgM), FA	Paired sera required for CF; cross-reactions with other flaviviruses Paired specimens required, acute 1 wk after symptoms Paired specimens required for both tests
Hepatitis A	RIA or EIA	Presence of IgM anti-HAV denotes acute infection
Hepatitis B	RIA or EIA	Detection of HBsAg, anti-HBs, and anti-HBe indicates stage/presence of infection
Hepatitis C	EIA	Tests for detection of anti-HCV widely used for blood-donor screening
	Immunoblot (RIBA)	Confirms EIA results and detects antibodies to specific viral gene products
Hepatitis D	RIA	Detection of HBsAg, anti-HDV, and IgM anti-HDV determines disease state and provides prognostic information
Hepatitis E	WB EIA	Detection of total anti-HEV and IgM anti-HEV determines disease state; reagents not commercially available in U.S.
HIV	EIA	Two of three positive results confirmed by WB or IFA; one of three considered nonreactive
	WB, immunofluorescence	Used to confirm EIA results
Measles virus	HI, EIA	Seroconversion or four-fold rise in titer required
	IgM by immunofluorescence, EIA, or RIA	Positive test indicates acute infection
Mumps virus	IgM by FA or EIA	Positive test indicates acute or recent infection; no cross-reaction with parainfluenza virus
Parvovirus B19	EIA (IgG, IgM)	Negative result does not rule out infection
	HAI, EIA, FA	Four-fold rise in titer suggestive of recent infection
Rubella virus	IgM by EIA, FA	Positive test indicates current infection
	Latex agglutination	Four-fold rise in titer suggestive of recent infection; rule out prozone in negative sera

Table continued on following page

fects. One such effect is the lysis of red blood cells in the presence of antibodies specific for the red blood cells. This reaction forms the basis of the indicator system used in the CF test, which consists of sheep red blood cells and rabbit anti-sheep red blood cells, the latter also called hemolysin.

In complement fixation tests, patient serum is mixed with antigen and guinea pig complement, usually in the wells of microtiter plates. If the antibody to the specific antigen is present, antigen-antibody complexes will be formed and complement will be bound. Thus, complement will not be available for binding to the

TABLE 57-20 ▶ INFECTIOUS DISEASE AGENTS THAT MAY BE DIAGNOSED BY SEROLOGIC TESTING *Continued*		
Agents[a]	Tests Typically Used[b]	Interpretation or Comments
Fungal Agents		
Coccidioides immitis	Complement fixation	Titers ≥1:16 usually indicative of infection
	Immunodiffusion	Results usually correlate with CF; used as a screening test; positive results should be confirmed by CF
Blastomyces dermatitidis	Immunodiffusion	Presence of 1–2 bands of identity considered positive for diagnosis
	Complement fixation	Titers of 1:8–1:16 are suggestive of infection; titers of >1:32 usually indicative of infection
	EIA	Positive tests determined by + optical density (O.D.) breakpoints as indicated by manufacturer
Histoplasma capsulatum	Immunodiffusion	H and M bands indicative of infection
	Complement fixation	Titers of 1:8 to 1:16 suggestive of infection; titers of >1:32 usually indicative
Paracoccidioides	Complement fixation	Titer >1:32 suggestive of disease; used to monitor efficacy of therapy; available through CDC
	Immunodiffusion, EIA	May require reference laboratory
Sporothrix	EIA	Titer 1:16 serum; 1:8 CSF considered diagnostic
	Latex agglutination	Titer >1:4 consistent with disease
Parasites		
Entamoeba histolytica (liver abscess)	Immunodiffusion	Not as sensitive as EIA or IHA
	EIA	Comparable to IHA
	Indirect hemaglutination	Titers ≥1:256 in 95% of patients with extra-GI tract infections; 70% with intestinal infection
Toxoplasma gondii	FA	Presence of IgG antibodies indicates current or past infection
	EIA	Presence of IgM antibodies suggests primary infection; useful in neonates
Others: *Echinococcus, Fasciola hepatica, Filaria* (nonresidents of endemic areas), *Leishmania, Paragonimus, Plasmodium* (blood donors at risk for infection), *Schistosoma, Strongyloides, Taenia, Toxocara, Trichinella, Trypanosoma*	EIA, FA, and CF in some cases	Useful in serologic diagnosis of several parasitic diseases infrequently encountered in the U.S.

[a]EEE = eastern equine encephalitis; WEE = western equine encephalitis; VEE = Venezuelan equine encephalitis; SLE = St. Louis encephalitis; AHF = Argentina hemorrhagic fever; BHF = Bolivian hemorrhagic fever; CEE = California equine encephalitis; VHF = Venezuelan hemorrhagic fever; LCM = lymphocytic choriomeningitis.
[b]FA = immunofluorescence, may be either direct or indirect; EIA = enzyme immunoassay, may include ELISA techniques; CF = complement fixation; HAI = hemagglutination inhibition.

sheep red blood cells–anti-sheep red blood cell complexes formed in the indicator system, when that reaction mixture is added. Consequently, the red blood cells will not be lysed, and the red cells will settle and form a button in the bottom of the wells. If the antibody sought is not present, complement will bind with the red blood cell–red blood cell antibody complex, the red cells will be lysed, and a button will not be formed in the bottom of the wells. Thus, there is an inverse relationship between the amount of complement-fixing antibody detected and the amount of lysis observed in the red blood cells.

The CF test is technically demanding, labor-intensive, and relatively insensitive compared to other tests currently available. For these reasons, the CF test has been replaced largely by other methodologies in clinical laboratories other than reference laboratories. However, it is still useful in the serodiagnosis of infections with *M. pneumoniae* and systemic fungi.

EIA (ELISA) Procedures

In *noncompetitive methods* of antibody detection by EIA, specific antigen is attached to a solid phase by passive adsorption or with antigen-specific antibody, if necessary. The test serum is added, and antibody to the adsorbed antigen, if present, will form complexes during incubation. In this case, the antigen serves to "capture" the antibody in question. After appropriate washing steps, an enzyme-labeled anti-immunoglobulin specific for the antibody in the serum is added followed by a chromogenic substrate. The amount of antibody detected is proportional to the amount of color development.

In the *competitive method*, test serum and labeled antibody specific for the antigen, which has been adsorbed to the solid phase, are added at the same time to the reaction mixture or wells. In this case also, the antigen serves to "capture" the antibody in question. After incubation and washing steps, the chromogenic substrate is added, and the amount of antibody present is inversely proportional to the color that develops. A class capture approach may also be used if a specific class of immunoglobulin is sought (i.e., IgM). Enzyme-labeled *antigen* is also used in some tests for IgM as in the serodiagnosis of Epstein-Barr virus (EBV), flaviviruses, and hepatitis A virus.

EIA antibody assays are frequently used in screening for immune status, such as in rubella testing, for CMV antibody, for antibodies to HBV antigens, and for detection of heterophil antibody in EBV infections. Third-generation EIAs are the preferred method for screening for HIV antibodies, positive results of which are confirmed by Western blotting (see later). EIA reagents for testing for HIV antibodies in serum are available from Abbott Laboratories and others. An EIA system that measures HIV antibody in oral mucosal transudate (OMT), collected from the lower gums and cheek, was approved by the FDA. This test (Orasure) is not a rapid or home test, and repeatedly positive results are confirmed by the Orasure HIV-1 Western Blot Kit (Epitope, Beaverton, OR). A follow-up serum EIA is not required. Other EIA test systems for detecting HIV antibodies include a home HIV test kit, the Express HIV-1 Test System, available from Home Access Health, Hoffman Estates, IL. The specimen for the test is collected by pricking a fingertip with a lancet and applying 3 drops of blood to a test card, which is mailed to the manufacturer for testing. Results are obtained through a phone call and the use of a code number for identification so that the patient remains anonymous. Positive results are confirmed by Western blotting or immunofluorescence. The Single Use Diagnostic System for HIV-1 or SUDS (Murex, Norcoress, GA) is a rapid EIA test system performed on serum or plasma and has been used successfully in cases of suspected occupational exposure to HIV. Reactive results are confirmed by Western blotting or immunofluorescence. EIA can also be used with specimens of urine for detection of HIV-1 (Calypte HIV-1 Urine EIA Kit), positive results of which are confirmed by a Western blot test performed on the urine specimen.[178]

Heterophil Agglutination

The most commonly used test for laboratory diagnosis of EBV mononucleosis is the heterophil test. Heterophil antibodies are those that are produced in response to infection by one agent (i.e., EBV) but that react with antigens from other species (i.e., beef red blood cells). Rapid hemagglutination assays and EIAs are commercially available. Both are 80% to 85% sensitive. For suspected cases of a false-negative reaction in the heterophil test, more specific tests for antibodies against antigenic components of EBV may be performed.

Immunofluorescent Antibody Procedures

To test for the presence of antibody, antigens are fixed on glass slides, dilutions of test serum are added, and the slides are incubated. After rinsing the slides, unlabeled anti-human immunoglobulin is added, followed by a fluorescein-labeled anti-immunoglobulin specific for the anti-human immunoglobulin.

Fluorescent assays for antibody conducted on glass slides are usually performed to detect antibodies to some bacterial and parasitic agents. Antibodies to viral agents are detected in an automated solid-phase method described as follows.

Solid-Phase Fluorescence Immunoassays

This procedure is similar in principle to the other FA tests described except that fluorescence is measured by a fluorometer, rather than by a fluorescent microscope. A commonly used version is the commercial system called FIAX (Whittaker Bioproducts).

In the FIAX system, antigens are immobilized on nitrocellulose disks attached to plastic strips, rather than to glass slides. The strips are placed in patient serum, and specific antibodies, if present, bind to the antigen on the strip. After incubation, the strips are placed in a solution of fluorescein-labeled anti-human IgG antibody, which binds to the patient's antibodies if bound to the antigen. The fluorescence is quantitated by a fluorometer.

Assays are available for detection of antibodies to CMV, EBV, measles, mumps, rubella, herpes simplex, and varicella viruses.

Hemagglutination Inhibition (HI, or HAI)

The HI test is based on the fact that some viruses are able to attach to receptors on certain species of erythrocytes and agglutinate them, a reaction inhibited in the presence of antibody. Serial dilutions of patient serum are allowed to react with a fixed amount of hemagglutinin (HA), which has been extracted from the virus in culture. Residual HA is detected by the addition of appropriate red blood cells. If antibody is present, it binds to the virus and prevents agglutination of the red blood cells.

A disadvantage to this procedure is that nonantibody inhibitors of HA must be removed from the patient's specimen as well as naturally occurring substance that may agglutinate the test red blood cells. The procedures for serum treatment vary among the viral agents tested, as do other details of the test.

Hemagglutination procedures may be used, primarily in reference laboratories, for testing antibody response to adenovirus and influenza, measles, mumps, and parainfluenza viruses.

IgM Assays

Indirect immunoassays in which viral antigen fixed to a solid support forms complexes with viral antibodies in patient serum followed by detection of the complexes with a labeled (fluorescent, enzymatic, radioactive) anti-IgM reagent have been widely used. However, these tests are subject to interference by rheumatoid factor (RF) and excessive levels of viral-specific IgG antibodies. The RF is an immunoglobulin, usually of the IgM class, that reacts with IgG. If the IgM RF binds with viral-specific IgG, tests to detect viral IgM may be falsely positive, since they will detect the RF IgM whether viral IgM is present or not. On the other hand, false-negative reactions may occur if high levels of viral-specific IgG antibodies competitively block the binding of IgM to viral antigen.

Methods of circumventing these problems include removal of RF and IgG by gel filtration, affinity chromatography, selective absorption of IgM to a solid phase, and removal of IgG with hyperimmune anti-human IgG, staphylococcal A, or recombinant protein G from group G streptococci. Fortunately, serum pretreatment methods are now included within the procedures of commercially available immunofluorescence and enzyme immunoassay.

Alternatively, a class capture or "reverse capture" solid-phase IgM assays may be used to avoid the problem of false-positive and false-negative results. In this procedure, antibody of the μ-chain of human IgM is adsorbed to a solid phase and used as the capture antibody. Patient serum is added, and IgM of all specificities is retained on the solid phase by the anti–μ-reagent. Washing steps remove unbound serum component so that when viral antigen is added, it binds to the specific IgM antibodies if they were present in the test serum. Labeled IgG antibodies to the viral antigen are added and bind to the antigen retained by the IgM antibodies. The label is then detected by isotope counting or the addition of substrate, depending on whether an RIA or enzymatic test format was used. Some systems utilize a labeled viral antigen, rather than viral antibody, in the final detection step.

Additional factors that should be taken into account in interpreting IgM results include possible delayed production of IgM, especially in suspected congenital infections, production of IgM in secondary or reactivated infections, the long persistence of IgM in some viral infections, and heterotypic IgM responses, as in EBV-induced cases of infectious mononucleosis producing CMV IgM antibody response.

Detection of IgM antibodies are particularly useful in the laboratory diagnosis of congenital CMV or *T. gondii* and for the diagnosis of hepatitis A virus.

Immunodiffusion

Immunodiffusion tests use precipitin reactions in agar to visualize antigen-antibody reactions. In the double-diffusion systems, such as those used for systemic fungal serology, both antigen and antibody are placed in separate opposing wells in agar plates and lines of precipitation occur at points of intersection where concentrations of antigen and antibody reach equivalence.

Latex Agglutination (LA)

Agglutination tests generally utilize polystyrene beads of uniform size that are coated with antigen for antibody detection. The test specimen is mixed with the suspension of latex particles in a tube or on a circular area of an appropriate slide, agitated mechanically, and examined for visible signs of clumping or agglutination. In some cases, the agglutination can be measured photometrically.

These tests are usually simple and rapid to perform, and there are several tests available for the detection of antibodies to viral agents, such as CMV, rubella, and HIV.

Microimmunofluorescence (Micro-IF)

The microimmunofluorescence (micro-IF) test may be useful in diagnosing diseases caused by *C. trachomatis*, such as trachoma inclusion conjunctivitis and genital tract infections, if appropriately timed acute- and convalescent-phase sera are obtained to allow detection of seroconversion or a four-fold rise in antibody titer. The detection of relatively high levels of IgM ($\geq$1:32) and IgG ($\geq$1:2,000) antibody in single specimens is suggestive of current disease in cases of LGV. Furthermore, high levels of IgM antibody are found in association with chlamydial pneumonia in neonates.

The micro-IF test is usually performed with antigen prepared from *Chlamydia* organisms grown in the yolk sac of chicken eggs. These antigens are available for research purposes only at the Washington Research Foundation and are available for specific serotypes of *C. trachomatis*.

TABLE 57-21 ▶ SUMMARY OF COMMONLY USED CONVENTIONAL SEROLOGIC TESTS FOR SYPHILIS

Type of Test	Name (Abbreviation) of Test	Specimen	Stage of Disease		
			1°	2°	Late
Nontreponemal	Venereal Disease Research Laboratory (VDRL) slide	Serum or CSF	70[a]	99[a]	56[b]
	Rapid plasma reagin (RPR) 18-mm circle card	Serum or plasma	80	99	56
Treponemal	Fluorescent-*Treponema*-antibody absorption (FTA-ABS)	Serum	85	100	98
	Microhemagglutination assay for antibodies to *T. pallidum* (MHA-TP)	Serum	65	100	95

[a]Percentage of patients with positive serologic tests in treated and untreated primary or secondary syphilis.
[b]Percentage of treated patients with positive serologic tests in late-stage syphilis.
Modified from Tramont ED: *Treponema pallidum* (syphilis). In: Mandell GL, Bennett JE, Dolin R (eds): Principles and Practice of Infectious Diseases, 4th ed. New York, Churchill Livingstone, 1995, p 2127.

Syphilis Serology

Several nontreponemal and treponemal antibody tests are used in an attempt to diagnosis syphilis. There are described in Tables 57–21 and 57–22 and the text that follows.

Nontreponemal Tests

FLOCCULATION AND AGGLUTINATION TESTS

All available nontreponemal tests utilize an antigen composed of an alcoholic solution containing measured amounts of cardiolipin, cholesterol, and purified lecithin. These nontreponemal or reagin tests measure IgM and IgG antibodies to lipoidal material that is released from damaged host cells as well as to lipids and lipoproteins produced by treponemes. An inherent nonspecificity of these tests results from the fact that antilipoid antibodies are produced not only as a consequence of syphilis and other treponemal diseases, but also in response to nontreponemal diseases of an acute and chronic nature in which tissue damage occurs.

As seen in Table 57–21, the most commonly used nontreponemal tests currently are the VDRL (Murex), a flocculation test read microscopically, and the RPR (MacroVue, Becton-Dickinson), an agglutination test that is read macroscopically. The VDRL is performed on a microscope slide, and the RPR on cards supplied by the manufacturer.

Nontreponemal tests can be used qualitatively, in which case a single dilution of patient specimen is screened for reactivity. More useful, however, is the quantitative approach in which serial two-fold dilutions are made and an end point (or titer) is determined as the last dilution exhibiting full reactivity. Baseline

TABLE 57-22 ▶ PERFORMANCE OF NEWER SYPHILIS SEROLOGY TESTS[a]

Reference	Test	N	Sensitivity	Specificity	Comments
Reisner et al[179]	Captia-RPR	1,288	100	99.8	Compared to RPR–MHA-TP
Young et al[180]	ICE	101,[b] 1,184	99	99.8	ICE sensitivity higher
	Captia		91.4	99.2	(*P* < .01) than Captia-
	FTA-ABS		92.4		RPR and FTA-ABS
	MHA-TP		97.1		ICE specificity higher (*P* < .02) than Captia-RPR
Young et al[182]	Syphilis Fast	114,[c] 1,518	95.6	99.9	No difference in sensitivity
	Captia		94.7	99.5	between Syphilis Fast and
	VDRL		43.9	99.4	Captia; both more
	TPHA		98.2		sensitive (*P* < .001) than
	FTA-ABS		95.6		VDRL
Ebel et al[181]	BioElisa	434,[d] 358	99.5	99.4	

[a]Results after discrepant analysis unless otherwise indicated.
[b]Sensitivity determined by testing 101 known positive sera from various stages of treated and untreated syphilis; specificity determined by testing 1,184 unselected sera undergoing routine testing.
[c]Sensitivity determined by testing 114 positive sera from various stages of treated and untreated syphilis; specificity determined by testing 1,518 unselected blood specimens.
[d]Sensitivity determined by testing 434 sera positive by FTA-ABS and MHA-TP from various stages of syphilis; specificity determined by testing 358 sera negative by VDRL, FTA-ABS, and TPHA.

specimens should be collected early in the disease and prior to antibiotic therapy. Specimens that are positive by nontreponemal tests should be tested by treponemal tests for confirmation.

Advantages of the nontreponemal tests include their simplicity, their ability to evaluate primary disease by detecting a four-fold or greater rise in titer between acute and convalescent specimens, their ability to detect reinfection or relapse by demonstrating an increase in titer in patients who are permanently positive by the treponemal tests, and their ability to monitor the effect of treatment by demonstrating a decline in titer from blood specimens or in CSF specimens by VDRL. The disadvantages of the nontreponemal tests include their rate of nonreactivity in cases of primary syphilis and late syphilis, their false-positive rates in pregnant patients or in those with autoimmune diseases, malignancy, aging or leprosy, and prozone reactions, which may be observed in 1% to 2% or patients with secondary syphilis.

Treponemal Tests

These tests are designed to detect antibodies, which have been produced in response to *T. pallidum*. All subspecies cross-react, however, and differentiation between venereal syphilis and other human infections with treponemes cannot be made serologically.

FTA-ABS Test

This test (Virgo FTA-ABS, Pharmacia Diagnostics) is an indirect fluorescent antibody technique that uses the Nichol's strain of *T. pallidum* subsp. *pallidum* as antigen. The patient's serum is diluted 1:5 in sorbent that is an extract from cultures of the nonpathogenic Reiter treponema to remove group treponemal antibodies that are produced in some persons in response to nonpathogenic treponemes.

The patient serum is layered on a microscope slide to which *T. pallidum* has been fixed and incubated. If the patient serum contains antibody, it coats the treponemes. FITC-labeled anti-human immunoglobulin is added and combines with the patient's antibody adhering to *T. pallidum*, resulting in FITC-stained spirochetes that are visible when examined with a fluorescent microscope. Interpretation is made by comparing the amount of fluorescence present with that of control slides which are nonreactive, reactive minimal (+1), or reactive.

A modification of the standard FTA-ABS test is the FTA-ABS double-staining test, which uses a tetramethylrhodamine isothiocyanate–labeled anti-human IgG globulin, which attaches to the antibody, if present, and a counterstain with FITC-labeled anti–*T. pallidum* conjugate, which binds to the organisms on the slide. The later was developed to eliminate the need to locate the treponemes on slides showing no reactivity.

MHA-TP Test

This test is a passive hemagglutination procedure that utilizes sheep red blood cells that have been sensitized (coated) with ultrasonicated material from the Nichol's strain of *T. pallidum*. Patient serum is mixed with adsorbing diluent, the serum is placed in a microtiter plate, and the sensitized sheep red blood cells are added. Serum-containing antibodies react with the red blood cells to form a smooth mat of agglutinated cells in the microtiter wells. If antibody is not present, the red blood cells form a button in the bottom of the well.

The advantages of the treponemal tests include their specificity in detecting an antibody response to infections by treponemes. This characteristic is useful in confirming positive results of the more nonspecific nontreponemal tests as well as for confirming a clinical impression of syphilis in which the nontreponemal tests are negative, as may be the case in early- or late-stage disease. The disadvantages of the treponemal tests are their cost and difficulty as well as the fact that they cannot be used to monitor the effects of treatment. Approximately 85% of patients who are successfully treated demonstrate reactive treponemal tests for many years, if not a lifetime.

Newer Tests for Syphilis Serology

Several currently available tests detect specific treponemal antibodies using an EIA format. The results of studies that have evaluated the performance of some of these more recent tests are presented in Table 57–22.

Reisner and coworkers[179] evaluated a combination of screening with Captia SelectSyph-G, an automated EIA system available from Centocore, and subsequent testing with RPR to detect active infection with an RPR screening and MHA-TP confirmation testing regimen. The sensitivity and specificity were 96.5% and 99.7%, respectively, before resolution of discrepant results by retesting or confirmation by FTA-ABS, and 100% and 99.8% after resolution of discrepant results. Although the use of the EIA procedure as the initial screening test produced an additional number of specimens requiring confirmation, the time per test was half that of RPR, which was previously used as the initial screening test in the authors' laboratory. The authors concluded that the Captia EIA is a reliable method by which to test for primary syphilis.

When the Captia system was compared to ICE, a novel immune capture EIA that uses three recombinant *T. pallidum* antigens, the ICE system was found to be statistically more sensitive and specific than Captia in detecting positive syphilis serology in patients with various stages of treated and untreated syphilis.[180] The ICE system was also found to be statistically more sensitive than FTA-ABS, but not more sensitive than MHA-

TP. The authors concluded that the high sensitivity and specificity of the ICE systems and its suitability for automation make it an ideal screening test for syphilis.

One other EIA test system recently reviewed[181] consists of a competitive test that uses human immunoglobulin antibodies as the competitor (BioElisa Syphilis). When compared to FTA-ABS and MHA-TP, the sensitivity and specificity were found to be 99.5% and 99.4%, respectively. The authors concluded that the BioElisa Syphilis test is a sensitive, specific, and simple assay for screening for syphilis.

A LA test (Syphilis Fast) that uses a pool of three

recombinant *T. pallidum* antigens was also found to be more sensitive and specific than the Captia system.[182] The authors concluded that the Syphilis Fast is a highly specific, simple and fast screening test with a sensitivity comparable to that of native antigen treponemal tests that should be considered as a frontline screening test for syphilis.

Western Blotting (Immunoblotting of Proteins)

Proteins that have been separated electrophoretically are transferred and immobilized on a solid support.

TABLE 57-23A ▶ SUMMARY OF DIAGNOSTIC APPROACHES FOR DISEASES CAUSED BY GRAM-NEGATIVE BACTERIA

Agent	Associated Clinical Syndrome	Preferred Specimens	Primary Diagnostic Method(s)	Other Diagnostic Methods/Factors
Bartonella henselae	Cat-scratch disease	Paired sera	Serology[1]	History of cat or dog bite
	Bacteremia, septicemia, encephalopathy in AIDS patients	Biopsy of skin lesions	Culture, histology	
	Bacillary angiomatosis			
Borrelia burgdorferi	Lyme disease	Paired sera	Serology	History of tick bite
Campylobacter	Diarrhea	Stool	Culture	
C. pneumoniae	Pneumonia	Paired sera	Serology	Amplification[1]
		BAL, lung biopsy	Culture	
Chlamydia trachomatis	Cervicitis	Cervical swab	Ag detection	Amplification, culture
	PID	Endometrial aspirate	DNA probe	
	Neonatal conjunctivitis, pneumonitis	Conjunctival swab		
		Throat swab		
C. granulomatis	Granuloma inguinale	Lesion biopsy	Wright's, Giemsa stain	
Escherichia coli	UTI	Urine	Gram stain, culture	
	Neonatal sepsis	Blood		
	Meningitis	CSF		
Enterotoxigenic *E. coli*	Diarrhea	Stool	Toxin testing by EIA	
Hemorrhagic *E. coli*	Hemolytic-uremic syndrome	Stool	Toxin testing by EIA, agglutination	Culture
		Serum		Serology
Francisella tularensis	Genital lesions	Aspirate	Culture	History of tick bite
		Paired sera	Serology	
Gardnerella	Bacterial vaginosis	Vaginal swab	Gram stain	Probe
Haemophilus ducreyi	Chancroid	Lesion aspirate	Gram stain, culture	
H. influenzae	Meningitis	CSF	Gram stain, culture	Ag detection
	Pneumonia	Sputum, BAL	Gram stain, culture	
Helicobacter pylori	Gastric ulcer	Expelled breath	Breath test	Culture
		Gastric biopsy	Urease test	Serology
		Stool		
		Paired sera		
Legionella pneumophila	Pneumonia	Sputum, BAL, lung	Ag detection	Culture
		Paired sera	Histopathology	Serology
Leptospira	Leptospirosis	Blood, urine	Culture	History of animal contact
Mycoplasma hominis	Pyelonephritis	Urine	Culture	
	PID	Endometrial aspirate		
	Postpartum infections	Blood, wound		
M. pneumoniae	Pneumonia	Paired sera	Serology	
		Sputum	Culture	
Neisseria gonorrhoeae	Cervicitis	Cervical swab	Ag detection	Probe
	PID	Endometrial aspirate	Culture	
	Neonatal conjunctivitis	Conjunctival swab		
	Sepsis	Blood		
N. meningitidis	Meningitis	CSF	Culture	Ag detection
	Neonatal sepsis	Blood		
Salmonella, Shigella	Diarrhea	Stool	Culture	
Treponema pallidum	Syphilis	Lesion fluid	Wet prep	Ag detection
		Serum	Serology	
Ureaplasma urealyticum	Chorioamnionitis, Postpartum fever	Amniotic fluid	Culture	
		Blood		

TABLE 57–23B ▶ SUMMARY OF DIAGNOSTIC APPROACHES FOR DISEASES CAUSED BY GRAM-POSITIVE BACTERIA

Agent	Associated Clinical Syndromes	Preferred Specimens	Primary Diagnostic Methods	Other Diagnostic Methods
Enterococcus	UTI	Urine	Culture	
	Pelvic infection	Endometrial aspirate		
	Wound infections, peritonitis	Wound aspirate Blood		
Listeria monocytogenes	Meningitis	CSF	Gram stain, culture	
	Neonatal sepsis	Blood		
Mycobacterium	Pneumonia	Sputum, blood	Acid-fast stain, culture	Amplification
	Cutaneous lesions	Lesion biopsy		
	Salpingitis	Menstrual blood		
Streptococcus agalactiae	Neonatal meningitis	CSF	Gram stain, culture	Ag detection
	Sepsis	Blood		
S. pneumoniae	Pneumonia	Sputum	Gram stain, culture	Ag detection
	Neonatal meningitis	Blood	Gram stain, culture	
	Sepsis	CSF		
		Blood		
S. pyogenes	Abscesses, wounds	Aspirate of abscess, wound, or endometrium	Gram stain, culture	Probe
	Postpartum endometritis		Culture	Ag detection
	Pharyngitis	Throat swab	ASO, DNase B culture	
	Glomerulonephritis, rheumatic fever	Blood for serology Vaginal swab		
	Toxic shock syndrome			
Staphylococcus saprophyticus	UTI	Urine	Gram stain, culture	
S. aureus	Wound	Wound aspirate	Gram stain, culture	
	Skin infections	Lesion aspirate		
	Toxic shock syndrome	Vaginal swab		

Serum specimen is applied, and the antibody in question, if present, will bind to the proteins in the support system. The bound antibody is detected by fluorescence-, enzyme-, or radionuclide-labeled anti-immunoglobulin specific for the test serum species and detected by appropriate methods. This technique is currently used primarily for detection of antibodies to *Borrelia burgdorferi*, the agent of Lyme disease, and confirmation of EIA tests in serum, oral mucosal transudate, and urine for HIV.

SUMMARY

The clinical syndromes and their causative agents described in this chapter are numerous. As indicated, different approaches are necessary, depending on the site of infection and the suspected pathogen. A general summary of the agents presented and suggested diagnostic procedures by agent is presented in Tables 57–23A–F. The array of testing procedures and technologies available is constantly expanding, and the clini-

TABLE 57–23C ▶ SUMMARY OF DIAGNOSTIC APPROACHES FOR DISEASES CAUSED BY ANAEROBIC BACTERIA

Agent	Associated Clinical Syndrome	Preferred Specimens	Primary Diagnostic Method	Other Diagnostic Methods
Gram-negatives:				
Bacteroides	Postpartum endometritis, abscesses	Endometrial aspirate, abscess aspirate, blood	Gram stain, culture	
Fusobacterium			Culture	
Prevotella				
Gram-positives:				
Actinomyces	IUD-associated PID	IUD	Gram stain, culture	
Clostridium sp.	Abdominal, other wounds; septicemia	Wound aspirate Blood	Gram stain, culture Culture	
C. difficile	Antibiotic-associated diarrhea	Stool	Toxin testing	Culture Ag detection
Peptostreptococcus	Postpartum endometritis, abscesses	Endometrial or abscess aspirate, blood	Gram stain, culture	

TABLE 57–23D ▶ SUMMARY OF DIAGNOSTIC APPROACHES FOR DISEASES CAUSED BY FUNGAL ORGANISMS

Agent	Associated Clinical Syndrome(s)	Preferred Specimens	Primary Diagnostic Method	Alternative Diagnostic Method
Blastomyces dermatitidis	Pneumonia, mucocutaneous or cutaneous lesions	Paired sera, sputum Lesion aspirate	Serology Culture	
Coccidioides immitis	Pneumonia, cutaneous lesions	Paired sera, sputum Lesion aspirate	Serology Culture	
Cryptococcus neoformans	Meningitis, mucocutaneous or cutaneous lesions	CSF Lesion aspirate	India ink prep Ag detection Culture	
Candida	Vaginitis, mucocutaneous or cutaneous lesions	Vaginal swab Lesion aspirate	Wet prep Culture	Probe, culture
Histoplasma capsulatum	Pneumonia, mucocutaneous or cutaneous lesions	Paired sera, sputum Lesion aspirate	Serology Culture	
Pneumocystis carinii	Pneumonia	BAL, lung biopsy	Toluidine blue stain	Ag detection Histopathology Amplification[1]
Saccharomyces	Vaginitis	Vaginal swab	Wet prep	Culture

TABLE 57–23E ▶ SUMMARY OF DIAGNOSTIC APPROACHES FOR DISEASES CAUSED BY PARASITIC AGENTS

Agent	Associated Clinical Syndrome	Preferred Specimens	Primary Diagnostic Method	Other Diagnostic Method/Factor
Cryptosporidium	Diarrhea	Stool	Modified AFB stain, Ag detection	
Cyclospora	Diarrhea	Stool, duodenal contents	Wet prep, modified AFB stain	
Entamoeba histolytica	Diarrhea Liver abscess	Stool Paired sera	Wet prep, iodine- or trichrome-stained prep Serology	Ag detection
Giardia lamblia	Diarrhea	Stool, duodenal contents	Wet prep, iodine- or trichrome-stained prep	Ag detection
Isospora	Diarrhea	Stool, duodenal contents, small bowel biopsy	Modified AFB stain	
Toxoplasma gondii	Encephalitis Neonatal pnemonitis	CSF, amniotic fluid, brain biopsy Blood for serology	Antigen detection, histologic staining IgM detection	Amplification
Trichomonas vaginalis	Vaginitis	Vaginal swab	Wet prep, antigen detection	Culture, probe

TABLE 57-23F ▶ SUMMARY OF DIAGNOSTIC APPROACHES FOR VIRAL DISEASES

Viral Agent	Associated Clinical Syndrome(s)	Preferred Specimens	Primary Diagnostic Method	Alternative Diagnostic Method
Adenovirus	Conjunctivitis Diarrhea Rash Upper respiratory tract Urinary tract Vaginitis	Conjunctival swab Stool Lesion, throat NP swab, nasal wash Throat Urine Vaginal swab	Antigen detection Virus isolation	Paired sera for serology: EM
Arbovirus: Alphaviruses Flaviviruses	Encephalitis	Paired sera and CSF for serology	Serology: IgM ELISA	Virus isolation from blood difficult
Arenavirus (LCM, Lassa fever)	Multi-system disease with fever, readily infects fetus	Paired sera	Serology	
CMV	Congenital, Neonatal cervicitis Infectious mononucleosis Ocular Upper, lower respiratory tract Urinary tract Hepatitis Post transplant	Throat, urine, buffy coat Cervical swab Throat, urine Conjunctival swab NP swab, BAL, sputum Urine Throat, buffy coat Throat, urine	Buffy coat: Hybrid capture Others: Virus isolation and IF using shell vial techniques	Urine: Antigen detection by ELISA, amplification
EBV	Mononucleosis Chronic EBV Burkitt's, post transplant, other lymphoma or carcinoma	Serum Serum Tumor biopsy	Heterophil Ab EBV antibody panel Assay for EBNA	EBV antibody panel Anti-EBNA 1 and 2 Assay EBV DNA or RNA
Enteroviruses	Meningitis Encephalitis Neonatal Enteritis Ocular Myocarditis Lesion, rash Upper respiratory Urinary tract	CSF, throat, feces CSF, throat, feces CSF, throat, feces Feces Conjunctival swab Pericardial fluid Throat, feces Throat, feces Urine	CSF, pericardial fluid: PCR Others: Virus isolation	
Filovirus (Marburg, Ebola)[2]	Hemorrhagic fevers	Paired sera	Serology	Send to reference laboratory
Hepatitis A–E	Hepatitis	Blood	Ag/AB assays by ELISA, RIA	Amplification for HBV, HCV
Herpes simplex	Meningitis Encephalitis Neonatal Genital Mononucleosis Ocular Lesions Post transplant	CSF Brain biopsy, CSF Throat, lesion, BC Lesion, cervical Buffy coat Conjunctival swab Aspirate Throat, urine	CSF: PCR[1] Others: Virus isolation and IF staining using shell vial	Antigen detection in cellular specimens
HIV	Congenital AIDS	Serum	Serology by EIA Western blot	Amplification
HPV	Venereal warts, congenital	Biopsy	In situ hybridization Hybrid capture	Dot blot or Southern blot hybridization
Human parvovirus B19	Asymptomatic or acute illness with rash and/or arthropathy, fetal hydrops and demise	Blood for serology	Serology by detection of IgM	Antigen detection DNA detection by hybridization, PCR[1]
Influenza	Upper, lower respiratory	NP or, throat swab, nasal washings, sputum Paired sera	Ag detection	Culture Serology

TABLE 57–23F ▶ SUMMARY OF DIAGNOSTIC APPROACHES FOR VIRAL DISEASES *Continued*				
Viral Agent	Associated Clinical Syndrome(s)	Preferred Specimens	Primary Diagnostic Method	Alternative Diagnostic Method
Molluscum contagiosum	Genital lesions	Biopsy	EM Histopathology	
Measles	Rash, upper respiratory	Paired serum Lesion, throat, urine	Serology Antigen detection	Virus isolation
Mumps virus	Meningitis encephalitis, genital, upper respiratory	Throat, urine, paired sera	Virus isolation	Serology
Norwalk agents	Enteritis	Stool	EM	
Parainfluenza	Upper, lower respiratory	NP swab, throat, BAL Paired sera	Ag detection	Culture Serology
Rotavirus	Enteritis	Stool	Antigen detection	EM
RSV	Upper, lower respiratory	Nasal washings, aspirates	Antigen detection	Virus isolation by shell vial Serology
Rubella	Congenital syndrome, rash	Blood, products of conception Paired sera	Virus isolation Serology, IgM	
VZV	Congenital syndrome, lesion	NP swab, urine Aspirate Paired sera	Antigen detection by IFA	Virus isolation Serology

¹Commercial kits currently not available, reagents available for in-house development and use.
²Specimens should be handled within maximum containment laboratory.

cian is encouraged to establish a close working relationship with the microbiology laboratory in order to keep abreast of the most current and, hopefully, improved diagnostic alternatives.

REFERENCES

1. Shearin RS, Boehike J, Karanth S: Toxic shock–like syndrome associated with Bartholin's gland abscess: Case report. Am J Obstet Gynecol 1989; 160:1073.
2. Lopez-Zeno JA, Ross E, O'Grady JP: Septic shock complicating drainage of a Bartholin gland abscess. Obstet Gynecol 1990; 76:915.
3. Frolich EP, Schein M: Necrotizing fasciitis arising from Bartholin's abscess: Case report and review of the literature. Isr J Med Sci 1989; 25:644.
4. Sweet RL, Gibbs RS: Postpartum infection. In: Sweet RL, Gibbs RS (eds): Infectious Diseases of the Female Genital Tract 3rd ed. Baltimore, Williams & Wilkins, 1995, pp 578–600.
5. Ledger WJ: Infection in the Female. Philadelphia, Lea & Febiger, 1986, p 270.
6. Rein MJ: Vulvovaginitis and cervicitis. In: Mandell GL, Bennett JE, Dolin R (eds): Principles and Practice of Infectious Diseases, 4th ed. New York, Churchill Livingstone, 1995, pp 1074–1089.
7. Miller JM: A Guide to Specimen Management in Clinical Microbiology. Washington, DC, ASM Press, 1996, p 37.
8. Miller JM: A Guide to Specimen Management in Clinical Microbiology. Washington, DC, ASM Press, 1996, p 90.
9. Eisenach K, Dyke J, Boehme M, et al: Pediatric blood culture evaluation of the BACTEC PEDS Plus and the Dupont Isolator 1.5 ml System. Diagn Microbiol Infect Dis 1992; 15:225.
10. Morello JA, Matushek SM, Dunne WM, et al: Performance of a BACTEC nonradiometric medium for pediatric blood cultures. J Clin Microbiol 1991; 29:359.
11. Pickett DA, Welch DF: Evaluation of the automated BacT/ Alert System for pediatric blood culturing. Am J Clin Pathol 1995; 103:320.
12. Miller JM: A Guide to Specimen Management in Clinical Microbiology. Washington, DC, ASM Press, 1996, p 92.
13. Woods G, Washington JA: The clinician and the microbiology laboratory. In: Mandell GL, Bennett JE, Dolin R (eds): Principles and Practice of Infectious Diseases, 4th ed. New York, Churchill Livingstone, 1995, pp 169–198.
14. Farrar WD: *Leptospira* species (leptospirosis). In: Mandell GL, Bennett JE, Dolin R (eds): Principles and Practice of Infectious Diseases, 4th ed. New York, Churchill Livingstone, 1995, p 2139.
15. Lennette DA: General principles for laboratory diagnosis of viral, rickettsial, and chlamydial infections. In: Lennette EH, Lennette DA, Lennette ET (eds): Diagnostic Procedures for Viral, Rickettsial, and Chlamydial Infections, 7th ed. Washington, DC, American Public Health Association, 1995, pp 3–25.
16. Fritsche TR, Smith JW: Diagnosis of parasitic infections: Collection, processing, and examination of specimens. In: Murray PR, Baron EJ, Pfaller MA, et al (eds): Manual of Clinical Microbiology, 6th ed. Washington, DC, ASM Press, 1995, pp 1141–1158.
17. Wisepelwey B, Scheld WM: Brain abscess. In: Mandell GL, Bennett JE, Dolin R (eds): Principles and Practice of Infectious Diseases, 4th ed. New York, Churchill Livingstone, 1995, pp 887–899.
18. Griffin DE: Encephalitis, myelitis, and neuritis. In: Mandell GL, Bennett JE, Dolin R (eds): Principles and Practice of Infectious Diseases, 4th ed. New York, Churchill Livingstone, 1995, pp 874–880.
19. Isenberg HD, D'Amato RF: Indigenous and pathogenic microorganisms of humans. In: Murray PR, Baron EJ, Pfaller MA, et al (eds): Manual of Clinical Microbiology, 6th ed. Washington, DC, ASM Press, 1995, pp 5–18.
20. Tunkel AR, Scheld WM: Acute meningitis. In: Mandell GL, Bennett JE, Dolin R (eds): Principles and Practice of Infectious Diseases, 4th ed. New York, Churchill Livingstone, 1995, pp 831–864.
21. Grishover BM, Ellner JJ: Chronic meningitis. In: Mandell GL, Bennett JE, Dolin R (eds): Principles and Practice of Infectious Diseases, 4th ed. New York, Churchill Livingstone, 1995, pp 865–873.

22. Miller JM: A Guide to Specimen Management in Clinical Microbiology. Washington, DC, ASM Press, 1996, p 85.

23. Steere AC: *Borrelia burgdorferi* (Lyme disease, Lyme borreliosis). In: Mandell GL, Bennett JE, Dolin R (eds): Principles and Practice of Infectious Diseases, 4th ed. New York, Churchill Livingstone, 1995, pp 2143–2154.

24. Weber DJ, Cohen MS: The acutely ill patient with fever and rash. In: Mandell GL, Bennett JE, Dolin R (eds): Principles and Practice of Infectious Diseases, 4th ed. New York, Churchill Livingstone, 1995, pp 549–560.

25. Portmore AC: Parvoviruses (erythema infectiosum, aplastic crisis). In: Mandell GL, Bennett JE, Dolin R (eds): Principles and Practice of Infectious Diseases, 4th ed. New York, Churchill Livingstone, 1995, pp 1439–1445.

26. Girshon AA: Measles virus (rubeola). In: Mandell GL, Bennett JE, Dolin R (eds): Principles and Practice of Infectious Diseases, 4th ed. New York, Churchill Livingstone, 1995, pp 1519–1525.

27. Chernesky MA, Mahony JB: Rubella virus. In: Murray PR, Baron EJ, Pfaller MA, et al (eds): Manual of Clinical Microbiology, 6th ed. Washington, DC, ASM Press, 1995, pp 968–973.

28. Whitely RJ: Varicella-zoster virus. In: Mandell GL, Bennett JE, Dolin R (eds): Principles and Practice of Infectious Diseases, 4th ed. New York, Churchill Livingstone, 1995, pp 1345–1350.

29. Miller JM: A Guide to Specimen Management in Clinical Microbiology. Washington, DC, ASM Press, 1996, pp 49–51.

30. Miller JM: A Guide to Specimen Management in Clinical Microbiology. Washington, DC, ASM Press, 1996, p 55.

31. Blaser MJ: *Helicobacter pylori* and related organisms. In: Mandell GL, Bennett JE, Dolin R (eds): Principles and Practice of Infectious Diseases, 4th ed. New York, Churchill Livingstone, 1995, pp 1956–1963.

32. Miller JM: A Guide to Specimen Management in Clinical Microbiology. Washington, DC, ASM Press, 1996, pp 47–48.

33. Baker CJ, Edwards MS: Group B streptococcal infections. In: Remington JS, Klein JO (eds): Infectious Diseases of the Fetus and Newborn Infant, 3rd ed. Philadelphia, WB Saunders, 1990, p 783.

34. Ingram DL, Pendergrass EL, Bromberger PI, et al: Group B streptococcal disease: Its diagnoses with use of antigen detection, Gram's stain, and the presence of apnea, hypotension. Am J Dis Child 1980; 132:754.

35. Miller JM: A Guide to Specimen Management in Clinical Microbiology. Washington, DC, ASM Press, 1996, p 47.

36. Miller JM: A Guide to Specimen Management in Clinical Microbiology. Washington, DC, ASM Press, 1996, p 52.

37. Miller JM: A Guide to Specimen Management in Clinical Microbiology. Washington, DC, ASM Press, 1996, pp 37–41.

38. Baron EJ, Cassell GH, Duffy LB, et al: Cumitech 17A Laboratory Diagnosis of Female Genital Tract Infections. Washington, DC, ASM Press, 1993.

39. Rein MR: Genital skin and mucous membrane lesions. In: Mandell GL, Bennett JE, Dolin R (eds): Principles and Practice of Infectious Diseases, 4th ed. New York, Churchill Livingstone, 1995, pp 1055–1062.

40. Ledger WJ: Infection in the Female. Philadelphia, Lea & Febiger, 1986, p 44.

41. Nolte FS, Metchock B: *Mycobacterium*. In: Murray PR, Baron EJ, Pfaller MA, et al (eds): Manual of Clinical Microbiology, 6th ed. Washington, DC, ASM Press, 1995, pp 400–437.

42. Sweet RL, Gibbs RS: Sexually Transmitted Diseases. In: Sweet RL, Gibbs RS (eds): Infectious Diseases of the Female Genital Tract, 3rd ed. Baltimore, Williams & Wilkins, 1995, pp 133–188.

43. Lambert DR, Yoider FW: Ectoparasites and molluscum contagiosum. In: Spagnna VA, Prior RB (eds): Sexually Transmitted Diseases: A Clinical Syndrome Approach. New York, Marcel Dekker, pp 333–355.

44. Sweet RL, Gibbs RS: Herpes simplex virus infection. In: Sweet RL, Gibbs RS (eds): Infectious Diseases of the Female Genital Tract, 3rd ed. Baltimore, Williams & Wilkins, 1995, pp 125–126.

45. Faro S: Sexually transmitted diseases. In: Faro S (ed): Diagnosis and Management of Female Pelvic Infections in Primary Care Medicine. Baltimore, Williams & Wilkins, 1985, p 74.

46. Sweet RL, Gibbs RS: Perinatal infections. In: Sweet RL, Gibbs RS (eds): Infectious Diseases of the Female Genital Tract, 3rd ed. Baltimore, Williams & Wilkins, 1995, pp 465–529.

47. Sweet RL, Gibbs RS: Intra-amniotic infection (intrauterine infection in late pregnancy). In: Sweet RL, Gibbs RS (eds): Infectious Diseases of the Female Genital Tract, 3rd ed. Baltimore, Williams & Wilkins, 1995, pp 548–563.

48. Hillier SL, Martius J, Krohn M: A case-control study of chorioamnionic infection and histologic chorioamnionitis in prematurity. N Engl J Med 1988; 319:972.

49. Martens MG, Faro S, Hammill HA, et al: Transcervical uterine culture with a new endometrial suction curette: A comparison of three sampling methods in postpartum endometritis. Obstet Gynecol 1989; 74:273.

50. Faro S: Sexually transmitted diseases. In: Faro S (ed): Diagnosis and Management of Female Pelvic Infections in Primary Care Medicine. Baltimore, Williams & Wilkins, 1985, p 17.

51. Sweet RL, Gibbs RS: Mixed anaerobic-aerobic infections. In: Sweet RL, Gibbs RS (eds): Infectious Diseases of the Female Genital Tract, 3rd ed. Baltimore, Williams & Wilkins, 1995, pp 189–230.

52. Mead PB: Infections of the female pelvis. In: Mandell GL, Bennett JE, Dolin R (eds): Principles and Practice of Infectious Diseases, 4th ed. New York, Churchill Livingstone, 1995, pp 1090–1097.

53. Sweet RL, Gibbs RS: Postpartum infection. In: Sweet RL, Gibbs RS (eds): Infectious Diseases of the Female Genital Tract, 3rd ed. Baltimore, Williams & Wilkins, 1995, pp 578–600.

54. Faro S: Sexually transmitted diseases. In: Faro S (ed): Diagnosis and Management of Female Pelvic Infections in Primary Care Medicine. Baltimore, Williams & Wilkins, 1985, p 177.

55. Faro S: Sexually transmitted diseases. In: Faro S (ed): Diagnosis and Management of Female Pelvic Infections in Primary Care Medicine. Baltimore, Williams & Wilkins, 1985, p 126.

56. Sweet RL, Gibbs RS: Pelvic Inflammatory Disease. In: Sweet RL, Gibbs RS (eds): Infectious Diseases of the Female Genital Tract, 3rd ed. Baltimore, Williams & Wilkins, 1995, pp 378–428.

57. Spirtos NJ: Sonography in acute pelvic inflammatory disease. J Reprod Med 1982; 27:312.

58. Cacciatore B, Leminen A, Ingman-Friberg S, et al: Transvaginal sonographic findings in ambulatory patients with suspected pelvic inflammatory disease. Obstet Gynecol 1992; 80:912.

59. Cleghorn AG, Wilkinson RG: The IUD-associated incidence of *Actinomyces israelii* in the female genital tract. Aust NZ J Obstet Gynecol 1989; 29:445.

60. Mueller-Helzner E, Gschwendtner A, Abfalter E, et al: *Actinomyces* and long-term use of intrauterine devices. Lancet 1990; 336:939.

61. Levson ME, Bush LM: Peritonitis and other intra-abdominal infections. In: Mandell GL, Bennett JE, Dolin R (eds): Principles and Practice of Infectious Diseases, 4th ed. New York, Churchill Livingstone, 1995, pp 705–739.

62. Miller JM: A Guide to Specimen Management in Clinical Microbiology. Washington, DC, ASM Press, 1996, p 89.

63. Donowitz GR, Mandell GL: Acute pneumonia. In: Mandell GL, Bennett JE, Dolin R (eds): Principles and Practice of Infectious Diseases, 4th ed. New York, Churchill Livingstone, 1995, pp 619–636.

64. Murray PR: Macroscopic and microscopic evaluation of respiratory specimens. Clin Lab Med 1982; 2:259.

65. Bartlett JG, Ryan KJ, Smith TF, et al: Cumitech 7A: Laboratory Diagnosis of Lower Respiratory Tract Infections. (Coordinating ed., JA Washington II.) Washington, DC, ASM Press, 1987.

66. Miller JM: A Guide to Specimen Management in Clinical Microbiology. Washington, DC, ASM Press, 1996, p 107.

67. Lennette DA: Collection and preparation of specimens for virological examination. In: Murray PR, Baron EJ, Pfaller MA,

et al (eds): Manual of Clinical Microbiology, 6th ed. Washington, DC, ASM Press, 1995, pp 868–875.

68. Minnich LL, Smith TF, Ray GC: Cumitech 24 Rapid Detection of Viruses by Immunofluorescence. (Coordinating ed., S Specter.) Washington, DC, ASM Press, 1988.

69. Gleaves CA, Hodinka RL, Johnston SLG, et al: Cumitech 15A. Laboratory Diagnosis of Viral Infections. (Coordinating ed., EJ Baron.) Washington, DC, ASM Press, 1994.

70. Miller JM: A Guide to Specimen Management in Clinical Microbiology. Washington, DC, ASM Press, 1996, pp 105–106.

71. Sweet RL, Gibbs RS: Postabortion infection, bacteremia, and septic shock. In: Sweet RL, Gibbs RS (eds): Infectious Diseases of the Female Genital Tract, 3rd ed. Baltimore, Williams & Wilkins, 1995, pp 372–373.

72. Lennette DA: Collection and preparation of specimens for virological examination. In: Murray PR, Baron EJ, Pfaller MA, et al (eds): Manual of Clinical Microbiology, 6th ed. Washington, DC, ASM Press, 1995, pp 868–875.

73. Sweet RL, Gibbs RS: Urinary tract infection. In: Sweet RL, Gibbs RS (eds): Infectious Diseases of the Female Genital Tract, 3rd ed. Baltimore, Williams & Wilkins, 1995, pp 429–465.

74. Sobel JD, Kaye D: Urinary tract infections. In: Mandell GL, Bennett JE, Dolin R (eds): Principles and Practice of Infectious Diseases, 4th ed. New York, Churchill Livingstone, 1995, pp 662–689.

75. Miller JM: A Guide to Specimen Management in Clinical Microbiology. Washington, DC, ASM Press, 1996, pp 69–70.

76. Sweet RL, Gibbs RS: Wound and episiotomy infection. In: Sweet RL, Gibbs RS (eds): Infectious Diseases of the Female Genital Tract, 3rd ed. Baltimore, Williams & Wilkins, 1995, pp 601–616.

77. Suman VJ, Ilstrup DM: Predictive value of viral diagnostic tests. In: Lennette EH, Lennette DA, Lennette ET (eds): Diagnostic Procedures for Viral, Rickettsial, and Chlamydial Infections, 7th ed. Washington, DC, American Public Health Association, 1995, pp 155–159.

78. Hadgu A: The discrepancy in discrepant analysis. Lancet 1996; 348:592.

79. Sewell DL, Schifman RB: Quality assurance: Quality improvement, quality control, and test validation. In: Murray PR, Baron EJ, Pfaller MA, et al (eds): Manual of Clinical Microbiology, 6th ed. Washington, DC, ASM Press, 1995, pp 55–66.

80. Norris SJ, Larsen SA: *Treponema* and other host-associated spirochetes. In: Murray PR, Baron EJ, Pfaller MA, et al (eds): Manual of Clinical Microbiology, 6th ed. Washington, DC, ASM Press, 1995, pp 636–651.

81. Spirochetal diseases. In: Koneman EW, Allen SD, Dowell VR Jr, et al (eds): Color Atlas and Textbook of Diagnostic Microbiology, 3rd ed. Philadelphia, PA, JB Lippincott, 1988, pp 765–783.

82. Hook EW III, Roddy RE, Lukehart SA, et al: Detection of *Treponema pallidum* in lesion exudate with a pathogen-specific monoclonal antibody. J Clin Microbiol 1985; 22:241.

83. Rein MF: *Trichomonas vaginalis*. In: Mandell GL, Bennett JE, Dolin R (eds): Principles and Practice of Infectious Diseases, 4th ed. New York, Churchill Livingstone, 1995, pp 2493–2497.

84. Chapin K: Clinical microscopy. In: Murray PR, Baron EJ, Pfaller MA, et al (eds): Manual of Clinical Microbiology, 6th ed. Washington, DC, ASM Press, 1995, pp 33–51.

85. Schwebke JR, Hillier SL, Sobel JD, et al: Validity of the vaginal gram stain for the diagnosis of bacterial vaginosis. Obstet Gynecol 1996; 88(4 Pt 1):573.

86. Paik G: Reagents, stains and miscellaneous test procedures. In: Lennette EH (ed in chief), Balows A, Hausler WJ Jr, Truant JP (eds): Manual of Clinical Microbiology, 3rd ed. Washington, DC, ASM Press, pp 1000–1024.

87. Lipsky BJ, Gates J, Tenover FC, et al: Factors affecting the clinical value for acid-fast bacilli. Rev Infect Dis 1984; 6:214.

88. Miller SE: Diagnosis of viral infections by electron microscopy. In: Lennette EH, Lennette DA, Lennette ET (eds): Diagnostic Procedures for Viral, Rickettsial, and Chlamydial Infections, 7th ed. Washington, DC, American Public Health Association, 1995, p 38.

89. Forghani B, Hagens S: Diagnosis of viral infections by antigen detection. In: Lennette EH, Lennette DA, Lennette ET (eds): Diagnostic Procedures for Viral, Rickettsial, and Chlamydial Infections, 7th ed. Washington, DC, American Public Health Association, 1995, pp 79–96.

90. Herrmann JE: Immunoassays for the diagnosis of infectious diseases. In: Murray PR, Baron EJ, Pfaller MA, et al (eds): Manual of Clinical Microbiology, 6th ed. Washington, DC, ASM Press, 1995, pp 110–122.

91. Perkins MD, Mirrett S, Reller LB: Rapid bacterial antigen detection is not clinically useful. J Clin Microbiol 1995; 33:1486.

92. Bhisitkul DM, Hogan AE, Tanz RR: The role of bacterial antigen detection tests in the diagnosis of bacterial meningitis. Pediatr Emerg Care 1994; 10:67.

93. Diamond RD: *Cryptococcus neoformans* infections. In: Mandell GL, Bennett JE, Dolin R (eds): Principles and Practice of Infectious Diseases, 4th ed. New York, Churchill Livingstone, 1995, pp 2331–2339.

94. Podorski RP, Persing DH: Molecular detection and identification of microorganisms. In: Murray PR (ed in chief), Baron EJ, Pfaller MA, et al (eds): Manual of Clinical Microbiology, 6th ed. Washington, DC, ASM Press, 1995, pp 130–157.

95. Tenover FC, Unger ER: Nucleic acid probes for detection and identification of infectious agents. In: Pershing DH, Smith TF, Tenover FC, White TJ (eds): Diagnostic Molecular Microbiology: Principles and Applications. Washington, DC, American Society for Microbiology, 1993, pp 3–25.

96. Cullen A, He L, Arthur P, et al: Comparison of the Digene GC-ID Hybrid Capture® II Test to conventional culture and ligase chain reaction for the detection of *Neisseria gonorrhoeae* in women. ASM Meeting, 1998.

97. Margiotta M, Forde A, Gallery F, et al: Comparison of three commercial kits for in situ detection of viral DNA. J Histotechnol 1996; 19:139.

98. Pershing DH: In vitro nucleic acid amplification techniques. In: Pershing DH, Smith TF, Tenover FC, White TJ (eds): Diagnostic Molecular Microbiology: Principles and Applications. Washington, DC, American Society for Microbiology, 1993, pp 51–87.

99. Forghani B, Erdman DD: Amplification and detection of viral nucleic acids. In: Lennette EH, Lennette DA, Lennette ET (eds): Diagnostic Procedures for Viral, Rickettsial, and Chlamydial Infections, 7th ed. Washington, DC, American Public Health Association, 1995, pp 97–120.

100. Moore SA, Sillekens P, Jacobs MV, et al: RNA amplification by nucleic acid sequence–based amplification with an internal standard enables reliable detection of *Chlamydia trachomatis* in cervical scrapings and urine samples. J Clin Microbiol 1996; 34:3108.

101. Smith JH, Buxton D, Cahill P, et al: Detection of *Mycobacterium tuberculosis* directly from sputum by using a prototype automated Q-beta replicase assay. J Clin Microbiol 1997; 35:1477.

102. Stepano JE, Genovese L, An Q, et al: Rapid and sensitive detection of *Chlamydia trachomatis* using a ligatable binary RNA probe and Q beta replicase. Mol Cell Probes 1997; 11:407.

103. Stone BB, Cohen SP, Breton GL, et al: Detection of rRNA from four respiratory pathogens using an automated Q beta replicase assay. Mol Cell Probes 1996; 10:359.

104. Hendrick DA, Stowe BJ, Hoo BS, et al: Quantitation of HBV DNA in human serum using a branched DNA (dDNA) signal amplification assay. Clin Microbiol Infect Dis 1995; 104:537.

105. Chernesky MA, Mahony JB, Castriciano S, et al: Detection of *Chlamydia trachomatis* antigens by enzyme immunoassay and immunofluorescence in genital specimens from symptomatic and asymptomatic men and women. J Infect Dis 1986; 154:141.

106. Baselski VS, McNeely SG, Ryan G, et al: A comparison of non–culture-dependent methods for detection of *Chlamydia trachomatis* infections in pregnant women. Obstet Gynecol 1987; 70:47.

107. Lefebvre J, Laprerriere H, Rousseau H, et al: Comparison of three techniques for detection of *Chlamydia trachomatis* in

endocervical specimens from asymptomatic women. J Clin Microbiol 1988; 26:726.

108. Skulnick M, Chua R, Simor AE, et al: Use of the polymerase chain reaction for the detection of *Chlamydia trachomatis* from endocervical and urine specimens in an asymptomatic low-prevalence population of women. Diagn Microbiol Infect Dis 1994; 20:195.

109. Clarke LM, Sierra MF, Daidone BJ, et al: Comparison of the Syva MicroTrak enzyme immunoassay and Gen-Probe PACE 2 with cell culture for diagnosis of cervical *Chlamydia trachomatis* infection in a high-prevalence female population. J Clin Microbiol 1993; 31:968.

110. Olsen MA, Sambol AR, Bohnert VA: Comparison of the Syva Microtrak enzyme immunoassay and Abbott Chlamydiazyme in the detection of chlamydial infections in women. Arch Pathol Lab Med 1995; 119:153.

111. Smith JW, Rogers RE, Katz BP, et al: Diagnosis of chlamydial infection in women attending antenatal and gynecologic clinics. J Clin Microbiol 1987; 25:868.

112. Thomas BJ, MacLeod EJ, Hay PE, et al: Limited value of two widely used enzyme immunoassay for detection of *Chlamydia trachomatis* in women. Eur J Clin Microbiol Infect Dis 1994; 13:651.

113. Blanding J, Hirsch L, Stranton N, et al: Comparison of the Clearview Chlamydia, the PACE 2 assay, and culture for detection of *Chlamydia trachomatis* from cervical specimens in a low-prevalence population. J Clin Microbiol 1993; 31:1622.

114. Warren R, Dwyer B, Plackett M, et al: Comparative evaluation of detection assays for *Chlamydia trachomatis*. J Clin Microbiol 1993; 31:1663.

115. Pasternack R, Vuorinen P, Kuukanorpi, et al: Detection of *Chlamydia trachomatis* infections in women by Amplicor PCR: Comparison of diagnostic performance with urine and cervical specimens. J Clin Microbiol 1996; 34:995.

116. Iwen PC, Blair TM, Woods GL: Comparison of the Gen-Probe PACE 2 system, direct fluorescent-antibody, and cell culture for detecting *Chlamydia trachomatis* in cervical specimens. Am J Clin Pathol 1991; 95:578.

117. Williams E, Moncada J, Cullen A, et al: Evaluation of Digene CT/GC Hybrid Capture® II Test for the identification of *Chlamydia trachomatis* and *Neisseria gonorrhoeae* in cervical specimens. ASM Meeting, 1998.

118. Girdner JL, Cullen AP, Salama TG, et al: Evaluation of the Digene Hybrid Capture® II CT-ID Test for the detection of *Chlamydia trachomatis* in female endocervical specimens. ASM Meeting, 1998.

119. Pasternack R, Vuorinen P, Pitkajarvi T, et al: Comparison of manual Amplicor PCR, Cobas Amplicor PCR, and Lcx assays for detection of *Chlamydia trachomatis* infection in women by using urine specimens. J Clin Microbiol 1997; 35:402.

120. Pasternack R, Vuorinen P, Miettinen A: Evaluation of the Gen-Probe *Chlamydia trachomatis* transcription-mediated amplification assay with urine specimens from women. J Clin Microbiol 1997; 35:676.

121. Puolakkainen M, Hiltunen-Back E, Reunala T, et al: Comparison of performances of two commercially available tests, a PCR assay and a ligase chain reaction test, in detection of urogenital *Chlamydia trachomatis* infection. J Clin Microbiol 1998; 36:1489.

122. Schepetiuk S, Kik T, Martin L, et al: Detection of *Chlamydia trachomatis* in urine samples by nucleic acid tests: Comparison with culture and enzyme immunoassay of genital swab specimens. J Clin Microbiol 1997; 35:3335.

123. Goessens WHF, Mouton JW, Van der Meijden W, et al: Comparison of three commercially available amplification assays, AMP CT, Lcx, and COBAS Amplicor, for detection of *Chlamydia trachomatis* in first-void urine. J Clin Microbiol 1997; 35:2628.

124. Stary A, Schuh E, Kerschbaumer M, et al: Performance of transcription-mediated amplification and ligase chain reaction assays for detection of chlamydial infection in urogenital samples obtained by invasive and non-invasive methods. J Clin Microbiol 1998; 36:2666.

125. Stary A, Najim B, Lee HH: Vulval swabs as alternative specimens for ligase chain reaction detection of genital chlamydial infection in women. J Clin Microbiol 1997; 35:836.

126. Hook EW III, Smith K, Mullen C, et al: Diagnosis of genitourinary *Chlamydia trachomatis* infections by using the ligase chain reaction on patient-obtained vaginal swabs. J Clin Microbiol. 1997; 35:2133.

127. Thomason JL, Gelbart SM, Sobieski VJ, et al: Effectiveness of Gonozyme for detection of gonorrhea in low-risk pregnant and gynecologic populations. Sex Transm Dis 1989; 16:28.

128. Donders GG, van Gerven V, de Wet HG, et al: Rapid antigen tests for *Neisseria gonorrhoeae* and *Chlamydia trachomatis* are not accurate for screening women with disturbed vaginal lactobacillary flora. Scand J Infect Dis 1996; 28:559.

129. Hale YM, Melton ME, Lewis JS, et al: Evaluation of the PACE 2 *Neisseria gonorrhoeae* assay by three public health laboratories. Clin Microbiol 1993; 31:451.

130. Vlaspolder F, Mutsaers JA, Blog F, et al: Value of a DNA probe assay (Gen-Probe) compared with that of culture for diagnosis of gonococcal infection. J Clin Microbiol 1993; 31:107.

131. Cullen A, He L, Arthur P, et al: Comparison of the Digene GC-ID Hybrid Capture® II Test to conventional culture and ligase chain reaction for the detection of *Neisseria gonorrhoeae* in women. ASM Meeting, 1998.

132. Crotchfelt KA, Welash LE, DeBonville D, et al: Detection of *Neisseria gonorrhoeae* and *Chlamydia trachomatis* in genitourinary specimens from men and women by a coamplification PCR assay. J Clin Microbiol 1997; 35:1536.

133. Smith KR, Ching S, Lee H, et al: Evaluation of ligase chain reaction for use with urine for identification of *Neisseria gonorrhoeae* in females attending a sexually transmitted disease clinic. J Clin Microbiol 1995; 33:455.

134. Stary A, Ching S-F, Teodorowicz L, et al: Comparison of ligase chain reaction and culture for detection of *Neisseria gonorrhoeae* in genital and extragenital specimens. J Clin Microbiol 1997; 35:239.

135. Buimer M, Van Doornum GJ, Ching S, et al: Detection of *Chlamydia trachomatis* and *Neisseria gonorrhoeae* by ligase chain reaction–based assays with clinical specimens from various sites: Implications for diagnostic testing and screening. J Clin Microbiol 1996; 34:2395.

136. Hook EW III, Ching SF, Stephaen J, et al: Diagnosis of *Neisseria gonorrhoeae* infection in women by using the ligase chain reaction on patient-obtained vaginal swabs. J Clin Microbiol 1997; 35:2129.

137. Adraanse AH, Muytjen HL, Kollee LA, et al: Sensitivity of intrapartum group B streptococcal screening and in vitro comparison of four rapid antigen tests. Eur J Obstet Gynecol Reprod Biol 1994; 56:21.

138. Simpson AJ, Mawn JA, Heard SR: Assessment of two methods for rapid intrapartum detection of vaginal group B streptococcal colonization. J Clin Pathol 1994; 47:752.

139. Hordnes K, Eide M, Ulstein M, et al: Evaluation of a rapid enzyme immunoassay for detection of genital colonization of group B streptococci in pregnant women: Own experience and review. Aust NZ J Obstet Gynaecol 1995; 35:251.

140. Park CH, Ruprai D, Vandel NM, et al: Rapid detection of group B streptococcal antigen from vaginal specimens using a new Optical ImmunoAssay technique. Diagn Microbiol Infect Dis 1996; 24:125.

141. Baker CJ: Inadequacy of rapid immunoassays for intrapartum detection of group B streptococcal carriers. Obstet Gynecol 1996; 88:51.

142. Andreu DA, Saleedo AS, Heredia PF, et al: Evaluation of three rapid methods for intrapartum detection of group B streptococcus. As Esp Pediatr 1997; 46:378.

143. Platt MW, McLaughlin JC, Gilson GJ, et al: Increased recovery of group B *Streptococcus* by the inclusion of rectal culturing and enrichment. Diagn Microbiol Infect Dis 1995; 21:65.

144. Greenberg DN, Ascher DP, Yoder BA, et al: Sensitivity and specificity of rapid diagnostic tests for detection of group B streptococcal antigen in bacteremic neonates. J Clin Microbiol 1995; 33:193.

145. Margiotta M, Forde A, Gallery F, et al: Comparison of three commercial kits for in situ detection of viral DNA. J Histotechnol 1996; 19:139.

146. Lorincz AT: Diagnosis of human papillomavirus infection by the new generation of molecular DNA assays. Clin Immunol Newslett 1992; 12:8.

147. Cope JU, Hildersheim A, Schiffman MH, et al: Comparison of the hybrid capture tube test and PCR for detection of human papillomavirus DNA in cervical specimens. J Clin Microbiol 1997; 35:2262.

148. Uberti-Foppa C, Origoni M, Maillard M, et al: Evaluation of the detection of human papillomavirus genotypes in cervical specimens by hybrid capture as screening for precancerous lesion in HIV-positive women. J Med Virol 1998; 56:133.

149. Clavel C, Bory JP, Rihet S, et al: Comparative analysis of human papillomavirus detection by hybrid capture assay and routine cytologic screening to detect high-grade cervical lesions. Int J Cancer 1998; 75:525.

150. Recio FO, Sahai Srivastava BI, Wong C, et al: The clinical value of digene hybrid capture HPV DNA testing in a referral-based population with abnormal Pap smears. Eur J Gynaecol Oncol 1998; 19:203.

151. Cox JT, Lorinsz AT, Schiffman MH, et al: Human papillomavirus testing by hybrid capture appears to be useful in triaging women with a cytologic diagnosis of atypical squamous cells of undetermined significance. Am J Obstet Gynecol 1995; 172:946.

152. Ferris DG, Wright TC Jr, Litaker MS, et al: Comparison of two tests for detecting carcinogenic HPV in women with Papanicolaou smear reports of ASCUS and LSIL. J Fam Pract 1998; 46:136.

153. McHugh TM, Vyas GN: Human immunodeficiency viruses. In: Lennette EH, Lennette DA, Lennette ET (eds): Diagnostic Procedures for Viral, Rickettsial, and Chlamydial Infections, 7th ed. Washington, DC, American Public Health Association, 1995, pp 407–421.

154. Uvin SC, Caliendo AM: Cervicovaginal human immunodeficiency virus secretion and plasma viral load in human immunodeficiency virus–seropositive women. Obstet Gynecol 1997; 90:739.

155. Thea DM, Steketee RW, Pliner V, et al: The effect of maternal viral load on the risk of perinatal transmission of HIV-1. New York City Perinatal HIV Transmission Collaborative Study Group. AIDS 1997; 11:437.

156. O'Shea S, Newell ML, Dunn DT, et al: Maternal viral load, CD4 cell count and vertical transmission of HIV-1. J Med Virol 1998; 54:113.

157. Lambert G, Thea DM, Pliner V, et al: Effect of maternal CD4+ cell count, acquired immunodeficiency syndrome, and viral load on disease progression in infants with perinatally acquired human immunodeficiency virus type 1 infection. New York City Perinatal HIV Transmission Collaborative Study Group. J Pediatr 1997; 130:890.

158. Delamare C, Burgard M, Mayaux MJ, et al: HIV-1 RNA detection in plasma for the diagnosis of infection in neonates. The French Pediatric HIV Infection Study Group. J Acquir Immune Defic Syndr Hum Retrovirol 1997; 15:121.

159. Alaeus A, Lidman K, Sonnerborg A, et al: Subtype-specific problems with quantification of plasma HIV-1 RNA. AIDS 1997; 11:859.

160. Coste J, Montes B, Reynes J, et al: Comparative evaluation of three assays for the quantitation of human immunodeficiency virus type 1 RNA in plasma. Med Virol 1996; 50:292.

161. Jackson JB, Parsons JS, Nichols LS, et al: Detection of human immunodeficiency virus type 1 (HIV-1) antibody by Western blotting and HIV-1 DNA by PCR in patients with AIDS. J Clin Microbiol 1997; 35:118.

162. Goldschmidt PL, Devillechabrolle A, Ait-Arkoub Z, et al: Comparison of an amplified enzyme-linked immunosorbent assay with procedures based on molecular biology for assessing human immunodeficiency virus type 1 viral load. Clin Diagn Lab Immunol 1998; 5:513.

163. Purcell R, Hoofnagle JH, Gerin JL: Parenterally transmitted hepatitis. In: Lennette EH, Lennette DA, Lennette ET (eds): Diagnostic Procedures for Viral, Rickettsial, and Chlamydial

Infections, 7th ed. Washington, DC, American Public Health Association, 1995, pp 331–359.

164. Hwang SJ, Lee SD, Lu RH, et al: Comparison of three different hybridization assays in the quantitative measurement of serum hepatitis B virus DNA. J Virol Methods 1996; 62:123.

165. Kapke GE, Watson G, Sheffler S, et al: Comparison of the Chiron Quantiplex branched DNA (bDNA) assay and the Abbott Genostics solution hybridization assay for quantification of hepatitis B viral DNA. J Viral Hepat 1997; 4:67.

166. Kessler HH, Pierer K, Dragon E, et al: Evaluation of a new assay for HBV DNA quantitation in patients with chronic hepatitis B. Clin Diagn Virol 1998; 9:37.

167. Pawlotsky J-M, Bastie AN, Lonjon I, et al: What technique should be used for routine detection and quantification of HBV DNA in clinical samples? J Virol Methods 1997; 65:245.

168. Levi MH, Torres J, Pinã C, et al: Comparison of the InPouch TV Culture System and Diamond's Modified Medium for detection of Trichomonas vaginalis. J Clin Microbiol 1997; 35:3308.

169. Beal C, Goldsmith R, Kotby M, et al: The plastic envelope method, a simplified technique for culture diagnosis of trichomoniasis. J Clin Microbiol 1992; 30:2265.

170. Draper D, Parker R, Patterson E, et al: Detection of Trichomonas vaginalis in pregnant women with the InPouch TV culture system. J Clin Microbiol 1993; 31:1016.

171. Schwebke JR, Morgan SC, Pinson GB: Validity of self-obtained vaginal specimens for diagnosis of trichomoniasis. J Clin Microbiol 1997; 35:1618.

172. Bickley LS, Krisher KK, Punsalang A Jr, et al: Comparison of direct fluorescent antibody, acridine orange, wet mount, and culture for detection of Trichomonas vaginalis in women attending a public sexually transmitted diseases clinic. Sex Transm Dis 1989; 16:127.

173. Ohlemeyer CL, Hornberger LL, Lynch DA, et al: Diagnosis of Trichomonas vaginalis in adolescent females: InPouch TV culture versus wet-mount microscopy. J Adolesc Health 1998; 22:205.

174. DeMeo LR, Draper DL, McGregor JA, et al: Evaluation of a deoxyribonucleic acid probe for the detection of Trichomonas vaginalis in vaginal secretions. Am J Obstet Gynecol 1996; 174:1339.

175. Briselden AM, Hillier SL: Evaluation of Affirm VP Microbial Identification Test for Gardnerella vaginalis and Trichomonas vaginalis. J Clin Microbiol 1994; 32:148.

176. Heine RP, Wiesenfeld HC, Sweet RL, et al: Polymerase chain reaction analysis of distal vaginal specimens: A less invasive strategy for detection of Trichomonas vaginalis. Clin Infect Dis 1997; 24:985.

177. Jespersen DJ, Drew WL, Gleaves CA, et al: Multisite evaluation of a monoclonal antibody reagent (Syva) for rapid diagnosis of cytomegalovirus in the shell vial assay. J Clin Microbiol 1989; 27:1502.

178. Weikersheimer PB: HIV testing: The new possibilities. Lab Med 1998; 29:531.

179. Reisner BS, Mann LM, Tholcken CA, et al: Use of the Treponema pallidum–specific captia syphilis IgG assay in conjunction with the rapid plasma reagin to test for syphilis. J Clin Microbiol 1997; 35:1141.

180. Young H, Moyes A, Seagar L, et al: Novel recombinant-antigen enzyme immunoassay for serological diagnosis of syphilis. J Clin Microbiol 36:913.

181. Ebel A, Bachelart L, Alonso JM: Evaluation of a new competitive immunoassay (BioElisa Syphilis) for screening for Treponema pallidum antibodies at various stages of syphilis. J Clin Microbiol 1998; 36:358.

182. Young H, Moyes A, de Ste Croix I, et al: A new recombinant antigen latex agglutination test (Syphilis Fast) for the rapid serological diagnosis of syphilis. Int J STD AIDS 1998; 9:196.

58 Placental Pharmacokinetics and Anti-HIV Compounds

BRIAN M. CASEY ▶ ROGER BAWDON

The placenta plays a significant role in the nutrition of the embryo and fetus, as well as in the development of secretory and regulatory functions for the maintenance of pregnancy. The placenta also plays an important role in hormone synthesis and drug biotransformation. Therefore, when prescribing any drug to a pregnant woman, a physician must consider physiologic changes or modifications in its pharmacokinetics that transpire across the maternal–fetal interface—the placenta. Clinicians must also be vigilant for any potential untoward fetal effects of drugs they prescribe. Finally, after pharmacokinetics and pharmacodynamics have been considered, practical concerns, such as route of administration and dosage, must be addressed.

To prescribe any medication in pregnancy, an understanding of the substance's ability to cross the placenta is necessary. However, it is difficult to elucidate pharmacokinetics in pregnancy because it is not technically feasible to obtain sequential serum drug concentrations in both mother and fetus over a prolonged period. Therefore, at present, our knowledge of placental transfer and kinetics for most drug compounds is grossly inadequate. The development of newer investigative techniques such as percutaneous umbilical blood sampling and fetoscopy has provided access to the intrauterine environment and made intrauterine therapy possible. Theoretically, this should improve our ability to evaluate placental pharmacokinetics in the future. Nonetheless, there currently are several study methods that provide important information on drug pharmacokinetics in pregnancy.

TECHNIQUES OF EVALUATING PLACENTAL PHARMACOKINETICS

In vivo studies for purposes of placental pharmacokinetics are encumbered by ethical considerations; the indications for violating the intrauterine environment are few, and such invasive measures would offer little information regarding pharmacokinetics. Many drug studies have measured maternal and cord blood at the time of delivery. These results are also of limited benefit because this "snapshot" view does not reflect the dynamic state that exists during pregnancy. Animal experiments, the logical alternative, offer a better reflection of the placental dynamics in pregnancy. However, the variability in placental structure among different species limits the number of usable animal models. Anatomically, no animal other than primates has a discoidal placenta, with a multivillous fetomaternal interdigitation and a hemomonochorial barrier. This makes use of pregnant animal models for drug pharmacokinetics across the placental barrier prohibitively expensive and time consuming.

Ex vivo perfusion of isolated placental cotyledons presents an exciting and powerful method for studying various aspects of human placental function. The advantages of such a system includes the elimination of hepatic biotransformation and renal clearance of study drugs. Also, this system enables the precise control of experimental conditions that might not otherwise be under the investigator's control. The weaknesses of such a system are related to the potential ischemic damage to the placenta at delivery, nonphysiologic oxygenation and perfusion of the selected cotyledon, and the elimination of maternal and fetal influences on regulation of placental functions. Despite these limitations, validation criteria for the perfusion of an isolated placental cotyledon have been proposed,[1–3] and limited animal data do not conflict with the data from the ex vivo human placental model.[4] Studies on placental transport of dideoxyinosine and stavudine in pigtailed macaques[5, 6] revealed similar results to those from studies in the ex vivo placental model.[7, 8] Consequently, *ex vivo* perfusion of an isolated placental cotyledon has gained acceptance as an accurate measure of pharmacokinetics in the human placenta. An example of such a system is briefly described in the following section.

Ex Vivo Placental Perfusion Model

Placentas are transferred from the labor and delivery suite to the laboratory in normal saline. On arrival in the laboratory, the truncal branches of the chorionic artery supplying a selected cotyledon along with the associated vein are cannulated using 3.0- and 5.0-French catheters. This re-establishes the fetal circulation. The cannulated cotyledon is then gently perfused with tissue culture media containing essential nutrients and bovine serum albumin (i.e., Eagle's Minimum Essential Medium [MEM] growth media). Those with preliminary vascular integrity are then transferred to a temperature-controlled chamber (37°C) and perfused for an additional period at a fetal flow rate of 3 to 4.5 mL/min. During this initial closed-system perfusion, the volume of fetal perfusate is monitored closely for further evidence of vascular leaks. Placental cotyledons with any evidence of vascular leakage are discarded.

"Maternal circulation" is re-established by inserting two 18-gauge needles into the intervillous space of the isolated cotyledon. The maternal flow rate is 17 mL/min. The reservoirs containing perfusion medium for both maternal and fetal circulation are continuously mixed and are equilibrated with a gas mixture of 95% oxygen and 5% carbon dioxide through fretted glass filters.

Placental membrane integrity, transport fraction (T_F), and clearance (C) are determined using the ^{14}C antipyrine reference method of Challier.[2] The use of antipyrine, a small, highly lipid-soluble molecule, as a marker substance determines the maternal–fetal match in the isolated cotyledon. Placentas are studied in a nonrecirculating (open) fashion for 60 minutes to determine T_F of ^{14}C antipyrine. The following formula is used:

$$T_F = \frac{(CFV - CFA)}{(CMA - CFA)}$$

where C = concentration, M = maternal perfusate, F = fetal perfusate, A = artery, and V = vein.

In the initial determination of maternal–fetal match, CFA is zero because the system is nonrecirculating. If the T_F is greater than 40%, the cotyledon is considered to be representative of a maternal–fetal circulating match. Clearance (C) of antipyrine is then calculated using the following formula:

$$C = T_F \times Q \text{ where } Q = \text{flow rate of fetal circulation.}$$

Placental perfusion studies can be done in an "open" fashion to determine "single-pass" pharmacodynamics, or may be performed in "closed" fashion, allowing recirculation of the perfusate and mimicking the physiologic state. Calculations of clearance index (Ci) are performed using the clearance of ^{14}C antipyrine as a reference within each perfusion experiment. The following formula is used:

$$Ci = \frac{C \text{ of test drug}}{C \text{ of antipyrine}}$$

Finally, accumulation of specific drug compounds in the fetal circulation or placental tissue can be calculated using specific assays for the compound tested. In this dual-perfusion model, a placental cotyledon can be maintained in a "viable" condition for several hours. Various aspects of placental pharmacology, such as drug transfer from maternal to fetal circulation and placental metabolism of a given compound, can be successfully studied using this technique. Increased use of this technique would undoubtedly replace some animal experiments and avoid the pitfalls of using different species. It also entails significant financial savings and provides more useful information than "snapshot" evaluations of placental metabolism at the time of delivery or percutaneous umbilical blood sampling.

PLACENTAL PHARMACOKINETICS

Therapeutic agents administered to pregnant women are variously distributed and undergo several maternal metabolic changes that may affect transport to the fetus. The placenta itself may also metabolize any maternally administered agent. Finally, once transported to the fetus, a particular drug or its intermediates may encounter fetal distribution and metabolic changes that also alter its effect.

Maternal Factors

Physiologic alterations that accompany pregnancy likely influence the pharmacokinetics of many agents prescribed to the gravid woman. These changes are evident before the end of the first trimester. They include an increase in body water, fat, and weight. There is a concomitant increase in blood volume, with a decrease in serum albumin. These changes are partly responsible for the increased cardiac output, renal plasma flow, and glomerular filtration rate representative of the pregnant state. Alterations in uterine vascular resistance, along with the aforementioned changes, translate into an increase in uterine blood flow. This increase in total body water and renal plasma flow and decrease in serum albumin, combined with an increased uterine perfusion, affects the amount of a therapeutic agent delivered to the placental bed.

Placental Factors

The placenta acts initially as a limited-permeability barrier to substances with a molecular weight greater than 1,000 daltons, but does not exclude molecules with a weight less than 600 to 800 daltons.[9, 10] As stated earlier, metabolic processes that may modify a particular drug also occur across the maternal–fetal interface. The metabolic capacity of the placenta has been well established for many years,[11] and our understanding of placental drug metabolism expands with more recent studies.[12, 13] Our comprehension of these modifications is complicated by the fact that, at any particular time, only a small fraction of maternal and fetal blood is in proximity.

The number of metabolic pathways that result in transformation or degradation of organic substances is relatively small. Oxidation, reduction, hydrolysis, and conjugation are the major conversion reactions responsible for the biotransformation of drugs by the placenta. Several different enzymes or enzyme systems may catalyze each reaction. The activities of some enzyme systems (i.e., cytochrome P-450) are significantly reduced in the placenta. Nevertheless, the metabolic capacity of the placenta has important implications for considering the formation of reactive metabolites so near to the fetus. Fortunately, most therapeutic agents that have been investigated do not exhibit appreciable placental metabolism.[14]

Fetal Factors

After placental transfer and metabolism of a particular agent occur, there are several anatomic and physiologic factors that potentially alter the fetal effects of maternally administered drugs. Much of the umbilical venous blood first bypasses the fetal liver by way of the ductus venosus, and then bypasses the lungs by way of the ductus arteriosus. This results in higher drug concentrations delivered to the fetal heart and central nervous system. Therefore, the pattern of fetal effects associated with a specific agent may vary according to fetal blood distribution.

Ultimately, any therapeutic agent administered to pregnant women is variously distributed and metabolized in the maternal circulation before exposure to the placental interface. Placental metabolism and transport of the agent then take place before distribution in the fetal compartment. Finally, fetal circulation and homeostasis effect the distribution of the particular agent and may dictate fetal effects. The *ex vivo* isolated placental cotyledon model enables investigators artificially to control many maternal and fetal factors and subsequently evaluate the equilibration dynamics and metabolism of a particular agent between mother and fetus.

PLACENTAL TRANSFER OF DRUGS

There are two major routes for transfer or exchange of substrates across the placental membrane: transcellular and extracellular. Extracellular transport is limited to passive diffusion of hydrophilic molecules through channels connecting the maternal and fetal blood streams. The extracellular transport rate of diffusion is much slower than the rate of transcellular transport for lipid-soluble compounds.

Transcellular transport also occurs through passive diffusion, but can be mediated by carrier systems with specific binding sites on the microvillous surface or the trophoblast basal membrane. Although specific transcellular transport systems are important for fetal supply of nutrients such as amino acids, vitamins, glucose, and immunoglobulins, most drugs cross the placenta into the fetal compartment by passive diffusion, both extracellular and transcellular, and the rate of transcellular transfer depends on the compound's lipophilicity.[15]

For extracellular passive transport of hydrophilic compounds to occur across the hemochorial placenta, the two layers of trophoblastic and endothelial cells of the fetal capillaries must be overcome. The trophoblast layer contains limited numbers of wide apertures that determine the trophoblasts' overall permeability. Also, the endothelium of the fetal capillaries contains numerous smaller intercellular pores that restrict diffusion of larger molecules. These two types of pores, both sized differently and arranged in series, are responsible for most of the placenta's permeability. Results from *in vivo* studies of term human placentas are compatible with this two-layered concept.[16]

According to Fick's law of diffusion, the net flux of a drug from mother to fetus or in the reverse direction can be calculated from the permeability, provided the transplacental concentration gradient is known. Data obtained from cord blood at the time of delivery are consistent with data obtained in *ex vivo* perfusion systems.[17] This further supports the expanded use of the dual-perfusion technique in future studies for developing drugs to be used in pregnancy.

Characteristics of particular drugs that determine the rate of their diffusion include molecular size, lipid solubility, ionization, and protein binding. Diffusion of a particular hydrophilic compound is inversely proportional to molecular size. Molecular weights as high as 5,000 daltons experience remarkably little stearic hindrance when crossing the placental barrier. The molecular weights of most drugs fall below this threshold. Therefore, the primary determinant of a drug crossing the placental barrier is maternal concentration. Maternal concentration is affected by many preplacental factors, including route and schedule of administration, volume of distribution, maternal metabolism, and maternal excretion.

The perfusion model has been used to demonstrate basic differences in exposure of the fetus to drugs depending on the mode of administration in the mother. Continuous infusion of a low-molecular-weight compound eventually results in equilibration between maternal and fetal circulation. However, by altering the maternal infusion rate in the dual-perfusion model to mimic the plasma concentration curve of a given drug after oral administration, maximal fetal concentrations and accumulations can be determined. This has been done with zidovudine (AZT)[18] and has been found to be consistent with *in vivo* data from maternal and cord blood samples obtained after intermittent oral intake.[19]

Zidovudine is one of only a few drugs that have been approved by the U.S. Food and Drug Administration (FDA) for use in treatment of acquired immunodeficiency syndrome. Furthermore, AZT has been studied most extensively with regard to treating HIV-infected pregnant women and reducing/preventing maternal–fetal human immunodeficiency virus (HIV) transmission. Placental perfusion studies using the dual-perfusion model permit evaluation of the effects of lamivudine, ritonavir, abacavir, and amprenavir, as well as AZT, on placental pharmacology and metabolism.

HUMAN IMMUNODEFICIENCY VIRUS INFECTION IN PREGNANCY

Heterosexual women represent the fastest-growing population of HIV-infected patients in the United States.[20] Therefore, a great concern in these HIV-infected women lies in the potential for perinatal transmission. Approximately 90% of all cases of HIV infection in children are the result of vertical transmission from an infected mother. Perinatal transmission principally occurs as a result of transplacental dissemination and intrapartum exposure to infected blood and genital tract secretions.[20] Without antiretroviral intervention, 15% to 40% of infants born to HIV-infected mothers will acquire the HIV infection.[21, 22]

Antiretroviral therapy during pregnancy requires consideration of maternal health as well as perinatal transmission. Antiretroviral regimens known to be of benefit to nonpregnant adults should not be withheld during pregnancy.[23] AZT, an inhibitor of reverse transcriptase, has been the mainstay of therapy for HIV infection in pregnancy. The effectiveness of AZT in preventing vertical transmission in mothers with CD4+ counts greater than 200 cells/mm^3 has been clearly demonstrated.[24] It has previously been shown that antepartum AZT treatment of the mother and treatment of her neonate can reduce transmission by up to 80%.[21] Despite the success of AZT monotherapy in preventing perinatal transmission, concerns for maternal health in HIV-infected women have led to treatment with multiple drugs, including protease inhibitors. The rapidity and magnitude of viral turnover in HIV infection are greater than previously appreciated, and current treatment focuses on early initiation of aggressive combination antiretroviral regimens.[25]

Treatment of nonpregnant adults consists of two nucleoside analogue reverse transcriptase inhibitors and a protease inhibitor. Pregnancy should not preclude the use of optimal therapeutic regimens, but recommendations for the treatment of infected pregnant women are subject to unique considerations.

Antiretroviral chemoprophylaxis to reduce the risk of perinatal transmission is based on maternal CD4+ count, HIV-1 RNA copy number, gestational age, and prior antiretroviral use. The three-part AZT chemoprophylaxis regimen recommended by the Pediatric AIDS Clinical Trials Group (PACTG) protocol 076 includes antepartum, intrapartum, and neonatal administration.[26] The combination of AZT chemoprophylaxis with additional antiretroviral drugs is recommended for women whose clinical, immunologic, and virologic status indicates the need for treatment. Regardless of the therapy used, informed consent of the patient is important and perinatal exposure to anti-HIV therapy should be reported to the Antiretroviral Pregnancy Registry.[27] Also, women who become pregnant while on combination therapy should be continued on therapy if they are beyond the first trimester. During the first trimester on a multiple-drug regimen, pregnant women should be counseled regarding potential risks and benefits. Should the woman decide to discontinue therapy, all medications should be stopped and reinitiated simultaneously beyond the first trimester.[28]

An increasing number of HIV-infected women will be receiving combination antiretroviral therapy for their own health during pregnancy. Preclinical evaluations of antiretroviral drugs for pregnancy-related and fetal toxicities should be completed for all existing and new drugs. Unfortunately, the development of newer drugs coupled with the obvious pressure to provide adequate therapy for this important population of infected women makes these evaluations even more difficult. Nevertheless, more data are needed regarding the safety and pharmacokinetics of antiretroviral drugs in pregnancy.

HUMAN IMMUNODEFICIENCY VIRUS REPLICATION AND INHIBITION

Human immunodeficiency virus is in the family Retroviridae, which encompasses a large number of infectious agents. One of the most important features of this family is its replication cycle. Retroviruses replicate from a single-stranded genome of polyadenylated RNA. The virion also contains several enzymes important in its replication, including reverse transcriptase, ribonuclease, and protease. The replication process includes encoding of the viral RNA into double-stranded DNA by reverse transcriptase and ribonuclease. The viral DNA is then integrated into the host DNA as a provirus, from which new viral RNA and viral proteins are synthesized to complete the cycle.[29]

The focus of anti-HIV therapy has been on the prevention of transcription by reverse transcriptase and the inhibition of protein cleavage by proteases at the termination of the virion's formation. Altering the structure of natural nucleotides may have an inhibitory effect, resulting in viral DNA chain termination. When these compounds are incorporated into growing chains, no further nucleosides can be added to viral DNA. Non-nucleoside inhibitors function as a phosphate group on the sugar structure of the nucleotide, which may inhibit reverse transcriptase. Finally, protease inhibitors affect HIV protease (aspartic proteinase) activity. These compounds bind competitively to the protease enzyme, resulting in immature virion production.

ANTIRETROVIRAL DRUGS

Nucleoside Analogue Reverse Transcriptase Inhibitors

Of the currently approved nucleoside analogue antiretrovirals (3'-azido-2'-3 dideoxyinosine [**AZT**]; 2'-3'-dideoxyinosine [**ddl**]; 2'-3'-dideoxycytidine [**ddC**]; 2'-3'-dehydro-3'-deoxythymidine [**d4T**]; 2'-dideoxy-3'-thiacytidine [**3TC**]; and 1S cis-4-2 amino-6-cyclopropyl-amino-9H-purin-9y-2-cyclopentane-1-methanol sulfate [**abacavir**]), the pharmacokinetics only for AZT and lamivudine (3TC) have been evaluated in clinical trials of pregnant women. AZT is well tolerated by pregnant women at the recommended adult doses (i.e., 200 mg three times a day) as well as by the neonate at the recommended doses (2 mg/kg orally every 6 hours). Initial studies done with AZT used the isolated single-cotyledon model with antipyrine as a freely diffusible marker.[7, 18, 30] These studies reported that the C_i of AZT was from 0.24 ± 0.04 to 0.29 ± 0.06. Furthermore, in vivo pharmacokinetic studies in three pregnant women at 19, 30, and 33 weeks' gestation resulted in no unusual side effects. Amniotic fluid levels were high, which suggests fetal renal excretion with accumulation in the amniotic fluid. Cord blood levels were also found to be 113% to 127% higher than maternal levels.[31] This confirms transplacental transport and fetal accumulation of AZT in human pregnancy. Ex vivo placental perfusion studies have also been performed on ddl, ddC,[7] d4T,[8] and 3TC.[32]

The results of these studies have shown that C_i's for these drugs are similar to that of AZT, and it is likely that they all reach therapeutic concentrations in the fetus rapidly. In addition, studies of these nucleoside inhibitors in combination with therapeutic doses of AZT revealed no change in C_i.

More recent studies have revealed that prolonged, continuous high doses of AZT administered to adult rodents are associated with the development of noninvasive squamous epithelial vaginal tumors in 3% to 12% of females.[33] The relevance of these animal data in humans is unknown. In January, 1997, an expert panel was convened by the National Institutes of Health to review these data and concluded that the proven benefit of reducing perinatal transmission outweighed the concern of transplacental carcinogenesis

raised by these animal studies. All of the nucleoside analogue antiretroviral drugs are classified as FDA Pregnancy Category C, except for ddl, which is classified as Category B. Abacavir is an investigational phase III drug that, on ex vivo placental perfusion analysis, was found to have a higher C_i than other nucleoside inhibitors.[34]

Non-nucleoside Analogue Reverse Transcriptase Inhibitors

Two non-nucleoside reverse transcriptase inhibitors have been approved by the FDA—**nevirapine** and **delaviridine**. The safety and pharmokinetics of nevirapine were evaluated in seven HIV-infected pregnant women and their infants. Equivalent blood concentrations were attained in all mothers and neonates. There were no short-term adverse effects observed in mothers or infants.[35] On the basis of these data, a phase III perinatal transmission prevention clinical trial is underway that is supported by the PACTG. Delaviridine has not been studied in phase I pharmacokinetic and safety trials of pregnant women. In premarketing clinical studies, seven women exposed to delaviridine before knowledge of their pregnancy were reported. Three pregnancies were ectopic, one infant was born prematurely and found to have a small muscular ventricular septal defect, and the remaining three infants were born healthy.[28] Long-term and transplacental animal carcinogenicity studies are not available for either drug. Both delaviridine and nevirapine are classified as FDA Pregnancy Category C.

The ex vivo human placental model was used to study another non-nucleoside reverse transcriptase inhibitor, **bisheteroarylpiperazine** (U-87201-E).[36] These studies revealed rapid transfer from mother to fetus with a C_i of 0.72 ± 0.17. This is twice the C_i of AZT. Placental tissue concentrations were similar to those of maternal blood, suggesting saturation.[36]

Protease Inhibitors

Phase I studies of HIV-infected pregnant women and their infants treated with several protease inhibitors (indinavir, ritonavir, nelfinavir, and saquinavir in combination with AZT and 3TC) are ongoing in the United States. Recent FDA approval of these four protease inhibitors for treatment of HIV infection represents a major advance in the management of HIV infection. However, these new drugs are not without adverse reactions because they all have significant side effect profiles and complicated drug interactions with other medications. Indinavir is metabolized through the cytochrome P-450 pathway and subsequently may interfere with the metabolism of other drugs through the same pathway. Saquinavir, ritonavir, and nelfinavir may also alter the metabolism of other drugs. Conversely, other medications may increase or decrease protease inhibitor bioavailability.[37]

Current information on the side effects of protease inhibitors is based on therapy in only a few thousand patients per drug, but each has a distinct dose-related side effect profile. Nephrolithiasis is the most important side effect of indinavir, with an incidence that ranges from 3% to 15%.[38] Nausea, vomiting, and abdominal pain are commonly reported by patients taking ritonavir, whereas saquinavir has few serious toxic effects. A newer formulation of saquinavir even has improved bioavailability, but is more likely to cause nausea and diarrhea. Patients taking nelfinavir are also subject to dose-limiting diarrhea.[38] All protease inhibitors have been approved under an FDA accelerated approval process; therefore, long-term safety of these drugs is unknown.[37] No data are available with regard to drug dosage, safety, and tolerance of the protease inhibitors in pregnant women or their newborn infants.

Because of these toxicity profiles and unknown teratogenic effects, there is a need for long-term *in vivo* studies in the nonhuman primate and pharmacokinetic studies on the *ex vivo* placental model. Only one ex vivo placental study has been completed using ritonavir. In this study, the Ci at therapeutic peak concentrations was 0.14 ± 0.04, suggesting that there is little transport across fetal membranes.[39] Another placental perfusion study performed on amprenavir, an investigational protease inhibitor, revealed a Ci of 0.38 ± 0.09 at peak concentrations (7 µg/mL) and a Ci of 0.14 ± 0.08 at trough concentrations (1.0 µg/mL).[34] Amprenavir crosses the placenta more readily than ritonavir in the *ex vivo* placental model. The clinical significance of these differences is unclear.

SUMMARY

An increasing number of HIV-infected women will be receiving antiretroviral therapy for their own health during pregnancy. Concomitantly, new anti-HIV drugs are under development. Preclinical evaluations of these drugs and those currently available should be performed for potential pregnancy-related toxicities and teratogenicity. Triple-drug combination therapy is recommended for nonpregnant adults infected with HIV. Although there is a paucity of information on the use of triple therapy in pregnant patients, it is important that new nucleoside and protease inhibitors be available for treatment in this growing population of HIV-infected patients. In addition, because there is a possibility that the use of three or more drugs in combination may completely suppress viral replication, the inclusion of combination therapy in the pregnant patient may be extremely important. In any case, AZT should be included in any regimen because it is the only drug that has been shown to reduce perinatal transmission. Results from several phase I studies should be available in the near future and will assist clinicians in making informed decisions regarding the treatment of HIV in pregnancy.

REFERENCES

1. Cannell GR, Karck RM, Hamilton SE, et al: Markers of physical integrity and metabolic viability of the perfused human placental lobule. Clin Exp Pharmacol Physiol 1988; 15:837.
2. Challier JC: Criteria for evaluating perfusion experiments and presentation of results. Contrib Gynecol Obstet 1985; 13:32.
3. Miller RK, Wier PJ, Shah Y, et al: Criteria for *in vitro* clinical perfusions in the human placental lobule: Perfusions in excess of 12 hours. In: Genbacev O, Klopper A, Beaconsfield R (eds): Placenta as a Model and a Source. New York, Plenum Press, 1989, p 27.
4. Bawdon RE: Ex vivo human placental transfer of antihuman immunodeficiency virus compounds. Infect Dis Obstet Gynecol 1998; 5:310.
5. Periera CM, Nosbisch C, Winter HR, et al: Transplacental pharmacokinetics of dideoxyinosine in pigtailed macaques. Antimicrob Agents Chemother 1994; 38:781.
6. Odines A, Nosbisch C, Keller RD, et al: In vivo maternal-fetal pharmacokinetics of stavudine (2′,3′ didehydro-3′-deoxy thymidine) in pigtailed macaques *(Macaca nemestuna)*. Antimicrob Agents Chemother 1996; 40:196.
7. Bawdon RE, Sobhi S, Dax J: The transfer of antihuman immunodeficiency virus nucleoside compounds by the term human placenta. Am J Obstet Gynecol 1992; 167:1570.
8. Bawdon RE, Kaul S, Sobhi S: The ex vivo human placental transfer of the anti-HIV nucleoside compound d4T. Gynecol Obstet Invest 1994; 38:1.
9. Boyd JD, Hamilton WJ: The Human Placenta. Cambridge, United Kingdom, Heffer and Sons, 1970.
10. Manson JN, Wise LD: Absorption, distribution and excretion of toxicants. In: Andur MO, Doull J, Klassen CD (eds): Casarett & Doulls Toxicology: The Basic Science of Poisons. New York, McGraw-Hill, 1997, p 67.
11. Juchau MR, Yaffe SH: Biotransformations of drug substrates in placental homogenetics. In: The Feto-Placental Unit. Amsterdam, Excerpta Medica, 1969, p 260.
12. Pasamen M, Pelkonen O: Human placental xenobiotic and steroid biotransformations catalyzed by cytochrome P450 epoxide hydrolase and glutathione s-transferase activities and their relationship to maternal cigarette smoking. Drug Metab Rev 1990; 21:427.
13. Barnea ER, Avigdor S, Boadi WY, Check JH: Effect of xenobiotics on quinolone reductase activity in first trimester explants. Hum Reprod 1993; 8:102.
14. Harbison RD, Borgert CH, Teaf CM: Placental metabolism of xenobiotics. In: Rama Sasty BV (ed): Placental Toxicology. Boca Raton, FL, CRC Press, 1995, p 213.
15. Schneider H: The role of the placenta in nutrition of the human fetus. Am J Obstet Gynecol 1991; 164:967.
16. Bain MD, Copas DK, Taylor A, et al: Permeability of the human placenta in vivo to four non metabolized hydrophilic molecules. J Physiol (Lond) 1990; 431:505.
17. Omarini D, Pistotti V, Bonatti M: Placental perfusion: An overview of the literature. J Pharmacol Toxicol Methods 1992; 28:6166.
18. Liebes L, Mendoza S, Wilson D, Dancis J: Transfer of zidovudine (AZT) by human placenta. J Infect Dis 1990; 161:203.
19. O'Sullivan MJ, Boyer P, Scott G, et al: A phase 1 study of the pharmacokinetics and safety of zidovudine in 3rd trimester HIV-1 infected pregnant women and their infants. Pediatr Res 1992; 31:173A.
20. Duff P: HIV infection in women. Prim Care Ob/Gyn 1996; 3:45.
21. Connor EM, Sperling RS, Gelber R, et al: Reduction of maternal-infant transmission of human immunodeficiency virus type 1 with zidovudine treatment. N Engl J Med 1994; 331:1173.
22. Dickover RE, Garratty EM, Herman SA, et al: Identification of

levels of maternal HIV-1 RNA associated with risk of perinatal transmission. JAMA 1996; 275:599.

23. Carpenter CJ, Fischl MA, Hammer SM, et al: Antiretroviral therapy for HIV infection in 1997. JAMA 1997; 277:1962.
24. Minkoff H, Augenbram M: Antiretroviral therapy for pregnant women. Am J Obstet Gynecol 1997; 176:478.
25. Perelson AS, Neumann AU, Markowitz M, et al: HIV-1 dynamics in vivo: Virion clearance rate, infected cell life-span, and viral generation time. Science 1996; 271:1582.
26. Centers for Disease Control and Prevention: Public Health Service Task Force on use of zidovudine to reduce prenatal transmission of human immunodeficiency virus. MMWR Morb Mortal Wkly Rep 1994; 43:1.
27. Centers for Disease Control and Prevention: MMWR Morb Mortal Wkly Rep 1998; 47:43.
28. Centers for Disease Control and Prevention: Public Health Task Force recommendations for the use of antiretroviral drugs in pregnant women infected with HIV-1 for maternal health and for reducing perinatal HIV-1 transmission in the United States. MMWR Morb Mortal Wkly Rep 1998; 47:1.
29. Levy J (ed): The Viruses: The Retroviridae, Vol. 1. New York, Plenum Press, 1992, p 190.
30. Schenker S, Johnson RF, King TS, et al: Azidothymidine (zidovudine) transport by the human placenta. Am J Med Sci 1990; 229:16.
31. Watts DH, Brown ZA, Tartaglione T, et al: Pharmacokinetic disposition of zidovudine during pregnancy. J Infect Dis 1991; 163:226.
32. Bloom SL, Dias KM, Bawdon RE, Gilstrap LC III: The maternal-fetal transfer of lamivudine in the ex vivo human placenta. Am J Obstet Gynecol 1997; 176:291.
33. Ayers KM, Clive D, Tucker E Jr, et al: Nonclinical toxicology studies with zidovudine: Genetic toxicity tests and carcinogenicity bioassays in mice and rats. Fundam Appl Toxicol 1996; 32:148.
34. Bawdon RE: The ex vivo human placental transfer of the anti-HIV nucleoside inhibitor abacavir and the protease inhibitor amprenavir. Infect Dis Obstet Gynecol 1998; 6:244.
35. Microchnick M, Sullivan J, Gagnier P, et al, and the ACTG Protocol 250 Team: Safety and pharmacokinetics (PK) of nevirapine (NVP) in neonates born to HIV-1 infected women. [Abstract.] In: Proceedings from the Fourth Conference on Retroviruses and Opportunistic Infections. Washington, DC, 1997, p 176.
36. Roberts S, Bawdon RE, Sobhi S, et al: The maternal-fetal transfer of bisheteroarylpiperazine (U-87201-E) in the ex vivo human placenta. Am J Obstet Gynecol 1995; 172:88.
37. Deeks SG, Smith M, Holodniy M, Kahn JO: HIV-1 protease inhibitors. JAMA 1997; 277:145.
38. Flexner C. HIV-protease inhibitors. N Engl J Med 1998; 338:1281.
39. Casey BM, Bawdon RE: Placental transfer of ritonavir with zidovudine in the ex vivo placental perfusion model. Am J Obstet Gynecol 1998; 179:758.

Index ■ ▼ ▶

Note: Page numbers in *italics* refer to figures; those followed by t refer to tables.

683

ISBN 0-7216-7379-1

90038

9 780721 673790